ENCYCLOPEDIA OF
BIOETHICS

Board of Editors

Area Editors

ENCYCLOPEDIA OF BIOETHICS

REVISED EDITION

Warren Thomas Reich

EDITOR IN CHIEF

Georgetown University

Volume 4

MACMILLAN LIBRARY REFERENCE USA

SIMON & SCHUSTER MACMILLAN

NEW YORK

SIMON & SCHUSTER AND PRENTICE HALL INTERNATIONAL

LONDON   MEXICO CITY   NEW DELHI   SINGAPORE   SYDNEY   TORONTO

Simon & Schuster Macmillan
866 Third Avenue, New York, NY 10022

PRINTED IN THE UNITED STATES OF AMERICA

printing number
   2   3   4   5   6   7   8   9   10

LIBRARY OF CONGRESS CATALOG-IN-PUBLICATION DATA

Encyclopedia of bioethics / Warren T. Reich, editor in chief. — Rev.
   ed.
      p. cm.
      Includes bibliographical references and index.
      ISBN 0-02-897355-0 (set)
      1. Bioethics—Encyclopedias.   2. Medical ethics—Encyclopedias.
   I. Reich, Warren T.
   QH332.E52   1995
   174′.2′03—dc20   94-38743
                                                            CIP

Lines from the poem "The Scarred Girl" by James Dickey, quoted in the entry on "Interpretation," originally appeared in *Poems, 1957–1967,* © 1978 by James Dickey, Wesleyan University Press, and have been reprinted here by permission of the University Press of New England.

The paper used in this publication meets the minimum requirements of American National Standard for Information Sciences—Permanence of Paper for Printed Library Materials, ANSI Z39.48-1984.

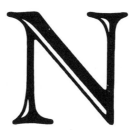

NARRATIVE

Human beings are a narrative species. We tell stories incessantly; we read and listen to them, watch them unfold on screen and stage. In making and absorbing narrative—news, gossip, fiction, drama, anecdotes, and history—we spin and untangle explanatory accounts of the way the world works and how we and our fellow human beings act in every conceivable circumstance. Memories of the past and ideas of the future are expressed in narrative accounts of how the world was and how it will, or should, become. Individual identities and self-conceptions are packaged in life stories, part (and heirs) of larger family, community, and national stories that shape the life events and choices to become the chapters that follow. There is even evidence that narrative, rather than simply a creative use human beings have found for language, is instead the motive for its acquisition: Young children learn to talk in order to give some account of occurrences in their daily lives (Bruner, 1990).

For the most part, the word "narrative" is used interchangeably with "story" to designate a more or less coherent written, spoken, or (by extension) enacted account of occurrences, either historical or fictional. "Story," however, is used more often, especially informally, to denote spoken and fictional accounts, while "narrative" emphasizes the inclusion of nonfiction or indicates a contrast with visual or numerical data, as in historiography or book production or computer science.

"Narrative" tends to be used generically in literary theory, perhaps following the Russian formalist and French structuralist distinction between "story" and "plot," where "story" designates the events, and "plot," the ordering of those events in the literary or historical account. Thus, the story of Oedipus begins with the prophecy his parents receive before his birth; the plot of Sophocles' play begins when, years later, he learns from the same oracle that the plague that afflicts his city is punishment for the unavenged death of the old king. Narrative refers to the whole and implies, for any particular telling, the inseparability of plot and story.

As it orders events, narrative asserts or connotes some causal relation among those events and imputes character and motives to the actors (Forster, 1927). Yet, despite this linearity, conclusions are never foregone. As narrative depicts events embedded in the lives and concerns of its protagonists, circumstances unfold through time in all their contingency and complexity (Ricoeur, 1988). Whether it is the life story essential to moral understanding (Burrell and Hauerwas, 1977; MacIntyre, 1981) or the political history of a nation (White, 1981), narrative explores the way cause and effect are entangled with the variables of human character and motivation, with luck and happenstance. When moral principles or political generalizations are abstracted from events without the use of narrative, those details are left behind as inessential, even though for those involved such particulars may represent what is most valued in a life or a history. Narrative remains mired in the particulars of human experience. From its designation of certain details as relevant "facts" and certain occurrences as "events" to the use of rhetorical strategies in the representation and description of those facts and events, narrative is concerned with the construction and interpretation of meaning.

Narrative and medical knowledge

Because narrative is the primary way of organizing and communicating the sense human beings make of the world, the interpretive process integral to shaping and understanding a story is at the heart of human knowing. Thus, the investigation of narrative forms and practices is a fruitful way of understanding how knowledge is acquired and transmitted. To understand medical knowledge—whether the patient's illness, the physician's practice, ideas of causality, issues of medical ethics, or activities of clinical research—it is helpful to look at the historical and explanatory narratives patients and practitioners tell themselves and each other (Charon, 1986, 1994; Hunter, 1991; Miles and Hunter, 1990).

Clinical medicine is a radically uncertain field of knowledge. Based on human biology, a science more complicated and multileveled than physics or chemistry, medicine has the task of applying scientific knowledge to the care of individual human beings. Not only does the living matter of biology change—the influenza virus mutates annually, tuberculosis and gonorrhea become drug-resistant, HIV gains purchase in the human community—but even more reliably, illness, that is, the manifestation of disease in human beings, varies unpredictably from person to person. Despite the triumph of the germ theory, "disease" remains a label given to a complicated interaction of physiological phenomena—none of which need be a necessary or sufficient cause—in circumstances identified and construed culturally, socially, and personally. Much about disease can be known scientifically, if not entirely predictably; but both the patient's illness and his or her response to treatment remain complex events with multiple causes occurring in circumstances that are impossible or immoral to replicate.

Given such uncertainty, narrative in its various guises is essential to the scientific practice of medicine. Patients relate the history of their illness when they present themselves for medical attention; disease plots make up the clinical taxonomy found in textbooks; their variant subplots are stored in physicians' memories; written accounts of medical care preserved in charts fill hospital basements; case reports contribute, one by one, to clinical research. In the physician's office where patients are well known and practice is solitary, narration may dwindle to a nearly invisible minimum. But in academic medical centers where medicine is taught and research carried out—just where one might expect to find narratives banished by the ever-present concern for scien-

tific objectivity—narrative flourishes. The clinical case is not only the record of care but the mainstay of clinical education and academic discourse. Cases are presented at morning report, at teaching rounds, patient-care conferences, grand rounds, ethics conferences, informally in halls and locker rooms, and around lunch tables. The case record is compiled in the hospital chart by several hands. When anomalies occur, the case becomes the vehicle for communication and further investigation that may lead to sustained clinical or laboratory research. As the translation and interpretation of the patient's account of illness, augmented by further investigation, the medical narrative enables clinicians to apply scientific knowledge and therapeutic judgment to the understanding and relief of illness in particular human beings.

The case thus constitutes the scientific data in the investigation and treatment of a patient's malady. Confronted with the signs and symptoms, guided by the patient's story, the physician asks questions, sorts the information into a list of possible diagnostic plots, and then sets to work to eliminate from consideration the least probable and most life-threatening and to confirm the most likely. The goals of this medical retelling of the patient's story are representational: fidelity to the clinical observation of the patient and minimalization of the observer's (and the patient's) subjectivity. To this end the conventions of the medical case are strict and almost inviolable. The narrator is all but effaced, appearing only as a signature authorizing the passive voice, while the patient's experience is subordinated to the medical retelling of illness events and physical signs, a version that resolutely ignores the fear and bewilderment, the loss of control, and the suffering that may attend the experience of illness. This is not meant to be cruel; it is meant to provide the patient with an objective gaze that is capable of establishing with some certainty what the matter is so that treatment may begin and, with luck, health may be restored.

The physician's familiarity with other cases grounds the investigation and, indeed, the whole interpretive, diagnostic circle. Whether read and heard about or, better, observed and directly experienced, these cases make up an intellectual storehouse backed by the myriad of information accumulated in publications and through consultation. Well understood and ready to hand, this body of practical knowledge enables physicians to apply physiological principles, textbook summaries, and clinical wisdom to signs and symptoms presented by individual patients, testing each particular case against those established, more abstract patterns. There are no all-encompassing laws of disease, and physicians must learn not only operative rules and their variants, but also the habits of perception that narrative enforces, habits that will stand them in good stead for a lifetime of practice in a field where knowledge and practice constantly change—and new diseases appear. The case narrative is the means by which such a store of exemplars is assembled both in formal education and in practice (Dreyfus and Dreyfus, 1987), and is the medium for the consultation, further investigation, and publication that are the hallmarks of modern academic medicine.

Narrative and bioethics

The centrality of narrative characteristic of clinical medicine is shared with other case-based disciplines of knowledge, such as law, moral theology, and criminal detection. In these domains, knowledge is not simply a "top-down," theory-driven activity. Research must be conducted retrospectively, and knowing is interpretive, accumulated from the experienced scrutiny of many individual instances in the light of general rules. The case—a term common to them all—functions as both exemplar and test of more general formulations: legislation, ethics, criminology, and biological science. In everyday practice, "in the trenches," these generalizations are extended or refined as they are applied, and practical expertise is developed in the continual search for more nearly adequate rules.

Narrative is also central to bioethics. Not only does it provide an opportunity for imaginative moral reflection for its audience, it is equally the proving ground of moral argument. Although the contemporary study of bioethics, especially medical ethics, until recently has focused almost exclusively on principles (Beauchamp and Childress, 1989; Pellegrino, 1993), the applicability of moral principles is inevitably gauged against the particular case, and cases regularly provoke the careful study and refinement of the rules. Indeed, the rehabilitation of casuistry—dealing with questions of right and wrong—has been the work of philosophers in bioethics (Toulmin, 1982; Jonsen and Toulmin, 1988; Jonsen, 1991).

The role of narrative in moral life is well established with regard to literature (Horace, 1960; Coles, 1979; Banks, 1994). Along with history, which is also strongly narrative, fictional narrative has long been regarded as a moral teacher—especially in that most narrative of eras, the nineteenth century. Both literary theory and historiography have struggled against this assumption of moral didacticism in the twentieth century. French historians of the *Annales* school and American cliometricians (mathematical and statistical analysts) have attempted to reduce the narrative element in history writing in favor of numerical data—the records of glacially slow and macroscopic social change for the former, and a microanalysis of economic statistics for the latter. In literature, from the "art-for-art's-sake" movement at the turn of the last century through Dadaist experimentation to the frequently reported "death" of

the novel, twentieth-century writers defied critics to draw morals from their stories. For much of the century, literary critics, too, eschewed moralism in favor of the aesthetics of "the work itself," relegating morals to a matter of folk tales. Thus, it was oddly fitting that when structuralists reanimated a critical concern with narrative it was necessary to turn to Vladimir Propp's *The Morphology of the Folktale* (1970; Todorov, 1977; Brooks, 1984). More recently, literary theorist Wayne Booth (1988) and philosopher Martha Nussbaum (1986) have made strong cases for literature as the medium of moral knowledge.

Literature's usefulness for moral reasoning lies not only in its themes and characters—those elements the McGuffey Readers drew upon for the "morals" that concluded their tales—but also in the interpretive reasoning it requires. As in clinical reasoning, narrative negotiates the application of general truths about human experience to the individual case. Readers know that murder is evil, but they turn to *Macbeth*, *Crime and Punishment*, or *Native Son* to reflect on precisely why and how. At the same time, narrative also tests such moral truths. Its representation of the particular instance asks implicitly whether circumstances can ever be extenuating; it negotiates on behalf of ethical inquiry, as it does for medical diagnostics, the imprecise and uncertain fit between general rule and particular instance.

The narrative that constitutes the bioethics case likewise plays a role in moral reasoning. The purpose of constructing and presenting a case in bioethics should not be limited to the illustration of a rule or principle any more than in medicine (Arras, 1991; Donnelly, 1992). It is rather to set out accounts of events in order to explore imaginatively their meaning for the people they affect and to determine what action should be taken. Because narrative's representation of subjective experience gives its audience access to the perception and judgment of other human beings, good ethics cases offer a means of thinking about the meaning of illness in the life of the patient, and about the role of the physician and the meaning of a patient–doctor interaction in the life of the physician. These are traditional themes of literature, and beyond literature—the themes of the unwritten stories, the gossip, and the self-revelation— that convey and test social values and give texture both to individual lives and to culture. To read and listen to stories and to watch them enacted on screen and stage is to open the understanding to the experience of other people, and to the meaning that experience has for them. Physicians do the former all the time, asking their patients about pain or the history of an illness, talking about the effects of disability or the likelihood of death. But imagining the meaning of experience for other people is very difficult and rarely undertaken (Kleinman, 1988; Waitzkin, 1991); for physicians, traditional, professional reticence and self-protection are obstacles (Katz, 1984). The desire for just this sort of understanding from another person, especially one pledged to a certain disinterested concern, informs both nostalgia for the legendary general practitioner and Anatole Broyard's request that his physician "spend five minutes thinking about my case" (1992). A longing for an interpreter who will both hear our stories in all their physical starkness and nevertheless see in us human subjects, people who create meaning in the story of our lives, may underlie the burgeoning interest in medical ethics. The public discussion of troubling cases—in the mass media, in the courts, in drama and film and autobiography, and in ethics courses—reveals a narrative hunger for meaning in the face of death. Indeed, Walter Benjamin (1936) has located in death's certainty the closure that narrative meaning requires.

As in clinical medicine, the use of narrative in bioethics is necessitated by the limits of human knowledge, and an attention to narrative enforces an awareness of these limits for both narrator and audience. Not only does the audience understand that the narrator's knowledge is limited, but, in addition, both narrator and audience know—or soon learn—that the knowability of the narrated is limited (Hunter, 1993). What happens next? Then? And then? The unfolding of narrative through time captures the contingencies of causation, the radical uncertainty of the most ordinary life, the uncontrolled variables that resist attempts to regularize and codify social knowledge. More questions may yield more information, yet uncertainty is best met not by the pursuit of every elusive clue, but by a sense of the balance of knowledge and tolerable ignorance sufficient for action. Although always accountable to social and cultural norms—indeed, these norms are operating in the framing and interpretation of narratives—moral knowledge is inevitably subjective, always open to question, discussion, elaboration, retelling, and reinterpretation.

In bioethics as in clinical medicine, narrative knowledge is always situated knowledge. Just as every malady has its patient, every tale has a teller—either the voice of an omniscient author or a character who has been witness to the events—and every narrator has an audience, imagined or real, to whom the story is addressed. Narratives are enmeshed in the circumstances of their telling, even when, as with clinical cases, the form is specially designed to extricate itself from those circumstances. Cases do not drop pure and untouched from the sky, nor do they contain a truth or essence that could be revealed if only the circumstances of their telling were stripped away. Instead, they are narratives constructed and presented by human beings who are making an effort to be understood—or to deceive, to impress an audience, or to reinterpret an event. Even stories meant to be perfectly transparent—medical cases, news re-

ports, ethics cases—are framed by their all-but-invisible tellers and interpreted by their audience. Though the narrator may be a disinterested and impartial observer, there is nevertheless a standpoint from which the story is told (Chambers). Some things will be emphasized or privileged, others will be out of the narrator's view. While norms exist and exert their force, they do so variously and unpredictably, and determining how they do so is one of the tasks that readers and listeners undertake. Narrators are revealed to their audience, in part, by the stands they take in relation to both the norms of society and the conventions of the narrative genre. This tension between tale and teller (or tale and the untold) is always a part of the narrative.

Where the sense of events offered by a narrative is contested or where its interpretation is in doubt, the narrative itself comes under scrutiny. The reader or listener begins to ask about the narrator and the narrative frame. Who is telling the story—the physician, the patient, a family member, an ethicist? Why is it told? In what circumstances? How does the teller frame the story to include or ignore culture, history, life stories, power relations, economic conditions, the history of the present question? Because an understanding of the problem turns upon the answers to these questions, this is where the study of ethical discourse must begin (Chambers, 1994). Cases may be narratively impoverished and morally inadequate even when bioethical principles are followed and apparently right conclusions are reached.

Through narrative, bioethics partakes of an ongoing dialogue among human beings perceiving and acting in the world. This is not a theoretical but a practical activity with strong resemblances to the clinical epistemology of which medical-case narrative is a part. As in medicine, the "facts" are sometimes of uncertain relevance and the circumstances may not be replicable, but the representation of experience through time acknowledges and puts to use the inevitable subjectivity of human understanding (Ricoeur, 1988). The subjectivity and apparent relativism unavoidable in narrative openly represents one of the conditions of moral discourse. There is no neutral position or Archimedean platform beyond nature from which a narrator, cleansed of bias, may see "truth" or "reality" in all its uncluttered purity. Indeed, narrative may be most valuable as a guarantee against this positivist assumption, for an awareness of narrative and its workings is a constant reminder that there is no absolute truth, no certainty. For the most part, stories are relatively straightforward about the conditions of their acquisition and telling. They make no pretense to objectivity—or when they do, the pretense is readily apparent as yet another storytelling genre. Narratives can be questioned: The potential prejudices of the narrator's situation beg to be understood. The interpretation of narrative may be one of the few ways human beings have of seeing our customary blind spots as both narrators and interpreters. As Ernst Hans Gombrich (1960) observed about the perception of art, there is no innocent, no "naked eye." And if there is no sight without a lens, it can become second nature to inquire into the character and quality of the lens in any particular instance—and to adjust it as needed.

Narrative exists in dialogue with other narratives, other interpretations—including the principles that, distilled from accounts of good and evil, have come to represent those accounts. Stories are not a substitute for norms and principles, just as clinical medicine does not replace medical research and case law does not render legislation irrelevant. Historians know well that every story implies an answering account, one that will surely—at last!—set the record straight. If the physician tells the patient's story, no one truly believes that it is the only story that matters; nor is the patient's story sufficient; otherwise the patient would not have sought medical help. The two are in dialogue. The goal is not a synthesis or a determination of a "truth" that will swallow up other accounts, but a sustainable representation of incommensurability, a consensus that may be acted upon. Ethics is practical knowledge, forged experientially and honed on circumstance. It is practiced in the negotiation of story and teller, story and listener, story and answering story. Because, in narrative, inquiry is inseparable from explanation, narrators and audiences must test the sources of our stories, compare versions, and sustain a healthy skepticism about answers. Thus, narrative represents the conditions of moral discourse, even as it is the principal medium of that discourse.

KATHRYN MONTGOMERY HUNTER

For a further discussion of topics mentioned in this entry, see the entries ETHICS, *article on* MORAL EPISTEMOLOGY; INTERPRETATION; LITERATURE; *and* VALUE AND VALUATION. *This entry will find application in the entries* CASUISTRY; DEATH: ART OF DYING; HEALTH AND DISEASE, *article on* THE EXPERIENCE OF HEALTH AND DISEASE; MEDICINE, SOCIOLOGY OF; PAIN AND SUFFERING; TECHNOLOGY, *article on* HISTORY OF MEDICAL TECHNOLOGY; *and* TRAGEDY. *For a discussion of related ideas, see the entry* METAPHOR AND ANALOGY.

Bibliography

ARRAS, JOHN D. 1991. "Getting Down to Cases: The Revival of Casuistry in Bioethics." *Journal of Medicine and Philosophy* 16, no. 1:29–51.

BAKHTIN, MIKHAIL M. 1981. *The Dialogic Imagination: Four Essays.* Translated by Michael Holquist. Austin: University of Texas Press.

BEAUCHAMP, TOM L., and CHILDRESS, JAMES F. 1989. *The Principles of Bioethics.* 3d ed. New York: Oxford University Press.

BENJAMIN, WALTER. 1968 [1936]. "The Storyteller: Reflections on the Works of Nikolai Leskov." *Illuminations: Essays and Reflections,* pp. 83–109. Translated by Harry Zohn. New York: Schocken.

BOOTH, WAYNE C. 1987. *The Company We Keep: An Ethics of Fiction.* Berkeley: University of California Press.

BRODY, HOWARD. 1987. *Stories of Sickness.* New Haven, Conn.: Yale University Press.

BROOKS, PETER. 1984. *Reading for the Plot: Design and Intention in Narrative.* New York: Alfred A. Knopf.

BROYARD, ANATOLE. 1992. *Intoxicated by My Illness: And Other Writings on Life and Death.* New York: Clarkson Potter.

BRUNER, JEROME S. 1990. *Acts of Meaning.* Cambridge, Mass.: Harvard University Press.

BURRELL, DAVID, and HAUERWAS, STANLEY. 1977. "From System to Story: An Alternative Pattern for Rationality in Ethics." In *Knowledge, Value and Belief,* pp. 111–152. Vol. 2 of *The Foundation of Ethics and Its Relationship to Science.* Edited by H. Tristram Engelhardt, Jr., and Daniel Callahan. Hastings-on-Hudson, N.Y.: Hastings Center.

CHAMBERS, TOD S. 1994. "The Bioethicist as Author: The Medical Ethics Case as Rhetorical Device." *Literature and Medicine* 13, no. 1:60–78.

———. "From the Ethicist's Point of View: The Literary Nature of Ethical Inquiry." In manuscript.

CHARON, RITA. 1986. "To Render the Lives of Patients." *Literature and Medicine* 5:58–74.

———. 1994. "Narrative Contributions to Medical Ethics: Recognition, Formulation, Interpretation, and Validation in the Practice of the Ethicist." In *A Matter of Principles? Ferment in U.S. Bioethics,* pp. 260–283. Edited by Edwin R. DuBose, Ronald Hamel, and Laurence J. O'Connell. Valley Forge, Pa.: Trinity Press International.

COLES, ROBERT. 1979. "Medical Ethics and Living a Life." *New England Journal of Medicine* 301, no. 8:444–446.

DONNELLY, WILLIAM J. 1992. "Hypothetical Case Histories: Stories Neither Fact nor Fiction." Presented at a meeting of the Society for Health and Human Values, Tampa, Fla., May 1.

DREYFUS, HUBERT L., and DREYFUS, STUART E. 1987. "From Socrates to Expert Systems: The Limits of Calculative Rationality." In *Interpretive Social Science: A Second Look,* pp. 327–350. Edited by Paul Rabinow and William M. Sullivan. Berkeley: University of California Press.

FORSTER, E. M. 1927. *Aspects of the Novel.* New York: Harcourt, Brace.

GLASER, BARNEY G., and STRAUSS, ANSELM L. 1967. *The Discovery of Grounded Theory: Strategies for Qualitative Research.* Chicago: Aldine.

GOMBRICH, ERNST HANS. 1960. *Art and Illusion: A Study in the Psychology of Pictorial Representation.* Bollingen Series, no. 35. New York: Pantheon.

HORACE. 1960. *The Ars Poetica of Horace.* Edited by Augustus S. Wilkins. New York: Macmillan.

HUNTER, KATHRYN MONTGOMERY. 1991. *Doctors' Stories: The Narrative Structure of Medical Knowledge.* Princeton, N.J.: Princeton University Press.

———. 1993. "The Whole Story." *Second Opinion* 19:97–103.

JONSEN, ALBERT R. 1991. "Of Balloons and Bicycles—or—The Relationship Between Ethical Theory and Practical Judgment." *Hastings Center Report* 21, no. 5:14–16.

JONSEN, ALBERT R., and TOULMIN, STEPHEN. 1988. *The Abuse of Casuistry: A History of Moral Reasoning.* Berkeley: University of California Press.

KATZ, JAY. 1984. *The Silent World of Doctor and Patient.* New York: Free Press.

KLEINMAN, ARTHUR. 1988. *The Illness Narratives: Suffering, Healing, and the Human Condition.* New York: Basic Books.

MACINTYRE, ALASDAIR C. 1981. *After Virtue: A Study in Moral Theory.* Notre Dame, Ind.: University of Notre Dame Press.

MILES, STEVEN, and HUNTER, KATHRYN MONTGOMERY. 1990. "Case Stories." *Second Opinion* 15:60–69.

NUSSBAUM, MARTHA C. 1986. *The Fragility of Goodness: Luck and Ethics in Greek Tragedy and Philosophy.* Cambridge: At the University Press.

PELLEGRINO, EDMUND D. 1993. "The Metamorphosis of Medical Ethics: A 30-Year Retrospective." *Journal of the American Medical Association* 269, no. 9:1158–1162.

PROPP, VLADIMIR. 1968. *The Morphology of the Folktale.* 2d ed., rev. Translated by Laurence Scott. Austin: University of Texas Press.

RICOEUR, PAUL. 1988. *Time and Narrative.* 3 vols. Translated by Kathleen McLaughlin Blamey and David Pellauer. Chicago: University of Chicago Press.

TODOROV, TZVETAN. 1977. *The Poetics of Prose.* Translated by Richard Howard. Ithaca, N.Y.: Cornell University Press.

TOULMIN, STEPHEN. 1982. "How Medicine Saved the Life of Ethics." *Perspectives in Biology and Medicine* 25, no. 4:736–750.

WAITZKIN, HOWARD. 1991. *The Politics of Medical Encounters: How Patients and Doctors Deal with Social Problems.* New Haven, Conn.: Yale University Press.

WHITE, HAYDEN. 1981. "The Value of Narrativity in the Representation of Reality." In *On Narrative,* pp. 7–23. Edited by W. J. Thomas Mitchell. Chicago: University of Chicago Press.

NATIONAL SOCIALISM

Most scholars trace the rise of the Nazi movement to the shallowness of German democratic traditions, the political polarization that followed Germany's defeat in World War I, and the economic collapse at the end of the 1920s. Adolf Hitler rose to power in 1933 amid optimism that he would put an end to the divisiveness of previous politics; he stressed the importance of "positive thinking," racial unity, and the celebration of all things German. Nazi ideology involved a complex dialectic of enlightenment and romance, modernism and antimodernism, the monstrous and the prosaic. A virulent racial hatred of Jews, Gypsies, and other purported "genetic inferiors" was at the core of the Nazi movement; the Nazis were also anticommmunist, antifeminist, and antidemocratic. Nazism also took root in a culture supporting the world's most advanced science, technology, and medicine. Nazism supported medicine and public health and, to a disturbing degree, physicians and scientists supported the Nazis.

Racial hygiene and Nazi ideology

The most important medical aspect of Nazi ideology was known as "racial hygiene." Racial hygiene (or eugenics, the English equivalent) responded to a set of fears: that "racial poisons" (such as alcohol or syphilis) were injuring the race, that the physically and mentally diseased were outbreeding healthier stocks, that the "struggle for existence" was being subverted by socialized medicine and other welfare state policies. Racial hygiene was supposed to provide long-run preventive medicine for the human genetic material, complementing personal hygiene (focusing on the individual) and social hygiene (focusing on public health, occupational safety and housing, clean air and water). Central to racial hygiene was biological determinism—the view that we are what we are exclusively by virtue of our biology, that it is our genes that ultimately determine whether we are rich or poor, criminal or law-abiding, homosexual or heterosexual, intelligent or stupid. In the Nazi version of the principle that emerged especially after 1933, certain groups of people were inherently worthless or "diseased." In 1934, Hans Weinert declared that "racial hygiene stands or falls with the recognition that peoples are neither of the same species [gleichartig], nor of the same value [gleichwertig]" (p.3). Racial hygienists were generally sympathetic to the Nazi movement when it gathered strength. In 1930 Fritz Lenz, the nation's first professor of racial hygiene, praised Hitler as "the first politician of truly great import who has taken racial hygiene as a serious element of state policy"; Lenz also was the first (in 1931) to characterize National Socialism as "applied biology."

One of the most disturbing things about medicine under the Nazis is how eagerly medical professionals embraced the new regime. In 1929, the National Socialist Physicians League was formed to coordinate Nazi medical policy and purify the German medical community of "Jewish Bolshevism"; nearly 3,000 doctors, representing 6 percent of the entire profession, joined the League by January 1933, before Hitler's rise to power. Doctors joined the Nazi Party earlier and in greater numbers than any other professional group: by 1942, more than 38,000 doctors had joined the party, representing about half of all doctors in the country. In 1937 doctors were represented in the SS seven times more often than was average for the employed male population. Younger physicians were especially eager joiners.

Hitler appreciated the efforts of physicians. In an early speech before the National Socialist Physicians' League the Führer argued that he could, if need be, do without lawyers, engineers, and builders, but that "You, you National Socialist doctors, I cannot do without you for a single day, not a single hour. If not for you, if you fail me, then all is lost. For what good are our struggles if the health of our people is in danger?" Consistent with his anti-Semitism, of course, it was only "German—not Jewish—physicians who could prove useful to the new regime. Early in the regime Jewish physicians were barred from government employment, and in 1938 they were forbidden to treat non-Jewish patients. "Cleansing" measures such as these earned Hitler a reputation as the "great doctor of the German people."

Sterilization

The 1933 Sterilization Law (Law for the Prevention of Genetically Diseased Offspring) was the first major triumph of Nazi racial hygiene. Modeled partly on American sterilization laws dating back to an Indiana law of 1907, the Nazi law allowed the forcible sterilization of anyone suffering from "genetically determined" illnesses, including feeblemindedness, schizophrenia, manic depression, epilepsy, Huntington disease, genetic blindness, deafness, and "severe alcoholism." Hundreds of "genetic health courts" and "appellate genetic health courts" were established to adjudicate the law. Doctors were required to register every case of genetic illness known to them, and could be fined for failing to do so. Physicians were required to undergo training in "genetic pathology" at one of the numerous racial institutes established throughout the country. The German Medical Association founded a journal, *Der Erbarzt* (The Genetic Doctor), to assist physicians in determining who should be sterilized: the journal included a regular column responding to physicians' queries about whether a particular patient with, say, a club foot or hearing impairment should be sterilized.

The 1933 sterilization law resulted in some 350,000 to 400,000 forced sterilizations by the end of the Nazi period. Compared with the demands of some racial hygienists, this was relatively modest: Franz Kallmann advised compulsory sterilization of all healthy, "heterozygous" carriers of the (supposedly dominant) gene for schizophrenia; Fritz Lenz argued that as many as 10–15 percent of the entire population ought to be sterilized. After the war, Occupation authorities never considered the Nazi sterilization program a criminal program; it would have been difficult for them to do so, given the multitude of compulsory sterilization laws in other countries—notably the United States.

Nuremberg Laws

A second major area of Nazi medical policy were the so-called Nuremberg Laws, enacted in the fall of 1935 further to cleanse the German populace from unwanted elements. The Reich Citizenship Law barred Jews from citizenship; the Blood Protection Law barred marriage and/or sexual relations between Jews and non-Jews; and the Marital Health Law required that couples pass a medical examination before marriage and forbade marriage between individuals suffering from venereal disease, feeblemindedness, epilepsy, or any of the genetic infirmities specified in the Sterilization Law.

When the Nuremberg Laws were announced in the fall of 1935, German medical journals applauded the sanctions as a much-needed response to public heath hazards. Health officials saw the prevention of human genetic disease, along with bans on racial miscegenation, as part of a single program of responsible public health policy. (The 1933 Castration Law, allowing the castration of certain criminals—notably sex offenders—was also viewed in this manner.) Several journals published charts indicating which individuals with a certain fraction of "Jewish blood" were fit to marry individuals of some other given fraction; the nation's leading medical journal, *Deutsches Ärzteblatt*, saluted the Blood Protection Law as a measure of historical importance that would help to "cleanse the body of our Volk." The journal greeted the Marital Health Law, passed shortly thereafter, as complementing the earlier Blood Protection Law, claiming that the Marital Health Law would "help secure the health and strength of the people for centuries to come." Physicians called on the government to construct a comprehensive genetic registry of the German population to assist in germ plasm management; proposals were also put forward that all German citizens be required to carry a "health pass" documenting their genetic and racial health. Genetic registries recording hundreds of thousands of individual traits were constructed; postwar scholars have pondered whether the genetic files compiled during the Nazi period (the recently rediscovered genealogies of thousands of Huntington disease carriers and their families, for example) should be opened for research and inspection.

The Nuremberg Laws resulted in an enormous expansion of marital and genetic counseling facilities. The Sterilization Law also required an increase in expenditures for public health. Despite the exclusion of Jews and communists, the total number of medical personnel actually increased throughout the Nazi period, from 287,000 in 1935 to 300,000 in 1939. Physicians' salaries also grew dramatically: in 1926 German lawyers earned about 18,000 RM per year, compared with only 12,000 RM for physicians. By 1936 doctors had reversed this, and now earned 2,000 RM more than lawyers. Physicians prospered under the Nazis, as Germans under Nazi guidance became increasingly obsessed with marital, genetic, and physical fitness.

Euthanasia and genocide

Wars have often provided either a rationale or a cloak for acts of criminal violence against civilians. During World War I, half of all German mental patients starved to death (45,000 in Prussia alone, according to one estimate) because they were low on the list to receive rations. In the Nazi period, the starvation of the mentally ill, the homeless, and other "useless eaters" became official medical policy after a prolonged propaganda campaign—in film, theater, and medical literature—to stigmatize the mentally ill and handicapped as "lives not worth living."

The euthanasia operation began in early October 1939, when Hitler issued orders that certain physicians be authorized to grant a "mercy death" (Gnadentod) to patients "judged incurably sick by medical examination." By August 1941, when the first phase of the "euthanasia" operation was brought to a close, more than 70,000 patients from German mental hospitals had been killed in an operation that provided the rehearsal for the subsequent destruction of the Jews, homosexuals, communists, Gypsies, Slavs, and prisoners of war.

The idea of the destruction of "lives not worth living" did not begin with the Nazis, but had been discussed in legal and medical literature since the end of World War I. Alfred Hoche and Karl Binding in their 1921 book, The Release and Destruction of Lives Not Worth Living, had argued in favor of forcible euthanasia for the mentally ill. Germans, however, were not the only ones entertaining such ideas. In 1935, the French-American Nobel Prize winner Alexis Carrel suggested in his book Man the Unknown that criminals and the mentally ill should be "humanely and economically disposed of in small euthanasia institutions supplied with proper gases." Six years later, as German psychiatrists were sending the last of their patients into the gas chambers, an article appeared in the Journal of the American Psychiatric Association calling for the killing of retarded children, "nature's mistakes."

The fundamental argument for forcible euthanasia was economic: killings were justified as a kind of "preemptive triage" to free up medical resources. This became especially important during the war, and in fact the onset of the euthanasia operation was timed to coincide with the invasion of Poland. The first gassings of mental patients took place at Posen (Poznan), in Poland, on October 15, 1939, just forty-five days after the invasion of that country, marking the beginning of World War II. In Germany itself, euthanasia became part of normal hospital routine after August 1941, when the first (gas chamber) phase of the euthanasia operation was brought to a close. Handicapped infants were thereafter regularly put to death; persons requiring long-term psychiatric care and judged "incurable" suffered a similar fate. Euthanasia operations were sometimes coordinated with bombing raids: elderly or otherwise infirm persons were killed to make room for the wounded (patients capable of productive work were usually spared). Psychiatrists eventually worried that their tireless efforts to eliminate Germany's mental defectives would render their own skills useless: Professor O. Wuth, chief physician for the army, pondered in the midst of the war years that with so many mental patients being eliminated by euthanasia, "Who will wish to study psychiatry when it becomes so small a field?"

Historians exploring the origins of the Nazi destruction of "lives not worth living" have only recently begun to stress the links between the euthanasia operation and the "final solution" of the "Jewish question." The most important theoretical link was what might be called the "medicalization of anti-Semitism," part of a broader effort to reduce a host of social problems—unemployment, homosexuality, crime, antisocial behavior—to medical or, ideally, surgical problems. In the course of the late 1930s, German scientists proposed a number of different solutions to the "Jewish question," ranging from deportation to Madagascar to sterilization of all Jews by X rays. Viktor Brack, a leading euthanasia physician, recommended sterilization of the 2 to 3 million Jews capable of work, who might be put to use in Germany's factories. During the early war years the official journal of the German Medical Association (Deutsches Ärzteblatt) discussed these various options in a regular column, "Solving the Jewish Question."

The ultimate decision to gas the Jews emerged from the fact that the technical apparatus already existed for the destruction of the mentally ill. In the fall of 1941, with the completion of the bulk of the euthanasia operation, the gas chambers at psychiatric hospitals were dismantled and shipped east, where they were reinstalled at Majdanek, Auschwitz, and Treblinka. Doctors, technicians, and nurses often followed the equipment. In this sense, there was a continuity in both therapy and practice between the destruction of the "lives not worth living" in Germany's mental hospitals and the destruction of Germany's ethnic and social minorities.

The euthanasia operation is yet another instance where physicians were willing pioneers rather than coerced pawns: there is no evidence of anyone ever having forced physicians to participate in the operation. Hans Hefelmann, another euthanasia expert, testified to this effect in 1964 at one of the post-war euthanasia trials: "No doctor was ever ordered to participate in the euthanasia program; they came of their own volition."

Medical experiments in concentration camps

The medical experiments carried out by Nazi doctors are probably the best-known examples of medical malfeasance under the Nazis. Several of the more grotesque experiments must be understood as part of the Nazi obsession with race, as when Josef Mengele injected concentration camp prisoners' eyes with dyes to see if he could thereby effect a permanent change in coloration. Most medical experiments, however, were designed to solve practical problems faced by military commanders in their eastward or southward expansion. At Dachau, Russian prisoners of war were immersed in ice water to find out what kinds of protective gear or rewarming techniques were most effective; prisoners were forced to drink seawater to see how long a pilot might survive if shot down at sea. Prisoners were placed in vacuum chambers to find out how the human body responds when forced to bail out at high altitudes. At Fort Ney, near Strasbourg, fifty-two prisoners were exposed to phosgene gas (a biowarfare agent) in 1943 and 1944 to test possible antidotes; at Auschwitz, physicians experimented with new ways to sterilize or castrate people (using X rays, for example, or fallopian tube scarification by means of supercooled carbon dioxide) as part of a plan to replace the population of eastern Europe with Germans. At Buchenwald, Gerhard Rose infected prisoners with spotted fever to test experimental vaccines against the disease; at Dachau, Ernst Grawitz infected prisoners with a broad range of pathogens to test homeopathic preparations. Nazi military authorities were worried about exotic diseases German troops might contract in Africa or eastern Europe; physicians in the camps reasoned that the "human materials" at their disposal could be used to develop remedies. In many of the experiments, death was the intended end point; many of those who survived lived with painful physical or psychological scars.

Criminal medical experiments were sometimes carried out in collaboration with prestigious university faculties. Heinrich Berning, at Hamburg, in 1941 allowed Russian prisoners of war to starve to study the effects of hunger on the body. Josef Mengele provided "experimental materials" from Auschwitz (including eyes, blood, and other body parts) to Otmar von Verschuer at the Kaiser Wilhelm Institute for Anthropology as part of a study on the racial specificity of blood types, funded by the Deutsche Forschungsgemeinschaft. This was one reason blood groups were so actively studied in the 1930s: Otto Reche had founded the German Society for Blood Group Research in 1926, ostensibly to see (by

his own admission) whether he could find a reliable means of distinguishing Aryans from Jews in the test tube.

As in the case of the euthanasia operation, doctors were never forced to perform such experiments. Physicians volunteered—and in several cases Nazi officials had to restrain overzealous physicians from pursuing even more ambitious experiments. The logic governing the use of prisoners for death-causing experiments was similar to that underlying efforts to eliminate "lives not worth living." In the Nazi view of the world there were superior and inferior races, worthies and unworthies, healthy and diseased. The Nazis assumed that the value of a Slav or a Jew was significantly less than that of a trained pilot in the German Luftwaffe. If it required the deaths of a hundred Russian prisoners to increase the chances of saving one German pilot, this was, on the Nazi scale of values, a justified investment. Concentration camp inmates were valued as slave labor, and when they were exhausted, they were not worth keeping alive. Doctors acting in such a manner were not without values: their values were clear (Nordic supremacy, total war demands extreme measures, Jews are vermin, etc.), and they acted in accordance with those values.

Postwar continuities

After the war, a handful of physicians accused of crimes against humanity were prosecuted by the American military Tribunal at Nuremberg. The Nuremberg Code, published in 1947 at the end of the trial, articulated standards for ethically permissible research. Although the code itself was never recognized as having legal standing, it stimulated decades of discussion about criteria for experimentation (Grodin and Annas, 1992). Abbreviated transcripts of the "Doctors' Trial" were published in 1949, though certain incriminating facts were deleted under political pressure from German medical authorities and the transcripts were not widely distributed (Mitscherlich and Mielke, 1949; Pross and Aly, 1989).

German physicians either ignored or downplayed medical involvement in Nazi crimes until the 1980s, when medical students and a number of "alternative" scholars accused medical authorities of suppressing the past (Baader and Schultz, 1983). Charges of failure to confront the past drew strength from the fact that, in many cases, Nazi affiliations were not a barrier to professional success: in 1973, for example, when Hans Joachim Sewering was elected president of the West German Chamber of Physicians, the fact that he had joined the SS in November 1933 apparently did not matter to his supporters. Nor did it matter that he had sent handicapped patients to the psychiatric hospital at

Eglfing-Haar, one of the euthanasia institutions established to eliminate Germany's "lives not worth living." Though forced to resign from West Germany's top medical post in 1978 (not for his Nazi connections, but for improper billing practices), he remained head of the Bavarian Physicians' Chamber and in the fall of 1992 was designated president-elect of the World Medical Association. International protests forced his withdrawal.

In recent years, a younger generation of critics (Christian Pross, for example) has gained substantial influence in the German medical community, prompting systematic historical investigations (Pross and Aly, 1989, for example). Memorial exhibits have been set up at several major euthanasia sites to commemorate the dead, and plaques have been placed at several eugenics institutions (the former Kaiser Wilhelm Institute for Anthropology, for example) to ensure that the past is not forgotten.

Significance

The significance of medicine under the Nazis lies less in the details of particular operations than in the fact that the medical profession became a willing partner to some of the most ghastly crimes of human history. Seldom have medical professionals acted with such cold-blooded cruelty on such a large scale. Under Nazi guidance, the German medical community became obsessed with the idea of distinguishing "superior" and "worthless" groups. There were occasional examples of resistance. A handful of Catholic physicians protested the euthanasia operation; socialist and communist physicians tried to organize resistance from outside the country or within the concentration camps. But effective acts of resistance were few and far between. In occupied Holland, Dutch physicians refused to send their psychiatric patients to their deaths in conformity with the German euthanasia operation; more than a hundred were arrested for resisting the regime.

Physicians commonly boasted that their profession had shown its allegiance earlier and in greater strength than any other professional group. But why? We should recall that the medical profession at this time was quite conservative. The profession was politicized and polarized after the economic collapse in the late 1920s and early 1930s. Physicians worried about their financial future moved from the political center to the left or (more often) to the right. By the end of 1932 the Nazi Physicians' League was twice as large as the Association of Socialist Physicians (3,000 vs. 1,500 members). The substantial Jewish representation in the medical field (60 percent of Berlin's physicians, for example, had been Jewish) meant that there was much room for opportunism. Jewish doctors were a convenient scapegoat for everything imagined to be wrong in German medicine,

from the impersonal routines of socialized medicine to the hazards of mandatory vaccination.

Nazi leaders recognized that medical collaboration was vital if they were to achieve their racial-political goals: Medical expertise was needed for sterilizations, for administering the Nuremberg Laws, for carrying out the euthanasia operation. Doctors were the ones who performed "selections" (of people to be killed) in the death camps, and on March 9, 1943, Heinrich Himmler, chief of the SS, ordered that henceforth only physicians trained in anthropology could perform selections at concentration camps. Physicians were needed to maintain racial and physical fitness; they responded readily, and were rewarded. Physicians achieved unprecedented power and prestige under the Nazis.

It would be wrong, though, to "demonize" Nazi health and social policy as something monstrous or otherworldly in comparison to policies elsewhere before or since. Nazi health policies were surprisingly modern in several respects. Consistent with their obsession with race and fitness, the Nazis supported extensive research into ecology, public health, cancer, behavioral genetics, and (of course) racial and social biology. Nazi physicians explored the effects of exposure to X rays, heavy metals, and asbestos; the Nazis were among the first to initiate bans on smoking in public buildings. Nazi leaders organized extensive support for midwifery, homeopathy, and a number of other areas of heterodox medicine. Nazi physicians recognized the importance of a diet high in fruit and fiber, and ordered German bakeries to produce whole-grain bread. Nazi physicians restricted the use of DDT and denied pregnant women tobacco ration coupons on the grounds that nicotine could harm the fetus. Racial hygiene was supposed to provide long-run, preventive care for the German germ plasm, complementing shorter-term social and individual hygiene.

The fact that crime existed alongside common sense is one of the most disturbing aspects of the Nazi medical phenomenon. Nazism took root in a culture possessing the greatest scientific talent in the world; this alone raises troubling questions concerning the ethics of science and medicine. It used to be argued that science is either inherently democratic or at worst apolitical; in the case of medicine under the Nazis, however, one can see how easily politics and science merged, with frightening consequences. The larger message is that ideologies of racial superiority and inferiority can have devastating human consequences when harnessed to a powerful state and a compliant profession.

ROBERT N. PROCTOR

Directly related to this entry is the entry EUGENICS. *For a further discussion of topics mentioned in this entry, see the entries* DEATH AND DYING: EUTHANASIA AND SUSTAIN-

ING LIFE, *articles on* HISTORICAL ASPECTS, *and* ETHICAL ISSUES; EUGENICS AND RELIGIOUS LAW; GENETIC ENGINEERING, *article on* HUMAN GENETIC ENGINEERING; GENETICS AND HUMAN SELF-UNDERSTANDING; GENETICS AND RACIAL MINORITIES; HEALTH SCREENING AND TESTING IN THE PUBLIC-HEALTH CONTEXT; HEALTH OFFICIALS AND THEIR RESPONSIBILITIES; POPULATION POLICIES, *section on* STRATEGIES OF FERTILITY CONTROL; *and* SOCIAL MEDICINE. *For a discussion of related ideas, see the entries* MINORITIES AS RESEARCH SUBJECTS; PRISONERS; RACE AND RACISM; RESEARCH, HUMAN: HISTORICAL ASPECTS; RESEARCH, UNETHICAL; *and* WARFARE, *article on* MEDICINE AND WAR. *Other relevant material may be found under the entries* ETHICS, *articles on* TASK OF ETHICS, NORMATIVE ETHICAL THEORIES, *and* SOCIAL AND POLITICAL THEORIES; FREEDOM AND COERCION; JUSTICE; LICENSING, DISCIPLINE, AND REGULATION IN THE HEALTH PROFESSIONS; MEDICAL CODES AND OATHS; PROFESSION AND PROFESSIONAL ETHICS; *and* VALUE AND VALUATION. *See also the* APPENDIX (CODES, OATHS, AND DIRECTIVES RELATED TO BIOETHICS), SECTION II: ETHICAL DIRECTIVES FOR THE PRACTICE OF MEDICINE, *and* SECTION IV: ETHICAL DIRECTIVES FOR HUMAN RESEARCH, *especially* THE NUREMBERG CODE.

Bibliography

ALEXANDER, LEO. 1949. "Medical Science Under Dictatorship." *New England Journal of Medicine* 241, no. 2:39–47.

ALY, GÖTZ; EBBINGHAUS, ANGELIKA; HAMANN, MATTHIAS; PFÄFFLIN, FRIEDEMANN; and PREISSLER, GERD. 1985. *Aussonderung und Tod: Die klinische Hinrichtung der Unbrauchbaren.* Berlin: Rotbuch Verlag.

BAADER, GERHARD, and SCHULTZ, ULRICH, eds. 1983. *Medizin und Nationalsozialismus: Tabuisierte Vergangenheit—Ungebrochene Tradition?* 2d ed. Berlin: Verlagsgesellschaft Gesundheit.

BAUR, ERWIN; LENZ, FRITZ; and FISCHER, EUGEN, eds. 1931. *Menschliche Erblichkeitslehre und Rassenhygiene (Eugenik).* 3d ed. Munich: J. F. Lehmann.

BOCK, GISELA. 1986. *Zwangssterilisation im Nationalsozialismus: Studien zur Rassenpolitik und Frauenpolitik.* Opladen: Westdeutscher Verlag.

CAPLAN, ARTHUR L., ed. 1992. *When Medicine Went Mad: Bioethics and the Holocaust.* Totowa, N.J.: Humana Press.

GRODIN, MICHAEL, and ANNAS, GEORGE J., eds. 1992. *The Nazi Doctors and the Nuremberg Code: Human Rights in Human Experiments.* New York: Oxford University Press.

KATER, MICHAEL H. 1989. *Doctors Under Hitler.* Chapel Hill: University of North Carolina Press.

KAUPEN-HAAS, HEIDRUN, ed. 1986. *Der Griff nach der Bevölkerung: Aktualität und Kontinuität nazistischer Bevölkerungspolitik.* Nördlingen: F. Greno.

KLEE, ERNST. 1983. *"Euthanasie" im NS-Staat: Die "Vernichtung lebensunwerten Lebens."* Frankfurt am Main: S. Fischer Verlag.

KOLLOQUIEN DES INSTITUTS FÜR ZEITGESCHICHTE. 1988. *Medizin im Nationalsozialismus.* Munich: R. Oldenburg Verlag.

KUDLIEN, FRIDOLF, and BAADER, GERHARD, eds. 1985. *Ärzte im Nationalsozialismus.* Cologne: Kiepenheuer und Witsch.

LIFTON, ROBERT J. 1986. *Nazi Doctors: Medical Killing and the Psychology of Genocide.* New York: Basic Books.

MITSCHERLICH, ALEXANDER, and MIELKE, FRED. 1947. *Das Diktat der Menschenverachtung.* Heidelberg: L. Schneider. Translated by Heinz Norden under the title *Doctors of Infamy: The Story of the Nazi Medical Crimes.* New York: Henry Schuman. 1949.

———. 1949. [1948]. *Medizin ohne Menschlichkeit: Dokumente des Nürnberger Ärzteprozesses.* Frankfurt am Main: S. Fischer Verlag. First published under the title *Wissenschaft ohne Menschlichkeit.* Translated under the title *The Death Doctors.* London: Elek Books. 1962.

MÜLLER-HILL, BENNO. 1988. *Murderous Science: Elimination by Scientific Selection of Jews, Gypsies, and Others, Germany 1933–1945.* Translated by George Fraser. New York: Oxford University Press.

PROCTOR, ROBERT N. 1988. *Racial Hygiene: Medicine Under the Nazis.* Cambridge, Mass.: Harvard University Press.

PROSS, CHRISTIAN, and ALY, GÖTZ, eds. 1989. *Der Wert des Menschen: Medizin in Deutschland 1918–1945.* Berlin: Edition Hentrich.

ROTH, KARL HEINZ, ed. 1984. *Erfassung zur Vernichtung, von der Sozialhygiene zum "Gesetz über Sterbehilfe."* Berlin: Verlagsgesellschaft Gesundheit.

SEIDELMAN, WILLIAM E. 1988. "Mengele Medicus: Medicine's Nazi Heritage." *Milbank Quarterly* 66, no. 2:221–239.

WEINDLING, PAUL. 1989. *Health, Race and German Politics Between National Unification and Nazism, 1870–1945.* Cambridge: At the University Press.

WEINERT, HANS. 1934. *Biologische Grundlagen für Rassenkunde und Rassenhygiene.* Stuttgart: F. Enke.

WEINREICH, MAX. 1946. *Hitler's Professors: The Part of Scholarship in Germany's Crimes Against the Jewish People.* New York: Yiddish Scientific Institute.

NATIVE AMERICAN RELIGIONS

Using the phrase "Native American" signals a recognition that there are indigenous peoples on the North American continent who retain distinct ethical perspectives within the mainstream cultures of the United States and Canada. Terms such as "First Peoples," "American Indian," and "Amerindian" are also used to refer to the indigenous peoples of the Americas. Each term has a history of use and limitations in its reference. For example, there are no actual people who call themselves Native Americans in their traditional language; rather, there are distinct ethnic groups who were on the North American continent prior to the arrival of Europeans, Africans, and Asians. Prior to contact with European settlers in the fifteenth century, it is believed, there were over 2,000 different native communities on the continent. Over 700 of these ethnic groups have survived repeated invasions, epidemic diseases, cultural genocide, and ideological exploitation. Thus, when we use the term "Native American," it is at a general level of understanding and reference that is fictional and conceptual. A deeper understanding of Native Americans must move to another level of reference, beginning with the names by which indigenous peoples know themselves.

In this entry the following system will be used. The indigenous name will be followed by the popular name in Canada and the United States. The peoples who call themselves Anishinabe are also known as Chippewa/Ojibwe, Ottawa, and Pottawatomi. In some instances, there are historical and sociological reasons for differentiating specific tribal names among a larger nation such as the Anishinabe. So also, the term Haudenosaunee, or "Long-House People," is the name of the northeastern North American peoples whom the French called Iroquois. Either term is often used to indicate individual nations within the Haudenosaunee political confederation, or "long house": Seneca, Cayuga, Onondaga, Oneida, Tuscarora, and Mohawk. Other examples can be listed: Apsaalooke/Crow; Tsistsistas/Cheyenne; Muskogee and Miccosukkee/Creek; Dine/Navajo; Ashiwi/Zuni; Tohono O'odham/Papago; and Skittagetan/Haida. This usage recognizes the right of a people to be known by the name by which they describe themselves.

The term "religion" raises a similar ethical concern; it carries associated references that can mislead an inquiry into Native American ways. The term "religion" derives from the Latin *religio*, "to bind fast." Traditionally this has carried associations from its Mediterranean-Atlantic heritage, namely, to be reunited, after a pilgrimage through life, with the personal, monotheistic, creator God who transcends earthly existence. The connotations of monotheism, the one deity as personal and transcendent, and a pilgrimage orientation to life are embedded in the term "religion" for many Euro-American Christians.

In contrast, the term "lifeway" emphasizes the road of life as indigenous people see it. Such a perspective can be associated with the concept "worldview," a distinct way of thinking about the cosmos and of evaluating life's actions in terms of those views. The Dakota/Sioux lawyer and professor of history Vine Deloria, Jr., speaks thus of an Indian ethical view of the universe: "In the moral universe all activities, events, and entities are related, and consequently it does not matter what kind of existence an entity enjoys, for the responsibility is always there for it to participate in the continuing creation of reality" (Deloria, 1993, p. 63). This view understands all life forms as having purpose, as being related, and as being cocreators of the world they oc-

cupy. The religious structure that flows from these views gives rise to a moral imagination in which the sacred is immanent, within the earth, and revealed in one's contemplation of natural occurrences. All life in one's local bioregion is both interdependent and participating in the act of creation evident, for example, in the changing seasons. The term "bioregion," is used here to suggest the Native American reverence and respect for all life forms in the local region. Indians have traditionally understood their local bioregion as filled with moral purpose, interrelated, and alive.

Cosmic interdependence

Moral actions in Native American lifeways are acts in harmony with a sacred power that is believed to pervade the world and is experienced most immediately in the local bioregion. While moral actors are not limited to the human community, any particular human is seen as integrated into the larger harmony by means of his or her community. Someone who has committed a crime is not made into an outsider by virtue of an isolated act. Rather, the one who is out of balance must be brought back, if possible, into the community by ritual treatment with that power believed to pervade the cosmos.

Native peoples in North America have articulated terms such as Wakan Tanka (Lakota), Kitche Manitou (Anishinabe), or Akbatatdia (Apsaalooke), which convey an understanding of the mysterious presence and fullness of pervasive cosmic power. These terms have often been used by nonnative missionary traditions to communicate ideas regarding the sacred, especially belief in a personal God. While such usage may be sanctioned by Christian native peoples, some traditional practitioners object to this interpretation as misleading. Sacred power, and the native terms used to evoke that mystery, do not indicate a patriarchal deity but emphasize the web of cocreative relationships throughout the spiritual realms and the ecological terrain, or bioregion. This pervasive power is experienced in a plurality of manifestations, or spirits, that relate to the presence of transformative power in distinct spiritual realms of the cosmos but especially to the local bioregion. Thus, Native American lifeways may be described as manifesting an "ethical naturalism" in which moral choices flow from the desires of individuals and communities to flourish within the limits and opportunities of nature as understood by the people and as typically observed within the particular bioregional conditions of a people (Lovin and Reynolds, 1985).

Synthetic ethics

Questions of the relation of ethics to ritual and myth are also analytical themes in the study of religion, but in

Native American traditions these questions are inextricably linked. This article will attempt to communicate this ethical wholeness by describing practices related to both ritual and the daily life of native North American peoples. One term used throughout this article, "synthetic ethics," refers to the Native American effort to bring people into the most immediate and profound encounter with resources for thought and for food: the bioregion, the animals hunted, the human community, the seasons, and the spiritual realm.

Synthetic ethics signifies the seamless whole of the Native American world in which personal actions affirm mythic values and in which ritual actions reflect relationships established with the surrounding bioregion. Rather than abstract principles, these ethical relationships correspond to moral metaphors transmitted in the myth stories. Such generative metaphors as the living earth and purposeful animals cause a person to contemplate, as ethical experiences, the seasons, or the hunt, or the eating of local foods at their harvest time. American Indian moral imagination arises from formal structures that are believed to govern personal and community life as well as the bioregion and the larger cosmos. Such a worldview implies integration of a situational ethic, which guides one in daily life, and a cosmological ethic, which flows from the harmonious rhythms of nature. Thus, the terms "lifeway," "synthetic ethics," and "bioethics" are used in this entry to suggest the wholeness or totality of a good life that is lived in thoughtful relationship to the seasons and the living bioregion.

Each particular native people has its own terms for such concepts as synthetic ethics and lifeway. For example, Winona LaDuke writes:

> The ethical code of my own Anishinabeg community of the White Earth Reservation in northern Minnesota keeps communities and individuals in line with natural law. "*Minobimaatisiiwin*"—it means both the "good life" and "continuous rebirth"—is central to our value system. In *minobimaatisiiwin*, we honor women as the givers of lives, we honor our *Chi Anishinabeg,* our old people and ancestors who hold the knowledge. We honor our children as the continuity from generations, and we honor ourselves as a part of creation. Implicit in *minobimaatisiiwin* is a continuous habitation of place, an intimate understanding of the relationship between humans and the ecosystem and of the need to maintain this balance. (LaDuke, 1992, p. 70)

It is possible to find similar expressions by elders from indigenous communities in North America that articulate the relationship between social justice and ecojustice in their lifeway. The range of indigenous terms need not be discussed here but, where appropriate, such terms will be introduced.

Land and the human presence

Three features of Winona LaDuke's description of Anishinabe/Ojibwe ethical naturalism—enduring habitation (land), cosmological understanding (lifeway), and ecological balance (synthetic ethics)—can be used to frame the Native American appreciation of land and the human presence. The Winter Dance among the Okanagan/Salish/Colville peoples of Washington State provides a unique insight into the relationships of land, lifeway, and synthetic ethics. The Winter Dance introduces us to a developed native North American lifeway in which ritual participation is believed to transform individuals, communities, and bioregions. Moreover, the Salish understand the relationships established during the ritual as historical, that is, they deepen as an individual matures in the ethical path.

While this ritual, from the interior Salish-speaking peoples of the Columbia River plateau, has been selected for discussion here, it should be emphasized that the themes discussed have parallels in many distinct native North American rituals. The Green Corn, or Busk, ceremony of the Muskogee in the Southeast, the Shalako and Winter Solstice rituals of the Ashiwi in the Southwest, the Ashkisshe, or Sun Dance, of the Northern Plains Apsaaloke and many more rituals throughout Indian country continue to be performed in sacred settings by traditional practitioners.

Okanagan/Salish/Colville Winter Dance. Among many Salish people the Winter Dance begins the annual ritual calendar. Rituals performed during the calendar year include individual and communal activities, such as sweat-lodge ceremonies, vision questing, stick gambling, curing rituals, and first fruits and harvest festivals for deer, salmon, and root crops. However, the major ritual, which draws together all of the old subsistence and healing rituals, is the Winter Dance. This dance is a complex renewal ritual convened by individual sponsors from late December through February. An abbreviated form of the ceremony can be performed at any time for someone in need. Simply by ritually establishing the center pole, the most significant symbol of the bioregion, in the middle of the dance house the curative and transformative powers of the Winter Dance can be evoked.

The Winter Dance ritual complex is especially focused on the singing of guardian spirit songs over the successive days of the ceremonial (Grim, 1992). Singing begins in the evening of each day and continues until dawn. "Ceremonial" also refers to the accompanying ritual activity that occurs during the day, such as feasting, sweat-lodge rituals (healings, purifications, petitions), giveaways, stick-game gambling, and storytelling. At the ritual heart of the Winter Dance, however, is the individual–guardian spirit relationship. Most important, this spirit–human exchange generates and reenacts the time of the traditional mythic stories, or cosmogony, in which the universe was created. The Salish moral imagination is established in this cosmogonic symbolism that is believed to renew community life and to regenerate plants and animals. Thus, individual–guardian spirit relationships form the core of the Salish synthetic ethics in which stories, songs, and symbolic actions bind individual, community, and bioregion together to generate a sacred cohesiveness and a spiritual empathy. This Native American ritual, then, provides an excellent example of the close relationship between land, lifeway, and synthetic ethics.

Prior to contact with mainstream America and the establishment of the reservation system in the nineteenth century, the Winter Dance provided the major impetus for independent villages to undertake ritual diplomacy with other villages. The ritual was the locus of interaction that smoothed individual conflicts and encouraged group cohesion. Thus, the multifaceted Winter Dance diminished aggressive rivalry between villages and brought them together for the shared task of world renewal. Just as the Winter Dance was the locus for negotiation between fiercely independent and self-governed villages, so this ritual continues to be the central place for negotiation between the human and spirit realms.

As a world renewal ceremony the Winter Dance calls the spirit powers of the bioregion into reciprocal relationship with the human communities. This ceremonial makes explicit the interdependence of minerals, plants, animals, and humans through the songs that are sung by those who have had visionary experiences of these spirits in special places of the bioregion. There is no explicit recitation of a cosmogony during the Winter Dance; however, during the days between the evening and all-night ritual activity, individuals are encouraged to tell stories. Coyote stories are especially popular on these occasions. While there is no single cosmogony among the Salish people, the cycle of Coyote stories has cosmogonic features that describe the formative activities in the time of mythic beginnings (Mourning Dove, 1933). The often humorous Coyote stories are ensembles of generative moral metaphors in which the ambiguous and mistaken actions of Coyote are narrated as examples of inharmonious behavior. Thus, the formal activities of singing vision songs and the giving of gifts, as well as the informal storytelling, serve to activate a ritual logic that informs participants of both the sources of motivation for a moral life and the purposive world around them.

The most significant symbol of land and the human presence is the center pole, a lodgepole pine ninety or so inches high. The center pole, symbolic of the bioregion, is set up in the middle of the dance hall. It is the most significant place for contact with, and communication from, guardian spirits. Songs and giveaways are the mode of the moral imagination during this ritual, and the singers are said to experience a spirit sickness because of their proximity to the cosmogonic powers. The singers go to that center pole to sing, speak in moral exhortation to the assembled community, and give gifts just as the ancient mythic spirits gave to humans. While dancing around the pole to the songs of the visionaries, the participants are said to be like the animals who "are moving around" during the snows of the Winter Dance season. The very structure of the Winter Dance as animals moving about the land is presented as having moral force in Salish thought. More than simply isolated ritual acts or symbolic gestures, it is understood as bringing a person and a community into the moral order established during the time of the cosmogonic events when the mythic plants, minerals, and animals decided to give their bodies to humans for food.

In the traditional Winter Dance singers renewed themselves in the centering experience of the ceremony, and by doing so re-created their village communities. Much has been lost due to the intrusion of the dominant Euro-American worldview, which has devalued the sacredness of the community of all life forms and has often misunderstood the visionary experiences of guardian spirits. Still, the Salish Winter Dance retains striking continuity with a traditional ethics of giving, evident in the giveaway features of the ritual, and of empathy, apparent in the spirit sickness. This is because of the evocation in the Winter Dance ritual of the ancient cosmogonic knowledge transmitted in the sacred power (*sumix*) of the mineral, plant, and animal persons, in the spirit sickness of the singers, and in the cosmic symbolism of the centering tree. This relationship between ritual and ethics can be labeled "synthetic" to signal the holistic character of the traditional lifeway of these people.

Health, sickness, and healing

Knowledge of health, reproduction, and death among particular native North American peoples developed in relation to their investigative exchange with bioregions, and in historical contacts among indigenous peoples long before the arrival of Europeans. One ancient religious practice, that of the healer, or shaman, still embodies traditional knowledge of bioregions accumulated over centuries of historical change. Comparative studies in shamanism suggest that Native American peoples brought healing practices with them in their transcontinental passages from Siberia as long as 40,000 years ago. The shaman, as a specialist in psychological and spiritual healing, can be contrasted in some native North American traditions with herbalists, who also sought to cure ills. Among the Winnebago of the western Great Lakes region of Wisconsin the following advice was given to young men who were about to seek a vision experience:

> There are individuals who know [the virtues and powers]. It is sad enough that you could not obtain [blessings from the more powerful spirits] during fasting; but at least ask those who possess plants to take pity on you. If they take pity on you, they will give you one of the good plants that give life [to man] and thus you can use them to encourage you in life. However, one plant will not be enough for you to possess. All [the plants] that are to be found on grandmother's hair, all those that give life, you should try to find out about, until you have a medicine chest [full]. Then you will indeed have great reason for being encouraged. (Blowsnake, 1920, p. 75)

Such advice not only emphasizes the disciplined attention given to the plant world and to those who know the healing properties of plants but also suggests the broad connections between religion, ethics, and bioregion.

The last 500 years of historical contacts with Eurasia have brought "virgin soil epidemics," diseases against which native peoples had no natural defense (Crosby, 1986), resulting in demographic devastation among Native American populations (Dobyns, 1983). The initial challenge to and decline in the ritual authority of Native American shamans due to disease during the seventeenth, eighteenth, and nineteenth centuries did not lead to the disappearance of these ritual practitioners. Rather, as epidemics subsided, traditional practices were often given full credit for effecting cures (Trigger, 1985). Currently, traditional healers are often found working with scientific medical practitioners on many reserves and reservations.

Mainstream American popularizations of surviving Native American healing practices resulted, during the nineteenth century, in misunderstandings of herbal healers or medicine persons (Albanese, 1990). This has led to romantic fictional accounts of shamans as creative individualists. One characteristic that courses through all of this interest in Native American health systems is the close connection between medicine and religion. As we have emphasized in the use of the term "lifeway," religion is a relational practice, and an indigenous shaman always stands in close connection with his or her bioregional community.

Ritual specialists capable of diagnosing disease, treating ailments, and guiding the dead are found in all traditional native North American settings (Hultkrantz, 1992). In many agricultural communities these specialists organized in priesthoods that transmitted traditional lore and ritual experiences that addressed specific sicknesses. Among the Ashiwi/Zuni in the Southwest, research on the human body was extensive and, during healing rituals, patterns symbolic of the somatic knowledge of Zuni healers were drawn on the patient (Hultkrantz, 1992). The physiology and anthropology informing this ritual, however, were not necessarily drawn from cadaver experiments or empirical observations of social structure. These healing societies typically abhorred cutting a dead body, for it still embodied ancestral animating principles in the process of release or dying. Often specialists in dreams, visions, and spiritual travel to other-than-human realms were believed to have acquired knowledge of the human body that could not have been obtained by observational means (Deloria, 1993).

The gathering-and-hunting societies of the period before the late nineteenth century, as well as many of these extant native communities, generally sanction individual shamans. Different from priests, who may be inducted into a healing cult through a personal healing or clan privilege to learn a traditional body of lore (Ortiz, 1969), shamans are usually called by vivid experiences of spirits that "adopt" them and enable them to respond to specific needs of their people (Grim, 1983). Myths among diverse native North American peoples, such as the Apsaalooke/Crow and the Dine/Navajo, often described a hero or heroine as someone who had been abandoned by the people and consequently, "adopted" by a spirit power (Eliade, 1964; Grim, 1983; Sandner, 1979; Sullivan, 1989).

Disease in a traditional Native American setting is usually attributed to transgression of a cosmological principle, performance of prohibited behavior, intrusion of an object "shot" into a diseased individual by witchcraft, or loss of a vital soul. Prohibitions in a native context often constitute a major ethical system involving hundreds of rules for the treatment of living organisms, handling the remains of organisms, and strategies for living with the spiritual powers in the bioregion. The Koyukon people of Alaska, for example, have an elaborate system of rules and regulations called *hutlanee* (Nelson, 1983). Disease and death can result from breaking these rules and disrupting the natural balance of *sinh taala*, the power of the earth. Koyukon shamans, *diyinyoo*, know the spiritual powers that reside in the bioregion and use their power to diagnose disease, to treat illness, and to restore *sinh taala*, the foundation of their medicine. Shamans and elders teach the wisdom needed to restore the power of the earth and to meet death with knowledge of the paths to those places in the bioregion where the dead one will live. These teachings are found in the stories from the Distant Time, or *Kk'adonts'idnee*, in which the origin, design, and functioning of nature were established. Instituted in Distant Time, the *hutlanee*, moral codes for conserving game animals and the environment, are not simply superstitions but the Koyukon synthetic ethics that governs life.

Disease that results from "object intrusion," or witchcraft, often implies a worldview in which balance or harmony between one's body and the local bioregion has been purposely broken by a malicious individual. Among the Dine/Navajo, the health of an individual is not an isolated case but a matter of the whole community of life. The "beauty," or *hozho*, inherent in the world can be put out of harmony by the malicious act of witchcraft. Cosmological ceremonies of great beauty, called chantways, are conducted by ritual specialists, or singers, to reestablish the diseased person's bodily harmony by removing the intruded object or retrieving lost vitality. The key relationship in Dine/Navajo rituals is that between the Holy People, *Diyin Dine'e*, who are potentially malevolent as numinous forces in the landscape, and the Dine themselves, as earth-surface people. To reestablish health, the ritual evokes the Holy People, who are the inner forms of the elements of nature. Through the narrative power of language, especially in a form of the chantway called Enemyway, which exorcises evil, the chaos of witchcraft can be transformed into order and beauty (Witherspoon, 1977). The synthetic ethics of the Dine/Navajo people does not expel malicious people from the community, where there would be no opportunity to undo their evil. Rather the hope is that they also can be restored to "beauty" and cosmic harmony.

In the Dine/Navajo Emergence Myth, the basic narrative source for the chantway stories, the beauty of the earth is evoked in the following chant to restore health: "Then go on as one who has long life, Go on as one who is happy, Go with blessing before you, Go with blessing behind you, Go with blessing below you, Go with blessing above you, Go with blessing around you, Go with blessing in your speech, Go with happiness and long life, Go mysteriously" (Sandner, 1979, p. vii). Through this repetitive language, the chanters amplify sacred power and control the inner forms of themselves, of their patients, and of the spiritual powers in the landscape that have been evoked into the sandpainting ritual. The chanter restores the blessedness of the one sung over by bringing the patient into the healing environment.

Current ethical perspectives

Major ethical issues involving native North American peoples have coalesced around the following three areas: ancestral bones, religious freedom, and sovereignty. The passage of the Grave Protection and Repatriation Act of 1990 has helped to slow the pillage of ancestral Native American gravesites. So also the itemization of Native American holdings in major museums will enhance the possibility of the return of sensitive religious material to native peoples from whom it was often improperly obtained.

Serious questions of trust and sovereignty between the American government and Native American peoples have arisen in the late twentieth century in a series of court cases in which indigenous religious freedom has been curtailed. The history of mainstream American cultural and legislative antagonism toward Native American lifeways had been momentarily reversed in the passage in 1978 of the American Indian Religious Freedom Act. However, a sequence of Supreme Court cases (especially *Lying* v. *Northwest Indian Cemetery Protection Association* and *Employment Division* v. *Smith*) has challenged the sovereignty of Native American lifeways and demonstrated an unwillingness to recognize their sacred relationships to land.

The emergence at the end of the twentieth century of a global voice of indigenous people comes as a result of such negative factors as the environmental crisis and the proximity of indigenous peoples to undeveloped areas on the globe. In the United States and Canada, native North American peoples, having been pushed onto reservations and reserves away from the majority populations of mainstream culture, now manage resources and undeveloped land. Native American peoples have increased their close contact with other indigenous peoples around the globe in an effort to protect themselves from environmental racism, the imposition of projects such as hydroelectric dams and toxic dump sites that destroy the environments of minority peoples. Gatherings such as the United Nations Earth Summit in Rio de Janeiro in 1992 and the meetings titled "Changing Ecological Values in the 21st Century" in Kyoto, Japan, in 1993 have included native North American representatives. Meetings have also brought together representatives from the world's religions to talk with elders from Native American lifeways about their traditional environmental ethics.

The remarkable resurgence of native North American peoples in the late twentieth century, after 500 years of suppression, derives from a complex process, but undoubtedly the knowledge transmitted in traditional ethics is a singular component of their endurance. Often dismissed as superstitious or derogatively labeled as primitive, the affective and holistic insights of native peoples are now recognized as ways of knowing grounded in close relationship with local bioregions. Those native teachers who still know this ethical system present their insights as a gift, a giveaway, to dominant America, which for so long juxtaposed the "nobility" of Enlightenment reason with the "contemptible character" of native thought. For traditional native North American peoples, the world is alive and, far from being a random collection of objects, is seen by some as our Mother and by many as a community of knowing subjects. Rather than a branch of knowledge, bioethics, in a native North American context, brings one to the heart of a way through life.

JOHN A. GRIM

Directly related to this entry is the entry ENVIRONMENT AND RELIGION. *For a further discussion of topics mentioned in this entry, see the entries* ABORTION; ANIMAL WELFARE AND RIGHTS; BODY; FERTILITY CONTROL; LIFE; NARRATIVE; *and* NATURE. *For a discussion of related ideas, see the entries* ENDANGERED SPECIES AND BIODIVERSITY; ENVIRONMENTAL ETHICS; *and* ETHICS, *article on* RELIGION AND MORALITY. *Other relevant material may be found under the entries* ETHICS, *article on* MORAL EPISTEMOLOGY; HEALING; *and* VALUE AND VALUATION.

Bibliography

ALBANESE, CATHERINE L. 1990. *Nature Religion in America: From the Algonkian Indians to the New Age.* Chicago: University of Chicago Press.

BLOWSNAKE, SAM. 1963. [1923]. *The Autobiography of a Winnebago Indian.* Edited and translated by Paul Radin. University of California Publications in American Archaeology and Ethnology, vol. 16, no. 7. New York: Dover.

CROSBY, ALFRED W. 1986. *Ecological Imperialism: The Biological Expansion of Europe, 900–1900.* Cambridge: At the University Press.

DELORIA, VINE, JR. 1993. "If You Think About It, You Will See That It Is True." *Noetic Sciences Review* no. 27 (Autumn): 62–71.

DOBYNS, HENRY F. 1983. *Their Number Become Thinned: Native American Population Dynamics in Eastern North America.* Knoxville: University of Tennessee Press.

ELIADE, MIRCEA. 1964. *Shamanism: Archaic Techniques of Ecstasy.* New York: Bollingen Foundation.

GRIM, JOHN A. 1983. *The Shaman: Patterns of Siberian and Ojibway Healing.* Norman: University of Oklahoma Press.
———. 1992. "Cosmogony and the Winter Dance: Native American Ethics in Transition." *Journal of Religious Ethics* 20, no. 2:389–413.

HOPPAL, MIHALY, and VON SADOVSZKY, OTTO, eds. 1989. *Shamanism: Past and Present.* 2 vols. Budapest: International Society for Trans-Oceanic Research.

HULTKRANTZ, AKE. 1992. *Shamanic Healing and Ritual Drama: Health and Medicine in Native North American Religious Traditions.* New York: Crossroads.

JILEK, WOLFGANG G. 1982. *Indian Healing: Shamanic Ceremonialism in the Pacific Northwest Today.* Surrey, B.C.: Hancock House.

KUNITZ, STEPHEN J. 1983. *Disease, Change, and the Role of Medicine: The Navajo Experience.* Berkeley: University of California Press.

LADUKE, WINONA. 1992. "Minobimaatisiiwin: The Good Life." *Cultural Survival Quarterly* 16, no. 4:69–71.

LOVIN, ROBIN W., and REYNOLDS, FRANK E., eds. 1985. *Cosmogony and Ethical Order: New Studies in Comparative Ethics.* Chicago: University of Chicago Press.

LYONS, OREN. 1987. "Communiqué No. 11." *Traditional Circle of Elders* (Denver), September 11.

MOURNING DOVE. 1990. [1993]. *Mourning Dove: A Salishan Autobiography.* Edited by Jay Miller. Lincoln: University of Nebraska Press.

NELSON, RICHARD K. 1983. *Make Prayers to the Raven: A Koyukon View of the Northern Forest.* Chicago: University of Chicago Press.

ORTIZ, ALFONSO. 1969. *The Tewa World: Space, Time, Being, and Becoming in a Pueblo Society.* Chicago: University of Chicago Press.

SANDNER, DONALD. 1979. *Navaho Symbols of Healing.* New York: Harcourt Brace Jovanovich.

STURTEVANT, WILLIAM C., ed. 1978–. *Handbook of North American Indians.* 20 vols. to date. Washington, D.C.: Smithsonian Institution.

SULLIVAN, LAWRENCE E., ed. 1989. *Native American Religions.* New York: Macmillan.

THORNTON, RUSSELL. 1987. *American Indian Holocaust and Survival: A Population History Since 1492.* Norman: University of Oklahoma Press.

TRIGGER, BRUCE G. 1985. *Natives and Newcomers: Canada's "Heroic Age" Reconsidered.* Montreal: McGill-Queen's University Press.

VOGEL, VIRGIL J. 1970. *American Indian Medicine.* Norman: University of Oklahoma Press.

WITHERSPOON, GARY. 1977. *Language and Art in the Navajo Universe.* Ann Arbor: University of Michigan Press.

NATURAL LAW

Natural law is perhaps the most ancient and historically persistent concept in Western ethics. Philosophers like Aristotle regarded nature as a ground of justice. Theologians like Thomas Aquinas distinguished between natural and supernatural sources of morality and law. By it Thomas Jefferson sanctioned a revolution. With it political reformers like Martin Luther King, Jr., justified civil disobedience. Upon it political philosophers like John Locke have built theories of the origin and limits of the civil state; and international lawyers, such as Hugo Grotius and Samuel Pufendorf, the order of justice between states. Despite disagreements about the theory of natural law, international bodies appeal to unwritten sources of rights to health care.

U.S. constitutional law has used natural law to clarify and sometimes amend the written law. Natural law undergirds the Thirteenth (1865) and Fourteenth Amendments (1868), which outlawed slavery and secured rights of U.S. citizens against state jurisdictions. Natural law also serves as a method of judicial interpretation, from which the judge looks beyond the written text of the Constitution in order to identify and vindicate rights of citizens. Today, constitutional debates have become the most public and controversial forum of natural-law discussion (Dworkin, 1985; Ely, 1980). Inasmuch as natural law is widely regarded as the moral basis for rights of privacy or personal autonomy, it is implicated in some of the most difficult biomedical issues, including abortion, reproductive technologies, and euthanasia.

The question of natural law emerges when we consider human laws and customs (Sokolowski, 1992). None is perfect, and some appear to be wicked. We then ask, What is the norm of reason in matters of morality and justice? Are moral norms merely the artifacts of human reason, devised to serve the circumstances of a particular culture? Or is there a ground that transcends cultures and histories? On what basis can laws be morally criticized and rectified?

Since these questions are fundamental to all ethical inquiry, what makes natural law different from other normative theories? There is no tidy answer. An array of moral theorists, using different theories, agree (1) that there are objective, though unwritten, moral grounds for right reason in the legislation and adjudication of human law, and (2) that moral reason must be guided by, and respect, certain values inherent in human nature (e.g., rationality and the capacity for free choice). If natural law means that moral and legal norms are grounded in reason, and that right exercise of human reason requires respect for goods inherent in human nature, then it would be exceedingly difficult not to hold a natural-law theory of one sort or another.

The health-care professional exploring natural-law issues will face a debate often abstract and bewildering. First, what starts as a debate over particular issues in law, politics, or health care often becomes a debate over the concept of natural law itself. Second, what distinguishes one natural-law theory from another is not always clear; there seem to be as many different theories of natural law as there are theorists. In any case, one must remember that the rubric "natural law" often hides important disagreements among its proponents, as well as significant agreements among those who dispute its particular formulations and applications. Third, until recently natural-law thinking for the most part has not directly addressed biomedical issues. A well-developed body of natural-law literature, as found in legal, moral, and political theory, does not yet exist for biomedical issues. Thus, it will be helpful to summarize some of the main historical and philosophical themes of natural law.

Ancient themes

Ancient Greek philosophers asked whether law and morality are due principally to nature or to convention. Aristotle, who is sometimes credited as the father of

natural law, contended that "[w]hat is just in the political sense can be subdivided into what is just by nature and what is just by convention. What is by nature just has the same force everywhere and does not depend on what we regard or do not regard as just" (*Nicomachean Ethics*, 1134b18). While Aristotle certainly held that there are standards for judging whether a law is "in accord with nature" (*Rhetoric*, 1373b6), whether he had a doctrine of "natural law" is much debated (Miller, 1991). The proposition that moral judgment is rooted in the soil of nature, and not merely in human artifice, does not necessarily mean that nature is a "law."

The form of natural-law theory that came to influence Western culture arose from the confluence of Stoic, biblical, and Christian Scholastic ideas. Cicero, the ancient authority most often cited by Christians, wrote:

> True law is right reason in agreement with nature; it is of universal application, unchanging and everlasting; it summons to duty by its commands, and averts from wrongdoing by its prohibitions. . . . It is a sin to try to alter this law, nor is it allowable to attempt to repeal any part of it, and it is impossible to abolish it entirely. . . . [there is] one master and ruler, that is, God, over us all, for he is author of this law, its promulgator, and its enforcing judge. (*De Re Publica*, 3.22.33)

Similarly, Thomas Aquinas said that "the participation in the eternal law by rational creatures is called the law of nature" (*Summa theologica*, 1947, I-II, q. 91, a. 2). Nature *as law* requires the notion that natural standards are promulgated by God. The human intelligence finds itself not merely in a natural order but under a divine commonwealth, which is a rule of law in the exemplary sense.

Aquinas and natural law

Since the theory of natural law as developed by Thomas Aquinas is widely regarded as the epitome of the premodern position, let us summarize his view. In the *Summa theologica*, Aquinas maintains that for something to be called law, it must be (1) reasonable, in the sense of directing action; (2) ordained to the common good; (3) legislated by the proper authority; and (4) duly promulgated (I-II, q. 90). The eternal law, whereby the world is ruled by divine providence, satisfies these criteria in an exemplary way (q. 91, a. 1). Natural law, however, is principally that part of divine reason accessible to the human intelligence. It is not to be confused with the order of the physical or biological world. Law is predicated only by a kind of similitude with the order found in nonrational entities (q. 91, a. 2 ad 3).

The first principle of the natural law is that "Good is to be done and pursued and evil avoided" (q. 94, a. 2). By nature, the human agent is inclined toward certain intelligible goods. Though Aquinas never claimed to provide an exhaustive list, these goods include life, procreation and care of offspring, entering into society, and knowing the truth about God. The first precepts of natural law take the form that something is to be done and pursued with respect to these goods, or resisted if contrary to them. Why call the precepts "natural"? Because the objectives of action are grounded in human nature antecedent to our deliberation and choice. In this sense, nature signifies the (human) essence directed to its specific operation. The term "natural" also indicates that the first precepts stand as the basic axioms of action, and are known naturally (*naturaliter*) rather than learned by study or by inference. Why call the objects of these inclinations "precepts" or "law"? Aquinas maintains that human agents are capable of seeing that certain goods are worthy of pursuit; they also grasp, in an elementary way, that in choices one is morally bound to act in accord with these goods.

The first precepts, however, are not a complete moral code. Aquinas holds that human reason must develop and apply them. First precepts are developed in terms of "secondary precepts," which spell out further implications for human action. For example, from the precept that one must act in accord with the good of life and resist what is contrary to it, we reason that murder is wrong. The first precepts also require "determinations," supplied by custom and positive laws. The "determinations" are ways that the natural law is made effective in the human community. Thus, while the care and education of offspring are enjoined upon humankind by a first precept of the natural law, how, where, and when the duty is discharged are determined by custom or positive law. Here, the virtue of prudence is paramount.

In the Thomistic scheme, the moral order in human law and politics is a kind of ecosystem, requiring for its proper function not only the universally binding precepts of natural law but also good customs, intelligently framed and emended positive laws, and acquired virtues, by which the laws are obeyed not just externally but also in the interior act of the will. It is therefore not advisable to isolate the doctrine of natural law in Aquinas from the rest of his account of moral agency. First, Aquinas flatly rejects the idea that human beings ever existed in a pure state of nature (I, q. 95, a. 1), unlike the ahistorical "state of nature" models of the modern era. Created in grace and wounded by sin, the concrete human condition, according to Aquinas, is in need of tutoring and, ultimately, of transformation by divine grace. Aquinas insists, for example, that the two great ends of the natural law—the love of God and of neighbor—obscured by sin and evil customs, require repromulgation by divine positive law (q. 100, aa. 5, 11). Second, the greater part of his *Treatise on Law* (I-II, qq. 90–108) puts the natural law in the double context of the divine positive law of the Old Testament (*lex vetus*) and the New Testament Law of Grace (*lex nova*). Biblical history shapes Aquinas's fully considered judgment and exposition of the natural law.

Aquinas can be absolved of the charge that he confuses moral and physical meanings of nature, as well as the charge that his account is ahistorical. Yet his theory of natural law does rely on a teleological conception of providence, and the historical cast of his thought is informed by the biblical narrative. These features are not accidental. To the extent that modern theorists reject the credibility of the teleological science of nature, and aim to provide an account of natural law that is neutral with respect to theological suppositions, the Thomist theory will be of more historical than systematic interest.

Modern theories

In modern times, the concept of natural law has undergone considerable doctrinal and institutional development. Although the theological framework of natural law was maintained as part of public rhetoric well into the nineteenth century, it was no longer the main interest of natural lawyers. As Lloyd Weinreb notes: "The puzzles with which Aquinas and others grappled when they tried to understand the place of humankind in nature appear in [modern] guise as part of the effort to describe the relationship of the individual to the state" (1987, p. 67). This shift of perspective and emphasis, from cosmological and theological themes to the more narrow political and legal issues of natural law, is complicated. Leo Strauss (1953) has argued that the ancient and modern theories are so radically different that they ought not to be confounded. Whether there is continuity or discontinuity between premodern and modern versions of natural law remains a disputed subject in the scholarly literature. While we cannot discuss this in detail, we can cite at least two problems that have shaped the modern approach.

Natural law and modern science. By the seventeenth century, the phrase "natural law" was expropriated by the modern sciences to denote purely descriptive or predictive aspects of natural bodies. In optics, astronomy, and physics, the relation between nature and law no longer expressed the *human* participation in divine providence but, rather, the intelligible, measurable, and predictable regularities in physical nature (Ruby, 1986). Teleological understanding was abandoned in favor of mechanistic explanations that relied exclusively upon material and efficient causes. The success and prestige of the physical sciences made it difficult thenceforth to interrelate the moral and physical meanings of natural law without falling into equivocation. How, for example, can law be predicated on nature without conflating physical and moral necessities? In the physical sciences, law denotes the measurable and predictable properties of things that have no freedom. But in the practical or moral sphere, law denotes principles that govern human freedom. These two meanings of natural law—nature as amenable to description and prediction, and nature as a prescriptive norm of freedom—present an ongoing theoretical difficulty in modern thought about the subject.

Natural law and the public order of rights. The humane focus of natural law concerns legal and political problems of the relationship between the individual and the state. In the seventeenth and eighteenth centuries, human nature rather than authority allegedly vested in churches or kings came to represent the legitimate origin of the state and its rule of law. Philosophers and jurists wrested natural law from the controversial settings of religion and custom, and attempted to reduce it to self-evident laws of reason sufficient to ground a public order of law and rights. While the well-known dictum by Hugo Grotius that the natural law would have validity even if God did not exist captures something of the modern temper, even more pertinent is his assertion that "[j]ust as mathematicians treat their figures as abstracted from bodies, so in treating law I have withdrawn my mind from every particular fact" (Grotius, 1925, Prolegomena nos. 11, 58). Modern natural-law theorists emphasize apodictic, nongainsayable propositions, and filter out anything dependent upon the mediation of culture and religion. These theories are expected to cut through religious and political controversy in order to secure that minimum of rational consensus needed for public purposes (Gewirth, 1984). In contrast with the ancients and medievals, the minimalistic bent of modern theories is not designed to mesh with the virtue of prudence.

Natural social necessities

Given the new scientific meanings of nature and law, as well as the practical need to devise principles of justice sufficient to limit the modern state, two approaches to natural law dominate the modern period. One tradition keys natural law to what is needed for survival and societal peace. By nature, human beings are vulnerable, and need a certain minimal protection of their interests. Thomas Hobbes set the pattern of this tradition. Other examples of this approach are David Hume's "circumstances of justice," Oliver Wendell Holmes's "can't helps," and H. L. A. Hart's "minimum natural law." Natural law sets a background for customs and laws prohibiting violations of life, limb, and property. The advantages of this approach are at least threefold. First, the desire to protect one's life and property, insofar as it can be described and predicted, comports with the physicalist model of nature and law favored by the modern sciences. Second, it picks out elementary goods and bads that are apt to win consensus. These basic needs do not seem to depend upon the idiosyncrasies of particular individuals and their private life plans. Third, at least in the Anglo-American world, issues of life, limb, and property are easily recognized and adjudicated within a system of positive law.

However, natural necessities provide little or no reason to recognize absolute moral norms or rights that might resist the utilitarian calculations of a political majority acting for its alleged interests in peace and security. As Oliver Wendell Holmes said in his famous essay on natural law: "The most fundamental of the supposed preexisting rights—the right to life—is sacrificed without a scruple not only in war, but whenever the interest of society, that is, of the predominant power in the community, is thought to demand it" (Holmes, 1918, p. 314). It is one thing to say that any system of positive law must work against the background of natural human necessities; it is quite another to hold that these pervasive natural facts about the human condition carry any prescriptive or moral force.

Natural right of autonomy

Another tradition, typified by Kant's dictum that one "[m]ust act as if the maxim of your action were to become through your will a universal law of nature" (Kant, 1981, no. 421, p. 30), emphasizes the autonomy of moral agents. This natural law can be expressed in the categorical imperative that humanity in one's person and in the person of others must be respected as an end in itself. As developed by many modern theorists, autonomy is a concept variously described as "moral independence" (Dworkin, 1985, p. 353), "the free choice of goals and relations as an essential ingredient of individual well-being" (Raz, 1986, p. 369), and "personal sovereignty" (Reiman, 1990, p. 43). Is autonomy a fact about human nature, or is it a moral ideal? There is disagreement about this (Schneewind, 1986). Reiman, for example, maintains that "Personal sovereignty [indicates] a natural fact about human beings, consideration of which will lead us to the natural ground of equality between human beings" (1990, p. 43). Put thus, autonomy embraces both a natural fact and a moral principle.

Some version of the autonomist theory is the preferred approach in much of contemporary natural-law theory, for the autonomist position emphasizes specifically moral principles of law rather than mere natural necessities. It seeks to tell us not what agents typically want or need, but how and why human beings must be respected. Moreover, it comports with the humanistic premise that human beings have a native dignity based upon a rational capacity to determine their conduct. It is the rational capacity that sets (at least some) human beings apart from other entities of nature, and constitutes the axioms of the moral world.

Despite its wide appeal, three problems routinely crop up in connection with the autonomist position. First, it is not always clear whether we are enjoined to respect the capacity for autonomy or the rightful exercise of that capacity. If we are enjoined to respect the capacity itself, are we thereby duty bound to respect the agent when he or she uses the capacity in a wicked way? In short, do agents have a moral right to do moral wrong? Second, the rights and obligations that flow from this "natural" fact of autonomy are difficult to formulate except in very general terms. What can a right to autonomy mean, except that persons ought not to be treated as mere objects; and what can this mean, except that a person ought to be treated according to sound moral considerations (Raz, 1986)? Hence, while autonomists emphasize a natural right to be treated equally, it is a humanist premise rather than the conclusion of moral reasoning (Raz, 1986). Third, we can ask whether the natural capacity for self-determination is adequate for moral reasoning about the status of other nonhuman species, prehuman entities (genetic material), incipient human life (embryos), and human beings whose autonomy is diminished.

Catholic natural-law theory

The Roman Catholic church is the only international institution to hold a natural-law doctrine in both the premodern and modern phases of the theory. Conciliar decrees, papal encyclicals, and canon law both reaffirm the natural law and have applied it across a range of moral issues (Fuchs, 1965; Finnis, 1980b). The encyclical Veritatis splendor (1993) gives considerable attention to natural law. Drawn chiefly from the work of Augustine and Aquinas, the papal formulation of natural law in Veritatis is traditional, emphasizing the status of natural law as real law, promulgated by God. Although there is only passing reference to biomedical issues, the encyclical represents perhaps the clearest exposition of the theoretical underpinnings of natural law by a modern pope. The concept of natural law has also recently been applied to natural rights. The new Code of Canon Law (1983) asserts the right of the church to address secular affairs insofar as such affairs pertain to "fundamental rights of the human person" (canon 747/2).

Over the past three decades natural-law debate has focused upon the encyclical Humanae vitae (1968), which condemned contraception as a violation of the natural law, not because it is artificial but because it is contrary to nature. The encyclical's premise is that marriage (apart from considerations of sacramental theology) naturally contains both a procreative and a unitive good. The moral question is whether these goods can be deliberately separated in the particular conjugal act. The natural-law reasoning of Humanae vitae has been interpreted in quite different, and sometimes contradictory, ways by moral theologians. A 1991 study finds that at least six natural-law positions have emerged in the de-

bate (Smith, 1991). This is because the encyclical is terse, and does not spell out its argument in the fashion of an academic exercise. But it is also due to the fact that the encyclical outlines an argument at three levels, each of which is open to debate: (1) that the conjugal act must preserve the intrinsic order toward the procreative end; (2) that the unitive and procreative goods of marriage must not be separated; (3) that the integrity of marriage cannot be maintained in its totality unless it is maintained in each and every conjugal act. Hence, its analysis of nature concerns not only the natural order of the sexual function but also the natural goods of marriage as well as the nature of the human sexual act itself. Whatever might be said about the document, it does not present a simple natural-law argument.

Critics like Charles Curran (1985) have charged that Humanae vitae confuses the physical and moral structures of human acts. Curran also charges the encyclical with adopting a "classicist worldview and methodology" that comports with neither the methods of the sciences nor the relativizing of nature by the history of salvation (1985). Bernard Häring raises objections similar to Curran's. Not only in matters of reproduction, but also more generally in biomedical issues, Häring notes that the physician no longer defines himself as a servant of "ordered potentialities and powers of nature." Rather, he "increasingly considers himself an architect and sculptor of the given stuff of nature" (Häring, 1973). So, too, the moral theologian, he argues, must emphasize the divine mandate to creatively mold and intervene in nature. As so often happens in debates about natural law, the practical issue at hand (in this case, contraception) quickly opens onto the more abstract philosophical and theological questions about the meaning of nature and how it relates to norms of conduct.

In 1987, Joseph Cardinal Ratzinger, prefect of the Congregation for the Doctrine of the Faith, issued Instruction on Respect for Human Life (Donum vitae). The Instruction addressed a number of biomedical issues, including experimentation upon human embryos; methods of prenatal diagnosis; and in vitro fertilization, both homologous (the meeting in vitro of the gametes of married spouses) and heterologous (the use of gametes coming from at least one donor other than the spouses). Whereas Humanae vitae contended that the procreative good cannot deliberately be suppressed in favor of the unitive good, Cardinal Ratzinger argued that the natural law also prohibits separating procreation from the unity and love of the spousal act. While the argument is similar to Humanae vitae, Cardinal Ratzinger makes it clearer that natural law is a moral law, not to be confused with a "set of norms on the biological level." By nature, the conjugal act is a "personal" act of love between spouses. This guarantees that the transmission of life is an act of procreativity rather than mere reproduction. The Instruction, therefore, maintains that in vitro fertilization, whether homologous or heterologous, is contrary to the personal and unitive meaning of the marital act.

With respect to human rights, Cardinal Ratzinger argues that in vitro fertilization violates not only the natural structure of the marital act but also the "inalienable rights" of the child. The child cannot be treated as an object serving the interests of the parents but, rather, must be treated as an end in itself. Parents have only the right to perform those acts that are per se ordered to procreation. Were parents to have a right to reproduce, by whatever means, then the child would be an object to which one has a right of ownership. At least on matters of bioethics, the *Instruction* represents an important development in the linkage between a traditional natural-law conception of the marital act with distinctively modern arguments concerning natural rights.

Natural-law theory is in a period of transition among Catholic scholars. Some scholars working in the Thomistic tradition now emphasize the role of the virtues rather than the juridical themes of natural law (Bourke, 1974; MacIntyre, 1988). Others, notably John Finnis (1980a) and Germain Grisez (1983), have developed a theory of the relationship between practical reason and "basic human goods" (e.g., life, knowledge, play, aesthetic experience, sociability, practical reasonableness, and religion). The aim of the theory is to identify moral norms governing how basic goods ought to be chosen. It was first undertaken by Germain Grisez (1964; 1983); John Finnis (1980a) has systematically applied Grisez's work to the whole field of jurisprudence. The natural-law component of the theory is much criticized. Some argue that it has no clear connection to the Thomistic doctrine of natural theology (Hittinger, 1987); others, particularly proportionalists, argue that absolute moral norms are not easily generated by such generalized forms of human well-being (McCormick, 1981). Although there is considerable agreement among Catholic philosophers and theologians that natural law is important, there is less agreement about how to deal systematically with the subject.

Natural law in law and bioethics

Constitutional and legal issues have occupied recent secular debates over natural law. It is noteworthy that the philosophical ground of the debate between natural lawyers and legal positivists continues to be revisited (see essays in George, 1992). At a more concrete level, however, discussion has focused upon civil liberties, particularly the right of privacy. Since this area of the law is the bellwether for many important biomedical questions, we will briefly outline the state of this discussion.

In *Griswold* v. *Connecticut* (1965), the Supreme Court invalidated a Connecticut statute forbidding the sale to and use of contraceptives by married people. The Court held that a zone of privacy protects marriage from intrusive governmental actions. Since the Constitution and its amendments do not mention the right of privacy, the Court was widely regarded as using natural law in constitutional interpretation. Indeed, the use of natural law was more controversial than the result in this particular case. In *Eisenstadt* v. *Baird* (1972), which invalidated a Massachusetts statute prohibiting the sale of contraceptives to unmarried people, Justice William Brennan reasoned that the right of privacy generally covers the decision of individuals, married or single, to make decisions about whether to "bear or beget" children. In *Roe* v. *Wade* (1973), the right to privacy was extended to abortion. Since then, it has been cited by lower courts as precedent for paternal refusal to allow the implantation of embryos. Other biomedical issues have also surfaced in the courts in terms of natural rights: "There is a fundamental natural right expressed in our Constitution as the 'right to liberty,' which permits an individual to refuse or direct the withholding or withdrawal of artificial death-prolonging procedures . . ." (*Cruzan* v. *Harmon*, 760 S.W.2nd 408, 434 [Mo. banc 1988] [Higgins, J., dissenting]).

It is unfortunate that some of the thorniest biomedical questions have been formulated legally in terms of a right to privacy. The moral substance of the right is often moved to the periphery in favor of the controverted issue of natural law as a tool of constitutional interpretation. Setting aside the legal questions, we can ask what are the ground and scope of a right to privacy. It is widely held that the moral basis of the right rests upon the natural autonomy of individuals to make decisions about their bodies, with respect not only to sexual conduct but also to many life-and-death concerns. The notion of the body as property has a long philosophical pedigree in the Anglo-American world (e.g., John Locke); the notion that there exists a field of private or self-regarding actions is traceable to a number of different moral theorists (e.g., John Stuart Mill). Moral and legal theorists generally have attempted to unite these themes under a right of autonomy or moral independence (surveyed in Hittinger, 1990). In *Planned Parenthood* v. *Casey* (1992), the U.S. Supreme Court reaffirmed its holding in *Roe* v. *Wade*. It is significant, however, that the Court discussed the right in the language of autonomy, and brought this language under the legal rubric of "liberty" (in section one of the Fourteenth Amendment), rather than "privacy." Because privacy has such disputable grounds in the positive law, this move from privacy to liberty in *Casey* can be read as an effort to find more secure grounds in the positive law for the moral right to autonomy.

Two problems attend the formulation of a right to autonomy. First, it is not clear that a natural right to autonomy can be applied with analytic precision. Even if we narrow the scope of autonomous actions to those that relate to use of the body, it would seem that contraception, abortion, and euthanasia are very different kinds of acts—not only materially but also morally. Hence, it can be objected that although autonomy is a necessary element in our consideration of these issues, it is not a sufficient condition for how they ought to be settled. Second, in Western history, the great tradition of natural rights has concerned the limitation of the coercive power of the state. In legislation and in public policy, a natural rights argument can be expected to shed light upon the principles that ought to govern the ends and the means of public force. But the right of autonomy provides only the most inchoate ground for distinguishing between legitimate and wrongful actions on the part of the state. Why, for example, should the state be prevented from intruding upon decisions about reproduction but not those concerning suicide or euthanasia? All these acts concern the body, and are plausible instances of the individual's interest in his or her autonomy. If the difference consists in the moral specifications of the acts (if, for example, abortion is adjudged morally licit or at least indifferent, while suicide and assisted euthanasia are deemed morally wicked), then autonomy needs to be augmented with other principles in order to draw a line between what belongs to the individual and what belongs to the state. If, on the other hand, one has a natural moral right to act autonomously regardless of the moral specifications of the acts, then one would seem to have a natural right to do wrong. While a government might have other reasons to tolerate wicked acts, it is unclear how a government can be bound to respect a right to do a moral wrong.

Since bioethics encompasses matters of physiological well-being, moral choice, and justice, some version of natural law might seem indispensable to how we should frame and resolve the issues. Despite theoretical problems and disagreements, nature stubbornly remains a standard for health (Kass, 1985). Until nature is exorcised, it will continue to invite natural law reflection on norms of medical practice. Modern technology urgently bids us to investigate the moral relevance of the contrast between nature and art. Furthermore, it would be hard to imagine a future in which citizens stop making claims about rights in the area of health care and the allocation of its resources. Natural law has become part of our repertoire of moral discourse about rights. Yet, as one critic of natural law has stated the problem: "Either the allegedly universal ends [of natural law] are too few and abstract to give content to the idea of the good, or they are too numerous and concrete to be truly universal. One has to choose between triviality and implausibility" (Ely, 1980, p. 51). The same can be said of any of the standard normative theories of ethics, whether deontological or utilitarian. With respect to any abstract theory, especially one as prodigious as natural law, one must look carefully at its different versions, and also take the applications of the theories on a case-by-case basis.

RUSSELL HITTINGER

Directly related to this entry are the entries HUMAN NATURE; ROMAN CATHOLICISM; *and* ETHICS, *especially the articles on* NORMATIVE ETHICAL THEORIES, *and* RELIGION AND MORALITY. *For a further discussion of topics mentioned in this entry, see the entries* ABORTION, *section on* RELIGIOUS TRADITIONS, *article on* ROMAN CATHOLIC PERSPECTIVES; AUTONOMY; FERTILITY CONTROL, *articles on* SOCIAL ISSUES, *and* ETHICAL ISSUES; LAW AND MORALITY; MARRIAGE AND OTHER DOMESTIC PARTNERSHIPS; PRIVACY IN HEALTH CARE; PUBLIC POLICY AND BIOETHICS; RIGHTS; *and* VIRTUE AND CHARACTER. *This entry will find application in the entries* EUGENICS AND RELIGIOUS LAW, *article on* CHRISTIANITY; GENETIC TESTING AND SCREENING, *articles on* PREIMPLANTATION EMBRYO DIAGNOSIS, *and* PRENATAL DIAGNOSIS; *and* REPRODUCTIVE TECHNOLOGIES, *article on* IN VITRO FERTILIZATION AND EMBRYO TRANSFER.

Bibliography

AQUINAS, THOMAS. 1947. *Summa theologica.* Translated by Fathers of the English Dominican Province. New York: Benzinger Brothers.

BOURKE, VERNON. 1974. "Is Thomas Aquinas a Natural Law Ethicist?" *Monist* 58, no. 1:52–66.

Code of Canon Law. 1983. Latin-English ed. Translated by Canon Law Society of America. Washington, D.C.: Canon Law Society of America.

CONGREGATION FOR THE DOCTRINE OF THE FAITH. 1987. *Instruction on Respect for Human Life in Its Origin and on the Dignity of Procreation: Replies to Certain Questions of the Day* (Donum vitae). Vatican translation. Boston: St. Paul Publications.

CURRAN, CHARLES E. 1985. "Natural Law." Ch. 5 in his *Directions in Fundamental Moral Theology.* Notre Dame, Ind.: University of Notre Dame Press.

DWORKIN, RONALD A. 1982. "'Natural' Law Revisited." *University of Florida Law Review* 34:165–188.

———. 1985. *A Matter of Principle.* Cambridge, Mass.: Harvard University Press.

ELY, JOHN H. 1980. *Democracy and Distrust: A Theory of Judicial Review.* Cambridge, Mass.: Harvard University Press.

FINNIS, JOHN. 1980a. *Natural Law and Natural Rights.* Oxford: At the Clarendon Press.

———. 1980b. "The Natural Law, Objective Morality, and Vatican II." In *Principles of Catholic Moral Life.* Edited by William E. May and William E. Baum. Chicago: Franciscan Herald Press.

FUCHS, JOSEF. 1965. *Natural Law: A Theological Investigation.* Translated by Helmut Reckter and John A. Dowling. New York: Sheed and Ward.

GEORGE, ROBERT P., ed. 1992. *Natural Law Theory: Contemporary Essays.* Oxford: At the Clarendon Press.

GEWIRTH, ALAN. 1984. "Law, Action, and Morality." In *The Georgetown Symposium on Ethics: Essays in Honor of Henry Babcock Veatch*, pp. 67–90. Edited by Henry Veatch and Rocco Porreco. Lanham, Md.: University Press of America.

GRISEZ, GERMAIN. 1964. *Contraception and the Natural Law.* Milwaukee, Wis.: Bruce.

———. 1983. *Christian Moral Principles.* Vol. 1 of *The Way of the Lord Jesus.* Chicago: Franciscan Herald Press.

GROTIUS, HUGO. 1925. *On the Law of War and Peace.* Translated by Francis W. Kelsey. Oxford: At the Clarendon Press.

HÄRING, BERNARD. 1973. *Medical Ethics.* Notre Dame, Ind.: Fides.

HART, HERBERT L. A. 1961. "The Minimum Content of Natural Law." In his *The Concept of Law*, pp. 189–195. Oxford: At the Clarendon Press.

HITTINGER, RUSSELL. 1987. *A Critique of the New Natural Law Theory.* Notre Dame, Ind.: University of Notre Dame Press.

———. 1990. "Liberalism and the American Natural Law Tradition." *Wake Forest Law Review* 25:429–499.

HOLMES, OLIVER WENDELL. 1918. "Natural Law." *Harvard Law Review* 32. In Holmes's *Collected Legal Papers*, pp. 310–316. New York: Harcourt, Brace and Howe, 1920.

KANT, IMMANUEL. 1981. *Grounding for the Metaphysics of Morals.* Translated by James W. Ellington. Indianapolis: Hackett.

KASS, LEON R. 1985. *Toward a More Natural Science: Biology and Human Affairs.* New York: Free Press.

MacINTYRE, ALASDAIR C. 1988. *Whose Justice? Which Rationality?* Notre Dame, Ind.: University of Notre Dame Press.

McCORMICK, RICHARD A. 1981. "Bioethics and Method: Where Do We Start?" *Theology Digest* 29, no.4:303–318.

MILLER, FRED D. 1991. "Aristotle on Natural Law and Justice." In *A Companion to Aristotle's Politics*, pp. 279–306. Edited by David Keyt and Fred D. Miller. Oxford: Basil Blackwell.

PASSERIN D'ENTRÈVES, ALESSANDRO. 1970. *Natural Law: An Introduction to Legal Philosophy.* 2d ed. London: Hutchinson University Library.

RAZ, JOSEPH 1986. *The Morality of Freedom.* Oxford: At the Clarendon Press.

REIMAN, JEFFREY. 1990. *Justice & Modern Moral Philosophy.* New Haven, Conn.: Yale University Press.

RUBY, JANE E. 1986. "The Origins of Scientific 'Law.'" *Journal of the History of Ideas* 47:341–359.

SCHNEEWIND, JEROME B. 1986. "The Use of Autonomy in Ethical Theory." In *Reconstructing Individualism*, pp. 64–75. Edited by Thomas C. Heller, Morton Sosna, and David E. Wellbery. Stanford, Cal.: Stanford University Press.

SMITH, JANET E. 1991. *Humanae Vitae: A Generation Later.* Washington, D.C.: Catholic University of America Press.

SOKOLOWSKI, ROBERT. 1992. "Knowing Natural Law." In *Pictures, Quotations, and Distinctions: Fourteen Essays in Phe-nomenology*, pp. 277–291. Notre Dame, Ind.: University of Notre Dame Press.

STRAUSS, LEO. 1953. *Natural Right and History.* Chicago: University of Chicago Press.

WEINREB, LLOYD L. 1987. *Natural Law and Justice.* Cambridge, Mass.: Harvard University Press.

NATURE

This entry will examine the historical origins of the modern concept of "nature" and of its various contrasting concepts. Then, in broad sweep, its transformation will be described, with an eye to how this transformation might influence ideas about science and technology as human culture moves into the twenty-first century.

The classical origins

When something is described as "natural," there is an implicit contrast involved. In the fifth century B.C.E., the classical Greeks developed contrasts between nature (*physis*) and custom (*nomos*), and between nature and art (*technē*). The contrasting concepts of custom and art both referred to products of human endeavor, while the Greek word that is translated "nature" is derived from a verb meaning "to bring forth." The natural is that which arises and persists on its own, in contrast to what results from human custom or craftsmanship. The earliest deliberately nontheological Western speculations about the cosmos were, according to our sources, titled "On Nature" (*Peri physeōs*), and their authors "naturalists" (*physikoi*).

Implicit in these contrasts, though not stressed, is a distinction between the natural and the artificial. An entirely different contrast, common among the early Greeks and still common, is that between the "natural" and the "unnatural." The latter does not mean "absence of nature" but, rather, "contrary to nature." An unnatural behavior, in this sense, presupposes that objects are members of "natural kinds." Objects that share a "nature" in this sense, share a set of properties that constitute their identity as members of that kind. Should they act in an *un*natural way, that is taken to be due either to an abnormal internal state of affairs (loss or distortion of a natural attribute) or to external forces interfering with their normal behavior. Finally, there is a contrast between the natural and the divine.

These distinct contrasts are illustrated nicely by Greek medicine (see the Hippocratic treatises *On Human Nature* and *On the Sacred Disease*, or Galen's *On the Natural Powers*. It can be argued that disease is both natural (meaning not due to a divine source) and unnatural (meaning that it is contrary to the proper balance of the humors, or the natural capacities, of human beings). The latter, in turn, constitute human nature (meaning the shared identity of humans). Medicine itself, on the other hand, is the most common example used to contrast "art" and "nature," since it cures by human interference in the natural course of events (how things would go on their own).

Plato (427–347 B.C.E.) and Aristotle (384–322 B.C.E.), the antipodal classical sources for the modern concept of nature, took attitudes profoundly different from those of their naturalist predecessors. Plato saw their views as metaphysically errant and morally pernicious. From the Platonic perspective, the "natural world" is in fact the product of divine, rather than human, craftsmanship. To claim that it was merely the sum of elemental objects necessarily acting in accordance with their natures was to admit that the universe was devoid of goodness, and thus of eternal standards upon which moral and political conduct could be based. If God, however, devised the universe according to such standards, then humans could search for them in the divine art and build their lives and cities in accordance with them (see *Laws*, X, 889a–890b; *Timaeus*, 27D–30c). This idea of the study of nature as a means to discover divine goodness was to have a profound and lasting impact on Western culture.

Like Plato, Aristotle found his predecessors' views about nature problematic. But in crucial respects he sided with the naturalists. He retained their contrast between "art" and "nature," and rested politics and ethics on a concept of *human* nature rather than divine craftsmanship (*Nicomachean Ethics*, I.7, 1097b24–1098a21). Political organization, he insisted, comes about by nature (*Politics*, I.1, 1252b28–1253a29).

His naturalist predecessors went wrong, he argued, in their view of what constituted the nature of things. Natural objects are not merely the material elements common to everything but, more fundamentally, the forms that differentiate one type of thing from another. Humans, hawks, and halibut are all flesh and blood, but when we wish to identify them precisely and fundamentally, we refer to their distinctive structures, and even more to the functions and activities for the sake of which those structures exist. Aristotle is quite clear that a natural being's material is part of its nature; but he is equally clear that its form is its primary nature (cf. *Physics*, II.1–2; *Parts of Animals*, I.1, 640b4–641a32).

On another fundamental issue—whether nature is created or eternal—Plato and Aristotle establish an enduring contrast. While Aristotle accepts the obvious fact that many natural things come to be and pass away, he argues that it is logically incoherent to extend this claim to nature as a whole, since one would then have to accept the idea that something comes to be from nothing. Up to this point, Plato would seem to agree, since in the *Timaeus* the divine craftsman creates a cosmos from a chaotic, unnameable something or other (see *Timaeus*, 48E–53c). But for Aristotle this precosmic state itself is incoherent: to be is to have a nature, a form, and that extends to the natural world as a whole. Specifically, the cosmos is a naturally, eternally revolving sphere (or nested set of spheres) within which are objects constituted of four elements, two of which "by nature" move upward, and two of which "by nature" move downward. The role of the divine in this natural philosophy remains controversial, but all agree it is not the creator, or even the shaper, of nature.

The triumph of Platonism

It is common to view the universe of the medieval Scholastic philosopher/theologians as a modified Aristotelianism, and on a superficial level this is correct. But in certain respects it is even more radically antinaturalistic than Plato's, since the cosmos was taken to be, on the prevailing interpretation of the Old Testament, not merely a divine craftsman's creation but a creation ex nihilo. To put it in an Aristotelian fashion, not only is the "formal nature" of the cosmos actually a work of art, but so is its "material nature." (It should be noted, however, that a minority of scholars continued to push for the view that God ordered, but did not create, the universe. For a fine review of these dissenters, and the Neoplatonic influence on them, see Sorabji, 1986, pp. 193–202.) Furthermore, not merely human products but also human beings themselves, insofar as they are bearers of a divine and immaterial soul, come to be contrasted with the rest of the natural world. In a cosmos divided between the natural and the supernatural, the material and the spiritual, humans are privileged. The human is now contrasted with the natural not only in the way that culture and artifice are, but also in the way that the divine is.

Many of the founding fathers of the "scientific revolution" of the seventeenth century worked firmly within the tradition of Christian Platonism. The "mathematical principles of nature" referred to in the title of Isaac Newton's *Principia* were taken to be the products of divine ordinance. Robert Boyle, in *A Disquisition About the Final Causes of Natural Things* (1772), explicitly invokes Plato's divine craftsman (*demiourgos*) as the designer of the exquisite mechanisms of eye and hand. Boyle's argument is with those who would revive the goalless (and godless) worldview of Lucretius's *De rerum natura*—*On the Nature of Things*—according to which the natural world consists of atoms in aimless motion in an infinite void. Like Plato, Boyle sees the natural world as a "mechanism" in no metaphorical sense. It is a device of divine craftsmanship, designed to subserve divine purposes.

In Great Britain this viewpoint became an integral feature in the union of theology and natural science that came to be known as "natural theology," embodied in the late eighteenth and the nineteenth centuries in the works of William Paley and the tracts by various authors known as the Bridgewater Treatises. In Catholic nations it was embodied in the Thomistic theory of the equal validity of natural and revealed truths. One of its central planks was that, at the deepest metaphysical level, the distinction between the artificial and the natural breaks down: nature is divine artifice, serving divine ends. God's nature is thus revealed, or evidenced, in nature's laws. One could argue from nature's designs to God's nature.

The hegemony of this view of nature as divine artifice began to crumble under the weight of a variety of forces: the theological skepticism of Enlightenment philosophes (Voltaire, Denis Diderot), in part motivated by a view of organized religion as the enemy of both scientific and social progress; the *Naturphilosophie* of the early Romantics (F. W. J. Schelling, Johann von Herder, Johann von Goethe, Jean-Jacques Rousseau) that tended to view "the natural" as spiritual and divine; and the various theories, devised in the same period and culminating in Charles Darwin's, that accounted for nature's designs by reference to natural law. Even certain forces from within were working against viewing nature as divine artifice. From the start there had been a distinction within the Newtonian camp between the designs of a "first cause"—God—and the empirically discernible "secondary causes" embodied in the laws of nature. In the works of Francis Bacon, Isaac Newton, René Descartes, Thomas Hobbes, and Baruch Spinoza, there are persistent warnings against admixing attempts to discover the laws of nature with the search for God's divine purposes. Science was the search for secondary causes alone, where the true road of induction could guide seekers to the truth. God's purposes should be left to the theologians. Science should be taken only as far back as the search for secondary laws will go.

Nature and the Darwinian revolution

That search soon began to go further back than was comfortable. Charles Lyell, having in volume 1 of his *Principles of Geology* presented overwhelming evidence for the continuous creation and extinction of organisms throughout Earth's history, opened volume 2 with a careful presentation of Jean-Baptiste Lamarck's theory of species transmutation, which aimed at explaining this evidence. Lyell would eventually reject Lamarck's evolutionary ideas, but only after making his sympathies

quite clear: "The theory of the transmutation of species, considered in the last chapter, has met with some degree of favour from many naturalists, from their desire to dispense, as far as possible, with the repeated intervention of a First Cause . . ." (Lyell, 1830–1833, vol. 2, p. 19). We know from his correspondence with astronomer and philosopher of science John F. W. Herschel that Lyell counted himself among the many naturalists with a predisposition to "dispense with the repeated intervention of a First Cause."

The works of Herschel and Lyell were the most profound influences on the young Charles Darwin. When Darwin returned to England in 1836 from his circumnavigation of the globe on board H.M.S. *Beagle*, he was convinced that new species were created by the slow transformation of previous species—a natural process. And in his search for the secondary causes of this transformative process, he was guided by Lyell's devastating critique of Lamarck. Darwin and Lyell became fast friends, and shortly after Darwin published *On the Origin of Species* (1964), Lyell conceded that the case had been made for a natural origin of new species—with the exception of humans. Lyell still could not accept the idea that God had not intervened on behalf of his own species.

Herschel, on the other hand, dismissed natural selection as "the law of Higgledy-Piggledy." The view of natural laws as God's creation brought with it views about the form such laws should take. They must be deterministic, productive of order, with God's design as their inevitable outcome. Darwin's argument, by contrast, undercut natural theology's strongest argument for viewing the natural world as a divinely crafted machine—the argument from design. The logic of this argument had, of course, been attacked before, most notably by the skeptic of the Scottish Enlightenment, David Hume. It was one thing, however, to have a skeptic argue that the inference from design to a designer was invalid, and quite another to have a theory that explained design in nature as the contingent outcome of chance variation and the struggle for existence. So long as no plausible natural mechanism could account for the incredible fact of organic adaptation, the analogy of a benevolent designer, a divine watchmaker, helped to make sense of it. Darwin provided such a natural mechanism.

He did not, however, ask his readers to abandon the idea that the laws governing the production of new species were "secondary" laws: "To my mind it accords better with what we know of the laws impressed on matter by the Creator, that the production and extinction of the past and present inhabitants of the world should have been due to secondary causes, like those determining the birth and death of the individual" (Darwin, 1964, p. 488). Why, then, did people take Darwin to be denying God as nature's craftsman? The answer lies in the fact that, on Darwin's account, which species have been produced or eliminated is largely a matter of chance. Further, his account treats adaptation as a relative affair—Darwin's God would have much in common with Rube Goldberg. From Herschel's standpoint, nature as Darwin described it could not be the product of an omnipotent creator.

At the same time, the distinction between the human and the natural was breaking down. The Judeo-Christian view of humans poised between the natural world and the spiritual world rested on a picture of human origins, and of the human soul, that was being challenged philosophically, psychologically, and biologically. To see human beings as the contingent outcome of natural selection among variations in an ancestral primate species seemed to do away entirely with the idea that humans were the inevitable and preordained result of divinely ordered natural laws.

Nature in the twentieth century

It might be thought that the logical extension of this way of thinking would be to view the distinctive features of human culture—scientific exploration, technological production, social experimentation, the fine arts—as natural activities, the characteristic behavior of a particular species. Whether logical or not, this has not been the dominant twentieth-century view of the relationship between nature and (human) culture. Rather, in the footsteps of certain Romantics (Rousseau, Henry David Thoreau, and Ralph Waldo Emerson), the dominant view has been one of a fundamental conflict between nature and culture.

On a variety of issues, the modern environmental movement has consistently argued that technological progress, especially since the union of applied science and capitalism in the nineteenth century, has led to the destruction of "nature": "The vision of the ecology movement has been to restore the balance of nature disrupted by industrialization and overpopulation. It has emphasized the need to live with the cycles of nature . . ." (Merchant, 1980, pp. xvi–xvii). Here "nature" excludes human culture, and refers rather narrowly to the organic and inorganic features of Earth, apart from the products of human technology. Its basis, then, is the traditional distinction between "art" and "nature." The current popularity of the idea of a conflict between technology and nature in Western cultures seems to have its origins in the counterculture of the 1960s, with its stress on getting "back to nature," "natural foods," "natural healing." The natural is the good, and is contrasted with products of human technology—and social conventions as well—which are viewed as having primarily negative consequences, one of which is destruction of "the nat-

ural." In popular culture one sees this morally loaded concept of nature in the constant use of the word "natural" to promote the sale of the products of technology. Most commentators identify the adoption, by the counterculture, of ideas in Rachel Carson's *Silent Spring* (1962) as a key event in the popularization of this view of technology as the enemy of nature.

Pollution of the soil, air, and water, loss of forests, destruction of the ozone layer, rising temperatures, extinction of species, various forms of cancers and other diseases in humans—all have been blamed on the unfettered application of scientifically based technology to improve the economic conditions of human beings. Until recently, the environmental movement has not been challenged either on its fundamental assumption that human technology is unnatural or on its one-sided emphasis on the negative consequences of technology. As one example, the environmental literature will specify in great detail the scientific evidence for the possible carcinogenicity of a pesticide but will seldom balance this by indicating either the economic or the health benefits of its use. DDT, for example, saved millions of human lives that would have been lost to malaria, and wiped out the gypsy moth in North America; both scourges are regaining a foothold since the ban on DDT. As another example, nuclear power, in comparison with any other form of electrical energy production, has a remarkable safety record, and produces none of the pollutants associated with the burning of fossil fuels (see Cohen, 1990). Yet the environmental literature presents it as an extremely dangerous and harmful technology, with a waste by-product that is both dangerous and impossible to get rid of (see Enger and Smith, 1989).

The moral underpinnings of the recent environmentalist literature can be divided broadly into two types. The first takes the quality of human life on Earth as the basic issue, and argues that specific technological developments do serious harm to aspects of the natural world upon which human life depends. Here technological harm to nature is wrong not in itself but because it interferes with the achievement of human values. The second sees "the natural" as good in itself, as a value to be preserved regardless of whether its preservation involves a cost to human life. Philosophers have tended to agree that the second viewpoint is extremely hard to defend; it is nonetheless popular within the environmental movement. Much of the literature of environmentalism mixes these two forms of argument (see Callicott, 1986).

A viewpoint that needs, but has not yet received, systematic development is one that defends human technological activity as natural, that is, as expressive of the essential character of an evolved species, differing from the building of dams by beavers or hives by bees only in degree, not in kind (a small step in this direction is suggested by Herbert Simon's *The Sciences of the Artificial* [1969]). The implications of this viewpoint may be seen if we apply it to a consideration of "genetic engineering," a form of human technology that most clearly raises the distinctively modern features of the traditional contrasts between art and nature. (Remember, the classical Greek word for "art" was *technē*, which included medicine and all forms of technology.)

Biotechnology takes to the ultimate extreme Francis Bacon's mandate to understand nature in order to control it. To quote the title of one popular presentation, its aim is to "improve on nature" (another euphemism for genetic engineering, a throwback to Platonism, is "playing God"). By its pervasive use of organic "tools" (the Greek for "tool" is *organon*) to craft new organisms for technological ends, it keeps violating all our intuitions about how to distinguish nature and technology, and since it finds pervasive application in the art of medicine, it is a fitting focus for this essay.

Between the unraveling of the structure of DNA in the early 1950s and the first successful attempts to splice a new genetic element into the DNA sequence of *E. coli* in the early 1970s, the science of genetics underwent a molecular revolution. That revolution was in part theoretical, involving unraveling of the genetic code, grasping the causal processes leading from DNA to protein, and understanding the complex interactions that take place between the various elements of an organism's genome and the other elements of its cells. But it was equally technological, in two distinct senses: early on, those involved saw the potential technological applications of their discoveries to agriculture, pharmacology, and medicine; and the laboratory technologies developed for theoretical purposes could, in principle, be used in realizing those technological applications (see Nichols, 1988).

If one views the genetic constitutions of organisms, including humans, as an important part of their nature, then altering the genetic constitution of a plant or animal by genetic engineering—to turn bacteria or other organisms into factories for the manufacture of drugs, or to make a fruit or vegetable frost-resistant—involves altering the natures of these organisms by technological means. Is this in principle different from what human beings have been doing for at least a few thousand years? Virtually all agricultural products, not to mention garden varietals and pets, are the (often radically) modified descendants of their "natural" ancestors. Indeed, it was the careful study of this process of "artificial selection" that led Charles Darwin to his idea of "natural selection." How, at the level of principle, do the new genetic technologies differ from the selective breeding performed for so long? At least two differences can be distinguished.

First, *the violation of "natural" boundaries.* It has surprised the geneticists that the genes of evolutionarily distant organisms can be spliced together and remain active. In the past, the actions of breeders were limited by (1) the available mutations and recombinations in an organism's own genetic material and (2) the recombinations possible through hybridization between closely related species or varieties. What the limits of biotechnology might be in this area are not at all clear, but they are certainly far fewer than those available when breeding was the only technology available.

Second, *the direct manipulation of the genetic code.* A related but different point is that genetic engineering need not "wait for nature"—it can actively engage in the creation of genetic variation. To put it another way, it is not restricted to selection—it can involve itself in creating the heritable variation. And since, given our understanding of the genetic code, we can infer genetic anomalies from their biochemical effects, the possibilities for treating genetic diseases by directly manipulating gene structure are limited only by current technology.

The implications of genetic engineering for the distinction between "art" and "nature" are profound. The distinction is in no small part based on the existence of a clear boundary between those features of the world that are as they are *independently* of human activity and those features of the world that are as they are *because* of human activity. Like other animals, human beings interact with their environment in an effort to satisfy their needs, and, as with other animals, that interaction has more or less significant consequences for other organisms and for themselves. A profoundly human form of interaction is based on a rational understanding of nature, followed by the use of that knowledge to produce values that the operation of natural processes alone would not.

Is this behavior natural? One clear way of answering that is to ask whether it is the expression of human nature, and from that perspective the answer is surely "yes." (This issue is at the heart of the debate over "sociobiology"—see Wilson, 1978; Kitcher, 1985.) Another way to answer it is to reconsider the original opposition between "the natural" and "the manmade"—in the form either of technology or of conventions and institutions. Do the Darwinian and molecular revolutions in biology call that distinction into question? If human beings are just recently evolved primates with their own form of cognition and behavior, why should that behavior and its effects be set in opposition to nature? Humans' ways of knowing—understanding and evaluating the world in conceptual terms—and their ability to fashion and refashion behavior, culture, and environment on the basis of that knowledge, certainly makes them unique. But not more unique than a monarch butterfly's transformation in its cocoon and its ability to travel 3,000 miles to mate in the same location as its parents.

The Darwinian and molecular revolutions in biology have called the distinction between the natural and the man-made into question, and this last question is one of the central questions for post-Darwinian humans to face, and to answer. That we can face, and answer, such questions is surely at the core of human nature—we must decide whether it is a perfectly natural thing to do.

JAMES G. LENNOX

Directly related to this entry are the entries LIFE; BIOLOGY, PHILOSOPHY OF; EVOLUTION; ROMAN CATHOLICISM; *and* NATURAL LAW. *For a further discussion of topics mentioned in this entry, see the entries* BIOTECHNOLOGY; ENVIRONMENTAL ETHICS, *especially the* OVERVIEW *and article on* DEEP ECOLOGY; EUGENICS; GENETIC ENGINEERING; GENE THERAPY, *article on* ETHICAL AND SOCIAL ISSUES; *and* HOMOSEXUALITY.

Bibliography

BOWLER, PETER J. 1989. *Evolution: The History of an Idea.* Rev. ed. Berkeley: University of California Press.

BOYLE, ROBERT. 1772. *A Disquisition About the Final Causes of Natural Things.* Vol. 5 of *The Works of the Honourable Robert Boyle.* Edited by Thomas Birch. London.

CALLICOTT, J. BAIRD. 1986. "On the Intrinsic Value of Nonhuman Species." In *The Preservation of Species: The Value of Biological Diversity,* pp. 138–172. Edited by Bryan G. Norton. Princeton, N.J.: Princeton University Press.

CARSON, RACHEL. 1962. *Silent Spring.* Boston: Houghton Mifflin.

COHEN, BERNARD L. 1990. *The Nuclear Energy Option: An Alternative for the 90s.* New York: Plenum.

COLLINGWOOD, ROBIN G. 1945. *The Idea of Nature.* Oxford: At the Clarendon Press.

DARWIN, CHARLES. 1964. [1859]. *On the Origin of Species by Means of Natural Selection: A Facsimile of the First Edition.* Cambridge, Mass.: Harvard University Press.

DURHAM, FRANK, and PURRINGTON, ROBERT D., eds. 1990. *Some Truer Method: Reflections on the Heritage of Newton.* New York: Columbia University Press.

ENGER, ELDON D., and SMITH, BRADLEY F. 1989. *Environmental Science: A Study of Interrelationships.* Dubuque, Iowa: William C. Brown.

FURLEY, DAVID J. 1987. *The Greek Cosmologists.* Cambridge: At the University Press.

JUDSON, LINDSAY, ed. 1991. *Aristotle's Physics: A Collection of Essays.* Oxford: At the Clarendon Press.

KITCHER, PHILIP. 1985. *Vaulting Ambition: Sociobiology and the Quest for Human Nature.* Cambridge, Mass.: MIT Press.

LENNOX, JAMES G. 1983. "Robert Boyle's Defense of Teleological Inference in Experimental Science." *Isis* 74, no. 271:38–52.

———. 1985. "Plato's Unnatural Teleology." In *Platonic Investigations,* pp. 195–218. Edited by Dominic J. O'Meara. Washington, D.C.: Catholic University of America Press.

LLOYD, GEOFFREY E. R. 1979. *Magic, Reason and Experience: Studies in the Origin and Development of Greek Science.* Cambridge: At the University Press.

LYELL, CHARLES. 1830–1833. *Principles of Geology.* 3 vols. London: John Murray.

McGUIRE, JAMES E. 1972. "Boyle's Conception of Nature." *Journal of the History of Ideas* 33:523–542.

MERCHANT, CAROLYN. 1980. *The Death of Nature: Women, Ecology, and the Scientific Revolution.* New York: Harper & Row.

NICHOLS, EVE K. 1988. *Human Gene Therapy.* Cambridge, Mass.: Harvard University Press.

SIMON, HERBERT A. 1969. *The Sciences of the Artificial.* Cambridge, Mass.: MIT Press.

SIMPSON, GEORGE GAYLORD. 1971. "Man's Place in Nature." In *Man and Nature: Philosophical Issues in Biology,* pp. 268–277. Edited by Ronald Munson. New York: Dell.

SORABJI, RICHARD. 1986. *Time, Creation, and the Continuum: Theories in Antiquity and the Early Middle Ages.* Ithaca, N.Y.: Cornell University Press.

WILSON, EDWARD O. 1978. *On Human Nature.* Cambridge, Mass.: Harvard University Press.

NATURE, HUMAN

See HUMAN NATURE.

NAZISM

See NATIONAL SOCIALISM.

NEONATAL CARE

See INFANTS.

NETHERLANDS

See MEDICAL ETHICS, HISTORY OF, *section on* EUROPE, *subsection on* CONTEMPORARY PERIOD, *article on* THE BENELUX COUNTRIES.

NEWBORN SCREENING

See GENETIC TESTING AND SCREENING, *article on* NEWBORN SCREENING.

NEW ZEALAND

see MEDICAL ETHICS, HISTORY OF, *article on* AUSTRALIA AND NEW ZEALAND.

NONMALEFICENCE, PRINCIPLE OF

See BENEFICENCE. *See also* HARM; *and* RISK.

NORMATIVE ETHICS

See ETHICS, *articles on* TASK OF ETHICS, *and* NORMATIVE ETHICAL THEORIES. *See also* OBLIGATION AND SUPEREROGATION; UTILITY; *and* VIRTUE AND CHARACTER.

NORWAY

See MEDICAL ETHICS, HISTORY OF, *section on* EUROPE, *subsection on* CONTEMPORARY PERIOD, *article on* NORDIC COUNTRIES.

NUCLEAR WARFARE

See WARFARE, *article on* NUCLEAR WARFARE.

NUREMBERG CODE

See NATIONAL SOCIALISM; RESEARCH, HUMAN: HISTORICAL ASPECTS; *and* RESEARCH, UNETHICAL. *For text of the Nuremberg Code, see the* APPENDIX (CODES, OATHS, AND DIRECTIVES RELATED TO BIOETHICS), SECTION IV: ETHICAL DIRECTIVES FOR HUMAN RESEARCH.

NURSING, THEORIES AND PHILOSOPHY OF

Philosophy has always involved reflective examination of the meaning of the ways in which human beings encounter the world. This reflection has raised some issues that are of particular interest to contemporary nursing. Philosophical issues of import to contemporary nursing are the meaning of good and evil, justice, and knowledge, but the issue that has most concerned nurses is the meaning of being. This issue has focused on the meaning of being a nurse and has led nursing scholars to explore the meaning of care and authentic being.

Following the movement from the quest for meaning in nursing to philosophy requires treatment of (1) why nursing has sought to define its own identity; (2) how reflecting on the meaning of nursing has led to philosophy; (3) how phenomenology has been appropriated in nursing's quest for meaning. This treatment needs to be supplemented by considering (4) other philosophical issues of concern to nurses, and (5) attempts to apply philosophy to nursing.

The quest for identity

The quest for the identity of nursing was fostered by several factors, including nursing education's move from the hospital to the academy, changes within nursing itself, and the feminist movement. Although there were nursing schools in a few universities before the 1950s, the movement to place nursing education and research in universities has accelerated since then. This move required nursing to establish its place in an academic setting. Usually nursing schools were placed in the natural or applied sciences, and consequently, nursing initially attempted to establish its identity as a science. The attempt to identify nursing with natural science led to scientific studies of nursing, but these studies, while important, did not show that nursing itself was a science. Recognition that nursing was a human practical activity led to use of the behavioral sciences to give a scientific account of nursing. In either case, nursing itself could, at best, be called an applied science. As such, scientific studies of nursing would lead to a theory of nursing; that theory would prescribe nursing practice. However, attempts to use theory to prescribe nursing practice were so far removed from the practice of nursing that these theories failed to give nursing an identity.

Involvement in an academic setting eventually broadened the meaning of nursing beyond that of applied science. The development of master's and doctoral degree programs in nursing fostered a movement away from the applied approach in nursing that had resulted from nurses taking graduate degrees in other fields and applying their methods and concepts to nursing.

Graduate study in nursing developed as nursing became more complex in ways that required nurses to make their own decisions concerning patient care. The development of intensive-care units in hospitals initiated the expansion of specialization and technical knowledge into nursing care. As this trend expanded, care for patients required nurses increasingly to make decisions without specific directives from physicians. As nurses became more responsible for patient care, they began to question the traditional control of nursing care by physicians and hospital administrators. Critical examination of their dependence on others encouraged nurses to seek an independent identity for nursing.

The feminist movement certainly enhanced the desire of nurses to be independent from control of physicians and hospital administrators. Feminist theorists pointed out that society, including health-care institutions, undervalued care and nurturing and overvalued command, technology, and hierarchical structure. Feminists enhanced the determination of nurses to become self-directing professionals rather than workers who followed the directions of physicians and administrators.

The quest for meaning

As nurses attempted to articulate their own practice, they became aware that nursing was focused on care rather than on science or applied science. Beginning in 1978, a series of annual conferences turned to the task of interpreting the meaning of caring as it related to nursing. The significance of this approach to nursing is evident in the following comment by a nurse who attended one such conference: "This is the first time I have ever heard nurses talk about caring or care as related to nursing care. I had nothing like these concepts in my nursing program, and yet they make sense and seem so logical and essential to nursing. In our classes, we were taught about curing medical diseases, understanding medical diagnostic techniques, and everything but caring" (National Caring Conference, 1981, p. vi). Published regularly, the proceedings of these conferences constitute a developing interpretation of caring as the source of identity for nursing. Philosophical interpretation of caring has also been fostered by the International Association for Human Caring and the Center for Human Caring at the University of Colorado.

Interpreting nursing as caring is central to the movement called the "new curriculum." This movement is an influential attempt to reform nursing education that developed in the last two decades of the twentieth century. Advocates of the new curriculum reject prescriptive approaches to nursing education in which nursing education is dictated by behavioral science or systematic philosophy. Nursing, they contend, is primarily caring. Nursing education should foster learning to care through clinical involvement and dialogical reflection on the meaning of clinical experience. Learning the meaning of nursing care in nursing education comes from cooperative efforts to discern the meaning of clinical practice by practitioners, faculty, and students. For example, Nancy Diekelmann contends that "knowledge is not . . . taught by the practitioners or the clinical faculty, because clinical knowledge cannot be taught; it can only be demonstrated, . . . and it can only be acquired through experience" (Diekelmann, 1988, p. 146). When clinical experience is interpreted, practice is "theory-generating," and it is "through practice that theories are refined, elaborated, and challenged" (p. 147). Thus the source of nursing theory, rather than being derived from the natural or social sciences, is nursing as practiced.

Phenomenology in the quest for meaning

In her phenomenological interpretation of nursing, Patricia Benner articulated the meaning of nursing by drawing exemplars of excellent nursing from concrete nursing practice. In sharp contrast to using theories to prescribe the meaning of nursing, Benner discloses the meaning of nursing excellence through descriptions of care for patients/clients in specific situations. These exemplars of excellence are interpreted to clarify and enhance the meaning evident in nursing practice. From the study of these exemplars, she identified seven domains of nursing practice with thirty-one distinct nursing competencies. For example, one of the domains is the helping role and two of the competencies of the helping role are (1) providing comfort measures and preserving personhood in the face of pain and extreme breakdown, and (2) maximizing the patient's participation and control in his or her own recovery (Benner, 1984). Rather than following the tradition in nursing of using definitions of good nursing to prescribe practice, Benner conveys the meaning of excellence through the work of excellent practitioners. Her study shows that knowledge of excellence gained from practice is essential to any adequate definition of nursing. Benner's work illustrates the use of hermeneutic phenomenological methodology in nursing in that she discloses the meaning of nursing excellence through exemplars in actual practice and interprets their significance for the identity of nursing.

Nursing is the practice of caring, according to Anne Bishop, a nurse, and John Scudder, a philosopher, who, like Benner, employ hermeneutic phenomenology to articulate the meaning of nursing (Bishop and Scudder, 1991). They contend that nursing is a practice, in that it is a traditional way of caring for patients that fosters the patient's well-being. This moral sense of nursing is inherent in the caring relationship between nurse and patient. Thus, ends and means are not separated from each other as they are in the applied-science approach. This approach imposes meaning on nursing, whereas the phenomenological approach discloses the meaning inherent in nursing practice.

Confused thought has been fostered by the tendency to use the term "nursing" to mean both care for patients and the study of that care. Bishop and Scudder call the study of nursing the discipline of nursing to distinguish it from the practice. They maintain that the discipline of nursing should be a human science because it studies how nurses care for the ill and debilitated. Furthermore, it is a practical human science since the discipline attempts to improve nursing practice as well as to study it. Practices, such as nursing, are expanded and enhanced by the realization of possibilities that are inherent in the practice.

Bishop and Scudder affirm the tendency to find the identity of nursing in caring. Although they articulate the meaning of care primarily from nursing practice, they find the discussions of care by feminists Carol Gilligan (1982) and Nel Noddings (1984) particularly helpful in their articulation. Gilligan's "web of connection" forms a context for the interpretation of nursing as being in between patient, physician, hospital administration, and family. Noddings's interpretation of care as engrossment in the situation of the other and shift of concern to the well-being of the other enhances their interpretation of nursing care as fulfillment of the moral sense of fostering the well-being of patients. They contend that the integral relationship between the moral sense and nursing practice is clearly evident in Benner's description of nursing excellence (1984). Nursing practice, as they interpret it, consists of two fundamental stances—the in-between stance that focuses on cooperative care, articulated by Bishop and Scudder (1990), and the stance of recognized nursing competence in which nurses are free to direct care, described by Benner. However, nursing's purpose is not to become autonomous, as is often stressed by nursing reformers, but instead to foster the patient's well-being. Since nursing has this fundamental moral sense, the primary purpose of ethical considerations of nursing should be to foster excellent care—a care that promotes wellness while respecting the dignity and rights of each person.

Unlike Benner and Bishop and Scudder, who seek the identity of nursing in nursing practice, Sally Gadow attempts to give nursing a new identity with her interpretation of nursing as "existential advocacy" (Gadow, 1980). She draws her conception of existential advocacy from the stress on authenticity that is central to the philosophy of existential phenomenology. Since being authentic entails choosing oneself, "freedom of self-determination is the most fundamental and valuable human right" (Gadow, 1980, p. 84). Since the primary meaning of being human is self-direction, it follows that nurses should become existential advocates who foster authentic human being for those facing illness, treatment, and possible death. The nurse becomes an existential advocate by "participating with the patient in determining the personal meaning which the experience of illness, suffering, or dying is to have for that individual" (Gadow, 1980, p. 97).

Other philosophical issues of concern to nurses

Philosophical inquiry in contemporary nursing has been fostered by three concerns other than the meaning of being a nurse. First, nurses are formulating an ethics appropriate for the difficult moral decisions that nurses must make in contemporary health care. Second, nurses are seeking justice for nurses who have been discriminated against because they are women and thus have been expected to support physicians and hospital administrators (mostly male). And finally, nurses are developing a theory of knowledge appropriate for a caring practice in a time that favors factual knowledge gained by scientific procedures.

As early as 1979, it became evident that the ethical issues being faced by nurses required a nursing ethics. In that year, a series of meetings attended by over 2300 persons in New York and New England brought together philosophers and nurses in an effort to "refine the [ethical] issues and illuminate ethics dilemmas in nursing" (Spicker and Gadow, 1980, p. xv). Since then, many books and articles on nursing ethics have attempted to apply philosophical understanding to the moral dilemmas faced by nurses. Those who arranged the encounter between nurses and philosophers did so because they believed that philosophers had focused on medical ethics to the neglect of ethical issues unique to nursing. Calls for a specific nursing ethics have continued since 1979. Many who believe that a medical ethics is not adequate for nursing point to the difference between nursing practice and medical practice. For example, physicians and patients usually select each other; nurses and patients rarely do. Nursing care is usually much more direct and continuous than medical care. Nurses regard care as central to their practice much more than physicians do. Nursing ethicists are increasingly calling for an interpretation of nursing ethics that is specifically appropriate to nursing care rather than one derived from medical ethics or from traditional philosophical ethics.

In developing a specific nursing ethic, a central issue concerns how to relate nursing, philosophy, and ethics. One approach to this relationship begins with the moral issues that arise in nursing care due to advances in biomedical science. These moral issues require ethical treatment that in turn leads nurses into philosophical inquiry and/or philosophical systems. A contrasting approach begins with a philosophical quest for identity that discloses the inherent moral sense of nursing, such as that of Benner (1984) and Bishop and Scudder (1990; 1991). Benner's concept of excellence and Bishop and Scudder's moral sense of nursing begin with the moral imperative inherent in nursing practice. From this perspective, the primary concern of nursing ethics is fulfillment of its moral sense. Hence, ethics concerns the primary thrust of nursing practice and not merely resolving moral problems that, although arising out of practice, are treated as adjunct to the practice.

The philosophers who took part in the aforementioned conference that brought nurses and philosophers together also asserted that "the long-standing concern of philosophy to assist in the process of emancipation" should be brought to bear on the "long subjugation of the nurse" by helping nursing move "away from its position of political and intellectual subordinance" (Spicker and Gadow, 1980, p. xiv). Nurses, who had long been impatient with being under the control of physicians and hospital administrators, were seeking greater individual and professional autonomy. The demand for greater autonomy was supported by feminist philosophy and by critical theory. Critical theory was used to disclose the hidden power structures in health care that denied nurses self-direction (Allen, 1987; Thompson, 1987).

Nurses also became interested in philosophy from their attempt to challenge the dominant scientific methodology and criteria for knowledge that prevailed when nursing first entered the academy. Recognition that nursing was primarily a human activity concerned with caring relationships between nurse and patient led nursing scholars to become involved in qualitative research and to use the methodology of the human sciences. A significant number of nurses became regular participants in the Society for Phenomenology and Human Sciences and the International Human Science Research Conference. Those nursing scholars who found the stress on empirical rational science too restrictive welcomed Barbara Carper's expanded conception of knowledge. She contended that nursing knowledge should include not only scientific empirical knowledge but three other ways of knowing in nursing—knowledge of how to make morally right choices; knowledge gained from personal experience; and knowledge of how to practice the art of nursing. Her patterns of knowing generated much interest among nurses who had long recognized that scientific knowledge alone was not adequate for nursing practice (Carper, 1978).

From philosophy to nursing

Interest in investigating nursing philosophy has come primarily from the quest for the identity of nursing and from encountering issues concerning ethics, knowledge, and justice within nursing itself. In contrast to this move from nursing practice to philosophy, there have been two major attempts to apply philosophy to nursing. The first is the attempt to foster the development of philosophy of nursing by the Institute for Philosophical Nursing Research at the University of Alberta, Canada. The institute invites nursing scholars with philosophical interests and talents to biannual conferences to discuss issues involved in developing a philosophy of nursing. The institute, through its conferences and publications, seeks to "establish common ground in nursing philosophy, accommodate diversity of thought in nursing phi-

losophy, and articulate a sound philosophy of nursing" (Kikuchi and Simmons, 1994, p. 4).

In contrast to the purposes of the institute, Martha Rogers attempted to develop a philosophy for nursing rather than of nursing. Centered on her conception of unitary human being, this philosophy drew heavily on theories in the physical and biological sciences. Her philosophy followed the evolutionary model of an organism adapting to the environment and rejected the separation of mind and body. Rogers herself did not claim to have developed a philosophy of nursing but rather an interpretation of what it means to be human from which nursing practice could be prescribed (Rogers, 1970). Rogers's thought has had considerable influence on nursing theory, but its relevance to nursing practice has often been questioned.

Conclusion

The development of an explicit philosophy of nursing is just beginning. To date, most nursing philosophy has developed out of nursing's quest for identity. Philosophizing about nursing has emerged from (1) the attempt to draw out the meaning of nursing from the practice of nursing; (2) the recognition and reaffirmation of the moral sense of nursing; (3) the enrichment of nursing from feminist reflection on nurture and care; and (4) the discovery of the essential meaning of nursing through a philosophy of care. Nurses also have been led into philosophy by concerns about ethics, justice, and knowledge that came from nursing practice itself. The direction this philosophical ferment will take is uncertain, but it is certain that philosophizing in nursing is expanding and developing rapidly. No doubt in the future, philosophy of nursing will become a part of the discipline of nursing, much as philosophy of education has become a part of the discipline of education. But as philosophy of nursing develops, it will have to face issues inherent in any philosophy. Will philosophy of nursing continue to move from nursing concerns to philosophical considerations or will it become oriented in philosophical issues and concerns that are applied to nursing? Furthermore, will philosophers of nursing become specialists who talk primarily to each other or will philosophy of nursing become an integral part of the development of a nursing discipline dedicated to the articulation and improvement of nursing practice?

JOHN R. SCUDDER, JR.
ANNE H. BISHOP

Directly related to this entry are the entries NURSING ETHICS; *and* NURSING AS A PROFESSION. *For a further discussion of topics mentioned in this entry, see the entries* CARE; FEMINISM; *and* WOMEN, *section on* WOMEN AS

HEALTH PROFESSIONALS. *For a discussion of related ideas, see the entries* AUTONOMY; COMPASSION; ETHICS, *article on* MORAL EPISTEMOLOGY; *and* JUSTICE.

Bibliography

ALLEN, DAVID G. 1987. "The Social Policy Statement: A Reappraisal." *Advances in Nursing Science* 10, no. 1:39–48.

BENNER, PATRICIA E. 1984. *From Novice to Expert: Excellence and Power in Clinical Nursing Practice.* Menlo Park, Calif.: Addison-Wesley.

BISHOP, ANNE H., and SCUDDER, JOHN R., JR. 1990. *The Practical, Moral, and Personal Sense of Nursing: A Phenomenological Philosophy of Practice.* Albany: State University of New York Press.

———. 1991. *Nursing: The Practice of Caring.* New York: National League for Nursing.

CARPER, BARBARA. 1978. "Fundamental Patterns of Knowing in Nursing." *Advances in Nursing Science* 1, no. 1:13–23.

DIEKELMANN, NANCY L. 1988. "Curriculum Revolution: A Theoretical and Philosophical Mandate for Change." In *Curriculum Revolution: Mandate for Change,* pp. 137–157. New York: National League for Nursing.

FRY, SARA T. 1989. "Toward a Theory of Nursing Ethics." *Advances in Nursing Science* 11, no. 4:9–22.

GADOW, SALLY. 1980. "Existential Advocacy: Philosophical Foundation of Nursing." In *Nursing: Images and Ideals: Opening Dialogue with the Humanities,* pp. 79–101. Edited by Stuart F. Spicker and Sally Gadow. New York: Springer.

GILLIGAN, CAROL. 1982. *In a Different Voice: Psychological Theory and Women's Development.* Cambridge, Mass.: Harvard University Press.

KIKUCHI, JUNE F., and SIMMONS, HELEN, eds. 1994. *Developing a Philosophy of Nursing.* Thousand Oaks, Calif.: Sage.

NATIONAL CARING CONFERENCE. 1981. *Caring: An Essential Human Need: Proceedings of Three National Caring Conferences.* Edited by Madeleine M. Leininger. Thorofare, N.J.: Charles B. Slack.

NODDINGS, NEL. 1984. *Caring: A Feminine Approach to Ethics and Moral Education.* Berkeley: University of California Press.

ROGERS, MARTHA E. *An Introduction to the Theoretical Basis of Nursing.* Philadelphia: F. A. Davis.

SPICKER, STUART F., and GADOW, SALLY, eds. 1980. *Nursing: Images and Ideals: Opening Dialogue with the Humanities.* New York: Springer.

THOMPSON, JANICE L. 1987. "Critical Scholarship: The Critique of Domination in Nursing." *Advances in Nursing Science* 10, no. 1:27–38.

NURSING CODES OF ETHICS

See NURSING ETHICS. *For text of nursing codes of ethics, see the* APPENDIX (CODES, OATHS, AND DIRECTIVES RELATED TO BIOETHICS), SECTION III: ETHICAL DIRECTIVES FOR OTHER HEALTH-CARE PROFESSIONS.

NURSING ETHICS

The development of nursing ethics has paralleled the development of nursing as a profession. As nursing has evolved from the use of rules of hygiene in the care of the sick (Nightingale, 1859) to a profession that defines its practice realm as the promotion of health, prevention of illness, restoration of health, and the alleviation of suffering (International Council of Nurses [ICN], 1973), so has nursing ethics evolved from following rules of conduct in attending the sick (Robb, 1921) to an identified field of inquiry within bioethics (Veatch and Fry, 1987).

Early interpretations of nursing ethics

Early interpretations of nursing ethics tend to be associated with the image of the nurse as a chaste, good woman in Christian service to others and as an obedient, dutiful servant. Florence Nightingale's good nurse was committed to the ideal of doing what was right and had responded to a religious calling to nursing. Being of the highest character, she was disciplined by moral training and could be relied upon to do her Christian duty in service to others.

This view of the good nurse as a good woman pervaded early textbooks on nursing ethics. In addition to being physically and morally strong, Isabel Hampton Robb thought that the nurse must be a dignified, cultured, courteous, well-educated, and reserved woman of good breeding. Like Nightingale, she considered the nurse's work as ministry, ". . . a consecrated service, performed in the Spirit of Christ . . ." (Robb, 1921, p. 38). Thus, moral virtue, moral duty, and service to others were established as important foundations upon which later interpretations of nursing ethics would be built.

At first, nursing ethics as practiced was virtually indistinguishable from nursing etiquette and the performance of duty. Nursing etiquette included forms of polite behavior such as neatness, punctuality, courtesy, and quiet attendance to the physician. The nurse demonstrated her acceptance of her moral duties by following rules of etiquette, and by being loyal and obedient to the physician (Robb, 1921). Early textbooks on the subject describe nursing ethics as the ideals, customs, and habits associated with the general characteristics of a nurse, and as doing one's duty with skill and moral perfection.

Some important distinctions were made between etiquette and ethics. Nurses learned proper ward etiquette in order to promote professional harmony in patient care; such etiquette became the foundation for all other nursing behaviors. Ethics, however, was taught to promote moral excellence and technical competence on the part of the nurse. Ethics was viewed as a science, the knowledge of which would enable the nurse to carry out prescribed duties with moral skill and technical perfection.

Following World War II, the nurse's role in patient care slowly shifted from that of the physician's obedient helper to that of an independent practitioner, held accountable for what had been done or not done in providing patient care. A shift in the understanding of nursing ethics accompanied this shift in roles. The nurse's moral responsibilities were no longer couched solely in terms of obedience to authority and institutional loyalty. Rather than someone who carried out the decisions made by others, the nurse now claimed authority for independent clinical decisions in patient care, including ethical decisions.

Contemporary nursing ethics began to develop in several directions. First, recently developed codes of nursing ethics were revised. Second, dramatic changes occurred in the teaching of nursing ethics. Third, nurses' attitudes and values, moral development, moral-reasoning abilities, and ethical practice or behavior were empirically studied. Fourth, the moral concepts of nursing practice were philosophically analyzed. Fifth, consideration was given to the development of theories of nursing ethics.

The development and revision of nursing codes of ethics

As professional nursing developed, nursing organizations discussed the need for a code of ethics for nursing practice. In the United States, the 1897 meeting of the newly constituted American Nurses' Association (ANA) was the first occasion for members of the profession to discuss a possible code of ethics for nursing. The ANA House of Delegates, however, did not accept a code of ethics until 1950. Revised in 1960, 1968, and 1976, the ANA Code for Nurses has served as a model for the development of nursing codes of ethics in other countries. Revised in 1985, the "interpretative statements" of the ANA Code delineate ethical principles that prescribe and justify nursing actions in the United States (ANA, 1985).

While the development of the ANA Code for Nurses was in process, the ICN, established in 1900, was developing an international code of ethics. A draft of an international code of nursing ethics was presented at the 1953 ICN Congress held in São Paulo, Brazil. The ICN Congress accepted the Code for Nurses and had it translated into several languages. The Code for Nurses was revised in 1965 and 1973 and reconfirmed in 1989. The ICN published guidelines on the use of the Code for Nurses in 1977 (ICN, 1973).

A significant number of national nurses' associations throughout the world have developed codes of ethics (Sawyer, 1989). Among the areas of agreement in nursing codes of ethics are nursing responsibility for practice competence; the need for good relations with co-workers; respect for the life and dignity of the patient; protection of patient confidentiality; and the nurse's ethical responsibility not to discriminate against patients on the basis of race, religious beliefs, cultural practices, or economic status (Sawyer, 1989). Like other professional codes of ethics, nursing codes provide important ethical standards that nurses can refer to when faced with questions of ethics or unethical practices on the part of co-workers and institutions. They are also an important historical record of the ethical concepts and principles considered important to nursing practice over time. Their periodic revisions have helped to shape the development of modern nursing ethics.

Codes of professional ethics are always hard to enforce. In the United States, the ANA Committee on Ethics encourages implementation of the elements of the Code for Nurses by supporting ethics education in nursing programs and by distributing copies of the Code for Nurses to nursing students. The ANA Committee on Ethics has also developed model policies and procedures that state nurses' associations can adopt in the processing of alleged violations of the Code for Nurses (Committee on Ethics, 1980).

Like all professional codes of ethics, nursing codes are hard to apply to patient-care situations. Since their statements represent moral ideals rather than specific action guides, professional nursing organizations have developed lengthy interpretations of nursing codes of ethics, or produced guidebooks with case applications of a code (Fry, 1994). In the United Kingdom, the Central Council for Nursing has published advisory documents to supplement its Code of Professional Conduct (United Kingdom Central Council, 1989).

Teaching ethics in nursing education

During the 1970s, models for nurses' ethical decision making taught in nursing education programs were critically examined. A study of ethics teaching in 209 accredited baccalaureate nursing programs in the United States revealed that general ethics content was integrated into the curricula of two-thirds of the programs surveyed (Aroskar, 1977). The majority of the programs also expressed a need for the teaching of more specific nursing ethics content. Several textbooks on nursing ethics helped define this content (Benjamin and Curtis, 1986; Davis and Aroskar, 1991; Jameton, 1984; Veatch and Fry, 1987). According to these textbooks, both the teaching of ethics in nursing curricula and the analysis of ethical conflicts as they occur in nursing practice could enhance nurses' ethical decision-making abilities. They also agreed that the ethical problems nurses most often experience involve balancing harms and benefits in patient care, protecting patients' autonomy, and distributing nursing-care resources.

As various approaches to teaching ethics in nursing education developed, a consensus emerged that the overall goal of teaching ethics to nurses is to produce an ethically accountable practitioner who is skilled in ethical decision making. Intermediate goals of ethics teaching are to (1) examine personal commitments and values in relation to the care of patients; (2) engage in ethical reflection; (3) develop skill in moral reasoning and moral judgment; and (4) develop the ability to use ethics for reflection on broader issues having policy implications and for research on the moral foundations of practice. These goals focus on the fact that ethics is a form of inquiry that is used by every nurse in clinical practice. Broad general acceptance of these goals in nursing education prompted research into nurses' ethical decisions and the types of ethical issues nurses confront in patient care.

Nursing ethics research

The earliest record of a nursing ethics research project was Rose Helene Vaughan's 1935 study of the diaries of ninety-five student and graduate nurses who recorded the ethical problems they encountered in nursing practice over a three-month period. Vaughan's analysis identified 2,265 moral problems, 67 problems of etiquette, and 110 questions about ethical behavior. The ethical problem the nurses faced most often was the lack of co-operation between nurses and physicians and among nurses in general. Other ethical problems noted were: duties to the nursing school, lying (including dishonest charting), duties to patients, lust, and problems of temperance. Vaughan concluded that the problem of lack of cooperation her subjects experienced signaled nurses' growing awareness of their responsibilities to society and the role they were playing in patient care. She recommended more emphasis on ethics education in nursing to ensure a high standard of individual morality, which she believed would "raise the nursing professional above and beyond the slightest suggestion of social disapproval . . ." (Vaughan, 1935, p. 105).

Despite this early interest in nurses' ethical problems, nursing ethics research did not begin in earnest until the 1980s. Research efforts initially focused on the ethical reasoning abilities and ethical behaviors and judgments among practicing nurses (Ketefian and Ormond, 1988). These studies focused on the ability of the nurse to make moral judgments, the hypothetical ethical behavior of the nurse, and nurses' perceptions of ethical problems. Methodologically, the studies were designed to document empirically the cognitive abilities of nurses to make moral judgments.

A few studies in nursing ethics have measured nurses' ethical decision-making styles, factors influencing nurses' ethical decisions, and the consistency of the way nurses make ethical decisions (Ketefian and Ormond, 1988). Nursing ethics research has also turned to the study of the attitudes and values of nurses concerning ethical issues (Davis and Slater, 1989), ethical conflicts nurses experience in the care of patient populations with severely disabling conditions (Norberg et al., 1987) and those receiving long-term tube feedings (Wilson, 1992). The use of nursing-care resources by do-not-resuscitate (DNR) patients in intensive-care units as well as the impact of the DNR order on nursing interventions has been the subject of another study (Lewandowski et al., 1985). Still another study has identified variables that are the best predictors of a DNR classification and the extent of nursing care required by the DNR patient (Tittle et al., 1991).

During the 1980s and early 1990s, the focus of nursing ethics research shifted from the study of nurses' ethical perceptions and behaviors, and how nursing ethics was taught, to the study of how nurses make ethical decisions and plan patient care when confronted with complex moral issues. Certain areas, however, remain unexplored. For example, the particular role of nurses in ethical decisions that affect patients is not very clear. Nurses' abilities to recognize moral values, make ethical decisions, and support patients' or family members' decisions are believed to be very important to the quality of patient care. However, little is known about the types of ethical decisions made by nurses and how they affect patient outcomes.

Another area that should be more carefully evaluated is the theoretical frameworks used to interpret study results in nursing ethics research. Since nursing is largely practiced by women, theoretical structures should include the process of ethical decision making by women as well as by men. Furthermore, researchers should use structures that can account for the nature and process of ethical decisions made by nurses in contrast to those of other health-care workers, such as physicians (Fry, 1989). This means that theoretical structures that are developed from the study of one gender alone or that consider ethical decisions as decisions made by physicians might not be appropriate for the study of nurses' ethical decisions. In considering appropriate theoretical frameworks, clarity about the moral concepts of nursing is very important.

Moral concepts of nursing ethics

Advocacy, accountability, collaboration, and caring are moral concepts that comprise the foundation for nurses' principled, ethical decision making (Fry, 1994). They are important because they enjoy a firm place in nursing standards and ethical statements throughout the history of the nursing profession and help define the ethical dimensions of the nurse–patient relationship.

Advocacy. Advocacy may be defined as the active support of an important cause (Fry, 1994). In nursing, it describes the nature of the nurse–patient relationship and has been interpreted as a legal metaphor for the nurse's role in relation to a patient's human and moral rights within the health-care system (Winslow, 1984). Others have interpreted advocacy as the ideal expressed when individuals are assisted by nursing in the exercise of self-determination (Gadow, 1980), or the moral concept that defines how nurses view their responsibilities to the patient (Lumpp, 1979).

Advocacy is said to be associated with courage (Winslow, 1984) and heroism (Lanara, 1981). It may also be understood as the means by which the nurse participates with the patient in determining the meaning that the experience of illness, suffering, or dying has for that individual (Gadow, 1980). Lumpp (1979) has even argued that two general, ethical principles—respect for human dignity and fidelity—are rooted in the advocacy concept. Some nurse ethicists have interpreted advocacy as the ethical principle that underwrites what nurses do to protect the human dignity, privacy, choice (when applicable), and well-being of the patient (Fry, 1994). This last view of advocacy seems most consistent with the values expressed in nursing codes of ethics and the primary ethical responsibilities of the nurse.

Accountability. The concept of accountability seems to have two major attributes: answerability and responsibility (Fry, 1994). Nurses are assumed to carry personal responsibility for nursing practice and are expected to justify or "give an account" of their nursing judgments and actions according to the profession's ethical standards or norms. Terms of legal accountability for nursing practice are contained in licensing procedures and state-regulated nursing practice acts, while terms of moral accountability appear as norms in codes of nursing ethics and other standards of nursing practice. By virtue of agreeing to perform nursing care, the nurse accepts accountability for performing such care according to these standards and norms.

Accountability is said to be a basic moral value in nursing practice (Fry, 1994) and a moral foundation for nursing practice (Yarling and McElmurry, 1986). A few codes of nursing ethics have focused on accountability as a central moral concept (ANA, 1985; United Kingdom Central Council, 1984), and at least one national nursing organization has provided documentation on the extent of nursing accountability in professional practice (United Kingdom Central Council, 1989).

Cooperation. Cooperation is active participation with others to obtain quality care for patients, collaboration in designing nursing care, and reciprocity to those with whom nurses professionally identify. It implies consideration for the values and goals of those with whom one works. The concept of cooperation encourages nurses to work with others toward shared goals, make mutual concerns a priority, and sacrifice personal interests to maintain the professional relationship over time.

Cooperation has been included in many codes of nursing ethics as a moral concept of nursing practice (Canadian Nurses' Association, 1989; ICN, 1973; New Zealand Nurses' Association, 1988). While early views on nursing ethics linked cooperation to a special loyalty shared by members of the professional group (Robb, 1921), later views linked cooperation to the need to compromise individual goals and interests in order to achieve a mutually determined and higher level of patient care (Benjamin and Curtis, 1986; Fry, 1994).

Caring. The moral concept of caring has long been valued in the nurse–patient relationship. Caring behavior is considered essential to the nursing role and is presumed to affect how humans experience health as well as life itself. Nurse caring is directed toward the protection of the health and welfare of patients and indicates a commitment to the protection of human dignity and the preservation of human health (Fry, 1994).

Recent feminist interpretations of human caring relate caring to the protection, welfare, or maintenance of another person (Noddings, 1984). Others have defined caring as a moral obligation or duty among health professionals (Pellegrino, 1985), and as a form of involvement with others that engenders concern for how they experience their world (Benner and Wrubel, 1989). These views indicate two attributes of the concept. First, caring is a natural, human sentiment and is the way all humans relate to their world and to each other (Noddings, 1984). It exists as a structural feature of human growth and development before caring behaviors actually commence. Second, caring is linked to moral or social ideals such as the human need to be protected from the elements or the need for love. Caring, in this sense, might be interpreted as a special duty that exists between individuals and an ethical obligation within a given context.

The concept of caring has been identified as an important moral foundation for a nursing ethic that protects and enhances the dignity of patients. Caring is said to be a moral art central to health-care practices (Benner and Wrubel, 1989); the moral foundation for the nurse–patient relationship (Huggins and Scalzi, 1988); and a moral virtue of nursing practices (Knowlden, 1990).

Theories of nursing ethics

Progress in the development of a theory of nursing ethics has been slow, partly because of the disputes about the relationship of nursing ethics to medical ethics and to the discipline of ethics itself. Some ethicists claim that there is little that is morally unique to nursing practice (Veatch, 1981). The same moral issues confront everyone in the health-care setting, regardless of whether one is a physician, nurse, or patient. This means that nursing ethics is a legitimate term only insofar as it refers to a subcategory of medical ethics. Since medical ethics is the ethics of all judgments made within the biomedical sciences, nursing ethics is simply the ethical analysis of those judgments made by nurses in much the same way that physician ethics is the ethical analysis of those judgments made by physicians. Any theory of nursing ethics will, therefore, be exactly like medical ethics theory. According to this view, a theory of nursing ethics may not even be necessary.

Others argue that nursing ethics is not just another form of applied ethics, especially medical ethics (Jameton, 1984). If the moral concepts and obligations inherent in nursing practice are different from (yet compatible with) those of other health professions, then nursing ethics may have a distinct voice in health care. If so, nursing ethics will use traditional and contemporary forms of philosophical analysis to describe the moral phenomena of nursing practices, to critically assess the language and conceptual foundations of nursing practice, and to raise normative claims about the aims of nursing practice within the health-care sphere. It will provide a perspective on what is good and bad, right and wrong in nursing practice and propose ethical principles to guide nursing judgments and actions. It will be nursing ethics theory and not medical ethics theory.

Regardless of its form, any theory of nursing ethics will need to address the relevance of the moral concepts of nursing practice in the years ahead. As the twenty-first century reveals new moral challenges in health care, nursing ethics must respond with conviction about the integrity of its moral concepts and methods of ethics teaching. If it is to claim its promise as a form of philosophical inquiry for the field of bioethics, it must also continue to move ahead on the expansion of nursing ethics research and the development of practice-based theories of nursing ethics.

SARA T. FRY

Directly related to this entry are the entries NURSING AS A PROFESSION; NURSING, THEORIES AND PHILOSOPHY OF; TEAMS, HEALTH-CARE; CARE, article on CONTEMPORARY ETHICS OF CARE; and WOMEN, section on WOMEN AS HEALTH PROFESSIONALS. For a further discussion of topics mentioned in this entry, see the entries AUTONOMY; BENEFICENCE; FEMINISM; FIDELITY AND LOYALTY; LICENSING, DISCIPLINE, AND REGULATION IN THE HEALTH PROFESSIONS; MEDICAL CODES AND OATHS; PROFESSIONAL–PATIENT RELATIONSHIP, article on ETHICAL ISSUES; PROFESSION AND PROFESSIONAL ETHICS; and TRUST. This entry will find application in the entries CLINICAL ETHICS, article on ELEMENTS AND METHODOLOGIES; and HOSPITAL, article on CONTEMPORARY ETHICAL PROBLEMS. See also the APPENDIX (CODES, OATHS, AND DIRECTIVES RELATED TO BIOETHICS), SECTION III: ETHICAL DIRECTIVES FOR OTHER HEALTH-CARE PROFESSIONS, CODE FOR NURSES of the INTERNATIONAL COUNCIL OF NURSES, CODE FOR NURSES of the AMERICAN NURSES' ASSOCIATION, and CODE OF ETHICS FOR NURSING of the CANADIAN NURSES ASSOCIATION.

Bibliography

AMERICAN NURSES' ASSOCIATION (ANA). 1985. *Code for Nurses with Interpretative Statements.* Kansas City, Mo.: Author.

———. COMMITTEE ON ETHICS. 1980. *Guidelines for Implementing the Code for Nurses.* Kansas City, Mo.: Author.

AROSKAR, MILA A. 1977. "Ethics in the Nursing Curriculum." *Nursing Outlook* 25, no. 4:260–264.

BENJAMIN, MARTIN, and CURTIS, JOY. 1986. *Ethics in Nursing.* 2d ed. New York: Oxford University Press.

BENNER, PATRICIA E., and WRUBEL, JUDITH. 1989. *The Primacy of Caring: Stress and Coping in Health and Illness.* Menlo Park, Calif.: Addison-Wesley.

CANADIAN NURSES ASSOCIATION (CNA). 1989. *Code of Ethics for Nursing.* Ottawa: Author.

DAVIS, ANNE J., and AROSKAR, MILA A. 1991. *Ethical Dilemmas and Nursing Practice.* 3d ed. Norwalk, Conn.: Appleton and Lange.

DAVIS, ANNE J., and SLATER, PATRICIA V. 1989. "U.S. and Australian Nurses' Attitudes and Beliefs About the Good Death." *Image* 21, no. 1:34–39.

FRY, SARA T. 1989. "Toward a Theory of Nursing Ethics." *Advances in Nursing Science* 11, no. 4:9–22.

———. 1994. *Ethics in Nursing Practice: A Guide to Ethical Decision Making.* Geneva: International Council of Nurses.

GADOW, SALLY. 1980. "Existential Advocacy: Philosophical Foundations of Nursing." In *Nursing: Images and Ideals,* pp. 79–101. Edited by Stuart F. Spicker and Sally Gadow. New York: Springer.

HUGGINS, ELIZABETH A., and SCALZI, CYNTHIA C. 1988. "Limitations and Alternatives: Ethical Practice Theory in Nursing." *Advances in Nursing Science* 10, no. 4:43–47.

INTERNATIONAL COUNCIL OF NURSES (ICN). 1973. *Code for Nurses: Ethical Concepts Applied to Nursing.* Geneva, Switzerland: Author.

JAMETON, ANDREW. 1984. *Nursing Practice: The Ethical Issues.* Englewood Cliffs, N.J.: Prentice-Hall.

KETEFIAN, SHAKE, and ORMOND, INGRID. 1988. *Moral Reasoning and Ethical Practice in Nursing: An Integrative Review.* New York: National League for Nursing.

KNOWLDEN, VIRGINIA. 1990. "The Virtue of Caring in Nursing." In *Ethical and Moral Dimensions of Care,* pp. 89–94. Edited by Madeleine M. Leininger. Detroit, Mich.: Wayne State University Press.

LANARA, VASSILIKI A. 1981. *Heroism as a Nursing Value: A Philosophical Perspective.* Athens: Sisterhood Evniki.

LEWANDOWSKI, WENDY; DALY, BARBARA; McCLISH, DONNA K.; JUKNIALIS, BARBARA W.; and YOUNGNER, STUART J. 1985. "Treatment and Care of 'Do-Not-Resuscitate' Patients in a Medical Intensive-Care Unit." *Heart and Lung* 14, no. 2:175–181.

LUMPP, FRANCESCA. 1979. "The Role of the Nurse in the Bioethical Decision-Making Process." *Nursing Clinics of North America* 14, no. 1:13–21.

NEW ZEALAND NURSES' ASSOCIATION. PROFESSIONAL SERVICES COMMITTEE. 1988. *Code of Ethics.* Wellington, New Zealand: Author.

NIGHTINGALE, FLORENCE. 1859. *Notes on Nursing: What It Is, and What It Is Not.* London: Harrison and Sons.

NODDINGS, NEL. 1984. *Caring: A Feminine Approach to Ethics and Moral Education.* Berkeley: University of California Press.

NORBERG, ASTRID; ASPLUND, KENNETH; and WAXMAN, HOWARD. 1987. "Withdrawing Feeding and Withholding Artificial Nutrition from Severely Demented Patients: Interviews with Caregivers." *Western Journal of Nursing Research* 9, no. 3:348–356.

PELLEGRINO, EDMUND D. 1985. "The Caring Ethic: The Relation of Physician to Patient." In *Caring, Curing, Coping: Nurse, Physician, Patient Relationships,* pp. 8–30. Edited by Anne H. Bishop and John R. Scudder. Tuscaloosa: University of Alabama Press.

ROBB, ISABEL HAMPTON. 1921. *Nursing Ethics: For Hospital and Private Use.* Cleveland: E. C. Koeckert.

SAWYER, LINDA M. 1989. "Nursing Codes of Ethics: An International Comparison." *International Nursing Review* 36, no. 5:145–148.

TITTLE, MARY BETH; MOODY, LINDA; and BECKER, MARK P. 1991. "Preliminary Development of Two Predictive Models for DNR Patients in Intensive Care." *Image* 23, no. 3:140–144.

UNITED KINGDOM CENTRAL COUNCIL FOR NURSING, MIDWIFERY, AND HEALTH VISITING. 1984. *Code of Professional Conduct for the Nurse, Midwife, and Health Visitor.* 2d ed. London: Author.

———. 1989. *Exercising Accountability: A Framework to Assist Nurses, Midwives, and Health Visitors to Consider Ethical Aspects of Professional Practice.* London: Author.

VAUGHAN, ROSE HELENE. 1935. "The Actual Incidence of Moral Problems in Nursing: A Preliminary Study in Empirical Ethics." Ph.D. diss., Catholic University of America, Washington, D.C.

VEATCH, ROBERT M. 1981. "Nursing Ethics, Physician Ethics, and Medical Ethics." *Law, Medicine, and Health Care* 9, no. 5:17–19.

VEATCH, ROBERT M., and FRY, SARA T. 1987. *Case Studies in Nursing Ethics.* Philadelphia: J. B. Lippincott.

WILSON, DONNA M. 1992. "Ethical Concerns in a Long-Term Tube Feeding Study." *Image* 24, no. 3:195–199.

WINSLOW, GERALD R. 1984. "From Loyalty to Advocacy: A New Metaphor for Nursing." *Hastings Center Report* 14, no. 3:32–40.

YARLING, ROLAND R., and McELMURRY, BEVERLY J. 1986. "The Moral Foundation of Nursing." *Advances in Nursing Science* 8, no. 2:63–73.

NURSING HOMES

See LONG-TERM CARE, *article on* NURSING HOMES.

NURSING AS A PROFESSION

Care for the ill or injured has existed since the beginning of recorded history, but modern nursing, as it is known in the twentieth century, had its beginnings in the nineteenth century with Florence Nightingale, who viewed nursing as a self-defining moral practice focused on caring. However, for decades after Nightingale established the school of nursing at St. Thomas Hospital in London, nursing made accommodations to other established institutions, especially medicine and hospitals—accommodations that dimmed Nightingale's original vision. Only after the nursing profession accomplished the tedious but necessary task of developing its craft and the institutions that any new venture must have in order to establish itself within a society did it engage in a concerted effort to establish its identity. Beginning in the 1960s, nursing attempted to gain recognition as a profession by applying science to nursing. Then in the 1980s, it began to identify itself as a caring practice, using qualitative methods of the human sciences to articulate the meaning of nursing practice.

Nightingale's vision

"A new art and a new science has been created since and within the last forty years. And with it a new profession—so they say; we say, *calling,*" wrote Florence Nightingale in 1893 to the meeting of the International Congress of Charities, Correction and Philanthropy in Chicago (Nightingale, 1949, p. 24). This congress initiated the organization of the nursing profession in the United States and Canada. Nightingale considered her "calling" a moral imperative from God (Woodham-Smith, 1983).

Nightingale preferred to designate nursing a "calling" rather than a "profession" to underscore its identity as a self-defining practice with a dominant moral sense. Nursing fulfilled its moral sense by putting "the patient in the best condition for nature to act upon him" (Nightingale, 1946); Nightingale regarded nursing as a way for women to make positive contributions to society. She recruited only women of the highest moral character, thus attempting to overcome the public impression that nurses were mostly drunks and prostitutes. In the male-dominated society of Nightingale's time, "refined" women did not work outside the home.

As medical science advanced, nurses increasingly came to be considered handmaidens of physicians, as Nightingale had feared. One reason she rejected the germ theory was that she feared it would lead to what eventually came to be called intervention medicine. She foresaw that intervention medicine would lessen the centrality of nursing care in health care (Rosenberg, 1979). Intervention medicine led to the belief that physicians cure by intervening in the development of disease, whereas nurses merely care for those being cured. Furthermore, science and applied science were regarded as masculine activities, whereas caring was believed to be a feminine activity.

The primary focus of caring was one's own family. Thus, in the early part of the twentieth century, much nursing care was given by young women who, for the most part, were waiting to fulfill what was seen as their primary calling: to care for family. While they were students, these young women were a cheap source of labor for hospitals. The few career nurses in hospitals directed these novice nurses, who gave most of the direct nursing care. Most nursing care in hospitals, then, was not given by nurses who could be called professionals in any sense of the word.

World War II required that large numbers of women enter the industrial work force for the first time, and nurses serving in the armed forces attracted greater attention to the importance of nursing. However, this apparent advance in women's professionalism merely implied that it was permissible for women to work outside the home when unusual circumstances demanded it. During the 1950s, nursing seemed not to progress as a profession except that married women were accepted into schools of nursing and allowed to practice in hospitals; the traditional view of women's vocation continued to prevail. Jo Ann Ashley (1976) has argued that hospital paternalism and sexist attitudes of physicians contributed to the exploitation of nurses, who were kept subservient. Susan Reverby has concluded that nurses were "so divided by class that their common oppression based on gender could not unite them" (1987, p. 6), and that nurses saw caring for patients as a duty that "constrained nursing's effort to control its own practice and occupational future" (1987, p. 199).

Throughout history, men, particularly in religious orders and in military service, provided nursing care for the ill and wounded. But since the development of modern nursing, few men have entered nursing as a vocation. Even with the encouragement of men to enter nursing in the last decades of the twentieth century, the percentage of male nurses in the United States has remained fairly constant at approximately 3 percent.

Nursing is mainly a woman's vocation throughout the world. One reason that few men enter nursing is that "the problems of nursing and nurses truly are universal: few well-prepared nurses, poor career structures, and lack of resources. It is only a question of degree" (Holleran, 1992, p. 3). Constance Holleran has observed

that hospitals in many countries have no budget for nursing and that in some countries there are many nursing administrators but few nurses who give direct care.

Gaining recognition as a profession

The question of whether nursing is a profession has concerned nursing organizations and scholars since the 1960s. Early attempts to gain recognition as a profession were based primarily on criteria drawn from disciplines outside of nursing. Using sociological criteria, Amitai Etzioni contends that although nursing had some of the characteristics of a profession, it could not be classified as a profession (Etzioni, 1969). In a major study to assess how far nursing had advanced in its attempt to become a profession between 1970 and 1980, researchers used six sociological criteria to determine its progress: a long and disciplined educational process; discretionary authority and judgment; an active and cohesive professional organization; acknowledged social worth; contribution and a strong level of commitment; and a unique body of knowledge and skill (Lysaught, 1981). These sociological criteria are helpful in understanding the controversy surrounding nursing's claim to be a profession.

A long and disciplined educational process. The first criterion has been one of the most difficult for nursing to meet because of the tension between hospital and collegiate programs. In the United States, nurses are prepared to be registered nurses in multiple ways: by diploma programs in hospitals; by associate degree programs, usually in community colleges and by baccalaureate degree and graduate degree programs in colleges and universities. Every major study of nursing in the twentieth century, however, has recommended that nursing education should be placed in the mainstream of collegiate education (Committee for the Study of Nursing, 1923; National Commission for the Study of Nursing and Nursing Education, 1970; National Commission on Nursing, 1983). As early as 1965, the American Nurses' Association recommended that all those licensed to practice nursing should be educated in institutions of higher education and that the baccalaureate degree in nursing should be the minimum preparation for beginning professional nursing practice. Although many hospital diploma programs have continued to educate nurses, the growing trend in the United States is toward preparation by associate and baccalaureate degree programs. Some graduate programs were developed for college graduates who originally studied in another field and wished to pursue a second career in nursing.

Like the United States, other countries have traditionally prepared nurses for practice in hospital schools of nursing. In many countries there continue to be no university-level basic or graduate (postbasic) programs for nurses (Holleran, 1992). In countries where university-level education for nurses is being sought, the United States has served as a model. However, progress toward collegiate education as the basic entry level has been varied. In Canada, for example, although nursing education is well established in the university system, only Prince Edward Island has the baccalaureate degree as the entry level for nurses (Thomas, 1993). In Japan, there are only twelve baccalaureate degree programs in nursing; other schools offer an associate degree or a diploma in nursing (Anders and Kanai-Pak, 1992). Sweden has its nursing education within regional colleges but not in universities (Gortner and Lorensen, 1989). New Zealand transferred all of its undergraduate nursing education programs from hospitals to technical institutes and community colleges between 1973 and 1987 (Chick, 1987).

Graduate education in nursing in the United States began to develop in the 1960s. Master's degree programs were established primarily in the specialties of nursing practice, such as adult health, maternal and child health, and psychiatric–mental health. Although doctoral programs in nursing in the United States originally developed slowly, they more than doubled, from twelve to twenty-seven, between 1974 and 1984 (Brodie, 1986), and by 1993 had doubled again. By 1989, there was one doctoral program in Norway and five in Finland (Gortner and Lorensen, 1989). Denmark initiated its first doctoral program in nursing in 1992. In Japan, there are five graduate nursing programs (Anders and Kanai-Pak, 1992). Of two university nursing programs in New Zealand that began to offer postbasic nursing courses in 1983, only one had developed graduate study by 1987 (Chick, 1987).

Discretionary authority and judgment. In the United States, regulation of nursing practice and enforcement of standards for practice and education first occurred at the turn of the twentieth century through the establishment of state boards of nursing. These boards, composed of members of the nursing profession, set criteria for the practice of nursing and established evaluation procedures to ensure that nurses are capable of practicing safely and effectively. In the 1950s, the state boards created standardized testing for licensure to practice.

The National League for Nursing (NLN), an organization of nurses and citizens concerned with improving nursing, has significantly influenced the standards of nursing by the development of voluntary accreditation for educational programs. The NLN has established criteria to determine the quality of nursing education and procedures for accreditation of all types of educational programs that meet their criteria.

State and national nursing associations have exercised their influence in the political arena since they first supported legislation to create state boards of nurs-

ing. In the 1980s and 1990s, they concentrated on developing a political agenda that sought a greater influence on state and national legislation affecting nursing practice, nursing education, and health issues. Prior to this time, nurses often had little influence in developing health-care policy. However, in 1992, two significant events demonstrated nursing's increased influence on health-care policy. First, the Community Health Accreditation Program (CHAP) of the NLN won "deemed status" from the federal government; this means that community health agencies that have met the standards of accreditation by CHAP will be considered to have met the federal government's conditions for participating in the Medicare program and can receive Medicare reimbursement. Second, the Joint Commission for Accreditation of Healthcare Organizations created an at-large nursing seat on its board of commissioners. This body is the official accrediting agency of hospitals and other health-care organizations, and consequently has a great influence on the standards of health care in hospitals.

As nursing education has advanced to the graduate level, specialized fields of practice have been established and nurses have banded together to establish standards of practice for these specialities. In order to ensure a high standard of practice, certification examinations for advanced levels of practice have been established.

In 1965, a new level of nursing practice was created with the establishment of the first nurse practitioner program at the University of Colorado. Nurse practitioners are nurses who have completed an additional specialized educational program that extends practice into areas of medicine such as pediatrics, maternity care, and family health. They focus mainly on the prevention of illness, maintenance of wellness, and dealing with acute and chronic health problems by interviewing, gathering health histories, and doing physical examinations and laboratory analyses. Nurse anesthetists and nurse midwives are also classified as nurse practitioners and function under the same standards of practice. Nurse anesthetists administer anesthesia during surgery, and nurse midwives provide prenatal and postpartum care and deliver babies.

Licensure for nurse practitioners is regulated through a variety of arrangements between boards of nursing and boards of medicine. Legislation has been passed in many states that gives nurse practitioners the authority to write prescriptions. Some states permit nurse practitioners and nurses in advanced practice to receive direct payment for services from third-party payers such as Medicare, Medicaid, and private insurance. Reimbursement from third-party payers is usually based on diagnoses for the patient/client. Since medical diagnoses are inappropriate for nursing practice, the North American Nursing Diagnosis Association was created in the 1980s to develop nursing diagnoses that would further standardize nursing practice and could serve as a basis for the establishment of a system of reimbursement for nurses.

In the 1980s and early 1990s, many nurses in the United States began to focus on providing primary health care. Nurse-managed centers for primary care were established across the country, often located in homeless shelters, housing projects, and other settings expressly to meet the needs of the poor, who have limited access to health care.

Active and cohesive professional organization. The lack of a cohesive professional organization in 1981 was evident in the statement, "What is needed for the professionalization of nursing is a new birth of leadership, individual and organizational, that can conceive of ways to unite the more than 20 associations that currently draw their membership from nurses" (Lysaught, 1981, p. 24). Activities promoted by the International Council of Nurses and the World Health Organization in the international arena would eventually bring nursing in the United States to a more cohesive union.

The International Council of Nurses (ICN), established in 1899 as an independent, nongovernmental federation of national nursing associations worldwide, is the only representative international body of the whole nursing profession. Its membership is composed of national nursing organizations. The World Health Organization (WHO), established in 1948 as a specialized agency of the United Nations, is an intergovernmental, interdisciplinary agency representing more than 160 countries. Nursing's involvement in the projects of WHO is administered by the chief nurse scientist, who maintains communications with the six regional offices of WHO and other international organizations related to nursing. There is a close working relationship between WHO and ICN, both of which are headquartered in Geneva, Switzerland.

In 1977, WHO set the year 2000 as the target date for the attainment of the highest possible level of health for all people and specified primary health care as the key to attaining optimal health. In keeping with WHO's goal, the ICN has encouraged its member associations around the world to prepare nurses to participate more fully in a primary health-care system.

Nursing in the United States has been moving toward primary care since the development of nurse practitioners. It has, however, needed political clout to achieve this and other reforms. Nurses gained greater political power in 1991 when the American Nurses' Association, the National League for Nursing, and the American Association of Colleges of Nursing joined to form the Tri-Council for Nursing Executives. The increasing influence of nursing in the political arena is evident in "Nursing's Agenda for Health Care Reform," developed by the Tri-Council and formally supported by sixty-four nursing organizations in early 1993 ("Additional Endorsements," 1993). The Tri-Council has led the effort to gain acceptance by the U. S. Congress of measures that would increase primary health care in community-based settings; foster community responsibility for personal health, self-care, and informed decision making in selecting health-care services; and facilitate utilization of the most cost-effective providers in the most appropriate settings ("58 Organizations," 1992).

Acknowledged social worth and strong level of commitment. The 1981 Lysaught study reported that the public had a high appreciation of nurses' social worth but that nurses ranked low in commitment since only 40 percent of licensed registered nurses were employed full-time. This was clearly an inappropriate use of quantitative criteria to measure commitment, which cannot be measured by the percentage of registered nurses in full-time employment. Commitment in nursing refers to the nurse's determination to foster the well-being of patients/clients. Using qualitative methods, Patricia Benner (1984) found that commitment to the patient's well-being was present to a high degree in those who were considered excellent nurses. Anne Bishop and John R. Scudder, Jr. (1990) also found that such commitment was evident in narratives in which nurses described their most fulfilling experiences as nurses.

Unique body of knowledge and skill. The development of a unique body of knowledge and skill depends in significant measure on funding for research. During the 1970s, the federal Division of Nursing, which is within the U.S. Public Health Service, focused its priorities for research on clinical studies that would determine the health problems needing nursing intervention, the effectiveness of nursing practice, and the means of appropriating researching findings into practice for the improvement of patient care. Funding for nursing research was enhanced with the establishment in 1986 of the National Center for Nursing Research within the National Institutes of Health.

The majority of nursing research in the United States in the 1960s and 1970s tended to use scientific models and to approach nursing knowledge as an applied science. Often theories were imported into nursing from the natural and behavioral sciences in an endeavor to create a credible body of knowledge concerning nursing that would enhance nurses' status in the academic community. This applied approach was perhaps predictable, given the fact that only one-third of nursing educators and scholars took their initial graduate degrees in nursing; the other two-thirds took their initial degrees in other fields (Moses, 1990). Since the mid-1980s, however, a growing number of nursing scholars have used the qualitative methodology of the human sciences to conduct research in the practice of nursing. The significant increase in nursing scholars holding doctorates continues to broaden the approaches to research in nursing, and the different approaches can be seen in the increasing number of nursing journals, including some devoted specifically to nursing research.

Enhancing the status of nursing

A review of the nursing literature demonstrates that nursing continues to seek its identity in almost all parts of the world. Everywhere, nurses face difficulties in establishing the authority of their own practice due to the elevated status of men and the lowered status of women.

Nurses are increasingly attempting to enhance their legitimate authority to direct nursing care by establishing the worth of their own practice. Margretta Styles, for example, has contended that nursing would be "better served by a set of internal beliefs about nursing than a set of external criteria about professions." She proposes the "bare necessities" (1982, p. 121) for professionhood: (1) nurses recognize the social significance of nursing by being certain about the nature and importance of their work; (2) nurses respond to the moral imperative of their work and perform to the utmost of their ability by being well prepared in knowledge, skill, and attitude; and (3) nurses realize that responsibility and authority are shared through collegiality and collectivity in order to preserve the wholeness of the profession (Styles, 1982).

Patricia Benner (1984) attempted to learn about nursing by studying its actual practice rather than applying theories from outside of nursing. Working with a team of nursing scholars, she used the qualitative research methods of narrative and interpretative phenomenology to describe the experiences of nurses in practice. She identified seven domains of nursing: the helping role, the teaching-coaching function, the diagnostic and patient-monitoring function, effective management of rapidly changing situations, administering and monitoring therapeutic interventions and regimens, monitoring and ensuring the quality of health-care practices, and organizational and work-role competencies. Furthermore, she identified the progression of nurses through five stages, from novice to expert, illustrating each stage with exemplars that reflect clinical knowledge (Benner, 1984). Benner's study is significant to the advancement of nursing knowledge because it illustrates, in part, that knowledge can be developed from nursing practice itself, as opposed to studies that attempt to reveal knowledge through the application of theories.

Like Benner, Anne Bishop and John R. Scudder, Jr. (1990, 1991) showed that phenomenological interpretation of nursing practice is appropriate to the study of nursing. They concluded that nursing is a practice with an inherent moral sense and is appropriately studied as a practical human science.

Benner, Bishop, and Scudder are part of a growing number of scholars—Jean Watson, Sally Gadow, Janet Quinn, Em Bevis, Nancy Diekelmann, Madeleine Leininger, Marilyn Ray, and many others—who are attempting to define nursing by using the concept of caring. They employ qualitative research methodology to clarify the meaning of nursing and to improve nursing.

Conclusion

In summary, those who are interpreting nursing from the inside of nursing approach the meaning of "profession" in a different way than those who follow the applied approach. The latter attempt to show that nursing is a profession by applying criteria for any profession to nursing. Using these criteria has helped to establish nursing as a profession; however, the criteria often function as norms to be achieved, and thus actually form, rather than merely assess, nursing. Those who interpret nursing from the inside are not primarily interested in demonstrating that nursing is a profession, although they are confident that it is when its identity is disclosed. They are attempting to articulate the meaning of nursing as it is practiced and are focused on improving that practice. The nursing practice they describe has advanced in ways that Nightingale could not have foreseen. However, it is the same self-defining moral practice focused on caring envisioned by Nightingale.

ANNE H. BISHOP

Directly related to this entry are the entries NURSING, THEORIES AND PHILOSOPHY OF; NURSING ETHICS; *and* ALLIED HEALTH PROFESSIONS. *For a further discussion of topics mentioned in this entry, see the entries* LICENSING, DISCIPLINE, AND REGULATION IN THE HEALTH PROFESSIONS; NARRATIVE; PROFESSION AND PROFESSIONAL ETHICS; *and* WOMEN, *section on* WOMEN AS HEALTH PROFESSIONALS. *For a discussion of related ideas, see the entries* AUTHORITY; RESPONSIBILITY; *and* VALUE AND VALUATION.

Bibliography

"Additional Endorsements for Nursing's Agenda." 1993. *American Nurse* 25 (March):8.

ANDERS, ROBERT L., and KANAI-PAK, MASAKO. 1992. "Karoshi: Death from Overwork: A Nursing Problem in Japan?" *Nursing & Health Care* 13, no. 4:186–191.

ASHLEY, JO ANN. 1976. *Hospitals, Paternalism, and the Role of the Nurse.* New York: Teachers College Press.

BENNER, PATRICIA E. 1984. *From Novice to Expert: Excellence and Power in Clinical Nursing Practice.* Menlo Park, Calif.: Addison-Wesley.

BISHOP, ANNE H., and SCUDDER, JOHN R., JR. 1990. *The*

Practical, Moral and Personal Sense of Nursing: A Phenomenological Philosophy of Practice. Albany: State University of New York Press.

―――. 1991. *Nursing: The Practice of Caring.* New York: National League for Nursing.

BRODIE, BARBARA. 1986. "Impact of Doctoral Programs on Nursing Education." *Journal of Professional Nursing* 2, no. 6:350–357.

CHICK, NORMA P. 1987. "Nursing Research in New Zealand." *Western Journal of Nursing Research* 9, no. 3:317–334.

COMMITTEE FOR THE STUDY OF NURSING (U.S.). 1923. *Nursing and Nursing Education in the United States.* Edited by Josephine C. Goldmark. New York: Macmillan.

ETZIONI, AMITAI. 1969. *The Semi-Professions and Their Organization: Teachers, Nurses, Social Workers.* New York: Free Press.

"58 Organizations Support Nursing's Reform Agenda." 1992. *American Nurse* 24 (February):24.

GORTNER, SUSAN R., and LORENSEN, MARGARETHE. 1989. "Development of Nursing Science in Scandinavia." *Nursing Outlook* 37, no. 3:123–126.

HOLLERAN, CONSTANCE. 1992. "Perspective of the International Council of Nurses." *Nursing Administration Quarterly* 16, no. 2:2–3.

LYSAUGHT, JEROME P. 1981. *Action in Affirmation: Toward an Unambiguous Profession of Nursing.* New York: McGraw-Hill.

MOSES, EVELYN B. 1990. *The Registered Nurse Population: Findings from the National Sample Survey of Registered Nurses, March 1988.* Washington, D.C.: U.S. Department of Health and Human Services, Public Health Service, Health Resources and Services Administration, Bureau of Health Professions, Division of Nursing.

NATIONAL COMMISSION ON NURSING. 1983. *Summary Report and Recommendations.* Chicago: Author.

NATIONAL COMMISSION FOR THE STUDY OF NURSING AND NURSING EDUCATION. 1970. *An Abstract for Action.* Edited by Jerome P. Lysaught. New York: McGraw-Hill.

NIGHTINGALE, FLORENCE. 1946. [1859]. *Notes on Nursing: What It Is, and What It Is Not.* Philadelphia: J. B. Lippincott.

―――. 1949. "Sick Nursing and Health Nursing." In *Nursing of the Sick* (1893), pp. 24–43. Edited by Isabel A. Hampton Robb. New York: McGraw-Hill.

Nursing's Agenda for Health Care Reform. 1991. Kansas City, Mo.: American Nurses' Association.

REVERBY, SUSAN M. 1987. *Ordered to Care: The Dilemma of American Nursing, 1850–1945.* Cambridge: At the University Press.

ROSENBERG, CHARLES E. 1979. "Florence Nightingale on Contagion: The Hospital as Moral Universe." In *Healing and History: Essays for George Rosen,* pp. 116–136. Edited by Charles R. Rosenberg. New York: Dawson Science History.

STYLES, MARGRETTA. 1982. *On Nursing: Toward a New Endowment.* St. Louis: C. V. Mosby.

THOMAS, BARBARA, and ARSENEAULT, ANNE-MARIE. 1993. "Accreditation of University Schools of Nursing: The Canadian Experience." *International Nursing Review* 40, no. 3:81–84.

WOODHAM-SMITH, CECIL. 1983. *Florence Nightingale, 1820–1910.* New York: Atheneum.

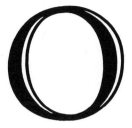

OATHS AND CODES, MEDICAL

See MEDICAL CODES AND OATHS; *and the* APPENDIX (CODES, OATHS, AND DIRECTIVES RELATED TO BIOETHICS), *especially* SECTION II: ETHICAL DIRECTIVES FOR THE PRACTICE OF MEDICINE.

OBLIGATION AND SUPEREROGATION

Much human behavior in the biomedical sphere is governed by moral principles. Due to their particular importance, medical relationships, in the wide sense of the term, have always been considered to be subject to evaluation in terms of justice, duty, obligation, and rights. Thus, the allocation of medical resources is weighed in terms of justice and fairness; the physician's professional role and powerful status define his or her professional duties; the contractual agreement and the special trust of patients places the doctor under a wide variety of obligations toward them; and the particularly urgent needs and interests of human beings (fetuses, handicapped persons, people in coma, and all sickly people included) grant them the right to be medically treated and respected. The regulation of medical practice under these terms of rights and duties has been acknowledged throughout history and formulated in a series of doctors' oaths. More recently there has been a growing trend to safeguard morally required behavior in medical practice under legal rules, on the one hand, and political (state) control, on the other. This institutionalization of medical relations has led to the effective enforcement of the moral rights and duties of patients and physicians, but also to the depersonalization, even dehumanization, of these relations.

Some forms of heroic sacrifice, volunteering, and beneficence have been traditionally treated as situated beyond the call of duty. This article seeks to establish the important (though limited) role of such behavior in the medical domain, especially against the background of the growing legislation, politicization, and commercialization of medical life. Eager to safeguard universal compliance, impartial distribution, and equal treatment, medical ethicists have tended to ignore the unique virtues of the morality of supererogation as a complement to the morality of duty.

The theological sources of supererogation

The term "supererogation" derives from the Latin verb meaning "to pay out more than is required." The first source for its use as an ethical concept goes back to the Latin version of the New Testament. In the famous parable, the Good Samaritan offers money to an innkeeper to care for a wounded man found on the road, and promises to repay the innkeeper "over and above" for any extra expenses (Luke 10:35). Consequently, Good Samaritanism has been closely associated with supererogatory behavior.

Yet the parable of the Good Samaritan does not distinguish explicitly between the obligatory and the supererogatory, but rather between the merely legally binding (to which the priest and the Levite in the biblical story seem to be exclusively committed) and moral or truly virtuous behavior (manifest in the deeds of the Good Samaritan). The explicit distinction between two types of moral norms, the commanded and the recommended, is better formulated in the contrast between keeping one's lawful riches and leading a life of total poverty (Matthew 19:16–24), or between lawful marriage and self-imposed chastity (1 Corinthians 7:25–28), or between ordinary religious faith and total commitment to a religious way of life.

Perpetual poverty, perfect chastity, and perfect obedience thus became the paradigm cases of evangelical counsels (consilia), which, in contrast with the religious commandments (praecepta), were considered by the church fathers and medieval theologians (from Augustine to Thomas Aquinas) to be truly meritorious. Other acts, by which one could freely choose to go beyond the religious precepts, included penance, patience, fasting, and martyrdom, as well as mercy (as opposed to justice) and beneficence (as in the bestowal of gifts). Living by the commandments guaranteed salvation, but following the counsels exemplified perfection.

Both the ideal of monastic life and the institution of sainthood were based on the gradually evolving two-level morality of duty and supererogation. Accordingly, two separate systems of norms applied to two categories of believers, ordinary people and those who had a special vocation or a particular moral capacity. In a later stage in the development of the idea of supererogation, it was claimed that the superabundant merit of the acts of those who belonged to the second category of believers (Jesus and the saints) was bequeathed to the spiritual treasury of the church, and could be dispensed by the pope to help sinners achieve salvation. Thus, the two systems of religious morality were linked by a mystical principle of transference of merit, from those who have a surplus to those who are in debt. The system of indulgences was based on the idea that the supererogatory merit of saintly people could compensate for the sins of ordinary folk. But the papal distribution of indulgences, gradually commercialized in the late Middle Ages, became one of the central targets of the reformers' attacks on the Roman Catholic church.

Martin Luther, John Calvin, and the Anglican Church questioned the theological foundations of the very idea of supererogation. If mortal human beings could not hope ever to carry out the religious precepts or commandments, how could they hope to do more than was required of them? The reformers' belief that salvation could be achieved only through God's grace, rather than through "good works," made the idea of supererogation absurd and blasphemous, a "superabomination." The denial of a two-tier religious morality directly challenged the ideas of sainthood, monasticism,

and indulgences. The metaphysical rejection of freedom of the will undermined the Catholic idea of licentia, that playroom for the virtuous exercise of free choice to do more than is required, which served as the condition and moral justification of supererogation conduct.

The theological debate over the concept of supererogation not only is the historical source for the parallel philosophical discussion in secular ethics, but also may serve as the model for this discussion. For despite the obvious differences between the two arenas (particularly on the objects of supererogatory acts, God and human beings, respectively), they share the basic features of the issue: the relation between goodness and duty, the limits of duty, the nature of free will, the place of virtue and perfection in a deontological theory, and the question of whether there are two categories of moral agents who are subject to moral requirements of different scope and stringency.

Supererogation in ethical theory

The subject of supererogation, rather surprisingly, did not receive much philosophical attention in ethical theory until the 1950s. In his pioneering article, James Urmson (1958) challenges the traditional tripartite classification of moral actions into the permissible (what one may do), the obligatory (what one ought to do), and the forbidden (what one ought not to do). Saintly and heroic acts are adduced as typical examples of actions that do not fall into any of these categories but still have a distinct moral value.

However, breaking the neat framework of the threefold division of moral action turns out to be a controversial enterprise. For example, it has to overcome the resistance of logicians, who try to draw a systematic analogy between the permissible and the possible, the forbidden and the impossible, and the obligatory and the necessary, thus creating a unified system of logic. If an act is morally good, how can it not be obligatory? And if there are good reasons for leaving it nonobligatory, cannot supererogation be analyzed in terms of the permissible? And finally, should supererogatory behavior not be considered forbidden, as a dangerous illusion of conceited and morally self-indulgent agents, who violate self-regarding duties and the principles of impartiality and fairness?

There are three kinds of answers to these questions regarding the seemingly paradoxical nature of supererogation: anti-supererogationism, qualified supererogationism, and unqualified supererogationism. Anti-supererogationism denies the existence of actions that go beyond the call of duty. Pure deontological theory, such as Kant's doctrine of the categorical imperative, is a typical example of this view. Obligatoriness (moral necessity) exhausts the moral sphere; duty is the only legitimate motive in morality; and universalizability is the ultimate test for the morality of actions. Hence there is no room for the nonobligatory, charity-based personal action that is typical of supererogation. Acts of beneficence or heroic self-sacrifice are either "imperfect duties" (which for Kant are no less binding than their "perfect" counterparts) or cases of moral fanaticism motivated by self-love.

Some forms of utilitarianism are no less anti-supererogationist. Thus, for the eighteenth-century utilitarian William Godwin, promoting the overall good (including the agent's) is the absolute and only moral duty (1971). This view leaves no room for supererogatory action (e.g., doing a favor), since either its beneficiary has a "complete right" over it or it is wrong ("unjust") to do it because of other people's rights (including the agent's). The derivation of "ought" statements from statements about the good (utility, happiness) leads George Edward Moore, too, to a straightforward denial of supererogation.

Modern utilitarian theorists point to the logical difficulty in distinguishing between utility-promoting actions that are obligatory and utility-promoting actions that are not obligatory, since such a distinction requires an appeal to a nonutilitarian principle. The common ground on which deontological and consequentialist anti-supererogationists rest their case seems to be the purely impersonal conception of morality, a conception typically expressed by the universalization principle or the classical utility principle of an agent-independent promotion of overall goodness "in the world." Impersonalism of this kind leaves no room for altruism, personal sacrifice, or the expression of individual preference.

Qualified supererogationism tries to do more justice to our common belief in the value of supererogatory conduct. It concedes that in some abstract or ideal sense every good action is obligatory, but highlights the circumstances that make such a morality too demanding, even absurd. Some utilitarians, like John Stuart Mill, distinguish between the prevention of harm (which is obligatory) and the altruistic promotion of the good (which deserves gratitude, honor, and moral praise). Henry Sidgwick is willing to distinguish between what a person ought to do and what people are justified in blaming him or her for not doing. Thomas Aquinas states that while the commandments apply to everyone, the counsels are directed only to the few who are capable of following them or who have made the life of perfection their special vocation. Rule utilitarians, as well as contract theorists like David Richards (1971), point to the possible decrease in overall happiness through the adoption of a general rule enforcing supererogatory action as a duty, and at the same time to the general social benefit derived from leaving it to individual discretion. Even Kant, in his later ethical writings, acknowledges

the existence of "duties of virtue" that "others cannot compel us (by natural means) to fulfill," as they are concerned with the adoption of ends, are binding only in the "internal" sense, and create no corresponding rights in the recipient. Finally, John Rawls (1971) and Joseph Raz (1975) analyze supererogation in terms of exemption: the exemption that "natural duty" allows in cases of high risk or loss to the agent (Rawls), or that granted by the second-order "exclusionary permission" not to act on the best balance of first-order reasons (Raz).

Qualified supererogationism is reductive in nature: it insists on accommodating supererogatory acts within a deontic framework (i.e., the language of duties and obligations). Every moral action is in principle required, though considerations of exemption, risk, disutility of enforcement, personal (in)capacity, excuses, difficult psychological circumstances, and rights define a supererogatory subcategory. Unqualified supererogationism, on the other hand, insists on placing the supererogatory "beyond duty" in the absolute, nonreductive sense (Urmson, 1958; Feinberg, 1968; Heyd, 1982). Supererogatory behavior is fully optional, that is, it lies beyond any kind of duty, under any condition, and for any moral subject. No excuse is needed for not acting heroically.

Definition and justification of supererogation

Most definitions of supererogation display the same general form, pointing to the asymmetry of commission and omission of actions. Thus supererogatory acts are said to be those acts that are good to do but not bad not to do, or right (just, virtuous, praiseworthy) to do but not wrong (unjust, vicious, blameworthy) to refrain from doing. These definitions, however, fail to capture either the special merit of supererogatory acts or their particular optional character. More sophisticated attempts retain the asymmetry but mix the contrasted pairs (e.g., "non-obligatory well doings," according to Roderick Chisholm [1963], or "meritorious non-duties," according to Joel Feinberg [1968]). Still, the definition of supererogation, at least of the unqualified version, must refer explicitly to the normative status of the acts in question, to their particular value, and to the person-relative features of these acts (the agent as well as the recipient).

A possible definition contains the following four conditions for an act to be supererogatory:

1. It is neither obligatory nor forbidden.
2. Its omission is not wrong and does not deserve sanction or criticism, either formal or informal.
3. It is morally good, both by virtue of its intended consequences and by virtue of its intrinsic value (being beyond duty).
4. It is done voluntarily for the sake of someone else's good, and is thus meritorious.

The first condition characterizes supererogatory acts in negative terms (being *non*obligatory), but the second emphasizes their purely optional nature. This distinction between the permissible and the optional points to the specific double value of the latter as opposed to the moral neutrality of the former: it is not only the good effect of supererogatory action that makes it praiseworthy; it is its motive, which is completely "free," that is, not even an "ought." This combination of desirable consequences and virtuous motive is the source of the moral merit ascribed to the agent of supererogatory acts.

It should be noted that the goodness of supererogation lies in its leading to consequences that are of moral value, that is, of the same type or on the same scale as those of obligatory action. This is clearly manifest in supererogatory transcendence of duty, such as "going the second mile" or doing more than one's job requires. In that respect, supererogation is continuous with the morality of duty. But the fact that the source of the value of a supererogatory act lies no less in the voluntariness of its motive points to its conceptual dependence on the idea of duty, that is, its being correlative to duty. It should be noted that there are ethical theories that are not based on the concept of duty at all (but rather on the idea of virtue, as in Aristotle). Such theories do not leave room for supererogation as it is defined here.

The general justification of supererogation is twofold: on the one (negative) hand, it has to do with the basic autonomy of individuals to lead their lives in ways not always subordinated to moral principles such as the overall good. On the other (positive) hand, it is associated with the supplementation of the impersonal and universal core of ethical theory with a personal dimension. This is expressed both by the agent's discretion and by the choice of the particular recipient of the beneficent act. Supererogation in that respect is highly important for social cohesion, trust, and friendship in society—values that cannot be fully achieved even in an ideally just society in which every person performs his or her duties and obligations. This justification for unqualified supererogationism is reminiscent of the debate about the legal enforcement of morality: in the same way that there are moral reasons for leaving some moral duties beyond the reach of the law, so there are moral reasons for leaving some morally good acts out of the system of moral duties and obligations. The Good Samaritan first took care of the wounded man (which was not his legal duty but certainly his moral duty); then he offered to pay the innkeeper "over and above," that is, for the expenses involved in housing and feeding the man (which was not even his moral duty).

Typical examples of supererogatory acts are saintly and heroic acts, which involve great sacrifice and risk for the agent and a great benefit to the recipient. However, more ordinary acts of charity, beneficence, and generosity are equally supererogatory. Small favors are a limiting case, because of their minor consequential value. Volunteering is an interesting case of supererogation, because it refers to the procedure by which the agent of an obligatory act is selected. That is to say, someone ought to do the act, but due to its particular difficulty or risk, it is hard to decide who. Finally, there are supererogatory forbearances, in which the agent refrains from taking a morally justified action that would have a negative impact on another. Forgiveness, pardon, and mercy are typical examples: we would have been justified in punishing a criminal, but we decided to exercise mercy or pardon.

Supererogation in medical ethics

The place of supererogation in medical ethics has been almost completely ignored, both in the theoretical discussions of supererogation and in the vast literature on medical ethics. This might be explained by the fact that both fields are relatively new, and by the tendency to bind the vital aspects of medical practice and relationship in a firm system of well-defined rights, duties, and obligations. The issues of confidentiality, informed consent, abortion, euthanasia, and allocation of scarce resources revolve around the debate on the rights of patients and the duties of doctors, the principles of justice, or the responsibilities of state and society to their members. However, there are some areas of medical practice in which supererogation has a central role to play, cases that could also help in understanding and justifying the theoretical distinction between obligation and supererogation: the collection and allocation of blood, organ donation, surrogate motherhood, and medical experimentation.

Antisupererogationists would tend to deny that some medical matters lie beyond the sphere of moral duty and social justice. In their attempt to reduce allegedly supererogatory conduct to one of three categories—the obligatory, the permissible, and the forbidden—they may, for instance, claim that blood donation is a moral duty, that surrogacy arrangements should be completely forbidden, or that participation in medical experiments should be left to the morally neutral (permissible) regulation of the free market. Grounding vital medical relationships in supererogatory altruistic motives offends our moral sense of equality, both in the access to treatment and in the undertaking of risks. Legislation and the market are two powerful alternatives that safeguard impartiality and personal neutrality, which are principal values in the ethics of duty and justice.

Qualified supererogationists would admit that ideally all medical practice should be subjected to universal deontic principles, especially since it deals with matters of life and death in which we want people to have equal chances, rights, and duties. But they point to the limit of what can be expected of individuals by way of giving and taking risks, particularly when the sacrifices required are of the same kind as the health needs of others that create the call for sacrifice. Therefore, when the health of a sick person requires an organ donation that would expose the donor to serious health hazards, one must leave the decision to the personal discretion of the donor. Institutional control or regulation under impersonal rules (such as legislation) is immoral, either because most people cannot make the required sacrifice ("ought" implies "can"), or because it could be counterproductive in utilitarian terms (the sacrifice of the donor being greater than the potential benefit to the recipient). Furthermore, the market mechanism, which is so efficient in much of our economic life, may lead to the exploitation of the poor by the rich or to other morally repugnant consequences related to the commercialization of human life and health.

The unqualified supererogationist shares many of these apprehensions but adds a positive justification for a "moral free zone" in medical life. Beyond the realm of relations of duties and rights, there is in medical practice some room for a totally free exercise of giving. It is a reflection of personal autonomy; it is grounded in a personal interest in another individual, and it creates personal relations; it strengthens social ties and cohesion. Blood donation is a typical example. Collection of blood for medical use in modern society can be based on a free-market system in which blood is freely bought and sold, or on a legally enforced system of duties (e.g., of young people to donate blood once a year), or on a fully voluntary system, as in Great Britain, in which people volunteer to give blood and patients get it free. Economists like Kenneth Arrow (1972) favor "the economy of charity," and believe that the market can better handle the needed balance of supply and demand of blood. Furthermore, they claim that altruism is itself a scarce resource, and therefore should be used only when necessary. Richard Titmuss (1973) and Peter Singer (1972), on the other hand, argue that the commercialization of blood donation is potentially destructive to society, especially because it concerns a "commodity" that has no price, that is, it is extremely valuable to the recipient and of almost no value to the donor. They add that altruism is not a scarce resource but, rather, a good that grows the more it is exercised. The supererogatory model is thus considered as superior both to the market mechanism and to the political (legal) arrangement of collection and allocation.

The donation of organs (like kidneys) is different in that it is much more costly to the donor than the donation of blood (particularly in the case of living donors). It is also more personal than the anonymous donation of a blood bank, as it usually involves someone personally close to the donor. Unlike blood donation (which may be considered morally obligatory though not legally enforceable), giving away a nonrenewable part of one's body is typically supererogatory, in the "saintly and heroic" sense. Ideals of personal responsibility, family ties, friendship, and particular emotional commitments make personal sacrifices like organ donation valuable beyond their sheer utility (which sometimes is tragically doubtful).

Surrogate motherhood can also be regulated by market mechanisms or left to voluntary, altruistic agreements. Beyond the controversial aspects of surrogacy (having to do with the interests of a third party, the child, and with the possibility of a change of mind by the surrogate mother), we may note that most legal systems prefer to leave it as a supererogatory matter. Thus, agreements on surrogacy are not considered criminal (forbidden) in many countries but are not enforced by the courts (in contrast with ordinary contracts). Commercialization is often treated as undesirable, even patently immoral and illegal.

Finally, medical experimentation on human subjects in most countries is now allowed only on the basis of volunteering. No person, sick or healthy, is required (legally or even morally) to take part in any experiment. On the other hand, participating in the enterprise of medical research and progress is definitely of great moral value. By altruistically giving our share to medical research, we express our gratitude to those in the past who made us beneficiaries of medical progress (Jonas, 1969). The supererogatory nature of participation in medical experimentation is typically connected to the case of volunteering, in which it is a moral "ought" that someone (in a group) do the job but no particular individual can be identified as having to do it. As opposed to any selection procedure based on substantive criteria (like merit), or formal criteria (like random devices, which are particularly attractive as a fair means of imposing burdens in risky situations), volunteering is completely supererogatory.

We may conclude, then, by pointing to the special status of supererogation in some aspects of medical ethics as combining the advantages of both morality and the market, as well as avoiding some of the dangers of both. A supererogatory system of blood collection is on the one hand of moral worth (no less, and even more, than its alternative regulation according to principles of duty fairness in a politically centralized system of collection and allocation), yet fully optional (as in the case of buying and selling in the market). On the other hand, it avoids the danger of exploitation, typical of the market mechanism, as well as the danger of compulsion, typical of often-abused political power or of social pressure. Supererogation can partly counter the undesirable trends of both commercialization and politicization of modern medical life by leaving an outlet for the autonomous and spontaneous exercise of supererogatory beneficence.

DAVID HEYD

Directly related to this entry are the entries BENEFICENCE; JUSTICE; *and* ETHICS, *article on* NORMATIVE ETHICAL THEORIES. *Also directly related is the entry* PATIENTS' RESPONSIBILITIES, *especially the article on* DUTIES OF PATIENTS. *For a further discussion of topics mentioned in this article, see the entries* ACTION; AUTONOMY; ETHICS, *article on* TASK OF ETHICS; FAMILY; FREEDOM AND COERCION; FRIENDSHIP; MEDICAL CODES AND OATHS, *article on* HISTORY; RIGHTS, *article on* SYSTEMATIC ANALYSIS; TRUST; UTILITY; *and* VIRTUE AND CHARACTER. *This entry will find application in the entries* BLOOD TRANSFUSION; ORGAN AND TISSUE PROCUREMENT, *especially the articles on* MEDICAL AND ORGANIZATIONAL ASPECTS, *and* ETHICAL AND LEGAL ISSUES REGARDING LIVING DONORS; ORGAN AND TISSUE TRANSPLANTS, *articles on* SOCIOCULTURAL ASPECTS, *and* ETHICAL AND LEGAL ISSUES; REPRODUCTIVE TECHNOLOGIES, *article on* SURROGACY; *and* RESEARCH POLICY, *articles on* RISK AND VULNERABLE GROUPS, *and* SUBJECT SELECTION. *Other relevant material may be found under the entries* AGING AND THE AGED, *article on* SOCIETAL AGING; CARE; CHILDREN, *article on* RIGHTS OF CHILDREN; FEMINISM; FIDELITY AND LOYALTY; HOSPITAL, *article on* MEDIEVAL AND RENAISSANCE HISTORY; LAW AND MORALITY; LOVE; RESPONSIBILITY; *and* VALUE AND VALUATION.

Bibliography

AQUINAS, THOMAS. *Summa theologica*, esp. I, q. 21; I, II, q. 108; II, II, q. 31, q. 32, q. 106, q. 184; and suppl., q. 25.

ARROW, KENNETH J. 1972. "Gifts and Exchanges." *Philosophy and Public Affairs* 1, no. 4:343–362.

CHISHOLM, RODERICK M. 1963. "Supererogation and Offence: A Conceptual Scheme for Ethics." *Ratio* 5, no. 1:1–14.

FEINBERG, JOEL. 1968. "Supererogation and Rules." In *Ethics*, pp. 391–411. Compiled by Judith J. Thomson and Gerald Dworkin. New York: Harper & Row.

GODWIN, WILLIAM. 1971. [1793]. *Enquiry Concerning Political Justice*. 3d ed. Oxford: At the Clarendon Press.

HEYD, DAVID. 1982. *Supererogation: Its Status in Ethical Theory*. Cambridge: At the University Press. A comprehensive monograph containing a detailed bibliography. For the theological origins of the concept of supererogation, see ch. 1.

JONAS, HANS. 1969. "Philosophical Reflections on Experimenting with Human Subjects." *Daedalus* 98, pp. 219–247.

KAMM, FRANCES MYRNA. 1985. "Supererogation and Obligation." *Journal of Philosophy* 82:118–138.

KANT, IMMANUEL. 1948. [1785]. *The Moral Law; or, Kant's Groundwork of the Metaphysic of Morals*. Edited and translated by John Paton. London: Hutchinson.

———. 1964. [1797]. *The Metaphysic of Morals*, Part II. Translated by Mary Gregor. New York: Cambridge University Press.

MILL, JOHN STUART. 1969. [1865]. "Auguste Comte and Positivism." In vol. 10, *The Collected Works of J. S. Mill*, pp. 261–368. Toronto: University of Toronto Press.

NEW, CHRISTOPHER. 1974. "Saints, Heroes and Utilitarians." *Philosophy* 49:179–189.

RAWLS, JOHN. 1971. *A Theory of Justice*. Cambridge, Mass.: Harvard University Press/Belknap Press.

RAZ, JOSEPH. 1975. "Permissions and Supererogation." *American Philosophical Quarterly* 12, no. 2:161–168.

RICHARDS, DAVID A. J. 1971. *A Theory of Reasons for Action*. Oxford: At the Clarendon Press.

SCHUMAKER, MILLARD. 1977. *Supererogation: An Analysis and Bibliography*. Edmonton, Alta.: St. Stephen's College.

SINGER, PETER. 1972. "Famine, Affluence, and Morality." *Philosophy and Public Affairs* 1, no. 3:229–243.

TITMUSS, RICHARD M. 1973. *The Gift Relationship: From Human Blood to Social Policy*. Harmondsworth, U.K.: Penguin. A classical comparative study of systems of blood donation.

URMSON, JAMES O. 1958. "Saints and Heroes." In *Essays in Moral Philosophy*, pp. 198–216. Edited by Abraham I. Melden. Seattle: University of Washington Press. The first article in analytic philosophy on supererogation.

OBLIGATIONS TO FUTURE GENERATIONS

See FUTURE GENERATIONS, OBLIGATIONS TO.

OCCUPATIONAL SAFETY AND HEALTH

I. Ethical Issues
   Charles Levenstein
II. Occupational Health-Care Providers
   Bailus Walker, Jr.
III. Testing of Employees
   Thomas H. Murray

I. ETHICAL ISSUES

The workplace setting presents unique problems for public health because, on the one hand, virtually all its hazards are environmental and can be prevented or controlled, while, on the other hand, it is a setting for social conflict with large economic stakes. Occupational injury and disease are economic phenomena resulting from social decisions about technology and the use of labor in the production of goods and services. The rights of property owners, even in state socialist systems; the economic obligations of managers to owners of enterprises; and the imbalance of power between labor and management present particular problems for occupational health. The position of health and safety professionals in industry is frequently problematic because of tensions between their responsibilities to employers and the ethical codes of their professions. The imperatives of production and profit frequently override other responsibilities for the health and welfare of employees.

Industrial hygiene is the principal profession applying scientific and engineering methods to the protection of workers from toxic chemicals, dust, other air contaminants, and job hazards. The basic industrial-hygiene approach to the work environment places engineering controls at the top of a hierarchy of methods for workers' health protection. This approach is enshrined in the ethical codes of the profession. A typical listing of industrial-hygiene approaches places substitution, process change, and isolation or enclosure at the top of the list. Methods that rely on personal protective equipment are considered less effective and are to be resorted to only when engineering controls are not feasible. The professional emphasis is on management's responsibility to provide a safe work environment rather than on workers' self-protection or adaptation to hazardous conditions.

Equity, or fairness in the distribution of society's material benefits, is not a primary concern in the economic theory or operation of the modern market. Public policy is predicated on the assumption that market mechanisms promote and reward efficiency. Policymakers presume that tax and/or subsidy policy will be used to cushion the effects on individuals or groups damaged in socially unacceptable ways, such as utter impoverishment. The market model minimizes the costs of factors of production, including labor, through entrepreneurial pursuit of profit. The role of government is restricted severely. Since consumer choice rules in the model, firms are guided in the production of goods and services by the willingness of consumers to pay, and resources are directed to consumers' financially expressed desires. Selfish motives are presumed of everybody, yet the model claims efficient results.

Even the strongest advocate of the market economy understands the limits of market efficiency. In the market model, collective consumption of goods and services, such as national defense, malaria control, road building, and the like, may be handled legitimately by the government. Further, where there are monopolistic imperfections in markets, where information is restricted or the mobility of labor and capital is impaired, the government may intervene. In addition, where costs or benefits are not internalized by the firm, air, water, wild animals, and the like are "free goods"; they cannot be considered in entrepreneurial calculations and "inefficient" solutions may result. For instance, a firm may use a process hazardous to human health if it will not bear the cost of worker illness that occurs years later. The existence of externalities is an argument for government intervention to force private parties to internalize these costs.

On what grounds does the government intervene to protect workers' health? Some would argue that imperfect information, imbalances in bargaining power, and other deviations from the perfect market model require that the state intervene on behalf of workers' health and safety. Others would argue that even if markets were working perfectly, the society has an overriding interest in the health of its members, including workers, and that it has a longer time frame than any of the market participants is willing to consider. Thus, market failure to deliver socially desirable ends, because of either imperfections or externalities, justifies state intervention.

Historical overview

Occupational health has rarely received much attention from the public. Historically, the commitment of the United States to economic advancement through technology has made its society myopic about its toll on workers' health. Through much of U.S. history, workers themselves have been too engaged in the pressing task of making a living for their families to pay much attention to widespread occupational safety and health problems. The labor movement has not been strong enough to force public attention to these issues on a continual basis.

In Europe, the tradition of occupational medicine is much greater. In the sixteenth century, the occupational health problems of miners and foundry and smelter workers were studied by Paracelsus. Bernardino Ramazzini (1633–1714) wrote a classic text on the occupational diseases of workers.

The industrial revolution brought a host of new health and safety problems to European workers. The social reform movements in England, for instance, sought protection for child labor and to restrict the working day to ten hours. Protective labor legislation was passed in 1833 (the Factory Act) and in 1842 (the Mines Act). Both occupational medicine and the trade union movement in Great Britain were launched in the nineteenth century as responses to awful conditions in many workplaces.

In the nineteenth century, the industrial revolution brought to the United States a host of safety problems and some public concern. Massachusetts created the first factory inspection department in 1867 and in subsequent years enacted the first job safety laws in the textile industry. The Knights of Labor, an early trade union, agitated for safety laws in the 1870s and 1880s, and by 1900 minimal legislation had been passed in the most heavily industrialized states.

After 1900, the rising tide of industrial accidents resulted in passage of workers' compensation laws; by 1920 virtually all states had adopted this no-fault insurance program. Previously, workers seeking financial compensation and medical care for industrial accidents had to sue their employers—and their employers had three extremely effective defenses. First, the courts accepted the notion that in a free market, workers assumed the responsibility for established occupational risks. Second, employers were absolved from responsibility for accidents to the extent that a worker's own actions contributed to the mishap. Third, in the eyes of the courts, employers were not financially responsible for injuries caused by fellow employees of the injured worker. In an economy of highly skilled artisans in which the labor process was controlled by the workers themselves, this defensive troika might have been reasonable; in an economy of mass production, high-speed assembly lines, and detailed division of labor, the illusion of worker autonomy fell of its own political weight. No-fault industrial accident insurance was the solution adopted by the states.

Throughout the 1920s, the rise of company paternalism was accompanied by the development of occupational medicine programs. Much attention was paid to preemployment physicals rather than industrial hygiene and accident prevention. Occasional scandals, like cancer in young painters of radium watch dials, reached the public attention, but until the resurgence of the labor movement in the 1930s, Congress did not pass important national legislation. The Walsh–Healey Public Contracts Act of 1936 required federal contractors to comply with health and safety standards, and the Social Security Act of 1935 provided funds for state industrial-hygiene programs. The Bureau of Mines was authorized to inspect mines.

After World War II, occupational health and safety again receded from public attention, as sympathy for the labor movement declined and the nation took a turn to the right. An exception to the general neglect of the field was passage of the Atomic Energy Act of 1954, which included provision for radiation safety standards. Not until the 1960s, when labor regained some political influence, did the issue reemerge. Injury rates rose 29 percent during the 1960s. A major mine disaster in 1968 at Farmington, West Virginia, in which seventy-eight miners were killed, captured public sympathy. In 1969, the Coal Mine Health and Safety Act was passed, and

in 1970, the broader Occupational Safety and Health Act became law.

Regulatory effects

A fundamental aspect of the new law was the unambiguous statement of employer responsibility for occupational health and safety. A new regulatory agency, the Occupational Safety and Health Administration (OSHA), was created in the U.S. Department of Labor. OSHA could require employers to provide safe and healthy workplaces and to promulgate and enforce safety standards. In addition, the OSHA Act established the National Institute for Occupational Safety and Health (NIOSH) as part of the U.S. Public Health Service, to do research and evaluate health hazards in the work environment.

Initially, OSHA adopted a host of so-called consensus standards. In addition to extending the Walsh–Healey regulations for government contractors to the rest of industry, the new agency adopted many of the voluntary guidelines developed by the American National Standards Institute and the American Conference of Government Industrial Hygienists. While this enabled OSHA to enter the field running, with standards to enforce, many of the guidelines were inappropriate as legal standards. Some were contradictory; others were overly detailed or anachronistic. For instance, OSHA adopted a requirement that toilet seats be split in the front, an idea that persisted from the day when people believed syphilis was caught from contaminated toilets. When Eula Bingham became head of OSHA in 1977, one of her earliest and most important tasks was standards simplification: throwing out inappropriate, ineffectual, or silly standards.

The process of developing new standards, however, was slow and cumbersome, involving substantial litigation before any new worker protection was extended. Perhaps the most tortuous path was that of the field sanitation standard for farm workers, which required that farmers provide clean water and toilet facilities for workers in the field. The standard took fourteen years to develop and ultimately was issued only because the courts required OSHA to do so. However, when OSHA, in a heroic effort to update its standards, adopted hundreds of new permissible exposure limits for air contaminants in the late 1980s, this wholesale revision was rejected by the federal courts as failing to meet the procedure required for standard development. In any case, since OSHA's inception, enforcement of standards has left much to be desired, largely because of understaffing.

While the OSHA Act covered most workers in the private sector, the Coal Mine Health and Safety Act established a special regulatory body to deal with the high-risk mining industry. Authority to regulate pesticide exposure of agricultural workers was assigned to the U.S. Environmental Protection Agency (EPA); OSHA bears responsibility for other aspects of farm employment, such as migrant-labor camp conditions and field sanitation.

The most important extensions of worker protection in recent years have been linked to growing public concern with general environmental issues. For instance, amendments to federal environmental laws in 1987 required both OSHA and the EPA to adopt safety and training requirements for a broad range of hazardous-waste workers and emergency personnel dealing with hazardous materials.

Federal government policy during the 1980s was characterized by a neoconservative, antiregulatory stance. Public-health advocates complained of the slow pace of OSHA standards promulgation, the federal ceding of enforcement authority to states, the failure to protect worker-complainants from employer discrimination, and the decimation of NIOSH's budget. The decline of the U.S. trade union movement has further weakened the political impetus for OSHA enforcement activity. In the early 1990s, efforts at legislative reform stress streamlining OSHA procedures for developing standards and enhancing workers' right to act.

Perhaps the most pressing problems in occupational health arise from the increasing integration of the world economy. In North America, the development of a continental free-trade agreement may threaten the work environment standards of Canada and the United States while bringing a host of new hazards to Mexico. The export of hazardous technologies, products, and waste represents increasing challenges for public health worldwide. On the one hand, our understanding of the nature of health hazards to workers has been improving; on the other hand, the restructuring of the world economy may undercut the political will to control these hazards.

The rights to know, to refuse, to act

Until the 1980s, workers in the United States did not have a legal right to know the names of hazardous materials to which they were exposed. This seems odd, since even market economists argue that good information is necessary if markets are to reflect working conditions correctly. Nevertheless, it was not until 1980, in the final days of the Carter administration, that OSHA promulgated a "right to know" regulation. The Reagan administration withdrew the proposed rule in 1981, and a political fight for this right ensued on state and local levels. Time and again, coalitions of workers' organizations and community environmental groups won state

and local laws mandating the right to know. Finally, OSHA came forth with the Hazard Communication Standard, which, although not as rigorous as some of the local ordinances, nevertheless extended a fundamental right to a wide range of workers across the country. This public-health regulation had to contend with competing property rights of corporations, such as the protection of trade secrets. Proposed legislation that would have required notification of workers discovered in NIOSH studies to be at high risk of occupational disease failed to pass Congress for such economic reasons. In addition, conservatives discovered that providing information involved economic costs to employers and sometimes to government. Companies argued that they should not be required to reveal essential substances or aspects of production processes because business competitors might obtain this information. OSHA was required to balance the protection of worker health with the protection of business's intellectual property rights.

Soon after the Hazard Communication Standard became law, labor advocates argued that the right to know was of little use as long as workers could not use such information to change hazardous working conditions. The OSHA Act made the violation of safety regulations an offense punishable by the government but gave workers only a very limited right to refuse hazardous work, and then only when there was objective evidence (not just fear) of imminent life-threatening danger. Moreover, the OSHA Act focused on the rights of individuals, not on collective worker action for health and safety. Health and safety advocates demanded an expanded right to refuse hazardous work, as well as the mandating of workplace health and safety committees with the right to act. Such committees, which already exist in countries other than the United States (Sweden, for instance), would mark a major departure in the regulatory approach in the United States. Worker empowerment is a substantially different approach from state regulation of the work environment.

Medical monitoring, reproductive hazards, and hazards to minority workers

Even though there is a long history of the use of preemployment examinations by occupational physicians in the United States, medical testing and monitoring remains a controversial area. Key ethical issues include confidentiality of medical records; inappropriate discrimination against minorities, women, and disabled or hypersusceptible employees; and "blaming the victim" vs. reducing exposures. Some OSHA standards require medical monitoring; perhaps one of the most distressing issues is the failure of OSHA and employers to analyze accumulated data systematically.

Because job segregation by gender continues to exist in the United States, women and men sometimes experience different health hazards. Perhaps the most controversial now concern reproduction. Some employers have sought to bar fertile women from jobs in which exposures to hazardous chemicals are within legal limits but may pose risks to a fetus. In some instances, where removal from such work involved serious income and/or opportunity loss, some women have agreed to sterilization in order to meet employer "fetal protection" requirements. Women's organizations and trade unions argue that such policies constitute unfair discrimination against women. The U.S. Supreme Court prohibited such policies in its decision in the case *Johnson Controls, Inc. v. UAW* in the spring of 1991 (110 S.Ct. 1522, 111 S.Ct. 1196).

Similarly, discrimination against and segregation of workers of color in the United States results in their having some of the most hazardous jobs. The situation of illegal immigrants exacerbates the problem, since they are fearful of turning to government for protection. Minority workers frequently have no union representation and are at the mercy of particularly exploitative employers. Migrant farm workers experience some of the most difficult conditions, in part because responsibility for their protection is split between the EPA, which regulates pesticides and related chemicals, and OSHA, which regulates labor camps. Domestic workers are another group largely composed of people of color who have little protection.

Workers' compensation, cost–benefit analysis, and the value of life

When workers are injured or killed on the job in the United States, workers' compensation programs at the state level are supposed to provide quick income support and medical care or a death benefit. These programs may provide a maximum of two-thirds of the average wage in the state, the rationale being that workers must have a financial incentive to return to work. No payment for pain or suffering is allowed. Workers are barred from suing their employers in this "no-fault" insurance scheme. There is no question that many workers suffer severe economic, as well as physical, hardship as a result of industrial injuries. Nevertheless, many employers complain about "cheaters" and fraud in the system, as well as about rising insurance premiums.

There is much debate about whether workers' compensation provides adequate compensation to workers who are injured on the job, and about the efficacy of the system for preventing injury; however, it seems evident that the system does not deal effectively with occupational diseases such as cancer and respiratory diseases. Workers have the burden of demonstrating that their ill-ness is job-related. Diseases of long latency and that may have multiple causes are rarely diagnosed as occupational and workers suffering from them are rarely compensated. Because the workers' compensation system failed to deal with asbestos-related disease, workers' attorneys initiated third-party liability suits in the 1970s and thereafter against asbestos suppliers, who, although they were not direct employers of the sick workers, had failed to warn asbestos product users about the hazards of the material. In this way, the inadequacies of the workers' compensation system have driven the occupational disease problem into the civil courts. Essentially, both the workers' compensation system and the civil courts place dollar values on worker health or life by making employers or suppliers pay monetary compensation for occupational disease or injury. Massachusetts, for instance, publishes a chart indicating the amount of money a worker will receive, under its workers' compensation regulations, for loss of different parts of the body. This system is not a satisfactory way to provide equitable compensation to sick workers because of the lengthy proceedings, the legal expenses, and the high probability that suits will fail.

Workers' compensation programs are not the only situations in which dollar values are placed on workers' health or life. Under the Reagan administration, all regulatory agencies had to calculate the costs and benefits of proposed government regulations. Thus OSHA was forced not only to estimate the costs to industry of compliance with new standards but also was required to place a dollar value on the lives and/or health saved. Economists have devised a variety of ways to estimate the value of a life through surveys of "willingness to pay" to save a life, analyses of apparent risk premiums (higher wages for higher risk jobs), in labor markets, and other techniques for evaluating human capital. Estimates range from as little as $28,000 to several million dollars per life saved.

Perhaps the most common approach is to imagine that a worker is a bond or security that will yield a return for some years in the future and that the stream of earnings a worker would receive is a reasonable measure of the worker's productivity. How much such a bond (or worker) would be worth now depends on the size of the earnings stream and on the interest rate that an investor could obtain on alternative bonds or securities. Thus, the present value of human capital can be calculated, and the value of lives saved or lost can be compared with the cost to industry of improvements in the work environment. It is important to note that economists always discount the future: economists believe that the gain or loss of a dollar ten years from now counts less than a gain or loss of a dollar now.

Another approach is to compare the wages of risky jobs with those that are less risky. Then the risk premium is considered to be the amount that workers themselves assign to their health. In a manner similar to the human capital approach, such calculations require us to assume that the markets work well and that wages are adequate measures of the value of labor and reflect the preferences of workers.

Some public-health advocates have argued that there is an inherent antiregulatory bias in such cost–benefit analysis because of the difficulties of placing dollar values on nonquantifiables such as pain, suffering, loss of loved ones, and the like. In addition, cost–benefit analysis attempts to equate economic losses of employers with health and life losses of workers, which critics argue is inappropriate. Another serious difficulty is the problem of discounting the future. What is the appropriate interest rate to use in calculating the present value of a stream of costs or benefits that extends into the distant future? Who should decide the worth of a health benefit twenty years from now?

Proponents of such economic approaches claim that there is really little choice in the matter, that public policy requires such calculation. People balance costs and benefits in an ongoing, practical way, even if exact calculations are not made. Certainly, companies must do such balancing. Thus, cost–benefit analysis utilizes market-based evaluation in situations brought about by the failure of the market to treat worker well-being adequately.

Society, by enacting laws and regulations through the political process, has decided to try to override the market. In the United States, as in other nations, worker health and safety appear to be attended to inadequately by employers and managers in charge of production. Even when workers have this information about occupational hazards, they frequently seem to lack the economic power to act to protect themselves. When government intervenes to protect workers, business interests have reasserted their belief in the primacy of economic concerns. Worker health and safety is an important arena in which the values of the market and the values of health and society are in conflict.

CHARLES LEVENSTEIN

Directly related to this article are the other articles in this entry: OCCUPATIONAL HEALTH-CARE PROVIDERS, *and* TESTING OF EMPLOYEES. *Also directly related are the entries* HAZARDOUS WASTES AND TOXIC SUBSTANCES; ENVIRONMENTAL HEALTH; JUSTICE; UTILITY; *and* GENETIC TESTING AND SCREENING, *articles on* PREDICTIVE AND WORKPLACE TESTING, *and* LEGAL ISSUES. *Other relevant material may be found under the entries* GENETICS AND ENVIRONMENT IN HUMAN HEALTH; HARM; HEALTH PROMOTION AND HEALTH EDUCATION; HEALTH SCREENING AND TESTING IN THE PUBLIC-HEALTH CONTEXT; INJURY AND INJURY CONTROL; LABORATORY TESTING; *and* TECHNOLOGY, *article on* TECHNOLOGY ASSESSMENT.

Bibliography

BAYER, RONALD, ed. 1988. *The Health and Safety of Workers: Case Studies in the Politics of Professional Responsibility.* New York: Oxford University Press.

LEVY, BARRY S., and WEGMAN, DAVID H., eds. 1988. *Occupational Health: Recognizing and Preventing Work-Related Disease.* 2d ed. Boston: Little, Brown.

MENDELOFF, JOHN M. 1988. *The Dilemma of Toxic Substance Regulation: How Overregulation Causes Underregulation at OSHA.* Cambridge, Mass.: MIT Press.

New Solutions: A Journal of Environmental and Occupational Health Policy. 1990–. Denver, Colo.: Alice Hamilton Memorial Library.

RAFFLE, P. A. B.; LEE, W. R.; McCALLUM, R. I.; and MURRAY, R. 1987. *Hunter's Diseases of Occupations.* Rev. ed. London: Hodder & Stoughton.

ROBINSON, JAMES C. 1991. *Toil and Toxics: Workplace Struggles and Political Strategies for Occupational Health.* Berkeley: University of California Press.

ROSNER, DAVID, and MARKOWITZ, GERALD E., eds. 1987. *Dying for Work: Workers' Safety and Health in Twentieth-Century America.* Bloomington: Indiana University Press.

II. OCCUPATIONAL HEALTH-CARE PROVIDERS

Occupational-health services—the focus of professional personnel, their health care and equipment, the programs offered for the prevention of disease and promotion of wellness—have become an increasingly important field in preventive medicine and public health during the twentieth century. The goal of these services is to develop and implement interventions that improve the health and safety of the workplace. They have advanced not only as a result of general developments in preventive medicine and public health but also because of increasing emphasis on the rights of employees and their overall welfare.

The occupational-health profession faces challenges represented by global economic competition, changes in labor force demographics, expanding markets, and new and different occupational and nonoccupational hazards to which workers are exposed. Occupational epidemiology is flourishing, and detailed studies of groups at risk are demonstrating previously unrecognized associations between work exposure and certain adverse health effects. Striking advances in molecular biology are bringing new tools and new insights into cellular aberrations induced by occupational exposure to physical and chemical agents, potentially offering the possibility of very early detection of occupational disease or risk, including risks to the fetuses or offspring of workers.

New rules and regulations are helping workers gain information on the toxicity of materials with which they are working and the precautions that must be taken to prevent excess exposure. Good translations of the technical literature into appropriate language ensure that previously guarded information becomes available to work groups. At the same time, the consumer movement has demanded and spread available data, and the Freedom of Information Act has brought disclosures of data not previously available. All these developments have significant ethical implications for the practice of occupational health, and therefore for those who engage in that practice: occupational-health professionals in occupational-health surveillance, specifically, screening programs. The ultimate goal of these services is to develop and implement interventions that improve some aspect or modify determinants of the health and well-being of people who work.

Before embarking on an overview of these ethical issues, it is well to consider the relationships of occupational-health professionals to industrial management, relationships that may have ethical implications. Occupational health services may be provided through (1) a complete in-plant health program with a full-time physician; (2) a partial in-plant health program with a physician in attendance for a portion of the day; (3) an out-of-plant medical program executed almost exclusively in the offices of private physicians; or (4) contract health programs.

In the complete in-plant health program, organizational placement of occupational-health professionals in the managerial structure may suggest to employees that the surveillance activities operate exclusively to protect the company. And although this situation has markedly improved, too often in the past many occupational-health professionals took the position that the company was always right. Such professionals ignored their responsibility to advise management on all matters pertaining to the health of employees, including deficiencies that required resolution or correction. The economic interest of the company may prompt management to pressure occupational-health professionals into a position of unilateral loyalty. This may lead to the expectation by managers that because the occupational-health physician is "one of them," some or all risk-assessment data, including information regarding chemical or other hazardous exposures for certain employees, will be shared irrespective of its confidential content. Unquestionably, the goal of a healthy company and the goal of healthy workers can collide, and when they do come into conflict, occupational-health personnel must be aware of their ethical responsibility to the health of the workers and to the principles of occupational medicine.

As industries seek to reduce the cost of health services, and as the social and scientific context of the workplace changes, less than full-time on-site occupational-health services may become more common. These arrangements can raise ethical issues of another kind, including questions about active advertising or direct solicitation of contracts for such services and about "self-referral"—the physician's referral of patients to an outside facility in which he or she has a financial interest. Growing evidence suggests that more and more physicians own health-care facilities to which they refer patients for services but at which they do not practice. The danger in occupational medicine is that part-time physicians may be strongly tempted to see their work as a golden opportunity to generate patients for off-site, private treatment facilities in which they own an interest, including services covered by workmen's compensation (Swedlow et al., 1992).

The principle that guides these relationships of service is that physicians and other occupational-health personnel cannot use their relationship with industry as a means to build their private practice. The American Medical Association's Council on Ethical and Judicial Affairs affirmed:

> However others may see the professional, the physicians are not simply business people with high standards. Physicians are engaged in the special calling of healing, and in that calling they are fiduciaries of their patients. They have different and higher duties than even the most ethical business purpose. There are some activities involving their patients that physicians should avoid whether or not there is evidence of abuse. (Council on Ethical and Judicial Affairs, 1992)

The Code of Ethical Conduct for Physicians Providing Occupational Medical Service emphasizes this principle in the following way: "Physicians should . . . avoid allowing their medical judgement to be influenced by any conflict of interest." Addressing the same issue, the *Guide to Developing Small Plan Occupational Health Programs* states:

> The plant physician should never use his industrial affiliation improperly as a means of gaining or enlarging his private practice. If he observes these ethical relationships, the plant physician should experience no difficulty in establishing cordial relationships with other physicians in the community and gaining mutual cooperation on the problem. (1983, p. 13)

Surveillance screening

Issues of privacy, confidentiality, and informed consent pervade almost every program activity for the assessment, preservation, restoration, and improvement of the health of workers at the place of employment. In screening programs especially, these issues are brought into bold relief. They may relate to the screening program itself or to the use of the results, which are designed to determine if the worker's health remains compatible with the job assignment and to detect any evidence of impaired health that may be attributed to employment.

Many such programs are ill-conceived from both a scientific and an ethical point of view. Problems of test validity and predictive values may weaken any appeal of beneficence. For example, some employers may insist on genetic testing even though the science of identifying genetic factors that may contribute to the occurrence of job-related illness is still in its infancy. The correlation of a genetic risk presumed to pose dangers (i.e., chromosomal damage) for the later occurrence of disease may not mean that all or most with the risk factor will become ill. Also, other genetic factors or environmental factors (such as smoking) may be necessary for the development of the disease. Thus, the use of genetic screening to identify and protect workers who might be at increased risk of disease in a workplace cannot be justified by the ethical principle of beneficence where there are low correlations between risk factors like genetic markers and disease. Just as there is uncertainty about who, or how many, could be harmed, so there is uncertainty about how industry should respond. There would be some physical risks associated with medical testing procedures.

Second, there would be risks to the worker from use of the screening information. These include the loss of a job or reassignment to a lower-paying or less desirable job, loss of self-esteem, and, possibly, stigmatization as "genetically inferior." Such a label conceivably could result in the person's exclusion from certain jobs in an entire industry. Historically disadvantaged groups—women and/or ethnic or racial minority workers—would be further disadvantaged. The use of such tests, in short, may provide no real benefit to the company and may cause harm to the worker.

The rapid growth of new molecular and biochemical tools in occupational medicine has resulted in the development of biological indexes or markers for predicting occupational diseases. Scientists hope that these biological indexes or markers will stand as early warnings of the occurrence of occupational risk and disease. Occupational medicine may use biological markers to enhance early detection and treatment of disease; occupational epidemiology may use them as indicators of internal exposure at the workplace or of potential health risks and the need for workplace monitoring. The use of these tools in workplace screening touches on areas of basic concern to most people: opportunity for employ-

ment, job security, health, self-esteem, and privacy. In the case of a biological marker known to reflect susceptibility, for example, should a worker who tests positive or has a higher measurement be removed from the workplace? If so, should the occupational-health professional recommend that the worker be offered an equivalent job in the same industry? Or should the occupational-health professional recommend that management clean up the workplace to protect the most sensitive worker? To complicate matters, most biological markers of occupational disease are presumed to predict group risks (increased rates of disease among workers), and these levels of risk are still sufficiently low as to not be reliable guides to which individuals are threatened. Therefore, it is important that workers be informed in advance that the results are interpretable only on the group level. Test results given to workers should be presented and discussed on the basis and in the context of the information that is available on the variability within groups of workers and between individuals (National Research Council, 1992).

Of equal importance is the treatment of the data generated by biological-marker testing. One concern of employees who have been screened would be to prevent the spread of embarrassing, damaging, or false information about themselves, particularly to potential employers. The Code of Ethical Conduct for Physicians Providing Occupational Medical Service provides that employers are entitled to receive counsel about the medical fitness of an individual in relation to work but are not entitled to diagnoses or specific details. No one in health care challenges the fact that the medical record is a confidential document. But many managers believe they should have access to it when there is interest in an individual employee. However, diagnostic information is not needed for placement of an employee or for changes in his or her workstation because of change in health status. The occupational-health physician can state that an individual is physically or emotionally capable for all work or that an employee should not work in areas where there are high concentrations of certain organic vapors. This information meets the needs of management and does not change the privilege of the medical information under the control of the occupational-health physician. The Code of Ethical Conduct of the American Occupational Medicine Association is clear on this issue:

> Treat as confidential whatever is learned about individuals served, releasing information only when required by law or by overriding public health considerations or to other physicians at the request of the individual according to traditional medical ethical practice and recognize that employers are entitled to counsel about the medical

fitness of an individual in relation to work but are not entitled to diagnoses or details of a specific nature.

Medical records usually need to be kept for a long time because of linkages between occupational exposure and disease or dysfunction with long latency periods. These are usually the kinds of disease (cancer, for example) that are most sensitive in terms of workers' feelings about privacy. Records become part of large data systems to which government regulatory agencies, courts, and law enforcement officials may have relatively easy access. Workers are concerned that leakage of sensitive information will affect their mobility and employability.

Confidentiality is seldom an absolute value. Information about patients may be revealed under certain circumstances, including those in which workers themselves give consent to provide it to insurance companies or other physicians. Because they are concerned about possible misuse of information from screening programs, or because they wish to know of risks to their health, employees may want access to their medical records. The ethical principle of autonomy implies a duty to provide employees with information about their health, even when it is not clear what the information means. The duty would be even stronger when the information is highly predictive of a risk of disease.

Autonomy would also appear to require that the workers be fully informed of the nature of any screening procedure to which they will be subjected. While the concept of informed consent would be most crucial in occupational-health research, it is also applicable to medical screening. In the latter case, even though the procedures are clearly beneficial, their application to work without informed consent is a paternalistic action.

Epidemiologic investigations

The results of screening programs may suggest the need for epidemiologic studies to provide additional information on adverse health effects from occupational exposure. These studies may be conducted by occupational epidemiologists. Even prior to the U.S. Occupational Safety and Health Act of 1970, companies involved in formulating and synthesizing chemicals had hired epidemiologists to conduct in-house studies. Such research is an important aspect of an employer's obligation to employees, consumers, and the public in general.

In conducting epidemiologic studies, occupational-health professionals have obligations to workers who are the study subjects as well as to the company's management, who ordered the study and will pay for it. Sometimes these obligations conflict, and the occupational-health professional must sort out ethical as well as scientific priorities. Depending on where the request for the study originates, for example, there may be con-

flict even in the initial decision as to whether the study should be undertaken. The analysis and interpretation of the data the study generates may be affected by its expected implications. Economic implications may be intertwined with political ones. Epidemiologic studies of workers who are occupationally exposed to neurotoxins or reproductive toxins, for example, may lead to political conflict between labor and management, with government as a possible third party. The dispute is essentially about the occupational environment rather than economic issues with political factors as a secondary concern. Here the company's epidemiologist may be under pressure to respond more fully to his or her responsibilities to the employer than to any professional obligation to the workers (Gordis, 1991).

As the research project proceeds, the subjects should be kept informed of its progress, subjects' privacy should be respected, and confidentiality of data should be maintained. This is an important task because the concept of research can be disquieting to workers and to management as well. When, in the course of the study, management and other investigators who are not part of the study ask that investigators share data on an individual basis, investigators face conflict between professional obligations and legal ones. Under the provisions of the Toxic Substances Control Act, for example, epidemiologists are required to communicate substantial risk to the U.S. Environmental Protection Agency within fifteen days after learning of such risk. This information is then made available to the public. Here the professional obligation is to make the best interpretation of the facts, perhaps even to the extent of realizing that the best interpretation cannot be made without additional facts. When there is no time for the investigator to gather additional data, he or she has an obligation to make the best interpretation of the data that is available (Bond, 1991).

Ethical guides for communicating potential health risk have not been defined. In this context occupational health personnel are often called on to distinguish between the significant and the trivial. The problem does not lie where real risk can be identified and effective action by the company can result in real benefit to the worker. The technical and ethical conflicts arise when the occupational-health specialist must decide whether a given risk is acceptable, or whether it must be disclosed when not enough is known to be able to measure the presumed risk, and when there are acceptable alternatives.

In such cases the occupational-health investigator must act judiciously, in the best interest of the health and well-being of the workers. Withholding pertinent information or providing unqualified, incomplete, or uncertain data may be detrimental to the worker and/or the company.

Conclusion

Economic performance is not the only responsibility of industry any more than educational performance is the only responsibility of a college or university. Unless economic performance is balanced with broader responsibilities for the health and safety of workers, industry will ultimately fail. The public's interest in health and safety, and its broader interest in the rights of workers, including the right to know of risks they face, seem a permanent feature of modern American capitalism. The demand for socially responsible industries and for workers' health and safety will not go away. These responsibilities involve concern about all factors that influence the health of employees, including assuring the availability of health services that are preventive and constructive. These services are not the work of any one group but depend on the cooperative activities of medicine, chemistry, toxicology, engineering, and many others. In this setting industry must recognize and respect the unique position of occupational-health-service providers and assist them in providing impartial, professional counsel to both management and employees. The occupational-health-service providers must be honest, consistent, courageous, and defenders of confidentiality.

Albert Jonsen states the case well:

> In a general way, the environment of modern industry comes about through investments from employer and employee alike, each making certain sorts of contributions. In our modern concept of relationship of those diverse contributions, we attribute right of ownership to employers and a variety of rights regarding wages and working conditions to employees. It is now common to consider that among these employees' rights is the right to know about hazards of the work environment.

They also have the right to know about interrelated elements of occupational safety and health. Ensuring those rights involves a great diversity and complexity of ethical responsibilities—interlocked with privacy, confidentiality, and professional and legal obligations—of the occupational-health service provider.

Anticipating these complex ethical issues and developing sound approaches for resolving them are significant challenges to those health-care professionals who have the responsibility to promote the health and well-being of people who work. Specifically, however, their responsibility is played out in the context of the workplace where many other health-care professionals have the responsibility to promote workers' health.

BAILUS WALKER, JR.

Directly related to this article are the other articles in this entry: ETHICAL ISSUES, *and* TESTING OF EMPLOYEES. *For a further discussion of topics mentioned in this article, see the entries* ALLIED HEALTH PROFESSIONS; AUTONOMY; BENEFICENCE; CONFIDENTIALITY; CONFLICT OF INTEREST; FETUS; GENETIC COUNSELING; GENETIC TESTING AND SCREENING, *article on* PREDICTIVE AND WORKPLACE TESTING; HAZARDOUS WASTES AND TOXIC SUBSTANCES; HEALING; HEALTH OFFICIALS AND THEIR RESPONSIBILITIES; INFORMED CONSENT; PRIVACY AND CONFIDENTIALITY IN RESEARCH; PRIVACY IN HEALTH CARE; PUBLIC HEALTH; RACE AND RACISM; RESPONSIBILITY; *and* SEXISM. *For a discussion of related ideas, see the entries* AIDS; ECONOMIC CONCEPTS IN HEALTH CARE; *and* ENVIRONMENTAL HEALTH. *See also the* APPENDIX (CODES, OATHS, AND DIRECTIVES RELATED TO BIOETHICS), SECTION II: ETHICAL DIRECTIVES FOR THE PRACTICE OF MEDICINE, *and* SECTION III: ETHICAL DIRECTIVES FOR OTHER HEALTH-CARE PROFESSIONS.

Bibliography

BOND, GREGORY G. 1991. "Ethical Issues Relating to Conduct and Interpretation of Epidemiologic Research in Private Industry." In *Industrial Epidemiology Forum's Conference on Ethics in Epidemiology,* pp. 295–345. Edited by William E. Fayerweather, John Higgenson, and Tom L. Beauchamp. New York: Pergamon.

BOND, M. B. 1971. "Occupational Medical Services for Small Employee Units." *Rocky Mountain Medical Journal* 68, no. 11:31–36.

COUNCIL ON ETHICAL AND JUDICIAL AFFAIRS. AMERICAN MEDICAL ASSOCIATION. 1992. "Conflict of Interest: Physician Ownership of Medical Facilities." *Journal of the American Medical Association* 267, no. 17:2366–2369.

GORDIS, LEON. 1991. "Ethical and Professional Issues in the Changing Practice of Epidemiology." In *Industrial Epidemiology Forum's Conference on Ethics in Epidemiology,* pp. 95–155. Edited by William E. Fayerweather, John Higgenson, and Tom L. Beauchamp. New York: Pergamon.

HIGGENSON, JOHN, and CHU, FLORA. 1991. "Ethical Considerations and Responsibilities in Communicating Health Risk Information." In *Industrial Epidemiology Forum's Conference on Ethics in Epidemiology,* pp. 515–565. Edited by William E. Fayerweather, John Higgenson, and Tom L. Beauchamp. New York: Pergamon.

JONSEN, ALBERT R. 1991. "Ethical Considerations and Responsibilities When Communicating Health Risk Information." In *Industrial Epidemiology Forum's Conference on Ethics in Epidemiology,* pp. 695–725. Edited by William E. Fayerweather, John Higgenson, and Tom L. Beauchamp. New York: Pergamon.

NATIONAL RESEARCH COUNCIL. 1992. "Biological Markers in Immunotoxicology." Washington, D.C.

ROSENSTOCK, LINDA, and HAGOPIAN, AMY. 1987. "Ethical Dilemmas in Providing Health Care to Workers." *Annals of Internal Medicine* 107, no. 4:575–580.

SWEDLOW, ALEX; JOHNSON, GREGORY; SMITHLINE, NEIL; and MILLSTEIN, ARNOLD. 1992. "Increased Costs and Rates in the California Workers' Compensation System as a Result of Self-Referral by Physicians." *New England Journal of Medicine* 327, no. 21:1502–1506.

III. TESTING OF EMPLOYEES

Employers are interested in obtaining information, including medical information, about their current or prospective employees. Their efforts raise three broad, ethical questions. First, what are the implications of the power imbalance in the employer–employee relationship for issues of justice? Second, what limits should exist on what an employer can know about its employees? Third, how much influence may an employer have over its employees' behavior outside of work? These three questions frame the debates over various forms of employee testing and screening.

The agreement between employee and employer to exchange labor for compensation is, in the absence of coercion, properly described as voluntary. The legal doctrine in U.S. law known as "employment at will" derives from this conception of the employment relationship (Blades, 1967). It views the parties as free, independent, equally situated partners to the agreement. But this notion of the employment relationship fails to acknowledge the often profound inequalities in financial resources, knowledge, and power between employer and employee. Such inequalities do not nullify the voluntariness of the employment relationship, but they may give employers a substantial advantage in setting the terms and conditions of employment. Testing has become one of the conditions that employees and prospective employees often have to accept in order to get work.

Employers may reasonably need certain information about their employees. They need to know, for example, whether employees are capable of doing the jobs for which they are hired. To the extent that previous work experience, education, and training are relevant to potential employees' qualifications, employers have a right to inquire about such factors. Similarly, employers have a right to know if employees are physically able to perform the tasks demanded by the job. But may employers seek and obtain any information whatsoever in which they might have some interest? Should employers be permitted to learn their employees' religious beliefs? Sexual practices? Political commitments? What of their medical circumstances, such as disabilities unrelated to the job, their risk of future disease, or the health of other family members?

Employers clearly have a right to limit some aspects of their employees' behavior. A trucking company, for example, can require that its drivers refrain from drinking alcohol or using mind-altering drugs while driving the company's vehicles. But how much control should employers be allowed to have over their employees' behavior off the job? Should employers be permitted to fire or refuse to hire people who smoke at home? Some employers have done exactly that.

The practice of medical examinations by employers began early in the twentieth century. It has expanded enormously since then, especially among large employers. At some firms, employees have been required to take written tests that purport to identify individuals likely to be dishonest. Employers have even used lie-detector tests for the same purpose. In addition, psychological profiles have been sought in the belief that they can detect desirable employees. Tests such as these may have questionable validity or relevance.

An important development in occupational testing of workers has been the expansion from testing to determine whether an employee can do the job competently and honestly to testing that may predict whether the individual is at elevated risk for nonoccupational disease (Rothstein, 1989). To the extent that the employer is responsible for employees' health-care costs, or is affected by other costs of illness and absence from work, employers have incentives not to hire people who are likely to become ill.

Why do employers test?

Employers test their employees for several different reasons, which vary greatly in their ethical defensibility. Three rationales may be offered.

For the worker's own good. First, employers may claim that they are testing workers for the workers' own protection. Tests intended to identify people with back problems before undertaking a job requiring strenuous lifting may be motivated, in part, by concern for the workers' health (although such screening tests also have financial implications for the employer). Genetic screening of workers, first proposed by the renowned geneticist J. B. S. Haldane in 1938, was conceived as a public-health measure. Workers congenitally susceptible to diseases like potter's bronchitis would be identified and steered away from occupational exposure to dust or chemicals that were especially risky for them. By avoiding the match between susceptible individual and workplace toxin, there would be fewer occupationally induced illnesses, and less illness in general. So at least ran the rationale.

When an employer refuses to hire someone on the grounds that he or she is at increased risk of harm, the rationale is paternalistic; that is, to protect the individual without regard for his or her own wishes. Most of the circumstances that justify paternalism—immaturity, incompetence, ignorance, coercion—would also undermine the moral justification—agreement between free, informed, competent adults—for the legitimacy of an employment contract. It is very difficult to say that a person, even a person at increased risk from occupational exposures, is better off without a job than with one, despite the risks. It is also ethically dubious to claim that the employer is justified in imposing judgments about what is best for the individual, or that the employer is better situated than the individual to judge what is in the individual's good. In general, the argument that employers should be allowed to test workers and exclude them from jobs for their own good is a weak one, rarely applicable in the employer–employee relationship.

To protect others.   A second ethical argument used to defend workplace testing is that it may protect third parties. In some occupations, airline pilot, for example, a physical or mental breakdown could be directly responsible for injuring or killing third parties. If medical testing could identify pilot candidates who were very likely to suffer catastrophic breakdowns, then the desire to protect third parties would be a cogent reason in favor of such testing. But the extreme nature of the example suggests the limited scope of this argument in occupational testing. Justifying medical testing by the need to protect third parties is only valid for jobs in which the safety of others is in someone's hands, in which there are medical conditions that can lead to sudden breakdowns, and in which there are medical tests that predict those conditions accurately.

More commonly, employee testing, such as for drug use by bank tellers, is justified by a rationale such as protecting customers against fraud by an employee desperate for money. The same reasoning could be used to justify other intrusive forms of surveillance to prevent employees from gambling, engaging in extramarital affairs, or doing anything else that might require the need for extra funds. Justifying testing on the grounds that it protects third parties is more ethically appealing than paternalism. Practically, though, it is usually not relevant to the workplace.

Workplace testing and screening to protect third parties takes a particularly interesting turn when the "third party" to be protected is a fetus and the employee a pregnant woman, or as some employer policies dictate, a "potentially pregnant female." This will be taken up later under the rubric of reproductive screening.

To protect the employer.   A third argument for testing workers is that the employer has a right to protect itself against avoidable costs. This is clearly relevant, but just as clearly an argument with limited force. There are many actions concerning the hiring and treatment of employees that companies could take to boost profits but that are forbidden. Laws requiring the control of occupational hazards trade profits for safety. Laws requiring fair hiring practices and forbidding discrimination against certain groups of prospective employees

such as women, people with disabilities, or religious, racial, or ethnic minorities, may result in additional costs to employers. Such laws embody ethical convictions that equal treatment and opportunity are valuable enough to override employers' liberty to hire whomever they please, and to warrant the cost such policies might incur.

In most instances, controversies over employee testing array employer liberty and concerns for cost against individuals' interests in liberty and privacy and society's concern to discourage discrimination.

Varieties of employer testing and screening

Employers screen prospective or current employees for a wide range of attributes like those detected by a conventional medical examination, disability evaluation, or test for genetic predisposition. Employees may be screened to determine if they smoke tobacco, use legal or illegal drugs, or are infected with the human immunodeficiency virus (HIV). Some employers have excluded all fertile women from certain workplaces on the grounds that occupational hazards may endanger any fetus such women might carry.

Medical examinations.   Physical examinations, often accompanied by laboratory tests, are done for at least two purposes. First, they may identify individuals who are physically unable to perform the tasks demanded in a particular job. Second, they may mark people who have or are likely to develop health problems. Employers have a right to ensure that the people hired can do what the job requires; however, genuine doubts persist as to whether the typical medical examination and accompanying tests yield valid information about the capacity to perform a particular job.

Economically concerned employers may try to avoid hiring workers who are likely to have greater needs for health care and more frequent absences. In countries where employers are responsible for the health-care costs of their employees, the incentive to avoid hiring workers who are likely to need extensive health care is powerful. A potential worker who is infected with HIV, for example, could incur very high health-care expenses.

Screening by medical examinations raises ethical questions of validity; of confidentiality, when employers seek personal information unrelated to the capacity to perform the job; and of discrimination, when prospective employees are excluded because of potential costs, especially health-care costs.

Genetic testing and screening.   Originally proposed as a public-health measure, there is little evidence that genetic screening of workers has been widely practiced by industry. This could change. With cheaper tests, rapidly increasing ability to detect genetic variations that might indicate susceptibility to nonoccupational diseases, and soaring health-care costs, genetic screening may become attractive to employers looking to save money.

Screening that leads to excluding workers from jobs provokes the strongest ethical objections. Screening for predisposition to occupational diseases such as heart disease or cancer does not have to lead to exclusion. It could be used to inform individuals with increased risks, leaving the decision whether to accept those risks in their own hands (Murray, 1983).

Smoking, drugs, and HIV.   Smoking, drugs, and HIV infection frequently are lumped together as "lifestyle" characteristics. In contrast to genetics, over which an individual has no control, the decisions to smoke cigarettes, use drugs, or engage in behaviors associated with risk of HIV infection have some level of voluntariness attributed to them. Probably for this reason, and because of the social disapproval attached to these decisions, testing for smoking, drug use, and HIV infection has not generated the intense opposition generated by genetic testing.

Drug use is blamed for a wide variety of workplace ills, from absenteeism and accidents to fraud, inefficiency, and theft. That drug use has a deleterious impact on the workplace seems plausible, though its magnitude is probably exaggerated (Zwerling et al., 1990). Drug testing, usually done with urine samples, raises a number of conceptual and moral difficulties. In countries where alcohol is legal, employers must decide whether to include it among the substances tested. Alcohol is by far the most common drug of abuse, and probably the greatest cause of workplace mishaps.

How intrusive should the testing program be? Some employers require urination to be witnessed to minimize the possibility of deception, but many workers experience this as an indignity and a violation of their privacy. The chemical assays of the urine reveal the presence of drugs or their metabolites; they do not show if the person is impaired or when the drug was taken (Rothstein, 1991). Marijuana metabolites persist for as long as three weeks; cocaine can be detected two or three days after it was last used (Council on Scientific Affairs, 1987). Workplace drug testing may punish individuals for behavior outside of work that has no impact on their job performance.

The urine tested for drugs also can be used to detect the metabolites of cigarette smoke. Smoking and secondary smoke inhalation have been linked to a wide variety of illnesses. As a result, many companies have curtailed or banned smoking in their facilities, and a few refuse to employ smokers, even those who smoke only off the job. Testing either for smoking or for drug use that does not impair workplace performance raises pointed questions about the legitimate extent of employers' efforts to be informed about and to control their employees' lives.

Screening for HIV infection has been defended with all three of the rationales mentioned above: protecting the worker, protecting third parties, and protecting the employer. There are some occupations that may be especially hazardous to HIV-infected persons, especially jobs involving exposure to infectious organisms. But paternalism is no more persuasive here than in other workplace contexts. Out of fear that HIV is communicable by casual contact, some employers have excluded HIV-infected persons in the mistaken belief that they were thereby protecting co-workers or the public. Other employers, recognizing that HIV is a chronic disease costly to treat, have wished to avoid that cost.

Bioethics has been concerned particularly with HIV-infected health-care workers. If any workers threaten to infect someone in the course of work, then surgeons, probing under patients' skin with sharp implements, or dentists, working with pointed tools in the confines of the human mouth among ruptured tissues, pose such a threat. Despite the apparent danger, actual transmission of HIV by health-care workers to patients seems to be extremely rare. Nonetheless, fear of HIV has prompted calls for screening and exclusion (from invasive procedures, at least) of infected health-care workers.

Patients do have a morally cogent interest in avoiding unnecessary risks. When the risk is extremely small, however, the public good may require that patients not be permitted to exercise that right—to know whether one's doctor is infected with HIV, for example—when in so doing everyone will be worse off (Daniels, 1992).

Screening for reproductive hazards.   Women have suffered employment discrimination in many countries. Given such a history, there can be little wonder that when women began to be excluded from traditionally male jobs on the grounds that any fetus they might carry was endangered by workplace exposures, some ethicists and other commentators wondered whether this was the old discrimination with a new pretext. Some substances, such as lead, do not appear to cause disease in adults at permitted workplace exposure levels but may harm developing fetuses. There is a dispute over whether substances that can harm fetuses through the mother's exposure might also harm fetuses through the father's exposure. Virtually all research on human reproductive hazards has examined the effects of exposing females to potentially harmful substances; very little is known about the effects of exposing males. But even if such damage occurred mostly through exposures of women, that does not serve as sufficient justification for excluding pregnant, or more generally, fertile women from hazardous jobs or workplaces. Many company policies excluded all nonsterilized women from such jobs, whether or not they were heterosexually active, infertile, or used birth control (U.S. Congress, Office of Technology Assessment, 1985).

The putative moral justification for so-called "fetal-protection policies" is to prevent harm to the children that at least some fetuses will become. Preventing such harms is a morally cogent and important consideration. To children suffering a lifelong illness or disability, it makes little difference to them whether their malady was caused by an exposure occurring before or after birth. Certainly, parents of born children have an important obligation to take reasonable measures to protect their children from harm. But parents remain moral agents who have obligations to other parties and who are permitted to consider their own interests as well. The moral mistake in fetal-protection policies is the presumption that the duty to prevent harm to fetuses overrides all other moral considerations pregnant women might have, including the need to feed and house other children, or to obtain health insurance for themselves and their families. People are not morally required to sacrifice all other interests and obligations to protect their children from remote risks of harm, and it makes no sense to compel women to do more for a fetus than fathers and mothers are obliged to do for their born children (Murray, 1987).

It is likely that fetal-protection policies rest more on a sentimentalized view of the relationship between a pregnant woman and her fetus than on any sound analysis of ethics or public policy. They may also reflect employers' concerns about legal liability for injuries to children that might have been caused by their mothers' exposure to workplace toxins.

As technologies for employee testing proliferate and employers' investments in their workers increase, the temptation to test current and prospective employees will grow. Careful scrutiny of the ethics of such policies must continue.

THOMAS H. MURRAY

Directly related to this article are the other articles in this entry: ETHICAL ISSUES, *and* OCCUPATIONAL HEALTH-CARE PROVIDERS. *Also directly related to this article are the entries* GENETIC TESTING AND SCREENING, *articles on* PREDICTIVE AND WORKPLACE TESTING, *and* LEGAL ISSUES; GENETICS AND THE LAW; *and* HEALTH SCREENING AND TESTING IN THE PUBLIC-HEALTH CONTEXT. *For a further discussion of topics mentioned in this article, see the entries* AIDS, *article on* PUBLIC-HEALTH ISSUES; CONFIDENTIALITY; *Fetus, article on* HUMAN DEVELOPMENT FROM FERTILIZATION TO BIRTH; HOMOSEXUALITY, *article on* ETHICAL ISSUES; *and* SUBSTANCE ABUSE, *articles on* SMOKING, *and* ALCOHOL AND OTHER DRUGS IN A PUBLIC-

HEALTH CONTEXT. *Other relevant material may be found under the entries* DISABILITY, *article on* LEGAL ISSUES; GENETICS AND ENVIRONMENT IN HUMAN HEALTH; HAZARDOUS WASTES AND TOXIC SUBSTANCES; LABORATORY TESTING; *and* WOMEN, *section on* WOMEN AS HEALTH PROFESSIONALS, *article on* CONTEMPORARY ISSUES.

Bibliography

BLADES, LAWRENCE E. 1967. "Employment at Will vs. Individual Freedom: On Limiting the Abusive Exercise of Employer Power." *Columbia Law Review* 67, no. 7:1404–1435.

COUNCIL ON SCIENTIFIC AFFAIRS. AMERICAN MEDICAL ASSOCIATION. 1987. "Scientific Issues in Drug Testing." *Journal of the American Medical Association* 257, no. 22:3110–3114.

DANIELS, NORMAN. 1992. "HIV-Infected Professionals, Patient Rights, and the 'Switching Dilemma.'" *Journal of the American Medical Association* 267, no. 10:1368–1371.

MURRAY, THOMAS H. 1983. "Warning: Screening Workers for Genetic Risk." *Hastings Center Report* 13, no. 1:5–8.

———. 1987. "Moral Obligations to the Not-Yet Born: The Fetus as Patient." *Clinics in Perinatology* 14, no. 2: 329–343.

ROTHSTEIN, MARK A. 1989. *Medical Screening and the Employee Health-Cost Crisis.* Washington, D.C.: Bureau of National Affairs.

———. 1991. "Workplace Drug Testing: A Case Study in the Misapplication of Technology." *Harvard Journal of Law and Technology* 5(Fall):65–93.

U.S. CONGRESS. OFFICE OF TECHNOLOGY ASSESSMENT. 1985. *Reproductive Health Hazards in the Workplace.* Washington, D.C.: Government Printing Office.

ZWERLING, CRAIG; RYAN, JAMES; and ORAV, ENDEL JOHN. 1990. "The Efficacy of Preemployment Drug Screening for Marijuana and Cocaine in Predicting Employment Outcome." *Journal of the American Medical Association* 264, no. 20:2639–2643.

OMISSION AND COMMISSION

See ACTION. *See also* DEATH AND DYING: EUTHANASIA AND SUSTAINING LIFE, *article on* ETHICAL ISSUES. *See also* DOUBLE EFFECT.

ORDINARY AND EXTRAORDINARY MEANS

See DEATH AND DYING: EUTHANASIA AND SUSTAINING LIFE, *articles on* HISTORICAL ASPECTS, *and* ETHICAL ISSUES.

ORGAN DONATION

See ORGAN AND TISSUE PROCUREMENT.

ORGANIZED MEDICINE

See MEDICINE AS A PROFESSION.

ORGAN AND TISSUE PROCUREMENT

I. Medical and Organizational Aspects
   Jeffrey Prottas
II. Ethical and Legal Issues Regarding Cadavers
   James F. Childress
III. Ethical and Legal Issues Regarding Living Donors
   Peter A. Ubel
   Mary B. Mahowald

I. MEDICAL AND ORGANIZATIONAL ASPECTS

Organ transplantation is high-technology medicine in one of its most extreme forms. It is very expensive, employs advanced biotechnologies, and requires large teams of highly trained specialists. It is used to intervene when the final stage of an illness is reached, and although it can save lives, it does not provide a "cure" or a return to a preexisting condition of health. Patients with transplants require constant, ongoing treatment with highly sophisticated and often quite dangerous medications.

But unlike most other advanced medical technologies, organ and tissue transplantation also depends on people. The only source of human organs and tissues is donations. In most instances these donations must be obtained from a young person who has died under sudden and tragic circumstances: by automobile accident, suicide, murder, and so forth. The organ procurement system's role is to provide a bridge between human tragedy and high technology.

The supply of organ donors

During the first half of the 1980s the supply of cadaveric organ donors grew continually and rapidly. In 1982 there were 3,681 cadaveric kidney transplants. In 1986 there were 7,089, an increase of almost 100 percent (or almost 25 percent a year). Since 1986, the rate of increase has slowed. In 1992, 7,579 cadaveric kidney transplants were performed, representing donations from about 4,000 donors. Although this was one of the largest num-

ber of organ donors in any year in U.S. history, the leveling out of the donor supply in the United States has caused much disquiet and debate over the efficacy of the organ procurement system and adequacy of the principles underlying it (Health Care Financing Administration, 1990).

While organs have been transplanted in most nations of western Europe, in Japan, and in some places in the Middle East, the infrastructure necessary to obtain organ donors routinely exists only in North America and western Europe. (While Japan certainly has the resources and expertise necessary, cultural factors, including discomfort with brain death and a strong commitment to intact burial, have militated against the development of such a system there.) Eurotransplant, serving Germany, Austria, and the Benelux nations, is the second largest organ procurement system in the world and the largest in Europe. In 1990, 3,171 kidneys were transplanted in the Eurotransplant region, as well as over 659 hearts and 575 livers. France and the United Kingdom have both operated national organ procurement systems since the 1980s, and each did about 1,900 kidney transplants in 1990. Scandia Transplant (serving Scandinavia) is an organization of long standing; it provided kidneys for almost 600 transplants in 1990. Since the early 1990s, both Italy and Spain have developed transplantation and organ procurement systems. Spain's program now provides over 1,200 kidneys. Italy has been much less successful, but in 1990 almost 550 kidneys were transplanted there. Almost 9,300 kidney transplants were done in western Europe in 1990, considerably more than in the United States. So, while the U.S. system remains the largest single system in the world, of the over 17,000 kidney transplants done worldwide in 1990, 54 percent were done in Europe (Eurotransplant Foundation, 1992).

Of course kidneys are not the only organs being transplanted. In 1990 over 4,700 livers and over 4,100 hearts were transplanted worldwide, along with more than 1,000 pancreas and 250 lungs or heart-lung combinations. In each case, a majority of these procedures occurred in the United States.

During the late 1980s, the total number of heart and liver transplants grew very rapidly, although the number of donors did not. This reflects an increase in multiple-organ donation. Donors who previously donated only kidneys were increasingly providing hearts, livers, and/or pancreas. In the United States, by 1992, 72 percent of all organ donors provided more than one organ (National Organ Procurement and Transplantation Network, 1991). While trustworthy data are difficult to obtain, it is probable that ten years earlier the percentage was less than 25 percent.

The number of actual donations must be understood in relation to the number of potential donors. In 1975 ground-breaking work done by Kenneth Bart for the Centers for Disease Control estimated that between 54.5 and 115.8 donors per million persons—about 25,000 to 26,000 potential donors—were available each year in the United States (Bart et al., 1981b). More recent work has applied more restrictive criteria to the examination of hospital death records. This work estimates a national donor pool of between 10,000 and 12,500 (Nathan et al., 1991). Although divergent, both estimates show that actual donation rates are not close to exhausting the potential supply of donors. They also indicate that the size of the donor pool is very sensitive to donor criteria, especially age. Medical criteria for acceptable donors are not fixed by immutable laws but change as transplant experience changes, and perhaps as the need for organs changes. The donor pool is itself a somewhat flexible and changing concept.

Criteria for donation. The one immutable medical criterion for organ donation has been brain death, or more exactly, the determination of death by brain-death criteria. Once the circulation ceases, an organ very rapidly becomes useless for transplantation unless it is cooled. For this reason organ donors must be kept on machines that maintain respiration and heartbeat after death. Because the heart must be kept pumping, death must be declared on the basis of total and irreversible cessation of brain function—brain death. The causes of death that are consistent with organ donation are therefore sharply limited to those involving damage to the central nervous system. Trauma is the most common cause of such damage. Over 55 percent of all donors in 1990 died of head trauma; about 25 percent died in auto accidents and about one-third of strokes (National Organ Procurement and Transplantation Network, 1991).

The need for organs is believed to be so severe that even the brain-death criterion is being questioned. Small-scale efforts are under way in a number of locations to test the feasibility of employing donors whose hearts are not beating for organ donation (i.e., donors who suffer cardiac arrest before organ retrieval). It is not clear what effect this might have on the supply of organs. The circumstances under which an organ can be preserved in such a donor are very limited, and actions to preserve must take place within minutes of death.

Other medical criteria also limit the potential supply of organs. Cancer, systemic infections, HIV, hepatitis, and structural organ abnormalities (e.g., abnormal blood vessels) can exclude a donor because of their possible transmission to the organ recipient. High blood pressure, diabetes, and many other conditions can render an organ unsuitable for transplantation by damaging it. The most general limiting factor is the age of the donor. There is little unanimity among transplant centers on acceptable donor age. In general the criteria for kidney donors is the least exclusive, and that for heart donors the most exclusive. Young donors are preferred; in the 1980s kidney donors over fifty-five were considered unsuitable, as were male heart donors over forty. Over time, age criteria have loosened noticeably. From 1978 to 1987 the percentage of kidney donors over fifty went from 5 percent to 10 percent, and the percentage over thirty grew from about 30 percent to 40 percent (Takemoto and Terasaki, 1988). Increases in acceptable donor age can enlarge the donor pool substantially, especially when combined with an increasing percentage of donors dying from causes other than trauma.

The supply of transplantable tissue

There is no shortage of corneas for transplantation. Each year about 43,000 corneal transplants are done in North America and an additional 45,000 to 50,000 corneas are used for nontransplant purposes, primarily research. The large supply of corneas reflects the fact that there are very few medical contraindications for corneal donation. In 1991 there were only about 6,800 people on eye bank waiting lists, and the average stay on such a list was less than two months—in contrast to an average 450-day wait for a kidney transplant (Prottas, 1991).

The supply of musculoskeletal tissue (bones, tendons, fascia, and related soft tissue) has more in common with organ supply than with corneal supply. While the data are very poor, informed estimates put the number of tissue donors at between 4,500 and 10,000 in 1990. Because a single tissue donor can provide tissue for many procedures, it is estimated that between 250,000 and 400,000 such procedures were done in 1990. The potential national supply of tissue donors has never been systematically studied. Medical criteria for musculoskeletal donation are much less restrictive than criteria for organ donation, so the potential supply of tissue donors certainly exceeds that of organ donors by a large margin.

The procurement systems

Local context. The earliest organ-procurement organizations (OPOs) in the United States were founded around 1970. They were purely local organizations that grew up around kidney transplantation teams and were meant to address those teams' needs for transplantable organs. By the mid-1980s, over ninety of these organizations had been formed; virtually no area of the nation was unserved.

While the organ-procurement system has undergone many changes since the early 1980s, the local components of organ procurement success have not changed. The central factor in successful organ procurement is timely information about potentially suitable donors. Only a very small percentage of deaths can lead to an organ donation, and the window of time available for action is short. Cooperation from hospital personnel, specifically doctors and nurses in intensive care units (ICUs), is essential. A referral from these professionals (i.e., notification that a potential donor is under treatment) is required for the donation process to begin. The average OPO spends more of its personnel's time encouraging doctors and nurses to make referrals than it does on organ procurement itself. This persuasion takes the form of in-service training sessions, one-on-one visits, and visits to the ICU itself. Success in obtaining referrals is the key determinant of successful organ procurement (Prottas, 1989).

A second factor of great importance is targeting appropriate hospitals. Not all hospitals are equally good sources of potential donors: Some see little trauma, and some lack the capacity to make brain-death determinations. OPOs that target their professional education efforts where the return can be the greatest are likely to be more successful than those that work with every hospital in their catchment area.

The final step in the procurement process is obtaining permission from families. This is a very delicate matter. Families of potential donors have suffered a terrible loss. Some OPOs prefer to have their own, experienced staff approach the family. Others depend more heavily on hospital staff. All depend on the physicians involved to inform the family that their relative has died. U.S. law forbids paying families to permit donation. All organ-donation decisions are therefore voluntary and altruistic.

The donation decision.   The American public, indeed the publics of all Western nations, appear to be very supportive of organ donation (Bergstrom and Gabel, 1991; Moore et al., 1976). Support levels for organ donation of 90 percent are routinely found in large-scale surveys. In the United States these rates vary by race/ethnicity and by education and income. White Americans, middle-class Americans, and well-educated Americans are more supportive of organ donation than are nonwhites and poorer and less educated citizens. However, the differences are all within the context of very high levels of support. African-American levels of support approach 80 percent (Prottas, 1994).

Actual willingness to donate is lower but still large. Survey data indicate that 75 to 80 percent of the population are willing to give permission for organ donation by a relative when they know that the person has been declared dead, even if they never discussed this issue with the deceased (Batten and Prottas, 1987). Here, too, there are significant differences across social class and ethnicities. Actual permission rates obtained are another measure of public willingness to donate—somewhat obscured by who is asked and the skills of those requesting permission. Permission rates vary among or-

gan-procurement organizations but generally lie between 55 percent and 65 percent.

There are two general categories of reasons that people give for being willing to donate the organs of a deceased relative. The more important is a desire to help another. Both families that have actually allowed a donation and the general public report that they support donation so that someone's life can be saved. The families of donors also assert that they permitted donation in order that something positive could come out of the death of their relative—this is only slightly less likely to be mentioned than the desire to save a life. The general public is less likely to give the solace of donation as a reason for its support of donation, but it, too, is the second most commonly given reason. Indeed, families and the general public agree that organ donation can help the families of the donor in the grieving process (Prottas and Batten, 1991; Batten and Prottas, 1987).

The reasons people give for their unwillingness to donate seem to reflect a mistrust of the medical establishment and the donation process. Among the most commonly given reasons is a fear that permission will compromise the care received or prolong the suffering of the relative. The second, closely aligned to the first, assumes that donation-related activities are occurring while the patient is still alive. From 45 to 65 percent of those unwilling to give permission for donation give answers of this sort as explanation for their unwillingness. Of this group, 60 percent will also say that they would not give permission because the donation process is too complicated. Finally, about a third attribute their unwillingness to expected resistance from other family members (Prottas and Batten, 1991).

Some of these reservations relate directly to the donation process itself and to the communication between OPOs and the public. Others may reflect more basic mistrustful or alienated attitudes toward medical institutions. In this regard the greater unwillingness to donate found among ethnic minorities and among poorer citizens becomes more comprehensible.

The donation process itself is generally well regarded by donors' families. There are many differences in detail in how different OPOs and hospitals manage the donation process, but the core elements always are the same. Once the medical suitability of a patient has been determined, the family must be approached with the patient's terminal prognosis and—then or somewhat later—with a request for donation. The fact of brain death must be presented by a physician, but the request for donation can be made by a doctor, a nurse, or a member of the local OPO. In different places the patterns vary. In some cases the organ-procurement specialists carry the main burden of talking with the families because they are trained and experienced in this kind of encounter. In other locales, nurses will assume the responsibility because they often have the best rapport with the family, developed while the patient was being treated.

The most common cause of death for an organ donor is accident trauma, and most donors are young—as a result, most family decision makers are parents. In recent years the age of donors has increased somewhat, and a larger percentage have died from cerebrovascular accidents. This has led to an increase in the percentage of decision makers who are spouses—most generally wives, since male donors outnumber female donors.

Donor families generally feel that the donation process was well handled, and almost 90 percent would make the same decision over again. The criticisms that do emerge usually regard the timing of the request and the clarity of the brain-death explanation. But it is impossible to say whether this reflects shortcoming in the donation process or the understandable difficulty families have in comprehending and accepting tragedy (Batten and Prottas, 1987).

System context.   Prior to 1986 the Southeastern Organ Procurement Foundation was the only regional OPO in the United States. It operated the United Network for Organ Sharing, a computer system listing most of the patients in the United States awaiting an organ. This computer list was simply a compilation of individual OPO lists, was readily accessible, and made inter-OPO organ sharing possible. However, the disposition of kidneys (few other organs were procured at that time) remained solely in the hands of the procuring agency.

Some OPOs were far more effective than others. Some procured forty kidneys per million population served; others, only eight. Cost per kidney also varied tremendously, from lows of $6,000 to $7,000 to highs of over $20,000. The percentage of organs not actually transplanted—in effect, wasted—was also very high and variable. In Europe 4–5 percent of the kidneys procured were discarded; in the United States the rate was almost 20 percent (a difference now virtually eliminated by improvements in the United States). Organ distribution criteria were different in different areas; often they were unwritten and inconsistently applied. Some transplant hospitals believed that when donor and recipient had similar immunological characteristics, the probability of successful transplantation was much higher. Others felt such matching was of little importance. Those who believed in matching offered to share organs more frequently than those who did not, and this tended to decrease access to transplants for their patients.

Public involvement.   The dual issues of system efficacy in organ procurement and equity in organ allocation induced Congress to become directly involved in organ-procurement and -transplantation matters. In 1972, Congress passed the End Stage Renal Disease (ESRD) Program as an amendment to the Social Security Act. Under this program, people suffering from renal failure automatically became eligible for Medicare coverage. Although most of the budget of this several-billion-dollar program pays for renal dialysis, renal-transplantation and organ-procurement costs are also covered. Under the ESRD Program, expenses of the nation's ninety OPOs were paid by the federal government. This financial involvement of the government, coupled with public concerns about efficacy and equity, led to major changes in the organ-procurement system in the late 1980s.

Starting in 1984 with the Organ Transplantation Act, Congress moved to restructure two key aspects of the organ procurement system by supporting the formation of a national organization to oversee the sharing of organs and by reforming the governance of OPOs themselves. By 1986 certain principles and structures were agreed upon that have come to define the organ procurement system of the nation. The most basic principle was that human organs are a public resource and that the organ procurement system was a steward of the public in its handling of organs. Each OPO and each transplant surgeon could be held accountable for organ allocation decisions. OPOs were now required to have public representatives on their boards.

A federally funded agency, the Organ Procurement and Transplantation Network (OPTN), was established to act as the public's agent in matters of organ allocation. This organization was given the authority to set rules controlling organ allocation at both the local and the interagency level, and to enforce those rules on all OPOs. Only member agencies of OPTN could procure organs; only member hospitals could transplant organs, on pain of losing Medicare reimbursement. OPTN was also given the authority to set membership standards, including those regarding personnel training and transplant outcomes. These standards had to be met if an OPO or a hospital was to be involved in organ procurement or transplantation. While OPTN has been very conservative in use of its powers, deferring to local practices and preferences whenever possible, in effect the federal government now has final say on how human organs are to be allocated to patients.

In the late 1980s, the Health Care Financing Administration (HCFA) exercised its right to set standards for the certification of OPOs, which included the definition of a service area for each OPO that was, to a large degree, the grant of a monopoly to procure organs in that area. Because HCFA rules precluded multiple OPOs in a single service area, there was a significant decrease in the number of OPOs in operation. As of 1994, the United States had some sixty-five certified OPOs.

The last major increase in government involvement was the passage of "required request" laws at both the federal and the state level. The philosophical underpinning of these laws is the belief that organ donation is a right that families have, and that medical institutions have an obligation to facilitate the exercise of that right. While there are differences among the various "required request" laws, they all share the same basic elements. Each requires that hospitals have a system in place to ensure that the family of every medically appropriate donor is asked if they wish to permit an organ or tissue donation. Reimbursement under Medicare can be denied to any hospital without such a system.

Donation rules.   Federal law defines the terms of exchange in organ donation. It is against federal law to buy or sell human organs and tissues. Organ and tissue donation requires explicit consent from the donor's family or a signed donor card. An alternative system exists called "presumed consent." This system reverses the burden of proof regarding family permission. Under it, if a family does not express an objection to organ donation, their permission is presumed. Austria, Belgium, Finland, France, Greece, Norway, Portugal, and Spain have "presumed consent" laws (Eurotransplant Foundation, 1992), but it is unclear how often they are implemented. Certainly some nations do not actually procure organs under these laws but insist on obtaining explicit permission from families. France and Spain, at least, are in this category.

In the United States, twenty-three states have some form of "presumed consent" laws with regard to cornea donations. According to these laws, corneas can be removed from cadavers under the jurisdiction of the medical examiner, based on permission from the medical examiner's office. Some states require a minimal effort to contact families, but others do not.

Tissue-procurement system.   The laws regarding organ procurement apply to tissue procurement in most ways. Tissue donation, too, must be voluntary and uncompensated, and families have the right to be given the option to donate when the medical circumstances are appropriate. However, the organizational structure of the tissue banking system is different from that of organ banking. Organ procurement is a closely regulated, federally financed system; tissue procurement is neither.

In fact, there are two quite distinct tissue-procurement systems. Eye banking is the largest and oldest system of human tissue procurement in the nation, unless one considers blood banking to be tissue procurement. There are about 120 eye banks in North America. Most of them belong to a professional association that gathers data about their activities and makes recommendations regarding matters such as quality control, cornea evaluation, cornea testing, and so forth (Eye Bank Associa-

tion, 1991). However, these eye banks are otherwise quite unregulated.

In the United States, eye banks differ markedly in terms of size and operating style. Some are large organizations that procure thousands of corneas a year, while others are staffed almost totally by volunteers. Some are members of multiple-facility organizations with banks spread across the entire nation; some are parts of teaching hospitals; others are supported by Lions Clubs; and still others are freestanding units with few outside organizational ties. The evidence indicates that the eye banking system meets the nation's need for corneas rather well, and this sufficiency has insulated eye banking from many of the questions of equitable allocation and local inefficiency that focused attention on organ procurement.

The system for procurement of musculoskeletal tissue (bone, tendons, fascia, ligaments) is virtually unregulated, except insofar as it falls under laws forbidding payments, certain FDA quality regulations, and "required request" laws. Only recently have shared professional and technical concerns begun to translate into discussion of procurement and distribution practices. Few rules have been agreed to, and there are no enforcement mechanisms. Government involvement in tissue banking is very recent and has occurred in response to public-health concerns about the spread of AIDS and hepatitis via transplanted tissue.

However, the organ- and tissue-procurement systems are increasingly overlapping at the operational level. Cooperation of hospitals and their medical staffs is central to the success of both, and there is overlap in terms of donor families as well. Because of this, OPOs and tissue banks have increasingly found themselves in conflict regarding access to hospital staff and to families. In some instances, OPOs have expanded their activities to include tissue banking, while in others, local agreements have generated cooperation. In many parts of the country, however, this has not been the case. The central organizational issue facing tissue banking is how to benefit from an association with the organ-procurement system, a well-funded, extensive, and governmentally sanctioned system, without being absorbed by it.

JEFFREY PROTTAS

Directly related to this article are the other articles in this entry: ETHICAL AND LEGAL ISSUES REGARDING CADAVERS, *and* ETHICAL AND LEGAL ISSUES REGARDING LIVING DONORS. *Also directly related are the entries* ORGAN AND TISSUE TRANSPLANTS; *and* XENOGRAFTS. *For a further discussion of topics mentioned in this article, see the entry* DEATH, DEFINITION AND DETERMINATION OF, *especially the articles on* CRITERIA FOR DEATH, *and* LEGAL ISSUES IN

PRONOUNCING DEATH. *For a discussion of related ideas, see the entries* ARTIFICIAL HEARTS AND CARDIAC-ASSIST DEVICES; ARTIFICIAL ORGANS AND LIFE-SUPPORT SYSTEMS; BLOOD TRANSFUSION; FAMILY; HEALTH-CARE FINANCING, *article on* MEDICARE; HEALTH-CARE RESOURCES, ALLOCATION OF, *article on* MICROALLOCATION; *and* KIDNEY DIALYSIS.

Bibliography

BART, KENNETH J.; MACON, EDWIN J.; HUMPHRIES, ARTHUR L., JR.; BALDWIN, ROBERT J.; FITCH, TERRY; POPE, RANDALL S.; RICH, MICHAEL J.; LANGFORD, DOROTHY; TEUTSCH, STEVEN M.; and BLOUNT, JOSEPH H. 1981a. "Increasing the Supply of Cadaveric Kidneys for Transplantation." *Transplantation* 31, no. 5:383–387.

BART, KENNETH J.; MACON, EDWIN J.; WHITTIER, FREDERICK C.; BALDWIN, ROBERT J.; and BLOUNT, JOSEPH H. 1981b. "Cadaveric Kidneys for Transplantation: A Paradox of Shortage in the Face of Plenty." *Transplantation* 31, no. 5:379–382.

BATTEN, HELEN LEVINE, and PROTTAS, JEFFREY M. 1987. "Kind Strangers: The Families of Organ Donors." *Health Affairs* 6, no. 2:35–37.

BERGSTRÖM, CHRISTINA, and GÄBEL, HÅKAN. 1991. "Organ Donation and Organ Retrieval Programs in Sweden, 1990." *Journal of Transplant Coordination* 1, no. 1:47–51.

EUROTRANSPLANT FOUNDATION. 1992. *Eurotransplant Newsletter* 91.

EVANS, ROGER W.; ORIANS, CARLYN E.; and ASCHER, NANCY L. 1992. "The Potential Supply of Organ Donors: An Assessment of the Efficacy of Organ Procurement Efforts in the United States." *Journal of the American Medical Association* 267, no. 2:239–246.

EYE BANK ASSOCIATION OF AMERICA. 1991. *Eye Banking Statistics.* Washington, D.C.: Author.

HEALTH CARE FINANCING ADMINISTRATION. 1990. *ESRD Program Highlights.* Washington, D.C.: Author.

MOORES, B.; CLARKE, G.; LEWIS, B. R.; and MALLICK, N. P. 1976. "Public Attitudes Towards Kidney Transplantation." *British Medical Journal* 1, no. 6010:629–631.

NATHAN, HOWARD, et al. 1991. "Estimation and Characterization of the Potential Organ Donor Pool in Pennsylvania." *Transplantation* 51, no. 1:112–149.

NATIONAL ORGAN PROCUREMENT AND TRANSPLANTATION NETWORK. 1991. *UNOS Update* 7, no. 11 (December).

PROTTAS, JEFFREY M. 1989. "The Organization of Organ Procurement." *Journal of Health Politics, Policy and Law* 14, no. 1:41–55.

——. 1991. "Study of Unmet Demand and Corneal Distribution in North America." Unpublished.

——. 1994. *The Most Useful Gift: Altruism and the Public Policy of Organ Transplants.* San Francisco: Jossey-Bass.

PROTTAS, JEFFREY M., and BATTEN, HELEN LEVINE. 1991. "The Willingness to Give: The Public and the Supply of Transplantable Organs." *Journal of Health Politics, Policy and Law* 16, no. 1:121–134.

TAKEMOTO, STEVEN, and TERASAKI, PAUL I. 1988. "Donor and Recipient Age." In *Clinical Transplants, 1988,* pp. 345–356. Edited by Paul I. Terasaki. Los Angeles: UCLA Tissue Typing Laboratory.

II. ETHICAL AND LEGAL ISSUES REGARDING CADAVERS

Several controversies in biomedical ethics revolve around the transfer and use, particularly in transplantation, of organs and tissues from cadavers. The language, concepts, and norms of cadaveric organ and tissue transplantation are matters of debate, in part because of complex beliefs, sentiments, and practices surrounding the dead body. Examples of problematic language include "harvesting," "salvaging," "procurement," and "retrieval" of organs, each of which has ambiguous and even controversial implications (Youngner, 1992). The widely used term "donor" itself presents problems, because it is used to refer to the cadaveric source of the organs as well as to the decision maker about donation. However, the first use is inappropriate unless the source of the organs also made the decision to donate. Thus, it is inappropriate to describe as "donors" deceased individuals who never had the capacity to decide or never decided to donate. Likewise, someone who sells an organ is not a "donor" but rather a "vendor" (Childress, 1989b).

Various laws and policies structure the transfer of organs and tissues from a cadaver to a transplant recipient. Assessments of actual or proposed laws and policies often appeal to general moral principles or values, such as respect for personal autonomy, voluntarism, altruism, and communal solidarity. They include judgments of ethical acceptability and ethical preferability, as well as of feasibility.

Debates about different ways to increase the supply of transplantable organs often involve disputes about the appropriateness of viewing human body parts as property (Andrews, 1986; Childress, 1992). Property is sometimes narrowly conceived in commercial terms, but even donation presupposes some conception of property in the broad sense of rights regarding cadaveric body parts. Thus, the society must determine who has rights and which rights they have over cadaveric body parts. For example, the possible owners include those to whom the decedent previously agreed to donate those parts, the decedent's family, or the larger community. And these persons could have rights to possess, to use, to exclude others from using, to destroy, or to transfer those parts by various means. In the nineteenth and twentieth centuries, several court decisions in Anglo-American common law construed the cadaver as "quasi-property" and recognized the family's "quasi-property" right in the corpse (Meyers, 1990). According to most of these court decisions, families have limited property rights in the corpse but lack full property rights to use or transfer body parts for commercial purposes. Different conceptions of personhood and embodiment pervade debates about limited or full property rights. For instance, those who identify an intimate relation between personhood and embodiment, often viewing the cadaver as symbolic of the person, tend to oppose the sale of organs (May, 1985; Murray, 1987).

Finally, a feasible policy for obtaining organs and tissues from cadavers presupposes a clear, compelling, and workable boundary between life and death. The development of the concept and criteria of brain death in the late 1960s was essential to the expansion of organ transplantation because of the need to obtain viable organs from heart-beating cadavers, whose cardiopulmonary function is maintained by machines. However, problems have emerged. First, there are difficulties in conceptualizing, operationalizing, and implementing conceptions of brain death, and uncertainty about brain death figures prominently in many of the stated reasons for individual and familial reluctance to donate organs. Second, some institutions in the early 1990s have attempted to enlarge the donor pool by including non-heart-beating cadavers declared dead by cardiopulmonary standards, which now often follows the deceased's decision to refuse further life-sustaining treatment. One concern is that such efforts will create a conflict of interest among professionals who have to manage the dying process in order to maximize the likelihood of viable transplantable organs without violating rules against killing patients or directly hastening their deaths (Arnold and Youngner, 1993). Third, the "dead donor rule" has been threatened by efforts to change the law to permit the removal of organs from anencephalic newborns, who lack most of their brain and whose deaths are inevitable and imminent but have enough of a brain stem to maintain spontaneous respiration at least briefly.

Methods of obtaining organs for transplantation

The major possible methods of transferring cadaveric organs and tissues include (1) express donation by the individual while alive or by the next of kin after his or her death; (2) presumed donation, with consent to donation presumed of the individual while alive and/or of the next of kin; (3) routine removal or salvaging; (4) expropriation or conscription; (5) abandonment; and (6) sale. These methods will be considered only from the standpoint of procurement, without any attention to distribution, even though procurement and distribution are morally connected. All of these methods play some role

in access to living or cadaveric organs, tissues, and fluids. For example, in the United States, express donation is virtually the only method of transferring solid organs, while presumed donation or routine removal is used in some states for corneas. Sale remains prevalent in the transfer of semen for artificial insemination, and abandonment has been common in the transfer of tissues for research purposes. Expropriation or conscription is rare and more controversial, but it appears in legally required autopsies and tests for the use of illicit drugs.

Express donation. Express donation laws operate in Australia, Canada, Denmark, the Netherlands, Japan, Sweden, Turkey, the United Kingdom, and most of Central and South America. In the United States, the legal framework for organ procurement in all fifty states and the District of Columbia is the Uniform Anatomical Gift Act (UAGA), which was adopted with modifications by the early 1970s (National Conference of Commissioners, 1968). The UAGA reflects the values of voluntarism and altruism (Caplan and Bayer, 1985). Within this legal framework, competent individuals can determine what will be done with their organs after their deaths; in the absence of a valid expression of the decedent's prior wishes, the family can decide whether to donate his or her organs. In practice the family, not the decedent while alive, has emerged as the primary donor of cadaveric organs (Prottas, 1985).

Individuals as donors. According to several opinion surveys, fewer than 50 percent of American adults are very or somewhat likely to donate their organs after their deaths (Gallup Organization, 1985, 1986, 1987), and even fewer actually sign donor cards. The reasons include lack of thought about donation and reluctance to face the prospect of death. Other significant reasons reflect distrust, or limited trust, of the system: Respondents worry that if they sign a donor card, physicians might take premature action to obtain their organs before they are really dead or even hasten their death. The stated willingness to become an organ donor is even lower among minority groups, such as blacks and Hispanics, who perceive themselves to be on the margins of the system and to have even less reason to trust it (Callender, 1992; Chapa, 1992).

Even when confronted with the decedent's signed donor card, a rare event, organ procurement teams still consult the family. And if the family opposes the decedent's wish to donate, the family tends to prevail, because of unwarranted fears of legal liability, legitimate fears of jeopardizing organ procurement and transplantation as a result of negative publicity, and the felt need to be sensitive to the family's wishes. However, conflicts between the decedent's expressed wish to donate and the family's opposition do not appear to preclude many transplants. In the final analysis, donor cards do not appear to be effective instruments of organ transfer, even though they may be important in intrafamilial discussion.

Several proposed policies of "encouraged voluntarism" have emerged (Caplan and Bayer, 1985). One that has been adopted in some places is "routine inquiry" directed at individuals in various settings. Concerns have arisen about the routine inquiry of patients entering the hospital, as recommended in the amended UAGA (National Conference, 1987) and enacted by some states, but few objections have surfaced about routine inquiry in other contexts, such as obtaining a driver's license. Another proposal is "mandated choice": individuals would have to indicate, perhaps when they obtain a driver's license or file income tax forms, whether they want to donate (or are undecided), and their choice would be entered into a national registry (Veatch, 1989). But, if forced to choose, many individuals would check no, because they are afraid of being on record as willing donors of organs, not because they oppose the donation of their organs after their deaths. Their no would preclude familial donation, and a policy of mandated choice would thus probably reduce rather than increase the number of donated organs. Both routine inquiry and mandated choice arguably concentrate too much on the donor card. Another possibility is to allow individuals to designate surrogate decision makers who can express their values after death (Areen, 1988). The rationale is that individuals may be more willing to designate a decision maker they trust than to sign a document of gift that might put them at risk at the hands of strangers in large, impersonal, bureaucratic institutions that appear eager to procure organs.

Families as donors. In the United States, as in most other countries, the family is the primary donor of cadaveric organs. Opinion surveys indicate that individuals are more willing to donate the organs of family members than they are to donate their own organs by signing donor cards, particularly if they know the decedent's wishes (Gallup Organization, 1985, 1986, 1987, 1993). The main bottleneck in obtaining cadaveric organs thus appears to be the failure of health-care professionals to ask families about donation when a relative has died. The problem has been construed as a shortage of askers rather than of familial givers. In this context, Arthur Caplan (1984) proposed "required request" directed at the decedent's next of kin; this policy has now been enacted in the United States by most state legislatures, is mandated in federal legislation for all institutions receiving Medicare or Medicaid funds, and is required by the Joint Commission on Accreditation of Health Care Organizations. Weak required-request statutes simply mandate that institutions develop protocols to ensure inquiries of families, while strong required-request statutes mandate that the request and its outcome be documented on the death certificate (Virnig and Caplan, 1992).

Even though required-request laws and policies may have contributed to increases in tissue donation, they do not appear to have increased the supply of donated organs—the number of acts of donation of solid organs each year remained relatively constant for several years, at 4,000 to 4,500, with most increases occurring as a result of changes in the criteria of donor eligibility (e.g., accepting donations from older persons whose organs would not have been used earlier). However, the overall donor pool has shrunk for various reasons, including the decline in automobile-related deaths, especially as a result of seat-belt laws, and the spread of infection by the human immunodeficiency virus (HIV), which causes AIDS. In this context, "Slow increases in the number of donors, or having the number of donors hold steady . . . suggest that the present level of donation may be higher than it would be without the laws" (Virnig and Caplan, 1992, p. 2156). Required-request policies may also have had positive indirect effects in making requests for donation more routine in hospitals (Virnig and Caplan, 1992). Nevertheless, the reluctance of physicians and other health-care professionals to make such requests may account for the modest direct effects. One proposal to overcome professional reluctance is routine referral or required referral, which would require that institutions and health-care professionals routinely notify a trained procurement team in circumstances where cadaveric organs and tissues might be available (Prottas and Batten, 1988).

Whatever legal and policy changes are enacted, public and professional education will remain crucial. For instance, some studies of the effects of required request indicate that familial refusal rates may be as high as 60 to 70 percent (Caplan et al., 1992). Effective educational programs will have to address individuals as members of families rather than merely as potential signers of donor cards, and to address confusions about brain death and attitudes of distrust that appear to pose obstacles to express donation.

Presumed donation or routine removal. Presumed donation or routine removal (frequently called "routine salvaging") laws have been adopted for corneas in several states in the United States and for organs and tissues in Austria, Belgium, Finland, France, Norway, Portugal, and Singapore. These laws authorize the removal of organs or tissues, usually without notification, in the absence of the decedent's prior and/or the family's current explicit dissent. They thus involve "opting out" rather than "opting in"—that is, individuals and their relatives must take action to stop the process of donation or removal rather than to initiate it.

Vigorous debate continues about how to construe and evaluate such laws. "Presumed donation" and "routine removal" are often considered interchangeable, but their moral bases are different. Presumed donation assumes that the individual (and/or the family) owns and has dispositional authority over cadaveric organs, and that the decedent's prior failure (or the family's current failure) to dissent constitutes consent. By contrast, routine removal presupposes that the society has a right of access to cadaveric organs and tissues because it owns them or because individuals and families have an enforceable social duty to provide them. Such a communitarian approach to organ removal may allow opting out for various reasons, such as conscientious objection (Nelson, 1992). To identify the operative moral basis of laws that authorize removal without express consent, it is necessary to look beyond the society's rhetoric to determine what occurs in practice. If the policy is presumed donation, then vigorous efforts should be undertaken to ensure public understanding and voluntariness; otherwise, a decedent's prior or a family's current failure to dissent may only indicate a lack of understanding of the opportunity or the means for dissent or of what will be done in the absence of dissent. If, however, the policy is routine removal, public understanding and voluntariness are superfluous, even though they may be sought for practical reasons.

The main objections to routine removal rest on what William May (1973) calls the "principle of extraterritoriality," which holds that even the deceased individual is not reducible to the needs of the social order. Many concede that presumed donation is ethically acceptable in principle but raise questions about its practice—for instance, ethically acceptable presumed donation, based on understanding and voluntariness, may actually be less cost-effective than enhanced and redirected educational efforts in the context of express donation. Furthermore, many view express donation as ethically preferable to presumed donation because it states and supports active altruism (Ramsey, 1970).

Objections to the presuppositions of routine removal may in part account for the prevalence of the rhetoric of presumed donation. And uneasiness about society's dispositional authority over cadavers, or about the meaning of an individual's or family's failure to dissent, may account for the similarity of practices in most countries, despite their different legal frameworks (Prottas, 1985; Caplan, 1984). For example, in most countries with what is termed "presumed consent," professionals regularly ask the family or follow the family's known wishes, just as they do in countries with express donation. Among European countries with presumed donation or routine removal, only Austria, with its long tradition of authorizing autopsies on all persons without requesting permission, does not in practice notify the next of kin (Land and Cohen, 1992).

Neither presumed donation nor routine removal appears to be politically feasible in many social contexts. In light of widespread public opposition in the United States to the removal of organs on the basis of presumed consent, such a policy would probably reduce rather than increase the number of donated organs. The attitudes of distrust that now obstruct express donations would probably lead individuals to remove themselves from the list of presumed donors and thereby preclude familial decisions to donate. However, supporters of presumed donation note that several states already have laws that authorize the removal of corneas, without consent, by medical examiners or coroners who examine bodies following accidents or homicides. These laws have survived constitutional challenges in some states, even when they do not require notification of or consent from the next of kin. Furthermore, they have been effective; for example, after Georgia adopted presumed donation, cornea transplants increased from 25 in 1978 to over 1,000 in 1984 (National Conference, 1987). Such laws may survive without major vocal opposition because of different views about different body parts (corneas versus solid organs), because brain death is usually required for the removal of solid organs while corneas can be removed following death by cardiopulmonary standards, or because the public is largely unaware of these laws, even in the states where they exist. If the last reason holds, critics charge that presumed donation is ethically invalid because of a lack of understanding on the part of the "donors," whose silence is construed as passive consent to donation. Under such circumstances, the policy touted as presumed donation is actually closer to routine salvaging or even to expropriation with a right to refuse.

Conscription or expropriation. Public-health considerations often justify autopsies to determine the cause of death, even against the conscientious objections of adherents of some religious groups. Strong communitarian views extend such arguments to justify conscription or expropriation of cadaveric organs (Silver, 1988). Some ethicists contend that the good of persons needing transplantable organs and the good of the community can justify the removal of organs even against the will of the decedent and the next of kin, because the cadaver lacks autonomy and cannot be harmed. Respect for the beliefs of the decedent while alive, and his or her sociocultural practices regarding burial, do not outweigh significant therapeutic benefits to recipients of organ transplants (Jonsen, 1988). Critics of organ conscription appeal to the principle of extraterritoriality, contend that individuals may be wronged (e.g., by having their will thwarted after their deaths) without being harmed, and note that sociocultural practices of disposing of bodies remain very important for various groups, including the family and religious communities. Furthermore, in a liberal society, respect for autonomous choices made prior to death should not be overridden if there are acceptable and effective alternatives. Finally, there is little reason to believe that this method of acquisition is politically feasible in most countries at this time.

Abandonment. Another possible mode of transfer of organs and tissues is abandonment, that is, a failure to claim bodies and their parts. For example, following some medical procedures, patients simply abandon their excised organs, tissues, blood, urine, and the like, which under some conditions may be used by researchers. This mode of transfer of body parts has been widely debated in the case of living sources, but it also appears to characterize statutes that authorize the removal and use of organs and tissues from unclaimed bodies. In principle, this mode of acquisition of cadaveric organs and tissues could be ethically acceptable, but it will not significantly increase the supply of organs or tissue for transplantation. Furthermore, strict rules are needed to ensure that the body is actually unclaimed.

Sales. While setting a legal framework for donation, the original UAGA did not prohibit the sale of organs because the Commissioners on Uniform State Laws did not want to establish an absolute barrier to sales and believed that this matter could be handled by local medical communities (Ramsey, 1970). Hence, for many years the sale of organs and tissues was arguably not illegal in most of the United States. Then, partly in response to a concrete proposal to broker human kidneys for transplantation, some states in the mid-1980s passed laws to prohibit the sale of organs, and the 1984 National Organ Transplant Act made it "unlawful for any person to knowingly acquire, receive, or otherwise transfer any human organ [defined as human kidney, liver, heart, lung, pancreas, bone marrow, cornea, eye, bone, and skin and any other human organ specified by the secretary of health and human services by regulation] for valuable consideration for use in human transplantation if the transfer affects interstate commerce." It is not illegal in the United States to sell blood, sperm, and ova. No country is reported to allow the sale of cadaveric organs, even though stories circulate about sales in some countries.

Two main arguments support the transfer of organs and tissues by sale. One is based largely on the principle of respect for autonomous choices; the other, largely on the principle of utility or maximization of human welfare. The first argument, a libertarian argument, holds that autonomous agents should have the liberty to dis-

pose of their body parts in whatever ways they choose, whether by donation or sale. The second argument, a utilitarian argument, holds that the society should accept transfers of cadaveric body parts by sale as the most effective and efficient way to increase the supply of organs that can save human lives. Libertarians tend to support only sales by individuals while alive for delivery after their deaths—for instance, a futures market (Cohen, 1989)—while utilitarians may also support sales by the next of kin following an individual's death. Many object to a market in human organs on the grounds that wealthy patients will receive priority for transplants; however, the society could purchase organs for distribution according to criteria other than ability to pay.

This objection about distribution aside, the main objections to the libertarian argument for sales rest on several moral claims: (1) there are risks to living vendors or to others whose parts may be transferred by vendors after being killed or allowed to die; (2) there are concerns about the vendors' lack of voluntariness, especially if they are poor, economically vulnerable, and subject to exploitation; (3) buying and selling organs involves commodification, that is, treating human body parts as commodities, and thus depersonalizes and degrades vendors and the society (May, 1985; Murray, 1987). According to defenders of sales, societal regulation rather than prohibition could reduce risks and establish voluntariness, and commodification is a vague and speculative concern. However, opponents contend that societal regulation itself, even if successful on the first two points, legitimates commodification and thus violates fundamental societal values.

The main rejoinders to the utilitarian argument hold that there are other effective, ethically acceptable, and even ethically preferable ways to increase the supply of organs. Shifting to sales would be costly, would probably drive out many donations, and could have serious negative effects through promoting commodification. In addition, critics question whether sales would actually increase the supply of organs. Proponents of markets stress that potential donors now fail to act because of inertia, inconvenience, mild doubts, and distaste in thinking about the transfer of their (or a relative's) cadaveric body parts, and that compensation will overcome these grounds of resistance (Hansmann, 1989). However, it is unclear whether fundamental attitudes of distrust will yield so easily to monetary incentives. Fears of being declared dead prematurely or having one's death hastened in order to provide organs for others can be expected to pose problems for a futures market. If people are now reluctant to sign donor cards because of fears that they may not receive proper care in the hospital, they will probably be afraid to accept money for the delivery of their organs upon their deaths. However, neither side can produce solid evidence for its claims.

The following question has emerged in recent years: Could financial and other tangible incentives strengthen the system of express donation through "rewarded gifting" without crossing the line into sales? Thomas Peters (1991) has proposed a pilot program to test the effects of providing a death benefit of $1,000 for recoverable donations. Critics contend that rewarded gifting differs very little from direct sales (May, 1991). However, a modified approach might provide effective financial incentives and yet preserve the meaning of the act of donation. As a regularized expression of gratitude for acts of donation of organs and tissues, the society could cover the decedent's funeral expenses up to a certain amount. In this way, the community would recognize with gratitude the decedent's and the family's act of donation and would pay respect to the donor/source of the organs and tissues by sharing in the disposition of the final remains, following the removal of donated parts (Childress, 1992).

Another proposal, already implemented in Singapore, is to give priority on the waiting list for organ transplants to individuals or family members who have indicated a willingness to donate their organs. While attractive in many respects, such a proposal needs to be assessed in light of defensible criteria for the just distribution of organs. In short, any particular proposal for rewarded gifting requires careful scrutiny, in part because organ donation is a highly sensitive activity, marked by complex beliefs, symbols, attitudes, and sentiments, as well as by ethical and political pitfalls.

Controversy about the use of cadaveric fetal tissue following deliberate abortions

In the late 1980s and early 1990s, controversy raged in the United States about the use of human fetal tissue following elective abortions. The debate has centered on the experimental transplantation of fetal neural tissue into patients suffering from Parkinson's disease. Fetal tissue is believed to be advantageous for such transplants because it is immunologically more naive than developed tissue, and it grows and differentiates rapidly. In addition, fetal tissue is amply available because over 1.5 million abortions occurred in the United States each year in the 1980s and early 1990s.

In most states the use of fetal tissue follows the pattern for the transfer and use of other transplantable cadaveric tissue. However, the Reagan and Bush administrations banned the use of federal funds in transplantation research using fetal tissue following deliberate abortions. The ban did not affect uses of aborted fetal tissue in other federally funded research, such as the de-

velopment of vaccines, nor did it affect transplantation research using tissue from spontaneously aborted fetuses, which may, however, not be usable because of medical problems. In 1988, the Human Fetal Tissue Transplantation Research Panel (HFTTRP), appointed by the National Institutes of Health, recommended lifting the ban on the use of federal funds, within guidelines and safeguards to separate as much as possible decisions about abortion and decisions about donation. But the ban remained in effect until the Clinton administration lifted it in 1993. The ban was a notable exception to the strong international consensus that it is permissible, within certain limits, to use human fetal tissue in transplantation research following deliberate abortions (Walters, 1990).

Opponents argue that the use of aborted fetal tissue in transplantation research constitutes complicity in the moral evil of abortion by signifying its approval through accepting the benefits of the transplanted tissue or through providing societal funds for the research (Burtchaell, 1988). Most supporters of the research concede that abortion is, at the very least, morally undesirable, but they deny that the use of aborted fetal tissue necessarily implies approval of abortion as long as certain guidelines are followed. After all, they note, it is possible to use organs and tissues from homicide and accident victims—and thus to accept significant benefits from those moral evils and tragedies—without approving of homicides and accidents and without reducing efforts to prevent their occurrence (HFTTRP, 1988).

Critics further contend that the use of aborted fetal tissue in transplantation research would lead to abortions that would not otherwise have occurred, especially if the transplant procedures become routine, by providing pregnant women, who are often ambivalent about abortion, with three additional incentives for abortions. The first possible incentive is to sell fetal tissue. However, defenders of the research generally agree that the sale of fetal tissue should be prohibited for various reasons—for example, to prevent additional abortions, to protect women from exploitation and coercion, to reduce moral controversy about abortion, and to prevent commodification of body parts. And if current legal rules do not clearly prohibit the sale of fetal tissue—the 1988 revision of the National Organ Transplant Act prohibits the sale of fetal organs or subparts of those organs—they can, and should, be modified to do so.

A second possible incentive for an abortion is specific altruism. Some women have volunteered to become pregnant in order to abort and donate fetal tissue to help a family member suffering from Parkinson's disease. The HFTTRP (1988) held that it is both desirable and feasible to prevent motives of specific altruism from leading to abortions by prohibiting women from designating the recipient of transplantable fetal tissue and by requiring anonymity between donor and recipient.

A third possible incentive for women to terminate their pregnancies is the most controversial. Opponents contend that the possibility of donating fetal tissue to benefit unrelated and unknown patients would encourage some women to have abortions they would not otherwise have had because they could rationalize that some good would come out of their decisions. By contrast, defenders argue that this risk is speculative and, in any event, is outweighed by the probable benefits of the research (HFTTRP, 1988). This debate hinges in part on empirical claims about the reasons women choose to have abortions, but neither side has solid evidence to support its position (Vawter et al., 1990). Defenders of the research emphasize that there is no evidence that the possibility of donating fetal tissue for research has played any role in abortion decisions since the mid-1960s. However, opponents contend that using fetal tissue as a therapy in transplantation is different from using fetal tissue to develop a therapy, such as a vaccine. In contrast to the incentives of financial gain and specific altruism, safeguards cannot completely eliminate the possibility that the opportunity to donate fetal tissue, based on general altruism, will play a role in some abortion decisions.

A final question concerns dispositional authority over fetal remains and acceptable modes of transfer. Fetal tissue has occasionally been viewed as abandoned or unclaimed following abortions, and then used without explicit maternal consent—perhaps sometimes based on presumed maternal consent (HFTTRP, 1988; Vawter et al., 1990). Within the current legal framework, donation by a woman choosing to have an abortion is the primary mode of transfer. However, critics insist, the woman choosing to have an abortion forfeits her role as "guardian" over the fetus and loses any right to donate fetal tissue (Burtchaell, 1988). By contrast, the HFTTRP held that a woman's choice of a legal abortion does not disqualify her legally, and should not disqualify her morally, from serving as "the primary decisionmaker about the disposition of fetal remains, including the donation of fetal tissue for research. . . . She still has a special connection with the fetus and she has a legitimate interest in its disposition and use. Furthermore, the dead fetus has no interests that the . . . woman's donation would violate" (HFTTRP, 1988, vol. 1, p. 6). According to the HFTTRP, discussion with the pregnant woman about the possibility of donating fetal tissue should not occur before her decision to abort, unless she specifically asks. And, finally, the timing and method of abortion should not be modified in order to secure more viable fetal tissue.

Religious and humanistic beliefs, attitudes, and practices

In contrast to religious traditions that view the human body as unreal, as evil, or as incidental, William May (1985) holds that the Jewish and Christian traditions affirm that the human body is real and good and is, furthermore, profoundly linked and identified with the spirit. Thus, the Jewish and Christian traditions tend to require consent to justify invasions of the living or dead body. They sympathize with natural human "aversions to tampering with a living body or corpse," but they also develop symbols and rituals to discipline those aversions (May, 1985). Jews and Christians affirm that human beings were created in the image of God (Gen. 1:26–27). This affirmation shapes fitting conduct toward the dead body, which is viewed as symbolic of the human person and his or her dignity, as well as toward the living body.

In Judaism, this affirmation is expressed in prohibitions against mutilating, deriving benefit from, or delaying the interment of the corpse and its parts. However, all prohibitions in Jewish law, except for those against murder, idolatry, and certain sexual offenses such as incest and adultery, can be overridden in order to save human life. Except where there are reservations about brain death, especially among the Orthodox, Judaism can accept nonexperimental cadaveric organ transplantation because of the high probability of immediate life-saving benefit (Rosner and Tendler, 1980). Even cornea transplants can be viewed as lifesaving, according to some rabbis, for blindness is a life-threatening condition because of the risk of fatal accidents. In addition, cornea transplants need not involve problems of brain death.

Within Christianity, Roman Catholicism has accepted the transplantation of cadaveric organs and tissues without the sorts of legal presumptions encountered in Judaism and also without worries about the resurrected body. It views the donation of cadaveric organs as praiseworthy, though usually not obligatory, and it does not require that the benefit of donation be as direct or as immediate as is often the case in Judaism. Protestant Christians tend to emphasize the principle of respect for persons and their consciences, and to justify and limit cadaveric organ donation according to the norm of love of neighbor (agape). Hence, the themes of voluntarism and altruism are prominent in both Roman Catholic and Protestant approaches to organ transplantation (Childress, 1989a).

Islamic religious and legal authorities have encountered obstacles in justifying cadaveric organ and tissue transplantation; these obstacles include beliefs in the bodily resurrection and norms of rapid burial and avoidance of mutilation and cremation of the corpse. As a result, Muslims have often gone to Western countries for organ transplants. And because of specific opposition to cadaveric organ donation by Islamic authorities, Muslims were not included in Singapore's law of presumed donation. However, the majority of Islamic authorities in various schools of thought now accept cadaveric organ donation, often appealing to the principles of saving human life and necessity, and requiring the decedent's or the relatives' permission (Sachedina, 1988).

Religious positions are often intermixed with social and cultural beliefs, practices, and superstitions to create complex views about the use of cadaveric organs and tissues in transplantation. And often the opposition to cadaveric organ transplantation, as in Orthodox Judaism, rests on dissatisfaction with the concept of brain death. In Japan, for instance, and in some Native American traditions, difficulties surrounding brain death, perhaps even more than attitudes and practices regarding the cadaver, have restricted cadaveric organ donations.

Debates can be expected to continue about effective ways to obtain more cadaveric organs and tissues for transplantation, particularly in view of the long waiting lists for transplants and the limited increases in donations. Religious beliefs, symbols, and practices, along with various other psychosocial forces, are important for determining the ethical acceptability and preferability, as well as the feasibility, of different laws, policies, and practices to obtain organs and tissues for transplantation. Some of the policy reforms in the United States in the 1980s may have been ineffective and perhaps even counterproductive because of inadequate sensitivity to such psychosocial factors. It is crucial that policymakers consider the whole range of relevant factors in order to ensure the effectiveness and minimize the negative consequences of organ-procurement policies.

JAMES F. CHILDRESS

Directly related to this article are the other articles in this entry: MEDICAL AND ORGANIZATIONAL ASPECTS, *and* ETHICAL AND LEGAL ISSUES REGARDING LIVING DONORS. *Also directly related are the entries* ORGAN AND TISSUE TRANSPLANTS, *and* XENOGRAFTS. *For a further discussion of topics mentioned in this article, see the entries* ABORTION; AIDS; ARTIFICIAL ORGANS AND LIFE-SUPPORT SYSTEMS; AUTONOMY; BEHAVIOR CONTROL; BENEFICENCE; BLOOD TRANSFUSION; BODY; CONFLICT OF INTEREST; DEATH, DEFINITION AND DETERMINATION OF; DEATH AND DYING: EUTHANASIA AND SUSTAINING LIFE; EASTERN ORTHODOX CHRISTIANITY; FAMILY; FETUS, *especially the article on* FETAL RESEARCH; FREEDOM AND COERCION; HUMAN NATURE; INFORMED CONSENT; ISLAM; JUDAISM; LAW AND BIOETHICS; LIFESTYLES AND PUBLIC HEALTH; OBLIGATION AND SUPEREROGATION; PERSON; PROTESTANTISM; PUBLIC HEALTH; RIGHTS;

ROMAN CATHOLICISM; TRUST; *and* UTILITY. *For a discussion of related ideas, see the entries* CONFLICT OF INTEREST; DEATH; *and* HARM.

Bibliography

ANDREWS, LORI B. 1986. "My Body, My Property." *Hastings Center Report* 16, no. 5:28–38.

AREEN, JUDITH C. 1988. "A Scarcity of Organs." *Journal of Legal Education* 38, no. 4:555–565.

ARNOLD, ROBERT M., and YOUNGNER, STUART J., eds. 1993. *Kennedy Institute of Ethics Journal* 3, no. 2. "Ethical, Psychosocial, and Public Policy Implications of Procuring Organs from Non-Heart-Beating Cadavers."

BURTCHAELL, JAMES T. 1988. "University Policy on Experimental Use of Aborted Fetal Tissue." *IRB* 10, no. 4:7–11.

CALLENDER, CLIVE O. 1992. "Organ/Tissue Donation in African Americans: A National Stratagem." In *The Surgeon General's Workshop on Increasing Organ Donation: Background Papers, Washington, D.C., July 8–10, 1991*, pp. 145–162. Washington, D.C.: U.S. Department of Health and Human Services, Public Health Service.

CAPLAN, ARTHUR L. 1984. "Ethical and Policy Issues in the Procurement of Cadaver Organs for Transplantation." *New England Journal of Medicine* 314, no. 15:981–983.

CAPLAN, ARTHUR L., and BAYER, RONALD. 1985. "Ethical, Legal and Policy Issues Pertaining to Solid Organ Procurement." New York: Hastings Center/Empire Blue Cross–Blue Shield.

CAPLAN, ARTHUR L.; SIMINOFF, LAURA; ARNOLD, ROBERT; and VIRNIG, BETH A. 1992. "Increasing Organ and Tissue Donation: What Are the Obstacles, What Are Our Options?" In *The Surgeon General's Workshop on Increasing Organ Donation: Background Papers, Washington, D.C., July 8–10, 1991*, pp. 199–232. Washington, D.C.: U.S. Department of Health and Human Services, Public Health Service.

CHAPA, JORGE. 1992. "Hispanics and Organ Donation: Prospects, Obstacles and Recommendations." In *The Surgeon General's Workshop on Increasing Organ Donation: Background Papers, Washington, D.C., July 8–10, 1991*, pp. 163–180. Washington, D.C.: U.S. Department of Health and Human Services, Public Health Service.

CHILDRESS, JAMES F. 1989a. "Attitudes of Major Western Religious Traditions Toward Uses of the Human Body and Its Parts." In *Justice and the Holy: Essays in Honor of Walter Harrelson*, pp. 216–240. Edited by Douglas A. Knight and Peter J. Paris. Atlanta: Scholars Press.

———. 1989b. "Ethical Criteria for Procuring and Distributing Organs for Transplantation." In *Organ Transplantation Policy: Issues and Prospects*, pp. 87–113. Edited by James F. Blumstein and Frank A. Sloan. Durham, N.C.: Duke University Press.

———. 1991. "Deliberations of the Human Fetal Tissue Transplantation Research Panel." In *Biomedical Politics*, pp. 215–248. Edited by Kathi E. Hanna. Washington, D.C.: National Academy Press.

———. 1992. "The Body as Property: Some Philosophical Reflections." *Transplantation Proceedings* 24, no. 5:2143–2148.

COHEN, LLOYD R. 1989. "Increasing the Supply of Transplant Organs: The Virtues of a Futures Market." *George Washington Law Review* 58, no. 1:1–51.

GALLUP ORGANIZATION. 1985–1987. *The U.S. Public's Attitudes Toward Organ Transplants/Organ Donation*. Princeton, N.J.: Author.

———. 1993. *The American Public's Attitudes Toward Organ Donation and Transplantation*. Boston: Partnership for Organ Donation.

HANSMANN, HENRY. 1989. "The Economics and Ethics of Markets for Human Organs." In *Organ Transplantation Policy: Issues and Prospects*, pp. 57–85. Edited by James F. Blumstein and Frank A. Sloan. Durham, N.C.: Duke University Press.

HUMAN FETAL TISSUE TRANSPLANTATION RESEARCH PANEL (HFTTRP). 1988. *Report of the Human Fetal Tissue Transplantation Research Panel*. 2 vols. Bethesda, Md.: National Institutes of Health.

JONSEN, ALBERT R. 1988. "Transplantation of Fetal Tissue: An Ethicist's Viewpoint." *Clinical Research* 36, no. 3: 215–219.

LAND, WALTER, and COHEN, B. 1992. "Postmortem and Living Organ Donation in Europe: Transplant Laws and Activities." *Transplantation Proceedings* 24, no. 5:2165–2167.

MAY, WILLIAM F. 1973. "Attitudes Toward the Newly Dead." *Hastings Center Studies* 1, no. 1:3–13.

———. 1985. "Religious Justifications for Donating Body Parts." *Hastings Center Report* 15, no. 1:38–42.

———. 1991. *The Patient's Ordeal*. Bloomington: Indiana University Press.

MEYERS, DAVID W. 1990. *The Human Body and the Law*. 2d ed. Stanford, Calif.: Stanford University Press.

MURRAY, THOMAS H. 1987. "On the Human Body as Property: The Meaning of Embodiment, Markets, and the Meaning of Strangers." *University of Michigan Journal of Law Reform* 20, no. 4:1055–1088.

NATIONAL CONFERENCE OF COMMISSIONERS ON UNIFORM STATE LAWS. 1968. *Uniform Anatomical Gift Act*. Chicago: Author.

———. 1987. *Uniform Anatomical Gift Act 1987*. Chicago: Author.

NELSON, JAMES LINDEMANN. 1992. "The Rights and Responsibilities of Potential Organ Donors: A Communitarian Approach." Washington, D.C.: Communitarian Network.

PETERS, THOMAS G. 1991. "Life or Death: The Issue of Payment in Cadaveric Organ Donation." *Journal of the American Medical Association* 265, no. 10:1302–1304.

PROTTAS, JEFFREY M. 1985. "Organ Procurement in Europe and the United States." *Milbank Memorial Fund Quarterly/Health and Society* 63, no. 1:94–126.

PROTTAS, JEFFREY M., and BATTEN, HELEN L. 1988. "Health Professionals and Hospital Administrators in Organ Procurement: Attitudes, Reservations, and Their Resolutions." *American Journal of Public Health* 78, no. 6: 642–645.

RAMSEY, PAUL. 1970. *The Patient as Person: Explorations in Medical Ethics*. New Haven, Conn.: Yale University Press.

ROSNER, FRED, and TENDLER, MOSHE D. 1980. *Practical Medical Halacha*. 2d ed. Jerusalem: Feldheim.

SACHEDINA, ABDULAZIZ. 1988. "Islamic Views on Organ Transplantation." *Transplantation Proceedings* 20, no. 1 (suppl. 1):1084–1088.

SILVER, THEODORE. 1988. "The Case for a Post-Mortem Organ Draft and a Proposed Model Organ Draft Act." *Boston University Law Review* 68, no. 4:681–728.

VAWTER, DOROTHY E.; KEARNEY, WARREN; GERVAIS, KAREN G.; CAPLAN, ARTHUR L.; GARRY, DANIEL; and TAUER, CAROL. 1990. *The Use of Human Fetal Tissue: Scientific, Ethical, and Policy Concerns*. Minneapolis: Center for Biomedical Ethics, University of Minnesota.

VEATCH, ROBERT M. 1989. *Death, Dying, and the Biological Revolution: Our Last Quest for Responsibility*. Rev. ed. New Haven, Conn.: Yale University Press.

VIRNIG, BETH A., and CAPLAN, ARTHUR L. 1992. "Required Request: What Difference Has It Made?" *Transplantation Proceedings* 24, no. 5:2155–2158.

WALTERS, LEROY. 1990. "Statement." In *Fetal Tissue Transplantation Research: Hearing Before the Subcommittee on Health and the Environment of the Committee on Energy and Commerce, House of Representatives, 101st Congress, April 2, 1990*, pp. 13–16. Washington, D.C.: U.S. Government Printing Office.

YOUNGNER, STUART J. 1992. "Psychological Impediments to Procurement." *Transplantation Proceedings* 24, no. 5:2159–2161.

III. ETHICAL AND LEGAL ISSUES REGARDING LIVING DONORS

This article identifies and discusses key factors for ethical assessment of procurement of tissue or organs from living donors. These factors are then applied to several problematic categories of donors and specific cases. Finally, the relevance of a distinction between related and unrelated donors is considered, along with the question of whether there is a special obligation to donate organs or tissue to relatives.

Factors to consider

In ethical decisions about cases and policies involving living human donors, at least four considerations are relevant: (1) risks and benefits to the donor; (2) risks and benefits to the recipient; (3) possibility and validity of consent for donation; and (4) donor privacy and confidentiality.

Risks and benefits to the donor. Living persons may donate a variety of organs and tissues to others, including sperm, ova, blood and blood products, bone marrow, kidneys, and portions of lungs, and liver, and the pancreas. One way of estimating risks to potential donors is to consider whether the body can replace the donated material. For example, the body continually produces bone marrow, blood products, ova, and sperm;

therefore, those who donate them do not lose irreplaceable tissue. While the liver is not a replaceable organ, it can regenerate over time. Thus, donating a lobe of one's liver does not lead to significant loss of liver function. Although the tissue remaining after donation of a kidney or part of one's pancreas or lungs adapts to the loss, the previous level of function does not return.

The invasiveness, discomfort, and risks of procedures used in obtaining tissue or organs must also be taken into account. Acquisition of sperm is noninvasive and painless; blood products are obtained through a slightly painful but risk-free procedure. Bone marrow or ova retrieval is more complex and painful, requiring anesthesia. In addition, ova donation is generally preceded by administration of superovulatory drugs. Removal of kidneys, liver segments, lobes of lung, and sections of pancreas involve major surgery, with the concomitant risk of general anesthesia. Although the risk of vital organ retrieval is still small in experienced centers, the procedures have on rare occasions resulted in donor death (Levey et al., 1986; Moore, 1988). A survey of U.S. kidney transplant centers shows 5 donor deaths in 19,368 live donor transplants (Najarian et al., 1992).

Not surprisingly, when live kidney donation was first undertaken, the benefits of the procedure to donors were not anticipated (McGeown, 1968). Both the medical community and the public viewed donation primarily as an act of altruism whereby a person, generally an adult related to the recipient, suffered the costs of donation in order to help another human being. As transplant centers gained experience with kidney donation, benefits to donors became evident. Psychological studies revealed significant increases in donors' self-esteem (Fellner and Marshall, 1968; Simmons et al., 1977). Initially, it was thought that this resulted from the near-hero status accorded the donor, but follow-up studies showed that the benefit of increased confidence and self-esteem remained nine years after the transplant, when others' appreciation of the donation had virtually vanished (Marshall and Fellner, 1977). The success of the transplant influenced the effect on the donor, but not greatly. Only 5 percent of those who donated kidneys regretted their decision or had any difficulties in relating to the recipient when the transplant was successful. In contrast, 10 to 18 percent of those donating an organ in an unsuccessful transplant regretted their decision (Kamstra-Hennen et al., 1981). Most individuals felt closer to the recipient, whether or not the treatment was successful.

Risks and benefits to the recipient.   The risks and benefits to recipients of organ or tissue transplants from living donors depend mainly on the organ, the prospects of success, and the possibility of alternative therapy, including cadaver donation. Liver transplanta-

tion, for example, is a lifesaving procedure with a high likelihood of success in many groups of patients, regardless of whether the grafts come from living donors or cadavers (Belle et al., 1992). Living-donor liver transplantation saves lives by shortening the time that patients have to wait for organs. Significant numbers of patients die while awaiting cadaver livers—as high as 25 percent in one series of children (Malatack et al., 1987). Although it is impossible to gauge whether a particular recipient would have survived until a cadaver organ became available, liver transplant candidates as a whole would benefit from a policy of allowing or encouraging live organ donation (Singer et al., 1989).

Other transplants do not carry as clear a benefit to recipients. Live-donor kidney transplants have a high likelihood of success, and can help reduce the shortage of kidneys available for transplant. However, because of the availability of dialysis, patients' lives do not depend on kidney transplants. Typically, the recipient's request for a transplant is associated with the desire for a better quality of life. Although kidney transplants are less costly than chronic dialysis, the difference in cost is not generally borne by the recipient. Because of donor risks, possible pressure on donors, and the overall success of cadaver donation, there is some question whether living-donor kidney transplantation should still be encouraged (Starzl, 1985).

Pancreas transplants may help some diabetic patients live better lives, with fewer complications, but the overall benefits are not well known. Because the benefits are uncertain, some conclude that live-donor pancreas transplantation is unjustifiable (Lantos and Siegler, 1992). Bone marrow transplantation can be used as part of treatment for a variety of malignancies, with a wide range of prognoses. Donation of bone marrow for treatment of a nearly hopeless malignancy is obviously less compelling than donation for one in which the transplant offers a significant chance of recovery.

Possibility and validity of consent.   As with many medical procedures, it is important to consider whether the tissue donor is able to provide informed consent to the procedure. Can a donor, under pressure to save another person, sufficiently understand the risks and benefits described above and arrive at a decision regarding donation without being coerced?

Courts have consistently allowed individuals who are not capable of informed consent, such as children and incompetent adults, to donate tissue only when both the donor and the recipient are likely to benefit (Fost, 1977). Typically, the recipient is a relative whose continued health is important to the donor. In *Strunk v. Strunk* (1969), for example, the Kentucky Court of Appeals determined that the state could permit removal of a kidney from a mentally incompetent ward for transplantation into his brother, who provided him with companionship and caregiving. Similarly, in *Hart* v. *Brown* (1972) and *Little* v. *Little* (1979), the courts allowed removal of solid organs from minors for their siblings. In the Hart case, the court based its decision on what it thought the donor would want done, or the donor's "substituted judgment." However, it makes little sense to refer to the substituted judgment of someone who has never had decision-making capacity. In contrast, the other two cases were decided on grounds of the donors' best interests.

Courts do not consider donation to a relative with whom there is little or no relationship to be in the potential donor's best interests. In *In re Richardson* (1973), for example, the Louisiana Court of Appeals found that a potential child kidney donor was so severely disabled that his best interests would not be served by providing a kidney to his sister. In *Curran* v. *Bosze* (1990) the court refused to require two three-and-a-half-year-old twins to undergo blood testing to see whether they would be suitable bone marrow donors for a half brother with whom they had no contact.

In a widely publicized case, Mary Ayala conceived a child because she and her husband hoped to provide a suitable bone marrow donor for their teenage daughter, who suffered from leukemia (Morrow, 1991). The "best interests" standard followed in the above cases would justify the transplant from the infant on grounds that an immediate family member needed it. However, this case is obviously different in that the primary reason for the donor's existence was the cure of her sister. Nonetheless, it may be argued that the benefit to the child is twofold: that of existence, and that of contributing to the health of another. The benefit of existence may be sufficient in its own right to justify the burden to the infant donor.

The woman who became pregnant, gestated, and gave birth to the potential donor should also be considered a donor in the Ayala case. The benefits and risks to her, as well as respect for her autonomy, are pertinent ethical considerations not only in this case but also in others in which women are significantly and essentially involved through pregnancy. There are obvious parallels between this issue and those of surrogate motherhood and fetal tissue transplantation.

Unlike young children, who are assumed to be incompetent unless proven otherwise, adults are potentially competent to decide whether they want to be donors. Thus, as with other important medical decisions, health-care workers need to assess prospective adult donors to see if they are competent to decide about donation. Incompetent adults should be dealt with in the same way outlined above for children.

Even with competent adults, some have questioned whether many donors reach their decision to donate in a manner that reflects genuine informed consent. A high percentage of adult donors decide to pursue donation immediately upon hearing of the possibility, even before they are aware of information relevant to their decision, or before they have time for rational reflection (Fellner and Marshall, 1968; Simmons et al., 1977). Even with time for reflection, many state that they could not have been dissuaded from donating, and that the decision to donate could not be compared with their normal decision-making process. One could conclude that such decisions, while not truly informed, are nonetheless free.

There are several possible ways of responding to immediate attempts to pursue donation. One is to distinguish between the decision and informed consent. Those who make an immediate (free) decision can subsequently become informed and then provide informed consent (or dissent) to the donation. Alternatively, one could regard living organ donation as a special case, in which one cannot and ought not to expect to attain the degree of informed consent that health care usually demands. Whether either response, potential donors should be given adequate time and information to reach informed decisions. The medical profession should not demand that all donors base their decisions on rational reflection, but should permit immediate decision making as an expression of autonomy. In contrast to either of these responses, one could argue that it is wrong to perform living-donor transplants if donors fail to utilize the time and information available in arriving at a rational decision. This last position seems to go beyond what a policy of informed consent should require.

Some cases involving adolescent donors raise questions about their ability to give informed consent. Studies of a group of kidney donors sixteen to twenty years old showed that many made instantaneous decisions to pursue donation (Bernstein and Simmons, 1974). A prevalent motive for donation was the desire to be recognized as an adult. One teenage donor expressed a desire for more access to the family car, while others, who viewed themselves as "black sheep," hoped to gain more acceptance by their families. Such motives suggest the importance of determining that the decision is truly free, that the best interests of the adolescent will be served by the donation, and that the donation is likely to benefit the recipient. As with the court cases described above, one does not necessarily need informed consent to justify donation from a minor. But as a child approaches adulthood, his or her opinion must be given increasing weight in deciding whether to allow donation. And there is no justification to force an adolescent to donate who does not want to.

Issues regarding donor privacy and confidentiality. Living-donor transplants raise special concerns regarding the privacy and confidentiality of potential donors. To identify and choose among appropriate related donors, transplant teams generally need to evaluate multiple members of the potential recipient's family. It is often difficult to keep such information and discussions private (Simmons et al., 1971). Lack of privacy and confidentiality can compromise the autonomy of potential donors. For example, while some family members vie over who will be allowed to donate, some undergo significant pressure to donate and others who wish to donate are sometimes pressured to refrain from donation.

Privacy and confidentiality are also threatened in cases involving unrelated potential donors. In *Head v. Colloton* (1983), for example, a man in need of a bone marrow transplant for his leukemia learned that the hospital's registry included the name of a potential donor. In accordance with hospital policy, she had been asked whether she would consider donating bone marrow to a nonrelative in need. On learning that the potential donor had no such interest, the patient asked to be informed of her identity so that he could make a direct appeal to her. The court refused to reveal the woman's identity on grounds that provision of such information would breach confidentiality.

Because violations of privacy and confidentiality may compromise autonomy, they are closely related to the preceding discussion of informed consent. Transplant teams evaluating potential donors must pay close attention to the factors influencing donors' decisions in order to ensure that those decisions are both informed and free.

Special groups

Potential living donors in whom the possibility of informed consent is absent or questionable deserve particular attention. Although fetuses may be considered in this group, it is generally assumed that only fetal remains, rather than living fetuses, may be used in transplantation. A related issue inevitably involves a living person, the pregnant woman whose fetus may be used in transplantation. Some have argued that a woman who has decided to terminate her pregnancy should not be considered a donor of fetal tissue provided through her abortion, because she "abandons her parental capacity to authorize research on that offspring." However, the majority of a federal panel considering this issue maintained that a woman's choice of abortion does not disqualify her "as the primary decisionmaker about the disposition of fetal remains" (Human Fetal Tissue Panel, 1988). If a woman is regarded as the donor of fetal tissue, the same ethical concerns that apply to other adult donors are applicable to her.

Anencephalic newborns are another problematic category of potential living donors. If an anencephalic newborn fulfills the criteria of brain death, the same ethical criteria apply to use of its vital organs and tissue as would apply to use of tissue from cadaveric donors for whom there are no advance directives. Unlike other potential living donors, however, anencephalics who do not fulfill the criteria of brain death have been considered a potential source of organs and tissues. In order for organs or tissue from anencephalic infants to be transplanted successfully, it is helpful to obtain them before the infants become brain dead (Peabody et al., 1989). However, society does not condone retrieval of vital organs from living donors because such retrieval is tantamount to homicide. Because anencephalic infants inevitably die within a short time, some have proposed considering these infants as a unique category of individuals for whom "brain absence" suffices as justification for retrieval of their vital organs before whole brain death occurs (Holzgreve et al., 1987). In fact, living anencephalic infants have some degree of functioning brain stem, despite the absence of cortical function; "brain absence" is therefore inaccurate.

Others have argued that society should permit vital organ donation from living anencephalics on the same grounds that it permits donation from brain-dead individuals: neither situation involves any expectation of sentient life or survival on the part of the donor (Truog and Fletcher, 1989). This proposal has drawn little support from those who develop public policy. In Germany, Japan, and the United States, living anencephalic infants may not be legally used as vital organ donors. Although Canada and the United Kingdom do not specifically exclude the use of living anencephalic donors, the practice is rarely attempted (Rothenberg, 1990).

Because anencephalics and persons in a persistent vegetative state lack the ability to think, communicate, and experience pain or pleasure, it is difficult to see what benefits or ill effects could accrue to them through donation of their organs or tissue. In contrast, the benefits of transplantation to recipients are clear and significant. Nonetheless, so long as death is legally defined as complete cessation of brain activity, it is highly unlikely that either of these groups will be used as a source of vital organs or tissue in the near future.

Additional categories of vulnerable patients include those whose capacity for informed consent may be compromised by institutionalization. Prisoners are an example in this regard. At the Peter Bent Brigham Hospital in Boston, the use of kidneys from prisoners was considered and rejected on two occasions (Moore, 1988). First, the hospital's transplant team discussed the payment of convicts for kidney donation. Their chief concern was that the prisoners would expect favorable treatment and decide to donate for spurious reasons. When the issue was broached a second time, a prisoner awaiting execution requested immunologic testing so that his organs could be made readily available. Here the team was concerned that society might unduly profit from the punishment. Possibly because these concerns have not been carefully scrutinized, no consensus has been reached on donation of organs from institutionalized populations.

Another category of living donors whose consent to donation may be questioned is women. The possibility of discrimination arises because of the disproportionate number of women who are donors. In the United States, 63 percent of kidneys donated to children by their parents came from the child's mother, despite the fact that paternal donations have a longer average graft survival (Koka and Cecka, 1991). At least two factors probably contribute to the disproportionality. First, women are more likely than men to be the primary caregivers of those in need of transplants. Donation of organs or tissue may be viewed as an extension of this role. Second, the incomes of women tend to be considerably less than those of men. Where either a man or a woman might serve as donor, the one with the higher income is more likely to continue working while the other donates. Women who are unemployed outside of the home may be particularly pressured to donate in such circumstances. Concerns about possible coercion must be addressed, but they do not provide an adequate argument for excluding women as donors. While transplant teams must attend to the possibility of compromised autonomy on the part of the donor, they also need to weigh the benefits as well as the burdens to her.

Payment of living donors. In general, economically disadvantaged people are vulnerable to exploitation. Although sale of solid organs is prohibited in the United States, sale of ova, sperm, and plasma is allowed. The difference in compensation rates reflects the difference in risk and discomfort, averaging $50 for sperm donation and $1,500 or more for egg donation (Brozan, 1988; Monarez, 1992). Not surprisingly, paid donors of gametes tend to be economically poorer than the recipients of their tissue. Poorer still are some who sell their plasma. If their blood type is unusual, such individuals may have a relatively reliable source of income. In all of these situations the autonomy of the donor may be compromised by economic need.

The impact of economic need is further dramatized by the prevalent sale of solid organs in Third World countries such as India (Moore, 1988) and Egypt (Hedges, 1992). Because such "donations" are ethically troubling, the Egyptian government banned kidney transplants from unrelated donors (Hedges, 1992). The question raised by the practice and the ban is whether a person who is unable to obtain adequate food, clothing, or shelter can freely decide to sell a kidney. Poverty is clearly a coercive factor in such situations, but whether it wholly negates the possibility that an individual can act autonomously is another matter. Moreover, even if poverty limits autonomy, individuals may have a moral right to sell their organs to obtain goods necessary for survival, or to improve the condition of their own or others' lives.

Concerns about justice inform arguments both for and against the sale of organs. Some argue that no solid organs should be sold, because once the practice is permitted, both the buying and the selling of organs will inevitably discriminate against the weakest members of society. Others argue that while we must address the injustices and economic realities that create such poverty, we should allow those caught in this situation to do what they can in the meantime.

Related versus unrelated donation

The vast majority of living-donor solid organ and bone marrow transplants involve relatives. Sperm and blood product donation, on the other hand, usually take place anonymously among unrelated persons. The riskier the donation, the greater the burden of finding lasting or significant donor benefits. The risk–benefit ratio seems to improve with related donation, because helping a close family member brings more direct benefits (Singer et al., 1989). Similar reasons underlie the court cases described above regarding whether to allow minors and incompetent adults to provide organs or tissue to others.

Related donation is even more compelling if it is assumed that we have special obligations toward those to whom we are related. Such obligations follow from an ethic of "filial duty" (Sommers, 1986). In contrast to an ethic of impartiality, an ethic of filial duty requires one to preferentially assist one's close relatives. Thus living donation to a parent may be morally obligatory, while donation to a stranger is altruistic or virtuous. One could take this approach one step further and argue that special responsibilities are not limited to family members, but also extend to close relationships such as friendships (Friedman, 1989). Either of these views supports the decision in *Head* v. *Colloton* (1983) that one is not obliged to donate one's bone marrow to a stranger. In addition, a filial or relation-based ethic is consistent with the phenomenon that some people feel compelled to donate to relatives and loved ones but are unwilling to donate organs or tissue to strangers.

Others argue that we ought to be more accepting of unrelated organ donation. Even unrelated donors may benefit from the donation, and thus their actions need not be understood solely as an extreme expression of altruism (Fellner, 1973). Transplant teams may look upon those willing to donate an organ to a stranger with suspicion, as if their motives cannot be as pure as those donating to a relative. Instead, one could recognize organ donation as an act of the highest morality. Whether related or unrelated, donors generally want to help another person, and will probably feel better about themselves in the future because of their donation.

A utilitarian approach to this question suggests that unrelated donation should be allowed when the risks of donation are low and the potential benefits of both donor and recipient are great (Levey et al., 1986). Prohibiting organ or tissue retrieval from living donors would be paternalistic toward donors, and would deny important benefits to recipients. To facilitate donation from nonrelatives, a national bone marrow registry has been established in the United States. Through use of the registry, clinicians who treat prospective recipients can find medically suitable, willing donors for their patients.

Conclusion

The factors identified above present an outline for examining the ethical parameters of cases and policies involving living-donor transplantation. Two general considerations are relevant in weighing these factors: first, that the donor's autonomy and privacy be maximized, and second, that there be adequate opportunity to reflect on the risks and benefits involved (Caplan and Siegler, 1985). Procedurally, the ethical assessment may be done by transplant teams, with recourse to ethics consultation, institutional review boards, or ethics committees when this seems necessary or helpful. Evaluation of the donor should ordinarily be conducted by someone who is an advocate for the donor and is not a member of the transplant team (Caplan and Siegler, 1985; House and Thompson, 1988). Although living donors are generally healthy, ethical obligations of beneficence and respect for autonomy apply to them as well as to the recipients.

PETER A. UBEL
MARY B. MAHOWALD

Directly related to this article are the other articles in this entry: MEDICAL AND ORGANIZATIONAL ASPECTS, *and* ETHICAL AND LEGAL ISSUES REGARDING CADAVERS. *Also directly related are the entries* ORGAN AND TISSUE TRANSPLANTS, *especially the article on* SOCIOCULTURAL PERSPECTIVES; INFORMED CONSENT, *article on* MEANING AND ELEMENTS OF INFORMED CONSENT; RISK; FREEDOM AND COERCION; CONFIDENTIALITY; PRIVACY IN HEALTH CARE; *and* OBLIGATION AND SUPEREROGATION. *This article will find application in the entries* BLOOD TRANSFUSION; *and* REPRODUCTIVE TECHNOLOGIES, *articles on* ARTIFICIAL INSEMINATION, *and* CRYOPRESERVATION OF SPERM, OVA, AND EMBRYOS. *Other relevant material may be found under* XENOGRAFTS.

Bibliography

BELLE, STEVEN H.; BERINGER, KIMBERLY C.; MURPHY, JANICE B.; PLUMMER, CHRISTINE C.; BREEN, TIMOTHY J.; EDWARDS, ERICK B.; DAILY, O. PATRICK; and DETRE, KATHERINE M. 1992. "Liver Transplantation in the United States: 1988 to 1990." In *Clinical Transplants, 1991*, pp. 13–29. Edited by Paul I. Terasaki and J. Michael Cecka. Los Angeles: UCLA Tissue Typing Laboratory.

BERNSTEIN, DOROTHY M., and SIMMONS, ROBERTA G. 1974. "The Adolescent Kidney Donor: The Right to Give." *American Journal of Psychiatry* 131, no. 12:1338–1343.

BROZAN, NADINE. 1988. "Rising Use of Donated Eggs for Pregnancy Stirs Concern." *New York Times*, January 18, p. A1.

CAPLAN, ARTHUR L. 1993. "Must I Be My Brother's Keeper? Issues in the Use of Living Donors." *Transplantation Proceedings* 25, no. 2:1997–2000.

CAPLAN, ARTHUR L., and SIEGLER, MARK. 1985. "Risk, Paternalism, and the Gift of Life." *Archives of Internal Medicine* 145, no. 7:1188–1190.

Curran v. Bosze. 1990. 141 Ill.2d 473. (S.C.).

FELLNER, CARL H. 1973. "Organ Donation: For Whose Sake?" *Annals of Internal Medicine* 79, no. 4:589–592.

FELLNER, CARL H., and MARSHALL, JOHN R. 1968. "Twelve Kidney Donors." *Journal of the American Medical Association* 206, no. 12:2703–2707.

FOST, NORMAN. 1977. "Children as Renal Donors." *New England Journal of Medicine* 296, no. 7:363–367.

FRIEDMAN, MARILYN. 1989. "Feminism and Modern Friendship: Dislocating the Community." *Ethics* 99, no. 2: 275–290.

Hart v. Brown. 1972. 29 Con. Supp. 368.

Head v. Colloton. 1983. 331 N.W.2d 870. (Iowa).

HEDGES, CHRIS. 1992. "Egyptian Doctors Limit Kidney Transplants." *New York Times*, January 23, p. A5.

HOLZGREVE, WOLFGANG; BELLER, FRITZ K.; BUCHHOLZ, BERND; HANSMANN, MANFRED; and KÖHLER, KURT. 1987. "Kidney Transplantation from Anencephalic Donors." *New England Journal of Medicine* 316, no. 17: 1069–1070.

HOUSE, ROBERT M., and THOMPSON, TROY L. 1988. "Psychiatric Aspects of Organ Transplantation." *Journal of the American Medical Association* 260, no. 4:535–539.

HUMAN FETAL TISSUE TRANSPLANTATION RESEARCH PANEL. 1988. *Report of the Human Fetal Tissue Transplantation Research Panel*, vol. 1, pp. 6, 47. Bethesda, Md.: National Institutes of Health.

KAMSTRA-HENNEN, L.; BEEBE, J.; STUMM, S.; and SIMMONS, R. G. 1981. "Ethical Evaluation of Related Donation: The Donor After Five Years." *Transplantation Proceedings* 13, no. 1, pt. 1:60–61.

KEARNEY, WILLIAM, and CAPLAN, ARTHUR L. 1992. "Parity for the Donation of Bone Marrow: Ethical and Policy Considerations." In vol. 1 of *Emerging Issues in Biomedical Policy: An Annual Review*, pp. 262–285. Edited by Robert H. Blank and Andrea L. Bonnicksen. New York: Columbia University Press.

KOKA, PRASAD, and CECKA, J. MICHAEL. 1990. "Sex and Age

Effects in Renal Transplantation." In *Clinical Transplants, 1990*, pp. 437–445. Edited by Paul I. Terasaki. Los Angeles: UCLA Tissue Typing Laboratory.

LANTOS, JOHN D., and SIEGLER, MARK. 1991. "Re-evaluating Donor Criteria: Live Donors." In *The Surgeon General's Workshop on Increasing Organ Donation: Background Papers*, pp. 271–290. Washington, D.C.: U.S. Department of Health and Human Services.

LEVEY, ANDREW S.; HOU, SUSAN; and BUSH, HARRY L. 1986. "Kidney Transplantation from Unrelated Living Donors: Time to Reclaim a Discarded Opportunity." *New England Journal of Medicine* 314, no. 14:914–916.

Little v. Little. 1979. 576 S.W.2d 493. (Tex. Civ.)

MALATACK, J. JEFFREY; SCHAID, DANIEL J.; URBACH, ANDREW H.; GARTNER, J. CARLTON, JR.; ZITELLI, BASIL J.; ROCKETTE, HOWARD; FISCHER, JOHN; STARZL, THOMAS E.; IWATSUKI, SHUNZABURO; and SHAW, BEYERS W. 1987. "Choosing a Pediatric Recipient for Orthotopic Liver Transplantation." *Journal of Pediatrics* 111, no. 4:479–489.

MARSHALL, JOHN R., and FELLNER, CARL H. 1977. "Kidney Donors Revisited." *American Journal of Psychiatry* 134, no. 5:575–576.

McGEOWN, MARY G. 1968. "Ethics for the Use of Live Donors in Kidney Transplantation." *American Heart Journal* 75, no. 5:711–714.

MONAREZ, PAULA. 1992. "Halfway There: Egg Donors Help Couples Solve the Conception Equation." *Chicago Tribune*, February 2, sec. 6, p. 4.

MOORE, F. D. 1988. "Three Ethical Revolutions: Ancient Assumptions Remodeled Under Pressure of Transplantation." *Transplantation Proceedings* 20, no. 1, supp. 1:1061–1067.

MORROW, LANCE. 1991. "When One Body Can Save Another." *Time*, June 17, pp. 54–58.

NAJARIAN, JOHN S.; CHAVERS, BLANCHE M.; McHUGH, LOIS E.; and MATAS, ARTHUR J. 1992. "20 Years or More of Follow-up of Living Kidney Donors." *Lancet* 340, no. 8823:807–810.

PEABODY, JOYCE L.; EMERY, JANET R.; and ASHWAL, STEPHEN. 1989. "Experience with Anencephalic Infants as Prospective Organ Donors." *New England Journal of Medicine* 321, no. 6:344–350.

Richardson, In re. 1973. 284 So.2d 185. (La. App.).

ROTHENBERG, L. S. 1990. "The Anencephalic Neonate and Brain Death: An International Review of Medical, Ethical, and Legal Issues." *Transplantation Proceedings* 22, no. 3:1037–1039.

SIMMONS, ROBERTA G.; HICKEY, KATHLEEN; KJELLSTRAND, CARL M.; and SIMMONS, RICHARD L. 1971. "Family Tension in the Search for a Kidney Donor." *Journal of the American Medical Association* 215, no. 6:909–912.

SIMMONS, ROBERTA G.; KLEIN, SUSAN D.; and SIMMONS, RICHARD L. 1977. *Gift of Life: The Social and Psychological Impact of Organ Transplantation.* New York: John Wiley and Sons.

SINGER, PETER A.; SIEGLER, MARK; WHITINGTON, PETER F.; LANTOS, JOHN D.; EMOND, JEAN C.; THISTLETHWAITE, J. RICHARD; and BROELSCH, CHRISTOPHER E. 1989. "Ethics of Liver Transplantation with Living Donors." *New England Journal of Medicine* 321, no. 9:620–622.

SOMMERS, CHRISTINA HOFF. 1986. "Filial Morality." *Journal of Philosophy* 83, no. 8:439–456.

STARZL, THOMAS E. 1985. "Will Live Organ Donations No Longer Be Justified?" *Hastings Center Report* 15, no. 2:5.

Strunk v. Strunk. 1969. 445 S.W.2d 145. (Ky.).

TRUOG, ROBERT D., and FLETCHER, JOHN C. 1989. "Anencephalic Newborns: Can Organs Be Transplanted Before Brain Death?" *New England Journal of Medicine* 321, no. 6:388–391.

ORGAN AND TISSUE TRANSPLANTS

I. Medical Overview
   Calvin R. Stiller
II. Sociocultural Aspects
   Renée C. Fox
   Judith P. Swazey
III. Ethical and Legal Issues
   Arthur L. Caplan

I. MEDICAL OVERVIEW

Since the first successful kidney transplant was performed in 1954 by Joseph Murray at the Peter Bent Brigham Hospital in Boston, remarkable advances have occurred in transplantation. In addition to kidneys, numerous other organs and tissues can now be transplanted. Better preservation of organs allows longer storage times so organs can be transported over greater distances. Antirejection drugs have dramatically improved success rates. Consequently, increasing numbers of patients are referred to waiting lists for transplant surgery. Certain areas remain problematic, however. Rejection of the transplanted organ and posttransplant complications, such as infection and cancer, can be monitored and treated but not necessarily prevented. The major obstacle remains the inadequate number of organs to meet the need of potential recipients.

Development of transplantation

Attempts to transplant a kidney from one person to another were made from the 1930s until the early 1950s. The initiative for these attempts was based on laboratory experiments by Alexis Carrel who had developed techniques for suturing blood vessels in 1902. These early transplants failed because every patient's immune system recognized that the transplanted organ (often called a graft) was a foreign substance. The immune system then attacked and destroyed the organ (rejection). Success was finally achieved in 1954 because the donor and recipient were identical twins. Because every healthy person has two kidneys, one kidney can be donated from a living person to another person. Identical twins have the same tissue type, so the recipient's immune system perceives the transplant organ as a part of its own body and does not reject the organ.

An organ or tissue that is transplanted between genetically identical twins is called an isograft. Allografts are organs or tissues that are transplanted between genetically nonidentical people, which occurs when organs or tissues are donated from a deceased person (cadaver donor). An autograft is a tissue transplanted from one part of a person's body to another part, for example, when a burn victim has healthy skin grafted from one area of the body to the burned area. A xenograft is an organ or tissue transplanted from a different species, for example, a baboon liver transplanted into a human.

During the 1950s, antirejection drugs had not yet been developed, so transplants were limited to kidneys from identical-twin donors. In 1959, however, Murray and his colleagues at Brigham Hospital again achieved a historical feat. They transplanted a kidney from a nonidentical twin to his brother who had undergone total body X-ray treatment. This patient lived twenty-six years. X-ray treatment (irradiation) had suppressed his immune response so that his body accepted the new organ. Irradiation was also tried with kidney transplants from cadaver donors. For most patients, however, the outcome was fatal because their immune systems were suppressed too much. Although they accepted the transplanted organ, patients died from infection because irradiation had reduced their natural defenses against bacteria and viruses. It seemed evident that irradiation for transplantation "was too dangerous to be practical" (Starzl, 1992).

During this time, chemical immunosuppression (drug therapy) was being studied. In 1960, René Küss in France achieved successful nonrelated kidney transplantation using a combination of total-body irradiation, steroids, and 6-mercaptopurine. Azathioprine (also called Imuran) was later derived from 6-mercaptopurine. The combination of azathioprine and prednisone (a type of steroid), suggested by Roy Calne, was a clinical milestone in 1962 as transplant results improved and fewer side effects occurred.

In 1967, the heart and the liver were each successfully transplanted—the heart by Christiaan Barnard in Capetown, South Africa, and the liver by Thomas Starzl in Denver, Colorado. These successful transplants were followed by a flurry of activity as hospitals worldwide rushed to perform transplant surgery. Lung, bowel, and pancreas transplants were attempted during the 1960s.

Most of these attempts failed and many transplant programs abruptly stopped.

By 1975, there were only two liver transplant programs in the world. Starzl was continuing to transplant in Denver, Colorado, and Roy Calne was leading a program in Cambridge, England. Lung transplantation was not tried for another fifteen years when the Toronto General Hospital in Canada established single-lung transplantation in 1983 and double-lung transplantation in 1986 as successful treatments.

Success with bowel transplantation was difficult to achieve. The intestine has a large number of cells called lymphocytes, which help trigger rejection and also react against the recipient (graft-versus-host disease). Bowel transplantation was not successfully performed until the late 1980s when a patient in Kiel, Germany, and another in Paris, France, had prolonged survival of small-bowel grafts. The first successful combined small-bowel and liver transplant took place at University Hospital (London, Canada) in 1988. Experience from these centers and from Pittsburgh, where more than fifty patients received intestinal grafts, showed that the bowel could be successfully transplanted. Patients who either had part of their bowel removed or had inadequate bowel function could resume eating a normal diet after their transplant without the need of special intravenous feeding solutions. The antirejection drug FK506 improved the success rate of bowel transplantation.

Transplantation of islet of Langerhans cells from the pancreas first occurred in the mid-1970s. Rather than transplanting the donor's whole pancreas, the insulin-producing islet cells were removed from the pancreas. The cells, injected into the liver's portal vein, adhered to the liver. The cells then began producing insulin. For diabetic patients who had to take insulin to stabilize their blood-sugar levels, islet-cell transplantation eliminated or reduced the need for daily insulin injections. It was not until 1990, however, that reports began to emerge of short-term and prolonged insulin independence (Tzakis et al., 1990; Scharp et al., 1990). Despite limited success, human islet-cell transplantation research continues. Because of the inadequate number of cadaver donors, the future may require using animal islet cells, probably from pigs.

In addition to islet cells, many other tissues can be successfully transplanted: the cornea from the eye, skin, bones and joints, heart valves, and bone marrow. Blood is the most frequently transplanted tissue, followed by bone; bone marrow is donated only from living donors.

The cadaver organ donor

Traditionally, death has been declared on the basis of cardiopulmonary criteria: The heart stops beating and the patient no longer breathes. Once the heart stops beating, oxygen-rich blood is no longer pumped to the body's organs, and the organs' cell functions begin to deteriorate. During the 1960s, organs came either from living donors (for kidneys) or from cadaver donors who were declared dead by the traditional cardiopulmonary criteria (nonheartbeating donors). The first successful liver and heart transplants in 1967 used organs from donors who were removed from ventilators (artificial breathing machines) and pronounced dead after the heart had stopped.

As medical technology progressed and it became possible to maintain bodies after death using mechanical support, doctors needed to determine when a patient could be declared dead. Accordingly, in 1968, an ad hoc committee comprising medical doctors, a lawyer, a philosopher, and a theologian convened at the Harvard Medical School to define acceptable criteria for brain death. They decided that death could be declared by neurologic criteria rather than the traditional cardiac criteria. Brain-dead donors, with the assistance of a ventilator, have oxygen circulating in their blood that maintains the usefulness of organs for transplant. Brain death is declared after a series of tests have been performed. The cause of death, such as trauma, intracerebral hemorrhage, hypoxia, or primary brain tumor, must be known. Patients with potentially reversible conditions, such as hypothermia or drug-induced coma, are not considered potential donors. The patient, therefore, is in an irreversible coma and does not respond to pain. There are no brain-stem reflexes so the patient does not breathe, swallow, or blink. Apnea testing shows that the patient cannot breathe when taken off the ventilator. After death, tests ensure that the deceased patient is a suitable donor, without disease or infection that could possibly be transmitted to the transplant patient.

In 1971, Finland became the first nation to accept brain-death criteria as legal. In most countries, brain-dead donors are preferred for transplant rather than nonheartbeating donors, because the former usually provide better quality organs. Most countries recognize the legal status of brain death, but if they do not have specific laws, they accept brain death as a medical basis to declare death.

When brain-death criteria are not recognized as a way to diagnose death, transplants are usually limited to tissues and kidneys. By the time the heart has stopped beating and death is declared through the absence of pulse and respiration, other organs are usually damaged. In Japan, for example, the public is equally divided between accepting brain-death criteria and accepting cardiopulmonary criteria for declaring death. Although the Japanese government issued a statement about brain death and organ transplantation in 1992, proposed legislation ensured that organs other than kidneys would be acceptable for transplant. In Japan, only about 30 per-

cent of kidneys are retrieved from cadaver donors with 70 percent of kidneys donated from living relatives. Although brain death had not been legally recognized, a nationwide survey found that one-third of cadaver kidneys were removed from brain-dead patients; the remainder were removed from nonheartbeating donors (Ota, 1991).

Nonheartbeating donors also have been used in Spain, The Netherlands, and the United States, although these countries have predominantly used brain-dead donors. Before 1988, when Sweden adopted its brain-death laws, transplant programs retrieved and transplanted livers from donors whose hearts had stopped beating. Because of the worldwide shortage of organ donors, many countries have explored the possibility of using nonheartbeating donors in addition to brain-dead donors.

The living organ donor

In many countries, living donors are used to a greater extent because of the limited number of cadaver donors. In Japan, as mentioned, approximately 70 percent of kidneys are donated from living donors who are genetically related to the recipients (living related donors). When the donor and recipient are genetically related, the kidney transplant is more likely to succeed (Gülay et al., 1989). In Turkey, living related donors are considered the primary source of kidneys, followed by cadaver donors and living donors who are not genetically related, such as a spouse, friend, or a stranger (living unrelated donors). In Central and South America, about 60 percent of kidneys are donated from living donors, although Cuba, Uruguay, Colombia, and Venezuela are mostly cadaver donors (Santiago-Delpin, 1991). Living unrelated donors are used routinely in Brazil and Peru and occasionally in Guatemala, Puerto Rico, Bolivia, and Mexico. In India, living donors are used exclusively and transplant programs are limited to kidneys. In countries that typically use cadaver donors, the rate of living donors varies: the United States, 26 percent; Canada, 15 percent; Europe, 11 percent; and Australia, 6 percent (Bonomini, 1991).

Living related donors are used for kidney and bone-marrow transplantation and, in a limited number of cases, for liver, lung, pancreas, and bowel transplants. Living unrelated donors are used for both kidney and bone-marrow transplants and have begun for liver transplants in children. For living donation of the liver, lung, pancreas, or bowel, only a small segment of the organ is removed. Given the severe shortage of donated cadaver organs, relatives, especially parents, may feel compelled to donate. The donor is informed of the risks and benefits of the donation. Although they place themselves at risk, donors may experience a greater psychological benefit from saving, or attempting to save, for instance, their child's life. The recipient does not have to wait as long for the transplant and will likely be healthier. This factor, combined with a reduced ischemic time—the length of time the organ has no blood supply—may provide greater success than transplants from cadaver donors. Because the donor and recipient operations can take place simultaneously and the organ does not have to be stored and transported, ischemia is reduced and organ function is not compromised.

Despite better long-term results than those achieved with cadaver organs, living kidney donation remains contentious. Some physicians and surgeons have questioned the justification for living donation that could potentially harm the donor. On the other hand, living donations are an important avenue to reduce the organ shortage. Without living donors, many patients would be denied transplantation. Consequently, some transplant programs accept living unrelated kidney donors who are fully informed of the potential risks, benefits, and alternatives. The donation must also be motivated by altruism rather than profit, because buying organs from living donors is prohibited in most countries. In India and other countries, organ buying occurs because cadaver donation either is not allowed or is very limited. If a patient does not have a suitable relative who can donate a kidney, then buying a kidney from a living donor is an alternative to dialysis or death.

Consent

For living donations, the donor must provide consent. For cadaver donations in North America, the next of kin provides consent, specifying which organs and tissues will be donated. This is often called an "opting-in" system because explicit consent must be given for donation to occur. Although a signed donor card from the deceased patient is a legal document, hospital staff follow the wishes of the next of kin. Hospital staff may fear litigation or a public backlash against transplantation if organs are removed without the next of kin's consent. In the United States, legislation requires hospital staff to inform families of potential donors about the opportunity to donate ("required request"). Initially, the practice of required request increased the number of organ and tissue donations, although increases were not sustained. Financial incentives for the families of potential cadaver donors have been explored in the United States. Incentives may encourage the next of kin to consent to organ donation. Incentives could, for example, be a payment for burial expenses or a tax rebate. Some transplant experts fear incentives would have a negative effect—the rate of donations could decline if people perceived this practice as buying the organs. In Canada, each province legislates on organ donation. Several

provinces have implemented required-request or similar legislation.

A few European countries—Britain, the Netherlands, Germany, and Turkey—have instituted opting-in systems. In most European countries, the next of kin's consent is not required, because this system presumes that potential donors would consent to organ donation unless they had specifically objected before their death ("presumed consent"). This has also been referred to as an "opting-out" system because explicit refusal must be given. Organs may be retrieved without the family's permission. However, in some of these countries medical personnel still approach family members to ensure that they have no objection. In the Scandinavian countries, Finland and Norway use presumed-consent legislation, whereas Sweden and Denmark follow an opting-in law. Some countries using presumed consent report a higher donation rate per capita than countries using a voluntary, opting-in system; other countries that use presumed consent have lower donation rates. There is no clear-cut relationship between presumed consent and high donation rates. The more recent trend in Europe is toward opting-in legislation and away from presumed consent.

Retrieval

Organ retrieval.   After patients are declared dead, they are transferred to an operating room where organs and tissues are removed. Sometimes, organs are removed, preserved, and sent directly to a transplant center. Often the transplant team travels to the hospital to remove and transport the organs. Surgical teams from different hospitals may be involved. Each team removes a different organ before returning by jet to its own transplant center.

In the operating room an incision is made on the donor that extends from the sternal notch (breastbone) to the pelvis. The rib cage is retracted so the organs can be seen easily. The organs are visually examined to check for damage or disease that perhaps was not detected by earlier tests. If the organ appears normal, the surgeon begins to carefully dissect, or cut away, the tissue surrounding the organ. If several organs will be removed, dissection takes approximately two hours. The aorta (the blood vessel through which blood flows from the heart to the rest of the body) is then clamped. A specially prepared, cold solution flushes blood out of each organ and lowers the organ's temperature, thereby helping to preserve the organ.

The heart or lungs are removed first; for heart-lung transplants, the heart and lungs are removed together. The liver and small bowel are usually removed next, followed by the pancreas and kidneys. The kidneys are removed together and then separated. The kidneys are preserved and packed separately so that two patients can be transplanted.

Each organ that has been removed is stored in a sterile container with a cold preservation solution, then surrounded by ice, and transported in another container, which looks like a picnic cooler. Because storage times are limited, the recipient is in surgery for immediate transplant when the organ arrives. When the ischemic time is shortened, initial organ function is better after transplant. When the donor and recipient are at the same transplant center, the surgeries can be done simultaneously so that organs do not have to be cold-stored for long periods.

Tissue retrieval. After organs have been removed, tissue recovery occurs if consent has been given. If rib bones are being donated, the chest remains open; otherwise, the kidney surgeons suture the abdomen and chest closed. The eyes or corneas are usually the first tissues removed. Often the entire eye is removed, placed in a sterile container with a solution, and sent to the nearest eye bank. The cornea of the eye is then removed, placed in a preservation solution, and usually transplanted within two or three days. Bones and joints as well as skin can be donated. A very thin layer of skin, similar to peeling from a sunburn, is removed.

Tissues can also be donated when organ donation does not occur. Eurotransplant in the Netherlands, for example, reported that only 8 percent of cornea donors, 32 percent of bone donors, and 84 percent of heart-valve donors also donated organs (de By, 1991). In most countries, organ donors are declared dead while connected to a ventilator, which helps to artificially support organ function. Without a ventilator, organs usually cannot be used for transplant but tissues can be donated within certain time limits. Tissue donors, therefore, can be referred from chronic-care facilities, emergency departments, and funeral homes.

Organ and tissue recovery is a delicate surgical procedure. Transplant staff are careful to prevent visible disfigurement so that usual funeral arrangements, including an open casket, are possible.

Preservation

Organ preservation. Preservation ensures adequate time to retrieve and distribute organs so that every suitable organ can be used. Various preservation solutions have been developed including Collins, Euro-Collins, HTK solution, and UW solution. Different solutions can be used for different organs removed from the same donor. These solutions slow down the organ's cell function through hypothermia. There are time limits that organs can be cold-stored ("cold ischemic time") before permanent cell damage occurs and the organ cannot be used for transplant. When the organ is removed

from the cold solution, the preservation solution is flushed out before the organ is transplanted into the recipient.

Advances in preservation, such as the UW (University of Wisconsin) solution, allow longer ischemia. Organs can be transported for greater distances while maintaining excellent function with fewer complications. In experiments, this solution has successfully preserved kidneys and pancreas for seventy-two hours and livers for forty-eight hours. Typically, however, kidneys are transplanted within thirty-six to forty-eight hours and livers are transplanted within twenty-four hours so as not to jeopardize organ quality by extremely long storage times. Heart, lung, and heart-lung preservation times remain limited to between four and six hours.

Whereas most organs are flushed and stored in a cold solution for transport, kidneys can be preserved by two methods: cold storage or machine perfusion. Most often, kidneys are stored in a sterile jar with a cold solution, surrounded by ice, and transported in a cooler. With perfusion, a machine periodically flushes a cold solution through the kidneys until they are transplanted. Some transplant centers using machine perfusion report that kidneys function better immediately after transplant. Over the long term, kidney transplants are equally successful whether they are cold-stored or machine perfused.

Tissue preservation. Tissues, unlike organs, can be removed for up to several hours after death. Tissues are not directly connected to the body's blood supply and are not as susceptible to damage from ischemia. Tissues must be removed within twelve to twenty-four hours depending on whether the donor had been cooled adequately following death. Tissue banks may recover, process, store, and distribute tissues for transplantation.

Techniques that include hypothermia, cryopreservation, deep freezing, and freeze-drying allow tissues to be preserved for future use. With hypothermia, tissues are stored in a cold solution between 2° and 8°C. This technique is useful for short-term storage, less than ten days. Cryopreserved tissues are frozen at a controlled rate for storage. Deep freezing occurs at temperatures below −70°C. Freeze-drying removes water from the tissue so it can be kept at room temperature and transported over long distances without special handling. Tissues are then rehydrated before transplant.

The preservation technique selected depends on the type of tissue and the tissue bank's technology. For example, corneas are usually stored in a preservation solution and transplanted within two to three days, whereas skin may be frozen and stored for as long as two years and bone for five years. Because of these techniques and prolonged storage times, tissue transplantation does not have the same urgency as organ transplantation. Blood-group matching does not play as important a role as it does with organ transplants. Often, tissues are matched based on their size (diameter or length).

Organ and tissue distribution

Potential transplant patients are assessed by transplant teams that evaluate each patient's health to determine if a transplant is needed and how quickly. Transplant centers may define their own specific criteria for patient acceptance on transplant waiting lists. Once on the list, each patient has an equitable chance of receiving an organ because policy guidelines for organ distribution are followed.

At times, selection criteria have included social factors. With many potential recipients and too few organs, bias results when selection criteria have included factors such as sex, race, marital status, number of dependents, age, education, and income (Kjellstrand, 1990). Cark Kjellstrand's study of kidney transplantation in the United States, Sweden, and Canada demonstrated that patients had a greater likelihood of receiving a transplant if they were in one of these four favored groups: rich (versus poor); male (versus female); white (versus black); or young (versus old). Nevertheless, studies demonstrate that when age restrictions are extended so that older patients are transplanted, these transplants can be as successful as those of younger recipients (Andreu et al., 1992; Pirsch et al., 1991; Miller et al., 1988). As the number of potential transplant patients increases—for example, by treatment of more diseases through transplantation and by extending age limits—patient selection criteria that ensure the focus remains medical usefulness of the organ rather than the purported social usefulness of the patient will be necessary.

When an organ becomes available, the most suitable recipient on the waiting list is usually identified through computer and telephone communication between transplant centers and organ-procurement agencies. In the United States, the United Network for Organ Sharing (UNOS) began a national, computerized list of potential recipients. After being informed of an available donor, the UNOS computer system could identify a list of suitable recipients.

Several factors may be considered in selecting the recipient: blood group; tissue type (for kidneys); size of donated organ; amount of time the patient has been waiting; proximity to the transplant center; and the patient's current health and "status rating." When their names are added to waiting lists, potential recipients are assigned a status code rating that describes their medical condition. For example, a rating of "1" could indicate that a patient's health is stable and that he or she is waiting at home. The highest number (4) indicates that the patient is on a life-support system in an intensive-care unit and may die within days without a transplant.

This number or rating changes as the patient's health changes so that the most needy patients can be transplanted first. Organs are usually distributed on a local or regional basis, then nationally. When organs cannot be transplanted to patients in the same region or country, they are offered to eligible patients, who are usually rated as urgent, in other countries.

In Scandinavia (Norway, Sweden, Finland, and Denmark), Scandiatransplant was established in 1969 to provide organ exchange. Exchange rules have evolved, but transplant organs generally cross these international boundaries easily. The UK Transplant Service serves all of Britain and is linked with other agencies in western Europe. In Europe, organ-matching agencies in Italy, France, Spain, and other countries arrange organ distribution according to agreed-upon rules. Eurotransplant, located in The Netherlands, registers potential recipients and distributes organs among The Netherlands, Belgium, Luxembourg, Germany, and Austria.

Tissues are distributed by local, national, or international tissue banks. In the United States, for-profit tissue banks have been established with distribution based on ability to pay for their services. In Canada, corneas are distributed through a not-for-profit eye bank that distributes them on a first-come-first-served basis. Eurotransplant has a subsidiary, Bio Implant Services, to distribute tissues among its member countries. There should be no shortage of tissues, such as corneas, skin, and bones, as the potential supply well exceeds the potential demand.

Rejection and immunosuppression

After the transplant, the body's attempt to reject the organ is normal; this is due to the function of the immune system, which recognizes and attacks foreign substances including the transplanted organ. Rejection can occur in three ways: immediate, hyperacute rejection; acute rejection; or long-term, chronic rejection. Hyperacute rejection occurs because the recipient's immune system has been presensitized by antibodies that immediately recognize the transplanted tissue as foreign. The organ is rejected within minutes. This type of rejection can be avoided if certain tests are performed before the transplant. Crossmatching tests determine if the recipient already has antibodies that would reject the new organ. The closer the match between donor and recipient tissues, the less likely the recipient's immune system will activate T cells and antibodies and the less likely rejection will occur. Although hyperacute rejection can be avoided, acute or chronic rejection may occur. Acute rejection is characterized by rapid onset, usually several days after the transplant. Chronic rejection develops more slowly over a longer time.

Transplant patients take drugs to suppress the immune response and prevent rejection. Drug therapy (immunosuppression) may be started prior to the transplant, during the transplant surgery, or following the transplant. If rejection occurs, the dosage of the patient's regular antirejection drugs may be increased temporarily. Alternatively, other immunosuppressants, such as OKT3, antilymphocyte globulin, or antithymocyte globulin, may be added to treat rejection episodes. New immunosuppressants continue to be investigated in clinical trials and animal studies to assess their effectiveness and side effects.

The antirejection drug cyclosporine was first used with transplant patients in 1978. These first clinical studies showed improved patient and organ survival. Until the 1990s, cyclosporine was the mainstay of immunosuppression. Nevertheless, a controversy emerged regarding its long-term use. Some members of the medical community believed that cyclosporine should be withdrawn after the critical first three months when rejection was most likely to occur. In this way, patients derived the benefit of cyclosporine while avoiding its potentially damaging effect on kidney function. On the other hand, there was evidence that cyclosporine should be continued because long-term patient and graft survival rates were better with its use (Heimbecker, 1985; Cyclosporin, 1986).

Immunosuppression varies among transplant centers although a combination of antirejection drugs, such as azathioprine, prednisone, and cyclosporine, has often been used. The drug dosage varies from patient to patient and depends on other antirejection drugs that the patient is taking, how well the transplant organ is functioning, and any side effects that the patient is experiencing. Immunosuppression requires a careful balance so that organ rejection is prevented and side effects are minimized. All immunosuppressive drugs, however, have some side effects because they affect the body's immune response just as irradiation did in the early days of transplantation. Fewer white blood cells are available to fight bacteria and infections. Immunosuppressive drugs may lower the body's resistance to infection, so infections may occur more frequently and be more difficult to treat. The more severe effects may include impaired kidney function, hypertension, or cancer. Some experts believe that patients have fewer adverse side effects when a combination of drugs is used because a large amount of a single drug is avoided. When large amounts of a single drug are given, negative side effects, such as impaired kidney function from cyclosporine or weight gain and hypertension from prednisone, may be more likely to occur.

Success of transplantation

Success rates vary according to organ type (Table 1). Usually, both patient and graft survival rates are measured. Patient survival rates may be higher because pa-

TABLE 1. Success Rates of Organ Transplantation

| Organ | One-Year Graft Survival | |
	United States†	Canada‡
kidney (cadaver donor)	79%	82%
kidney (living donor)	91%	91%
liver	67%	77%
heart	81%	83%
heart-lung combination	55%	72%
lung	66%	58% (single) 72% (double)
pancreas	73%	56%

†United Network for Organ Sharing (UNOS), Richmond, Virginia: UNOS Scientific Registry data as of November 1992. Includes all transplants from October 1, 1987, to December 31, 1991.

‡Canadian Organ Replacement Register (CORR), Toronto, Ontario: Registry data as of November, 1993. Includes all transplants from January 1, 1987, to December 31, 1992.

tients may survive even though the transplant fails. This is true especially for kidney recipients, who can depend on dialysis machines to perform the kidney's functions artificially, and pancreas or islet-cell transplant patients, who may resort to insulin injections. For other organs, patients may live if another organ is available immediately. Success rates for a second or third transplant, if a patient is fortunate enough to receive one, are lower. Once the body has already rejected an organ, it is more likely to quickly recognize subsequent grafts and rejection may occur again.

Transplant patients have been asked to rate their quality of life—their "life satisfaction," "well-being," and "psychological affect." The average scores reported by kidney, heart, liver, and pancreas recipients are similar to scores reported by the public, indicating a comparable quality of life (Table 2). This major transplant study in the United States also reported that 80 to 90 percent of kidney, heart, liver, and pancreas recipients were physically active. Less than one-half of kidney, liver, and heart recipients were employed, but this employment rate is similar to that of other patients who have experienced life-threatening illness and surgery. Other studies have confirmed patients' improved quality of life by showing that 85 to 93 percent of patients with a successful kidney, liver, or heart transplant are rehabilitated and eventually able to work or return to school (Bismuth et al., 1993; Morel et al., 1991; Slavis et al., 1990; Shimon et al., 1989).

Transplant recipients are encouraged to follow good health habits, including regular exercise and appropriate weight with attention to diet. Transplant patients take

TABLE 2.   Quality-of-Life Assessment

	Life Satisfaction[1]	Well-Being[2]	Psychological Affect[3]
kidney recipient	5.25	11.01	5.23
heart recipient	5.11	11.11	5.49
liver recipient	6.70	not available	6.40
pancreas recipient	5.40	11.03	5.35
general population	5.55	11.77	5.68

[1]Range of values, 1.0 to 7.0 where 7.0 = positive satisfaction
[2]Range of values, 2.1 to 14.7 where high score = positive well-being
[3]Range of values, 1.0 to 7.0 where 7.0 = positive affect
Source: Evans, Roger W. 1991. *Executive Summary: The National Cooperative Transplantation Study.*
Seattle, Wash.: Battelle-Seattle Research Center, p. 20. Reprinted with permission.

immunosuppressive drugs to prevent organ rejection for the rest of their lives. Lack of compliance is considered one of the most common causes for graft loss in the long term. Despite the need for multiple medications, the increased incidence of life-threatening infection and cancer, and the threat of organ rejection, patients report remarkable life satisfaction and well-being.

Transplantation costs and reimbursement

Transplantation is expensive, as are many other medical therapies and surgical treatments. Data gathered in 1988 by the Battelle-Seattle Research Center in Washington show that the median, or average, costs for transplants—including hospital, professional, and organ-retrieval fees—in the United States were $40,000 for a kidney, $67,000 for a pancreas, $91,000 for a heart, $135,000 for a heart-lung combination, and as high as $145,00 for a liver (Evans, 1991). Because of other costs incurred before the transplant and after discharge from the hospital, total costs were higher. In view of limited health-care resources, these costs must be considered as society determines the extent of its willingness to fund transplantation. However, the number of years and quality of life attained from transplantation must also be considered. Numerous studies have documented the cost savings of kidney transplantation when compared to its alternative—dialysis (Kiberd, 1992; Croxson and Ashton, 1990; Eggerss, 1988). Heart and liver transplants can be as cost-effective as many other medical and surgical treatments.

In the United States, federal funding (Medicare) and state funding (Medicaid) have provided coverage for many kinds of transplants at approved transplant centers. Approved centers must have performed at least a specified number of transplants with a certain level of success. Medicare has been the primary provider of kidney-transplant coverage, although coverage has

also been provided for certain patients requiring bone-marrow, cornea, heart, or liver transplants. Medicaid coverage has varied from state to state, but usually bone-marrow, cornea, kidney, and liver transplants have been covered. Heart transplants have been widely available, but coverage for heart-lung, lung, and pancreas transplants has been limited. Most states have covered the cost of organ retrieval, and every state has paid for antirejection drugs for the first year after the transplant. During the 1990s, drug coverage increased so that new transplant patients would have coverage for three years.

Private insurance and the patient's own financial resources are often necessary. Even when public and private insurance covers transplantation, patients may only be partially reimbursed. The total costs for organ retrieval, surgery, and follow-up health care may not be reimbursed, so the patient may have substantial medical bills to pay.

In Canada, provincial health programs cover the costs of organ retrieval, transplant surgery, and medical care. The major cost for recipients is transportation to the transplant center, which may be located in another province. The antirejection drug cyclosporine is paid for all transplant recipients by a government-sponsored program. Costs are paid as long as patients take the drug, regardless of the socioeconomic status of patients. If patients take other immunosuppressive drugs, these costs may be completely or partially reimbursed by work benefits or private insurance. Long-term, follow-up care is covered by the patient's provincial health-care plan.

In Europe, according to European Economic Community (EEC) agreements, patients may be eligible for transplant in other countries, and their own governments would pay the costs. Patients from countries outside the EEC may also be transplanted but they would have to pay the costs themselves. As more programs have developed, however, fewer patients need to travel to other countries for their transplants.

The lack of cadaver donors and alternatives

Given the success of transplants, more patients are being referred for transplant surgery. The inadequate supply of organs, however, limits the number of transplants, so waiting lists continue to grow. Transplant programs, therefore, continue to expand their criteria for acceptable organs and to try innovative ways to procure more organs. Organs from older cadaver donors have been accepted and studies have shown that their organs function as well as organs from younger donors (Wall et al., 1990). Kidneys from pediatric donors have been transplanted into adult recipients. Unsuitable hearts, which would not usually be used, have been transplanted as "biological bridges" in urgent situations until a suitable heart has been found. Livers have been split in two for transplant into two patients, with results comparable to whole-liver transplantation. This technique has been researched for kidney transplantation. "Domino transplantation" has allowed a recipient's healthy organ to be removed and transplanted into another patient. For example, when a patient needs a double-lung transplant, he or she may receive a heart-lung transplant because of the technical ease of the combined graft. In this situation, the healthy heart is transplanted into another patient rather than being discarded.

Organs and tissues have also been retrieved from infants born with anencephaly, and used for transplant. Anencephaly is a lethal, congenital malformation in which a major portion of the brain and skull is missing. The brain stem is developed so these infants have reflexes, such as breathing and sucking. Because these infants survive no longer than a few weeks, they could potentially be organ donors for other infants. They cannot be declared dead until all brain-stem activity ceases. Anencephalic infants have been investigated by some centers as a source of organs, but research has indicated that these infants may not provide a significant supply of usable organs (Medearis et al., 1989; Medical Task Force on Anencephaly, 1990; Peabody et al., 1989).

Patients in Mexico, England, Sweden, the United States, and Canada have received brain cells from aborted fetuses for treatment of Parkinson's disease. Patients with Parkinson's disease take drugs that stimulate their brain cells to produce dopamine. Even with drug therapy, however, their brain cells continue to die. Patients experience loss of muscle control, progressing from tremors to rigidity and paralysis. Fetal tissue, injected into the brain, produces dopamine and replaces the patient's dying brain cells. Fetal-cell implants have enabled patients with severe Parkinson's disease to resume walking and caring for themselves. In addition to Parkinson's disease, fetal tissue could potentially treat diabetes, Alzheimer's disease, and Huntington's disease. Clinical researchers in Sweden, Germany, Hungary,

Australia, China, and the United States have injected or implanted fetal pancreas tissue to provide insulin and prevent diabetic complications.

Fetal tissue, widely available from elective abortions, may be less prone to rejection and graft-versus-host disease than tissue obtained from cadavers. Fetal cells have not yet developed antigens that would activate the recipient's immune system. However, because of its association with abortion, use of fetal tissue has generated ethical and legal debates. Opponents state that fetal tissue transplantation encourages abortion and that the timing and method of abortion may be influenced by the need for tissue. Proponents state that the abortion and use of fetal tissue are separated, so women are not encouraged to abort. Separation between the abortion clinic and the transplant facility by a not-for-profit organization has been considered as a required safeguard for the ethical practice of fetal-tissue transplantation. Although it has been proposed that tissue could be obtained from ectopic pregnancies, spontaneously aborted or stillborn fetuses, these are not alternatives; tissues from these fetuses are often abnormal. Also, the time between fetal death and being spontaneously aborted or stillborn means the tissue has been ischemic and therefore is unsuitable.

Xenografts are another potential source of transplant organs. Although attempts to transplant animal organs into humans took place at the beginning of the twentieth century, most attempts began during the 1960s. In 1964, the first heart-transplant patient received his organ from a chimpanzee donor. The longest survival time has been nine months, when a woman was transplanted with a chimpanzee's kidney in 1964. Newborn infant Baby Fae was the first xenograft patient treated with cyclosporine. She received a baboon's heart in 1984 and lived for twenty days, dying from kidney failure. During 1992 and 1993, two patients were transplanted at Pittsburgh. In one case, a patient with hepatitis B disease (which would recur in a human liver) was successfully transplanted with a baboon liver. The patient died seventy-one days later from a brain hemorrhage, with the liver still working. The second patient, who also received a baboon liver, died twenty-six days after the transplant.

Rejection is less of a problem when species are closely related, such as a primate-to-human transplant. Some primates, such as chimpanzees and apes, are considered to be ethically unacceptable. Baboons, which are not endangered and in many countries are considered an environmental pest, appear to be acceptable as a "first step" in xenotransplantation. Many problems, however, remain. Safe and effective immunosuppression is unknown. Zoonosis (the transfer of infectious organisms between species) may occur after transplant whereby undetected viruses in the baboon may cause disease and infection in humans. In baboon-to-human liver transplants, as in all liver transplants, patients depend on the proteins manufactured by the liver for many physiological functions in other parts of the body. The long-term effects of baboon products on human patients are not known.

These clinical experiences, however, show that animal organs can support human life and that rejection of xenografts can be successfully treated. New antirejection drugs may allow long-term survival. A genetically manipulated animal, such as a pig, could be developed to provide organs. To overcome rejection, genetic engineering could either insert new genes into the animal ("transgenic animals"), or make the animal's existing genes nonfunctional ("genetic knockout animals"). As a result, the human immune system would accept the xenograft.

There are, however, ethical concerns. Opponents of xenotransplantation believe that humans should not use animals to save human lives. If animals have rights equal to humans, then our moral obligation extends beyond the humane use and sacrifice of animals ("animal welfare"). In contrast, some traditional ethical theories give precedence to human needs so that the use of animals is justified when it is in the best interest of humans. These are some of the ethical issues debated in this controversial area.

Increasingly, alternative means to obtain human organs are being explored, including the use of nonheart-beating donors. After these donors are declared dead by traditional cardiopulmonary criteria, a tube must be inserted quickly so organs can be cooled and preserved to prevent injury from warm ischemia. If the next of kin are not available, this procedure would take place without their prior consent. Another scenario for using nonheartbeating donors occurs when continuation of life-support measure is considered futile and the patient or family decides to forgo life-sustaining treatment. In this situation, with premortem consent for organ donation, the patient would be observed when the life-support system is withdrawn in the operating room. When the heart stops beating, the organs would be cooled and removed. These practices clearly challenge some of the guidelines that govern organ procurement.

Another proposed method is the use of "vicarious living-related donors." Some family members who want to donate a kidney to a relative cannot because of blood-group (ABO) incompatibility or a positive crossmatch test. Another family with a similar situation could easily be identified. Each family member could then donate a kidney to the unrelated recipient, so each patient would receive a kidney from the other family's donor. This practice could increase significantly the number of kidney transplants done, but again, this borders on accepted medical practice. Few countries have routinely used living unrelated kidney donors. Until the 1990s, these donors did not provide better transplant outcomes than those from cadaver donors, whereas living related donors have been acceptable because of the superior results based on tissue matching. Vicarious living related donors would, therefore, change traditional practice, making unrelated donations more common.

Each time a new surgical procedure is described to and performed on patients who are desperate for life, many unknowns exist and mortality and morbidity rates are often high. Nevertheless, the shortage of organs will extend the current limits of medical practice as new, innovative procedures are tried. Patients who are desperate for organs should be considered patient pioneers. Consequently, medical and ethical supervision is required to provide guidelines during the search for new life for more patients.

CALVIN R. STILLER

Directly related to this article are the other articles in this entry: SOCIOCULTURAL ASPECTS, *and* ETHICAL AND LEGAL ISSUES. *Also directly related are the entries* ORGAN AND TISSUE PROCUREMENT; CRYONICS; DEATH, DEFINITION AND DETERMINATION OF; *and* XENOGRAFTS. *For a discussion of related ideas, see the entries* JUSTICE; *and* TECHNOLOGY. *For a discussion of related medical technologies, see* ARTIFICIAL HEARTS AND CARDIAC-ASSIST DEVICES; ARTIFICIAL ORGANS AND LIFE-SUPPORT SYSTEMS; BLOOD TRANSFUSION; *and* KIDNEY DIALYSIS. *Other relevant material may be found under the entry* SURGERY.

Bibliography

ANDREU, J.; DE LA TORRE, M.; OPPENHEIMER, F.; CAMPISTOL, J. M.; RICART, M. J.; VILARDELL, J.; TALBOT, R.; and CARRETERO, P. 1992. "Renal Transplantation in Elderly Recipients." *Transplantation Proceedings* 24, no. 1: 120–121.

AUCHINCLOSS, HUGH, JR. 1988. "Xenogeneic Transplantation: A Review." *Transplantation* 46, no. 1:1–20.

BARKER, CLYDE F., and MARKMANN, JAMES F. 1992. "Xenografts: Is There a Future?" *Surgery* 112, no. 1:3–4.

BENENSON, ESTHER, ed. 1992. "Transplantation in Europe." *UNOS Update* 8, no. 10:17–30.

BISMUTH, H.; AZOULAY, D.; and DENNISON, A. 1993. "Recent Developments in Liver Transplantation." *Transplantation Proceedings* 25, no. 3:2191–2194.

BONOMI, VITTORIO. 1991. "Ethical Aspects of Living Donation." *Transplantation Proceedings* 23, no. 5:2497–2499.

CAPLAN, ARTHUR L. 1992. *If I Were A Rich Man Could I Buy a Pancreas? and Other Essays on the Ethics of Health Care.* Bloomington: Indiana University Press.

CERILLI, G. JAMES, ed. 1988. *Organ Transplantation and Replacement.* Philadelphia: J. B. Lippincott.

CHURCHILL, LARRY R., and PINKUS, ROSA LYNN B. 1990. "The Use of Anencephalic Organs: Historical and Ethical Dimensions." *Milbank Quarterly* 68, no. 2:147–169.

CROXSON, B.E., and ASHTON, T. 1990. "A Cost Effectiveness Analysis of the Treatment of End-Stage Renal Failure." *New Zealand Medical Journal* 103:171–174.

"Cyclosporin for Ever?" 1986. *Lancet* 1:419–420. Editorial.

DE BY, T. 1991. "Tissue Banking." *Transplantation Proceedings* 23, no. 5:2665–2666.

DOSSETOR, JOHN B.; MONACO, ANTHONY P.; and STILLER, CALVIN R., eds. 1990. "Ethics, Justice, and Commerce in Transplantation: A Global View." *Transplantation Proceedings* 22, no. 3.

EGGERS, PAUL W. 1988. "Effect of Transplantation on the Medicare End-Stage Renal Disease Program." *New England Journal of Medicine* 318:223–229.

EVANS, ROGER W. 1991. *Executive Summary: The National Cooperative Transplantation Study*. BHARC-100-91-020. Seattle, Wash.: Battelle-Seattle Research Center.

EVANS, ROGER W.; ORIANS, CARLYN E.; and ASCHER, NANCY L. 1992. "Potential Supply of Organ Donors: An Assessment of the Efficiency of Organ Procurement Efforts in the United States." *Journal of the American Medical Association* 267, no. 2:239–246.

FLYE, M. WAYNE, ed. 1989. *Principles of Organ Transplantation*. Philadelphia: W. B. Saunders.

FOX, RENÉE C., and SWAZEY, JUDITH P. 1992. *Spare Parts: Organ Replacement in American Society*. New York: Oxford University Press.

GARRY, DANIEL J.; CAPLAN, ARTHUR L.; VAWTER, DOROTHY E.; and KEARNEY, WARREN. 1992. "Are There Really Alternatives to the Use of Fetal Tissue from Elective Abortions in Transplantation Research?" *New England Journal of Medicine* 327, no. 22:1592–1595.

GÜLAY, H.; ARSLAN, G.; SERT, S.; HABERAL, M. 1989. "Successful Living-Unrelated Donor Kidney Transplantation." *Transplantation Proceedings* 21, no. 1:2196.

HEIMBECKER, RAYMOND O. 1985. "Transplantation: The Cyclosporine Revolution." *Canadian Journal of Cardiology* 1, no. 6:354–357.

KEARNEY, WARREN; VAWTER, DOROTHY E.; and GERVAIS, KAREN G. 1991. "Fetal Tissue Research and the Misread Compromise." *Hastings Center Report* 21, no. 5:7–12.

KIBERD, BRYCE A. 1992. "Equitable Allocation Versus Best Outcome: Competing Economic and Ethical Strategies in Renal Transplantation." *Annals of the Royal College of Physicians and Surgeons of Canada* 25, no. 7:446–448.

KILNER, JOHN. 1990. *Ethical Criteria in Patient Selection: Who Lives? Who Dies?* New Haven, Conn.: Yale University Press.

KJELLSTRAND, CARL. 1990. "The Distribution of Renal Transplants—Are Physicians Just?" *Transplantation Proceedings* 22, no. 3:964–965.

McCULLAGH, PETER. 1987. *The Foetus as Transplant Donor: Scientific, Social, and Ethical Perspectives*. Chichester, U.K.: Wiley Medical Publishing.

MEDEARIS, DONALD N., and HOLMES, LEWIS B. 1989. "On the Use of Anencephalic Infants as Organ Donors." *New England Journal of Medicine* 321, no. 6:391–393.

MEDICAL TASK FORCE ON ANENCEPHALY. 1990. "The Infant with Anencephaly." *New England Journal of Medicine* 322, no. 10:669–674.

MILLER, LESLIE W.; VITALE-NOEDEL, NANCY; PENNINGTON, GLENN; McBRIDE, LAWRENCE; and KANTER, KIRK R. 1988. "Heart Transplantation in Patients Over Fifty-Five Years." *Journal of Heart Transplantation* 7:254–257.

MOREL, P.; ALMOND, P. S.; MATAS, A. J.; GILLINGHAM, K. J.; CHAU, C.; BROWN, A.; KASHTAN, C. E.; MAUER, S. M.; CHAVERS, B.; NEVINS, T. E.; DUNN, D. L.; SUTHERLAND, D. E. R.; PAYNE, W. D.; and NAJARIAN, J. S. 1991. "Long-Term Quality of Life After Kidney Transplantation in Childhood." *Transplantation* 52, no. 1:47–53.

NATIONAL INSTITUTES OF HEALTH. 1988. *Report of the Human Fetal Tissue Transplantation Research Panel*. Bethesda, Md.: National Institutes of Health.

OTA, K. 1991. "Present Status of Kidney Donation in Japan." *Transplantation Proceedings* 23, no. 5:2512–2513.

PEABODY, JOYCE L.; EMERY, JANET R.; and ASHWAL, STEPHEN. 1989. "Experience with Anencephalic Infants as Prospective Organ Donors." *New England Journal of Medicine* 321, no. 6:344–350.

PETERS, THOMAS G. 1991. "Life or Death: The Issue of Payment in Cadaveric Organ Donation." *Journal of the American Medical Association* 265, no. 10:1302–1305.

PIRSCH, J. D.; KALAYOGLU, M.; D'ALESSANDRO, A. M.; VOSS, B. J.; ARMBRUST, M. J.; REED, A.; KNECHTLE, J. J.; SOLLINGER, H. W.; and BELZER, F. O. 1991. "Orthotopic Liver Transplantation in Patients 60 Years of Age and Older." *Transplantation* 51, no. 2:431–433.

SANTIAGO-DELPIN, E. A. 1991. "Organ Donation and Transplantation in Latin America." *Transplantation Proceedings* 23, no. 5:2516–2518.

SCHARP, DAVID W.; LACY, PAUL E.; SANTIAGO, JULIO V.; McCULLOUGH, CHRISTOPHER S.; WEIDE, LAMONT G.; FALQUI, LUCA; MARCHETTI, PIERO; GINGERICH, RONALD L.; JAFFE, ALLAN S.; CRYER, PHILIP E.; ANDERSON, CHARLES B.; and FLYE, M. WAYNE. 1990. "Insulin Independence After Islet Transplantation into Type 1 Diabetic Patient." *Diabetes* 39:515–518.

SCHNEIDER, ANDREW, and FLAHERTY, MARY PAT. 1985. *The Challenge of a Miracle: Selling the Gift*. Pittsburgh, Pa.: Pittsburgh Press.

SHIMON, DOV V.; ADMON, DAN; ZILBERMAN, SHALOM; GOTSMAN, MERVYN S.; and BORMAN, JOSEPH B. 1989. "Heart Transplantation—State of the Art." *Israel Journal of Medical Sciences* 25:575–582.

SIGARDSON-POOR, KATHERINE M., and HAGGERTY, LINDA M., eds. 1990. *Nursing Care of the Transplant Recipient*. Philadelphia: W. B. Saunders.

SINGER, PETER. 1992. "Xenotransplantation and Speciesism." *Transplantation Proceedings* 24, no. 2:728–732.

SINGER, PETER A.; SIEGLER, MARK; WHITINGTON, PETER F.; LANTOS, JOHN D.; EMOND, JEAN C.; THISTLETHWAITE, J. RICHARD; and BROELSCH, CHRISTOPH E. 1989. "Ethics of Liver Transplantation with Living Donors." *New England Journal of Medicine* 321, no. 9:620–622.

SKELLEY, LUKE, ed. 1989. "Organ and Tissue Transplantation." *Nursing Clinics of North America* 24, no. 4.

Slavis, S. A.; Novick, A. C.; Steinmuller, D. R.; Streem, S. B.; Braun, W. E.; Straffon, R. A.; Mastroianni, B.; and Graneto, D. 1990. "Outcome of Renal Transplantation in Patients with a Functioning Graft for 20 Years or More." *Journal of Urology* 144, no. 1:20–22.

Starzl, Thomas E. 1992. *The Puzzle People: Memoirs of a Transplant Surgeon.* Pittsburgh, Pa.: University of Pittsburgh Press.

Stiller, Calvin. 1990. *Lifegifts: The Real Story of Organ Transplants.* Toronto: Stoddart.

Turcotte, Jeremiah G., and Benjamin, Martin, eds. 1989. "Patient Selection Criteria in Organ Transplantation: The Critical Questions." *Transplantation Proceedings* 21, no. 3.

Tzakis, Andreas G.; Ricardi, Camillo; Alejandro, Rodolfo; Zeng, Yijun; Fung, John J.; Todo, Sataru; Demetris, Anthony J.; Mintz, Daniel H.; and Starzl, Thomas E. 1990. "Pancreatic Islet Transplantation After Upper Abdominal Exenteration and Liver Replacement." *Lancet* 336:402–405.

Virnig, B. A., and Caplan, A. L. 1992. "Required Request: What Difference Has It Made?" *Transplantation Proceedings* 24, no. 5:2155–2158.

Wall, William; Mimeault, Richard; Grant, David; and Bloch, Michael. 1990. "The Use of Older Donor Livers for Hepatic Transplantation." *Transplantation* 49:377–381.

Wolfslast, Gabriele. 1992. "Legal Aspects of Organ Transplantation: An Overview of European Law." *Journal of Heart and Lung Transplantation* 11, no. 4, part 2:S160–S163.

II. SOCIOCULTURAL ASPECTS

Transplantation has been defined by the medical profession and society at large as a "gift of life" since the first human organ grafts were performed in the mid-1950s. Initially, the notion of the gift was used metaphorically, with little awareness or analysis of its implications. Only gradually, through clinical experience and interpretative input from psychiatrists, social workers, and social scientists, did the psychological, social, and cultural meanings and repercussions of the gift-exchange aspects of transplantation become more apparent and better understood (Fox and Swazey, 1978).

Despite all the biomedical and social changes that have ensued within and around the field of organ replacement, the "gift of life" aspects of seeking, giving, and receiving a human organ remain intrinsic to the dynamics and meaning of transplantation. For this reason organ transplantation continues to be one of the most sociologically intricate and powerfully symbolic events in modern medicine. The increased frequency of organ transplants, and their greater routinization in certain regards, have not eliminated the gift elements from these surgical and medical acts, or reduced their effects on donors, recipients, and their families (Fox and Swazey, 1992).

Marcel Mauss's gift-exchange paradigm

"The theme of the gift, of freedom and obligation in the gift, of generosity and self-interest in giving reappear in our society like the resurrection of a dominant motif long forgotten," wrote the renowned French sociologist Marcel Mauss in his classic essay *The Gift* (Mauss, 1954, p. 66). To a remarkable degree, organ transplantation has been shaped by the triple set of "symmetrical and reciprocal" obligations that, according to Mauss, govern all gift exchange, no matter how spontaneous and expressive it may appear to be. These are the entwined obligations to offer and give, to receive and accept, and to seek and find an appropriate way to repay. Failure to live up to any of these obligations, Mauss pointed out, produces major social strains that affect the giver, the receiver, and those associated with them.

Mauss also emphasized that gifts have "emotional" and symbolic as well as "material" value and meaning. In this sense, he said, the gift and the obligations attached to it are "not inert." Rather, "the spirit of the thing given" and received is "alive and often personified." It "pertains to a person," and because it does, it creates a "sort of spiritual bond" between donor and recipient (Mauss, 1954, pp. 10–11). Anthropomorphic and magical connotations of the gift have proved to be as characteristic of the modern medical, scientific, and technological milieus in which the giving and receiving of organs through transplantation take place, as of the settings in "primitive" and "archaic" societies that were the contexts of Mauss's study.

Obligations to give organs

The gift-exchange paradigm illuminates many of the distinctive psychological and social phenomena that donors, recipients, their families, and the transplant team encounter. To begin with, even though the U.S. organ donation system has been organized around the cardinal societal principles of voluntarism and freedom of choice, the situations in which transplants are performed subject prospective donors and their families to strong inner and outer pressures to make such a gift. This is most apparent in the case of live organ transplants, which usually involve the donation of a kidney to a parent, sibling, or child who is gravely ill with end-stage disease. Most transplant teams scrupulously try to avoid urging close biological kin to offer themselves as donors. Nevertheless, they do inform patients and their families that a live kidney transplant from a relative who is a "good tissue match" is likely to have a better prognosis than a cadaver transplant from a nonrelated donor. In addition to the biomedical reasons that favor a live kidney donation, its symbolic meaning virtually obliges every family member at least to consider making such a gift. The integrity, intimacy, and generosity of the family and each of its members are involved in their individual and collective willingness to give of themselves to a terminally ill relative in this supreme, life-sustaining way (Simmons et al., 1977).

It would be easy to assume that because cadaver organs come from persons who are unrelated and unknown to recipients, such donations are relatively free from inner and outer gift-giving pressures. Nevertheless, under the circumstances in which the option of donating cadaver organs arises, families may feel emotionally and spiritually constrained to make such a gift of life when this prospect is presented to them by an organ procurement team. Most cadaver organs are obtained from young, healthy persons who have been fatally injured in a vehicular accident or a homicide, or who have taken their own lives. These sudden and unexpected deaths are especially tragic and fraught with problems of meaning. In the face of this sort of death, the grief-stricken family may be motivated to donate their young relative's organs by their intense need to make redeeming sense out of what they would otherwise experience as morally and existentially absurd.

Obligations to receive organs

The candidate-recipient who is offered a live or cadaver organ is subject to strong, complementary pressures to receive it. Whatever the potential recipient's reservations may be about a transplant, great reluctance or outright refusal to accept the lifesaving gift that is offered symbolically implies a rejection of the donor and of the donor's relationship to the recipient.

There are several recurrent sets of reasons why recipients may be reluctant to accept the kind of gift of life that a donated organ represents. First, the recipient may not want a living, related donor exposed to the degree of discomfort, danger, or sacrifice that a transplant entails. Second, the recipient may feel that receiving an organ from this individual would make the relationships between them too emotionally complicated and difficult. Third, whether the proffered organ comes from a live relative or a deceased stranger, the recipient may be heavily burdened by the realization that it is such an extraordinary gift that he or she will never be able to repay it. Fourth, the recipient may have great concern or apprehension about absorbing a donated part of another known or unknown individual into his or her body, person, and life.

The reactions of recipients to the prospect and to the actual experience of receiving a donor's organ illustrate some of the forms in which transplantation has evoked buried, often animistic feelings that many people have about their vital organs and the integrity of their body. Among the preconscious sentiments that these recipients seem to share is the belief that some of the psychic and social, as well as physical, qualities of the donor are transferred with his or her organ into the person in whom it is implanted. The characteristic interest that recipients of cadaver organs and their kin express in knowing what kind of person the donor was (for example, the donor's sex, age, ethnicity, marital status, education, occupation, religion, character, and life history), and what sort of family he or she belonged to, is related to this same phenomenon. So, too, is the eagerness of donor families to learn something about the persons to whom living parts of their deceased relatives have been given, and about their families.

In the early years of human organ transplants, during the 1950s to mid-1960s, medical teams were inclined to reveal the identities of the donors of cadaver organs, their recipients, and their families, and to provide details of their backgrounds and lives. Physicians believed that these intimate participants in the acts of giving and receiving that transplantation entails were entitled to such knowledge. They also thought it would enhance the meaning of the transplant experience for the recipient and recipient's family, and afford consolation and a sense of completeness to the donor's family.

However, with the passage of time and increased clinical experience, transplant teams became more wary about the information they conveyed. The transplanters were discomfited by the way in which recipients, their kin, and donor families personified cadaver organs, and by how many of them not only arranged to meet but also tried to become involved in each other's lives, as if they were indebted and related to one another. These interactions were major factors that led most transplant units to establish the normative practice of not telling the recipient about the donor, or the donor's family about the recipient. Above all, this little-discussed policy of confidentiality developed out of the desire of transplanters to reduce the stresses and burdens that the obligation to repay this symbolically charged gift entails.

Obligations to repay the "gift of life" and the "tyranny of the gift"

At the center of organ transplantation is a gift of surpassing significance—in the words of philosopher Hans Jonas, a "supererogatory gift . . . beyond duty and claim" (Jonas, 1970, p. 16). Paradoxically, it is an offering that so perfectly epitomizes one of the ultimate Judeo-Christian values of our society—the injunction to give of ourselves in ways that include strangers as well as our brothers and sisters—that it transcends what is ordinarily asked or expected of us. The sublime meaning of what is exchanged, along with the literal and figurative sense in which a living part of the giver comes to reside and function inside the recipient, usually creates a very strong bond between the donor, the recipient, and their families. The sense of oneness and ennoblement that a donor or donor's family and a recipient often experience as a result of the life-giving and life-receiving acts in which they have participated can greatly enrich them, emotionally and spiritually.

But as Marcel Mauss could have foretold, what recipients believe they owe to donors, and the sense of obligation they feel about repaying "their" donor for what has been given, weigh heavily upon them. This psychological and moral burden is especially onerous because the gift the recipient has received from the donor is so extraordinary that it is inherently nonreciprocal. It has no physical or symbolic equivalent. As a consequence, the giver, the receiver, and their families may find themselves locked in a creditor–debtor vise. We have called these aspects of the gift-exchange dimensions of transplantation "the tyranny of the gift" (Fox and Swazey, 1978, ch. 1).

Alterations in the theme of the gift

The 1980s brought a number of significant changes in the ways the medical community and the American public thought about the gift of a transplantable organ, and in how they acted in relation to their conception of it. In part, this was due to the latent assumption that because transplantation had become more commonplace and routinized in some respects, it was no longer evoking the powerful positive and negative gift-associated reactions in donors, recipients, and their families that it had in the past.

Changes also were wrought by the growing preoccupation with the shortage of transplantable organs, and the ways that this shortage could be ameliorated. The decade was marked by a substantial expansion in the number and types of transplants and retransplants, in the number of hospitals doing these procedures, and in the number of patients on waiting lists. The discovery and pervasive use of cyclosporine, a more effective immunosuppressive drug for managing the rejection reaction triggered by transplanted organs, was a key biomedical factor that contributed to this transplant "boom." To the mounting distress of organ procurement agencies and transplanters, these increases occurred in the face of a plateauing of cadaveric donors and a slight decline in living donors. The "alarming number of patients who die waiting" for a transplant led members of the transplant community and their advocates to define the organ shortage as a "public health crisis" (Peters, 1991, p. 1302; Randall, 1991, p. 1223). In the context of various sociomedical policy strategies that were deployed to combat this growing "crisis," the concept and

theme of transplantation as a gift of life underwent a number of alterations.

Efforts to augment the supply of organs included, first, a renewed and increased interest in the use of living donors. This resulted in an expansion of the kinds of live donor transplants that surgeons were willing to perform, and significant redefinitions by the transplant community of how, for purposes of giving and receiving an organ, donors and recipients can be nonbiologically "related" to each other. Second, there were increasingly active and large-scale campaigns to recruit future donors, urging people to "make a miracle" by giving a gift of life through the provisions of the Uniform Anatomical Gift Act. (Promulgated in 1968 and adopted in some form by every state by 1973, the act enables individuals legally to signify their willingness to have their bodily parts used for transplantation after their death; if the deceased's wishes are unknown, the act grants the next of kin the right to make this decision.) Third—in addition to public appeals—those concerned about an organ shortage, the reasons for it, and the means by which more organs could be obtained directed their attention to the medical professionals involved in the procurement process, focusing on how doctors' and nurses' attitudes and behaviors that were seen as hampering donations could be altered.

The fact that the supply of cadaver kidneys was not great enough to meet the growing demand for them emboldened a number of medical centers to undertake transplants of kidneys from unrelated live donors in the 1980s. In effect, until then, something akin to a collective taboo against performing this type of graft had existed among transplant physicians. A new term appeared in the medical literature: "emotionally related donors," meaning persons whose relationship to recipients, though not biological, was analogously close. In 1985 the Council of the Transplantation Society issued a set of "guidelines for the donation of kidneys by unrelated living donors" that legitimated their use in exceptional circumstances "when a satisfactory cadaver or living related donor cannot be found." These normative recommendations expressed continuing concern about the motives of such donors, about the recognition and protection to which they were entitled for such "a gift of extraordinary magnitude," and about the ever-present danger "in the current climate of commercialization" that, particularly in the case of "living stranger donors," the covert buying and selling of organs might be involved (Council of the Transplantation Society, 1985, p. 716).

In the atmosphere produced by the acceleration in the number and range of transplants performed, the mounting sense of crisis over the organ shortage, and the increased support given to live-donor kidney transplants, liver and lung transplantation from living donors was tried for the first time in the United States. The initial liver recipients, in 1989, were two infants with biliary atresia, a congenital, usually fatal condition. Each of them was surgically implanted with a liver lobe from a parent. In 1991, a nine-year-old girl received two successive live-donor lung-lobe transplants: first from her father and then, when this did not provide enough lung capacity, another transplant from her mother. During the second procedure, the child died of heart failure.

Another form of live donation, employed since 1984, is generating even greater uncertainty and debate about "the permissible limits of one of our most powerful instincts, the one that leads us to fight for the life of our children" (Quindlen, 1991). These cases involve conceiving and giving birth to a baby in order to provide a bone marrow donor for one's dying child when no donor with a compatible tissue type can be located. The case that has received the most attention, because of the decision to go public, is that of the Ayala family, whose nineteen-year-old daughter, Anissa, was slowly dying of chronic myelogenous leukemia. In 1990 her parents announced that they had conceived a child on the one-in-four chance that the baby's tissue type would be compatible with Anissa's. There was a tissue match, and at age fourteen months the baby had her bone marrow withdrawn and infused into her sister.

The Ayalas' story was viewed by many as an act of love as well as of science—all the more so because the parents made it clear that they never considered aborting the fetus if its tissue type did not match Anissa's. But pervading all the discussion that this case evoked was an underlying uneasiness about how morally acceptable it was to bring a baby into the world to serve in this way (Morrow, 1991). Questions also were raised about the impact this act might eventually have on the sense of identity and reason for being of the donor child, who did not consent to be used in this way and might not have agreed to the transplant if she had been able to make this choice (Kearney and Caplan, 1992).

By the mid-1980s, emphasis also was being placed on how the knowledge and skills, sentiments, and role behavior of physicians and nurses involved in the procurement process hampered organ donation, and what could be done to remedy these problems. Attention focused particularly on what was viewed as the frequent "failure" of physicians and nurses to approach families of patients potentially qualified to become organ donors, to inform them of the possibility and right they had to donate their relatives' organs, and ask them if they were willing to do so. In response to what was now defined as this "main bottleneck" to organ donation, bioethicist Arthur L. Caplan proposed that "required request" procedures be established in hospitals to ensure that the next of kin or the legal guardians of every potential donor be notified of the transplantation option, and asked to make a donation of their relatives' organs for this purpose (Caplan, 1984a, 1984b).

Caplan's idea was rapidly drafted into law. By the end of the 1980s, required request had been enacted by most state legislatures, mandated in federal legislation for all institutions receiving Medicare or Medicaid funds, and incorporated into hospital accreditation standards. Yet despite the almost bandwagon-like conviction and speed with which the "required request" principle was translated into laws and procedures, preliminary studies suggested that its influence was minor at best (Annas, 1988; Caplan, 1988).

The inability of the "required request" legislation to provide a "legal fix" for the problems of organ procurement and supply, and the recalcitrance that it engendered in some physicians, were associated with one of its most important though largely unanticipated consequences. Its enactment helped to bring to the surface and underscore the pervasive conceptual confusion over defining and declaring "brain death," and the disquietude about some of its implications for the medical management of the organ donor and for organ retrieval that existed among physicians and nurses (Darby et al., 1989; Youngner et al., 1989; Wikler and Weisbard, 1989).

During the 1980s, in western Europe more than in the United States, increasingly serious attention was given to the use of "presumed consent" or "opting out" as a way to increase the number of cadaver organs procured for transplantation. This system, in which body parts can be harvested unless a person has stipulated an objection prior to death, was legally implemented in Austria in 1982 and Belgium in 1987, with notable increases in kidney procurement rates. However, there is evidence suggesting that if the "opting out" system requires the next of kin to be informed about organ removal from their deceased relative before it is done, physicians may be less inclined to initiate the procurement process and families more likely to object to the donation. Additionally, opinion polls in the Netherlands, Great Britain, and the United States consistently have shown that there is strongly held and widely distributed resistance to establishing a presumed-consent basis for organ and tissue procurement (Kokkedee, 1992). The social and cultural factors that account for these patterns have not been systematically investigated.

From "gifts of life" to market commodities?

The growing imbalance between the demand for transplantable organs and their supply in the United States and in other countries has fueled long-simmering concerns about black markets in body parts, and debate about the pros and cons of various forms of regulated payment for organ donations. Issues concerning the buying, selling, and brokering of solid organs and tissues has evoked strong responses from many medical groups; from ethicists, lawyers, economists, legislators, and policy analysts; from a variety of local, national, and international political and governmental bodies; and from the mass media. Reactions to the concept of legalized payment for organs, and to their brokerage, went beyond spirited discussion and debate in the 1980s. On the one hand, special guidelines and resolutions were drafted by an array of medical societies and health organizations, and a number of new laws proscribing buying and selling organs were passed (Childress, 1989; Council of the Transplantation Society, 1985). On the other hand, somewhat paradoxically, a number of individuals concerned with public policy aspects of transplantation began to advocate and develop proposals for the regulated compensation of donors and for dealing with bodily parts as market commodities.

To begin with, there were persistent voices, like that of health-policy analyst Jeffrey M. Prottas, arguing that organ donation and procurement were more than "a moral enterprise" and "a mechanism for giving reality to altruism" (Prottas, 1989, p. 42). In his view, it should also be defined as a not-for-profit "industry" engaged in "selling altruism" (Prottas and Batten, 1991, p. 131).

Prottas's marketing and business approach remained within the "gift of life" and "encouraged altruism" concept of organ donation endorsed by the National Task Force on Transplantation. But from the mid-1980s on, especially in the United States, an increasing number of persons writing about the scarce supply of transplantable organs, and about how donation rates might be augmented, moved beyond such a gift-exchange framework. They argued that many of the problems in obtaining and distributing organs could be ameliorated by the adoption of one or more systems of financial incentives or "regulated compensation" to those providing their organs or to their next of kin. Some of these far-reaching proposals involve creating a market in organs by methods that are much more sophisticated than simply permitting organs to be bought and sold on the open market. For example, since 1986 proposals have been set forth for creating a "futures market" in cadaver organs. In these proposals, "the right to harvest a person's organs upon death must be purchased from him while still alive and well" (Hansmann, 1989, p. 63). If at the time of the "vendor's" death, organs are successfully harvested and transplanted, a contractually agreed-upon sum of money would be paid to his or her designee (Cohen, 1989).

The chief spokespersons for shifting from a gift to a market model of organ donation and procurement include North American economists, lawyers, and health-policy analysts and managers who share a set of assumptions. They believe that an "organ market" would be a more effective mechanism for increasing the supply of organs than "[t]he altruistic 'gift relationship' [that] may be inadequate as a motivator" (Trucco, 1989, p. C1). Although they recognize that markets are driven by the competitive self-interests of buyers and sellers, they also view the market as a social policy instrument that would reduce the "social costs" of transplantation by fostering greater efficiency and coordination in the process of exchange and distribution. Even if the commercial sale of organs were ethically wrong (which they do not believe is the case), "it may nevertheless be preferable to accepting the suffering and death of patients who cannot otherwise obtain transplants" (Trucco, 1989, p. C1). Advocating that organs be exchanged for compensation in a market transfer is compatible with what such thinkers regard as a "moral canon": namely, that people's bodies are their own "private property," which they have the right to dispose of as they see fit (Cohen, 1989).

Whether human organs will, in fact, become societally legitimated market commodities rather than "gifts of life" is an open question as the twentieth century ends. The answer will depend as much on larger social, political, and ideological forces at work on the American scene as on the magnitude of the organ shortage. It is more than coincidental that a market approach to organ donation gained momentum during the 1980s, a decade when a certain view of the market became more prominent and "attractive" not only in the economic sector of American society, but in its "moral and social spheres as well" (Wolfe, 1989, p. 76). This market vision—permeated by supply-side economic and neoconservative political thinking—is grounded in the conviction that both economic and social relations should ideally be organized around and guided by the maximization of rational, self-interested, free choices, and that "moral obligations to others can be satisfied [best] . . . by first satisfying obligations to the self" (Wolfe, 1989, p. 33).

In its most extreme laissez-faire form, a market-based outlook is considered to be just as applicable to the procuring of human organs for transplantation, and to paying for them, as it is to economically driven decisions about any other "commodity." Furthermore, it ignores or minimizes some of the deeper reasons why people feel reluctance about donating their organs. These reasons include the fear of being prematurely pronounced dead; anxiety about the disfigurement or dehumanization of donors; religiously based concern about the fate of persons who enter the afterlife with organs or tissues removed from their bodies; and, among African-Americans, apprehension about the medical community's intentions and trustworthiness in dealing with black patients and their families (Callender, 1987).

Above all, many are morally and socially troubled by the failure of this economically deterministic, individualism-based market approach to recognize the more-than-materialistic meaning represented by the giving of ourselves to others through organ and tissue donation. For proponents of the gift-exchange framework for donation, this act is integrally related to the nonpecuniary values of altruism, community, and solidarity so vital to what it means to belong to human society that it is perilous to disregard or tamper with them.

RENÉE C. FOX
JUDITH P. SWAZEY

Directly related to this article are the other articles in this entry: MEDICAL OVERVIEW, *and* ETHICAL AND LEGAL ISSUES. *Also directly related are the entries* ORGAN AND TISSUE PROCUREMENT; INTERPRETATION; OBLIGATION AND SUPEREROGATION; *and* BLOOD TRANSFUSION. *For a further discussion of topics mentioned in this article, see the entries* BENEFICENCE; *and* ECONOMIC CONCEPTS IN HEALTH CARE.

Bibliography

ANNAS, GEORGE J. 1988. "The Paradoxes of Organ Transplantation." *American Journal of Public Health* 78, no. 6: 621–622.

CALLENDER, CLIVE O. 1987. "Organ Donation in Blacks: A Community Approach." *Transplant Proceedings* 19, no. 1, pt. 2:1551–1554.

CAPLAN, ARTHUR L. 1984a. "Ethical and Policy Issues in the Procurement of Cadaver Organs for Transplantation." *New England Journal of Medicine* 311, no. 15:981–983.

———. 1984b. "Organ Procurement: It's Not in the Cards." *Hastings Center Report* 14, no. 5:9–12.

———. 1988. "Professional Arrogance and Public Misunderstanding." *Hastings Center Report* 18, no. 2:34–37.

CHILDRESS, JAMES F. 1989. "Ethical Criteria for Procuring and Distributing Organs for Transplantation." In *Organ Transplantation Policy: Issues and Prospects,* pp. 87–113. Edited by James F. Blumstein and Frank A. Sloan. Durham, N.C.: Duke University Press.

COHEN, LLOYD R. 1989. "Increasing the Supply of Transplantable Organs: The Virtues of a Futures Market." *George Washington Law Review* 58, no. 11:1–51.

COUNCIL OF THE TRANSPLANTATION SOCIETY. 1985. "Commercialisation in Transplantation: The Problems and Some Guidelines for Practice." *Lancet* 2, no. 8457: 715–716.

DARBY, JOSEPH M.; STEIN, KEITH; GRENVIK, AKE; and STUART, SUSAN A. 1989. "Approach to Management of the Heartbeating 'Brain Dead' Organ Donor." *Journal of the American Medical Association* 261, no. 15:2222–2228.

FOX, RENÉE C., and SWAZEY, JUDITH P. 1978. *The Courage to Fail: A Social View of Organ Transplants and Dialysis.* 2d ed., rev. Chicago: University of Chicago Press.

———. 1992. *Spare Parts: Organ Replacement in American Society.* New York: Oxford University Press.

HANSMANN, HENRY. 1989. "The Economics and Ethics of Markets for Human Organs." In *Organ Transplantation Policy: Issues and Prospects,* pp. 57–85. Edited by James F. Blumstein and Frank A. Sloan. Durham, N.C.: Duke University Press.

JONAS, HANS. 1970. "Philosophical Reflections on Experimenting with Subjects." In *Experimentation with Human Subjects,* pp. 1–31. Edited by Paul A. Freund. New York: George Braziller.

KEARNEY, WARREN, and CAPLAN, ARTHUR L. 1992. "Parity for the Donation of Bone Marrow." In vol. 1 of *Emerging Issues in Biomedical Policy: An Annual Review,* ch. 19. Edited by Robert H. Blank and Andrea L. Bonnicksen. New York: Columbia University Press.

KOKKEDEE, WILLIAM. 1992. "Kidney Procurement Policies in the Eurotransplant Region: 'Opting In' Versus 'Opting Out.'" *Social Science and Medicine* 35, no. 2:177–182.

MAUSS, MARCEL. 1954. *The Gift: Forms and Foundations of Exchange in Archaic Societies.* Translated by Ian Cunnison. Glencoe, Ill.: Free Press.

MORROW, LANCE. 1991. "When One Body Can Save Another." *Time,* June 17, pp. 54–58.

PETERS, THOMAS G. 1991. "Life or Death: The Issue of Payment in Cadaveric Organ Donation." *Journal of the American Medical Association* 265, no. 10:1302–1305.

PROTTAS, JEFFREY M. 1989. "The Organization of Organ Procurement." In *Organ Transplantation Policy: Issues and Prospects,* pp. 41–55. Edited by James F. Blumstein and Frank A. Sloan. Durham, N.C.: Duke University Press.

PROTTAS, JEFFREY M., and BATTEN, HELEN L. 1991. "The Willingness to Give: The Public and the Supply of Transplantable Organs." *Journal of Health Politics, Policy, and Law* 16, no. 1:121–133.

QUINDLEN, ANNA. 1991. "The Heart's Reasons." *New York Times,* June 6, p. A25.

RANDALL, TERRI. 1991. "Too Few Human Organs for Transplantation, Too Many in Need . . . and the Gap Widens." *Journal of the American Medical Association* 265, no. 10:1223, 1227.

SIMMONS, ROBERTA G.; KLEIN, SUSAN D.; and SIMMONS, RICHARD L. 1977. *The Gift of Life: The Social and Psychological Impact of Organ Transplantation.* New York: John Wiley. Reprinted with new introduction and new subtitle, *The Effect of Organ Transplantation on Individual, Family, and Societal Dynamics,* by Roberta G. Simmons, Susan Klein Marine, and Richard L. Simmons. New Brunswick, N.J.: Transaction Books.

TRUCCO, TERRY. 1989. "Sales of Kidneys Prompt New Laws and Debate." *New York Times,* August 1, pp. C1, C6.

WIKLER, DANIEL, and WEISBARD, ALAN J. 1989. "Appropriate Confusion over 'Brain Death.'" *Journal of the American Medical Association* 261, no. 15:2246.

WOLFE, ALAN. 1989. *Whose Keeper? Social Science and Moral Obligation.* Berkeley: University of California Press.

YOUNGNER, STUART J.; LANDEFELD, SETH; COULTON, CLAUDIA J.; JUKNIALIS, BARBARA W.; and LEARY, MARK. 1989. "'Brain Death' and Organ Retrieval: A Cross-sectional Survey of Knowledge and Concepts Among Health Professionals." *Journal of the American Medical Association* 261, no. 15:2205–2210.

III. ETHICAL AND LEGAL ISSUES

No modern medical technology raises more ethical, legal, and policy questions than transplantation. Since World War II, most nations capable of performing transplants have obtained organs and tissues from both living persons and the dead, on the basis of voluntary consent motivated by altruism. In the case of the deceased, consent is obtained either through a written advance directive, often a "donor card," or on the basis of proxy consent by next of kin. The values of voluntarism and altruism have come in for much critical scrutiny and debate in recent years as the supply of organs and tissues has not kept up with the capacity to perform these operations.

The scarcity of organs and tissues available for transplantation has forced those in the field to articulate policies and criteria for allocating what are often life-saving resources. Disputes about equity in the distribution of organs and tissues have elicited a great deal of discussion about the relevance of such factors as age, mental and physical disabilities, ability to pay, psychosocial variables, and patient compliance in organ and tissue allocation. Transplants are often very expensive. Issues of fairness in terms of covering the exorbitant costs of transplants by third-party payers continue to dominate debates about access to and coverage for transplants. Questions of fairness also arise with respect to which centers and teams can and should perform various types of transplants, and whether too many fiscal and human resources are being devoted to the creation of a greater capacity to perform transplants, given both the scarcity of organs and the need to provide other forms of healthcare services. Questions about the proper moral foundation for obtaining organs and tissues and how best to allocate the limited supply have swirled about the field of organ transplantation since the first successful transplants were performed.

The early years: The 1950s and 1960s

The modern age of organ transplantation began in 1954 with the successful transplantation of a kidney from a young boy to his identical twin brother at the Peter Bent Brigham Hospital in Boston, Massachusetts. The early surgical pioneers and their patients faced tremendous technical challenges. Organs could be taken only from living donors, since it was not known whether cadaver organs would function. Even if cadaver organs did function, it was unclear how to remove, store, and handle them. There were no effective drugs available to prevent or to treat the rejection of a transplanted organ from a nonidentical biological source. Knowledge about the biology of the human immune system was spotty. Identical twins or closely related siblings were the only feasible donor–recipient pairs since their bodily organs possessed

the same or very similar genetic information. In the middle and late 1950s, the only organs transplanted were kidneys. Surgeons believed this was the only organ that could be removed from a human being without compromising the health of the donor (Murray, 1992).

Because of the dubious efficacy of transplantation during this period, moral concerns focused more on the rights and interests of prospective donors than on those of prospective recipients. A person with chronic renal failure with no other hope of survival would, doctors assumed, accept the risks and uncertainties associated with kidney transplantation. Physicians were deeply concerned, as were many religious leaders, that those doing transplants make every effort to minimize the risk of serious harm to donors (Wolstenholme and O'Connor, 1966). Some worried that removing a kidney from a healthy person solely to benefit another came uncomfortably close to violating the principle of nonmaleficence, or "do no harm," which permeates and continues to dominate the ethic of Western medicine.

The moral means that emerged for not violating the principle of nonmaleficence by risking the health of one person to aid another were informed consent and altruism. Those doing transplants felt they were not harming prospective donors if they were certain that the risk of doing harm was very low and fully disclosed and if the decision to make a kidney available was freely and voluntarily chosen. Voluntary altruism became the central tenet of transplantation ethics. This ethos did not emerge because giving was seen as morally preferable to either allowing organs to be sold or granting the state or doctors the right simply to take organs when someone was in need. Rather, physicians and theologians felt that the act of removing a kidney did not violate the strict prohibition against doing harm when procurement took place with the informed and altruistic concurrence of the donor.

The desire to respect the principle of nonmaleficence in the earliest days of transplantation was reinforced by Jewish and Christian religious traditions, which saw a person's relationship to his or her body as the stewardship of a gift from God. The key moral challenge raised by living donation, especially within the Catholic and Jewish traditions, was whether removing a kidney to give to another constituted immoral self-mutilation of the body (Wolstenholme and O'Connor, 1966). It was not until the 1960s that a consensus emerged among religious authorities in North America and Europe that if the act of organ donation were freely and voluntarily entered into from the motive of love and the desire to help another human being (beneficence), then donation was morally licit.

The most problematic moral cases during this period concerned prospective donors who were young children or mentally incompetent persons. The pool of possible kidney donors was so small that those in need of transplants had no alternative but to turn to family members, some of whom were clearly not competent to make voluntary, altruistic choices.

When approached about the prospect of using minor or incompetent donors, U.S. courts followed two principles. Some judges argued that it was in the best interest of a child or cognitively impaired person to be permitted to try to save the life of a relative. Thus, they approved donation on behalf of such persons on the grounds that it was in their interest. Other U.S. courts insisted that guardians or surrogate decision makers, frequently parents, be appointed to exercise surrogate informed consent for the minor or incompetent prospective donor (Scott, 1981). In the United States, a number of donations by children and incompetent adults did occur with the proxy consent of parents. In most nations in Europe, however, children under the age of eighteen and mentally incompetent persons were ruled out as possible donors on the grounds that they could not freely consent, thereby undermining the moral basis for violating the nonmaleficence principle.

From experiment to therapy: The 1970s and 1980s

A number of technological innovations revolutionized the world of organ transplantation in the late 1960s and early 1970s. The widespread dissemination of ventilators and other life-support machines raised the possibility of utilizing cadavers as sources of organs. This newly emerging technology could prevent immediate damage to vital organs even though the patient had died.

The ability to artificially support organ function even though a person had died called into question the medical profession's criteria for pronouncing death. There were no agreed-upon legal or clinical criteria for determining death in a person whose vital organ functions were being maintained by machines. Heated debates broke out among physicians and others concerning the need to redefine or expand the definition of death to include those whose brains had irreversibly ceased to function, even though their hearts and lungs continued to do so. These debates culminated in the addition of brain death to the long-accepted definition of cardio-pulmonary death in U.S. state laws and in the laws of other nations such as Great Britain, Australia, France, and Canada (Scott, 1981).

The ability to preserve the organs of cadavers opened the door to the possibility of using cadaver organs for transplantation. This possibility became a reality when breakthroughs were made in the fields of immunology and pharmacology. Scientists began to unlock the mysteries of the immune system. They discovered key chemicals in each cell—antigens—that triggered the body's natural defenses against foreign tissue. The more closely related two people are, the more likely it is that they have the same antigens in their cells. Testing for antigens in a given organ made it possible to match those who were not immediate biological relatives but who, by chance, happened to have similar antigen types. Breakthroughs in the development of immunosuppressive drugs allowed transplant teams to use organs from donors who were not precise biological matches by suppressing the rejection phenomena in recipients. With the development of successful techniques for preserving, handling, and shipping organs outside the body using cryopreservation and various preservative solutions, the world of transplantation underwent a revolution.

By the early 1980s, it was commonplace to use cadavers as sources of organs. Not only kidneys, but hearts, livers, lungs, and combinations of these organs were being transplanted successfully. Organs from cadaver sources were routinely shipped hundreds of miles to recipients who bore no biological relationship to donors. The rates of success in transplants using cadaver organs started to approximate those associated with living donors. This rapid evolution in the field of transplantation raised a host of new ethical problems and challenges about using cadavers as the primary source of organs.

The shift to cadaver sources

The earlier emphasis on voluntary choice and altruism as the moral basis for permitting living donors to assume risks in the face of uncertain benefits carried over to cadaver donation in the 1970s and 1980s. Public concern about the importance of altruistic, voluntary choice was reinforced when it was revealed that, during the late 1960s, some physicians had surreptitiously removed pituitary glands from cadavers in order to obtain growth hormone to help children born with congenital dwarfism (Caplan, 1984).

In the United States, both the public and the Congress expressed outrage over the removal of tissues from cadavers without prior consent from either the deceased via wills or from their families. This reaction indicated that the desire to guarantee individuals the right to control their own bodies was thought to extend to the disposition of their remains after death. The great value placed on personal autonomy in the United States led to professional and public discussions about the need to design a system of advance directives that would allow each individual to control the disposition of his or her bodily remains (Scott, 1981; Meyers, 1990). The Uniform Anatomical Gift Act, which created the donor-card system, emerged from the moral concern about individual choice.

In the late 1960s, various model statutes were advanced proposing a brain-death standard (Scott, 1981). By 1975, some form of brain-death legislation had been adopted in more than thirty states (Meyers, 1990). These states recognized the total and irreversible cessation of all brain function as a criterion of death that could be used along with the older definition of death, that is, the irreversible cessation of cardiopulmonary function.

The ability to use cadavers as sources of transplantable organs led to heated debate about whether public policy with respect to organ and tissue procurement should be changed. Some analysts argued that the impressive success of transplantation justified abandoning the prerequisite of informed consent in favor of laws based on the presumption of consent, thereby permitting the routine salvaging of cadaver organs (Sanders and Dukeminier, 1968). Others argued that the time had come to allow financial rewards to those willing to make organs and tissues available after their deaths (Scott, 1981).

Critics of presumed consent and routine salvaging argued that it was unfair to imperil the rights of those who opposed cadaveric organ and tissue donation for religious reasons (Ramsey, 1970). Those holding minority points of view about cadaver donation would feel powerful social pressure to abandon their religious beliefs. Others who opposed any change in the moral foundation of procurement were concerned that public policies that allowed either the routine removal of organs and tissues from cadavers or permitted financial incentives would corrode social attitudes toward the dignity of the body and the sanctity and worth of the individual. The moral argument that ultimately prevailed was that public policy should be based on voluntary choice and altruism, because these values were consistent with the need to respect individual autonomy. Public policies based on these values might permit an adequate supply of organs and tissues to be obtained from cadaver sources if adequate educational efforts were made to inform the public about the importance of cadaver-organ donation (Caplan, 1984).

State and federal laws pertaining to cadaver donation. The ethical concern that the donation of organs and tissues be voluntary and altruistic was reflected in the earliest U.S. legislation dealing with cadaver donation. In 1968, the National Conference of Commissioners on Uniform State Laws adopted the Uniform Anatomical Gift Act (UAGA). By 1972, versions of this law had been passed in all fifty states. These laws recognized a signed card as completely sufficient for donation as long as family members did not object. Health-care professionals who made a good-faith effort to locate next of kin prior to relying on a donor card to remove organs and tissues were immunized against legal action (Meyers, 1990). In order to ensure that decisions to donate were altruistic, laws explicitly prohibiting the sale of organs and most tissues were subsequently enacted in some states; and in 1984, federal legislation, the National Organ Transplant Act, became law.

If a deceased person did not complete a donor card, the UAGA permits donation based on the consent of relatives or guardians. In such circumstances, immediate family members have the right to veto donation. The law clearly recognizes family members' legitimate interest in the fate of bodily remains but does not assign the family a property interest in the body (Caplan, 1984).

In the 1980s, as the demand for cadaver organs increased and waiting lists began to grow, another legislative reform was introduced—"required request." Legislation was enacted requiring that a request be made to family members for organ donation at the time of death. This legislation was based on the ethical argument that mandating requests would not be coercive to families but would afford them the opportunity to choose to donate. Oregon and New York enacted the first required-request laws in 1985. By 1992, forty-seven states and the District of Columbia had enacted some form of required-request legislation governing cadaver sources (Caplan, 1992). In 1986, the U.S. Congress enacted legislation requiring hospitals to institute required-request policies. Shortly thereafter, the Joint Commission on Accreditation of Health-Care Organizations ordered that request policies be in place as a condition of hospital accreditation.

The only exception to the requirement of voluntary consent in U.S. public policy concerns the disposition of bodies in the custody of the state. Ten states and a small number of municipalities have enacted legislation granting authority to medical examiners and coroners to procure organs and tissues from unclaimed bodies undergoing autopsy. The states of Louisiana, Texas, Florida, and Ohio and the cities of San Francisco and Denver are among the localities that permit procurement from bodies under the control of medical examiners or coroners when no family members can be found and there is no reason to assume any prior objection to procurement. In 1992, Texas enacted a modification of the UAGA whereby family members are not allowed to object to donation when the deceased has signed a donor card.

The problem of scarcity

Scarcity in the supply of organs emerged in the 1990s as the single most frustrating problem for those involved in transplantation. At the end of 1987, the United Network for Organ Sharing (UNOS), the semiprivate entity created to help distribute organs among the nation's transplantation centers, reported that 13,396 people were waiting to receive kidneys, hearts, livers, or lungs. In 1989, there were 19,173 names on the waiting list. One year later, there were 22,008 names on the list, an increase of more than 60 percent over three years. Despite the fact that more and more transplants are performed each year, the list has continued to grow. Similar gaps between supply and demand exist in every other nation where transplants are done.

A key factor in the expansion of waiting lists is that, as surgical skill has improved, the criteria have relaxed for considering people with end-stage organ disease as potential transplant recipients. Age limits that prevailed in the 1970s—no one older than fifty-five for heart and liver transplants, for example—have since been extended to include persons in their late sixties and early seventies. Diabetes is no longer an absolute contraindication for kidney transplantation. Persons suffering liver failure resulting from alcohol abuse have had successful transplantations (Caplan, 1992).

As the pool of potential recipients has grown, so have the numbers of those who die while on waiting lists. Between one-third and one-half of all Americans on waiting lists for hearts, livers, lungs, and multiple-organ combinations die before transplantable organs are found. The shortage of organs for newborns and very young children is especially acute. UNOS reports that 25 percent of those waiting for liver transplants are children less than ten years old and that in 1993, more than 400 infants born with congenital defects of the heart died because there were no donor hearts available for them.

The demand for organs is likely to continue to increase at a rapid rate. Success rates associated with all forms of transplantation have improved. The shift in the demographics of the United States, Europe, and Japan toward an older population means that more individuals will need transplants. Continuing improvements in immunosuppressive drugs, combined with a better understanding of the genetics of the immune system that the Human Genome Project is providing, mean that success rates will continue to improve for various types of transplants, making an even larger segment of those suffering from organ failure potential candidates for transplants.

Since the early 1960s, the number of medical centers and hospitals capable of performing transplants has steadily increased. This increasing capacity to do transplants, and the high costs involved, have also increased the pressure to find more organs and tissues.

Other factors promise further increases in the demand for transplants. These include improvements in techniques for "bridging"—temporarily keeping those in acute organ failure alive—such as the use of Left Ventricular Assist Devices (LVADs), bioartificial livers, or xenografts of pig or primate organs; the ability to maintain patients with end-stage organ failure using new technology, such as the insulin pump and extracorporeal membrane oxygenation; and the modification of the immune systems of donor and recipient through genetic engineering.

Moral choices in the face of scarcity. In many countries, national policies for allocating organs emerged after a series of complaints and media accounts concerning the inequitable distribution of organs at individual transplant centers. For example, in the early 1980s the media in the United States, Italy, and the United Kingdom carried many reports about wealthy foreigners who paid high sums of money for priority placement on transplant center waiting lists. That wealthy noncitizens could move to the top of waiting lists seemed to many to be unfair and immoral. The U.S. government threatened to take over the allocation of cadaver organs unless the transplant community established a publicly accountable national network to distribute organs to those in need. This resulted in the development of UNOS during the late 1980s.

UNOS resolved the question of access by declaring that no more than 10 percent of any center's transplant population could be foreigners. But other problems quickly boiled to the surface as UNOS and other agencies, such as U.K. Transplant and Eurotransplant, which handles organ distribution in Germany and the Benelux nations, began to grapple with how best to allocate an increasingly scarce supply of organs.

Traditionally, transplant programs around the world had given great weight in their allocation policies to such factors as tissue type, the physical size of donor and recipient, blood type, medical urgency, and how much time the recipient had spent on the waiting list. But doubts began to surface in some circles about the fairness of biological criteria (Kjellstrand, 1988). The use of the closest match of tissue types may increase the success of a transplant, but it puts minorities at a disadvantage. Asian-Americans, Pacific Island peoples, and aboriginal peoples living in the United States or other nations with large caucasian populations are less likely than whites to find close matches in a pool of cadaver donors that is largely white. Decisions about the importance of biology in allocating organs involve trade-offs between the desire to maximize the outcome of a transplant and the desire to ensure that each person in need has a fair chance of receiving a transplant.

Organs obtained from cadaver donors are distributed among transplant centers according to criteria that include blood type, geographic location where organs are obtained, tissue-matching, patient waiting time, and medical urgency (Caplan, 1992). Most transplant centers follow a policy of "share one, keep one" where locally obtained cadaver kidneys are concerned. With few exceptions, organs go to those who have been waiting the longest at centers near where the donor is. Consortiums in other nations use similar criteria to share organs.

Some critics maintain that giving top priority to the sickest patients on a national waiting list skews the allocation of valuable organs to those who are least likely to survive (Ubel et al., 1993). Those who need a second, third, or even fourth transplant because their initial transplant failed gain top priority for the next available kidney, heart, or liver even though the odds of a successful retransplant are lower than they are for first-time transplants. Similarly, assigning top priority to those who have received an artificial organ or a xenograft as a temporary bridge has elicited much criticism as an unfair and inefficient use of scarce cadaver organs (Annas, 1993).

Macroallocation and morality.   Despite the fact that there are national criteria for allocating organs to ensure fair access to those who need transplants, there are still reasons for concern about the overall fairness of the current system. Primary among these is the role played by money in determining not who gets a transplant at a particular hospital, but who is referred for consideration and gains admission to a transplant center.

Transplantation is an expensive procedure. In 1992, a kidney transplant cost around $35,000; a heart transplant, between $60,000 and $100,000; and a liver transplant, anywhere between $150,000 and $250,000 (Caplan, 1992). These figures presume a procedure that goes relatively well, without complications requiring longer hospital stays or further surgery. They do not include costs such as travel, time lost from the job, or day care, which can be enormously burdensome to transplant candidates and their families since these costs are not covered by medical insurance.

In order to be considered for a transplant, a person must be able to meet these costs. He or she must also have access to a physician who is capable of recognizing that the medical problem is amenable to a transplant. In the United States and many other nations, insurance to cover primary medical care and to pay the costs of a transplant is pivotal in determining who gains access to transplant centers for evaluation and, if appropriate, placement on a waiting list.

Many insurance programs do not cover the costs of certain kinds of transplants. This is especially true for newer, more innovative forms of transplantation such as lung, pancreas, or intestinal transplants; xenografts; or multiple-organ transplants. Whether or not government insurance programs, such as Medicaid, will cover the costs of transplants depends on where an individual lives and whether or not he or she has been disabled for a significant period of time. Access to transplantation is very much a function of access to good primary medical care and the right kind of insurance coverage (Caplan, 1992).

Some people would argue that the ability to pay is a fair basis for allocating an expensive service such as organ transplants, and that societies do not have an obligation to provide access to every possible form of medical care, especially when organ failure is the result of voluntary behavior such as smoking and drug or alcohol abuse (Moss and Siegler, 1991). Others maintain that, while money might be an unfair method for determining who has access to transplant services, equity requires limiting rather than increasing access. If there are large numbers of persons in a particular society who do not have access to basic health-care services, then allowing a tiny number access to expensive forms of treatment such as transplantation seems inherently unfair (Fox and Swazey, 1992).

There is no consensus about how to evaluate the overall equity of a health-care system or the provision of particular services such as transplantation. However, most theories of justice hold that if the provision of a particular service using public money places an undue burden on the services that are available to others, then those who have access to such a service ought to pay the costs involved out of their own resources. Few would want to defend publicly funded provision of procedures that lack efficacy, or are capable of providing only marginal benefits, when other procedures are known to be far more efficacious and beneficial. The debate about the equity of transplantation services available in a given society, or how much a society ought to spend on these services relative to other types of medical or public-health interventions, requires attention not only in terms of justice, but also in terms of the efficacy and benefit associated with particular kinds of treatments.

International responses to the problem of scarcity.   Most nations in the Western world maintain a strong commitment to voluntarism and altruism as the basis of obtaining organs from both cadaver and living sources. But the lack of organs for transplant has led some nations to pursue public policies such as routine salvage or presumed consent, which rest upon different values. France, using the argument that the needs of society outweigh the rights of the individual to control bodily remains after death, enacted a presumed-consent law in 1976. For many decades, Austria has had what amounts to a routine salvage policy, in which the state assigns dominion over bodies to physicians to use them for important social purposes. In 1988, Singapore instituted a donation policy based upon reciprocal altruism: Those willing to serve as donors receive priority for transplants.

A small increase in kidney donation followed the enactment of the presumed-consent law in France. Most of the increase, however, was used to decrease the number of kidney transplants involving living donors (Kokkedee, 1992). Other nations such as Austria and

Belgium, which have placed societal needs ahead of individual autonomy and voluntarism, have not, according to Eurotransplant officials, seen any improvement as of 1994 in the supply of organs.

A few nations, including India, Turkey, Haiti, the former Soviet Union, the Philippines, and Brazil, permit—or have at least tolerated—the offering of financial incentives to living donors or to the families of cadaver donors. These practices have provoked heated debate about the morality of markets in body parts, both within and outside the countries in which they occur. No nation appears to allow financial rewards with respect to cadaver donation; however, reports of payment for cadaver kidneys obtained from prisoners have emerged from China and Hong Kong. The moral justification for allowing financial incentives is rooted in the claim that individuals should be free to sell bodily organs if they wish to do so, as long as they do so without pressure or coercion (Blumstein and Sloan, 1989; Peters, 1991). Counterarguments hinge on the view that the body ought not be made an object of commerce; that more potential donors will be repelled by monetary rewards than will be attracted by them; and that the quality of organs obtained through policies that permit financial compensation will be lower, since those who are paid will have a motive to conceal their health status (Caplan et al., 1993).

The ongoing ethics challenge of scarcity

Regardless of the public policy adopted, the number of potential cadaver organ sources is very small (Novello, 1992). One possible strategy for increasing the number of organs and tissues available is to encourage more educational efforts to persuade individuals and families to donate organs. Despite public-opinion polls showing widespread support for organ donation, family refusal is a real barrier to procurement. It is not clear whether this is a failure of voluntarism, or the failure of health-care professionals to explain carefully and thoughtfully the reasons for organ donation. Without adequate empirical information, it is impossible to determine whether the appropriate public-policy response is more educational training for health-care professionals; more public education; changes in the timing, setting, or identity of those making requests; or abandoning the moral framework of altruistic voluntarism altogether.

Revisions in the UAGA suggest that hospitals ask all patients about their organ-donor status upon admission. Some states, such as New Jersey, have enacted this requirement into law. The *Patient Self-Determination Act of 1990* mandates that all prospective patients be apprised of the importance of having a living will; many of the standard forms used with this document contain a provision regarding organ donation.

Another strategy to alleviate the problem of scarcity is to broaden the criteria of age and health status used to determine both living- and cadaver-donor eligibility. However, broadening the definition of who can be a donor raises important moral and legal questions. Most living donors have a biological relationship with those in need of a transplant. Some programs have begun to explore the option of recruiting strangers to serve as living donors for those in need. The moral justification for such a strategy is that it is the individual who can best weigh the risk associated with donating a kidney or part of another organ against the benefits to be gained. Reliance on individual autonomy is the rationale for expanding the pool of persons who are considered potential organ donors (Spital and Spital, 1985).

Another way to increase the supply of organs is to permit the elective use of mechanical ventilation solely to permit organ donation in persons who otherwise would die without life support. In persons dying from cerebrovascular accidents, where life support has not been used, families could be asked for their consent to the use of mechanical ventilation in order to make organ donation possible (Arnold and Youngner, 1993). A similar strategy for expanding the cadaver-donor pool involves obtaining organs from persons who die in emergency rooms or hospitals by preserving them using special fluids as soon as death has been pronounced (Novello, 1992).

It may also be possible to make more efficient use of the cadaver-donor pool than is currently the case. For example, if allocation rules on waiting lists were to place less emphasis on severity of illness and waiting time and more on likely prognosis, the same number of cadaver organs might be able to save more lives. If more selective criteria were used in determining eligibility for transplants, including discouraging or prohibiting retransplantation, overall posttransplant survival might be increased (Fox and Swazey, 1992).

There has been some discussion of broadening the definition or the criteria used to determine death. For example, some commentators have suggested permitting the use of different criteria for determining brain death in anencephalic infants to facilitate their use as organ donors. Others suggest that the concept of donor be expanded to include persons in permanent vegetative states or those for whom brain death cannot be determined but whose hearts have stopped (Arnold and Youngner, 1993).

Another strategy to increase the size of the pool of organs available for transplant is to turn to animal sources. There are obvious ethical, psychosocial, and public-policy issues involved in pursuing this alternative. Many people believe that it would be immoral to kill animals, particularly primates, for the sole purpose of harvesting their organs. Others note that the use of animals is currently so experimental that the informed-consent procedures of recipients must be especially rigorous and peer review exceedingly conscientious before any potential recipients can be recruited (Caplan, 1992). The ethics of using animals as routine sources of organs must be carefully examined, since breakthroughs in genetic engineering and immunology are likely to facilitate cross-species transplants.

Scarcity will characterize the field of transplantation for the rest of the twentieth century. The key moral questions are whether the framework of values that has dominated U.S. attitudes toward the procurement of human organs and tissues is consistent with expanding the pool of cadaver and living donors; whether the pressing need for organs justifies abandoning these values; and whether the symbolic and social cost of shifts in these values would come at an ethical price that is too high to pay (Fox and Swazey, 1992).

ARTHUR L. CAPLAN

Directly related to this article are the other articles in this entry: MEDICAL OVERVIEW, *and* SOCIOCULTURAL ASPECTS. *Also directly related to this article are the entries* ORGAN AND TISSUE PROCUREMENT; *and* XENOGRAFTS. *For a further discussion of topics mentioned in this article, see the entries* ANIMAL WELFARE AND RIGHTS, *article on* ETHICAL PERSPECTIVES ON THE TREATMENT AND STATUS OF ANIMALS; AUTONOMY; BENEFICENCE; BODY; CHILDREN; DEATH, DEFINITION AND DETERMINATION OF; EASTERN ORTHODOX CHRISTIANITY; FAMILY; FREEDOM AND COERCION; HARM; HEALTH-CARE FINANCING; HEALTH-CARE RESOURCES, ALLOCATION OF; HEALTH POLICY; INFANTS; INFORMED CONSENT; JUDAISM; JUSTICE; LOVE; MEDICAL ETHICS, HISTORY OF, *section on* EUROPE, *subsection on* CONTEMPORARY PERIOD; MENTALLY DISABLED AND MENTALLY ILL PERSONS; PROTESTANTISM; RIGHTS; RISK; ROMAN CATHOLICISM; SUBSTANCE ABUSE; SURGERY; *and* TECHNOLOGY. *For a discussion of related ideas, see the entries* ADOLESCENTS; AGING AND THE AGED, *articles on* SOCIETAL AGING, HEALTH-CARE AND RESEARCH ISSUES, *and* OLD AGE; AIDS; ARTIFICIAL HEARTS AND CARDIAC-ASSIST DEVICES; *and* UTILITY.

Bibliography

ANNAS, GEORGE J. 1993. *Standard of Care: The Law of American Bioethics.* New York: Oxford University Press.
ARNOLD, ROBERT M., and YOUNGNER, STUART J. 1993. "Non-Heart-Beating Donors." *Kennedy Institute of Ethics Journal* 3, no. 2:1–12.
BLUMSTEIN, JAMES F., and SLOAN, FRANK A., eds. 1989. *Organ Transplantation Policy: Issues and Prospects.* Durham, N.C.: Duke University Press.
CAPLAN, ARTHUR L. 1984. "Organ Procurement: It's Not in the Cards." *Hastings Center Report* 14, no. 5:9–12.
———. 1992. *If I Were a Rich Man Could I Buy a Pancreas? and Other Essays on the Ethics of Health Care.* Bloomington: Indiana University Press.
CAPLAN, ARTHUR L.; TILNEY, NICHOLAS L.; and VAN BUREN, CHARLES T. 1993. "Financial Compensation for Cadaver Organ Donation: Good Idea or Anathema?" *Transplantation Proceedings* 25, no. 4:2740–2742.
FOX, RENÉE C., and SWAZEY, JUDITH P. 1992. *Spare Parts: Organ Replacement in American Society.* New York: Oxford University Press.
KJELLSTRAND, CARL M. 1988. "Age, Sex and Race Inequality in Renal Transplantation." *Archives of Internal Medicine* 148, no. 6:1305–1309.
KOKKEDEE, WILLIAM. 1992. "Kidney Procurement Policies in the Eurotransplant Region: 'Opting In' Versus 'Opting Out.'" *Social Science and Medicine* 35, no. 2:177–182.
MEYERS, DAVID W. 1990. *The Human Body and the Law.* 2d ed. Stanford, Calif.: Stanford University Press.
MOSS, ALVIN H., and SIEGLER, MARK. 1991. "Should Alcoholics Compete Equally for Liver Transplantation?" *Journal of the American Medical Association* 265, no. 10: 1295–1298.
MURRAY, JOSEPH E. 1992. "Human Organ Transplantation: Background and Consequences." *Science* 256, no. 5062: 1411–1415.
NOVELLO, ANTONIA C. 1992. *The Surgeon General's Workshop on Increasing Organ Donation.* Washington, D.C.: Department of Health and Human Services, Public Health Service, Surgeon General of the United States.
PETERS, THOMAS G. 1991. "Life or Death: The Issue of Payment in Cadaveric Organ Donation." *Journal of the American Medical Association* 265, no. 10:1302–1305.
RAMSEY, PAUL. 1970. *The Patient as Person: Explorations in Medical Ethics.* New Haven, Conn.: Yale University Press.
SANDERS, DAVID, and DUKEMINIER, JESSE, JR. 1968. "Medical Advance and Legal Lag: Hemodialysis and Kidney Transplantation." *UCLA Law Review* 15:357–413.
SCOTT, RUSSELL. 1981. *The Body as Property.* New York: Viking.
SPITAL, AARON, and SPITAL, MAX. 1985. "Donor's Choice or Hobson's Choice." *Archives of Internal Medicine* 145, no. 7:1297–1301.
UBEL, PETER A.; ARNOLD, ROBERT M.; and CAPLAN, ARTHUR L. 1993. "Rationing Failure: The Ethical Lessons of the Retransplantation of Scarce Vital Organs." *Journal of the American Medical Association* 270, no. 20:2469–2474.
U.S. TASK FORCE ON ORGAN TRANSPLANTATION. 1986. *Organ Transplantation: Issues and Recommendations.* Rockville, Md.: U.S. Department of Health and Human Services, Office of Organ Transplantation.
WOLSTENHOLME, GORDON E. W., and O'CONNOR, MAEVE, eds. 1966. *Ethics in Medical Progress: With Special Reference to Transplantation.* London: Churchill.

ORGAN TRANSPLANTATION

See ORGAN AND TISSUE TRANSPLANTS; *and* XENOGRAFTS.

ORTHODOXY IN MEDICINE

See UNORTHODOXY IN MEDICINE. *See also* ALTERNATIVE THERAPIES.

OSTEOPATHY

See ALTERNATIVE THERAPIES, *article on* HISTORICAL ASPECTS. *See also* MEDICINE AS A PROFESSION.

OVA DONATION AND BANKING

See REPRODUCTIVE TECHNOLOGIES, *article on* CRYOPRESERVATION OF SPERM, OVA, AND EMBRYOS.

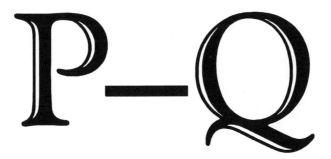

PAIN AND SUFFERING

Suffering demands explanation and relief. Some appear to suffer in excess of their actions, the innocent suffer as the evil do, and the best suffer with the worst. Theologies and theodicies attempt to cope with the paradox of a holy, omnipotent, omniscient, just god and the presence of suffering. Healers and systems of medicine arise in every culture in response to suffering. Yet what suffering is, where in the human condition it originates, and in what direction its solution is, remain poorly understood.

Pain is the most commonly considered source of suffering, so much so that the two terms are commonly linked—as in "pain and suffering." They are, however, distinctly different forms of distress. Understanding what pain is and how it is related to but different from suffering, provides an introduction to the topic.

How the nervous system is involved in pain—the nociceptive apparatus

The nervous system pathways—the nociceptive apparatus—involved in the transmission of noxious stimuli, do not simply transfer information from an injured part to the central nervous system. They are part of a system in which the information can be either enhanced, diminished, or suppressed. The modulation of the noxious sensation occurs as part of the process of perception where meaning influences the original message.

Skin, muscles, and internal organs are supplied with nerve endings that come from several types of nerve fibers. Some are specifically responsive to mechanical, thermal, and chemical stimuli that give rise to the noxious physical sensation called nociception. These nociceptive nerve fibers enter the spinal cord and make complex connections with the spinal nerves that ascend to the thalamus and from there to areas of the cortex of the brain. Neural pathways from the higher centers, in what is called the endogenous pain control system, descend to make connections in the dorsal horn of the spinal cord in the area where the pain fibers make their initial central connections. These descending tracts are able to modulate the nociceptive signal by exerting an inhibitory effect specifically on pain-transmission neurons.

In addition to neural pathways, which do not merely transmit noxious sensations but change their character, chemical messengers and their receptors within the nervous system also have an influence on the message. Naturally occurring brain peptides such as enkephalin and beta-endorphin, collectively known as endorphins, exert analgesic effects in different areas of the nervous system by binding to specialized receptors. These same receptors also bind drugs such as morphine or meperidine, allowing them to provide pain relief. Other neurotransmitters, such as serotonin and dopamine, also have effects that temper the transmission of nociceptive messages.

Pain as perception

Historically, knowledge about nociception as neural transmission of noxious stimuli predated knowledge about the modulation of the nociceptive process. This simplified view of nociception fits the mechanical understanding of the nervous system that has held until recent times. This view accounts for the fact that the noxious sensation that is nociception is so commonly confused with pain and that the two terms, although distinct, are often used interchangeably. Nociception provides the noxious sensation resulting from extremes of mechanical pressure or temperature that is interpreted by the organism as pain.

Because pain is a perception based on sensory information from the nociceptive apparatus—just as seeing something is a perception based on information from the visual apparatus—it involves a cognitive effort that requires judgment. The place of cognition in the process may be questioned in acute, severe, or momentary pain, but most pain is longer lasting and more ambiguous in source and meaning.

Nociception is usually followed by aversive action. The reflexive withdrawal of a burned hand, however, has little applicability to understanding human pain. The actions of humans in response to pain generally take into account the location, severity, cause, and anticipated course of the pain. Knowledge and judgment are required. Reactions to pain range from the momentary to well-laid future plans. While the former may depend on reflexes, the latter do not. *Pain is the entire process of sensing, interpreting, and modulating the nociceptive process, assigning cause, anticipating course, and determining response.* As a consequence, it is obvious why it is a source of confusion that human pain does not exist without sentience. Unconscious or comatose persons may demonstrate nociceptive reactions such as reflex withdrawal from noxious stimuli or elevations in pulse and blood pressure. Consciousness, however, is required for the full experience of pain. This is why a useful working definition of pain is experience reported in the statement "it hurts."

Attempts to refute the subjective nature of pain may take the form of statements that pain is usually accompanied by physiologic changes in, for example, pulse and blood pressure, but the body and its physiology are part of the person and nothing happens to one part that does not happen to all. Confusions such as this are residua of the mind–body dichotomy that has ruled medical science for centuries and still disorders understanding. The fact that pain cannot be measured has been a source of great frustration to investigators. Noxious stimuli and nociceptive responses can be quantified, but pain cannot. The difficulty of understanding pain is part of the age-old conundrum of how a physiological event be-comes a feeling or a thought and how thoughts and feelings are translated into physiology.

Chronic pain

Chronic pain—by definition, pain lasting more than six months—represents a greater challenge to understanding than acute pain. What is known about the nociceptive system does not explain the phenomenon of chronic pain. There is evidence that the reparative response that occurs after damage to peripheral nerves may alter their function in a manner that perpetuates or exaggerates their response to noxious stimuli. Similar modifications of the whole nociceptive apparatus, including the function of its neuroendocrine component (for example, endorphins), may provide some basis for pain that continues after the initial stage of tissue damage. Nonetheless, paucity of solid evidence to resolve the enigma of chronic pain has led to speculation and hypothesis based more on belief than on knowledge. For example, various schemata have been developed that explain chronic pain in many ways: as a result of continued tissue damage (e.g., rheumatoid arthritis); because of psychic perpetuation of organic pain (e.g., phantom limb pain); or from emotional factors believed to precipitate the organic (e.g., duodenal ulcer); as well as to hypothesized states of psychogenic pain arising from psychic conflicts experienced in a somatic manner (Whitehead and Kuhn, 1990).

The problem has also been framed as a conflict between peripheralists and centralists. The peripheralist believes that there must be continued nociceptive input and that treatment should be directed toward blocking the presumed nociceptive process with analgesics or nerve blocks and by other means. Centralists believe that although some peripheral pathology with nociceptive consequences initiated the pain, under some circumstances it can be continued "as a self-perpetuating physiological generator mechanism within the central nervous system" (Crue, 1985).

The role of meaning

Human pain, acute or chronic, involves the constant and interactive contribution of both psychic and physical determinants. The most important psychological component of pain is its meaning, that is, its significance and its importance. Significance denotes the event as a this or a that: "Chest pain (of this type) signifies a heart attack." Importance evaluates the event: "A heart attack will be the end of my active life." These two functions of meaning are always intertwined and arise from the concepts (e.g., heart attacks) to which they refer. The interpretation of a pain as arising from, for example, cancer, contains within it ideas of process: "Cancer comes from . . . and goes on to become . . ."

as well as to ideas of the impact on the person: "Cancer pain is terrible and heralds death." Things have affective, physical, and spiritual as well as cognitive meanings. People act on their interpretation of the consequences of the distress, doing what is necessary on their part for it to improve. For example, a person who develops unexpected chest pain while walking may stop because it is impossible to continue. But the person may also walk more slowly in the future, deny the pain's significance, go to an emergency room, worry, panic, take nitroglycerin, or any of a variety of actions, in response to what the person believes the symptom means.

The distinction between pain and suffering

Suffering is closely related to pain because pain is a common cause of suffering, but they are distinct forms of distress. People may report suffering when a pain, such as that caused by a dissecting aortic aneurysm, is overwhelming. Or they may tolerate even extremely severe pain if they know what it is, know that it can be relieved, or know that it will soon end. Less intense pain may be a source of suffering if the person does not know its source or believes that it has a dire cause (e.g., cancer), cannot be controlled, or will be "never-ending." Suffering can sometimes be controlled merely by changing the meaning of the pain. Clinicians working with terminally ill patients frequently see suffering patients grunting with pain who cannot be comforted. When their pain has been adequately relieved and it has been demonstrated that such relief will be forthcoming if the pain should return, they will frequently tolerate the same level of pain (by their report) without requesting medication. Once assured that relief is possible, suffering often subsides although the pain remains. It is difficult to relieve the suffering of patients who are frightened without also relieving their fear.

People may suffer from pain even when the pain is not present. Some who have had severe pain will suffer from the fear of the pain's return even when they are pain-free. People with severe and frequent migraine may suffer from their fear of a return of the headache. These headaches have repeatedly ruined what would otherwise have been pleasurable or important experiences: Family relationships, jobs, sports, and virtually everything that is dear to the person may have been negatively influenced by the headaches. Not surprisingly, such patients may be obsessed with their headaches and their attempts at relief virtually to the exclusion of other aspects of life. They suffer when they do have the actual pain and also when they do not.

The distinction between pain and suffering is clarified by the case of the pain of childbirth. Different kinds of pain relief, some more effective than others, are popular in different parts of the United States. The more important issue seems to be the degree to which the woman is in control of her own labor and delivery, rather than the absolute control of pain. Control of the process of childbirth does not relieve pain, but appears to prevent suffering. In other cases, symptoms such as dyspnea (labored respiration), choking, or even diarrhea may be sources not of pain but of suffering if they are sufficiently severe. In fact, suffering may be present in the absence of any symptoms. Parents, particularly if they are helpless in the situation, commonly suffer at the sight of their children in pain. Grinding poverty may be a source of suffering, as well as betrayal or the loss of one's life work.

The role of the future

The role of the future in these situations of suffering is crucial. In cases of overwhelming pain, in long-continued ("never-ending") pain accompanied by fear of the inability to continue to "take it," and in the situation where the pain is suspected of having terrible meaning, a sense of future is necessary in order to suffer. In each of these instances—when at the moment the pain is not overwhelming, the person is "taking it," and the fact of a dreadful disease does not yet exist—the body cannot worry; it knows no future. The body cannot supply information about the future because at any moment, for the body, the future does not yet exist. Only imagination, beliefs, memories, or ideas can supply the information necessary to provide a "future." In other words, in order to suffer, there must be a source of thoughts about possible futures.

To summarize thus far: Although suffering may attend pain, they are distinct. There may be pain without suffering. There may be suffering without pain. There seems to be no suffering without an idea of the future. Bodies do not have the beliefs, concepts, ideas, or fantasies necessary to create a future—only persons do. One can conclude that although bodies may experience nociception, bodies do not suffer. Only persons suffer.

Suffering defined

Suffering is a specific state of severe distress induced by the loss of integrity, intactness, cohesiveness, or wholeness of the person, or by a threat that the person believes will result in the dissolution of his or her integrity. Suffering continues until integrity is restored or the threat is gone. The whole person does not mean solely the whole biological organism or the solid-bounded object, although it may be the object of the threat. Persons, while they may be identified with their bodies, cannot be whole in body alone. Nor should the threat to the whole person be understood as solely a quantitative matter (i.e., that persons subjected to more than X amount of pain or Y amount of tissue destruction suffer, even if this amount of pain or tissue destruction may virtually always cause suffering), since one individual may suffer from pain considered unimportant by another. Suffering may occur in relationship to any part of a person.

Wholeness, self, and person defined

Suffering helps define the concept of person. Person is not mind, body, or self, although persons have all of these things. The word "self," as employed here, denotes that aspect of the person that is an object of the consciousness of a person—the person's own consciousness or that of another. It has cohesive characteristics and it exists over time. Persons cannot be known in their entirety and they cannot be known by reducing them to their parts. As one does that, the person disappears. A topography, however, is possible. A person is the composite entity made up of its body, its selves, its history, its collected beliefs, its believed-in future, unconscious, incorporated society and culture, associations with others including the family, the family's history, its political dimension, secret life, and transcendent dimension.

Persons are also constructed by their ideas and beliefs, by the past, the present, and a sense of the future, as well as by a sense of some level of stability in the environment. Suffering may thus be initiated by profound changes in the person's physical, political, or social world. Clinical observation suggests that the suffering of some patients is initiated by their inability to explain what has happened to them. "What did I do that made this happen to me?" is not merely a question but a metaphysical statement about how the world works. If the person's beliefs and demand for explanations are too rigid and the person cannot accept fate or uncertainty, then the integrity of the person is violated by the unexplained injury.

If physicians focus on the sick person, as necessitated by suffering, they will require knowledge of persons in the way that they presently have knowledge of the body. Persons, however, are different from other objects of science and so they pose difficulties for twentieth-century understanding. Considering persons as ahistorical, atomistic individuals, in which the body is separate from the mind—largely the stance of the sciences, the law, and some schools of philosophy—is not supported by a knowledge of suffering. The sciences of humankind, including psychology and the social sciences, have followed the lead of the physical sciences in employing reductive methodologies, but these lead to a distorted understanding. Similarly, division of the sciences of humankind into the physical, psychological, and social leads away from an understanding of persons and therefore of suffering. Virtually everything that is social is also ultimately physical and psychological. A person is not an object with physical or temporal boundaries, but

rather he or he she is a process in a trajectory through time. The challenge to a scientific understanding of persons lies in accepting these characteristics.

Suffering is unique and individual

Suffering is always individual because it can arise in relation to any aspect of a person, and persons are necessarily unique and particular. If the suffering of two people is initiated by an identical physical insult (e.g., the same kind of severe burn or similar overwhelming pain), the suffering of each will be unique and particular because it becomes suffering by virtue of its effect on a particular dimension or characteristic of the suffering person. No one can know with certainty why another person suffers. One can know that someone is suffering, but not what it is about this specific person that leads to the suffering. Sufferers themselves may not know. What threatens the loss of wholeness of one person is not necessarily the same as that which jeopardizes another. In chronic illness this distinctiveness is more easily seen. Here, suffering can arise because the sick person may not be accepted by, feel at home in, or be able to meet the expectations of others. The way these feelings affect the person will be unique to that person. These difficulties may evoke loneliness, anger, or feelings of unfairness, abandonment, or hurt. The suffering person will be focused on the feeling and the external source that is seen as its cause, not on suffering per se. This is because the same feelings may cause suffering in one person but not in another, and the suffering itself is the result of the disruption of the person arising from the discomfort. Even when suffering is caused by physical pain, the person feels pain, not suffering.

Purpose

To be whole and able to suffer is to have aims or purposes. One of these purposes, central purpose, is the preservation and continued evolution of myself as I know myself. Purposes entail actions. When suffering exists, the identity that the sufferer fears will disintegrate is an identity expressed in purposeful action—legs walk, hands grasp, eyes see, minds have ideas. Purposes and their enabling actions may not require anything from consciousness, but they are nonetheless "self"-defining. Illness and other sources of suffering interfere with actions that may be conscious, below awareness, or habitual, and thus contribute to damaging the integrity of the person and lead to suffering.

The suffering of the chronically ill may start with the inability to accomplish their previously important purposes. It may actually begin when it finally dawns on the chronically ill person that the life of illness that has been held off for so long and with such effort and determination is now truly imminent. Again, notice that suffering begins not merely when persons cannot do something but when they become aware of what the future holds, even though at the time of recognition their function has not yet worsened. The task of the person, of identity, indeed of wholeness, is the centralization of purpose, while disease, pain, and suffering may contribute to the defeat of such purpose. Pain or other symptoms may focus the person's attention on the distressed body part so completely that central purpose is lost (Bakan, 1968). This is probably always true of suffering, which arises with the loss of the ability to pursue purpose and also defeats purpose. It is one of the wonders of humanity, on the other hand, to see how a central purpose, exemplified in the biblical story of Job, may overcome suffering as well as disease and pain.

Suffering always involves self-conflict

The source of suffering is usually seen as outside the sufferer. What is usually identified as the origin of the suffering is the thing that causes the pain, or the pain itself, the life circumstances, or the stroke of fate. In fact, however, suffering always involves self-conflict. Thinking about acute pain, one wonders how this can be. The clue lies in the fact that meaning is essential to suffering. The threat to the person's intactness or integrity resides in the meaning of the pain or beliefs about its consequences. The book of Job provides an illustration of the place of self-conflict in suffering. That there is a God and that God is just are not merely facts for Job; they are part of his self-understanding. Job is a righteous man, but his friends taunt him: If Job is righteous as he says, God would not punish him. Job responds, "Yet does not God see my ways and count my every step?" (31:4). On the other hand, he wants to defend himself before God: "I would plead the whole record of my life and present that in court as my defense" (31:37). If God knows his every step and God is just, why would he have to defend himself? The suffering of Job, generally identified with the awful things that happen to him, has as its deeper source the conflict between that part of him that knows that God is aware of his every step and is a just God, and that part of him that believes (with his friends) that only the wicked are punished. Either he *is* wicked when he knows he is not, or God is not just.

The saints offer a contrary example. Reaching toward Christ by sharing the bodily suffering of others or through punishments imposed on the body are familiar aspects of early Christianity. Denial of bodily needs, tolerance of awful afflictions, and self-inflicted torture are commonplace in the histories of the saints. Adversities and pains are seen as allowing the holy person to identify with the suffering of Christ. Conflict with the body and the tolerance of the pain do not cause conflict within the person because they permit reaching a desired goal.

If there were no Christ with whom to identify, then suffering would follow.

The sick, especially the chronically ill, are often unable to do what they need to do to ensure their self-esteem and their ability to be like others and be admired by others, to excel. But they do not stop wanting to meet these standards, which they usually picture as existing outside of themselves. The resulting internalized conflict of the sick person with the external world becomes self-conflict.

Confrontations between the person and his or her body, as well as dissension within the various aspects of the individual, can threaten to destroy the integrity of the person. This is most easily seen when the demands of the body conflict with the needs of the person. Pain or other symptoms, disabilities, medical care, or other needs may require attention to the body that deters the person from pursuits or purposes considered vital, or they may require attention to the body that the person finds extremely onerous. The body may become an untrustworthy "other" that fails the sick person when it is most needed. It may be a source of humiliation because of, for example, loss of bowel or bladder control. The body's needs, sexual or otherwise, may force the person to engage in behaviors that lead to social failures. Conflicts between the person and the body may cause suffering when no illness is present. The internal struggle that may occur in regard to sexual desire is notorious. Even in acute pain, self-conflict is present. If the person did not care about the pain or its consequences, did not resist its overwhelming force, and instead became completely passive or resigned to the injury, suffering would not occur. This represents extreme self-discipline. People want to live, to resist the pain, to fight back, and therein is the genesis of the suffering.

Suffering is a lonely state

Because the individual is ultimately unknowable and suffering is unique and individual, involving a withdrawal of purpose from the social world and marked by self-conflict, suffering is inevitably a lonely condition. The inability to know with certainty why someone is suffering, and thus to identify truly with the sufferer, creates difficulties for its treatment. The treatment and relief of suffering, *even when pain cannot be relieved,* is often best accomplished by attempting to overcome its loneliness. This is illustrated in Tolstoy's superb story about sickness and suffering, *The Death of Ivan Ilych*. Virtually the only relief from his suffering that Ilych experiences late in his illness is the constancy and compassion of the servant, Gerasim, who stays with him when all others have effectively abandoned him (Reich, 1989).

Persons are communal in origin and by nature. They cannot be known or understood apart from their social being. As a consequence, the sufferer's inherent loneliness furthers the suffering. Because the sufferer's loss of connection with the group is one of the most important aspects of suffering both from the standpoint of its origins and its opportunities for relief, the loneliness of the sufferer is not only the feeling of being alone but an absence from the general "we-ness" of the world, from a shared participation in spirit. The idea of spirit reaches back into the history of both philosophy and religion. The word has many meanings in different traditions, but fundamentally, spirit has to do with the relationship of individuals to the group and to an overriding belief in the existence of God, Nature, or other transcendency. For the purposes of understanding suffering, spirit in a Hegelian sense is useful: some sort of general consciousness that unites all persons (Solomon, 1972).

Pain or suffering in special groups

Until recently, minor surgical procedures were performed on newborns and very young infants without anesthesia in the belief that they did not feel pain. Whether their perception is of pain in the manner of fully functioning adults, where other psychological factors such as meaning play a part, is not as important as the understanding that newborns and very young infants (as known from neuroanatomic criteria, psychophysiologic measures, and their behaviors) experience nociception and resulting sensory pain and thus require anesthesia and analgesia. The situation is not as clear for fetuses, but they also exhibit aversive responses to nociceptive stimuli, suggesting the need for analgesia (Anand and Carr, 1989).

Depending on the depth of coma, patients in coma may or may not experience nociception as shown by whether they react to nociceptive stimuli. Reaction to painful stimuli is employed as a measure of the depth of coma and is often the first sign of recovery of central nervous system function. Nociception does not appear to be present in persons in a persistent vegetative state (Katayama et al., 1991).

By definition, comatose patients and patients in a persistent vegetative state cannot suffer. Since suffering involves persons and their appreciation of their own intactness or threats to it, and requires a sense of identity, of the past, and of the future, these features must be present for suffering to occur. The applicability of these criteria to fetuses and neonates is unknown, but young children have the capacity to suffer.

Philosophical issues

The history of medicine, like much of philosophy, has been marked by the dichotomy between empiricism and rationalism. In medicine, empiricism has also been identified with vitalism, the belief that there exist forces for health within the patient—the *physis* of the Hippocratics. For more than 150 years, medicine has been dominated by rationalist thought that has focused on disease as known by the objective criteria of pathoanatomic or pathophysiologic alterations. Diagnostic and therapeutic interventions and the actions of physicians have been based on the science of medicine and its conviction that all illness and pathophysiology would be explained by the laws of physics and chemistry. Symptoms and the reactions of sick persons to their diseases have been treated as epiphenomena, matters of less importance than science, and given over to the art of medicine, which was ranked lower than that of science.

In recent decades, however, the sick person has become more important. This is largely the result of vitalist-empiricist beliefs expressing themselves as a desire for a more "holistic" medicine, as well as changes in the social context of medicine since the 1960s. During the period of the civil-rights movement and the women's movement in the United States, patients (and more recently persons with disabilities) have achieved the social status of full personhood. The rise of bioethics in the United States during this period has played an important part in this social transformation. Recent interest in pain and suffering can be attributed both to the fact that they defy explanation on purely physicochemical grounds and to the increased attention being given to the experience of the sick person.

The concept of patient autonomy has been of central importance in bioethics, but suffering can put the sufferer's autonomy in question, creating ethical dilemmas. Autonomy implies a self-directed individual with consistent goals and intentions springing from a rational evaluation of situations and norms. Reasoning about choices is coupled here with coherence of purpose—central purpose. The ability to remain autonomous requires that things over which one has no control do not remove all of one's choices or the ability to choose. For the suffering person, autonomy is removed when purposes are directed by the immediate needs of the sick body or by the compulsion to address what is perceived to be the source of suffering. This creates difficulties for an ethics that relies heavily on the principle of autonomy. The exercise of authentic choice in this circumstance requires the help of others, individuals who can represent suffering persons to others and, perhaps, to themselves. The difficult task in these situations is to help the sufferer make choices and act as if suffering were absent. But suffering is marked by loneliness that can deny the help of others. The loss of autonomy following severe illness is usually obvious, while the fact that autonomy is no longer present because of suffering may not be apparent. Actions that are beneficent or even nonmaleficent in relation to the suffering person, in contrast to the ill person, may not be obvious. Thus, what is known about suffering casts doubt on the usefulness of an ethics of principle such as that advocated by Tom Beauchamp and James Childress. In contrast, the nature of suffering suggests the importance of a communitarian view of ethics where the relations of individuals to each other as members of a community guide notions of the right and the good. Stanley Hauerwas has raised questions about the obligations of physicians to relieve suffering—if, in fact, medicine could remove all suffering—in view of the importance often placed on the benefit of suffering. Rather, the duty to alleviate suffering highlights the physician's classical responsibility to have compassion for the suffering person, as in the story of the Good Samaritan, even in the absence of the ability to lift the burden of the sufferer (Hauerwas, 1979).

Theological perspectives on suffering

Suffering as a result of human sin. A commonly employed explanation of suffering is to see it as the fault of human beings, as punishment or retribution for individual or group actions or sins. The idea that God keeps tabs on individual actions and punishes sinners is widespread. This corresponds to the conviction of one of Job's friends: "As I have seen, those who plow iniquity and sow trouble reap the same" (Job 4:8). Yet, it is obvious that the innocent as well as the evil are made to suffer. In the New Testament (Luke 13:1 and John 9), Jesus indicates the mistake of interpreting each evidence of suffering as the consequence of someone's sins. A recent Apostolic Letter of Pope John Paul II (1984) on the Christian meaning of suffering acknowledges the Old Testament writings that show suffering as punishment inflicted by God for human sins, but goes on to disavow such a simple understanding.

Suffering as educational and evidentiary. Where would we be without suffering to tell us what is important, make us better, to lead us back into the paths of righteousness? Suffering, in this view, offers the opportunity to learn humility.

> My son, do not spurn the Lord's correction
> or take offence at his reproof;
> For those whom he loves the Lord reproves,
> and he punishes a favorite son. (Proverbs 3:11, 12)

But it could not provide such opportunities in the absence of a God of grace and love. The prophets provide many examples of this view of the importance of human suffering. But suffering also reveals to the sufferer a greater depth of human experience and meaning. After the experience of suffering, the person is led to a richer understanding of the meaning of being human, a greater concern for the suffering of others, and away from the superficialities that too often characterize daily existence.

Suffering as sacrificial and leading to some greater good. Both on a religious and a secular basis, it is not unusual for suffering persons to believe that their suffering is a form of selfless service to others. Through the acquisition of meaning in this fashion, the suffering is alleviated. It should be remembered that suffering occurs when the intactness or integrity of the person is threatened or disrupted, and it can be relieved when the person is reconstituted even if the agency of its occurrence continues. Giving the distress meaning, which is what occurs in sacrificial suffering, is one way the person can be made whole again. The suffering of one may benefit many. The suffering of the prophets in the service of Israel is such an example. Another is the crucifixion of Jesus, an evil done by others, turned by God into Christianity's central saving act and a demonstration of the power of love over suffering.

Suffering resulting from the forces of evil or chaos. This view suggests that God is not the only supernatural force and that there exist powers that are specifically evil. Satan is such an example, although he is specifically mentioned only three times in the Old Testament; the best known of these mentions appears in Job. In the New Testament, the Devil, Satan, demons, or evil spirits are frequently mentioned as sources of suffering. Modern peoples are frequently uncomfortable with such images, yet suffering on a huge scale has occurred so often in recent times that it seems necessary to draw on some other source of evil while keeping God a positive, loving, and just force. Another variant, non-demoniac, implies that there is a limit to the power of God and that he is just one force in the universe. God, in this view, should be called on for what he can do, but one should realize his limitations. A popular book employs this explanation for the problem raised in its title, *When Bad Things Happen to Good People* (Kushner, 1981). The mystical tradition of Judaism denies these limitations, insisting that to speak of God as one ("Hear, O Israel, the Lord is God, the Lord is One" [Deut. 6:4]) is to speak of the unity of all. Everything is God, good and evil, joy and suffering. "And know today and bring it home to your heart that the Lord, He is God, in the heavens above and on the earth below—there is none other" (Deut. 4:39) (Luzzatto, 1982).

Suffering as mysterious or meaningless. For the classical Greeks, fate and the actions of the gods are indifferent to humankind's ideas of good or justice. Unconcerned fate has, however, a beginning, a middle, and an end and what starts must ultimately be realized. In the Greek tragedies, the terrible end is foretold in the beginning, the middle is the attempt of the hero to live the heroic existence, while in the end the suffering and tragedy that had been foretold must necessarily occur. Suffering and tragedy, then, have their origins in meaningless fate, but they follow from initial actions of humans. A somewhat similar conclusion is reached in the reincarnation religions such as Buddhism and Hinduism: Suffering in this life is inherent in existence, following, in part, from desire in a previous existence that determines the current behavior that leads to suffering. Since one cannot know what transpired in the previous animation, suffering in this life appears to be the result of capricious fate. Deliverance can only come by escape from individual personality, and ultimately, by giving up desire.

The Old Testament, particularly in Job and Ecclesiastes, explores the problem of suffering in depth, ultimately concluding that it is beyond the ability of ordinary mortals to explain. Explanation itself, and the reasoning on which it is based, may be the problem. In their early speeches, Job's counselors know that he must have transgressed, otherwise he would not be punished. Simple explanation—the connection of logically related, but largely unexamined, premises leading to a conclusion—particularly of the facile type presented by Job's counselors, prevents any deeper understanding. If, for example, Job's privations are not punishment directed at him, but occur as part of the natural order of God's universe, then the search for the explanation itself prevents an acceptance of the mystery. Yet the acceptance of mystery, of the fundamentally unsolvable, points the way to changes in fundamental presuppositions and to the relief of suffering. Religion for the Preacher of Ecclesiastes and for Job represents the general, not simple, truths, including the goodness of God, that have the capacity for transforming character and relieving suffering when they are sincerely held and vividly apprehended, even in the painful void of evidence for their truth. It belongs to the depth of religious spirit to have felt forsaken by God (Whitehead, 1974).

A consideration of the nature of suffering opens possibilities for reflection and study about the nature of persons, the relation of persons to their bodies, the goals of medicine, relationships between persons and within communities, and the place of spirit in the lives of individuals. It is little wonder that consideration of suffering and its place in the human condition and in the relationship of God to humankind has occupied human thought throughout the ages—and still the questions remain.

ERIC J. CASSELL

Directly related to this entry are the entries HARM; HEALTH AND DISEASE, *article on* THE EXPERIENCE OF HEALTH AND ILLNESS; *and* TRAGEDY. *For a discussion of related ideas, see the entries* BODY, *article on* EMBODIMENT: THE PHENOMENOLOGICAL TRADITION; DEATH, *articles on* EASTERN THOUGHT, *and* WESTERN RELIGIOUS THOUGHT; DEATH, ATTITUDES TOWARD; DEATH AND DYING: EU-THANASIA AND SUSTAINING LIFE; *and* LIFE, QUALITY OF. *Other relevant material may be found under the entries* CARE; CHRONIC CARE; COMPASSION; HEALING; *and* HOSPICE AND END-OF-LIFE CARE.

Bibliography

ANAND, K. J. S., and CARR, D. B. 1989. "The Neuroanatomy, Neurophysiology, and Neurochemistry of Pain, Stress, and Analgesia in Newborns and Children." *Pediatric Clinics of North America* 36, no. 4:795–822.

BAKAN, DAVID. 1968. *Disease, Pain, and Sacrifice: Toward a Psychology of Suffering.* Chicago: University of Chicago Press.

BEAUCHAMP, TOM L., and CHILDRESS, JAMES F. 1994. *Principles of Biomedical Ethics.* 4th ed. New York: Oxford University Press.

CASSELL, ERIC J. 1982. "The Nature of Suffering and the Goals of Medicine." *New England Journal of Medicine* 306, no. 11:639–645.

———. 1991. *The Nature of Suffering and the Goals of Medicine.* New York: Oxford University Press.

CLEARY, FRANCIS X. 1974. "Biblical Perspectives on Suffering." *Hospital Progress* (December):54–58.

CRUE, BENJAMIN L. 1985. Chapter in *Evaluation and Treatment of Chronic Pain.* Edited by Gerald M. Aronoff. Baltimore: Urban and Schwarzenberg.

FRANKL, VIKTOR E. 1962. *Man's Search for Meaning: An Introduction to Logotherapy.* Translated by Ilse Lasch. Boston: Beacon Press.

HAUERWAS, STANLEY. 1979. "Reflections on Suffering, Death, and Medicine." *Ethics in Science and Medicine* 6:229–237.

JOHN PAUL II. 1984. "Salvifici doloris." *Acta Apostolica Sedis* 76 (March 1):201–250. Translated under the title "Salvifici doloris: On the Meaning of Christian Suffering." *The Pope Speaks* 29 (Summer):105–139.

KATAMAYA, YOICHI; TSUBOKAWA, TAKASHI; YAMAMOTO, TAKAMITSU; HIRAYAMA, TERUYASU; MIYAZAKI, SHUHEI; and KOYAMA, SEIGON. 1991. "Characterization and Modification of Brain Activity with Deep Brain Stimulation in Patients in a Persistent Vegetative State: Pain-Related Late Positive Component of Cerebral Evoked Potential." *Pacing and Clinical Electrophysiology* 14, no. 1:116–121.

KUSHNER, HAROLD S. 1981. *When Bad Things Happen to Good People.* New York: Schocken.

LOEWY, ERICH H. 1991. *Suffering and the Beneficent Community: Beyond Libertarianism.* Albany, N.Y.: State University of New York Press.

LOVEJOY, ARTHUR O. 1961. *Reflections on Human Nature.* Baltimore: Johns Hopkins University Press.

LUZZATTO, MOSHE HAYYIM. 1982. *The Knowing Heart: The Philosophy of God's Oneness.* Translated by Shraga Silverstein. Jerusalem: Feldheim.

REICH, WARREN T. 1989. "Speaking of Suffering: A Moral Account of Compassion." *Soundings* 72, no. 1:83–108.

SCARRY, ELAINE. 1985. *The Body in Pain: The Making and Unmaking of the World.* New York: Oxford University Press.

SIMUNDSON, DANIEL J. 1980. *Faith Under Fire: Biblical Interpretations of Suffering.* Minneapolis, Minn.: Augsburg.

SOLOMON, R. C. 1972. "Hegel's Concept of 'Geist.'" In *Hegel: A Collection of Critical Essays*. Edited by Alasdair C. MacIntyre. Notre Dame, Ind.: University of Notre Dame Press.

WHITEHEAD, ALFRED NORTH. 1974. *Religion in the Making.* New York: New American Library.

WHITEHEAD, WILLARD, III, and KUHN, WOLFGANG F. 1990. "Chronic Pain: An Overview." In vol. 1 of *Chronic Pain*, pp. 5–48. Edited by Thomas W. Miller. Madison, Conn.: International Universities Press.

PARAGUAY

See MEDICAL ETHICS, HISTORY OF, *section on* THE AMERICAS, *article on* LATIN AMERICA.

PASSIVE EUTHANASIA

See DEATH AND DYING: EUTHANASIA AND SUSTAINING LIFE. *See also* INFANTS.

PASTORAL CARE

Pastoral care normally refers to the help given by ordained ministers, priests, and other persons with designated religious roles (such as deacons and members of Roman Catholic religious orders) to suffering, troubled, or perplexed persons. In the simplest and most profound sense, pastoral care has been defined from a Christian perspective as "the attempt to help others, through words, acts, and relationships, to experience as fully as possible the reality of God's presence and love in their lives" (Holst, 1985, p. 46). The term is primarily Christian, but it is sometimes used analogously in other faith traditions (e.g., the rabbi's care in Judaism). When pastoral care is provided in hospitals or other health-care facilities by pastors or rabbis sponsored by the institution, it is known as "health-care chaplaincy." Because health-care chaplaincy is the primary way in which contemporary pastoral care becomes involved with the issues of bioethics, this entry focuses on it.

Historically, pastors have extended their care to a wide range of personal needs and concerns, from struggles of faith, doubt, moral failure, and problems of conscience to marriage and family conflict and the suffering involved in illness, tragedy, and death. In Christian care the historic "means of grace"—sacrament, scripture, prayer—continue to be important, meaningful, and in some traditions essential "resources" of pastoral care, especially in situations of crisis (e.g., dying) and tragedy. But in many situations, conversational methods predominate. Pastoral conversation emphasizes the caregiver's psychological understanding and ability to foster a therapeutic or healing mode of relationship and style of conversation with the person receiving care. This includes empathic listening, the ability to form emotionally honest, trusting relationships, and the care receiver's active participation with the pastor in the search for healing and wholeness. At the root of their care, pastoral caregivers help persons find the kind of faith and value commitments that can sustain, enrich, and give redemptive meaning to their lives, and "to experience as fully as possible the reality of God's presence and love in their lives."

Pastoral care and its specialized form, health-care chaplaincy, are often distinguished from another ministerial specialization—pastoral counseling. When this distinction is made, pastoral counseling is commonly defined as a specialized form of ministry characterized by an intentional contract between the pastoral caregiver and the person or family seeking help for a series of prearranged sessions focused on the person or family's concern. This structured form of care contrasts with the more casual and varied forms of caring relationships that parish pastors and health-care chaplains typically form. Though many parish ministers, priests, rabbis, and health-care chaplains provide short-term counseling of the more formal kind, pastoral counseling as a specialized ministry is devoted entirely to this work. To a large extent it is a form of psychotherapy or family therapy (and is often called "pastoral psychotherapy"), and usually involves a number of sessions and the payment of a fee. Pastoral counselors, like health-care chaplains, have specialized training requirements, professional organizations (principally, the American Association of Pastoral Counselors), and standards of certification. They serve on the staffs of larger churches, in pastoral counseling centers, and in other professional settings, and are often licensed by state governments as pastoral (or other) counselors, psychologists, or marriage and family therapists.

Pastoral care in health-care settings: The health-care chaplain

Functions and role. Much of what health-care chaplains do involves helping persons and families (of all faiths) with the emotional and spiritual dimensions of the healing process, offering support and therapeutic care in situations of crisis and grief, helping to resolve conflicts and communication difficulties, and consulting in situations of bioethical and other decision making. Most chaplains also develop an extensive ministry with nurses, physicians, aides, administrators, and others in the medical setting who carry significant emotional burdens and moral concerns. Chaplains promote communication between patients, families, and staff concerning religious and cultural traditions that may bear upon medical decisions (e.g., concerning blood transfusion, abortion, and the use of life-support technologies). They often become involved in discussions with all parties involved in health-care decisions. In addition, health-care chaplains form educational relationships with local clergy and congregations, function as liaisons between the health-care institution and the community, and serve on the boards of related community organizations. As more health care is provided on an outpatient basis, and as more congregations develop health-care emphases and programs, these aspects of their work are expected to increase.

Chaplains often play a significant role in hospital ethics committees; in many instances, they helped to organize these committees in the late 1970s and 1980s. The chaplains' role in ethics committees, as in their consulting with patients and families on bioethical decisions, consists largely in promoting good communication and mutual understanding, interpreting religious and cultural traditions, resolving conflicts, clarifying moral issues, and facilitating free and responsible moral decision making. It is a basic principle of the College of Chaplains, the National Association of Catholic Chaplains, and similar national certifying organizations that health-care chaplains respect the belief and value systems of others and refrain from proselytizing or trying to impose their own convictions on them.

Many health-care institutions sponsor professional training programs in pastoral care called "clinical pastoral education" (C.P.E). These programs train not only future chaplains in pastoral care, but also large numbers of theological students, pastors, and members of religious orders not seeking specialized ministry certification. C.P.E. students minister under the supervision of a highly trained and certified chaplain supervisor with whom they meet individually and as a group to analyze and reflect on their work. Such reflection involves intense examination of detailed case reports, personal reflection on the trainees' ways of caring for other persons, and consideration of the psychological, social, cultural, theological, and ethical questions involved in their experiences. Pastoral supervision has evolved in the second half of the twentieth century into a distinct and important specialization within health-care chaplaincy.

Relation of health-care chaplaincy to other health-care professions. Most pastors who serve in health-care settings hold a broad, liberal understanding of themselves and their ministries that enables them to cooperate easily with the medical profession and to work pastorally with a wide range of persons. They do not limit their ministries to persons with problems that are explicitly defined in religious or moral terms, but seek to become related to persons in supportive and thera-

peutic ways whatever the immediate, presenting needs or issues may be.

Thus their work often closely resembles, in certain respects, that of psychiatrists, psychologists, psychiatric nurses, social workers, and patient representatives. This makes the chaplain a valuable member of the health-care team. He or she is "cross trained" in a variety of institutionally valuable skills usefully integrated into a single profession: "psychosocial and spiritual counselor, clinical ethicist, patient representative and ombudsperson, cultural anthropologist and religious scholar, gatekeeper of community resources and public relations expert, and health promoter" (Burton, 1992, p. 2). But the chaplain's range of competencies also raises questions of vocational distinctiveness and identity for other professionals and sometimes for themselves. The situation is made more problematic by the fact that pastoral identity in health-care facilities is usually not defined primarily in terms of the performance of religious rituals or counseling on a narrowly conceived range of "religious" problems.

What then gives the chaplain's wide-ranging work comprehensive definition and focus? The answer to this question is much debated within the profession. In general terms, however, it seems clear that pastoral identity in health-care settings has two poles of concern: healing and health, and religion (Burton, 1992). Chaplains are significantly identified with each. The distinctiveness of the profession lies in the way these two poles are held together in an ambiguous but creative unity in the actual performance of the chaplain's professional function.

At one pole there is a concern for and participation in the processes of health and healing. While health-care chaplains do not practice medicine or psychiatry, they believe that the meanings and values by which people live, and the quality of personal relationships, play an important role in the organic processes of illness and health. They also believe that a comprehensive concern for human well-being, including a concern for health and healing, is integral to the faith traditions they represent. Thus chaplains believe that religion supports the fundamental aims of medicine and health care. And they see their ministries as essentially involved in the process of healing, which they understand in comprehensive terms as healing of the whole person—body, mind, and spirit. Consequently, they view themselves as significant members of the health-care team, and increasingly are being viewed in that way by the medical professions.

At the other pole, health-care chaplains are committed to representing religious meanings and values that include but transcend the values of health and healing. They seek to enable people to find and experience that which ultimately can fulfill their lives and redeem them from the threats of meaningless shame, guilt, and death that pervade all of life, in illness as well as in health. And they set health and healing as values into an encompassing faith perspective that affirms the meaningfulness of life whether or not healing occurs. For the health-care chaplain, this larger context is ultimately rooted in the reality and loving power of God, who at times makes health possible, but who also makes meaning, hope, and love possible in every circumstance of life, in illness and adversity as well as in health and wholeness.

Thus pastoral identity is bipolar, committed to both healing and religious faith and to their essential interrelationship. It is the ambiguous but disciplined interplay of these polar commitments that constitutes the distinctive orientation of health-care chaplaincy.

Education, certification, and licensure. Virtually all specialized health-care chaplains today hold college and seminary degrees or have other appropriate theological education, and have been ordained or otherwise endorsed by their religious denominations. Health-care chaplains are not licensed by state governments as chaplains, though some who also practice specialized pastoral counseling are licensed as pastoral counselors, psychologists, or marriage and family therapists.

Nearly all full-time, professional health-care chaplains have trained for their ministries through clinical pastoral education as described above. C.P.E. is sponsored mainly by the Association for Clinical Pastoral Education, the National Association of Catholic Chaplains, the Canadian Association for Pastoral Education, and similar bodies in other countries. Various national professional associations also exist for specialized health-care chaplains, principally as the College of Chaplains, the National Association of Catholic Chaplains, and the National Association of Jewish Chaplains. These organizations set high standards for professional practice, enforced through rigorous certification and review procedures. A consortium of these and related organizations publishes the *Journal of Pastoral Care*. There is also a large umbrella organization in the United States and Canada, the Congress on Ministry in Specialized Settings (COMISS), that sponsors joint meetings of pastoral-care organizations in which issues of the profession are intensively discussed.

In 1994, there were 348 C.P.E. training centers accredited by the Association for Clinical Pastoral Education and 882 certified C.P.E. supervisors. Similar organizations and C.P.E. programs exist in Canada and a number of other countries; an international organization closely related to the movement, the International Congress of Pastoral Care, meets quadrennially.

History of health-care chaplaincy in the United States. Hospital chaplaincy, like the hospital itself, had its origin in the ancient and medieval Christian church. The rise of the modern secular hospital in the late nineteenth century, however, was not immediately accompanied by the presence of chaplains as members of hospital staffs. Such pastoral ministry as occurred in secular hospitals was usually provided by retired clergy, often on a voluntary and/or part-time basis, who had no special training for the work beyond general parish experience. This pattern has continued in some smaller institutions, but for the most part health-care chaplaincy has become fully established as a specialized ministerial profession, and chaplains are employed as regular staff members by most large health-care institutions.

The turn toward specialized, highly trained, professional health-care chaplaincy had its roots in the "religion and health" movement early in the twentieth century, in which a positive relation between religion and modern medicine was first seriously explored (Holifield, 1983). This led in the 1920s to the first attempts to train theological students in clinical settings (Thornton, 1970). Notable was the groundbreaking work of a physician, William S. Keller, who placed theological students in a general hospital in Cincinnati in 1923, and Anton T. Boisen, a Congregational minister who began what became the "clinical pastoral training movement" with his pioneering program relating religion to mental disorders at Worcester State Hospital in Massachusetts in 1925. Boisen had the key support of two physicians, the distinguished Boston medical educator, Richard C. Cabot, and the progressive superintendent of Worcester State Hospital, William A. Bryan. Shortly thereafter, another physician, Flanders Dunbar, noted for her research in psychosomatic medicine, became a major leader of the movement. These and other early innovators were convinced that it was not books but intensive clinical experience—learning to interpret the experience of real human beings, to read the "living human documents" through clinical encounters—that held the key to developing a realistic and profound theological understanding of human nature and the art of effective pastoral care (Boisen, 1971, p. 248). The movement developed rapidly in the 1930s and especially in the postwar period, when many training centers were organized, chaplain supervisors certified, and staff chaplaincy positions brought into existence in mental and general hospitals.

Partly for pedagogical reasons related to the abundance of pastoral opportunities in hospitals, and partly for practical, financial reasons—hospitals were better able to pay for these programs than churches or seminaries—clinical pastoral education was seldom undertaken in congregational settings. Most programs were sponsored by hospitals, and C.P.E. programs remained largely unrelated to the formal curricula of the theological seminaries until the late 1950s and 1960s. C.P.E.

thus acquired a somewhat nonecclesiastical, "secular" style and appearance, and there has always been a concern that C.P.E. students would develop a confused professional identity as a result of C.P.E.'s close ties to the medical establishment and its models and methods of care.

Today, however, C.P.E. is widely embraced by the "mainline" Protestant and Catholic churches, and C.P.E. programs are a common, and often required, component of Protestant, Catholic, and some Jewish theological education. Health-care chaplaincy itself is similarly established as a highly specialized, professionally trained and certified form of ministerial practice. Most hospital administrations require staff chaplains to have completed a year or more of C.P.E., or its equivalent. The national College of Chaplains, the National Association of Catholic Chaplains, and similar organizations require C.P.E. in their certification standards.

Philosophical and cultural orientations

Relation of religion and health. The high degree of professional cooperation existing today between pastoral caregivers and medical professionals represents a remarkable and relatively recent development in both medicine and religion. In ancient and medieval times medicine and religion often enjoyed a close relationship; healing rites, exorcisms, pilgrimages, and health cults flourished. Beginning with the Protestant Reformation and in the seventeenth century with the rise of modern science and scientific medicine, however, Christian ministry began a long retreat from its tradition of involvement in healing, and theology grew increasingly wary of making scientific, empirical claims about the natural world. An intellectual and professional schism between religion and medicine resulted. As medicine became scientific and ministry became confined to matters of God and the soul, corresponding spheres of professional influence were delineated: physicians cared (scientifically) for the body; clergy cared (spiritually) for the soul. Medical science assigned mental and emotional disorders, traditionally considered problems of the "soul," to the "body" as organically caused, and regarded them as at least potentially treatable by physical (i.e., medical) means.

Beginning with the development of dynamic psychiatry and the religion and health movement in the early twentieth century such distinctions began to blur. Psychoanalysis and related developments in psychiatry revealed psychogenic factors in many psychiatric disorders, while empirical studies in psychosomatic medicine demonstrated the profound effects of emotional and spiritual attitudes on physical health and healing. At the same time, theology began to recover biblical, "wholistic" conceptions of human personhood, salvation, and the healing potential of religious ministry. In this theology the welfare of the whole person, physical, mental, and spiritual, was regarded as a profound unity. The result was a gradual closing of the theoretical gap between medicine and religion and the emergence of a more collaborative style of work between physicians and pastoral caregivers.

Influence of therapeutic psychology. Prior to the twentieth century, pastoral care was dominantly concerned with problems that could be clearly or outwardly identified as religious and moral in nature or as having religious significance, such as faith, doubt, sin, repentance, and the mysteries of suffering, illness, death, and dying. Contemporary pastoral care, however, at least as practiced in the larger Christian denominations (sectarian churches being the usual exception), holds to broader conceptions of Christian ministry, human welfare, and the meaning of salvation. In these conceptions, physical welfare and emotional health play prominent parts in the overall meaning of salvation; ministry's sphere of concern has been enlarged to include the total health and welfare of persons and families "in this world." Often this understanding gives prominence to psychology as an adjunctive discipline, and ministry acquires a distinctly psychotherapeutic style and orientation. This has been especially evident in the mainline Protestant denominations, but it is increasingly true of Roman Catholic and some conservative Protestant traditions. A strong affirmation of human health and welfare has generally been a strong emphasis in Judaism.

With respect to pastoral care's relation to bioethics, this therapeutic style of ministry has important ethical and professional consequences. Typically, it seeks to broaden moral discussion in health-care settings from a focus on the content of moral decisions—what to do—to a focus on the process and quality of the decision making itself. Health-care chaplains try to foster the psychological conditions that will facilitate free and responsible moral judgment and decision. These conditions include relationships of trust that permit open, honest communication among all parties concerning feelings as well as ideas and opinions. Though facilitating such conditions is not usually thought of as a form of moral guidance, it obviously has important moral value. One leading Protestant authority, however, while affirming this approach, has also urged pastoral caregivers to engage the substantive questions of ethics more directly in their caring ministries (Browning, 1976, 1983).

Affinities with situation ethics and character ethics. Pastoral care, including health-care chaplaincy, has not been highly articulate concerning the traditions of philosophical and theological ethics out of which it has operated. Most pastoral theologians have concentrated instead on theological questions of human nature and the relation of religion to health (Browning, 1983; Holifield, 1983). However, much of the informal ethical reflection in the field has probably been influenced chiefly by "situation ethics" of one kind or another. Situation ethics holds that fixed laws and rules are inadequate for moral decision making; decisions must be reached through a careful assessment of the particulars of each situation, guided by very general principles such as love, justice, and responsibility. Pastors with therapeutic training often exemplify this orientation since they tend to be concerned more about the specifics of situations than the application of abstract moral rules and principles (Poling, 1984b). Their typical ethical question is likely to be: "What is the appropriate, responsible, loving, or just thing to do in this situation, given its many complexities and dynamics?"

Pastoral care has also had a close affinity with what is called the "ethics of character and virtue," though this connection has seldom been recognized (Poling, 1984a). Psychological conceptions of personality often function as secular character ideals for pastoral care that is influenced by therapeutic psychology. For example, health-care chaplains commonly assume that psychological self-knowledge and the ability to experience oneself and others fully, without the distorting effects of emotional defensiveness, is desirable as a moral good, as an aspect of mental health in general, and as a basis for free and responsible moral action.

The practical significance of this orientation is important. In many situations, as a matter of principle, health-care chaplains are likely to be as concerned about the emotional health and maturity of the persons exercising moral judgment—their capacities as moral agents for making free and responsible decisions—as about the particular decisions that are reached. Their commitment to an ethic of character and virtue thus easily complements the field's general tendency to support situational or contextual forms of ethical reasoning.

Relation of theory and practice. Much of the way pastors have ministered to troubled and suffering persons over the centuries may be regarded as a practical implementation of the ethical principles of the pastors' religious communities and traditions. Insofar as they have attempted to represent official moral and religious teachings in the lives of their parishioners and counselees (e.g., through practices of confession and absolution or forgiveness), pastoral caregivers have expressed and enacted prevailing moral norms. Practice has followed theory, "applying" it.

But human needs and problems do not always fit neatly into prescribed categories and practices, and so-

cial and cultural forces change over time; contemporary problems of bioethics provide many cases in point. In such situations, pastoral care cannot operate as a straightforward application of established moral theories and principles. A degree of conscientious improvising becomes necessary, especially in times of rapid social, cultural, and technological change.

Thus moral theory does not always easily or clearly guide practice; in fact, to some degree it reflects practice and is changed by practice. To this extent pastoral experience over time, in concert with other social and cultural factors, gradually helps moral theory to evolve. The Jewish *responsa* literature, representing the accumulated moral debates and evolving traditions of Judaism's encounter with novel problems over many centuries, provides massive evidence of this process in one tradition (Meier, 1990). A similar process, though often less explicit and legally constructed, has occurred in Christian pastoral care (Browning, 1976). This can be seen in changing contemporary pastoral attitudes in the mainstream Protestant churches on issues like divorce, remarriage, abortion, and artificial life support. Pastoral caregiving is thus culturally innovative as well as conservative, and represents (as Browning argues) a practical form of "moral inquiry."

Issues in health-care chaplaincy

Like other health-care professions, health-care chaplaincy faces a number of challenges as the technology and institutional forms of health care undergo rapid and extensive developments. With minimal elaboration, four challenges may be particularly noted:

1. Multiculturalism and minority concerns constitute an increasingly visible and important feature of the social landscape in which health-care chaplaincy functions. This fact presents novel professional issues for health-care chaplains, including difficult questions such as how to help persons of non-Western cultural and religious traditions relate to the social values and practices of advanced Western health-care facilities. Increasingly, health-care chaplains must understand a wide range of religious and ethnic cultures and find ways of relating their ministries with appropriateness and integrity to persons with religious faiths and social customs very different from their own.

2. The expanding cultural diversity and overlap of professional roles in contemporary health-care settings intensify the problem of defining the health-care chaplain's pastoral identity. This question is becoming urgent. As institutional budget pressures increase, many health-care chaplains and pastoral departments have been forced to define their identities and defend the value of their ministries to health-care administrators,

often in quantifiable, cost-benefit terms that are alien to traditional meanings of ministry.

3. A further dimension of the identity question is whether and how health-care chaplains can maintain a specific theological identity for themselves as representatives of particular religious and moral traditions in the often secular, religiously "value-neutral," humanistic world of the health-care institution. Focusing on "process" rather than "content" of moral decision making, and maintaining an institutionally proper value-neutral stance on specific questions, is clearly an important and organizationally facilitating stance in many health-care institutions. But such public neutrality may beg important questions. For example, how (in theory or practice) can chaplains maintain an institutionally appropriate neutrality yet remain significantly committed to their particular traditions of faith? Is there any way the ethical commitments and insights of particular religious traditions can contribute to contemporary moral reflection in institutional health-care decision-making and policy setting? Can health-care chaplains represent their traditions without imposing themselves inappropriately on others or abusing their institutional positions?

4. Increasingly, health-care chaplains are being drawn beyond pastoral care as the direct delivery of service to individuals and families and into issues of health-care policy in their institutions and society at large. This expanded arena offers new opportunities to witness to their moral commitments in the face of institutional, economic, and political injustice in health care, for example, by questioning unjust policies and practices and advocating the rights of the poor. But it also raises difficult questions. How far and in what way—if at all—should health-care chaplaincy develop this expression of ministry's moral integrity in place of or in addition to its healing work of care and compassion?

RODNEY J. HUNTER

For a further discussion of topics mentioned in this entry, see the entries ALLIED HEALTH PROFESSIONS; CASUISTRY; CLINICAL ETHICS; ETHICS, *especially the articles on* TASK OF ETHICS, *and* RELIGION AND MORALITY; HEALING; HEALTH-CARE DELIVERY, *article on* HEALTH-CARE INSTITUTIONS; HEALTH-CARE RESOURCES, ALLOCATION OF, *article on* MACROALLOCATION; HOSPITAL; JUDAISM; MENTAL HEALTH, *article on* MENTAL HEALTH AND RELIGION; PROTESTANTISM; ROMAN CATHOLICISM; TEAMS, HEALTH-CARE; *and* VIRTUE AND CHARACTER. *For a discussion of related ideas, see the entries* BENEFICENCE; CARE; COMPASSION; TRUST; *and* VALUE AND VALUATION. *Other relevant material may be found under the entries* BIOETHICS EDUCATION; DEATH, *article on* WESTERN RELIGIOUS THOUGHT; *and* LICENSING, DISCIPLINE, AND REGULATION IN THE HEALTH PROFESSIONS.

Bibliography

BOISEN, ANTON T. 1971. [1936]. *The Exploration of the Inner World.* Philadelphia: University of Pennsylvania Press.

BROWNING, DON S. 1976. *The Moral Context of Pastoral Care.* Philadelphia: Westminster Press.

———. 1983. *Religious Ethics and Pastoral Care.* Philadelphia: Fortress Press.

BURCK, J. RUSSELL. 1983. "The Chaplain amid Dilemmas of Health-Care Ethics." *American Protestant Hospital Association Bulletin* 47, no. 3:69–76.

BURTON, LAUREL ARTHUR, ed. 1992. *Chaplaincy Services in Contemporary Health Care.* Schaumburg, Ill.: College of Chaplains. The official publication of the College of Chaplains.

HAYES, HELEN; VAN DER POEL, CORNELIUS J.; and NATIONAL ASSOCIATION OF CATHOLIC CHAPLAINS. 1990. *Health-Care Ministry: A Handbook for Chaplains.* New York: Paulist Press. The current Roman Catholic handbook.

HOLIFIELD, E. BROOKS. 1983. *A History of Pastoral Care in America: From Salvation to Self-Realization.* Nashville, Tenn.: Abingdon Press.

HOLST, LAWRENCE E., ed. 1985. *Hospital Ministry: The Role of the Chaplain Today.* New York: Crossroad.

HUNTER, RODNEY J., gen. ed. 1990. *Dictionary of Pastoral Care and Counseling.* Associate editors: H. Newton Malony, Liston O. Mills, and John Patton. Nashville, Tenn.: Abingdon Press. The major reference work, covering every theoretical and practical aspect of the field; includes bibliographies and cross references.

Journal of Health-Care Chaplaincy. 1987–. New York: Haworth Press. Biannual.

LAPSLEY, JAMES N. 1990. "Moral Dilemmas in Pastoral Perspective." In *Dictionary of Pastoral Care and Counseling,* pp. 752–755. Edited by Rodney J. Hunter; associate editors H. Newton Malony, Liston O. Mills, and John Patton. Nashville, Tenn.: Abingdon Press.

MARTY, MARTIN E., and VAUX, KENNETH L., eds. 1982. *Health/Medicine and the Faith Traditions: An Inquiry into Religion and Medicine.* Philadelphia: Fortress Press. See also the Crossroad series of interfaith books on particular traditions, "Health and Medicine in the Faith Traditions."

MEIER, LEVI. 1990. "Medical-Ethical Dilemmas, Jewish Care and Counseling In." In *Dictionary of Pastoral Care and Counseling,* pp. 696–698. Edited by Rodney J. Hunter; associate editors H. Newton Malony, Liston O. Mills, and John Patton. Nashville, Tenn.: Abingdon Press.

MITCHELL, KENNETH R. 1972. *Hospital Chaplain.* Philadelphia: Westminster Press.

POLING, JAMES N. 1984a. "Ethical Reflection and Pastoral Care: Part I." *Pastoral Psychology* 32, no. 2:106–114.

———. 1984b. "Ethical Reflection and Pastoral Care: Part II." *Pastoral Psychology* 32, no. 3:160–170.

Second Opinion. 1986–. Park Ridge, Ill.: Park Ridge Center. The primary journal for the relation of bioethics and religious concerns.

THORNTON, EDWARD E. 1970. *Professional Education for Ministry: A History of Clinical Pastoral Education.* Nashville, Tenn.: Abingdon Press.

PATENTING ORGANISMS

Patents provide inventors with the right to exclude others from making, using, or selling their inventions for a limited term. Historically, some nations have justified their patent systems under "natural law" principles as a means of recognizing the inherent rights of inventors to their discoveries. The U.S. Constitution, however, justifies the patent system as a means of promoting technological progress (U.S. Constitution, Article I, Section 8, Clause 8). The U.S. patent system promotes technological progress through the financial incentives it creates for innovation and through its disclosure requirement. In exchange for exclusive rights, patent applicants must disclose their inventions in terms that are adequate to enable others who are skilled in the field to make and use them (U.S. Patent Act, §112). When a patent is issued, this broad disclosure becomes freely available to the public, and when the patent term expires, the public is free to use the patented invention itself.

Background and history

As commercial interest in biological products and processes has grown, inventors have turned to the patent laws seeking rights to inventions involving living materials. They have encountered a number of difficulties under traditional patent doctrine. It has long been established that products of nature and phenomena of nature are not patentable under U.S. law, even if newly discovered (*Funk Brothers Seed Co. v. Kalo Inoculant Co.*, 1948). But judicial decisions prior to the explosion of modern commercial biotechnology minimized the significance of this obstacle to patent protection by permitting patents on materials derived from natural sources through human intervention, such as purifications of naturally occurring products, so long as the patent claims did not cover the product in its natural state. Under this interpretation of the law, courts have upheld the validity of patents on purified prostaglandins (*Bergstrom*, 1970), purified acetylsalicylic acid (*Kuehmsted v. Farbenfabriken*, 1910), purified adrenalin composition (*Parke-Davis & Co. v. H. K. Mulford & Co.*, 1911), and even a purified bacterial strain (*Bergy*, 1977). Prior to 1980, living things were generally considered unpatentable, either because they were thought to be products of nature or because they were not amenable to written description as required by the patent statute (*Funk Brothers Seed Co. v. Kalo Inoculant Co.*, 1948).

The U.S. Congress explicitly provided for exclusive rights in living materials in two statutes designed to promote agricultural research and development. The Plant Patent Act of 1930 extended protection to new and distinct asexually propagated plant varieties (U.S. Patent Act, §§161–164). This statute relaxed the disclosure requirement for plant varieties, specifying that the disclosure need only be "as complete as is reasonably possible" (U.S. Patent Act, §162). The Plant Variety Protection Act of 1970 extended patentlike protection, administered by the Department of Agriculture rather than the Patent and Trademark Office (PTO), to new sexually reproduced plant varieties, but made protection subject to limitations not present in the patent statute. These limitations include a research exemption that allows use of protected varieties to develop new varieties (U.S. Plant Variety Protection Act, §2544), and a farmer's exemption that allows farmers to save protected seed for use on their farms or for sale to other farmers (U.S. Plant Variety Protection Act, §2543).

Pharmaceutical firms have long obtained U.S. patents on processes for using bacterial strains for such commercially valuable purposes as producing antibiotics, but the strains themselves were generally assumed to be unpatentable until the 1980 decision of the U.S. Supreme Court in *Diamond v. Chakrabarty*. In that case the Court held that a living single-celled bacterium, transformed with DNA plasmids (small circles of bacterial DNA) through human intervention to give it the capacity to break down multiple components of crude oil, could be patented as a "manufacture" or "composition of matter." In arriving at this decision, the Supreme Court stated that the patent statute allows patents to issue on "anything under the sun that is made by man" (*Diamond v. Chakrabarty*, 1980, p. 309).

With this broad directive from the Supreme Court, the PTO quickly expanded the categories of living subject matter that it considered eligible for patent protection. In 1985 the PTO held that corn plants were eligible for standard utility patents, as opposed to the more limited plant variety protection (*Hibberd*, 1985), and two years later it held that polyploid oysters fell within the range of patentable subject matter (*Allen*, 1987). Shortly thereafter the Commissioner of Patents issued a notice stating that the PTO "now considers nonnaturally occurring nonhuman multicellular living organisms, including animals, to be patentable subject matter" (U.S. Patent and Trademark Office, 1987). Any claim covering a human being would not be considered patentable, however, because "the grant of a limited, but exclusive property right in a human being is prohibited by the Constitution." The first patent on a genetically altered animal (U.S. Patent No. 4,736,866) was issued in April 1988 to Harvard University for the development of a mouse harboring a human oncogene that makes it susceptible to cancer. The decision to extend patent protection to animals has generated considerable public controversy and has been the focus of numerous hearings in the U.S. Congress. Restrictive legislation has been proposed, including a moratorium on animal patenting (Adler, 1988; Dresser, 1988; Moga, 1994: U.S. Congress, Office of Technology Assessment, 1988).

While national patent laws vary somewhat, as a general rule the range of biotechnology inventions that may be patented outside the United States is more restricted than it is under U.S. law. Patent protection is widely available for microorganisms, and many nations offer various forms of patentlike rights to plant breeders. The European Commission (the executive body responsible for carrying out the activities agreed to by the member states of the European Economic Community) has twice proposed uniform patent protection for biotechnology products throughout Europe, but the proposal has been opposed by religious and environmental groups and plant breeders (Crespi, 1993; MacKenzie, 1992). Two provisions of the European Patent Convention have presented obstacles to the issuance of standard utility patents covering plants and animals in Europe (Dickson, 1989). Article 53(b) of the European Patent Convention states that European patents will not be issued for plant or animal varieties and essentially biological processes for the production of plants or animals, with the exception of microbiological processes or the products thereof. Article 53(a) of the European Patent Convention bars the issuance of a patent on an invention if its publication or exploitation would be contrary to public order or morality. The European Patent Office (EPO) concluded that neither of these provisions barred the issuance of a European patent to Harvard University on its transgenic mouse (HARVARD/Onco-Mouse, 1991). The EPO reasoned that the claims in the patent application were not excluded from protection under the prohibition of Article 53(b) against patenting "animal varieties" because the claims were drafted broadly to cover non-human "mammals" and "rodents," which constitute taxonomic classification units of a much higher order than "animal variety." This would seem to lead to the paradoxical result that broad patent claims to animals are permitted whereas more narrowly worded claims are not. The EPO also stated that the invention was not excluded from protection under Article 53(a) as contrary to public order or morality, citing its usefulness to humankind as a means for studying cancer and its tendency to reduce the number of animals needed for cancer research.

Objections to patenting organisms

Some of the objections to patenting living organisms that have emerged in the wake of these legal developments are better understood as objections to the underlying technology itself, rather than to its protection under the patent laws (Adler, 1988; Dresser, 1988; Merges, 1988). Objections of this character include concerns about the hazards of genetic engineering to public health and to the environment, concerns that transgenic animal research involves cruelty to animals or reveals an arrogant human disregard for the integrity of other species, and warnings from religious organizations that scientists who tamper with the genetic blueprint for life forms are "playing God" or somehow violating the sanctity of life (U.S. Congress, Office of Technology Assessment, 1989; World Council of Churches, 1982). Closely related are concerns that genetic technology might be put to ethically questionable uses.

One might question whether these sorts of objections are properly the concern of the patent laws, or whether they might be better met through other sorts of regulation such as containment guidelines for the conduct of laboratory research, animal rights legislation, or outright prohibition of certain types of research or of certain applications of new knowledge of genetics. On the other hand, withholding commercial rewards may be an effective means of slowing the pace of such research without prohibiting it altogether. Outright bans on research raise troubling questions about the proper role of government in research science that might be avoided by taking the less restrictive step of denying patent protection (Kass, 1981).

Other objections speak more directly to the effects of patenting itself, rather than viewing patent rights as a symbolic imprimatur on the underlying research or its applications. One recurring set of concerns has to do with the impact of patents on the conduct of research science, particularly in biomedical research (Eisenberg, 1987). Patents could retard scientific progress by allowing patent holders to withhold important discoveries from their competitors. Moreover, by encouraging researchers to be alert to the potential commercial value of their work, the patent system may retard scientific progress by inducing interim secrecy. The patent system may also distort the research agenda and distract universities from their mission of expanding the knowledge base in favor of pursuing potentially lucrative patent rights. Some of these distortions arguably arise from the commercial potential of the underlying research rather than from the availability of patent rights. Indeed, in the absence of patent rights, one might expect greater interference with scientific communication as researchers seek to preserve exclusivity in their discoveries through trade secrecy. On the other hand, the prospect of obtaining patents may increase commercial interest in certain fields of research and thereby aggravate tension between scientific norms and commercial imperatives.

Another set of arguments concerns the impact of patents on various economic interests. For example, some people have argued that the higher cost of patented livestock or seed could bankrupt small farms or lead to further concentration in markets for agricultural products (U.S. Congress, Office of Technology Assessment, 1989). Others have argued that the present patent system undervalues the contributions of less developed countries to biological diversity (McGowan, 1991; World Resources Institute, 1993).

More broadly, some have argued that patenting of life forms promotes an unwholesome or irreverent materialistic conception of life (Hoffmaster, 1989). A strong version of this argument holds that characterizing a life form as a patentable manufacture or composition of matter reduces a patented organism to nothing more than a material object (Kass, 1981). A more attenuated version would stress the potential for commercial interests to debase our attitudes toward life when life forms are treated as commodities to be bought and sold in the market (Murray, 1987).

These concerns are particularly salient when the organisms to be patented have been altered to possess human traits (Dresser, 1988). The creation and patenting of animal-human hybrids may seem to call into question assumptions about the unique character of the human species and thereby to threaten human dignity. The patenting of species with human characteristics also triggers concerns about the effectiveness of the PTO's policy of excluding humans from the category of patentable subject matter as scientists move toward creating genetically engineered humans (Hoffmaster, 1989).

REBECCA S. EISENBERG

Directly related to this entry is the entry BIOTECHNOLOGY. *For a further discussion of topics mentioned in this entry, see the entries* ANIMAL RESEARCH; COMMERCIALISM IN SCIENTIFIC RESEARCH; GENETIC ENGINEERING, *article on* ANIMALS AND PLANTS; *and* LIFE. *Other relevant material may be found under the entries* AGRICULTURE; ANIMAL WELFARE AND RIGHTS, *articles on* ETHICAL PERSPECTIVES ON THE TREATMENT AND STATUS OF ANIMALS, *and* ANIMALS IN AGRICULTURE AND FACTORY FARMING; *and* ENVIRONMENTAL ETHICS.

Bibliography

ADLER, REID G. 1988. "Controlling the Applications of Biotechnology: A Critical Analysis of the Proposed Moratorium on Animal Patenting." *Harvard Journal of Law and Technology* 1:1–61.

Allen, ex parte. 2 U.S.P.Q.2d 1425 (PTO B.d Pat. App. & Interf. 1987).

ARMITAGE, ROBERT A. 1989. "The Emerging U.S. Patent Law for the Protection of Biotechnology Research Results." *European Intellectual Property Review* 11, no. 2:47–57.

Bergstrom, In re. 1970. 427 F.2d 1394, 57 (C.C.P.A.) 1240, 166 U.S.P.Q. (BNA) 256.

Bergy, In re. 1977. 563 F.2d 1031, 195 U.S.P.Q. (BNA) 344, *vacated sub nom. Parker v. Bergy,* 438 U.S. 902 (1978), *on remand, Bergy, In re,* 596 F.2d 952, *cert. granted sub nom. Parker v. Bergy,* 444 U.S. 924 (1979), *vacated and remanded with instruction to dismiss as moot sub nom. Diamond v. Chakrabarty,* 444 U.S. 1028 (1980).

CRESPI, R. STEPHEN. 1993. "Protecting Biotechnological Inventions." *Chemistry and Industry,* May 17.

Diamond v. Chakrabarty. 1980. 447 U.S. 303, 65 L. Ed. 2d 144, 100 S. Ct. 2204.

DICKSON, DAVID. 1989. "Europe Tries to Untangle Laws on Patenting Life." *Science* 243, no. 4894:1002–1003.

DRESSER, REBECCA. 1988. "Ethical and Legal Issues in Patenting New Animal Life." *Jurimetrics Journal* 28, no. 4: 399–435.

EISENBERG, REBECCA S. 1987. "Proprietary Rights and the Norms of Science in Biotechnology Research." *Yale Law Journal* 97:177–231.

Funk Brothers Seed Co. v. Kalo Inoculant Co. 1948. 333 U.S. 127, 192 L. Ed. 588, 68 S. Ct. 440.

HARVARD/Onco-Mouse Application No. 85 304 490.7. 1991. European Patent Office Reports 525.

Hibberd, Ex parte. 1985. 227 U.S.P.Q. 473 (PTO B.d Pat. App. & Interf.).

HOFFMASTER, BARRY. 1989. "The Ethics of Patenting Higher Life Forms." *Intellectual Property Journal* 4:1–24.

KASS, LEON R. 1981. "Patenting Life." *Commentary* 72, no. 6: 45–57.

Kuehmsted v. Farbenfabriken. 1910. 179 F. 701 (7th Cir.), *cert. denied,* 220 U.S. 622, 55 L. Ed. 613, 31 S. Ct. 724.

MACKENZIE, DEBORA. 1992. "Europe Debates the Ownership of Life." *New Scientist* 133, no. 1802:9–10.

McGOWAN, JANET. 1991. "Who Is the Inventor?" *Cultural Survival Quarterly* 15, no. 3:20.

MERGES, ROBERT P. 1988. "Intellectual Property in Higher Life Forms: The Patent System and Controversial Technologies." *Maryland Law Review* 47:1051–1075.

MOGA, THOMAS T. 1994. "Transgenic Animals as Intellectual Property (or the Patented Mouse That Roared)." *Journal of the Patent and Trademark Office Society* 76:511–545.

MURRAY, THOMAS H. 1987. "On the Human Body as Property: The Meaning of Embodiment, Markets, and the Meaning of Strangers." *University of Michigan Journal of Law Reform* 20, no. 4:1055–1088.

Parke-Davis & Co. v. H. K. Mulford & Co., 1911. 189 F. 95 (S.D.N.Y. 1911), *aff'd,* 196 F. 496 (2d Cir. 1912).

U.S. CONGRESS. HOUSE. COMMITTEE ON THE JUDICIARY. 1988. *Patents and the Constitution: Transgenic Animals.* Hearings Before the Subcommittee on Courts, Civil Liberties and the Administration of Justice. 100th Cong., 1st Sess.

———. OFFICE OF TECHNOLOGY ASSESSMENT. 1989. *"New Developments in Biotechnology: Patenting Life—Special Report."* Washington, D.C.: U.S. Government Printing Office.

U.S. Constitution, Article 1, Section 8, Clause 8. United States Code Annotated (West Publishing Co., 1987).

U.S. Patent Act. 35 United States Code Annotated §§101, 112, 161–164 (West Publishing Co., 1984 & Supp. 1992).

U.S. PATENT AND TRADEMARK OFFICE. 1987. Commissioner's Notice, Animal Patentability. *Official Gazette of the Patent and Trademark Office* 1077:24 (April 21).

U.S. Plant Variety Protection Act of 1970. Pub. L. No. 91-577, 84 Stat. 1542, codified at 7 United States Code Annotated §§2321–2583 (West Publishing Co., 1988 and Supp. 1992).

WORLD COUNCIL OF CHURCHES. CHURCH AND SOCIETY. 1982. *Manipulating Life: Ethical Issues in Genetic Engineering.* Geneva: Author.

WORLD RESOURCES INSTITUTE. 1993. *Biodiversity Prospecting: Using Genetic Resources for Sustainable Development.* Washington, D.C.: Author.

PATERNALISM

Paternalists maintain that restricting the autonomy of persons is justified if these persons would be likely to cause serious harm to themselves or fail to secure an important benefit for themselves. The main ethical issue is whether paternalistic interventions are morally justified, and if so, under what conditions. In bioethics, rightful authority in the patient–physician relationship and public-health interventions have been the focus of the discussion. For health policy, paternalism is central to questions concerning the government's role in promoting healthy lifestyles and preventing self-caused injury and illness.

Many actions, rules, and laws are commonly justified by appeal to some paternalistic principle. Examples include laws that protect drivers by requiring seat belts; restrictions on the availability of drugs; rules prohibiting a healthy subject of biomedical research from voluntarily undergoing a high-risk procedure; overriding adult refusals of treatment; disclosing confidential information about a patient to protect the patient's health; involuntary commitment to hospitals; interventions to prevent suicides; and denial of an innovative therapy to someone who wishes to receive it. Laws are the usual vehicle for translating paternalistic beliefs into public policy, but individual actions and institutional policies can also have paternalistic roots.

Early history in ethical theory

In an eighteenth-century discussion, the philosopher Immanuel Kant denounced paternalistic government ("imperium paternale") for its benevolent cancellations of the freedoms of its subjects (Kant, 1974, pp. 58–59). However, it was the nineteenth-century English philosopher John Stuart Mill who presented the first systematic attack on paternalism, a term he avoided, in his 1859 monograph *On Liberty:*

> The only purpose for which power can be rightfully exercised over any member of a civilized community, against his will, is to prevent harm to others. His own good, either physical or moral, is not a sufficient warrant. He cannot rightfully be compelled to do or forbear because it will be better for him to do so, because it will make him happier, because in the opinions of others, to do so would be wise, or even right. These are good reasons for remonstrating with him, or reasoning with him, or persuading him, or entreating him, but not for compelling him. . . . In the part which merely concerns himself his independence is, of right, absolute. (p. 223)

Mill thus articulated a principle that properly restricted social control over individual liberty, regardless of whether such control is political, religious, or of some other type. He defended his principle with the utilitarian argument that granting people liberty rather than subjecting them to paternalism produces the best possible conditions for social progress and for the development of individual character and talent. Independent of his commitment to utilitarianism, Mill's *On Liberty* has played a more important role in discussion of paternalism than any treatise in ethical theory.

Neither Mill nor Kant anticipated that a paternal model of justified intervention into the affairs of competent adults might be extended to interventions with adult persons who, like children, have only a restricted or compromised capacity to choose autonomously. Yet this latter and broader model has become the most widely defended account of paternalism.

Definitions of paternalism

The word "paternalism" refers loosely to acts of treating adults as a benevolent father treats his children, but the term has been given both a narrow and a broad meaning in ethical theory. In the narrow sense, paternalism refers to acts or practices that restrict the autonomy or liberty of individuals without their explicit consent; justification for such actions is either the prevention of some harm they stand to do to themselves, or the production of some benefit for them that they would not otherwise secure. This conception of paternalism leads to the following definition: Paternalism is the intentional limitation of the autonomy of one person by another, where the person who limits autonomy justifies the action exclusively by the goal of helping the person whose autonomy is limited (Dworkin, 1992; Beauchamp-McCullough, 1984). Following this definition, an act of paternalism overrides the value of respect for autonomy on some grounds of beneficence. Paternalism seizes decision-making authority by preventing persons from making or implementing their own decisions.

Many writers object to this analysis of paternalism because it does not comprehend the meaning of the term as it has descended from common usage and venerable legal precedent, where the notion is linked to guardianship, surrogate decision making, and government intervention to protect the vulnerable. The root sense of paternalism in ordinary language ("government as by a benevolent father") is joined with the law's wide-ranging use of terms such as *parens patriae* to produce a broad meaning that includes interventions into both autonomous and nonautonomous actions. Those who follow this broad vision recommend the following definition: Paternalism is the intentional overriding of one person's known preferences by another person, where the person who overrides justifies the action by the goal of benefiting the person whose will is overridden. Under this second definition, if a person's stated preferences do not derive from a substantially autonomous choice, overriding his or her preferences can still be paternalistic. The only essential condition of paternalism is beneficent treatment that overrides a known preference; a condition of substantial autonomy is not essential (VanDeVeer, 1986; Kleinig, 1983).

Defenders of the first definition argue that there are compelling reasons for resisting this second definition. First, paternalism originates in ethical theory as an issue about the valid limitation of freedom and autonomy. To include cases involving persons who lack substantial autonomy, such as drug addicts or the mentally disabled, broadens the term in a way that obscures the central issue, which is how, whether, and when liberty or autonomy can be justifiably limited. Second, the legal concept of *parens patriae* powers has its own subtleties and complexities. Courts do not apply this notion across the same range of thought and conduct that paternalistic literature treats as problematic. To incorporate a marginal legal doctrine together with the vagueness of ordinary language might prove more confusing than instructive in the end.

These two definitions are currently contested in literature. However, defenders of these two definitions need not disagree on all controversies about the meaning of paternalism. For example, it has sometimes been said that the term "paternalism" is inherently pejorative because it implies that authorities may treat adults such as hospital patients as if they were children lacking considered preferences of their own; therefore, they reason, the term is tainted by illegitimate authoritarianism or repressive dominance (Feinberg, 1980, 1986; Sherwin, 1992). Proponents of the above two definitions are free either to accept or to resist this interpretation. For example, they can both resist this pejorative meaning by arguing that paternalism suggests nothing beyond an analogy to respectable parental benevolence, in which parents act in the best interests of their children for good reason.

Weak (soft) paternalism and strong (hard) paternalism

Joel Feinberg's distinction between weak and strong paternalism has profoundly affected literature on the subject. Although he switched to the language of "soft" and "hard" paternalism in his later work (1986), the terms "weak" and "strong" seem to have more deeply influenced the bioethics literature and will be used here.

In weak paternalism, one "has the right to prevent self-regarding harmful conduct only when it is substantially nonvoluntary or when temporary intervention is necessary to establish whether it is voluntary or not" (Feinberg, 1971, p. 113). This type of paternalism confines permissible limitations of autonomy to substantially nonautonomous (or nonvoluntary) behaviors. For example, it is permissible to pick up injured, partially incoherent victims of automobile accidents who refuse ambulance service and to admit against their will mentally ill persons who are dangerous to themselves. In strong paternalism, however, it is proper to protect or benefit a person by autonomy-limiting measures even if the person's contrary choices are autonomous. This paternalism supports interventions that protect competent adults against their will; that is, it controls or restricts substantially autonomous behaviors. For example, refusing to release a competent hospital patient who will die outside the hospital but requests the release knowing the consequences is an act of strong paternalism.

Weak paternalism is built on conditions of compromised ability or dysfunctional incompetence. When conduct that affects only the actor is restricted, some degree of autonomy may be present in the restricted actor, but the action must be substantially nonautonomous. Conditions that can significantly compromise the ability to act autonomously include the influence of psychotropic drugs, painful labor while delivering a child, and a blow to the head that affects memory and judgment. In medical situations, a patient's illness can be so devastating that it affects decision-making capacity. As the patient becomes weaker, less aware, or less alert, his or her dependence on the physician increases. A member of the medical profession who overturns the preferences of a substantially nonautonomous patient in the interests of the person's medical welfare acts paternalistically and justifiably by the standards of weak paternalism. For this reason, weak paternalism has been widely accepted in law, medicine, and moral philosophy as an appropriate basis for intervention.

Strong paternalism, by contrast, supports some interventions intended to benefit a person whose choices and actions are informed and autonomous. Strong paternalism usurps autonomy by either restricting the information available to a person or overriding the person's informed and voluntary choices. These choices may not be fully autonomous or voluntary, but in order to qualify as strong paternalism the choices of the beneficiary of paternalistic intervention must be substantially autonomous or voluntary. For example, a strong paternalist would prevent a patient capable of autonomous choice from receiving diagnostic information that might lead to suicide. Unlike weak paternalism, strong paternalism does not require any conditions of compromised ability, dysfunctional incompetence, or encumbrance as the basis of intervention (although strong paternalists of course accept the justifiability of weak paternalistic interventions as well).

Justification of paternalism and antipaternalism

Defenders of paternalism in ethical theory have paid more attention to the justifying grounds for paternalism than to the type of paternalism justified. Some justifications range widely and defend both strong and weak paternalism. Typically, however, a condition in the argument states or hints that only weak paternalism is justified, although strong paternalism is the most controversial and interesting type of paternalism and may be the only type worth the effort of justification.

Justified paternalism.   Defenders of paternalism often appeal to either a principle of rational consent or a principle of welfare or beneficence in order to justify their position. In one prominent justification, Gerald Dworkin argues that paternalism should be regarded as a form of "social insurance policy" that fully rational persons would take out for their protection (Dworkin, 1972, p. 65). That is, paternalism is justified under conditions to which an impartial rational agent would consent if he or she were to appreciate the possibility of being tempted at times to make decisions to commit acts that are potentially dangerous and irreversible. The agent might at other times be driven to do something that would be considered too risky if he or she could objectively assess the situation—for example, smoking or drinking so heavily that health and life are endangered. A paternalistic health policy would remove or severely restrict the availability of tobacco and alcohol. In other cases, persons might not sufficiently understand or appreciate the dangers of their conduct, or might distort information about their circumstances. Seat-belt laws and motorcycle-helmet laws have often been enacted on this paternalistic basis.

Dworkin argues that a paternalistic act that denies a person an immediate liberty may paradoxically protect deep autonomy (i.e., the person's deeper values and preferences about the principles and standards on which he or she ought to act). A physician might lie to a patient, for example, in order to prevent a suicide, if the physician knows that the patient really wants to live and will later calm down and not commit suicide, although the patient is presently in no position to appreciate this fact. Dworkin argues that rational consent (consent that would be given) is the only acceptable way to express the conditions of justified paternalism. Many philosophers subsequently agreed with this thesis and made some form of consent a necessary condition of justified paternalism. However, justifications on bases other than consent have also been attempted (Dworkin, 1972; see VanDeVeer, 1986; and Kleinig, 1983).

A justification based on consent may do more to obscure than to clarify the issues. If the paternalist's objective is to protect or improve the welfare of another, then intervention can be justified by harm-avoidance or benefit-production, as is the case in the justification of parental actions that override the wishes of their children. Children are treated paternalistically not because they will subsequently consent or would have consented were they rational, but because they will have better lives. This justification rests on providing for their welfare, not on respecting their autonomy.

The justification of antipaternalism.   Some believe that paternalism is never justified. Mill supported this position, but with the important qualification that we are justified in restricting a person's liberty temporarily in order to ensure that the person is acting intentionally with adequate knowledge of the consequences of the action; once warned and informed, the person must be allowed to choose whatever course he or she desires. One need not be a follower of Mill's utilitarianism to defend this antipaternalism. For example, it can be defended by appeal to principles of respect for autonomy and privacy. Perhaps the most widely shared reason antipaternalists oppose (strong) paternalism is that it interferes with the authority of the individual, insults autonomous agents, and fails to treat them as moral equals (Childress, 1982).

The antipaternalist permits an initial, temporary infringement of liberty and privacy in the belief that persons who have a well-formed, autonomous resolution to do something harmful to themselves will have ample opportunity to perform the action after the temporary intervention has occurred. Intervention, in this limited respect, need not be a deep moral offense. Defenders of weak paternalism, however, view this qualified antipaternalism as insufficient because it disallows some highly desirable forms of intervention, such as long-term involuntary hospitalization for those in need of medical attention. Who, they reason, would not support altruistic beneficence directed at confused cardiac patients, ignorant consumers, frightened clients, and young persons who know little about the dangers of alcohol, smoking, drugs, and motorcycles? No caring and decent person would leave these individuals unprotected, and no reasonable philosopher would defend a normative thesis that permits such outcomes.

Weak paternalists thus project the appearance of steering a moderate and reasonable course between two radical and excessive extremes, strong paternalism and antipaternalism. The solution to the problem of paternalism, from their perspective, is to present the most defensible form of weak paternalism. But a severe stumbling block lies in the path of this tempting resolution of the issues: Weak paternalism has no clear substantive moral disagreement with antipaternalism, and therefore there is no reason to choose one over the other. Protection from harm caused to an individual by conditions beyond his or her knowledge and voluntary control—for example, by conditions beyond his or her self—is not an intervention that antipaternalists either criticize or disallow; they deny only the acceptability of intervention with substantially autonomous, self-caused harm. Weak paternalists too condemn such actions as an unjustifiable form of strong paternalism.

Weak paternalism, then, seems to be a defensible but noncontroversial position that virtually everyone accepts in some form. As Feinberg notes, it is "severely misleading to think of [weak paternalism] as any kind of paternalism," because weak paternalism is not "'paternalistic' at all, in any clear sense" (Feinberg, 1986, pp. 12–14). Both weak paternalism and antipaternalism agree on the following critical claims:

(a) It is justifiable to interfere in order to protect persons against harm from their own substantially nonautonomous decisions; and
(b) it is unjustifiable to interfere in order to protect persons against harm from their own substantially autonomous decisions.

Weak paternalism is thus not a form of paternalism that can be distinguished in any morally important respect from antipaternalism. Weak paternalism does not seem to rest on a liberty- or autonomy-limiting principle independent of some moral principle of beneficence that supports prevention of harm to others (see Feinberg, 1971, pp. 107f., 124, and Feinberg, 1986, p. 13). Feinberg sarcastically suggests that the label "soft antipaternalism" seems to mean the same as "soft paternalism" (1986, p. 15).

The weak paternalist and the antipaternalist also join hands in opposition to the strong paternalist, who alone allows interventions that override and violate substantially autonomous actions.

The justification of strong paternalism.   Although substantial autonomy is necessarily overridden in strong paternalism, conditions can be specified by a strong paternalist to restrict severely the range of justifiable interventions. For example, the strong paternalist might maintain that interventions are justified only if: no acceptable alternative to the paternalistic action exists; a person is at risk of serious harm; risks to the person that are introduced by the paternalistic action itself are not substantial; projected benefits to the person outweigh risks to the person; and any infringement of the principle of respect for autonomy is minimal.

Strong paternalism, so interpreted, will stand or fall on the strength of the argument that major welfare interests under some specifiable conditions legitimately override relatively minor autonomy interests. Many cases can be found that fit this model. For example, when healthy persons with no heart disease volunteered as subjects in a research study to have an artificial heart transplanted at the University of Utah, it was entirely reasonable that a review committee declared that the risk relative to benefit for a healthy subject is morally unacceptable and that they should not be allowed to undergo the procedure (Beauchamp and Childress, 1994).

Issues of paternalism in bioethics

Many examples of controversial paternalistic justifications are found in bioethics. Only a few general topics are treated here.

Overriding refusals of treatment.   It is sometimes controversial whether procedures should be withheld or withdrawn even when the patient refuses the procedures. Justifications for overruling a patient's refusal of therapy need not be paternalistic, but they often are paternalistic because their objective is to prevent harm that would be caused by the patient's refusal. The issue is not whether a physician actually knows what is best for the patient, but whether the patient has a right to refuse treatment even if the refusal is harmful and the treatment beneficial.

Persons of questionable competence who refuse therapy present delicate moral problems and difficult conceptual issues about whether interventions are paternalistic. For example, do schizophrenic patients have a right to refuse a therapy for dehydration if a physician determines it to be safe and efficacious, and would an intervention after a refusal be paternalistic? Similarly, do children who understand what is being done to them have a right to refuse therapies when their parents and physicians judge these therapies to be essential, and are such interventions paternalistic?

Overriding requests for treatment.   Patients or their legal representatives occasionally request medical procedures that physicians believe are harmful, ineffective, or futile. The physician may then refuse to act on these requests for paternalistic reasons. If the requests by patients are incompatible with accepted standards of care or conflict with the physician's conscientious beliefs about standards of care, a physician's refusal to comply may be justified for these apparently nonpaternalistic reasons of appropriate physician conduct. Nonetheless, the interventions are paternalistic whenever the primary ground of noncompliance with the request is that the treatment is not in the patient's best interests. Moreover, setting professional standards of practice is itself often a paternalistic attempt to protect patients' interests, and as such may be either justified or unjustified paternalism (Childress, 1982; Brett and McCullough, 1986). The same argument can be applied to drug policies of a government agency that refuses to accept requests for experimental therapies on grounds of risk to patients.

Partial disclosures to prevent harm.   Physicians and families often argue that a particularly devastating diagnosis or prognosis should not be disclosed to a patient. The concern is that bad news might adversely affect the patient's health or lead the patient to commit suicide. If the patient asks for the information or expects a truthful disclosure, it is paternalistic to withhold the truth. Physicians also occasionally make difficult medical decisions without consulting the parents of seriously ill newborns. These actions too are paternalistic if the objective is to prevent anguish to the parents. Other examples extend beyond serious patient illness. For example, genetic counselors sometimes use potential marital conflict for a patient as a reason not to disclose a condition such as nonpaternity, thereby depriving a patient of information generated in part by materials the patient provided.

In a much-quoted article on medical ethics, L. J. Henderson claimed that "the best physicians" use the following as their primary guide: "So far as possible, 'Do No Harm.' You can do harm by the process that is quaintly called telling the truth. You can do harm by lying. . . . But try to do as little harm as possible, not only in treatment with drugs, or with the knife, but also in treatment with words" (Henderson, 1935, p. 823). The premise that some information may legitimately be withheld or disclosed only to the family for the patient's good is a clear instance of this rule and an equally clear case of paternalism. Why the family, rather than the competent patient, is given the information without the patient's prior permission is itself an important issue concerning paternalistic medical practices.

Invoking the therapeutic privilege.   Therapeutic privilege is a legally recognized privilege of the physician to withhold information from a patient if disclosure would cause serious deterioration in the physical, psychological, or emotional condition of the patient. This privilege has long been used in clinical settings to justify not obtaining consent and has elicited a particularly furious exchange over whether autonomy rights can be validly overridden for paternalistic reasons.

The courts have yet to develop a standard for appropriate use of the therapeutic privilege that renders it coherent with requirements of informed consent. If stated broadly, physicians can withhold information when disclosure would cause any countertherapeutic deterioration, however slight, in the physical, psychological, or emotional condition of the patient. If stated narrowly, physicians can withhold information if and only if the patient's knowledge of the information would have serious health-related consequences—for example, by jeopardizing the success of the treatment or harming the patient by critically impairing relevant decision-making processes. Confusion has also surrounded appropriate measures of rationality, psychological damage, and emotional stability under the standard of therapeutic privilege. Loose standards can permit physicians to climb to safety over a straw bridge of speculation about the psychological consequences of information, and this threat of abuse has made the therapeutic privilege highly controversial.

Health policy for excessive risk.   Antipaternalists argue that paternalistic standards for policy would authorize too much intervention. Paternalism could in principle prohibit smoking, drinking, and hazardous recreational activities such as hang-gliding, mountain-climbing, and white-water rafting, making such activities subject to criminal sanctions. Careful defenses of paternalism would disallow these extreme interventions, and at best antipaternalist arguments establish only a rebuttable presumption against paternalistic intervention. Nonetheless, antipaternalists are convinced that an unacceptable latitude of judgment would remain in contexts in which power is subject to abuse. Strong paternalism suggests that it would be permissible and perhaps obligatory to restrain and punish those who violate paternalistic rules. If so, antipaternalists argue, the state would be permitted to coerce morally heroic or valiant citizens if they act in a manner "harmful" to themselves. More generally, the state would be empowered to take away from persons the right to make decisions about their lives whenever officials view risks as excessive.

Government agency restrictions.   Some government bureaus can be viewed, at least in part, as paternalistic guardians. For example, the Food and Drug Administration (FDA) in the United States is chartered to restrict persons from purchasing foods, drugs, and medical devices that are unsafe or inefficacious. A controversial decision by the FDA in 1992 to severely restrict the use of silicone-gel breast implants exemplifies paternalistic controversies that have beset the FDA. Women had elected implants for over thirty years, either to augment their breast size or to reconstruct their breasts following mastectomies. Over two million women in the United States had had these implants (three million worldwide) when, in April 1992, the FDA restricted the use of silicone-gel breast implants until additional studies could be conducted to establish their safety. Concerns centered on the implants' longevity, rate of rupture, and link with various diseases. Those who defended complete prohibition contended that no woman should be allowed to take a risk of unknown but potentially serious magnitude because her consent could not be informed. The FDA defended a restrictive policy, rather than prohibition, holding that patients with breast cancer and others have a legitimate need for breast reconstruction. The FDA distinguished sharply between reconstruction candidates and augmentation candidates, arguing that the favorable risk–benefit ratio is confined to reconstruction candidates (Kessler, 1992).

Critics of this decision charge that the government's decision is inappropriately paternalistic, especially in contrast to the more permissive public decisions reached in European countries. These critics argue that subjective benefits for many women outweigh the identified risks, and opinion surveys indicate that 90 percent of women receiving the implants are satisfied with the results (see Parker, 1993). Critics argue that the only defensible policy is to permit the continuing use of silicone-gel breast implants while requiring adequate disclosure of information about risks. Raising the level of disclosure standards is, from this perspective, more appropriate than raising the level of paternalistic restraints on choice.

The model of paternal authority.   The term "paternalism" has often been criticized as sexist and in need of correction to "parentalism." However, some feminists in bioethics as well as some critics of paternalistic medical practices have argued that this usage is a rare case in which gendered language should be retained on grounds that an appropriate link is made between the privileges of a father in a patriarchical family and the privileges of physicians in an authoritarian medical system. The thesis is that just as hierarchical arrangements have long been the norm in the family, so paternalism has been the norm in medicine; to appreciate the need to revise authority structures in the family should similarly point to the need to revise the model of rightful authority in medicine (see Sherwin, 1992).

This criticism extends beyond analysis of the meaning of paternalism. It assumes the persistence among physicians, male and female, of the belief that a paternal model of authority is requisite in clinical practice be-

cause of compromised reasoning abilities in patients, the essential need for technical information in medical decision making, and the needs many patients have for an authority figure as healer. Susan Sherwin (1992) and other writers in bioethics have argued for replacing this traditional paternalistic model with a radically different model of the physician–patient relationship, such as a model based on friendship or on contract.

However, those who support justified paternalism in medicine believe that paternalism, properly understood, fits coherently with our normal expectations of altruistic beneficence and fiduciary responsibility in professional health-care relationships. Their model is that of a dedicated professional who possesses superior knowledge, experience, and skills and who seeks to further a patient's best interest. Whether pieces of these two starkly different models can be joined consistently is a matter of widespread controversy in bioethics.

Suicide intervention.   Many views about reporting, preventing, or intervening in suicide are paternalistic. Because of the extreme and irreversible effects of suicide, some defenders of intervention believe that a principle of respect for life creates an obligation to prevent suicide that overrides obligations based on the principle of respect for autonomy. A weaker account relies on Mill's strategy: Intervention is justified to establish autonomy in the person; but after it is determined that the person's decisions are substantially autonomous, further intervention would be unjustified. (Kleinig, 1983, discusses several other paternalistic arguments for suicide intervention.)

Both this weaker account and stronger accounts have been defended on grounds that others do sometimes know our best interests with more insight and foresight than we do. It is often difficult to know how much ability persons have to act autonomously or how much insight they have into their "best interests." The stronger account is also defended on grounds that many suicidal persons are under intense strain or the influence of drugs or alcohol, clinically depressed, destabilized by a crisis, or simply wish to end their pain, and that these persons can be helped with their problems by health professionals. Another defense is that failure to intervene symbolically communicates to potential suicides an absence of communal concern and diminishes a feeling of communal responsibility. Finally, some argue that it is a justified form of paternalism for friends and health-care professionals to infringe confidentiality by reporting suicide threats to those who may be in a position to help prevent the acts. Some even defend a paternalistic obligation to report suicide threats (Bloch, 1987).

Involuntary institutionalization.   Finally, a vast literature surrounds the involuntary hospitalization of persons who have never harmed others or themselves but are thought to stand in danger of inflicting such harm or of being vulnerable to harm by others. A major part of the contemporary rationale for use of police powers for the emergency detention and civil commitment of those dangerous to themselves is a paternalism supported by the knowledge that treatment has often helped persons over a momentary crisis. These interventions can involve a double paternalism: a paternalistic justification for commitment and a paternalistic justification for forced therapy (e.g., psychotherapy) after commitment.

Conclusion

Bioethics in the 1970s and 1980s exhibited a strong tendency to reject paternalism as an unjustified tampering with autonomy. However, from the mid-1980s through the mid-1990s many voices began to be heard that were more sympathetic to various paternalistic appeals. Paternalism seems likely to continue to be a viewpoint that will gain or lose adherents as the issues and larger social context shift. We may never again see the concentrated flurry of scholarly interest in this subject that was exhibited from the mid-1970s to the mid-1980s, but paternalism is not likely to be an issue that will soon disappear.

TOM L. BEAUCHAMP

Directly related to this entry are the entries AUTONOMY; BENEFICENCE; FREEDOM AND COERCION; AUTHORITY; INFORMED CONSENT; PROFESSIONAL–PATIENT RELATIONSHIP, *article on* ETHICAL ISSUES; HARM; *and* PUBLIC POLICY AND BIOETHICS. *This entry will find application in the entries* ADOLESCENTS; AUTOEXPERIMENTATION; COMMITMENT TO MENTAL INSTITUTIONS; INFORMATION DISCLOSURE; INSTITUTIONALIZATION AND DEINSTITUTIONALIZATION; SUBSTANCE ABUSE, *article on* ALCOHOL AND OTHER DRUGS IN A PUBLIC-HEALTH CONTEXT; *and* SUICIDE. *Other relevant material may be found under the entries* BEHAVIOR CONTROL; FEMINISM; LAW AND BIOETHICS; MEDICAL CODES AND OATHS; MEDICINE AS A PROFESSION; RIGHTS; *and* UTILITY. *See also the* APPENDIX (CODES, OATHS, AND DIRECTIVES RELATED TO BIOETHICS), SECTION II: ETHICAL DIRECTIVES FOR THE PRACTICE OF MEDICINE, *and* SECTION III: ETHICAL DIRECTIVES FOR OTHER HEALTH-CARE PROFESSIONS.

Bibliography

BEAUCHAMP, TOM L., and CHILDRESS, JAMES F. 1994. *Principles of Biomedical Ethics,* 4th ed. New York: Oxford University Press.

BEAUCHAMP, TOM L., and McCULLOUGH, LAURENCE B. 1984. *Medical Ethics: The Moral Responsibilities of Physicians.* Englewood Cliffs, N.J.: Prentice-Hall.

BLOCH, KATE E. 1987. "The Role of Law in Suicide Prevention: Beyond Civil Commitment—a Bystander Duty to Report Suicide Threats." *Stanford Law Review* 39, no. 4:929–953.

BRETT, ALLAN S., and McCULLOUGH, LAURENCE B. 1986. "When Patients Request Specific Interventions: Defining the Limits of the Physician's Obligation." *New England Journal of Medicine* 315, no. 21:1347–1351.

BUCHANAN, ALLEN. 1978. "Medical Paternalism." *Philosophy and Public Affairs* 7, no. 4:371–390.

CHILDRESS, JAMES F. 1982. *Who Should Decide? Paternalism in Health Care.* New York: Oxford University Press.

DWORKIN, GERALD. 1972. "Paternalism." *Monist* 56, no. 1: 64–84.

———. 1992. "Paternalism." In *Encyclopedia of Ethics,* pp. 939–942. Edited by Lawrence C. Becker. New York: Garland.

FEINBERG, JOEL. 1971. "Legal Paternalism." *Canadian Journal of Philosophy* 1:105–124. Revised in *Social Philosophy.* Englewood Cliffs, N.J.: Prentice-Hall 1973. Recast in *Harm to Self* (below).

———. 1980. "The Child's Right to an Open Future." In *Whose Child? Children's Rights, Parental Authority, and State Power,* pp. 124–153. Edited by William Aiken and Hugh LaFollette. Totowa, N.J.: Rowman and Littlefield.

———. 1986. *Harm to Self.* Vol. III, *The Moral Limits of the Criminal Law.* New York: Oxford University Press.

HENDERSON, L. J. 1935. "Physician and Patient as a Social System." *New England Journal of Medicine* 212, no. 18: 819–823.

KANT, IMMANUEL. 1974. [1793]. *On the Old Saw: That May Be Right in Theory But It Won't Work in Practice.* Translated by E. B. Ashton. Philadelphia: University of Pennsylvania Press.

KESSLER, DAVID A. 1992. "Special Report: The Basis of the FDA's Decision on Breast Implants." *New England Journal of Medicine* 326, no. 25:1713–1715.

KLEINIG, JOHN. 1983. *Paternalism.* Totowa, N.J.: Rowman & Allanheld.

MILL, JOHN STUART. 1977. [1859]. *On Liberty.* In *Collected Works of John Stuart Mill,* vol. 18. Toronto: University of Toronto Press.

PARKER, LISA S. 1993. "Social Justice, Federal Paternalism, and Feminism: Breast Implants in the Cultural Context of Female Beauty." *Kennedy Institute of Ethics Journal* 3, no. 1:57–76.

PELLEGRINO, EDMUND D., and THOMASMA, DAVID C. 1988. *For the Patient's Good: The Restoration of Beneficence in Health Care.* New York: Oxford University Press.

PURDY, LAURA M. 1992. *In Their Best Interest: The Case Against Equal Rights for Children.* Ithaca, N.Y.: Cornell University Press.

SARTORIUS, ROLF, ed. 1983. *Paternalism.* Minneapolis: University of Minnesota Press.

SHERWIN, SUSAN. 1992. *No Longer Patient: Feminist Ethics and Health Care.* Philadelphia: Temple University Press.

VanDeVEER, DONALD. 1986. *Paternalistic Intervention: The Moral Bounds on Benevolence.* Princeton, N.J.: Princeton University Press.

PATIENTS' RESPONSIBILITIES

I. DUTIES OF PATIENTS

Today, popular culture in the United States seems to be stressing health promotion and disease prevention; it is easy to get the impression from many sources that if one does not exercise regularly, eat the proper foods, and avoid tobacco and other dangerous substances, one has failed in a fundamental duty. In medicine and nursing, a vast literature has accumulated on "patient compliance"; despite some reminders that patients ought to be viewed as autonomous agents—the wisdom of the term "compliance" has been called into question—much of this literature assumes that the patient has a duty to follow advice given by the health professional. By contrast, eighteenth- and nineteenth-century codes of medical ethics, which listed responsibilities that patients owed to their physicians in order to balance the responsibilities that physicians were said to owe to their patients, have been condemned by most modern authors as paternalistic and self-serving. Whether patients owe any duties to health professionals and to others, and the extent of those duties if they exist, remain problematic. The topic has been much less studied in bioethics than the duties owed by professionals to patients and to society.

Duties owed to health professionals

Many helpful models of the professional–patient relationship are based on some variant of social contract or covenant; and those models would imply that patients owe at least some duties to the professionals. These models deny the assumption that underlies most eighteenth- and nineteenth-century codes of medical ethics, namely, that professional ethics is a matter to be decided solely by professionals themselves, with no necessary role for patients in determining the rights and responsibilities that constitute professional ethics. It is this exclusion of patients from defining professional ethics, and not the idea of patient responsibilities per se, that permits the criticism that the alleged responsibilities of patients are paternalistic.

Are there any duties patients themselves would agree they owe to health professionals? Duties that would reasonably fall under this heading are so closely linked to the adequate carrying out of the professional role that their violation would make it impossible for the professional to provide the patient with the care the patient expects and demands. Such duties, properly circumscribed, cannot pose a threat to any patients' rights, because all such rights exist within a relationship whose purpose is to provide the patient with health care from a professional. Indeed, Meyer (1992) argues that the very notions of patients' rights and autonomy presuppose such a relationship.

Martin Benjamin (1985) proposes two such patient responsibilities: (1) honoring commitments, including compliance with a treatment regimen one has consented to carry out; and (2) disclosing relevant information, especially data needed to reach an accurate diagnosis and management plan for the illness. He is careful to insist that no patient has a duty to adopt any treatment plan merely because a professional recommends it; otherwise, there would be no patient right to informed consent. However, once the patient has agreed to try a plan, the patient has an obligation either to continue with the treatment or to inform the professional in a timely manner if circumstances (such as medication side effects) have made it impossible to do so. In this way, we acknowledge both the patient's right to autonomous choice and the professional's need to rely on disclosure of information and honoring of commitments in carrying out the assigned role.

Duties owed to identified others

In general, duties owed to identified others are justified by the nature of the relationship between the patient and that other party. For example, as an extension of the duty to protect the interests of and to avoid harm to members of one's family, patients could have a duty to disclose health information (such as information about communicable diseases and genetic conditions) that would otherwise be protected by the right of confidentiality.

Where it is difficult to specify the precise nature and scope of the relationship, there will be a corresponding disagreement about the duties one owes. For instance, there is controversy about the duties that a pregnant woman owes to the fetus or the unborn child, in avoiding behaviors that might pose a health risk to herself or to the fetus and, in some instances, in either seeking or failing to seek an abortion. Such controversy will be resolved at least in part by more satisfactory conceptions of the precise relationship between the pregnant woman and the fetus or child. For instance, viewing the mother and fetus as two strangers with a conflict of basic interests hardly seems to do justice to the actual nature of their bond.

Duties owed because of specific contractual relationships are much easier to understand and to justify.

For example, if an insurance policy does not cover a particular laboratory test unless it is required to diagnose a specific condition, the patient has a duty not to ask the physician to falsify the claim form and say that he or she suspects the condition, when in fact the patient merely wants to know the laboratory value as a screening measure.

Duties owed to other patients generally

A patient in a modern technological society receives many benefits because of sacrifices made by patients in the past. I could not receive a medication for an infection unless that drug had been tested in research subjects. I could not receive care from a highly qualified physician or nurse unless that professional, as a student, had practiced on other patients, under supervision. It would seem at first glance that I would have a corresponding duty to serve as a research subject or as "teaching material" when I could do so with relatively little risk and inconvenience. But the health-care system generally regards such participation as fully voluntary, not as arising out of any duty. The difference between these two views may be a result of differences in the level of moral analysis—one may acknowledge that one owes a moral duty as an individual, even if as a policy matter the institution is unwilling or unable to enforce any such duty. A full analysis of the duties, if any, that patients owe in such circumstances may nonetheless hinge upon the general theory of justice one adopts.

Duties owed to society

An important debate centers upon whether one's entitlement to health-care services, or the portion of the cost of care that one bears, should hinge on the extent to which one has adhered to a healthy, low-risk lifestyle—an increasingly difficult task, as science regularly uncovers previously unappreciated health risks.

One proposal to fund expanded health-care coverage and benefits in the United States, for instance, includes a substantial increase in the tax on cigarettes. This could be justified purely as a matter of public health, since empirical evidence suggests that a number of people will stop smoking as a result of the tax. In turn, the public-health agenda could be justified in part by referring to a patient's duty to himself or herself to avoid serious health risks (though some analytic philosophers would claim that a duty to oneself is incoherent, since if someone owes a duty to me, I can always voluntarily release him or her from that duty), or to the duty that an individual owes to close family members not to abandon them or decrease one's ability to support them by running unnecessary and substantial health risks. Alternatively, the tax could be justified as a matter of justice, with those who voluntarily adopt unhealthy behaviors

having some responsibility to pay for a larger share of the overall health costs. According to this latter line of analysis, the tax is therefore justified even if it fails to persuade any current smokers to stop.

Some of the debate about a duty to avoid health risks centers upon the addictive nature of some undesirable behaviors. Addiction implies a loss of voluntary control, suggesting that any duty not to engage in that behavior is correspondingly weakened, assuming that I cannot have a duty to do what I cannot do. On the other hand, a careful analysis of most addictive behavior patterns reveals certain actions that do appear to be under voluntary control, even if other aspects of the pattern seem to be characterized by loss of control. For instance, smokers may elect not to sign up for smoking-cessation counseling, and may socialize in settings where they know the temptation to smoke will be high.

To some extent, linking entitlement to care with a duty to remain healthy depends on where one stands on a spectrum between individualistic and communitarian conceptions of health-care justice. On a purely individualistic approach, I have no responsibility to help pay for the health needs of anyone else; on a communitarian interpretation, we all have a shared responsibility to provide decent care for all, and that sense of shared responsibility is undermined by efforts to assign differential duties to pay to different citizens on the basis of their personal behaviors. Also, a duty to avoid health risks seems more justifiable when it is applied evenhandedly rather than being used to condemn those whose lifestyles differ from one's own. Finally, a policy based on a duty to avoid health risks seems justifiable in inverse proportion to its personal intrusiveness. Thus a tax on the sale of cigarettes appears more justifiable than refusing health care to those whose diseases are caused by smoking, or spying on citizens in their homes to be sure that they really have stopped smoking.

HOWARD BRODY

Directly related to this article is the companion article in this entry: VIRTUES OF PATIENTS. *Also directly related is the entry* PATIENTS' RIGHTS. *For a further discussion of topics mentioned in this article, see the entries* AUTONOMY; BEHAVIOR CONTROL; CONFIDENTIALITY; FAMILY; FETUS, *especially the article on* PHILOSOPHICAL AND ETHICAL ISSUES; HARM; MATERNAL–FETAL RELATIONSHIP; PATERNALISM; PROFESSIONAL–PATIENT RELATIONSHIP; PROFESSION AND PROFESSIONAL ETHICS; *and* SUBSTANCE ABUSE. *This article will find application in the entry* AIDS. *For a discussion of related ideas, see the entries* ACADEMIC HEALTH CENTERS; FIDELITY AND LOYALTY; FRIENDSHIP; HEALTH PROMOTION AND HEALTH EDUCATION; INFORMATION DISCLOSURE, *article on* ETHICAL ISSUES; *and* JUSTICE. *Other relevant material may be found under the entries* ADVERTISING; HEALTH SCREENING AND TESTING IN THE PUBLIC-HEALTH CONTEXT; PRIVACY IN HEALTH CARE; *and* PRIVILEGED COMMUNICATIONS. *See also the* APPENDIX (CODES, OATHS, AND DIRECTIVES RELATED TO BIOETHICS), SECTION I: DIRECTIVES ON HEALTH-RELATED RIGHTS AND PATIENT RESPONSIBILITIES.

Bibliography

BENJAMIN, MARTIN. 1985. "Lay Obligations in Professional Relations." *Journal of Medicine and Philosophy* 10, no. 1: 85–103.

GATENS-ROBINSON, EUGENIE. 1992. "A Defense of Women's Choice: Abortion and the Ethics of Care." *Southern Journal of Philosophy* 30, no. 3:39–66.

GOROVITZ, SAMUEL. 1984. "Why You Don't Owe It to Yourself to Seek Health." *Journal of Medical Ethics* 10, no. 3: 143–146.

MEYER, MICHAEL J. 1992. "Patients' Duties." *Journal of Medicine and Philosophy* 17, no. 5:541–555.

SIDER, ROGER C., and CLEMENTS, COLLEEN D. 1984. "Patients' Ethical Obligation for Their Health." *Journal of Medical Ethics* 10, no. 3:138–142.

STIMSON, GERRY V. 1974. "Obeying Doctor's Orders: A View from the Other Side." *Social Science and Medicine* 8, no. 2:97–104.

WIKLER, DANIEL. 1987. "Personal Responsibility for Illness." In *Health Care Ethics: An Introduction*, pp. 326–358. Edited by Donald VanDeVeer and Tom Regan. Philadelphia: Temple University Press.

II. VIRTUES OF PATIENTS

Although considerable attention has been given to virtues in medicine (Drane, 1988; Pellegrino and Thomasma, 1993), most writings focus on the virtues of caregivers rather than on those of care receivers. Patients writing about their experiences of illness (Abram, 1982; Sacks, 1984; Scott-Maxwell, 1968) often struggle with questions of virtue and character, but they tend not to express those questions in systematic or theoretical form. Little has been written on patients' virtues per se.

Several commentators suggest that virtues of different people involved in medicine have to be correlated with the goals or purposes of the medical encounter (Drane, 1988; Pellegrino and Thomasma, 1993). For example, in *For the Patient's Good*, Edmund Pellegrino and David Thomasma (1988) suggest that the virtues of a good patient include truthfulness, probity (or an effort to uphold one's end of the healing relationship), justice, tolerance, and trust (which includes some elements of gratitude and friendship). These virtues arise out of the model of obligations appropriate to the internal goods of the practice of medicine. In *The Virtues in Medical Prac-*

tice, Pellegrino and Thomasma add benevolence, humility, and courage. These virtues, which apply to practitioners as well as patients, "dispose both parties to act well in relation to the ends of medicine" (1993, p. 194).

However, Edmund Pincoffs (1985) argues that virtues cannot be reduced simply to qualities related to the internal goods of a practice. If virtues are correlative to role-specific duties, as Tom Beauchamp and James Childress (1989) suggest, then patients might be expected to exhibit the virtues correlative to their duties of truthfulness, compliance with treatment regimen, and respect. However, such a view would neglect important virtues, such as gratitude, that are not readily identified with action guides.

Both Karen Lebacqz (1985) and William F. May (1991) address the virtues of patients as qualities that emerge in response to the situation of illness or limitation, but not specifically as qualities having to do with the doctor–patient or caregiver–care receiver relationship and not specifically as correlated with duties. Drawing on both fictional (Solzhenitsyn, 1969) and real-life (Abram, 1982; Fox, 1959; Scott-Maxwell, 1968) stories of patients, Lebacqz addresses the virtues of patients generally. May treats the virtues of the elderly within the general context of their confrontation with limitation, adversity, and death.

In line with other commentators (Drane, 1988; Hauerwas, 1985; Pellegrino and Thomasma, 1988), Lebacqz argues that virtue, which can be defined as a unity of the self, is not the same as specific *virtues*. Virtues are qualities or traits of character judged to be excellent. They emerge as general stances toward the world or as responses to situations. The situation of patients is generally characterized by bodily change, threats to self-identity and understanding, and the assumption of a new social role—that of "patient," with all its indignities, loss of control, and powerlessness. The virtues of patients are "excellences" in response to these situational changes.

Using classical virtue theory (Pieper, 1966), Lebacqz proposes that two "cardinal" virtues and one "theological" virtue are particularly appropriate to the situation of patients. Fortitude, or courage in the face of fear, is the first virtue for patients, who often wonder whether they have the strength to do what is needed. Fortitude includes both endurance and attack: both accepting limits and railing against limitation.

Prudence, or acting in accord with the real, is crucial for patients, who must learn to deal with new realities in their lives. The first aspect of prudence is perception; the second aspect is the willingness to act on what is perceived. Perception includes both listening, or contemplation, and removing hardness from the heart in order to value the little things in life.

Finally, Lebacqz suggests that hope in the sense of trust in the attainment of ends is crucial for patients (cf. Hauerwas, 1985, who argues that hope forms every virtue). In the face of despair and even terror, hope keeps patients from falling into despair. Humor is a central component of such hope.

Lebacqz stresses that there is no single pattern of virtue for patients and no one way of expressing relevant virtues. While she follows the Aristotelian pattern of assuming virtue to be a mean between extremes, she notes that virtues are culturally conditioned and, hence, what is considered virtuous in one culture may not be in another. For example, patient waiting might be prized in some cultures while aggressive resistance would be in others. Whereas Pellegrino and Thomasma (1988) note that health-care providers often consider the "good patient" to be the one who is willing to suffer (1988), Lebacqz rejects long suffering as a central virtue for patients. Similarly, virtues might be assessed differently for men and women in different cultures.

May's (1991) treatment of virtues of the elderly stresses several of those noted by Lebacqz. May also puts courage at the head of the list, and includes in it both endurance and attack. He places the virtue of prudence into the broader category of wisdom, and uses traditional categories to propose that prudence includes *memoria*, or learning from the past; *docilitas*, or the capacity to be silent and thus to perceive; and *solertia*, a readiness for the unexpected and an openness to the future. He does not list hope per se, but does include humor or *hilaritas* ("celestial gaiety") as a virtue related to wisdom.

May also adds some virtues of the elderly in situations of illness. Since patients are "receivers," May argues that humility is a crucial virtue for them. It removes the sting from the humiliations that they must endure. While Lebacqz argues that patience is not always a virtue, May suggests that purposive waiting and taking control of one's own spirit under circumstances of adversity is a virtue. For the elderly, May adds the virtues of benignity, letting go of one's possessions in openhanded love, and simplicity, learning to travel unencumbered. Finally, he suggests that integrity is a virtue that expresses unity of character and implies both uprightness and wholeness. Although May does not list theological virtues per se, he does suggest that integrity points to the transcendent dimension.

These different treatments of patients' virtues suffice to indicate that there is no single list of virtues appropriate to patients and no agreed mechanism for deriving such a list. Nonetheless, using Pincoffs's (1985) sorting scheme, we might suggest that patients need both instrumental and noninstrumental virtues.

Instrumental virtues are geared toward the goal of restoring health. These fit best with the view that virtues are qualities intrinsic to the goods of an institution or practice such as medicine. In the case of patients, such instrumental virtues would include complying with appropriate treatment regimens (probity) and telling the truth about one's situation (honesty). These virtues support the goal of working toward the patient's health.

Patients also need noninstrumental virtues. In these, Pincoffs includes (1) aesthetic qualities such as serenity, which comes close to May's virtue of simplicity; (2) meliorating qualities such as tolerance and tactfulness, which come close to notions of humor utilized by both Lebacqz and May; and (3) moral virtues such as fairness and honesty, akin to virtues urged by Pellegrino and Thomasma.

There is general agreement, then, that virtues are qualities of persons generally admired or praised in a culture, and that certain qualities are particularly important for patients: courage (or fortitude), wisdom (especially prudence), humor, hope, truthfulness, and faithfulness to the task of healing, whether through long-suffering endurance or through attack and resistance. In spite of this agreement, the assessment of what constitutes a virtue will be culturally conditioned and will likely reflect the biases of dominant groups in a culture.

KAREN LEBACQZ

Directly related to this article is the companion article in this entry: DUTIES OF PATIENTS. *Also directly related is the entry* VIRTUE AND CHARACTER. *For a further discussion of topics mentioned in this article, see the entries* BENEFICENCE; DEATH: ART OF DYING; DEATH, ATTITUDES TOWARD; FEMINISM; FIDELITY AND LOYALTY; FRIENDSHIP; JUSTICE; NARRATIVE; PAIN AND SUFFERING; PROFESSIONAL–PATIENT RELATIONSHIP; TRUST; *and* VALUE AND VALUATION. *For a discussion of related ideas, see the entries* AUTHORITY; AUTONOMY; BODY, *especially the article on* SOCIAL THEORIES; COMPASSION; DISABILITY; HEALING; HEALTH AND DISEASE, *especially the article on* THE EXPERIENCE OF HEALTH AND ILLNESS; *and* INFORMATION DISCLOSURE. *See also the* APPENDIX (CODES, OATHS, AND DIRECTIVES RELATED TO BIOETHICS), SECTION I: DIRECTIVES ON HEALTH-RELATED RIGHTS AND PATIENT RESPONSIBILITIES.

Bibliography

ABRAM, MORRIS B. 1982. *The Day Is Short: An Autobiography.* New York: Harcourt Brace Jovanovich.

BEAUCHAMP, TOM L., and CHILDRESS, JAMES F. 1989. *Principles of Biomedical Ethics.* 3d ed. New York: Oxford University Press.

BRODY, HOWARD. 1994. "Patients' Responsibilities." In *Encyclopedia of Bioethics.* Edited by Warren T. Reich. New York: Macmillan.

DRANE, JAMES F. 1988. *Becoming a Good Doctor: The Place of Virtue and Character in Medical Ethics.* Kansas City, Mo.: Sheed and Ward.

FOX, RENEE C. 1959. *Experiment Perilous: Physicians and Patients Facing the Unknown.* Glencoe, Ill.: Free Press.

HAUERWAS, STANLEY. 1985. "Virtue." In *Powers That Make Us Human: The Foundations of Medical Ethics,* pp. 117–140. Edited by Kenneth Vaux. Urbana: University of Illinois Press.

LEBACQZ, KAREN. 1985. "The Virtuous Patient." In *Philosophy and Medicine,* vol. 17, *Virtue and Medicine: Explorations in the Character of Medicine.* Edited by Earl E. Shelp, pp. 275–288. Dordrecht, Netherlands: D. Reidel.

MAY, WILLIAM F. 1991. *The Patient's Ordeal.* Bloomington: Indiana University Press.

PELLEGRINO, EDMUND D., and THOMASMA, DAVID C. 1988. *For the Patient's Good: The Restoration of Beneficence in Health Care.* New York: Oxford University Press.

———. 1993. *The Virtues in Medical Practice.* New York: Oxford University Press.

PIEPER, JOSEF. 1966. *The Four Cardinal Virtues: Prudence, Justice, Fortitude, and Temperance.* Notre Dame, Ind.: University of Notre Dame Press.

PINCOFFS, EDMUND L. 1985. "Two Cheers for Meno: The Definition of the Virtues." In *Philosophy and Medicine,* vol. 17, *Virtue and Medicine: Explorations in the Character of Medicine.* Edited by Earl E. Shelp, pp. 111–131. Dordrecht, Netherlands: D. Reidel.

SACKS, OLIVER W. 1984. *A Leg to Stand On.* New York: Summit.

SCOTT-MAXWELL, FLORIDA. 1968. *The Measure of My Days.* New York: Knopf.

SOLZHENITSYN, ALEKSANDR ISAVICH. 1969. *Cancer Ward.* Translated by Nicholas Bethell and David Burg. New York: Bantam.

PATIENTS' RIGHTS

I. Origin and Nature of Patients' Rights
George J. Annas
II. Mental Patients' Rights
Louis E. Kopolow

I. ORIGIN AND NATURE OF PATIENTS' RIGHTS

In most industrialized countries it is taken for granted that citizens have a right *to* medical care, but there is much less recognition of rights *in* medical care. In the United States, in contrast, concentration has historically been on rights that individuals may exercise in the medical-care context, whereas only in the mid-1990s has discussion begun to focus on rights to medical care (or at least the right to medical insurance). From "informed consent" to the "right to abortion" to the "right to die," patients' rights have become both a political slogan and a part of broader political agendas.

Although initially the trend toward recognizing patients' rights concentrated on the institutional setting in which medical care was delivered, and focused on issues such as natural childbirth and informed consent, by the 1990s the trend was visible throughout the health-care system in the United States and was spreading internationally.

The doctor–patient relationship has historically been described as based on trust rather than on the monetary considerations evident in the more typical business transaction. Nevertheless, increased expectations and increased cost have contributed to patients' views of themselves as "consumers," and by the 1980s hospitals began considering themselves private businesses. U.S. courts and legislatures had previously moved to protect the weaker party from abuses of power in areas formerly unregulated, such as landlord–tenant, seller–buyer, creditor–debtor, employer–employee, police–suspect, and warden–prisoner relationships. The law has now also come to the aid of patients asserting their rights in medical situations.

The recognition of patients' rights flows from two fundamental premises: (1) The health-care consumer possesses certain interests, many of which may properly be described as rights, that are not automatically forfeited by entering into a relationship with a physician or a health-care facility; and (2) many physicians and health-care facilities fail to recognize the existence of these interests and rights, fail to provide for their protection or assertion, and frequently limit their exercise without recourse (Annas and Healey, 1974).

History

In 1969, the Joint Commission on Accreditation of Hospitals (JCAH)—a private, voluntary accreditation organization composed of members from the American Hospital Association (AHA) and the American Medical College of Surgeons—issued its proposals for revisions in its standards. The National Welfare Rights Organization (NWRO), a grass-roots consumer organization spawned during the activist 1960s, responded in June 1970 by drafting a document containing twenty-six demands; this was the first comprehensive statement of "patients' rights" from the consumers' perspective. Included were provisions for such things as grievance procedures, community representation on hospital governing boards, nondiscrimination on the basis of source of payment, restrictions on transfers, provisions on privacy and confidentiality, and prompt attention to patients' requests for nursing assistance (Silver, 1974). After months of negotiation, a number of these items were specifically written into the revised standards of the JCAH. By the late 1980s, issues of access to care, of respect and dignity, privacy and confidentiality, consent, refusal of treatment, and patient transfer to another facility were specifically addressed in a new section of their accreditation manual called "Rights and Responsibilities of Patients" (Annas, 1989).

In late 1972, the American Hospital Association adopted a Patient Bill of Rights based on the premise that "[the] traditional physician–patient relationship takes on a new dimension when care is rendered within an organizational structure . . . the institution itself also has a responsibility to the patient." The text of the AHA bill of patient rights called for acknowledgment of the rights to (1) respectful care; (2) current medical information; (3) information requisite for informed consent; (4) refusal of treatment; (5) privacy; (6) confidentiality; (7) response to requests for service; (8) information on other institutions touching on the patient's care; (9) refusal of participation in research projects; (10) continuity of care; (11) examination and explanation of financial charges; and (12) knowledge of hospital regulations. In 1992, items on access to medical records and use of advance directives were added. Although the listing remains vague and incomplete, and there is no enforcement mechanism, it moves in the direction of more adequately informing patients of their rights.

Between 1974 and 1988, many states, including Arizona, California, Illinois, Kentucky, Maryland, Massachusetts, Michigan, Minnesota, New Hampshire, New York, Pennsylvania, Rhode Island, and Vermont, adopted a patients' bill of rights by regulation or statute (Annas, 1989). All fifty states have adopted some form of advance health-care directive document, such as a living will or durable power of attorney, in which people can express their wishes regarding medical care should they become incompetent. Both former President Nixon and Jacqueline Kennedy Onassis used such documents in 1994.

The American Medical Association (AMA), probably because of its traditional paternalistic philosophy, did not seriously consider adopting its own version of the patients bill of rights until 1989. Five of the six provisions of its proposal—the rights of patients to access information in the medical record and to make treatment decisions and the rights to respect, to confidentiality, and to continuity of care—seem to have been uncontroversial. The bill of rights was rejected by the AMA House of Delegates, however, because of its sixth provision: "The patient has the right to essential health [medical] care." In the absence of some national health-care program, or unless the patient has a preexisting relationship with a physician or insurance program or is experiencing an emergency medical condition, there is no "right to medical care" in the United States (although opinion polls taken since 1948 show that most physicians and Americans believe this right either exists or should exist).

International scope of the movement

Although "rights talk" is uniquely American (as are the Bill of Rights and Declaration of Independence), the patients' rights movement should not be viewed as unique to any one country. In 1975, for example, the Parliamentary Assembly of the Council of Europe submitted a draft recommendation to its sixteen member-nations recommending that all necessary action be taken to ensure that the sick can receive relief from their suffering and that people can prepare adequately for death; that commissions be established to study the issue of euthanasia; and that physicians be impressed "that the sick have a right to full information, if they request it, on their illness and the proposed treatment, and to take action to see that special information is given when entering hospitals as regards the routine, procedures and medical equipment of the institution." By 1990, work on a European Declaration of the Rights of Patients was well under way (Westerhall and Phillips, 1994; Leenen et al., 1993). In 1991, a national conference on patients' rights was held in Japan, and at the impetus of tort lawyers and some physicians, a trend toward recognizing patients' rights is developing in that country as well.

The worldwide trend toward recognizing human rights in health should be viewed in context of the worldwide trend toward recognizing human rights in general. Recognition of rights to bodily integrity in general, for example, translates into a right to refuse treatment in the medical context. In this regard documents such as the Nuremberg Code (1947), the United Nations Universal Declaration of Human Rights (1948), and the United Nations International Covenant on Civil and Political Rights (1966) should be viewed as foundational (Annas and Grodin, 1992; Sieghart, 1983).

Patients' rights in context

Historian Paul Starr discusses the patents' rights movement in the United States as part of the "generalization of rights," distinguishing the movement to recognize health care as a basic human right (still unfulfilled) from the movement to work for rights in health care. In his words, "The new health care rights movement went beyond traditional demands for more medical care and challenged the distribution of power and expertise" (Starr, 1982, p. 389). Grass-roots consumer organizations in some states, such as Oregon, have begun to influence health policy, as have activist groups such as ACT-UP. Courts, of course, have contributed greatly to this trend, especially through decisions defining the doctrine of informed consent and by upholding treatment refusals as an individual's right to the exercise of liberty. But no one should have to go to court to have rights vindicated. Some have suggested the establishment of ethics committees to help patients enforce their rights, but such committees usually represent institutional interests more than the rights of individual patients (Annas, 1993). There is a need for an effective enforcement mechanism and an efficient dispute-resolution mechanism. Institutional and professional interests have made agreement on these issues difficult, and legal requirements to adopt such mechanisms may be needed.

One effective method of protecting patients' rights would be the establishment, either by the government under a national health-care system or by health-insurance plans, of a patients' rights advocate program. The advocate should have the authority, under the direction of the patient, to exercise the patient's rights and powers on behalf of the patient. Such individuals could operate at the institutional level, but they are more likely to be effective in health plans, multi-institutional settings, and, of course, under any national health plan (Annas and Healey, 1974).

GEORGE J. ANNAS

Directly related to this article is the companion article in this entry: MENTAL PATIENTS' RIGHTS. *Also directly related are the entries* RIGHTS; AUTONOMY; *and* PROFESSIONAL–PATIENT RELATIONSHIP. *For a discussion of specific rights of patients, see the entries* CONFIDENTIALITY; DEATH AND DYING: EUTHANASIA AND SUSTAINING LIFE, *article on* ADVANCE DIRECTIVES; INFORMED CONSENT, *especially the articles on* MEANING AND ELEMENTS OF INFORMED CONSENT, *and* LEGAL AND ETHICAL ISSUES OF CONSENT IN HEALTH CARE *(with its* POSTSCRIPT*); and* PRIVACY IN HEALTH CARE. *Other relevant material may be found under the entries* MEDICAL ETHICS, HISTORY OF, *section on* THE AMERICAS, *article on* UNITED STATES IN THE TWENTIETH CENTURY; PATIENTS' RESPONSIBILITIES; RESEARCH, HUMAN: HISTORICAL ASPECTS; *and* RESEARCH ETHICS COMMITTEES. *See also the* APPENDIX (CODES, OATHS, AND DIRECTIVES RELATED TO BIOETHICS), SECTION I: DIRECTIVES ON HEALTH-RELATED RIGHTS AND PATIENT RESPONSIBILITIES; *and* SECTION II: ETHICAL DIRECTIVES FOR THE PRACTICE OF MEDICINE, *especially the* PRINCIPLES OF MEDICAL ETHICS *and selected* CURRENT OPINIONS *of the* AMERICAN MEDICAL ASSOCIATION, *and the* DECLARATION OF GENEVA *of the* WORLD MEDICAL ASSOCIATION.

Bibliography

ANNAS, GEORGE J. 1989. *The Rights of Patients: The Basic ACLU Guide to Patient Rights.* 2d ed. Carbondale, Ill.: Southern Illinois University Press. Contains a model patients' bill of rights.

———. 1993. *Standard of Care: The Law of American Bioethics.* New York: Oxford University Press.

ANNAS, GEORGE J., and GRODIN, MICHAEL A., eds. 1992. *The Nazi Doctors and the Nuremberg Code: Human Rights in Human Experimentation.* New York: Oxford University Press.

ANNAS, GEORGE J., and HEALEY, JOSEPH M., JR. 1974. "The Patient Rights Advocate: Redefining the Doctor–Patient Relationship in the Hospital Context." *Vanderbilt Law Review* 27, no. 2:243–269.

INLANDER, CHARLES B., and PAVALON, EUGENE I. 1990. *Your Medical Rights: How to Become an Empowered Consumer.* Boston: Little, Brown.

LEENEN, HENK; GEVERS, SJEF; and PINET, GENEVIEVE. 1993. *The Rights of Patients in Europe: A Comparative Study.* Deventer, Netherlands: Kluwer.

SIEGHART, PAUL. 1983. *The International Law of Human Rights.* Oxford, U.K.: At the Clarendon Press.

SILVER, LAURENS H. 1974. "The Legal Accountability of Nonprofit Hospitals." In *Regulating Health Facilities Construction,* pp. 183–200. Edited by Clark C. Havighurst. Washington, D.C.: American Enterprise Institute.

STARR, PAUL. 1982. *The Social Transformation of American Medicine.* New York: Basic Books.

WESTERHALL, LOTTA, and PHILLIPS, CHARLES, eds. 1994. *Patient's Rights: Informed Consent, Access and Equality.* Stockholm: Nerenius & Santérus.

II. MENTAL PATIENTS' RIGHTS

The strength of a society's commitment to justice and humanity can often be assessed by examining its treatment of its most vulnerable and/or disliked citizens. Few individuals have been as disliked, feared, persecuted, or stigmatized as have the mentally ill. Briefly reviewing the treatment of the mentally ill can provide a useful perspective in addressing present issues in mental patients' rights.

This article will examine mental patients' rights, including legal rights (judicial decisions, legislative and administrative enactments); human wants (basic human rights and entitlements); and clinical needs (the mental-health view of the right of every citizen to be free of the pain and limitations of mental illness).

In the United States, the mentally ill have historically experienced deprivation of many rights enjoyed by other citizens. Since colonial times there has been essentially a two-tier system distinguishing the treatment of the rich from that of the poor. The insane rich were usually kept at home—or more recently, in private institutions—and concealed from society to protect the reputation of their families, while the insane poor were left to the care of local communities. If the insane poor were seen as harmlessly deranged, society's main fear was that they would become public charges and drain the community's resources. To prevent this from happening, the mentally ill were often subjected to whipping and banishment, forced to wander from village to village. If they refused to leave their home community, their "treatment" frequently was incarceration in the local jail or poorhouse (Deutsch, 1948).

During the nineteenth century "moral treatment" was brought to America by a Quaker clergyman, the Rev. Thomas Scattergood. Great success, as high as 90 percent improvement in conditions, was reported by its early practitioners. The treatment was accomplished by removing patients from their family and community and placing them in a peaceful rural retreat—the asylum—where, under the absolute control of the physician, they lived a highly disciplined existence and engaged in useful employment (Rothman, 1971). "Moral treatment" represented an improvement in the conditions under which the mentally ill were treated. While still deprived of the legal and civil rights enjoyed by other citizens, they were at least given humane and hopeful treatment. This improvement, however, did not last long. By the end of the nineteenth century, as the result of a large influx of immigrants and a growing population of chronic patients, the asylums became overcrowded and inadequately staffed. Overcrowding and disorder created justification for mechanical restraints and punishments that grew in usage and severity; hospitals became human warehouses instead of treatment centers.

The failings and increasing harshness of public asylums did not lead to their dismantlement. Loose commitment laws facilitated the expulsion of the mentally ill from an increasingly urban society less willing to tolerate them. Efforts to improve conditions were sporadic, and progress was slow and uneven. Despite numerous books and exposés, including Clifford Beers's *A Mind That Found Itself* (1930), Albert Deutsch's *The Shame of the States* (1948), and Mary Jane Ward's *The Snake Pit* (1946, later made into a movie), the period of incarceration without adequate treatment continued well into the first half of the twentieth century.

By the mid-1950s, the mental-health community began to express its discontent with the situation in state mental hospitals. The resident population soared to 550,000, and approximately 40 percent of hospital beds were in state and county mental hospitals. The president of the American Psychiatric Association declared in 1958, "I do not see how any reasonably objective view of our mental hospitals today can fail to conclude that they are bankrupt beyond remedy" (Solomon, 1958, p. 7).

Public concern about the plight of the nation's mentally ill led Congress to establish the Joint Commission on Mental Illness and Health in 1955. The commission advocated the goal of community-based mental-health care accessible and responsive to the needs of all citizens. Community mental-health centers would provide the mentally ill with treatment close to their homes and jobs, and would reduce the need for prolonged or repeated hospitalization. As the result of the development of psychotropic medicine (medications that therapeutically affect an individual's mood or cognitive thoughts), expansion of community-based care, increased public concern about civil rights, and some greater tolerance of alternative behaviors, the population of the hospitalized mentally ill dropped to 220,000 during the 1960s and 1970s. This process of deinstitutionalization, however, did not always proceed smoothly. Frequently, patient discharges from hospitals occurred precipitously and without adequate aftercare. In addition, communities protested that they were becoming "dumping grounds" for patients unprepared for the demands of community living and for whom no adequate support system had been established (*Stone v. Miller,* 1974).

Despite the increased willingness of the public to support improved care for the mentally ill within their home communities, the plight of those treated in large state hospitals was still characterized by dehumanization, inadequate facilities, and insufficient staff. Such conditions provoked a flurry of lawsuits during the 1960s and 1970s, which led to increased attention to the rights of the mentally ill. These cases fit into three broad categories: the right to treatment; the right to refuse treatment; and the right to be placed in the least restrictive alternative. A fourth right, the right to liberty, represented by the U.S. Supreme Court's *O'Connor v. Donaldson* decision (1975), has aspects that encompass the three other categories.

Right to treatment and right to liberty

During the 1960s, mental-health litigation reflected the increased activism of many civil-rights attorneys who turned their attention to mental patients' rights. In a parallel development, courts that had previously refused to rule on matters of medical treatment began, during the same period, to question whether conditions that would enable treatment to occur actually existed in facilities to which the mentally ill were committed. The concept of a right to treatment was first enunciated by Morton Birnbaum, who wrote the following in an *American Bar Association Journal* article:

> The fact that a person has a mental ailment is not a crime. Therefore, if anyone is voluntarily restrained of his liberty because of mental ailment, the state owes a duty to provide him reasonable medical attention. If medical attention reasonably adjusted to the needs is

not given, the person is not a patient, but . . . virtually a prisoner. (Birnbaum, 1960, p. 499)

As a result of such thinking, a number of lawsuits were filed under the rationale of a constitutional right to treatment. Facilities in which widespread abuses and violation of clinical and legal rights were common were excellent targets for such litigation. Such was the situation that existed in certain hospitals in 1971, when the *Wyatt* v. *Stickney* lawsuit was brought against the Alabama Mental Health System. It was established during the trial that the state legislature had seriously underfunded Parlow and Bryce hospitals, leading to severe understaffing, deterioration in services and facilities, and limitation on treatment and basic care for the patients there. As a result of the rights violations described in the trial, the judge promulgated minimum standards for nearly every aspect of institutional care and a detailed program for implementation.

The minimum standards promulgated by the court include the following: a provision against institutional peonage; a number of protections to ensure a humane psychological environment; minimum staffing standards; provision for a human-rights committee at each institution; detailed physical standards; minimum nutritional requirements; a provision for individualized evaluations of patients, habilitation plans, and programs; minimum staff/patient ratios; and a requirement that every mentally impaired person has a right to the least restrictive setting necessary for treatment (*Wyatt* v. *Stickney*, 1971).

The courts have felt justified in moving into the vacuum caused by a lack of national standards to assure the treatment rights of involuntarily committed psychiatric patients. In the *O'Connor* decision, for example, the Supreme Court dismissed as "unpersuasive" the argument that the court should not be involved, noting: "Where treatment is the sole asserted ground for depriving a person of liberty it is plainly unacceptable to suggest that courts are powerless to determine whether the asserted ground is present" (*O'Connor* v. *Donaldson*, 1975, p. 574, n. 10). In other cases, such as *Wyatt* v. *Stickney*, the judges have consulted with various professional organizations, taken expert testimony, and come up with what they considered minimum standards. These standards tend to be more of the mortar-and-brick and staff-to-patient-ratio variety than to pertain directly to the quality of treatment. The basis behind the right-to-treatment issues as reflected in *Wyatt* and other cases is the expectation that if a psychiatric patient is to be involuntarily confined in order to be treated, then the facility in which he or she is placed should at least have the minimum capacity to deliver such treatment as will assure the patient's recovery and release. To do other

than this is to "warehouse" patients and thus violate their constitutional right to liberty. The limited holding of the Supreme Court's *O'Connor* decision emphasized this point: "A state cannot constitutionally confine without *more* [emphasis added], a nondangerous individual who is capable of surviving safely in freedom by himself or with the help of willing and responsible family members or friends" (*O'Connor* v. *Donaldson*, 1975, p. 576).

Changing perspectives on patient–physician relationships

The Supreme Court's decision in *O'Connor* v. *Donaldson* reflects an evolving philosophy about the rights of the mentally ill in relation to society and to mental-health practitioners. For hundreds of years, many concerned with care and treatment of the mentally ill believed that their condition categorically prevents them from accurately perceiving reality and making reasoned judgments. Therefore it was considered the state's duty, according to the principle of *parens patria* (the state acting as a good parent to the nation's citizens) to take care of such afflicted individuals, and to prevent them under the state's police power from harming themselves or others, or disturbing the peace and safety of the community (Fowlkes, 1978).

Consistent with these commitment perspectives has been the psychiatric view that life and health or physical and emotional well-being are at the pinnacle of any hierarchy of values and should be maintained at any cost—even if the cost is a considerable loss of liberty for the individual whose health is at stake (Kopolow, 1976). A corollary to this position is the belief that mental illness is a disease of processes that impairs an individual's judgment and capacity for responsible action in relation to self and others. In refusing hospitalization and treatment, therefore, the patient's wishes might very well be discounted and viewed as symptoms of his or her mental illness (Sadoff and Kopolow, 1977).

A countervailing philosophy was reflected in the civil-liberties perspective and shared by a growing number of lawyers and mental-health professionals concerned with human rights. This view maintains that although a person's physical and mental health are important they are not necessarily of the highest value, and that freedom of the individual to place a higher value on other things should be respected. Those espousing this view maintain that what is called "mental illness" is not a process that necessarily interferes with or invalidates a person's will or lessens responsibility for his or her behavior (Szasz, 1961). Even psychotic individuals should have their wish to live at home rather than in a state mental hospital taken into consideration by the judges and psychiatrists who determine their fate.

Increasingly, states have abandoned the *parens patria* doctrine as being intrusive into the lives of individuals and have begun to utilize a more limited criterion of dangerousness as the justification for the use of "police power" for commitment. The *O'Connor* court seemed to sanction a definition of dangerousness as applied to civil commitment when it declared:

> Of course, even if there is no foreseeable risk of self injury or suicide, a person is literally dangerous to himself if for physical or other reasons he is helpless to avoid the hazards of freedom either through his own efforts or with the aid of willing family members or friends. (*O'Connor v. Donaldson*, 1975, p. 574, n. 9)

As a result of such court decisions, the test for commitment in many states now requires that the person be harmful to self or others by reason of mental illness and that no less restrictive alternative exists (Stone, 1975).

Initially, right-to-treatment decisions such as *Wyatt v. Stickney* and the right-to-liberty case of *O'Connor v. Donaldson* were welcomed by some mental-health professionals who viewed litigation as a potentially effective means for obtaining the release of patients who were receiving only custodial care or should not have been institutionalized in the first place. Others considered litigation as an intrusion into clinical practices that would produce great disruption in the mental-health system and no long-term benefit for patient care. While this debate continues, it does seem clear that litigation did focus public attention on the plight of the hospitalized mentally ill and, at least in the short term, resulted in pressure on legislatures to increase mental-health appropriations in order to avoid litigation or to avert increased court intervention.

Traditionally, the decisions about therapies and medical procedures have been within the domain of the treating professional responsible for the patient. In many states, patients who were hospitalized involuntarily were considered incompetent to make decisions on their own behalf. As a result of these medical and legal perspectives, patients frequently were denied the rights of other citizens when they were hospitalized. They were not permitted to vote; often they could not make phone calls or correspond without censorship of their mail. Additionally, they were not told what was happening to them or the consequences of the treatment imposed on them.

In the past, patients within an institution experienced a double limitation on their rights—one created by their disabilities and the other by the inherent organization of an institutional system. Even now, the prevailing atmosphere in many hospitals and especially psychiatric facilities perpetuates dependency and helplessness (Goffman, 1961).

While the actual disabilities that require institutional care limit a patient somewhat, the prejudging of his or her capacities by the staff may constitute an even greater obstacle. Even at the most enlightened institution, there will inevitably be a strain between the needs of the individual to live a life free of outside control and the institution's need to deliver care efficiently and effectively. Within a mental-health institution or any long-term-care facility, such organizational factors can be dehumanizing and promote frustration, regimentation, and despair. In addition, the stigmatization of mentally ill patients throughout history has seriously hampered attempts to protect their rights, meet their clinical needs, and advance their basic human wants.

Right to refuse treatment

The right to refuse treatment in many ways encompasses virtually all other rights of patients and raises fundamental questions as to the extent of control that can be exerted by a treater over a person who may not wish to participate in treatment. The issues raised by this right include the right to privacy, personal sovereignty, inviolability of one's thoughts, freedom from harm, freedom from cruel and unusual punishment, and the issue of the least restrictive alternatives to institutionalization (Perlin, 1979).

From the legal perspective, the right to refuse treatment arises from a composite of postulated constitutional sources including the constitutional right to freedom from harm and the constitutional right to privacy. While the courts and legislatures in recent years have been active in assuring patients the right to refuse such intervention as electroconvulsive therapy and psychosurgery, they have been slower to recognize the right to refuse psychotropic medication (Clayton, 1987).

Many individuals with mental illness wish to avoid psychotropic medication because of the potential side effects, which range from merely unpleasant (dry mouth, tiredness, blurry vision) to permanent and disfiguring (tardive dyskinesia, involuntary muscle movement). In addition, some mentally ill patients refuse medication not for the side effects but because the medication works well and therefore forces them to surrender the positive defensive adaptation of the psychotic state. Such adaptations may include an increased sense of importance and power, an ability to shut out problems that exist in the real world, and the support offered by hospitals and physicians (Appelbaum, 1988).

In various jurisdictions, including Massachusetts (*Rogers v. Okin*, 1979), New York (*Rivers v. Katz*, 1986), New Jersey (*Rennie v. Klein*, 1978), and the nation (*Washington v. Harper*, 1990), mental-health attorneys have sought to expand and clarify issues related to the right to refuse treatment, especially medication. Among the issues examined have been questions such as the right to protect all mental processes (thoughts, feelings, beliefs) from governmental interference; the right to protect autonomy over one's own body; the effectiveness of involuntary treatment versus voluntary treatment; and the questions of whether the potential benefits of drug treatment are worth the risks and who should be permitted to make this decision (Perlin, 1979).

The courts in the cases cited above sought to establish various procedures to protect patient autonomy and decision making in refusing antipsychotic medication. While these court decisions and subsequent legislative statutes have attempted to make the right to refuse treatment a legal and clinical reality, recent studies have revealed serious practical complications in applying these principles. One such study examined the assumption by the courts that patients' refusals of treatment are based on autonomous decision making. The study concluded that for most patients the decision to refuse psychotropic medication is a manifestation of their illness and does not reflect autonomous functioning or consistent beliefs about mental illness or its treatment (Schwartz et al., 1988).

A study done by Paul Appelbaum noted that while refusal of treatment was not uncommon, ultimately most of the patients received treatment during their hospitalization (Appelbaum, 1988). Some clinicians have studied the cost of implementing court-mandated protection programs in the wake of the Rogers decision. On the basis of the studies' results, these clinicians have concluded that from the economic perspective, such programs are not cost-effective (Schouten and Gutheil, 1990). Furthermore, some authors have noted that the right to refuse treatment may infringe on the constitutionally based right to treatment for involuntarily committed mental patients (Blais, 1975). Thus the battle continues to be fought. On one side is concern for patients' autonomy and for protection from intrusive and potentially dangerous procedures. On the other side is concern for the clinical needs of patients and the necessity of interventions that can restore them to mental and physical freedom. The future evolution of this right will need to take into consideration not only legal and psychiatric perspectives but also the reality of the consequences of court intervention.

Right to the least restrictive alternative to hospitalization

A third important right that has received increasing judicial and psychiatric attention is the right to the least restrictive alternative to hospitalization. Many mental-health departments have seen deinstitutionalization as an effective way to reduce the cost of mental-health care; unfortunately, clinical services have not always followed patients to their communities.

The trend toward community-based services (least restrictive alternative to hospitalization) was initially heralded as the answer to improved quality and more responsive services. However, it has only partially addressed the need to protect mental patients' rights in the community. In place of the neglect by large institutions, many ex-patients now suffer from the despotic control of boardinghouse managers; in place of "voluntary work with token rewards," they now face long hours of inactivity; in place of even rudimentary treatment plans, they now receive larger doses of tranquilizers administered by untrained persons. These patients also face the continuing threat that unless they conform and follow the rules, they will be rehospitalized (Kopolow, 1979). While community-based services are less restrictive than institutional care, services are only as good as a community is willing to make them.

In the case of Dixon v. Weinberger (1974), Judge Aubrey Robinson ruled that patients in the District of Columbia have a statutory right to treatment in the least restrictive alternative to institutionalization. Responsibility was placed on the District of Columbia and the federal government to prepare a plan to identify and transfer patients to newly created community facilities. It is significant to note that twenty years later, the court's orders still have not been fully implemented. This case clearly shows the limitation of the courts in establishing rights when a community is resistant to, or incapable of, compliance. Another important judicial decision that has relevance to least restrictive treatment is O'Connor v. Donaldson. In this decision, the court acknowledged that states have a legitimate interest in providing care and assistance to patients, but it also declared that the patients' preferences should be recognized as well:

> The mere presence of mental illness does not disqualify a person from preferring his home to the comforts of an institution. Moreover, while the States may arguably confine a person to save him from harm, incarceration is rarely if ever a necessary condition for raising the standards of those capable of surviving safely in freedom. (O'Connor v. Donaldson, 1975, p. 575)

The court's movement toward a standard of ability to survive and the expectation that the least drastic means of treatment will have to be used put increased pressure on communities to develop an adequate range of services. To have such a range of services, however, requires commitment of resources that, as the Dixon case so clearly pointed out, may be slow in coming. The right to the least restrictive alternative will become meaningful only when communities invest adequate resources to develop such alternatives and provide mechanisms such as patient advocates to protect and advance patients' rights within the community or within an institution.

Advocacy

Advocacy has many meanings, depending on the interests and priorities of the various groups using it: mental-health professionals, consumers, attorneys, citizens' organizations. In its classic sense it means "to summon to one's assistance, defending, or calling to one's aid." The present-day connotation of conflict or antagonism is not inherent in the basic concept of advocacy, but results from the manner in which some advocates pursue their duties.

The mentally ill, as noted previously, suffer from prejudice and stigmatization that make it difficult for them to advocate their own causes. In addition to these factors, the complexity of the support and treatment programs and the need for change agents in what is essentially a conservative system make the need for advocates especially important. Advocacy, as related to patients' rights, is the responsibility of many individuals and professionals, including lawyers, psychiatrists, social workers, and concerned citizens. While it is obvious that it is the responsibility of the legal profession to advocate for legal rights of patients, the term also has other useful meanings within the mental-health service delivery system. After pure legal rights have been established and attorneys are available to patients to ensure their protection, other issues remain that cannot and should not be resolved through the legal system. Such issues, including staff attitudes, environmental conditions, and alternative treatment services, which influence the quality of the day-to-day life of mental patients, can be more effectively dealt with through administrative and legislative actions.

It is clear that no one approach or even one professional group can perform all the necessary tasks of mental-health advocacy. Advocacy functions can be divided into three broad categories:

1. Education and training of hospital staff regarding the nature of patients' rights and the best way to assure their protection.
2. Establishment of procedures to allow the speedy resolution of problems, questions, or disagreements that may or may not be legal rights. Such procedures would enable quick and efficient resolution outside the courtroom of legal and nonlegal rights issues.
3. While functions (1) and (2) can be properly handled by appropriate state agencies, a final category requires the use of independent outside lawyers and agencies: provision for independent and readily available legal support when it is necessary to litigate for protection of patients' rights after internal procedures have failed.

A major controversy in advocacy is whether the predominant emphasis should be on internal or external rights-protection programs. An external advocacy program system would be implemented by individuals who are totally independent of the mental-health system. An internal advocacy program would be implemented by employees of the service system. Arguments for external programs relate to the concept that the advocate is ultimately loyal and responsible to the client. An advocate who is an employee of a department or agency of state government may have divided loyalty. An alternative perspective is that not all state employees are equally subject to that conflict—for example, someone working in an independent section or agency of the state government.

Internal rights-protection or advocacy programs, however, frequently tend to be highly efficient in solving complaints about daily living and in planning for future patients'-rights needs. They have easier access to patient records, can participate in program policy development, have a more collegial relationship with administrators that engenders trust and greater cooperation, and have the ability to identify problems to be corrected without outside pressures or publicity. Unfortunately, such programs suffer from the double danger of co-optation and replacement at the discretion of administrators.

An external advocacy program can use persuasion, and when persuasion fails, litigation is always a backup position. Such a program can bypass administrative changes for quick action; however, court cases may move slowly. Therefore, while external advocacy may have a limited range of action, it nonetheless can be powerful and decisive in producing change in a system now receptive to patients' rights protection.

This analysis of internal and external advocacy programs clearly illustrates a patient's need for the availability of both programs. Such comprehensive advocacy programs can go far in assuring that patients'-rights concerns do not become mere rhetoric or window dressing, but are permitted to make substantive changes necessary to create a more responsible mental-health system.

Conclusion

In answering the question "What rights do mental patients have?" it is important to go beyond judicial decisions, administrative actions, or legislative statutes, and look at the status of the mentally ill in American society. The rights of mental patients have historically been disregarded and denied. The mentally ill were frequently viewed as incompetent to make decisions, and society's concern was to place them in institutions where they would cause neither themselves nor others harm and where they might receive treatment for their conditions.

The patients'-rights movement, made up of civil-rights attorneys, enlightened mental-health professionals, and former patients, has waged a struggle in courts, in legislatures, and in local communities to stop patient abuse, end stigmatization, increase needed community services, and empower patients to exert their full civil rights. Major patients'-rights litigation in the areas of right to treatment, right to refuse treatment, right to least restrictive alternatives, and right to liberty have led to increased recognition of the existence of these rights. But it is clear, when one examines the plight of the mentally ill down through history, that "something else" is needed if there is to be no recurrence of the cycle of abuse, exposé, improvement, neglect, and abuse again.

This "something else" that can safeguard patients' rights is the advocate. Mental patients already have extensive rights under the Constitution. The problem is not simply granting or recognizing rights but protecting them. Only through the continuing efforts of the advocates will the mentally ill truly have the rights enjoyed by other citizens. In the case of patients, as in the case of other citizens, "the price of freedom is eternal vigilance." The advocate provides the vigilance that helps assure that the legal rights, human wants, and clinical needs of the mentally ill are protected and promoted.

LOUIS E. KOPOLOW

Directly related to this article is the companion article in this entry: ORIGIN AND NATURE OF PATIENTS' RIGHTS. *Also directly related are the entries* RIGHTS; AUTONOMY; INFORMED CONSENT, *article on* ISSUES OF CONSENT IN MENTAL-HEALTH CARE; PATERNALISM; *and* PROFESSIONAL–PATIENT RELATIONSHIP. *For a further discussion of topics mentioned in this article, see the entries* COMPETENCE; INSTITUTIONALIZATION AND DEINSTITUTIONALIZATION; *and* VALUE AND VALUATION. *For a discussion of related ideas, see the entries* COMMITMENT TO MENTAL INSTITUTIONS; FREEDOM AND COERCION; MENTAL-HEALTH THERAPIES; MENTAL ILLNESS; PSYCHOPHARMACOLOGY; *and* PSYCHOSURGERY. *See also the* APPENDIX (CODES, OATHS, AND DIRECTIVES RELATED TO BIOETHICS), SECTION I: DIRECTIVES ON HEALTH-RELATED RIGHTS AND PATIENT RESPONSIBILITIES, A PATIENT'S BILL OF RIGHTS *of the* AMERICAN HOSPITAL ASSOCIATION, *and* RIGHTS OF MENTALLY RETARDED PERSONS *of the* GENERAL ASSEMBLY OF THE UNITED NATIONS; *and* SECTION III, ETHICAL DIRECTIVES FOR OTHER HEALTH-CARE PROFESSIONS, *especially the* ETHICAL PRINCIPLES OF PSYCHOLOGISTS *and* CODE OF CONDUCT *of the* AMERICAN PSYCHOLOGICAL ASSOCIATION.

Bibliography

APPELBAUM, PAUL S. 1986. "The Rising Tide of Patients' Rights Advocacy." *Hospital and Community Psychiatry* 37, no. 1:9–10.

———. 1988. "The Right to Refuse Treatment with Antipsychotic Medications: Retrospect and Prospect." *American Journal of Psychiatry* 145, no. 4:413–419.

BEERS, CLIFFORD W. 1930. *A Mind That Found Itself: An Autobiography.* Garden City, N.Y.: Doubleday.

BIRNBAUM, MORTON. 1960. "The Right to Treatment." *American Bar Association Journal* 46, no. 5:499–505.

BLAIS, NORMAN N. 1975. "Forced Drug Medication of Involuntarily Committed Mental Patients." *Saint Louis University Law Journal* 20:100–119.

CLAYTON, ELLEN WRIGHT. 1987. "From Rogers to Rivers: The Rights of the Mentally Ill to Refuse Medication." *American Journal of Law and Medicine* 13, no. 1:7–52.

COURNOS, FRANCINE; MCKINNON, KAREN; and ADAMS, CAROLE. 1988. "A Comparison of Clinical and Judicial Procedures for Reviewing Requests for Involuntary Medication in New York." *Hospital and Community Psychiatry* 39, no. 8:851–855.

DEUTSCH, ALBERT. 1948. *The Shame of the States.* New York: Harcourt, Brace.

Dixon v. Weinberger. 1974. No. 74285 (C.D.D.C. Feb. 14).

FOWLKES, E. OLIVER. 1978. "Mental Patients Rights." In *Proceedings: Symposium on Safeguarding the Rights of Recipients of Mental Health Services.* Washington, D.C.: U.S. Government Printing Office.

FREDDOLINO, PAUL P., and APPELBAUM, PAUL S. 1984. "Rights Protection and Advocacy: The Need to Do More with Less." *Hospital and Community Psychiatry* 35, no. 4:319–320.

FREDDOLINO, PAUL P.; MOXLEY, DAVID P.; and FLEISHMAN, JOHN A. 1989. "An Advocacy Model for People with Long-Term Psychiatric Disabilities." *Hospital and Community Psychiatry* 40, no. 11:1169–1174.

GOFFMAN, ERVING. 1961. *Asylums: Essays on the Social Situations of Mental Patients and Other Inmates.* Chicago: Aldine.

KOPOLOW, LOUIS E. 1976. "A Review of Major Implications of the O'Connor v. Donaldson Decision." *American Journal of Psychiatry* 133, no. 4:379–383.

———. 1979. "The Challenge of Patients' Rights." *Advocacy Now* 1, no. 1:19–21.

MILLER, ROBERT D.; RACHLIN, STEPHEN; and APPELBAUM, PAUL S. 1987. "Patients' Rights: The Action Moves to State Courts." *Hospital and Community Psychiatry* 38, no. 4:343–344.

O'Connor v. Donaldson. 1975. 95 S.Ct. 2486.

PERLIN, MICHAEL L. 1979. "The Right to Refuse Treatment: A New Right Emerges. *Advocacy Now* 1, no. 1.

———. 1993. "Decoding Right to Refuse Treatment Law." *International Journal of Law & Psychiatry* 16, nos. 1–2: 151–177.

Rennie v. Klein. 1981. 653 F. 2d. 83 (3d Cir.); vacated 458 U.S. 1119 (1982).

Rivers v. Katz. 1986. 67 N.Y. 2d. 485 N.E. 2d. 337, 504 N.Y.S. 2d. 74.

Rogers v. Okin. 1979. 478 F. Supp 1342 (D.Mass.).

ROTHMAN, DAVID J. 1971. *The Discovery of the Asylum: Social Order and Disorder in the New Republic.* Boston: Little, Brown.

SADOFF, ROBERT, and KOPOLOW, LOUIS E. 1977. "The Mental

Health Professional's Role in Patient Advocacy." In *Mental Health Advocacy: An Emerging Force in Consumer Rights,* pp. 36–41. Edited by Louis Kopolow and Helene Bloom. Washington, D.C.: U.S. Government Printing Office.

SCHOUTEN, RONALD, and GUTHEIL, THOMAS G. 1990. "Aftermath of the Rogers Decision: Assessing the Costs." *American Journal of Psychiatry* 147, no. 10: 1348–1352.

SCHWARTZ, HAROLD I.; VINGIANO, WILLIAM; and PEREZ, CAROL BEZIRGANIAN. 1988. "Autonomy and the Right to Refuse Treatment: Patients' Attitudes After Involuntary Medication." *Hospital and Community Psychiatry* 39, no. 10:1049–1054.

SOLOMON, HARRY C. 1958. "Presidential Address: The American Psychiatric Association in Relation to American Psychiatry." *American Journal of Psychiatry* 115, no. 1:1–10.

STONE, ALAN A. 1975. *Mental Health and the Law: A System of Transition.* Washington, D.C.: U.S. Government Printing Office.

Stone v. Miller. 1974. 373 F. Supp. 177 (E.D.N.Y.).

SZASZ, THOMAS S. 1961. *The Myth of Mental Illness: Foundations of a Theory of Personal Conduct.* New York: Hoeber-Harper.

VEATCH, ROBERT M. 1981. *A Theory of Medical Ethics.* New York: Basic Books.

WARD, MARY JANE. 1946. *The Snake Pit.* New York: Random House.

Washington v. Harper. 1990. 494 U.S. 210.

Wyatt v. Stickney. 1971. 325 F. Supp. 781 (M.D. Ala.).

ZIEGENFUSS, JAMES T., JR. 1986. "Conflict Between Patients' Rights and Patients' Needs: An Organizational Systems Problem." *Hospital and Community Psychiatry* 37, no. 11:1086–1088.

PERSIA

See MEDICAL ETHICS, HISTORY OF, *section on* NEAR AND MIDDLE EAST, *articles on* ANCIENT NEAR EAST, *and* IRAN.

PERSISTENT VEGETATIVE STATE

See DEATH, DEFINITION AND DETERMINATION OF; *and* DEATH AND DYING: EUTHANASIA AND SUSTAINING LIFE.

PERSON

Bioethical debates often center on determination of whether specific individuals are persons. It may be argued, for example, that elective abortion is morally wrong because the fetus is a person, or that termination of life support for an individual in persistent vegetative state is morally permissible because the individual is not a person. Or vice versa in either case. To understand the positions supported by different sides on such issues, it is

important to consider different definitions of person or personhood.

Although the terms "person," "human being," "man," and "self" are sometimes used interchangeably, "person" may be construed either more narrowly or more broadly than the others. The term "self" usually connotes identity or continuity and is applicable to nonhuman as well as human entities, and even at times to inanimate entities. The term "man" may be used to signify all of the members of the human species or specific human individuals. Even among those who purport to use the term generically, "man" often applies exclusively to males (Mahowald, 1983). "Person" is both broader and narrower than "human being." It is broader because not only human but nonhuman entities such as angels or other extraterrestrial beings may be considered persons (Doran, 1989); it is narrower because some human beings, such as fetuses and those who are permanently comatose, may not be considered persons in the context of law, public policy, or ethics.

Humans whose personhood is questionable and controversial include those whose capacity for rational activity is absent, undeveloped, or severely compromised. Although some authors claim otherwise (Feinberg, 1984), many view determination of personhood as crucial to resolution of long-standing issues that arise in caring for such individuals (Macklin, 1983). This entry examines historical and current concepts of person and relates these to decisions about the beginning and end of life, criteria for moral agency, and personal identity.

Classical philosophical and religious sources

In ancient times, the term "person" was applied to those who fulfilled a particular role in theater or in life. The term is derived from the Latin *persona,* meaning a mask worn by a player (Danto, 1972). Although the *dramatis personae,* or list of characters in a drama, reflect this etymology, the theatrical usage of the term is uncommon today. Instead, it is typically used to signify the role that any human being, as human, plays. Theologically, the meaning of person was and is associated with the role or roles played by God. The Christian doctrine of the Trinity, for example, maintains that there are three persons in one God (Pegis, 1945). Although each of these possesses the same divine nature, the work of creation may be attributed to the father, the work of redemption to the son, and the work of sanctification to the spirit (Nolan, 1987).

Boethius's (ca. 480–524) classical definition of person, "an individual substance of a rational nature," in his *The Consolation of Philosophy,* embodies elements of both Platonic and Aristotelian concepts of human nature. The emphasis on rationality, ignoring bodiliness or materiality, is consistent with Plato's concept of the human being as essentially immaterial, a soul imprisoned in a body. In Plato's *Republic,* the human being is tripartite; reason, the highest part, controls the other two parts, spirit and appetite. Plato's denial of the reality or intelligibility of the world of physical objects and images, and his view that immaterial forms such as the soul are eternal, support a positive attitude toward death as liberation of the soul from the body. But his concept of death as the soul's release from the prison of the body into the immaterial world of universal forms implies that the soul is not an individual substance, as Boethius maintains. Plato's teachings about reincarnation and knowledge by recollection give further support to this position.

Aristotle also stresses rationality in his account of human nature, but contends in *On the Soul* that body and soul are an essential or inseparable union in living human beings. Death, as separation of soul and body, is then seen as the demise of the human being. Because of their capacity for expressing rationality through intellect and will, human souls, for Aristotle, are distinct from and superior to the souls of living plants or nonhuman animals. Rationality is expressed through the body, which is the principle of individuation and the means through which the immaterial soul is substantiated. The soul is the form that unites with the matter of a particular body. This account includes all of the elements of Boethius's definition of person.

Both Plato and Aristotle envisage human beings as citizens. For Plato, good citizenship involves the role of social critic. For Aristotle, human beings are political animals, whose good as individuals should be subordinated to the good of the community. Since a person is one who thus has a political role to play, this definition also reflects the etymological meaning of the term.

Platonic and Aristotelian views have been utilized by religious scholars to provide a philosophical basis for their beliefs. Augustine, for example, relates the Platonic concept of humans as souls to his belief that God created human beings according to the divine image. The immateriality of the human soul allows it to live forever when the soul is separated from the body through death. While on earth, one's role is to live as if one is already in the "City of God" (Bk. 19).

Thomas Aquinas couples his belief in the supernatural origin and destiny of human beings with an Aristotelian view of human nature as an essential union of body and soul (*Summa Theologica* I, Q 76). The religious doctrine of the resurrection of the body provides a context for explaining human immortality despite the termination of life that death presents. Like Aristotle, Aquinas imputes to individual human beings a role within the state to promote the common good above their own. His concept of human beings is consistent with the notion of persons as role players. Through their rationality, human beings have a special role to play on the world's stage.

In general, classical concepts of person, particularly those of Aristotle and Aquinas, have been influential in the development of natural law and virtue theory. Their account of nature and the relation between soul and body, joined with Aquinas's supplementary account of the divine origin and destiny of human beings, laid the groundwork for later applications to bioethics. Catholic theologians, for example, have drawn heavily on Aquinas in support of their views about reproduction and sexual ethics. Philosophers such as Alasdair MacIntyre (1984) and Martha Nussbaum (1986) have used Aristotle to develop an ethics of virtue or character. Only persons as such are capable of virtue or of vice.

Modern concepts

Reacting critically to the outward focus of classical thinkers, modern philosophers turned inward to provide an account of person that emphasized self-consciousness. René Descartes (1596–1650) offered a Platonic version of this emphasis by defining human beings as "thinking things." Although many scholars interpret this concept as barren for ethics and social philosophy, Annette Baier has argued that Descartes paid due regard to the embodiment and sociality of human beings. The "Cartesian person," she maintains, is "one who acts and seeks its good in this world, does speak and engage in other activities whose norms, like those of speech, derive from a human community . . ." (Baier, 1985, pp. 79–80). She compares Descartes's need to posit a divine mind to ground the reliability of his own thoughts with Peter Strawson's thesis on the necessity of consciousness of others for establishment of self-consciousness (Strawson, 1959). One develops a sense of oneself through comparison with other selves.

Following Descartes, John Locke (1632–1704) distinguished between man and person, holding that the former is a corporeal being while the latter is not. In his *Essay Concerning Human Understanding* (1689) he describes a person as a connected flow of consciousness. Memory is the glue that links discrete episodes of consciousness to one another, leading to a sense of a perduring self or personal identity. The continuity thus perceived provides a basis for imputing moral responsibility to individuals for deeds previously performed. In light of this linkage, Locke views "person" as a "forensic" term, belonging "only to intelligent agents, capable of a law, and happiness, and misery" (Ford, 1988, p. 69).

Although other rationalists and empiricists elaborated distinct concepts of person, man, and self, Immanuel Kant (1724–1804) has been most influential in this regard. Kant's metaphysical view is comparable to Plato's in its affirmation of a duality between things-as-they-appear (phenomena) and things-in-themselves (noumena), but his epistemology contrasts with that of Plato in its insistence on experience as the source of human knowledge. For Kant, although we know the world of appearances through experience, we only grasp reality—noumena—through postulates of reason. His idea of freedom is one such. Freedom is the necessary condition of the universal experience of moral obligation; we know *that* freedom is without knowing *what* it is.

A person, according to Kant, is the rational agent who alone is capable of exercising freedom as autonomy. In contrast with a heteronomous will whose choices are driven by extrinsic purposes, an autonomous will acts solely in accordance with duties that it defines for itself. Autonomy, as self-determination, is "the supreme principle of morality" (Kant, 1990, p. 53). From Kant's view that each moral self is an end-in-itself, his second formulation of the categorical imperative emerges: Persons must always be treated as ends and never only as means. His sense of a moral community of persons is expressed in a third formulation of the imperative: Through the laws that they enact, persons acknowledge a "reign of ends," that is, "a whole of all ends in systematic connection" (Kant, 1990, p. 50).

By emphasizing the self-consciousness of the individual, modern writers take the concept of person as role player to a different level than did their predecessors. The role to be played by a person as such is unique rather than generic; it is not a role that can be repeated by other players or in other plays. Personhood thus reveals *who* rather than *what* someone is. This concept is evident in existentialist writers who, like Kant, define the person in terms of autonomy. Jean-Paul Sartre, for example, identifies human nature with freedom, claiming that individuals define their own nature through their choices (Sartre, 1957). Gabriel Marcel's characterization of a person as a mystery rather than a problem is reminiscent of Kant's distinction between things and persons. A problem, for Marcel, is subject to analysis because it is abstracted from reality. A mystery is not subject to such analysis because it is dynamic and relational (Marcel, 1976). In the medical context, this distinction is exemplified by the difference between a cadaver to be studied and a patient to be treated. Just as Kant imputes dignity to persons, Marcel regards the proper attitude toward persons as one of reverence.

Contemporary views

Contemporary writers on personhood often address the concept in the context of ethical decisions, laws, and policies about the beginning and end of a right to life. Because rights are usually associated with duties or responsibilities, the attribution of personhood usually entails an assumption of moral agency, at least on the part of those whose duty it is to respect others' lives or rights. In other words, today's scholars tend to emphasize moral concerns rather than metaphysical considerations. Whether or not the two are ultimately separable remains a matter of debate. Questions of personal identity and moral agency are inseparable from the concept of autonomy, a paramount consideration in contemporary bioethics.

Like their classical forebears, some philosophers claim that the meaning of person is to be discovered rather than decided. Baruch Brody, for example, follows the Aristotelian method of observing what is special about living human beings, coupling this with what we now know about brain development in utero. In an article recommended as required reading "by every freshling in every course on contemporary moral issues" (Goodman, 1988, p. 21), Brody arrives at a formulation of what constitutes "the essence of humanity"—namely, brain activity, occurring at about six weeks' gestation (Goodman, 1988). Once brain activity is initiated, he claims, the human fetus has a full set of rights, even equal to those of the pregnant woman on whose support it depends for continued existence (Goodman, 1988). Although Brody's argument here addresses the onset of a full right to life, his view is equally applicable to the demise of that right through death. Legal and clinical definitions of death as cessation of brain activity are well supported by this argument.

Lawrence Becker undertakes to discover what constitutes human beings as distinct from human becomings and from parts or products of human beings. Through an analogy with insect metamorphosis, he tracks the course of human development from zygote to mature fetus. Until morphological and histological development is virtually complete at about seven months' gestation, Becker maintains, the organism is a "human becoming" rather than a "human being." His account also distinguishes between humans that are beings and those that have been human beings. He stops short of equating human beings with persons, however, denying that mature fetuses have a right to life even while attributing to them the status of human beings. Persons, as "self-conscious subjects of experience," can "make claims on us which nonpersons cannot make" because nonpersons lack self-consciousness (Goodman, 1988, p. 70). Nonetheless, persons may have duties toward nonperson human beings such as fetuses. He does not consider whether human becomings and former human beings can make claims on us.

In contrast to Brody and Becker, Daniel Dennett is skeptical about ever discovering the essential meaning of person, even while acknowledging that the term may be "an ineliminable part of our conceptual scheme" (Goodman, 1988, p. 146). He argues that the concept is not only normative but at least partially arbitrary. The latter admission does not prevent him from proposing and defending six necessary conditions for personhood. Three of these are commonly stipulated by others: rationality, consciousness, and self-consciousness (Feinberg, 1984; Goodman, 1988). Intentionality figures centrally in Dennett's understanding of consciousness. Two further conditions are proposed: "stance" and "reciprocity." By stance Dennett means that attitudes taken toward specific entities are constitutive of their personhood. Reciprocity means that "the object toward which this personal stance is taken must be capable of reciprocating in some way" (Goodman, 1988, p. 148). To be a person, in other words, is to treat others as persons. Another condition that Dennett proposes is both unique and problematic: the capacity for verbal communication. He claims that this condition, which excludes nonhuman animals from full personhood, underlies all social-contract theories of ethics.

As already suggested, many authors develop their concepts of person by examining who among possible claimants possess a right to life. Not all use the term "person" to identify rights holders. In an article "In Defense of Abortion and Infanticide," for example, Michael Tooley develops criteria for imputing a right to life to any being, human or nonhuman, without using the term "person" to identify those who have such rights (Feinberg, 1984). He argues that an entity "cannot have a right to life unless it is capable of having an interest in its own continued existence," and that this in turn requires "the concept of a continuing self, or subject of experiences and other mental states" (Feinberg, 1984, p. 132). Since neither fetuses nor newborns have such a capacity, neither have, in this view, a right to life.

Mary Anne Warren provides a more extended list of criteria, but her concept is essentially the same as that of Tooley, and she uses the term "person" in elaborating it. "A fetus," she claims, "is not a person, and hence not the sort of entity to which it is proper to ascribe full moral rights" (Feinberg, 1984, p. 102). The criteria Warren requires for personhood are five: consciousness, reasoning, self-motivated activity, the capacity to communicate, and the presence of self-concepts and self-awareness. Unlike Dennett, she does not require that persons be capable of verbal communication. Consistent with her criteria, she does not consider newborns persons, but argues nonetheless that infanticide is much more difficult to justify than abortion. In other words, determination of personhood does not settle questions about the morality of killing.

A few authors specify but one condition as sufficient and necessary for personhood. Robert Joyce and John Noonan, for example, regard the conception event as triggering the onset of a right to life. Noonan (Feinberg, 1984) bases his view on conception by human parents; Joyce bases his on a notion of "natural potential." For the latter,

every living individual being with the natural potential, as a whole, for knowing, willing, desiring, and relating to others in a self-reflective way is a person. But the human zygote is a living individual (or more than one

such individual) with the natural potential, as a whole, to act in these ways. Therefore, the human zygote is an actual person with great potential. (Goodman, 1988, p. 199)

Although other authors concur that the potential for full human development that the human fetus represents is morally relevant, few impute as strong a rights claim to the early embryo or zygote as they do to mature fetuses or newborns. For some, such as Norman Ford and Richard McCormick, developmental individuality rather than genetic identity is crucial to the establishment of personhood. Developmental individuation is not determined until about the end of the second week after fertilization, when implantation is underway. Only then has a single body axis begun to form, ending the possibility of recombination or twinning (Ford, 1988; McCormick, 1991).

Harry G. Frankfurt and Annette Baier also posit a single criterion for personhood, but they demand much more of the entities to which they impute that designation than do Ford, McCormick, Joyce, or Noonan. Frankfurt, for example, proposes second-order volitions as the defining characteristic (Goodman, 1988); by second-order volitions he means effective desires to oppose one's own first-order desires. To be a person thus means to have freedom of will as control of one's inclinations. For example, a drug addict who confronts her habit and takes steps to change it exhibits personhood as second-order volitions. Obviously, this definition excludes human beings who have not yet developed or have lost their capacity to counter first-order desires. Although Frankfurt's view also excludes most nonhuman animals from personhood, his position is applicable to those who appear to act against self-interest in support of other members of their species.

Baier's cryptic definition of persons is "second persons" (Baier, 1985). By this she means that persons are and can only be constituted by their relationships to other persons. Citing "the exercise of cultural skills, in particular linguistic ones," that Dennett and others impute to persons, Baier observes that these are "acquired during our drawn-out dependency on other persons" (Baier, 1985, p. 84). Interdependence is thus perceived as historical as well as relational:

The fact that a person has a life history, and that a people collectively have a history, depends upon the humbler fact that each person has a childhood in which a cultural heritage is transmitted, ready for adolescent rejection and adult discriminating selection and contribution. Persons come after and before other persons. (Baier, 1985, p. 85)

Although her definition may be criticized as circular, Baier's view presents a broader and more accurate sense of the developmental context of personhood than is found in other authors. Her concept necessarily involves psychosocial as well as biological elements of human development. Rather than define a specific cut-off point between personhood and nonpersonhood, she insists on the continuity of various stages in the life of a human being.

Similarly, several authors maintain that there are degrees of personhood, and some distinguish between senses or kinds of personhood. W. R. Carter, for example, argues that persons are not essentially persons, because their existence antedated their achievement of personhood. A human fetus, he maintains, "is not a person from the moment of its conception" (Goodman, 1988, p. 187), but it becomes such over time. As it does so, it acquires more and more of a right to life, the full extent of which coincides with undeniable personhood. Personhood is manifestly present in individuals who possess the capacity to think and reason. "Moral weight" is attributable to nonpersons, whether these be human fetuses, infants, or nonhuman animals, but only to the extent that they approximate fulfillment of that standard. The approximation leaves us with "marginal persons," whose moral weight can never be greater than that of "full-fledged persons" (Goodman, 1988).

H. Tristram Engelhardt, Jr., distinguishes between strict personhood and social personhood. Concurring with Kant's definition of person, he applies a strict definition of personhood only to those who are clearly moral agents, who as such are "individual, living bearers of rights and duties" (Goodman, 1988, p. 175). So strict a standard obviously excludes many of those to whom we clearly have moral obligations in the health-care context: infants and young children, the comatose, the profoundly retarded, and those whose mental competence is temporarily or permanently severely compromised. In an account that is reminiscent of the definition of person as role player, Engelhardt describes how infants play the role of persons even though they lack the rationality and self-consciousness required for actual personhood. Through the parent–child relationship, he maintains,

> the infant is treated as if it had the wants and desires of a person—its cries are treated as a call for food, attention, care, and so on, and the infant is socialized, placed within a social structure, the family, and becomes a child. The shift is from merely biological to social significance. (Goodman, 1988, p. 176)

Engelhardt insists, however, that even though normal infants are only social persons rather than strict persons, they are able to engage in a minimum of social interaction. In contrast, anencephalic infants "may not qualify for the role *person*, just as brain dead adults would fail to qualify" (Goodman, 1988, p. 176). While he views the mother–child relation as conferring social personhood on the newborn, he does not accord the same capacity to the relationship between the pregnant woman and her fetus.

Moral agency and personhood

The meaning of moral agency is often equated with those definitions of person that involve maximal criteria. Among the preceding accounts, Dennett, Frankfurt, Tooley, and Warren all articulate conditions necessary for the exercise of responsibility as well as rights, imputing to such rights-holders the capacity for moral agency. Noonan, Joyce, Brody, Ford, McCormick, and Becker, on the other hand, attribute personhood or full humanhood to entities that have rights without responsibility, namely, fetuses and newborns. This attribution would logically extend also to humans who are profoundly retarded, comatose, or persistently vegetative. Writers who emphasize the developmental character of personhood, such as Carter and Baier, are likely to see moral agency as a concurrent developmental accomplishment. In this context, personhood is a necessary but insufficient condition for moral agency.

Moral agency is also distinguishable from moral status or moral standing because the latter concepts are applicable to entities whose personhood is questionable or absent. Moral status refers to a continuum of values ranging from nothing to that of a normal human adult who is unquestionably a person and a moral agent. Moral standing specifies the point along the continuum at which a particular entity stands (Sumner, 1981). Consider, for example, human embryos or profoundly retarded humans. The fact that such entities are not capable of exercising moral agency does not imply that they have no moral status or standing, or that those who are moral agents have no moral responsibility toward them. Moral agency is a more demanding concept than moral status or moral standing because it imputes both rights and responsibility to the agent.

A useful concept of moral agency may be derived from Alan Gewirth's definition of morality as "a set of categorically obligatory requirements for action that are addressed at least in part to every actual or prospective agent, and that are concerned with furthering the interests, especially the most important interests, of persons or recipients other than or in addition to the agent or the speaker" (Gewirth, 1978, p. 1). For Gewirth, the "most important interests" or necessary goods to be promoted by persons are well-being and freedom (Gewirth, 1978). Following Kant, he insists that the freedom and well-being of others as well as oneself must be supported. Morality is thus a social enterprise.

Gewirth analyzes the generic structure of human action as dependent on purposiveness and voluntariness. Purposiveness embraces the cognitive element of agency, requiring that an individual act for some intended end. As intended, the end must be known *by,* and known to be related in some way *to,* the individual who selects it. Moreover, the end pursued always appears good to the pursuer. An action is voluntary, Gewirth claims, if an individual "unforcedly chooses to act as he does, knowing the relevant proximate circumstances of his action" (Gewirth, 1978, p. 27). Voluntariness is thus tied to rationality, precluding the possibility that sheer impetuosity or spontaneity is truly voluntary.

What then is moral agency? Synthesizing the crucial elements of Gewirth's view, it involves two components: the capacity for voluntary and purposeful actions, and recognition that such actions influence the well-being or freedom of others. The first element refers to agency and generally assumes personhood. The second element refers to the social context or content of agents' choices, determining whether their choices are in fact moral or immoral as opposed to amoral. While all moral agents are persons, not all of the actions of persons as such are moral actions.

Personal identity

Beyond the problem of defining personhood is the problem of personal identity, which is also related to the concept of moral agency. Agents, after all, are not accountable for previous acts unless they are the same individuals who committed those acts. Whether they indeed are the same—given the psychological, physiological, and circumstantial changes that characterize the lives of individuals—remains debatable.

Locke proposed memory as the determinant of whether an individual preserves identity over time. Only to the extent that someone recalls having performed a specific act is he or she responsible for it. An obvious flaw in this rationale is its suggestion that a perpetrator's subsequent forgetfulness constitutes grounds for absolution. David Hume also views memory as the source of a concept of personal identity, but adds a role for the imagination in fashioning the concept. Consistent with his analysis of causality, he denies that the sense of a continued self can be rationally proved. In the following passage, Hume reminds us again of the role-player meaning of person:

> The mind is a kind of theatre, where several perceptions successively make their appearance; pass, re-pass, glide away and mingle in an infinite variety of postures and situations. There is properly no *simplicity* in it at one time, nor *identity* in different, whatever natural propension we have to imagine that simplicity and identity. (Hume, 1888, p. 253)

Personal identity is thus a fiction of the imagination.

Among contemporary philosophers, Derek Parfit has been a leading contributor to discussions of personal identity. Logically, he claims, personal identity is either totally present or totally absent in each individual. Psychologically, however, continuity and connectedness are morally more important than identity, and these occur in degrees along the spectrum of development (Parfit, 1984). Parfit's view has implications not only for decisions about patients but also for societal decisions based on distributive justice. As Loren Lomasky suggests, an assessment of the justice involved in distributing benefits and burdens to individuals over the course of their lives may be impossible "if the fact of personal identity over time is not a 'deep' further fact beyond continuity and connectedness" (Lomasky, 1992, p. 955).

Discussions of personal identity are also related to issues involving advance directives (Dresser, 1989), definitions of death (Green and Wikler, 1980), and transplantation of brain tissue (Mahowald, 1992). The legitimacy of obtaining and respecting advance directives (instructions from competent patients about treatment or nontreatment when they are no longer competent) is challengeable on grounds that "the very circumstances which would bring an advance directive into play are often those in which one of the necessary conditions for personal identity is not present" (Buchanan and Brock, 1989, p. 155). Because a given individual's goals and desires change throughout the life course, how one would feel and decide in circumstances never experienced cannot be anticipated. By such an account, an ill or comatose patient truly is a different person than he or she was when well and conscious.

Definitions of death and transplantation of brain tissue are related to personal identity because brain function is essential to the rational and volitional activities that appear unique to human beings as persons. Since death marks the end of a life process, it assumes that that life has perdured through some previous stretch of time, no matter how brief. Definitions of death thus assume personal identity. For those who subscribe to a minimalist concept of personhood, personal identity is defined solely in those terms; for example, if a person is defined as any living, genetically distinct human organism, personal identity refers simply to the ongoing existence of that organism. If a person is someone capable of higher brain function, and death is cessation of that function, personal identity refers to the ongoing existence of the organism in which such activity occurs.

In addition to defining death as cessation of brain function, Michael Green and Daniel Wikler equate brain function with personal identity. If the entire brain of one individual were transplanted into another, they claim, the other would then be that individual (Green and Wikler, 1980). This notion of personal identity necessarily includes a psychological history not attributable to fetuses at the onset of brain development. The use of fetal brain tissue for treatment of severe neurological disorders of adults provides a clinical context in which concerns about personal identity are theoretically relevant but probably unwarranted. Even if a whole human fetal brain were transplanted into an adult, the difference in size between fetal and adult brain minimizes such concerns. Moreover, even if personal identity were transformed through brain grafts, an individual faced with severe morbidity or death unless the treatment is undergone might well calculate that life as someone else is preferable to the only available alternatives.

As indicated at the start, the concept of person is of great significance to a variety of issues in contemporary bioethics. As illustrated throughout this discussion, the concept is nonetheless subject to a variety of interpretations and justifications, with different implications for the issues. Careful bioethical analysis demands not only recognition of the relevance of the concept but clarification of its meaning in arguments for alternative positions.

MARY B. MAHOWALD

Directly related to this entry are the entries LIFE; NATURE; HUMAN NATURE; *and* BODY, *article on* EMBODIMENT: THE PHENOMENOLOGICAL TRADITION. *For a discussion of related ideas, see the entries* AUTONOMY; BIOLOGY, PHILOSOPHY OF; EMOTIONS; ETHICS; FREEDOM AND COERCION; NATURAL LAW; RESPONSIBILITY; RIGHTS; *and* VIRTUE AND CHARACTER. *The topics in this entry will find application in the entries* ABORTION, *section on* CONTEMPORARY ETHICAL AND LEGAL ASPECTS, *article on* CONTEMPORARY ETHICAL PERSPECTIVES; DEATH AND DYING: EUTHANASIA AND SUSTAINING LIFE; FETUS; *and* REPRODUCTIVE TECHNOLOGIES, *articles on* IN VITRO FERTILIZATION AND EMBRYO TRANSFER, *and* CRYOPRESERVATION OF SPERM, OVA, AND EMBRYOS.

Bibliography

AUGUSTINE. 1963. *The City of God.* Edited by Vernon J. Bourke. Garden City, N.Y.: Image Books.

BAIER, ANNETTE. 1985. *Postures of the Mind: Essays on Mind and Morals.* Minneapolis: University of Minnesota Press.

BUCHANAN, ALLEN E., and BROCK, DAN W. 1989. *Deciding for Others: The Ethics of Surrogate Decision Making.* New York: Cambridge University Press.

DANTO, ARTHUR C. 1972. "Persons." In *Encyclopedia of Philosophy,* vol. 6, pp. 110–114. Edited by Paul Edwards. New York: Macmillan.

DORAN, KEVIN. 1989. *What Is a Person? The Concept and the Implications for Ethics.* Lewiston, N.Y.: Edwin Mellon Press.

DRESSER, REBECCA S. 1989. "Advance Directives, Self-Determination, and Personal Identity." In *Advance Directives in Medicine,* pp. 155–170. Edited by Chris Hackler, Ray Moseley, and Dorothy E. Vawter. New York: Praeger.

FEINBERG, JOEL, ed. 1984. *The Problem of Abortion.* 2d ed. Belmont, Calif.: Wadsworth.

FORD, NORMAN M. 1988. *When Did I Begin? Concept of the Human Individual in History, Philosophy, and Science.* Cambridge: At the University Press.

GEWIRTH, ALAN. 1978. *Reason and Morality.* Chicago: The University of Chicago Press.

GOODMAN, MICHAEL F., ed. 1988. *What Is a Person?* Clifton, N.J.: Humana Press.

GREEN, MICHAEL B., and WIKLER, DANIEL. 1980. "Brain Death and Personal Identity." *Philosophy and Public Affairs* 9, no. 2:105–133.

HUME, DAVID. 1888. [1739–1740]. *A Treatise of Human Nature.* Edited by L. A. Selby-Bigge. Oxford: At the Clarendon Press.

KANT, IMMANUEL. 1990. *Foundations of the Metaphysics of Morals* and *What Is Enlightenment?* Rev. 2d ed. Translated and with an introduction by Lewis White Beck. New York: Macmillan.

LOCKE, JOHN. 1894. *An Essay Concerning Human Understanding.* Oxford: At the Clarendon Press.

LOMASKY, LOREN E. 1992. "Person, Concept of." In *Encyclopedia of Ethics,* vol. 2 (L-Index), pp. 950–956. Edited by Lawrence C. Becker and Charlotte B. Becker. New York: Garland.

MacINTYRE, ALASDAIR. 1984. *After Virtue: A Study in Moral Theory,* 2d ed. Notre Dame, Ind.: University of Notre Dame Press.

MACKLIN, RUTH. 1983. "Personhood in the Bioethics Literature." *Milbank Memorial Fund Quarterly/Health and Society* 61, no. 1:35–57.

MAHOWALD, MARY B., ed. 1983. *Philosophy of Woman: An Anthology of Classic to Current Concepts.* 2d ed. Indianapolis, Ind.: Hackett.

———. 1992. "Brain Development, Personal Identity, and Neurografts." In *Emerging Issues in Biomedical Policy,* vol. 2, pp. 232–246. Edited by Robert H. Blank and Andrea L. Bonnicksen. New York: Columbia University Press.

MARCEL, GABRIEL. 1976. *Being and Having: An Existentialist Diary.* Gloucester, Mass.: Peter Smith.

McCORMICK, RICHARD A. 1991. "Who or What Is the Preembryo?" *Kennedy Institute of Ethics Journal* 1, no. 1:1–15.

NOLAN, BRIAN M. 1987. "Person, Divine." In *The New Dictionary of Theology,* pp. 757–759. Edited by Joseph A. Komonchak, Mary Collins, and Dermot A. Lane. Wilmington, Del.: Michael Glazier.

NUSSBAUM, MARTHA C. 1986. *The Fragility of Goodness: Luck and Ethics in Greek Tragedy and Philosophy.* Cambridge: At the University Press.

PARFIT, DEREK. 1984. *Reasons and Persons.* Oxford: Oxford University Press.

PEGIS, ANTON C., ed. 1945. *Basic Writings of Saint Thomas Aquinas,* vol. 1. New York: Random House.

RORTY, AMÉLIE OKSENBERG, ed. 1976. *The Identities of Persons.* Berkeley: University of California Press.

SARTRE, JEAN-PAUL. 1957. *Existentialism and Human Emotions.* New York: Philosophical Library.

STRAWSON, PETER. 1959. *Individuals: An Essay in Descriptive Metaphysics.* London: Methuen.

SUMNER, L. W. 1981. *Abortion and Moral Theory*. Princeton, N.J.: Princeton University Press.

PERU

See MEDICAL ETHICS, HISTORY OF, *section on* THE AMERICAS, *article on* LATIN AMERICA.

PETS AND COMPANION ANIMALS

See ANIMAL WELFARE AND RIGHTS, *article on* PETS AND COMPANION ANIMALS.

PHARMACEUTICS

I. Pharmaceutical Industry
   John F. Beary, III
II. Issues in Prescribing
   David T. Lowenthal
   George J. Caranasos

I. PHARMACEUTICAL INDUSTRY

The research-based pharmaceutical industry develops cures or incremental therapeutic advances for unconquered or inadequately treated diseases. While this article focuses on the research-based industry, there are two other pharmaceutical industry sectors, the generic and nonprescription sectors. The generic sector copies commercially successful molecules with expired patents and is not engaged in discovery research. The nonprescription sector manufactures and markets "over the counter" products, or diagnostic and therapeutic products that the U.S. Food and Drug Administration (FDA) deems safe for use without a prescription.

There are approximately 100 research-based pharmaceutical firms in the United States that develop about twenty-five new medicines and vaccines per year. These firms spent $12.6 billion on research and development during 1993 (Beary, 1994).

Drug development is a lengthy and risky process. Of every 5,000 compounds screened in chemical and receptor testing, 250 are further evaluated in animals; five progress to human testing; and only one of these five molecules is approved for marketing.

Patents provide the incentive to risk the large sums of private capital that finance the industry. In the United States, the term of a patent is seventeen years, during which time the patent holder has exclusive use of the discovery. For drugs, the actual market time available to recover the average investment of $360 million per new medicine is considerably less than seventeen

years because of the ten-year lag from the initial synthesis of the new chemical (and concurrent patent filing) to FDA approval of the New Drug Application (NDA). This decade is consumed by the animal testing, human testing, and regulatory review needed to prove the safety and efficacy of the new medicine.

Since only about seven years are available to market a new medicine before generic competition begins, all new medicines have relatively high prices. Only three of ten new medicines pay back their research and development (R&D) investments, which means that one successful product is at times carrying the entire pharmaceutical firm.

The profits generated by the patent incentive system are sometimes said to be justified because they have motivated great productivity in the drug industry. Since World War II, researchers in the pharmaceutical industry have discovered and marketed drugs such as beta-blockers and angiotensin converting enzyme (ACE) inhibitors (pioneering drugs for hypertension); the first biotechnology products; the first antivirals for the acquired immunodeficiency syndrome (AIDS); clot dissolvers for heart attack; cholesterol-lowering agents; new anticancer agents; and important new vaccines directed against hepatitis B and *Hemophilus* meningitis.

Drug price issues

The tensions about drug prices are part of the overall debate in the United States about whether health care ought to be seen as a public good or a private market economy. Most industrialized countries have health-care systems that reflect the former model, and because they are larger purchasers, are able to negotiate lower prices.

Prescription drugs are one of the few health-care expenses that most patients pay for out of their own pocket. This engenders criticism concerning prices and profits, especially from the elderly who have more diseases and use more prescription drugs, and are often on fixed and limited incomes.

Critics argue that drug prices in the United States are too high compared with those in developing countries like Mexico or in most European countries. A 1992 study showed that certain drugs were as much as five times less expensive in Mexico than in the United States. Industry argues that the hourly wage of U.S. workers is eight times the average wage in Mexico, which means that the products in the study are actually more affordable in the United States, even though U.S. prices are higher. Mexico performs hardly any new drug research.

A January 1994 U.S. General Accounting Office (GAO) study of seventy-seven drugs compared U.S. and U.K. wholesale prices and found U.S. prices to be about 60 percent higher than prices in the United Kingdom. The industry response is that U.K. price controls deny new medicines and technologies to British patients and are enforced by a system based on conflict-of-interest, where physicians are penalized if they exceed their annual prescribing budgets although certain expensive medicines would be best for individualized therapy. The U.K. market is also small, only 3 percent of the world market compared with 30 percent for the U.S. market, so the U.K. price controls do not have much impact on global pharmaceutical research. However, it is unfair that the U.K. government policies in effect "cost-shift" global research costs onto U.S. consumers.

Economists have tried to ascertain how much profit margin is really necessary to stimulate innovation, but there is no consensus on the answer. Some feel that scientists would strive for new discoveries without as much of a promise of profit, such as in academia. The U.S. industry argues that the current level of profit is necessary to sustain our global leadership in this area.

The U.S. industry view is that the long-term solution is to persuade other countries to abandon price controls so that global prices will reflect local economic conditions including differences in relative per capita incomes. Thus, citizens of wealthier countries would pay more than citizens in developing countries and would continue to support global pharmaceutical R&D, but in a way that shares the burden.

The industry also argues that prescription drugs are not a significant factor in driving up health-care costs. For the last twenty-five years, pharmaceutical prices have remained virtually constant at less than 1 percent of the U.S. Gross Domestic Product (GDP). Total health-care costs on the other hand, have been increasing steadily, and today, account for more than 14 percent of the GDP. Retail outpatient prescription drugs are responsible for only five cents of each health-care dollar spent, compared with twenty cents for physicians and forty cents for hospitals.

Regulatory issues

The U.S.–European drug lag was first identified in the 1970s and refers to the fact that most new medicines become available in Europe first. Recent data show that about 70 percent of all new medicines are first approved abroad. The pharmaceutical industry became global during the 1980s and often simultaneously submits marketing applications to U.S. and European authorities. Western Europe has high scientific and regulatory standards and a tradition of more efficient regulatory reviews.

FDA review times for new medicines have averaged thirty months in recent years. Following collaboration of the U.S. Congress, industry, and the FDA, the User Fee Act of 1992 was passed. Reviews by the FDA should be more timely as a result of the $327 million in new

resources that the research-based pharmaceutical industry will pay in user fees during 1993–1997. These funds will be used to hire scientific and medical reviewers to reduce FDA review backlogs. FDA has committed to reducing review times for drugs for life-threatening and serious diseases to six months or less, and to twelve months for all other new drugs and biologic products.

One restraint on global diffusion of new drug discoveries is the duplication of research effort required by some governments. Even when a pivotal study showing the safety and efficacy of a new medicine has already been replicated in a major developed country, governments require additional animal or human research. Why? Motivation ranges from national pride to the desire to generate more work for local scientists. The U.S. pharmaceutical industry is one of the six regulatory and industrial parties involved in the harmonization of new drug registration requirements in Europe, Japan, and the United States. Ninety-five percent of global pharmaceutical R&D is conducted in these three regions. The first International Conference on Harmonization (ICH) was held in Brussels in November 1991, and announced agreements on geriatric clinical trials and toxicology testing. The purpose of these ongoing conferences is to increase harmonization of government requirements, while ensuring that high-quality, safe, and effective medicines are developed and registered in the most efficient and cost-effective manner. These activities should prevent unnecessary duplication of clinical trials and minimize the use of animal testing, without compromising the regulatory obligations of safety and effectiveness.

Marketing, promotion, advertising, and gifts

Marketing activities and the related topics of marketing codes and continuing medical education (CME) guidelines are important issues. This discussion will focus on recent controversies involving gifts and print advertisements.

The availability of a drug is of little value unless the prescriber of the product is aware of its existence and has the scientific and medical information to use it effectively. By definition, a prescription drug is not considered safe for unsupervised use by the ultimate consumer (the patient), and information about the drug must be provided to an educated intermediary (the prescribing physician). In the United States, promotion of drug products must be confined to the content of the FDA-approved product label.

The promotional practice of pharmaceutical firms giving gifts to physicians has recently been reviewed by Mary-Margaret Chren (Chren et al., 1989). She argues that the gift relationship may adversely affect the character of a prescriber by shifting the balance between self-interest and altruism and that it is unjust to give physicians gifts when patient-derived revenues are the ultimate source of funding for gifts. Chren notes that the acceptance of a gift establishes a relationship between the donor and recipient with "vague but real obligations." Such obligations are minimized when gifts are institutional rather than personal.

Therefore, Chren argues, it is acceptable for pharmaceutical firms to give money to institutions for educational activities, books, and journals. This situation is not ethically hazardous because no personal relationship is formed, and there is no obligation for the individual physician to respond in any way to the company. For those concerned that institutions can also be corrupted, Chren argues that full disclosure, avoidance of extravagance, and a goal of improving patient care make such activities ethically acceptable. In addition, several CME programs in small communities have no source of support other than the industry. Stopping such programs would hurt patient care, not advance it.

The industry has responded to such criticisms by adopting an updated marketing code in 1990 that addresses the major concerns of Chren and other industry critics. In addition, some physicians have recently raised questions about print advertising. In an *Annals of Internal Medicine* article (Wilkes et al., 1992), the authors concluded that many advertisements are deficient in regard to FDA standards on promotion.

This study assumed that advertisements should be judged by the same criteria as peer-reviewed journal articles. The industry replied that advertisements are not journal articles; they are commercial communications that—unlike journal articles—are regulated by the government. By their nature, advertisements are designed to attract attention to a particular product and should never be the sole source of prescribing information.

Industry marketing codes.   To provide ethical guidance to members, the industry has a Code of Pharmaceutical Marketing Practices that was amended in 1990 (Pharmaceutical Manufacturers Association, 1990). The code endorsed the American College of Physicians (ACP) position statements on promotion, adopted the American Medical Association (AMA) Guidelines on Gifts to Physicians from Industry, and also endorsed the Accreditation Council for Continuing Medical Education (ACCME) Standards for Commercial Support of Continuing Medical Education.

The industry's code states that gifts, hospitality, or subsidies offered to physicians by the pharmaceutical industry should not be accepted if acceptance might influence or appear to others to influence the objectivity of clinical judgment. A useful criterion to determine acceptable activities and relationships is: "Would you be willing to have these arrangements generally known?" The guidance also provides that firms should follow the

guidelines of various professional societies that discourage excessive industry-sponsored gifts and hospitality to physicians at meetings.

In summary, the industry marketing code of 1990 eliminates gifts to physicians or students unless the gifts are modest and contribute in some way to patient care. Finally, the rise in managed health-care systems in the United States has moved the focus of marketing away from individual physicians to the powerful institutions that manage the drug benefit in health plans.

Continuing medical education (CME) guidelines.   CME is required in many states for medical license renewal. In order to award CME credit to attendees, industry sponsors of CME activities must meet the guidelines of the independent ACCME. The ACCME Guidelines, endorsed by the pharmaceutical industry, stress that program sponsors are responsible for the content, quality, and scientific integrity of programs and materials. Presentations must give a balanced view of all therapeutic options. Commercial exhibits should not influence planning nor interfere with the presentation of CME activities. Subsidies for hospitality should not be provided outside of modest meals or social events that are held as a part of the activity. Commercial support must be disclosed in printed announcements and brochures, but without reference to specific products. Finally, an accredited sponsor should have and follow a conflict-of-interest policy for CME activities.

Special populations

The study of special populations in clinical trials is an important subject, and questions have been raised about adequate representation of women, children, and the elderly in clinical studies.

Concerns about the extent of women's participation in clinical trials focus on equal access for women to the benefits of health research. The issue exposes a conflict between two public policy positions: protectionism and access. Injuries caused by thalidomide and diethylstilbestrol in the 1960s resulted in restrictive regulations governing the clinical study of women who were pregnant or in their child-bearing years.

The Institute of Medicine (IOM) completed an extensive study of women and health research in 1994. The IOM Committee organized its analysis around principles of justice and recommended the following three principles in regard to gender and the conduct of clinical research. First, the scientific community must ensure that advances in research benefit fairly all people regardless of gender, race, ethnicity, and age. Second, where it is established that specific health interests of women have not received a fair allocation of research attention or resources, preferential treatment may be required to remedy a past injustice. Third, volunteers for clinical study should be recruited without regard to gender so that research yields scientific results applicable to both genders.

There are also special challenges involved in testing drugs in children. These include finding a sufficient number of parents who will consent to enrolling their children in trials, concerns for the safety of children who are often fragile trial subjects, and the increasing cost of pediatric clinical trials related to legal liability exposure until the child reaches age 21.

Following U.S. Congressional hearings in 1989, the FDA reviewed the issue of adequate representation of the elderly in clinical trials and has concluded that present-day clinical trials do involve appropriate numbers of elderly subjects. In addition, a harmonized clinical trial guideline on geriatric studies was formally adopted in 1993 by the European Union, the United States, and Japan.

International issues

Three major global issues are harmonization of animal testing and human testing requirements, international drug price differences, and international drug labeling differences. The first two topics were discussed earlier.

Drug labeling in both developing and developed countries is ultimately determined by national regulatory authorities, not pharmaceutical companies. Drug labeling does differ from one country to another, due primarily to differences in local health conditions and prescribing practices. This is an accepted fact among international health authorities, including the World Health Organization (WHO). The preface of the WHO Model Prescribing Information states that, "It is appreciated that it is not possible to develop an informational sheet on a specific drug that is appropriate to the circumstances prevailing in each of the WHO's member states" (World Health Organization, 1991, p. 1).

Summary

Society has two important concerns pertaining to pharmaceuticals that should not be in conflict, namely the need for research advances that generate new therapies and vaccines for poorly treated diseases, and the need for patient access to these products. There remain important ethical tensions because of the marketplace issues of the private for-profit industry that produces these medications and the limits to out-of-pocket expenditures by many citizens, and lack of support for continued growth of publicly supported health insurance.

The prescription drug access issue in the United States will be addressed during the 1990s as the United States reforms its health-care system and designs an outpatient drug benefit that is equitable and based on sound therapeutic principles.

JOHN F. BEARY, III

Directly related to this article is the companion article in this entry: ISSUES IN PRESCRIBING. *Also directly related is the entry* PHARMACY. *For a further discussion of topics mentioned in this article, see the entries* ADVERTISING; AGING AND THE AGED, *article on* HEALTH-CARE AND RESEARCH ISSUES; ANIMAL RESEARCH; ANIMAL WELFARE AND RIGHTS, *article on* ETHICAL PERSPECTIVES ON THE TREATMENT AND STATUS OF ANIMALS; CHILDREN, *article on* HEALTH-CARE AND RESEARCH ISSUES; CLINICAL ETHICS, *article on* INSTITUTIONAL ETHICS COMMITTEES; COMMERCIALISM IN SCIENTIFIC RESEARCH; CONFLICT OF INTEREST; ECONOMIC CONCEPTS IN HEALTH CARE; HARM; MEDICAL CODES AND OATHS; MEDICAL ETHICS, HISTORY OF, *section on* EUROPE, *subsection on* CONTEMPORARY PERIOD, *especially the article on* UNITED KINGDOM; RISK; *and* WOMEN, *articles on* HEALTH-CARE ISSUES, *and* RESEARCH ISSUES. *For a discussion of related ideas, see the entries* ACADEMIC HEALTH CENTERS; AIDS, *article on* HEALTH-CARE AND RESEARCH ISSUES; FRAUD, THEFT, AND PLAGIARISM; INTERNATIONAL HEALTH; RESEARCH, HUMAN: HISTORICAL ASPECTS; RESEARCH METHODOLOGY; *and* RESEARCH POLICY. *See also the* APPENDIX (CODES, OATHS, AND DIRECTIVES RELATED TO BIOETHICS), SECTION II: ETHICAL DIRECTIVES FOR THE PRACTICE OF MEDICINE, SECTION IV: ETHICAL DIRECTIVES FOR HUMAN RESEARCH, *and* SECTION V: ETHICAL DIRECTIVES PERTAINING TO THE WELFARE AND USE OF ANIMALS.

Bibliography

AVORN, JERRY; CHEN, MILTON; and HARTLEY, ROBERT 1982. "Scientific Versus Commercial Sources of Influence on the Prescribing Behavior of Physicians." *American Journal of Medicine* 73, no. 1:4–8.

BEARY, JOHN F., III. "Profits and Research Spending." *American Medical News* 37:27.

BEARY, JOHN F., III; WIERENGA, DALE E.; COPMANN, T.; and EATON, C. ROBERT. 1992. "Drug and Biologic Product Approvals During 1991." *Journal of Pharmaceutical Medicine* 2:175–182.

CHREN, MARY MARGARET; LANDEFELD, SETH; and MURRAY, THOMAS H. 1989. "Doctors, Drug Companies and Gifts." *Journal of the American Medical Association* 262, no. 24:3448–3451.

D'ARCY, PATRICK F., and HARRON, D. W. G., eds. 1992. *Proceedings of the First International Conference on Harmonisation, 1992.* Belfast: Queen's University of Belfast. A

590-page book summarizing key presentations on preclinical and clinical pharmaceutical testing.

DiMasi, Joseph A.; Hansen, Ronald W.; Grabowski, Henry G.; and Lasagna, Louis. 1991. "Cost of Innovation in the Pharmaceutical Industry." *Journal of Health Economics* 10, no. 2:107–142.

Iber, Frank L.; Riley, W. Anthony; and Murray, Patricia J. 1987. *Conducting Clinical Trials.* New York: Plenum Medical.

Kaitin, I. Kenneth; Manocchia, Michael; Seibring, Mark; and Lasagna, Louis. 1994. "The New Drug Approvals of 1990, 1991, and 1992: Trends in Drug Development." *Journal of Clinical Pharmacology* 34, no. 2:120–127. Statistics on the "drug lag."

Mastroianni, Anna C.; Faden, Ruth R.; and Federman, Daniel D., eds. 1994. *Women and Health Research: Ethical and Legal Issues of Including Women in Clinical Studies.* 2 vols. Washington, D.C.: National Academy Press.

Pharmaceutical Manufacturers Association. 1990. *Code of Pharmaceutical Marketing Practices.* Washington, D.C.: Author.

Porter, Roger J.; Malone, Thomas E.; and Vaughan, Christopher C., eds. 1992. *Biomedical Research: Collaboration and Conflict of Interest.* Baltimore, Md.: Johns Hopkins University Press.

Scherer, F. M. 1993. "Pricing, Profits, and Technological Progress in the Pharmaceutical Industry." *Journal of Economic Perspectives* 7, no. 3:97–115.

Spilker, Bert. 1989. *Multinational Drug Companies: Issues in Drug Discovery and Development.* New York: Raven.

U.S. Congress. House of Representatives. Committee on Energy and Commerce. 1992. *Prescription Drug User Fee Act of 1992: Report to Accompany H.R. 5952.* Washington, D.C.: U.S. Government Printing Office.

———. House of Representatives. Select Committee on Aging. Subcommittee on Human Services. 1989. *Drug Misuse Among the Elderly and Its Impact on Community-Based Care: Hearing.* Washington, D.C.: U.S. Government Printing Office.

———. Office of Technology Assessment. 1993. *Pharmaceutical R&D: Costs, Risks and Rewards.* Washington, D.C.: Author. A 354-page government report on pharmaceutical R&D.

U.S. Food and Drug Administration (FDA). 1992. "Statement: Women in Clinical Trials." October 29.

U.S. General Accounting Office. 1992. *Prescription Drugs: Companies Typically Charge More in the United States Than in Canada.* GAO/HRD-92-110. Washington, D.C.: Author.

Wilkes, Michael S.; Doblin, Bruce H.; and Shapiro, Martin F. 1992. "Pharmaceutical Advertisements in Leading Medical Journals: Experts' Assessments." *Annals of Internal Medicine* 116, no. 11:912–919.

Woosley, Raymond L. 1994. "Centers for Education and Research in Therapeutics." *Clinical Pharmacology and Therapeutics* 55, no. 3:249–255.

World Health Organization. 1991. *WHO Model Prescribing Information Series: Drugs Used in Mycobacterial Diseases.* Geneva: Author.

II. ISSUES IN PRESCRIBING

Medicines, in addition to their pharmacologic actions in treating diseases or conditions, have symbolic aspects that serve cultural, sociological, and psychological purposes. The act of prescribing satisfies a deep human need: a need for the physician to know what is wrong and to show knowledge about what to do, and a need for the patient's symptoms to be legitimated and treated (Fessel, 1981).

The act of prescribing represents a modern laying on of hands. Prescribing has both a scientific (medical) and a nonscientific (sociocultural) base (Frølund, 1978). In the traditional medical model of rational prescribing, the patient presents challenging symptoms that the physician investigates and then diagnoses a disease. Based on this diagnosis, the appropriate drug and/or nondrug treatment—for example, physical therapy—is prescribed. Emphasis is placed on accurate diagnosis and application of pharmacologic principles, which govern the use of safe and effective drugs to treat a disease (O'Hagan, 1984).

Current realities of prescribing

Prescribing of medication occurs in an estimated 90 percent of patient encounters. Our society is programmed to accept the concept of a pill for every ill (Morgan and Weintraub, 1974; O'Hagan, 1984). The most significant reasons are (1) patient expectation—a friend or a family member may be gaining relief through a medication given for the same symptom the patient is experiencing; (2) radio, television, newspaper, and periodical advertisements plant the powerful seeds of suggestion, raising patients' expectations; (3) lack of physicians' efforts to speak at length with the patient and initially advise nondrug regimens; (4) pressure on the physician by the pharmaceutical industry to prescribe the most current (and probably most expensive) medication(s) for symptom relief, bypassing patient understanding as to the cause of the symptom, any explanation of the expected duration of treatment, and likelihood of recurrence of symptom(s).

As an example, mild hypertension (high blood pressure) can be treated with a regimen including low-salt diet, weight reduction by means of calorie restriction and exercise, and alcohol intake restricted to less than two ounces per day. If this is ineffective, then prescription of a medication can be based on mutual consent and understanding.

Clearly, it is more difficult not to prescribe than to prescribe. Medicines are viewed as good, and prescribing as a beneficent act. If taking a medicine has a positive value, then discontinuing a medicine or not giving any—by implication—may have a negative value. As a result, physicians are often reluctant to stop medicines that may no longer be needed, and thus patients continue to take unnecessary drugs prescribed in the distant past. This continued drug consumption leads to an increased drug load and drug exposure, which are major causes of adverse drug reactions. The proper action for physicians is to discontinue unneeded medicines, explaining to patients the potentially harmful consequences of taking them.

Certain physician–patient issues may influence prescribing behavior. The physician may be responding to the expectation of the patient that something can and will be done about a symptom. With a prescription a patient feels confident that something concrete has been offered (Fessel, 1981). This reflects the public's high expectations from scientific medicine coupled with a decreased tolerance for discomfort (Schwartz et al., 1989). However, physicians, by imputing a desire for medicine among patients, may be overestimating the actual desire (Frølund, 1978).

Prescribing fulfills the physician's need to feel powerful and to be an interventionist (Fessel, 1981; O'Hagan, 1984). It also allays the concern that the patient may be unhappy if not given a prescription and go elsewhere for the medicine believed to be necessary (Schwartz et al., 1989). In addition, a prescription symbolizes the physician's mystical healing power. Presumably only the physician knows which drug to choose and how it works. Since physicians have this special power, they use it at times to prescribe medicines they know may be ineffective in order to achieve a placebo effect (O'Hagan, 1984).

Many patients have nonspecific symptoms resulting from minor, self-limited illnesses or from psychosocial stressors. Consequently, physicians often prescribe drugs for symptomatic treatment without fully understanding the diagnosis or prognosis—for instance, treating psychosocial stress with psychoactive drugs (O'Hagan, 1984). Physicians often may not have the time, knowledge, or interest to provide counseling for psychosocial problems and instead resort to a "quick fix" by prescribing a psychoactive drug (Schwartz et al., 1989).

The nonspecific presenting complaints of many patients create uncertainty for physicians about the diagnosis. A prescription reassures the patient that the doctor knows what is wrong even if the doctor is uncertain (O'Hagan, 1984). Prescriptions can act as temporizing measures, fulfilling the patient's expectations for treatment while waiting for a firm diagnosis or spontaneous remission of a self-limited illness (Fessel, 1981).

In some instances a prescription may help define the disease in situations where the diagnosis is uncertain (O'Hagan, 1984). "I prescribe an antibiotic, therefore the patient has a bacterial infection." Or "I prescribe a tranquilizer, so the symptoms must be due to anxiety."

Reimbursement requirements of insurers reinforce this attitude, since often a diagnosis must be written even if the physician is uncertain.

Regardless of how trivial the complaint may be, the patient's sick role is legitimated by a prescription. It validates the doctor visit and allows future visits for vague symptoms (Stimson, 1976; O'Hagan, 1984; Ryde, 1976). Yet some physicians feel guilty for charging a patient if they have not done "something." Writing a prescription is doing "something." Advice and counseling tend to be given little value.

Ethics in prescribing

Conflicts arise around giving a prescription when there is disagreement between the physician's authority and the patient's wish to choose. Some common situations include the physician who acts in what he or she considers the patient's best interest but with either no patient consent or only presumed patient consent. If informed consent is obtained from the patient, the physician explains the disease and treatment and expects the patient to comply with the treatment regimen. Conversely, the patient can decide not to take prescribed medicine even though this may not be in his or her best interest. The ideal interaction between physician and patient is the collaborative relationship in which a consensus is reached by an informed negotiation between the two parties. In dealing with patients, physicians must assume many roles, choosing the style that best meets each individual patient's needs. A prescription can fulfill a patient's unspoken expectation or explicit demand, which results from societally sanctioned high expectations from medicine and low tolerance for discomfort (Frølund, 1978; O'Hagan, 1984).

Ethical restraints on appropriate prescribing practices

There are many considerations with regard to the ethics of prescribing. For every protagonist view there will always be an antagonist opinion. Thus, for every item listed as a restraint there can be a rebutting response against the item listed.

Examples of issues that pose restraints on prescribing are listed below.

1. The prescribing of psychotropic drugs not by physicians but by surrogate physicians, specifically social workers who fill out blank prescriptions and get the physician to sign. Is this a means to save the physician time, or a means to prevent direct communication and interaction between patient and physician? True, there is a movement of the chronically ill patient from institutional to outpatient care. Thus, the responsibility for the maintenance of this population

has shifted to nonphysician community health providers. Social workers, however, are not in a position to be able to detect adverse reactions or drug interactions, as might a physician or a nurse practitioner (Miller et al., 1980).

2. What is the ethical responsibility of a physician for prescribing to an underage woman involved in unlawful sexual intercourse? What is the legal or ethical position of a doctor who knows or has reason to suspect that he or she is being asked for a prescription for oral contraceptives by or for a woman under the age of sixteen? If the physician prescribes the birth-control pills for a minor, is he or she liable for drug-related problems, fostering promiscuity, and possible immoral behavior? On the other hand, it is not the doctor's behavior that has encouraged the minor to engage in sexual activity. It is, however, the physician's obligation to help determine whether the patient is mentally defective and under coercion to submit to sexual intercourse (Brahams, 1982).

3. Double-blind, controlled, randomized clinical trials including placebos are the gold standard by which therapeutic design mandates studies for experimental therapy. Specifically, the referral of cancer patients for participation in randomized clinical trials elicits a multiplicity of ethical considerations. Robert Levine (1986) contends that there should be referral of these patients for clinical trials and asserts that the physician–patient relationship would not be broken, since the patient ultimately could benefit. Patient well-being and the ability of the patient to make a decision come first. Such trials have been championed for patient access to experimental therapy for the treatment of AIDS. Amid a major ethical dilemma, U.S. Food and Drug Administration officials and AIDS researchers repeatedly raise arguments to justify denying access to experimental therapy. The arguments suggest that patients need to be protected from their own desperate outlook, the experimental drugs may be more harmful than beneficial, and that public access (through the black market) to experimental drugs might prevent adequate conduct of clinical trials because it would be easier to procure the drugs without participation in a legitimate randomized study. It is possible that both science and patient can be better served by a system that allows access to unapproved drugs for life-threatened patients while allowing scientists funds and facilities to monitor such therapy in order to detect where risk outweighs benefit (Levine, 1986; Delaney, 1989).

4. In geriatric medicine the issue extends beyond ethical restraints on appropriate prescribing to restraining the physician from overprescribing. In the United States, 12 percent of the population is over age sixty-five, and 35 percent of the prescriptions written are for people over age sixty-five. At least four prescriptions are taken by ambulatory elderly persons, six by those in hospitals, and more than eight by those residing in extended-care facilities (nursing homes). On the average, people over age sixty-five may have five or six chronic illnesses concomitantly. Only in certain instances might long-term drug therapy be indicated. Examples are hypertension, diabetes, atrial fibrillation, chronic lung disease, and degenerative joint disease, all of which may coexist in one patient. The physiological changes associated with age, plus the various diseases, added to the myriad medications pose a triple threat with regard to patient safety (Lowenthal et al., 1990). Ethically, the physician may want to treat; practically, overmedication can add to the list of disease entities, resulting in iatrogenic illness.

Ethical nondrug therapeutic considerations

Placebos.   Placebos can have a powerful positive psychological effect on patients and their families. They are easily prescribed by physicians who feel it part of their duty to please patients, and therefore regard it as ethically correct to use them (Schwartz et al., 1989). Conversely, a strong case can be made that placebos should never be prescribed because their use is a form of deception (Bok, 1974).

Long-term placebo treatment will divert attention from the cause of a patient's complaints, possibly resulting in a serious medical problem's going unrecognized. In addition, the patient will lose trust in the physician upon recognizing the deception (Schwartz et al., 1989).

Truth-telling, the ethical principle involved in the use of placebos, creates a situation in which the patient feels better without the production of harm. In such an instance the physician would regard beneficence as outweighing truth-telling. When a placebo is used to create the image that a physician knows what he or she is doing or to fulfill the patient's presumed explicit demand for medicine, the requirement for truth-telling is suppressed, the potential risk is low, and the chance of patient satisfaction is high.

Patient participation.   Increased patient participation in selection of therapeutic agents has important ethical implications (Fessel, 1981). The physician and patient must share information that allows the patient to make an informed decision. This is dependent on the patient's having adequate knowledge of the disease, available drugs that can be helpful, potential side effects, alternative modes of treatment, and potential risks and benefits. These are complex ethical issues that test a physician's skill and time to provide explanations and a patient's intellectual and psychological makeup to understand and weigh alternatives.

The sharing of information by the physician is an expression of beneficence. Decision making by the patient maintains patient autonomy, the overriding principle in any physician–patient interaction.

DAVID T. LOWENTHAL
GEORGE J. CARANASOS

Directly related to this article is the companion article in this entry: PHARMACEUTICAL INDUSTRY. *Also directly related are the entries* PHARMACY; PLACEBO; PSYCHOPHARMACOLOGY; *and* SUBSTANCE ABUSE, *article on* LEGAL CONTROL OF HARMFUL SUBSTANCES. *For a further discussion of topics mentioned in this article, see the entries* FREEDOM AND COERCION; INFORMATION DISCLOSURE, *article on* ATTITUDES TOWARD TRUTH-TELLING; INFORMED CONSENT; *and* TRUST. *Other relevant material may be found under the entries* COMMUNICATION, BIOMEDICAL, *article on* MEDIA AND MEDICINE; *and* HEALTH-CARE FINANCING, *article on* PROFIT AND COMMERCIALISM.

Bibliography

BOK, SISSELA. 1974. "The Ethics of Giving Placebos." *Scientific American* 231:17–23.

BRAHAMS, DIANA. 1982. "Prescribing for Unlawful Sexual Intercourse." *Practitioner* 226, no. 1368:1025–1026.

COUNCIL ON SCIENTIFIC AFFAIRS. 1982. "Drug Abuse Related to Prescribing Practice." *Journal of the American Medical Association* 247, no. 6:864–866.

DELANEY, MARTIN. 1989. "The Case for Patient Access to Experimental Therapy." *Journal of Infectious Diseases* 159, no. 3:416–419.

FESSEL, W. JEFFREY. 1981. "Strategic Aspects of Prescription Writing." *Postgraduate Medicine* 70, no. 1:30–34, 37.

FRØLUND, FLEMING. 1978. "Better Prescribing." *British Medical Journal* 2, no. 6139:741.

LEVINE, ROBERT. J. 1986. "Referral of Patients with Cancer for Participation in Randomized Clinical Trials: Ethical Considerations." *CA* 36, no. 2:95–99.

LOWENTHAL, DAVID T.; LEVY, G.; LAVY, N. W.; McMAHON, F. GILBERT; SELLERS, E. M.; VIDT, DONALD G.; WHITSETT, THOMAS L.; FORD, GARY A.; BLASCHKE, T. F.; and BRATER, D. C. 1990. "That None Should Be Denied." *Clinical Pharmacology and Therapeutics* 47, no. 3:422–423.

MILLER, ROSALIND S.; WIEDEMAN, GEORGE H.; and LINN, LOUIS. 1980. "Prescribing Psychotropic Drugs: Whose Responsibility?" *Social Work in Health Care* 6, no. 1: 51–61.

MORGAN, JOHN P., and WEINTRAUB, MICHAEL. 1974. "A Course on the Social Functions of Prescription Drugs: Seminar Syllabus and Bibliography." *Annals of Internal Medicine* 77, no. 2:217–222.

O'HAGAN, J. J. 1984. "What Influences Our Prescribing?—Some Nonpharmacological Issues." *New Zealand Medical Journal* 97, no. 756:331–332.

RYDE, DAVID. 1976. "Does the Patient Really Need a Prescription?" *Practitioner* 216, no. 1295:557–559.

SCHWARTZ, R. K.; SOUMERAI, S. B.; and AVORN, J. 1989.

"Physician Motivations for Nonscientific Drug Prescribing." *Social Science and Medicine* 28, no. 6:577–582.

STIMSON, G. V. 1976. "Doctor–Patient Interaction and Some Problems for Prescribing." *Journal of the Royal College of General Practitioners* 26 (suppl. 1):88–96.

TEELING-SMITH, G. 1968. "Advertising and the Pattern of Prescribing." *Proceedings of the Royal Society of Medicine* 61:748–750.

WESSON, DONALD R., and SMITH, DAVID E. 1990. "Prescription Drug Abuse: Patient, Physician, and Cultural Responsibilities." *Western Journal of Medicine* 152, no. 5:613–616.

WILFORD, BONNIE B. 1990. "Abuse of Prescription Drugs." *Western Journal of Medicine* 152, no. 5:609–612.

PHARMACY

Since the 1960s, the purpose and functions of pharmacy practice have progressed in the United States and other industrialized countries from the mere supplying of drugs to include involvement with the patient and other health-care professionals to design, implement, and monitor a drug therapy plan that will produce therapeutic outcomes. The context of practice and education has also changed. The majority of pharmacists still practice in community pharmacy settings, although a significant number practice in hospitals, long-term care facilities, and ambulatory care. Pharmacy education has experienced a shift from bachelor degree programs to the single, entry-level Doctor of Pharmacy degree. Recognizing the diversity in practice settings and educational preparation, professional pharmacy organizations in the United States have agreed on a uniform mission statement for pharmacy: "The mission of pharmacy is to serve society as the profession responsible for the appropriate use of medications, devices, and services to achieve optimal therapeutic outcomes" (American Pharmaceutical Association [APhA], 1990).

To fulfill this mission, pharmacy practitioners and educators in the United States have espoused a practice philosophy called "pharmaceutical care." Pharmaceutical care is the responsible provision of drug therapy for the purpose of achieving patient outcomes that improve a patient's quality of life (Hepler and Strand, 1990). It restores emphasis on the pharmacist's direct obligations to the individual patient, grounded in a covenantal relationship. The pharmacist must participate as an equal with other health professionals in patient care and protect the patient from the harmful effects of "drug misadventuring," morbidity, or mortality resulting from the misuse of drugs (Manasse, 1989a, 1989b).

These changes in practice philosophy lead to ethical problems unique to pharmacy. Technological advances in drug development and delivery systems are beginning to raise ethical questions regarding such concerns as the use of very expensive drugs with narrow therapeutic applications (such as human growth hormone) or the relative benefits of two drugs that vary significantly in cost (such as streptokinase versus tissue plasminogen activator [TPA] for opening occluded coronary arteries). Factors external to the profession, such as state pharmacy practice laws, federal and state regulations of certain drugs, and case law, have generated additional ethical challenges.

Ethical problems in pharmacy practice

Ethical problems in pharmacy have not received a great deal of systematic attention (Lowenthal, 1988; Haddad, 1991). The pharmacy literature has touched on diverse ethical concerns, from the common, such as the use of drugs for nonapproved indications (Veatch, 1983), to the exotic, such as distributing soon-to-expire medications to the former Soviet Union (Poikonen et al., 1992). The ethical problems discussed below are important for two critical reasons: They are commonly encountered, and they reflect pharmacy's range of responsibilities, from the individual to the societal level.

The pharmacist–patient relationship.   Pharmacists are struggling with an essential question: Whom do I serve? The relationship between the pharmacist and patient is characterized by trust and commitment, yet most frequently their relationship is predicated on a financial transaction. Pharmacists may owe more to patients who are loyal customers. It is not always clear whether or not they owe patients advice regardless of where drugs are purchased. These issues underlie the need to separate reimbursement for cognitive pharmacy services, such as counseling, from dispensing fees (i.e., an amount paid to the pharmacist for the preparation of the drug beyond the cost of the drug product). This issue requires pharmacists to prove to reimbursement sources that they offer a service that makes a significant difference in a patient's health, such as preventing an unnecessary side effect or even a hospitalization.

The duty to protect patients from drug misadventuring involves respect for the patient as a person who has the right to make personal decisions about drug therapy. It also involves beneficence, the practice of pharmacy in the best interests of the patient. Patients can make poor decisions or merely disagree with the professional's proffered advice. Pharmacists must be willing to accept that once patients have been fully informed of the benefits and risks of a certain therapeutic regimen, they then have the right to refuse treatment (Buerki and Vottero, 1991).

Patient-centered care does not allow pharmacists to bow out of conflicts with noncompliant patients by passing their professional responsibilities to physicians; nor will it tolerate unjustifiable paternalism. Rather, it de-

mands a response that respects autonomy while protecting patients from certain harm.

Addictive drugs.   Whether or not to dispense potentially addictive drugs in the case of suspected or incipient abuse is the most common and most difficult problem in pharmacy practice (Haddad, 1991). However, it obscures the more compelling conflict between pharmacists' personal gain from selling addictive drugs and their ethical duty to prevent drug misuse.

Informed consent and disclosure.   For a variety of reasons, patients often arrive at a pharmacy with little information about prescribed medications. Pharmacists must then determine how much a patient knows about his or her medical problem and medications without compromising the physician–patient relationship. Prior to 1981, the APhA code of ethics did not include the duty to provide information to patients (APhA, 1985). Since the Omnibus Budget Reconciliation Act (OBRA) was passed in 1990, pharmacists have had a federally mandated responsibility to inform and counsel patients.

The question of whether or not fully to disclose information to the patient regarding a medication is particularly problematic in the area of placebo therapy, where the pharmacist is being asked by a physician intentionally to deceive the patient, ostensibly for the patient's good. Similar ethical problems exist in double-blind clinical drug trials. In such cases, the pharmacist-researcher does not know which drug is the active agent and which is the placebo. The pharmacist-researcher is called upon to be concerned not only for the welfare of individual patients but also for the interests of the broader society and its scientific concerns (Veatch, 1991).

Confidentiality.   In the course of their work, pharmacists routinely learn private information about their patients. A dilemma arises when pharmacists are called upon to make judgments regarding when and to whom private information about their patients should be provided without patient consent. For example, should the pharmacist inform a patient's spouse about the action or side effects of a prescription? Should the parents of a minor be informed about their daughter's prescription for oral contraceptives (Haddad et al., 1992)? The 1981 APhA code of ethics allows pharmacists to disclose confidential information if the patient's interests are best served, but does not provide guidance as to what constitutes the patient's best interest.

Conflicts between personal values and patient welfare

Pharmacists often find themselves caught between fulfilling their professional obligations (e.g., properly dispensing and labeling a prescription) and their own personal values and beliefs. Medications that commonly elicit this type of response include contraceptives, abortifacients, fertility drugs, and drugs used in the treatment of acquired immunodeficiency syndrome (AIDS). Pharmacists serve as intermediaries who supply medications to the community. But they may be unwilling to dispense medications that violate their personal moral values, since they believe that doing so would be tantamount to cooperating in an immoral action. Yet pharmacists recognize that they cannot abandon patients who require service. Pharmacists can look to their religious beliefs, the pharmacy code of ethics, and institutional ethics committees, when available, for assistance in resolving conflicts of this type.

Conflicts between physicians and pharmacists

Pharmacists and physicians disagree about the status and functions of the pharmacy profession. Patients find pharmacists the most accessible of health-care professionals and seek their advice about common ailments, a function previously performed by family physicians. Pharmacists maintain that their most important function is to design, implement, and monitor a drug therapy plan that will produce positive therapeutic outcomes. Doing so requires a greater involvement of pharmacists with patients, which could threaten physicians' relationships with their patients and widen the existing schism between the professions. Pharmacists must educate physicians about their expanded functions to justify the need for sharing information about their patients' medical histories.

The profession of pharmacy is responding to these various problems in several ways. Its code of ethics is under revision to incorporate the responsibilities inherent in the expanded role of contemporary pharmacists. Further, ethics instruction has been identified as a core component of pharmaceutical education.

Trends in pharmacy practice

Several trends in pharmacy portend ethical problems. For example, the accessibility of pharmacists places them in an ideal position to participate in public health education on a variety of topics, from the prevention of AIDS to the harms of alcohol and tobacco use. Yet pharmacists may own or work in community pharmacies that sell liquor and cigarettes, creating a conflict between the business and professional components of pharmacy.

There have also been changes among the people who choose pharmacy as a career. In 1950, only 4 percent of active pharmacists in the United States were women. By 1988, that proportion had risen to over 26 percent, a trend expected to continue. Sixty-three percent of the students enrolled in pharmacy schools in 1992 were women (American Association of Colleges of Pharmacy, 1992). The percentage of minorities in pharmacy remains relatively stable at approximately 10 percent, faring somewhat better than nursing (8.5 percent), dentistry (2.6 percent), and medicine (7 percent). As the gender, race, and educational statuses of the profession change, we can expect changing attitudes toward the power and role of pharmacists among persons both within and without the pharmacy profession.

Finally, the public debate regarding physician-assisted suicide will involve the pharmacist. What will be pharmacy's involvement, if any, in the preparation of medications to end a patient's life?

The challenges pharmacy faces arise simultaneously with the profession's growing opportunities to provide ethical leadership in the evolving process of medication use.

AMY MARIE HADDAD

Directly related to this entry are the entries PHARMACEUTICS, *articles on* PHARMACEUTICAL INDUSTRY, *and* ISSUES IN PRESCRIBING; ALLIED HEALTH PROFESSIONS; PSYCHOPHARMACOLOGY; *and* PLACEBO. *For a further discussion of topics mentioned in this entry, see the entries* INFORMATION DISCLOSURE, *article on* ETHICAL ISSUES; INFORMED CONSENT, *article on* LEGAL AND ETHICAL ISSUES OF CONSENT IN HEALTH CARE; *and* PROFESSIONAL–PATIENT RELATIONSHIP, *article on* ETHICAL ISSUES. *Other relevant material may be found under the entries* FERTILITY CONTROL, *article on* LEGAL AND REGULATORY ISSUES; HOSPITAL, *article on* CONTEMPORARY ETHICAL PROBLEMS; SUBSTANCE ABUSE, *article on* LEGAL CONTROL OF HARMFUL SUBSTANCES; *and* TEAMS, HEALTH-CARE.

Bibliography

AMERICAN ASSOCIATION OF COLLEGES OF PHARMACY. 1992. "Academic Pharmacy's Vital Statistics." Alexandria, Va.: Author.

AMERICAN PHARMACEUTICAL ASSOCIATION (APhA). 1985. The codes of ethics of the association (1852, 1922, 1952, 1969, 1981) have been collected in the appendix of *The Challenges of Ethics in Pharmacy Practice*, pp. 60–64. Edited by Robert A. Buerki. Madison, Wis.: American Institute of the History of Pharmacy.

———. 1990. "Mission Statement for the Pharmacy Profession." Washington, D.C.: Author.

BUERKI, ROBERT A., and VOTTERO, LOUIS D. 1991. "The Changing Face of Pharmaceutical Education: Ethics and Professional Prerogatives." *American Journal of Pharmaceutical Education* 55, no. 1:71–74.

COCOLAS, GEORGE, ed. 1984. "Can a Professional Ethos Be Taught?" *American Journal of Pharmaceutical Education* 48, no. 4:395–408. Special section.

HADDAD, AMY M. 1991. "Ethical Problems in Pharmacy Practice: A Survey of Difficulty and Incidence." *American Journal of Pharmaceutical Education* 55, no. 1:1–6.

HADDAD, AMY M.; OBERMEIER, KARLA K.; and BROWN, KATE H. 1992. "Confidentiality and Pharmacy Practice: Urban Versus Rural Perspectives." *American Journal of Pharmaceutical Education* 56, no. 1:16–20.

HEPLER, CHARLES D., and STRAND, LINDA M. 1990. "Opportunities and Responsibilities in Pharmaceutical Care." *American Journal of Hospital Pharmacy* 47, no. 3:533–543.

LOWENTHAL, WERNER. 1988. "Ethical Dilemmas in Pharmacy Practice." *Journal of Medical Humanities and Bioethics* 9, no. 1:44–49.

MANASSE, HENRY R., JR. 1989a. "Medication Use in an Imperfect World: Drug Misadventuring as an Issue of Public Policy, Part 1." *American Journal of Hospital Pharmacy* 46, no. 5:929–944.

———. 1989b. "Medication Use in an Imperfect World: Drug Misadventuring as an Issue of Public Policy, Part 2." *American Journal of Hospital Pharmacy* 46, no. 6:1141–1152.

"Pharmacy Ethics." 1989. *American Journal of Hospital Pharmacy.* A quarterly discussion of complex cases beginning in vol. 46, no. 1:116–119; with analysis and commentary by Robert M. Veatch.

POIKONEN, JOHN C.; VINSON, MICHAEL C.; and VEATCH, ROBERT M. 1992. "Distributing Soon-to-Expire Medications to the Commonwealth of Independent States." *American Journal of Hospital Pharmacy* 49, no. 11:2773–2777.

SMITH, MICKEY; STRAUSS, STEVEN; BALDWIN, H. JOHN; and ALBERTS, KELLY T., eds. 1991. *Pharmacy Ethics.* New York: Pharmaceutical Products Press.

VEATCH, ROBERT M. 1983. "Ethics of Drugs for Non-Approved Uses." *U.S. Pharmacist* 8, no. 7:69–72.

———. 1991. "Professional Prerogatives: Perspectives of an Ethicist." *American Journal of Pharmaceutical Education* 55, no. 1:74–78.

PHENOMENOLOGY

See BODY, *article on* EMBODIMENT: THE PHENOMENOLOGICAL TRADITION; *and* HEALTH AND DISEASE, *article on* THE EXPERIENCE OF HEALTH AND ILLNESS. *See also* INTERPRETATION.

PHILIPPINES

See MEDICAL ETHICS, HISTORY OF, *section on* SOUTH AND EAST ASIA, *article on* SOUTHEAST ASIAN COUNTRIES.

PHILOSOPHY OF BIOLOGY

See BIOLOGY, PHILOSOPHY OF.

PHILOSOPHY OF MEDICINE

See MEDICINE, PHILOSOPHY OF.

PHILOSOPHY OF SCIENCE

See SCIENCE, PHILOSOPHY OF.

PHYSICAL DISABILITY

See DISABILITY; *and* REHABILITATION.

PHYSICIAN-ASSISTED SUICIDE

See DEATH AND DYING: EUTHANASIA AND SUSTAINING LIFE; *and* SUICIDE.

PHYSICIAN–NURSE RELATIONSHIP

See HEALTH-CARE TEAMS. *See also* MEDICINE AS A PROFESSION; *and* NURSING AS A PROFESSION.

PHYSICIAN–PATIENT RELATIONSHIP

See PROFESSIONAL–PATIENT RELATIONSHIP.

PLACEBO

"Placebo" and "placebo effect" are quite difficult to define. Most commonsense definitions contain serious inconsistencies. For example, one commonly hears placebo defined as an "inert remedy"; but if a placebo were totally inert, there would be no point in giving it.

Placebo in Latin means "I shall please," but the effects of placebo can be either positive or negative (the term *nocebo*, roughly "I shall harm," is sometimes used to designate negative effects). Adolf Grünbaum (1989) has emphasized that whether or not a remedy is a placebo is always relative to some biomedical theory. A sugar pill is a placebo for a migraine only because the biomedical theory agreed upon by all discussants denies any pharmacologic efficacy of small amounts of oral glucose in altering the pain of vascular headache.

Some find it useful to locate the species "placebo" under the genus "nonspecific therapy," by which they mean a therapy that strengthens the general resistance of the organism to disease of many sorts (as opposed to a therapy that removes the specific cause of a single disease or class of diseases). But the latter term may be as hard to define precisely as "placebo." Moreover, there may be an unspoken assumption that nonspecific therapies are synonymous with "therapies that operate through psychological rather than biological mechanisms." But this is clearly false; some psychological therapies may be very specific for certain diseases according to established psychiatric theories, and some biological therapies, notably diet and exercise, seem to be good candidates for "nonspecific" status.

For purposes of ethical analysis, "placebo effect" may be defined generally as the change in a patient's condition that results from the symbolic aspects of the encounter with a healer or with a healing setting, and not from the pharmacological or physiological properties of any remedy used. "Symbolic" alludes not only to the psychological processes that occur within the patient but also to the social and cultural belief systems that form a background to the patient's thoughts and feelings, and give meaning to the healing process. A placebo, then, is a remedy administered either for purposes of eliciting the placebo effect or as a control in an experimental situation. Virtually any modality, including surgery and psychotherapy, can function as a placebo; the term is not confined to pills, capsules, or injections.

The practical goal of defining "placebo effect" as precisely as possible is to distinguish the changes it produces in the patient's condition from changes produced by other causes. In treatment, the two factors likely to be confused with placebo effects are the pharmacological or physiological effects of the therapy employed, and the natural history of the illness. For example, if a patient with gastritis visits a physician, who recommends antacids, and the patient improves, the relief could have come from the pharmacological properties of the antacids, the natural tendency of gastritis to heal over time, the soothing symbolic effects of the physician consultation, or some combination of the three. The two-group design in a controlled experimental trial ("active" treatment vs. placebo) allows the investigator to distinguish pharmacological or physiological effects from the placebo effects and the natural history of the illness. It does not allow a distinction to be made between natural history and placebo effects.

It is also helpful to distinguish a pure placebo, thought to have no pharmacological potency under any circumstances whatever, from an impure placebo, which has pharmacological potency under some circumstances. Common examples of impure placebos are vitamins administered to patients who have no documented deficiency, and antibiotics administered to patients who have viral illnesses. In today's medical practice, impure placebos are probably used much more commonly than pure placebos.

In the traditional use of placebos, a pharmacologically inert pill might be administered to a patient under circumstances that encourage the belief that a powerful drug is being given. Many patients—on the average, one-third—will experience some degree of positive response under such circumstances (White et al., 1985). This traditional use is ethically questionable because the patient is deceived. Therefore, an ethical analysis of

placebo use might proceed with two questions. First, is deception necessary to produce the patient benefit promised by the placebo effect? Second, are there nondeceptive uses of placebos?

Recent research has begun to identify some of the factors that explain placebo effects. At the biochemical and cellular level, organ changes may come about due to the release of catecholamines, endorphins, or immunoactive cells; all three have been shown to be very sensitive to the psychological or emotional state of the patient. At the social and psychological level, one must identify aspects of the setting or of the human interaction that cause the patient to perceive the situation as a healing one, thereby releasing whatever biochemically active substances might be involved. It appears safe to claim that a positive change in the patient's health status is most likely to occur when at least three things happen: the patient receives a satisfying explanation of the illness and treatment; the patient feels cared for and supported; and the patient feels an enhanced sense of mastery and control over symptoms.

If, therefore, one wishes to utilize placebo effects for the benefit of patients, one can simply work to enhance those aspects of the patient encounter that stimulate these positive feelings. One can show care, offer explanations, and enhance perceived mastery and control in many ways that require no deception whatever. Since, in the traditional use of placebos, the deception is justified by appeal to patients' benefit (Rawlinson, 1985), it is important to see that in almost all patient encounters, a nondeceptive alternative can produce the same result. Sissela Bok (1978), moreover, argues that the defender of the deception entailed in the traditional use of placebos makes two miscalculations: ignoring possible short-term harm (e.g., missing a diagnosis of serious disease because a placebo has temporarily relieved the patient's complaints) and failing to see how apparently trivial acts build up into collectively undesirable practices (e.g., overreliance on medication).

One may conclude that the traditional use of placebos in therapy can be justified only by very unusual circumstances (in which the use of a dummy pill is the only way to encourage the desired psychological state, for instance). By contrast, since reassuring patients and offering explanations and emotional support are part and parcel of good clinical care, one may argue that a physician has a positive ethical duty to try to enhance the placebo effect in every patient encounter (Connelly, 1991).

Counterarguments in defense of the traditional use focus upon the claim that the deception is apparent rather than real (Spiro, 1986). It might be argued, for example, that if one gives the patient a placebo and says, "There, this will make you feel a lot better," one has not really lied. Perhaps the best reply to these counterarguments was proposed by Richard Cabot (1903): "A true impression, not certain words literally true," is what the physician is obligated to promote in the patient.

Besides the traditional use, placebos may be employed in other ways that do not entail deception. These other uses may therefore be fully licit, since deception is usually the only ethical objection raised to the use of placebos.

In controlled studies, it is generally possible to obtain a fully informed consent, in which the nature of the study design and the possibility that the patient will receive either a placebo or the study drug are made clear. As no individual patient knows whether he or she is receiving the placebo or the investigational treatment, the disclosure does not invalidate the double-blind conditions for a sound scientific study, but it does eliminate any unethical deception. In a much smaller class of studies, the only way to achieve the desired scientific information is to conceal from patients that placebos are being used. (Ironically, many studies designed to learn more about the placebo effect fall into this category.) The ethical question, then, is the extent to which deception can be justified in research upon human subjects.

It is also possible to use placebos in the therapy of individual patients in a way that avoids deception. One formal procedure for doing so has been termed the "N of 1 Trial," since it is basically a double-blind, controlled research trial performed on a single subject. The usual purpose of an N of 1 trial is to see whether a patient really needs a potentially toxic medication that appears to be controlling a troublesome symptom. A nurse or pharmacist administers placebo or drug capsules on alternate days or weeks according to a prearranged code, and the patient records daily levels of the symptom. If the symptom relief is as great during placebo use as during medication use, both patient and physician will discover this fact when the code is broken.

HOWARD BRODY

For a further discussion of topics mentioned in this entry, see the entries AIDS, *article on* HEALTH-CARE AND RE-SEARCH ISSUES; HEALING; INFORMATION DISCLOSURE; INFORMED CONSENT; PHARMACEUTICS, *article on* ISSUES IN PRESCRIBING; *and* RIGHTS IN BIOETHICS. *This entry will find application in the entries* RESEARCH, UNETHICAL; *and* RESEARCH METHODOLOGY. *For a discussion of related ideas, see the entries* FIDELITY AND LOYALTY; FREEDOM AND COERCION; *and* TRUST. *Other relevant material may be found under the entries* HEALTH POLICY, *article on* HEALTH POLICY IN INTERNATIONAL PERSPECTIVE; PHARMACEUTICS, *article on* PHARMACEUTICAL INDUSTRY; RE-SEARCH, HUMAN: HISTORICAL ASPECTS; RESEARCH BIAS; *and* RESEARCH ETHICS COMMITTEES. *See also the* APPENDIX (CODES, OATHS, AND DIRECTIVES RELATED TO BIOETHICS), SECTION IV: ETHICAL DIRECTIVES FOR HUMAN RESEARCH.

Bibliography

BOK, SISSELA. 1978. *Lying: Moral Choice in Public and Private Life.* New York: Pantheon.

BRODY, HOWARD. 1980. *Placebos and the Philosophy of Medicine: Clinical, Conceptual, and Ethical Issues.* Chicago: University of Chicago Press.

———. 1982. "The Lie That Heals: The Ethics of Giving Placebos." *Annals of Internal Medicine* 97, no. 1:112–118.

CABOT, RICHARD C. 1903. "The Use of Truth and Falsehood in Medicine: An Experimental Study." *American Medicine* 5, no. 9:344–349. Reprinted in *Ethics in Medicine: Historical Perspectives and Contemporary Concerns,* pp. 213–220. Edited by Stanley J. Reiser, Arthur J. Dyck, and William J. Curran. Cambridge, Mass.: MIT Press, 1977.

CONNELLY, ROBERT J. 1991. "Nursing Responsibility for the Placebo Effect." *Journal of Medicine and Philosophy* 16, no. 3:325–341.

GRÜNBAUM, ADOLF. 1989. "The Placebo Concept in Medicine and Psychiatry." In *Non-Specific Aspects of Treatment,* pp. 7–38. Edited by Michael Shepherd and Normal Sartorius. Bern, Switzerland: Hans Huber.

GUYATT, GORDON; SACKETT, DAVID; TAYLOR, D. WAYNE; CHONG, JOHN; et al. 1986. "Determining Optimal Therapy—Randomized Trials in Individual Patients." *New England Journal of Medicine* 314, no. 14:889–892.

RAWLINSON, MARY C. 1985. "Truth-Telling and Paternalism in the Clinic: Philosophical Reflections on the Use of Placebos in Medical Practice." In *Placebo: Theory, Research, and Mechanisms,* pp. 403–418. Edited by Leonard White, Bernard Tursky, and Gary E. Schwartz. New York: Guilford Press.

SPIRO, HOWARD M. 1986. *Doctors, Patients, and Placebos.* New Haven: Yale University Press.

WHITE, LEONARD; TURSKY, BERNARD; and SCHWARTZ, GARY E., eds. 1985. *Placebo: Theory, Research, and Mechanisms.* New York: Guilford Press.

PLAGIARISM

See FRAUD, THEFT, AND PLAGIARISM. *See also* COMMU-NICATION, BIOMEDICAL, *article on* SCIENTIFIC PUBLISHING.

POLAND

See MEDICAL ETHICS, HISTORY OF, *section on* EUROPE, *sub-section on* CONTEMPORARY PERIOD, *article on* CENTRAL AND EASTERN EUROPE.

POLLUTION, ENVIRONMENTAL

See ENVIRONMENTAL ETHICS; *and* HAZARDOUS WASTES AND TOXIC SUBSTANCES.

POPULATION ETHICS

I. ELEMENTS OF POPULATION ETHICS

A. DEFINITION OF POPULATION ETHICS

Population studies deal with fertility, mortality, and migration. Fertility refers to human reproduction, mortality to death, and migration to the movement of people from one region to another. The articles on population ethics and population policies in this *Encyclopedia* take up only those aspects of fertility and migration with close links to health care and the life sciences, that is, to bioethics.

Population ethics has two main foundations: moral principles and factual information. Moral principles come from religious traditions, philosophy, declarations of human rights, and other sources. Factual information derives from careful analysis of what is happening or has happened in a given place or situation. Judgments about the ethics of population policies require the application of moral principles to cases based on solid, factual information. Vague principles or a poor understanding of how population programs really operate lead to questionable judgments about population ethics.

The articles on normative approaches and on religious traditions show similarities and differences in the moral principles applied to population policies. One major normative framework, accepted in principle by most countries, includes the universal statements on human rights developed by the United Nations. By endorsing and defining rights such as life, liberty, and welfare, the United Nations has established ethical standards applicable to all social programs, including those dealing with population. The major religious traditions of the world also have their own perspectives on fertility control and migration. Many of these are fully compatible with U.N. statements on human rights, but some are not. The main conflicts over population ethics arise when governments, most of which have officially accepted U.N. standards on human rights, violate those rights in their own population programs.

The articles on population policies apply moral principles to strategies used in fertility control, health standards required in that field, ethical issues in programs involving migration and refugees, and the work of donor agencies dealing with fertility control and migration and refugees. Strategies of fertility control can range from the application of force to information campaigns aimed at voluntary changes in attitudes and behavior. They include compulsion, which has been used to force China's one-child-per-couple policy; strong persuasion, such as the application of heavy government and community pressure on potential users of fertility control; financial incentives and disincentives given to users, field workers, and communities; and educational or information campaigns aimed at promoting greater acceptance of fertility control. The ethical issues are most serious with the use of compulsion and least serious, though still significant, with information campaigns.

Debates over whether rapid population growth poses problems for human societies also show the need for clear moral principles and solid factual understanding. Advocates enter those debates with different principles and factual information.

The moral principles guiding discussions about population problems include preventing environmental pollution (Ehrlich and Ehrlich, 1990); keeping population size within the carrying capacity of the world (Hardin, 1993); and promoting economic growth (World Bank, 1984). Each principle leads to a different focus on factual information. Those concerned with pollution analyze data about global warming, acid rain, and depletion of the ozone layer. Those proposing to keep population size within the carrying capacity of the world look, for example, at figures on population density. Students of economic growth consider the many links between birthrate and economic development, including relationships among fertility, education, and health care.

Because each concern leads to a different meaning of a population problem and a different selection of information, it is difficult to compare one problem definition with another.

Two research practices have held back the development of an adequate factual base for population ethics. One practice begins with conclusions and then selects only those facts consistent with them. Analysts claiming that rapid population growth has had negative consequences for economic development often cite facts supporting that conclusion and leave out contrary evidence (World Bank, 1984). Those claiming benefits from rapid population growth do the same (Simon, 1990).

The second practice involves assigning more or less weight to population conditions than objective research would support. Some advocates of fertility control claim that rapid population growth has caused starvation and political instability in the developing countries. Such simple interpretations overlook the many other influences leading to those conditions, such as the lack of food in poor countries, corruption among political leaders, and ethnic conflicts.

The strategies countries use to control fertility have provoked the sharpest debates about population ethics. China and India have used outright coercion to promote sterilization or abortion. In China, women found to be pregnant with unauthorized children have been forced to undergo abortions (Aird, 1990). Between 1975 and 1977, police in some parts of India rounded up eligible men and required them to be sterilized (Gwatkin, 1979). Indonesia's use of strong community pressures to increase use of contraceptives has also been controversial. To gain new users the Indonesian government has relied on such methods as repeated visits to eligible women from village heads, family-planning workers, and members of Acceptors Clubs; pressure to accept intrauterine devices during "safaris" attended by prominent public officials; and promoting a positive image of small families. Those defending coercion and heavy social pressures argue that countries such as China, India, and Indonesia require vigorous methods of fertility control to curb swelling populations. Voluntary methods, they say, will work too slowly to prevent damage to the economy and create impossible demands for a nation's schools and other public services. Critics respond that applying force and heavy pressure violates human rights and disregards international agreements on fertility control, such as the 1974 World Population Plan of Action (United Nations, 1975).

Policies on migration and refugees also raise questions of ethics. Under what conditions, if any, do residents of one country have the right to enter another? Are the moral claims of potential migrants stronger when they are facing starvation, persecution, or violence? Do countries have the right to bar or expel immigrants they see as harmful to their national interest, as the United States did with Haitian immigrants in the early 1990s? What obligations, if any, does a government have to undocumented aliens within its borders? Can it deny them health-care services regularly available to its own citizens? What kinds of aid should donor agencies, such as the World Food Program or the International Committee for the Red Cross, provide to migrants, refugees, and displaced persons? And how should that aid be distributed?

Issues of medical risks and proper standards of health care arise in fertility control as well as migration and refugee programs. Family-planning programs sometimes put more emphasis on achieving numerical targets for clients than on safeguarding the freedom and health of users. Field workers may promote medically unsafe methods of fertility control, fail to disclose the risks of a given method, or be unavailable to deal with the side effects that do occur. Or they may insert the subdermal contraceptive Norplant and then refuse to remove it at the client's request (Ubinig, 1991). Fertility-control programs also differ in the health support they provide to users, such as local clinics to deal with minor problems or hospitals to handle serious complications.

Questions about standards for health care also arise in programs for refugees. Program managers often have to decide whether refugees should be sent back to countries from which they fled, where they may be tortured, imprisoned, or killed. If they are kept in camps, what should be done to prevent the high rates of illness sometimes seen in those settings? Possible preventive measures include providing adequate food, safe water, suitable shelter, sanitation, immunization of vulnerable groups, and a primary health-care system.

International donor agencies, such as the World Bank, the United Nations Population Fund, and the U.S. Agency for International Development, also face moral choices in their assistance to fertility-control programs. Among those choices are whether donors should support programs known or thought to involve coercion, such as that in China; whether those organizations funding a variety of projects, such as the World Bank, should put pressure on countries to initiate fertility-control programs as a precondition for other aid; and how far and in what ways they should ensure that recipients of their funds provide honest explanations of methods to clients and adequate health support for complications or side effects.

In migration and refugee programs, ethical principles affect decisions about who receives assistance and who does not. Are those decisions based mainly on the health and welfare needs of those to be served or on other criteria, such as racial or ethnic politics? This question is particularly salient in countries where the government controls donor access to areas in which its political opponents want to be evacuated. Donors must likewise make moral choices in designing programs for migrants or refugees. In interventions for disaster relief, they must often choose between strategies providing rapid action by outsiders, such as building homes, or slower methods of educating residents in how to become more self-sufficient (Parker, 1994). Instead of constructing new homes after an earthquake, donors might show community members how to build their own homes using earthquake-resistant methods of construction. The result could be greater self-sufficiency and better protection against future disasters.

Population ethics thus involves the application of moral principles to what are often complex empirical situations. Its greatest challenges are to select principles that are broadly applicable to population issues, rather than those that advance some specific interest, and to explore their implications with an adequate factual understanding of the circumstances involved.

DONALD P. WARWICK

While all the articles in the other sections of this entry are relevant, see especially the companion articles in this section: IS THERE A POPULATION PROBLEM?, *and* HISTORY OF POPULATION THEORIES. *Directly related to this article is the entry* POPULATION POLICIES. *For a further discussion of topics mentioned in this article, see the entries* ABORTION; ADVERTISING; AUTONOMY; BEHAVIOR CONTROL; DEATH; ENVIRONMENTAL ETHICS; ETHICS, *articles on* NORMATIVE ETHICAL THEORIES, *and* RELIGION AND MORALITY; FERTILITY CONTROL; FREEDOM AND COERCION; LIFE; *and* MEDICAL ETHICS, HISTORY OF, *section on* SOUTH AND EAST ASIA, *article on* INDIA, *and sub-section on* CHINA, *article on* CONTEMPORARY CHINA. *For a further discussion of related ideas, see the entries* BIOETHICS; DEATH, ATTITUDES TOWARD; DEATH AND DYING: EUTHANASIA AND SUSTAINING LIFE; ENVIRONMENTAL POLICY AND LAW; FOOD POLICY; FUTURE GENERATIONS, OBLIGATIONS TO; RACE AND RACISM; *and* WOMEN, *article on* HISTORICAL AND CROSS-CULTURAL PERSPECTIVES. *Other relevant material may be found under the entries* HEALTH POLICY, *article on* HEALTH POLICY IN INTERNATIONAL PERSPECTIVE; INTERNATIONAL HEALTH; *and* VALUE AND VALUATION.

Bibliography

AIRD, JOHN SHIELDS. 1990. *Slaughter of the Innocents: Coercive Birth Control in China.* Washington, D.C.: AEI Press.
EHRLICH, PAUL R., and EHRLICH, ANNE H. 1990. *The Population Explosion.* New York: Simon and Schuster.
GWATKIN, DAVIDSON R. 1979. "Political Will and Family Planning: The Implications of India's Emergency Experience." *Population and Development Review* 5, no. 1:29–59.
HARDIN, GARRETT JAMES. 1993. *Living Within Limits: Ecology, Economics, and Population Taboos.* New York: Oxford University Press.
PARKER, RONALD S. 1994. *The Achievement of Educational Objectives: A Study of the A2Z Relief and Development Agency's Projects and Procedures Under Emergency Conditions.* Doctoral Dissertation, Harvard Graduate School of Education, Harvard University.
SIMON, JULIAN LINCOLN. 1990. *Population Matters: People, Resources, Environment, and Immigration.* New Brunswick, N.J.: Transaction Publishers.
UBINIG. 1991. "'The Price of Norplant Is TK. 2000! You Cannot Remove It.' Clients Are Refused Removal in Norplant Trial in Bangladesh." *Issues in Reproductive and Genetic Engineering: Journal of International Feminist Analysis* 4, no. 1:45–46.
UNITED NATIONS. 1975. *Report of the United Nations World Population Conference, 1974.* E/CONF.60/19. New York: United Nations.
WORLD BANK. 1984. *World Development Report 1984.* New York: Oxford University Press.

B. IS THERE A POPULATION PROBLEM?

Policy analysts, the popular press, and scholars often speak of "the population problem." This phrase usually means that the existence of too many people on the planet will cause difficulties or even catastrophes for individuals, couples, countries, or the world. It can also mean that a country or region has too few people for its economic, social, or political welfare.

The first definition argues that rapid population growth, large population size, or high population density can bring widespread poverty, famine, air pollution, poor public health, drought, more children than can be educated in national school systems, overcrowded cities, or other serious harms. Under the second definition, too few people can reduce a country's population below the number that the government wants, decrease the size of the labor force, change the size and mix of ethnic groups in ways that can cause conflict, or create a population with few young and many old people. In either case the location of the problem can be the world, geographic regions such as sub-Saharan Africa, single countries, cities, or other regions within a country.

Those stating that there is a population problem base their assertions on three elements: perceived threats to social, moral, or political values; factual evidence; and theories explaining how population creates the conditions that threaten values. Much of the confusion in discussion of population problems arises from ambiguity or disagreement about these three elements.

Every statement of a population problem explicitly or implicitly expresses concern about values such as preventing famine, having an adequate number of workers and jobs, and giving couples the opportunity to determine their family size. Whether the concern is with too many or too few people, those stating that there is a problem always mention or allude to some moral, social, or political value. They also directly cite factual evidence to support their case or imply that this evidence exists. The evidence may be quantitative, such as figures on the relationship between population size and the number of teachers and schools in a country, or qualitative, such as the judgments of political scientists on a country's strength in foreign affairs, or a combination of the two. And every claim that there is a population problem involves a theory or conceptual scheme showing the links between too many or too few people and indicators of the values at stake in the discussion. Economic theories, for example, may try to show how, specifically, rapid population growth has created or will create unemployment.

Confusion about whether there is a population problem arises when analysts are vague about the values advanced or threatened by population size; omit relevant factual evidence; or use theories that have little validity. Advocates are vague about values advanced or threatened when they state that there is a population problem without indicating the social, moral, or political goods affected by population size. Some writers simply take it for granted that the world is now too crowded and go on to say what should be done about it. Omitting relevant factual evidence leads to charges of bias in statements about population problems. So does the use of theories that aim more at making the case for a problem than at objectively weighing the influence of population conditions.

Whether or not there is a population problem is critical to the ethics of population control. If rapid or limited population growth, population size, and population density do indeed cause serious damage, societies and governments will have some ethical justification for trying to change those conditions. If, on the other hand, pronouncements about population problems fail to state the values affected, are selective in their choice of factual evidence, or rely on dubious theories, the ethical justification for policies to deal with those problems will be tenuous.

The following discussion illustrates the complexity of making statements about population problems by comparing four approaches: those of Paul and Anne Ehrlich, the World Bank, the U.S. National Academy of Sciences, and Julian Simon. It reviews the values at stake in each approach, the completeness of the factual evidence cited, and the theories invoked to link popu-

lation conditions to outcomes reflecting the values of concern.

Approaches to the population problem

In *The Population Bomb* Paul Ehrlich made this statement about population growth:

> The battle to feed all of humanity is over. In the 1970s and 1980s millions of people will starve to death. . . . Although many lives could be saved through dramatic programs to "stretch" the carrying capacity of the earth by increasing food production and providing for more equitable distribution of whatever food is available . . . these programs will only provide a stay of execution unless they are accompanied by determined and successful efforts at population control. (1971, p. xi)

During the 1970s and 1980s, high birthrates did not produce the levels of starvation Ehrlich predicted, in part because of the Green Revolution, which led to much higher food production than in the 1960s. Nonetheless, in their 1990 book *The Population Explosion* Paul and Anne Ehrlich continued to argue that the human race would face starvation and widespread disease unless societies immediately controlled their birthrates.

> Human inaction has already condemned hundreds of millions more people to premature deaths from hunger and disease. The population connection must be made in the public mind. Action to end the population explosion *humanely* and start a gradual population *decline* must become a top item on the human agenda: the human birthrate must be lowered to slightly below the human deathrate as soon as possible. (Ehrlich and Ehrlich, 1990, pp. 22–23)

The authors blame overpopulation for starvation in Africa, homelessness and drug abuse in the United States, global warming, holes in the atmosphere's ozone layer, fires in tropical forests, sewage-blighted beaches, and drought-stricken farm fields.

The World Bank has taken a different approach to the population problem. The *World Development Report 1984* (World Bank, 1984) acknowledges that the evidence on this subject is complex but concludes that "population growth at the rapid rates common in most of the developing world slows development" (p. 105). This statement echoes the remarks of the Bank's president in the foreword: "What governments and their peoples do today to influence our demographic future will set the terms for development strategy well into the next century" (p. iii). In the World Bank's view, high fertility and rapid population growth bring on a problem by creating conditions, such as lower-quality education, that block economic development.

In 1971 the National Academy of Sciences (NAS) claimed that rapid population growth causes serious harm to economic development in sixteen ways. It holds down growth in per capita income; leads to unemployment and underemployment; creates mass poverty; distorts international trade; aggravates political, religious, linguistic, and ethnic conflicts; retards the mental and physical development of children; and has other negative consequences.

Fifteen years later the NAS (National Research Council, 1986) issued a report that backs away from the earlier conclusions. According to that report, slower population growth may benefit developing countries, but there is little evidence for judging whether its impact will be large or small. Furthermore, the results of population growth will depend not only on numbers of people but also on the effectiveness of government administration, social institutions, and the resources of specific countries. Thus, over a decade and a half the NAS shifted from a negative to a more neutral assessment of the impact of demographic growth.

Julian Simon (1990) gives a much more optimistic view of population growth than do the Ehrlichs, the World Bank, and the NAS. He first questions what he calls myths about population and resources. For example, while some say that the food situation in developing countries is worsening, Simon holds that per capita food production has been increasing about 1 percent each year. Responding to arguments that higher population growth means lower per capita economic growth, Simon states: "Empirical studies find no statistical correlation between countries' population growth and their per capita economic growth, either over the long run or in recent decades" (1990, p. 45). Simon also offers evidence challenging statements that the world is running out of natural resources and raw materials and that energy is becoming more scarce.

Simon argues that having additional children improves productivity in the more developed countries and raises the standard of living in less developed countries. Over a period of thirty to seventy years in the more developed countries, each additional person contributes to increased knowledge and technical progress by "inventing, adapting, and diffusing new productive knowledge" (1990, p. 48). Over the same time period in the less developed countries, more children lead to more work done by parents, stimulate agricultural and industrial investment, and bring other benefits. Simon calls people "the ultimate resource" and holds that population growth increases that resource.

The four approaches have different notions of how population growth affects economies and societies. The Ehrlichs are consistently gloomy about the impact of population growth on human societies. The World Bank

is seriously concerned about its effects, and generally negative in its conclusions, but willing to consider different points of view and some evidence challenging its position. Like the World Bank, the NAS focuses on population growth and economic development, but comes to very different conclusions in its 1971 and 1986 reports. Simon plays down the harms and underscores the advantages of population growth for economic development and social welfare.

Values, evidence, and theories

The statements just reviewed show the difficulty of having a coherent discussion about "the population problem." The main reason is that the authors are concerned about different values, do not use all available factual evidence, and base their conclusions on different conceptual schemes and theories.

For Paul and Anne Ehrlich, central values include avoiding starvation, protecting the environment, preserving the world's resources, and maintaining public health: "*The Population Explosion* is being written as ominous changes in the life support systems of civilization become more evident daily. It is being written in a world where hunger is rife and the prospects of famine and plague ever more imminent" (Ehrlich and Ehrlich, 1990, p. 10). The World Bank shows greater concern with promoting economic growth, providing the world with adequate food supplies, having public services such as health and education, and protecting the environment. Both reports of the NAS address similar values. The values guiding Julian Simon's work include showing the benefits of population growth for human welfare and economic development; removing or reducing popular fears about population growth and the availability of resources; and convincing the public that "life on earth is getting better, not worse" (1990, p. 21).

What evidence do these writers use, and how representative is that evidence of all that was available? In *The Population Bomb*, Paul Ehrlich does not try to be objective. He opens his first chapter with these words:

> I have understood the population explosion intellectually for a long time. I came to understand it emotionally one stinking hot night in Delhi a few years ago. My wife and daughter and I were returning to our hotel in an ancient taxi. The seats were hopping with fleas. The only functional gear was third. As we crawled through the city we entered a crowded slum area. The temperature was well over 100, and the air was a haze of dust and smoke. The streets seemed alive with people. People eating, people washing, people sleeping. People visiting, arguing, and screaming. . . . People defecating and urinating. People clinging to buses. People herding animals. People, people, people, people. (1971, p. 5)

Ehrlich goes on to specify the nature of the problem, summarize what is being done to deal with it, state what needs to be done, and tell readers what they can do to help. The book makes its case more by an appeal to the moral and political concerns of its readers than by presenting factual evidence.

The Population Explosion has a more scholarly tone, but still limits the findings presented to those that would be widely interpreted as supporting the authors' claims about overpopulation. It has chapters on shortages of food in developing countries; the difficulties facing agriculture; greenhouse warming, acid rain, and other damages to Earth's ecosystems; and urban air pollution, crowding, and hazards to public health. The Ehrlichs adduce no evidence challenging or qualifying their conclusions. They conclude with a chapter showing what readers can do to stop the population explosion.

Like the Ehrlichs, Simon gives a one-sided presentation of his findings. He contrasts popular views of bad news about population with the "unpublicized, good-news truth" (1990, p. 42) deriving from his own analysis. He summarizes commonly cited statements, such as that the food situation in developing countries is growing worse, and then offers his own view under the heading of *fact*. Instead of presenting a balanced summary of research findings, he tries to attack the popular belief with as many findings as he can assemble that will be widely interpreted as contrary.

The World Bank (1984) admits that judging the evidence about the consequences of population growth is not easy and summarizes some conflicting views on that subject. But it does not mention dozens of cross-national studies that contradict its main conclusion, including work by Simon Kuznets (1974) and Ester Boserup (1965, 1981). This research shows no relationship between the rates of growth of population size and the growth rates of per capita income. Nor does the Bank's report explore the possibility, put forth by Boserup and Simon, that population size, population growth rate, and population density contribute to technological progress. According to one reviewer, "the Report can be evaluated from two different perspectives: as a position paper making the best case for a point of view; or as a summary of current knowledge. It is clearly much more successful as the first than as the second" (Lee, 1985, p. 129).

The two reports by the NAS are also mainly concerned with economic growth, but they differ in their approach to the studies they cite. The 1971 report selects evidence that supports its conclusions about the negative consequences of population growth and neglects research whose findings challenge or contradict those conclusions. The 1986 study is much better balanced in its coverage of the evidence and more cautious in arriving at conclusions. The authors draw a clear distinction, for example, between conditions caused by population growth and those only associated with such growth.

The four approaches also differ in their use of theories and conceptual schemes. In *The Population Bomb*, Paul Ehrlich has no social-scientific theory; he argues almost entirely by assertion. He assumes that the connections between population growth and conditions such as starvation are evident and therefore need no conceptual or theoretical justification. As is the case with their choice of evidence, in *The Population Explosion* Paul and Anne Ehrlich select only those conceptual frameworks showing the negative consequences of population growth. The World Bank recognizes the diversity of theories about the impact of population growth, but chooses a model that eliminates the possibility of any positive effects, such as those mentioned by Julian Simon. The 1971 NAS report also relies heavily on conceptual models showing the harms done by population growth. The 1986 NAS report applies concepts and theories allowing for a fairer evaluation of the relationships between population growth and economic development.

Much of the debate about whether there is a population problem and what it means stems from the different values and concerns behind statements of problems; selective use of evidence; and choosing theories to support preestablished conclusions rather than to arrive at impartial conclusions. Until analysts remove the ideology and biases commonly found in discussions about population problems, the confusion will continue.

The population problem: Where and when?

Most discussions of the population problem focus on the world at large or regions such as developing countries. It is also possible to examine the impact of population growth, size, and density on single countries. This is the focus of the work done by the Population Division of the Department of International Economic and Social Affairs (DIESA) of the United Nations (Chamie, 1994). The Population Division assumes that, whatever the impact of population size, density, and growth across the world, single countries will have different views on what those concepts mean to them. Since the mid-1970s DIESA has maintained the Population Policy Data Bank to assess the perceptions and policies of governments regarding fertility.

At the end of the 1980s, 44 percent of U.N. member countries reported that their fertility levels were too high and 12 percent that they were too low (Chamie, 1994). If one defines a population problem as a government's perception that its fertility is either too high or too low, then 56 percent of U.N. member countries had a problem. The response to that problem depended on whether the governments thought that their fertility was too high or too low.

The first group, usually in countries with low per capita incomes, often set up programs of birth control. Countries reporting that their fertility is too low, such as France, Greece, Hungary, and Switzerland, adopt financial incentives and other policies to encourage more births (McIntosh, 1986). Singapore has been unusual in shifting from the perception that it would have too many people to its current view that it requires higher fertility. These differing perspectives show the importance of asking where and why population is a problem. While many studies focus on the world or on developing countries, the research done by DIESA underscores the importance of opinions and policies in single nations.

The single countries mentioned show agreement on the definition of a population problem. The value of most concern is the government's perception of whether it has too many, too few, or the right number of people. This may be a limited way of defining a population problem, but it does have a consistent point of reference: the views of the government. The evidence used is also the same: the information collected for the Population Policy Data Bank. Conceptual frameworks and theories differ about the reasons for governments' perceptions of a population problem and about why they do or do not take action on population issues. But consistency in the value behind the data and in the evidence used makes it much easier to compare definitions of population problems than in the four approaches outlined earlier.

Another critical question about population growth, size, and density is how they will affect the future. Paul Ehrlich's *The Population Bomb* and William and Paul Paddock's *Famine 1975* (1967) show that confident predictions of disasters are often wrong. But that experience does not mean students of population problems should stop looking to the future. Instead, they should make their predictions but be modest enough to indicate that, because they do not know everything that will happen between the time of writing and the time of the predicted event, they may be mistaken about the predicted events.

A related question concerns the obligations of the present generation to future ones. Do people living now have a duty to preserve the world so that future societies and individuals will have the resources and health conditions currently available? There is no simple answer. Over time, serious problems, such as the pollution of London a century ago, have been resolved and new problems, such as the depletion of water supplies in some regions, have arisen.

Two principles can help reflection on this topic. First, U.N. organizations and governments should pay explicit attention to the long-term consequences of pop-ulation policies. Rather than taking a passive stance in debates on this topic, they should encourage and, if necessary, subsidize research on how population growth, population size, and population density affect the future. Second, the present generation has no right to adopt or accept population policies likely to damage the health and welfare of future generations. These might include actions leading to widespread environmental pollution, deforestation, and poor conditions of public health.

Recommendations

How can students of population policy reduce the bias now seen in many discussions of population problems and provide a solid basis for comparing different statements of those problems?

First, commentators should explicitly state the geographic focus of their analysis. Is it the universe? All the countries in the world? Some region of the world, such as sub-Saharan Africa or South America? A single country? Regions within a single country, such as cities or rural areas? Or some combination of those options, such as a country as a whole and its urban and rural areas? Given the great differences in population, economic, social, and political conditions across nations, specifying the geographic focus would immediately help observers to see similarities and differences across the territory covered. Tables such as those in the World Bank's annual *World Development Report* would be helpful for that purpose.

Second, those discussing population problems should indicate the moral, social, or political values of concern in their analysis. This recommendation should apply whether the observer claims that the region being analyzed has too many, too few, or an adequate number of people. Values often found, explicitly or implicitly, in such analyses include promoting economic growth; preserving the environment; preventing a decline in the region's population; increasing the size of the dominant ethnic group or changing the sizes of ethnic minorities; and maintaining the availability of schools and other social services for the region's inhabitants.

Third, scholarly analyses of population problems should use all relevant evidence rather than just studies that support the author's point of view. Discussions of population growth and economic development should make full use of the numerous cross-national comparisons on that subject. When, as often happens, the sources of evidence lead to different conclusions, that situation should be mentioned.

Fourth, those discussing population problems should specify the theories or conceptual frameworks guiding their analysis. It is particularly important to indicate how population conditions, such as growth rates and size, influence conditions such as economic growth or the availability of schools. Many publications have used conceptual models that attribute more influence to population than it deserves, partly because other relevant influences are not considered. Such is the case with the 1971 NAS study on the consequences of rapid population growth. By using a more thorough conceptual framework and considering a broader range of evidence, the 1986 NAS study in effect retracts many of the conclusions in the 1971 report.

Fifth, conclusions should be based on the results of careful conceptual or theoretical analysis and the weight of the evidence rather than on a priori judgments by the authors. Following this recommendation will often mean reporting contradictory or inconsistent evidence and arriving at qualified judgments. The greatest single source of confusion in present statements on population problems is a strong ideological bias in writing. This bias has led to vagueness about the values at stake, use of incomplete theories and conceptual schemes, citation only of those parts of the evidence consistent with the authors' preconceptions, and conclusions based more on ideology than on a fair assessment of the evidence.

Sixth, policy recommendations in statements about population problems should be based on the evidence presented rather than on the personal preferences of the authors or the donors who have supported them. For example, after a lengthy discussion of the links between population growth and economic development, the 1986 NAS report suggests that governments should establish family-planning programs. This recommendation has little to do with the main lines of the report, which says nothing about family planning. This practice is intellectually misleading, for it suggests that the policy suggestions flow directly from the scholarly analysis, which in this case they do not.

Conclusions

Is there a population problem? When the focus is on single countries, when the source of information is the Population Policy Data Bank maintained by the United Nations, and when the definition of the population problem is the government's opinion on whether it has too many, too few, or the right number of people, it is possible to answer that question. But when the focus is on the world as a whole, and authors are concerned with different values, use different theories and sources of evidence, and become advocates for a particular point of view, there is and can be no answer.

To have more comparable notions of population problems, authors must clearly identify the geographical region they are discussing; indicate the values of concern to them; use all available evidence; apply theories or conceptual schemes that consider all relevant influences; weigh the evidence objectively; and draw only

those conclusions supported by their analysis. The ideological discourse seen in current discussions of population problems must give way to scholarly analysis. When these criteria are met, more accurate, less biased, and more comparable discussions of population problems will be available.

DONALD P. WARWICK

While all the articles in the other sections of this entry are relevant, see especially the companion articles in this section: DEFINITION OF POPULATION ETHICS, *and* HISTORY OF POPULATION THEORIES. *Directly related to this article is the entry* POPULATION POLICIES. *For a further discussion of topics mentioned in this article, see the entries* ENVIRONMENTAL HEALTH; ENVIRONMENTAL POLICY AND LAW; FOOD POLICY; FUTURE GENERATIONS, OBLIGATIONS TO; UTILITY; *and* VALUE AND VALUATION. *For a discussion of related ideas, see the entries* ABORTION; AGING AND THE AGED, *especially the articles on* LIFE EXPECTANCY AND LIFE SPAN, *and* SOCIETAL AGING; CHILDREN; CLIMATIC CHANGE; ENDANGERED SPECIES AND BIODIVERSITY; ENVIRONMENTAL ETHICS; ENVIRONMENT AND RELIGION; EPIDEMICS; FERTILITY CONTROL; GENETICS AND ENVIRONMENT IN HUMAN HEALTH; HAZARDOUS WASTES AND TOXIC SUBSTANCES; INTERNATIONAL HEALTH; MEDICAL ETHICS, HISTORY OF, *section on* SOUTH AND EAST ASIA, *and section on* EUROPE, *subsection on* CONTEMPORARY PERIOD; *and* PUBLIC HEALTH.

Bibliography

BOSERUP, ESTER. 1965. *The Conditions of Agricultural Growth: The Economics of Agrarian Change Under Population Pressure.* Chicago: Aldine.

———. 1981. *Population and Technological Change: A Study of Long-Term Trends.* Chicago: University of Chicago Press.

CHAMIE, JOSEPH. 1994. "Trends, Variations, and Contradictions in National Policies to Influence Fertility." *Population and Development Review* 20 (supp.):37–50. Reprinted in *The New Politics of Population: Conflict and Consensus in Family Planning.* Edited by Jason L. Finkle and C. Allison McIntosh. New York: Population Council.

EHRLICH, PAUL R. 1971. [1968]. *The Population Bomb.* Rev. ed. New York: Ballantine.

EHRLICH, PAUL R., and EHRLICH, ANNE H. 1990. *The Population Explosion.* New York: Simon and Schuster.

KUZNETS, SIMON SMITH. 1974. *Population, Capital and Growth: Selected Essays.* New York: Norton.

LEE, RONALD. 1985. "World Development Report 1984: Review Symposium." *Population and Development Review* 11, no. 1:127–130.

McINTOSH, C. ALLISON. 1986. "Recent Pronatalist Policies in Western Europe." *Population and Development Review* 12 (supp.):318–334.

NATIONAL ACADEMY OF SCIENCES (U.S.). OFFICE OF THE FOREIGN SECRETARY. 1971. *Rapid Population Growth: Conse-*

quences and Policy Implications. Baltimore: Johns Hopkins University Press.

NATIONAL RESEARCH COUNCIL (U.S.). COMMISSION ON BEHAVIORAL AND SOCIAL SCIENCES EDUCATION. COMMITTEE ON POPULATION. WORKING GROUP ON POPULATION GROWTH AND ECONOMIC DEVELOPMENT. 1986. *Population Growth and Economic Development: Policy Questions.* Washington, D.C.: National Academy Press.

PADDOCK, WILLIAM, and PADDOCK, PAUL. 1967. *Famine 1975!* Boston: Little, Brown.

SIMON, JULIAN L. 1990. *Population Matters: People, Resources, Environment, and Immigration.* Brunswick, N.J.: Transaction.

WORLD BANK. 1984. *World Development Report 1984.* New York: Oxford University Press.

C. HISTORY OF POPULATION THEORIES

Ancient and medieval theories

Like most general theories of Western civilization, those concerning population evolved first in ancient Greece. Both policies and their conceptual frameworks varied in their details, but there was much consistency from one city-state to another. The typical pronatalist policies were intended not to induce a growth in numbers but to prevent their decline (Stangeland, 1904, chap. 1; Hutchinson, 1967, chap. 2). In the ideal city-state that Plato pictured in *Laws,* the population was to be kept stable at 5,040 (the product of $1 \times 2 \times 3 \times 4 \times 5 \times 6 \times 7$) by encouraging or inhibiting fertility or by infanticide. If the population grew much beyond this optimum, the community was to establish colonies. To neglect measures that would keep the population more or less fixed, according to Aristotle, would "bring certain poverty on the citizens, and poverty is the cause of sedition and evil" (*Politics,* 2.9).

Greek thought on population, in sum, was characterized by an overriding concern with policy, and thus a relative indifference to empirical or conceptual analysis. Policy was to be applied, moreover, to aggregates ridiculously small by present-day standards. And whether the meaning of "population" was in accord with the modern sense is often not clear; in most instances the term may have referred only to citizens, thus omitting females, children, slaves, and aliens.

In its far larger arena, Rome's policy was more consistently pronatalist. As imperial hegemony spread from Italy throughout the Mediterranean basin and beyond, the center was troubled by moral decay, the dissolution of the family, and a slower growth of population. Successive pronatalist measures culminated in three enactments under Augustus (63 B.C.E.–14 C.E.), which punished celibacy and adultery and rewarded prolific couples (Stangeland, 1904, pp. 30–38). Since they had little apparent effect, the laws were repeatedly amended and finally repealed under Constantine (ca. 288–337).

As the empire gradually disintegrated, many came to believe that the end of the world was imminent, and various sects offered competing dogmas appropriate to the apocalypse. The early Christian church gradually developed its own doctrine with a compromise between libertine and ascetic, but emphasizing the latter (Noonan, 1965). Catholic thought reached its apogee in the *Summa Theologica* of Thomas Aquinas (ca. 1224–1274). For him, a marriage between Christians is not merely a means of obeying the injunction to replenish the earth but also a spiritual bond, a sacrament. The function of intercourse is procreation (Bourke, 1967).

Early modern theory

The dominant theme of the early modern period was the view that population growth is precarious and has to be fostered. Just as the mercantilist state hoarded gold, so it hoarded people, and for the same reason—to increase its economic, political, and military power. If rapid population growth resulted in what was termed "overcrowding," the mercantilist solution was to ship the surplus to colonies, where the settlers and their progeny could continue to aggrandize the state's power in another quarter of the globe.

Modern demography began with the efforts of mercantilist states to keep track of their populations (Glass, 1973). William Petty (1623–1687) was the first exponent of what he called "political arithmetic." John Graunt (1620–1674) constructed the first crude life table. Gregory King (1648–1712) calculated population estimates based on local enumerations, which he corrected for technical errors. On the Continent, Johann Peter Süssmilch (1707–1767) used Protestant parish records to estimate Prussia's fertility and mortality. Richard Cantillon (ca. 1680–1734) held that internal migration, deaths, and especially marriages (and therefore births) varied according to the prevailing standard of living and the structure of the demand for labor. François Quesnay (1694–1774), who founded what was later called physiocratic thought, analyzed the implicit bounds to population growth.

The philosophes of eighteenth-century France varied greatly on many issues, but most also found reason to favor policies stimulating population growth. Charles-Louis de Secondat, Baron Montesquieu (1689–1755), believed that the entire world had undergone depopulation and recommended pronatalist decrees. According to Voltaire (1694–1778), a nation is fortunate if its population increases by as much as 5 percent per century. Louis de St.-Just (1767–1794) held that one can usually depend on nature "never to have more children than teats," but to keep the balance in the other direction requires the state's assistance. By this notion of an equitable family law, as inspired by Jean-Jacques Rousseau (1712–1778), marriages should be encouraged by state loans, and a couple that remained childless after several years ought to be forcibly separated.

The two utopians that Thomas Robert Malthus opposed in the first edition of his *Essay on the Principle of Population,* William Godwin (1756–1836) and Marie-Jean Caritat, Marquis de Condorcet (1743–1794), focused their attention on the wholly rational age they discerned just over the horizon. According to them, in a world from which diseases had been wholly eliminated, the span of life would have no assignable upper limit. People would devote themselves to more important tasks than, in Condorcet's words, "the puerile idea of filling the earth with useless and unhappy beings."

Malthus

Malthus summarized or contravened earlier ideas so effectively that, for more than a century and a half, subsequent theorists have generally taken him as a benchmark. Unfortunately, many references to "Malthusian" thought are based, at best, on the first edition of *Essay on the Principle of Population* rather than on the much enlarged and thoroughly revised later editions—or, at worst, on a total misunderstanding of what he stood for (Petersen, 1979, chap. 4).

Thomas Robert Malthus (1766–1834) was a professor at the newly founded East India College, occupying Britain's first chair in the new discipline of political economy. He spent much of his life collecting data on the relation between population and its social, economic, and natural environments, bringing his theory into accord with these facts and adjusting it to criticism. There were seven editions of the *Essay* in all.

According to the principle of population as expounded in the *Essay*, population, "when unchecked," doubles once every generation. Among "irrational animals" this potential is realized, and its "superabundant effects are repressed afterwards by want of room or nourishment." But rational human beings can consider the consequences of their reproductive potential and curb their natural drive. With humans, thus, there are two types of control of population growth: "preventive checks," the chaste postponement of marriage, and "positive checks," the deaths resulting from too large a population relative to its subsistence. Tension between numbers and food can have a beneficial effect: A man who postpones marrying until he is able to support a family is goaded by his sex drive to work hard, thus contributing to social progress. For this reason Malthus opposed contraceptives, for their use permits individual sexual gratification with no benefit to society.

Through the successive editions of the *Essay*, Malthus increasingly stressed the negative correlation between station in life and size of family. This, in his view, was the principal clue to solving what later became known as "the population problem." In order to bring the lower classes up to the self-control and social responsibility exercised by those with more money and education, Malthus asserted, the poor should be given more money and education. "The principal circumstances" that induce prospective parents to have fewer children are "liberty, security of property, the diffusion of knowledge, and a taste for the comforts of life." Those that tend to increase procreation are "despotism and ignorance." The thesis that upward mobility into the middle class effects a decline in fertility, though it is far less familiar than that relating population growth to food, is in retrospect Malthus's most important contribution.

For many decades Malthus's reputation was far below that of lesser social analysts. Recently it has become apparent that much of present-day demography was at least partly stimulated by Malthus and that those who denounced him as a false prophet had typically begun by misrepresenting his ideas.

Population optima

Most of the populations that Malthus discussed tended to grow too rapidly relative to the available resources, and he recommended institutional checks to their fertility. But the extraordinarily rapid growth of the American colonies, whose population was doubling every twenty-five years, he held to be of great benefit. In other words, each country has an optimum size and rate of growth, depending on the social and economic conditions. Malthus neither used the term "optimum" nor developed the concept beyond an implicit statement, but he planted the seed of the theory. Malthus's principle that the population tends to increase by a geometrical ratio and food by an arithmetical ratio can be reformulated as a law of diminishing returns. If to a fixed acreage of land more and more labor is added, return per person may first rise but then will decline as the work force increases beyond its most efficient size. The first definition of "the optimum" was based on this schema: It is that population which under given conditions produces the highest per capita economic return.

Soon, however, the optimum came to mean simply "the best population," with each analyst furnishing a particular yardstick of what is "good." By this route the theory of population optimum could be regarded as a version of social choice theory, with a wide variety of open questions (Dasgupta, 1987). Should the population be related to the present institutional structure or to some supposed future ("socialism," for instance)? Should the criterion of "good" be economic welfare, military strength, the conservation of resources, or some combination of these? This conundrum is aggravated by the fact that optima vary greatly, according to the goal that society sets. And should the standard relate exclusively to the number of people or also to their age structure, rate of growth, level of skill, and other characteristics that affect how efficiently the society can operate?

Obviously, no judgment concerning "the optimum" can be very precise. Whether a country of western Europe, say, is underpopulated or overpopulated is less a demographic-economic measurement than a more or less arbitrary opinion. The norm can be applied meaningfully only at the extremes. The colonies that became the United States were definitely underpopulated, as Malthus pointed out. And in some of today's less developed countries, by the judgment of most demographers, the rapidly growing populations impede a rise in the people's well-being.

Migration

We are all born and we all die, but only some of us move from one place to another. Unlike fertility and mortality, migration is not a biological process. Indeed, many determinants of migration are political: Movements are subsidized, restricted, or forced, and the status of migrants in their new homeland depends on the state's laws on aliens. If we conceive of migration following the usual definition—as the relatively permanent movement of persons over a significant distance—the specifications "permanent" and "significant" must be set by more or less arbitrary criteria. Partly for this reason, migration statistics are generally imprecise and subject to capricious interpretation.

Migration changes the size of population and the rate of growth in the two areas involved, but usually not in the simple fashion that common sense suggests. Most migrants are young adults, and their movement changes the age structure, and thus the birth and death rates, in both areas. Given a sedentary population and a stimulus to emigrate, typically some leave and some do not. There is self-selection by age, sex, family status, and occupation, as well as possibly by intelligence, mental health, and independence of character. Since migration is not unitary, it cannot be analyzed in supracultural terms but must be differentiated even at the most abstract level with respect to the social conditions obtaining. Generalizations about migration, thus, developed mostly outside of standard population theories.

Demographic transition

The number of people in the world is increasing at an unprecedented rate to unprecedented totals, and the basic reason is no mystery: Mortality has fallen sharply, and in many areas fertility has not. As originally formulated (e.g., Landry, 1934), this so-called demographic transition was conceived as taking place in three broad stages: (1) preindustrial societies, with high fertility more or less balanced by high mortality and a consequent low natural increase; (2) societies in transi-

tion, with continuing high fertility but declining mortality and a consequent rapid natural increase; and (3) modern societies, with both fertility and mortality stabilized at low levels and a consequent more or less static population. In its barest form this theory is one of the best-documented generalizations in the social sciences.

Collapsing the whole of human history into these three demographic types means, of course, that not only details but also important distinctions are passed over. When actual populations are reconstituted, so simplistic a theory often proves to be less a guide to research or policy than an invitation to misunderstanding. And this has been so concerning each of the three stages (Chesnais, 1986).

It is assumed that the mortality of primitive peoples was high relative to that in advanced societies, but estimates of the longevity in ancient times can hardly be very precise. Whether or not preindustrial peoples were warlike, lived in a favorable climate, developed cultural norms promoting cleanliness, and so on certainly influenced their death rates. And the usual formula—that since the mortality of primitive humans was high, their fertility must have been close to the physiological maximum if the group was to survive—is also questionable. From an early survey of contemporary primitive cultures, Alexander Carr-Saunders (1922) concluded that *all* of them included customs intended to restrict the increase of population. There is no reason a priori to postulate that all prehistoric peoples reproduced like unthinking animals, incurring the cost of a subsequent unnecessarily high mortality.

In stage 2, the first steps toward a modern industrial society bring about a decline in mortality—but also often, contrary to the theory, a rise in fertility. Improved health can result in greater physiological ability to reproduce. Whatever means had been used to reduce population growth, such as infanticide in Tokugawa Japan, may not survive modernization. If the age at marriage had been set well past puberty, as in early modern western Europe, the institutions bolstering this norm often became less effective. Religious practices or taboos unintentionally inhibiting fertility, such as the one prohibiting the remarriage of widows in Hindu India, may dissipate. Most remarkably, family-planning programs can result in a rise in fertility, for if women are able to depend on controls later in their reproductive life, many begin childbearing at an earlier age. In short, the effect of modernization is partly to increase fertility and partly to decrease it (Heer, 1966).

Moreover, the early analysts of the demographic transition failed to forecast the decline of mortality in less-developed countries. Over the past two centuries or so, as the main advances were applied in medicine, surgery, public sanitation, agriculture, and nutrition, Western populations gradually improved in health and longevity. During the last several decades, however, some of the most recent techniques have been transferred to areas lacking most prior scientific controls; peoples cared for until recently by witch doctors acquired access to antibiotics. In Ceylon (now Sri Lanka), to take one striking example, the estimated expectation of life at birth increased from forty-three years in 1946 to fifty-two in 1947; the gain achieved in this one year had taken half a century in most Western countries.

Efforts to reduce fertility

Because of the continuing high fertility and the sharp decline of mortality in less-developed countries, their populations have grown at rates high enough to stimulate widespread control measures. Some of these programs have been successful, but many have achieved far less than their proponents hoped they would, in part because none has an appropriate theory underlying it.

Is a large and rapidly growing population indeed a problem? Leaders of the independence movements of pre-1940 European colonies held that their countries' poverty derived not from excessive procreation but from imperial misrule, and this view often persisted after independence. The very slow start of India's programs to check its population growth, for instance, was due in part to Jawaharlal Nehru's initial ambivalence. Among those who accept the thesis that too many people can impede modernization, proponents have often advocated *either* birth control *or* industrialization, as though one or the other were the sole relevant factor.

The theories underlying birth-control programs, often implicit rather than spelled out in papers, reports, or books, can be summed up in the following propositions:

1. *Elements of "traditional" society constitute the principal impediment to the spread of contraception.* But, as we have noted, most traditional cultures include anti-natalist tendencies and, on the other hand, modern nationalism is often strongly pronatalist.
2. *The most important variable in any program is the contraceptive means to be used.* But the history of the West suggests that, given the will to reduce fertility, people will make effective use of whatever means are available to them—coitus interruptus and illegal abortion in France, postponed marriage or nonmarriage in Ireland, and so on.
3. *The agency through which contraception can be most effectively disseminated is the state.* But this contradicts, again, the history of the decline of Western fertility, where officialdom typically opposed the private neo-Malthusian leagues and their successors.
4. *Population policy can be equated essentially with family policy: That is, zero population growth can be realized by inducing each pair of parents to have an average of only*

two children. But the rate of growth depends also on the proportion of the population that is of childbearing age, and in less-developed countries that is generally very high.

5. *It is so important that the population crisis be solved that policy-oriented action and knowledge-oriented research must be collapsed into a single operation.* This procedure violates the scientific canon that truth can be effectively sought only in a setting made as value-free as possible. As a consequence, field workers and analysts are encouraged to accept spurious results as valid, for it is very difficult to ascertain the actual sentiments and behavior patterns of respondents.

In sum, the many attempts to reduce fertility in less-developed countries have typically been made with little regard to what had been learned from the prior decline in family size in the industrial West. Perhaps the best link between the two is the wealth-flow theory, so designated by John Caldwell. The crucial factor is whether children are productively useful to their parents and care for them in their old age; if so, as in African cultures he studied, the incentive is to procreate to the maximum feasible. If, however, parents incur net costs for the long-term care and education of their children, who generally contribute little to household finances, the inevitable tendency is to reduce the number brought into the world. By concentrating on the family budget, Caldwell (1982) was able to elucidate both the historical decline of fertility in the West and the partial success of family-planning programs in less-developed countries.

Theories of population in totalitarian countries

A focus on economic or cultural factors can mean that political influences on fertility are bypassed. More generally, theories developed in the democratic West are in many respects ill suited to analyze such past totalitarian societies as the Soviet Union and Nazi Germany. Though their cultures differed greatly, these two countries had certain features in common, many of which related to population theory and its application.

1. The Nazi party and the Communist party were defined as omnipotent, able to cope with any increase in population. According to the first Soviet delegate to the U.N. Population Commission, "I would consider it barbaric for the Commission to contemplate a limitation of marriages or of legitimate births, and this for any country whatsoever, at any period whatsoever. With an adequate social organization it is possible to face any increase in population" (quoted by Sauvy, 1952, vol. 1, p. 174; cf. Petersen, 1988).
2. Population theory had the same purpose as any other science—to bolster the power of the party in power

(Besemeres, 1980). In particular, the need of the totalitarian state for labor was reflected in theories on how to maintain a high rate of population growth and in such applications as family subsidies.

3. Efforts to stimulate the birthrate, however, were hampered by the ruling party's hostility to the family, which by its legal and emotional links between generations helps to maintain a traditional opposition to radically new ideas and practices. Both Nazi Germany and the Soviet Union tried to establish institutions that could replace the family, such as brothels in which SS men could impregnate young women certified as racially pure, or the Soviet children's homes in which the state could convert orphans and the offspring of political dissidents into reliable instruments of the Community party. But such substitutes never produced a large enough crop, and policy toward the family therefore vacillated in both countries.

4. The need for a high fertility was enhanced by the recklessness with which sectors of the population designated as hostile or inferior were killed off. The terror most closely associated with the Nazis was the mass slaughter of Jews, based on the outpouring of writings on *Rassenkunde* (race science). More often Communists defined their victims as class enemies (though antagonism to ethnic minorities was also a constant element of Soviet life), but the difference was not fundamental: The slaughter began in different sectors of the population and was sometimes concentrated there, but in both cases it spread to the whole society (Hilberg, 1973; Conquest, 1990).

5. Totalitarian ideology was based on what in German is called *Stufenlehre*, a doctrine of stages. All analysis, all planning, began not in the empirical present but in the inevitable perfect future, homogenized into a "classless" (*Judenfrei*, "Jewless") sameness. The road to this paradise could be seen clearly only by the Nazi party and the Communist party, whose function was to move the rest of the population toward its destiny. The ruthless terror that was often needed was warranted, thus, by the glorious community that would ensue.

Conclusions

Intellectual history includes few population theories in the narrow sense; most theories were developed as usually minor adjuncts to systematic statements about the society or the economy. Even this thin conceptual framework, however, may have profound ethical implications, for long before anything scientific was known about the determinants and consequences of population growth, statesmen, theologians, and scholars proposed—and their societies sometimes adopted as policies—rules of behavior allegedly suitable to their environment.

Until the modern era, the usual policy orientation was pronatalist, for it was generally assumed both that more people were better than fewer and that realizing a faster growth required state aid. Though not the first to take a contrary position, Malthus was by far the most important. Paradoxically, the greatly increased concern with policy in recent decades has not been accompanied by a more precise definition of goals. The judgment of whether a population is too large or too small obviously depends on a reasonably precise designation of the optimum, which has remained perhaps the most controversial concept in demography.

In past times, tyrants and conquering armies slaughtered many aliens, variously defined, but the combination of ruthless nationalism with scientific means of disposing of "inferior" sectors of the population is an innovation of the twentieth century. Partly because of a reaction against totalitarian genocide, demographers have given less systematic attention than warranted to such population characteristics as health or skill, though in many contexts these may be more important than mere numbers.

In recent decades the most striking characteristic of demography has been the attempt to dispense with theory in the solution of population problems widely recognized as critical. The substitution of "concern" for competence has not led, however, to many successes. In spite of the proliferation of antinatalist programs in less-developed countries and of the numbers of potential parents who accept the contraceptives made available, the world's population continues to grow at a rapid rate.

WILLIAM PETERSEN

While all the articles in the other sections of this entry are relevant, see especially the companion articles in this section: DEFINITION OF POPULATION ETHICS, *and* IS THERE A POPULATION PROBLEM? *Directly related to this article is the entry* POPULATION POLICIES. *For a discussion of topics mentioned in this article, see the entries* EUGENICS; FAMILY; FERTILITY CONTROL; INFANTS, *article on* HISTORY OF INFANTICIDE; MARRIAGE AND OTHER DOMESTIC PARTNERSHIPS; NATIONAL SOCIALISM; PUBLIC HEALTH, *article on* DETERMINANTS OF PUBLIC HEALTH; SEXUALITY IN SOCIETY; *and* WOMEN, *article on* HISTORICAL AND CROSS-CULTURAL PERSPECTIVES. *For a discussion of related ideas, see the entries* ABORTION, *especially the sections on* CONTEMPORARY ETHICAL AND LEGAL ASPECTS, *and* RELIGIOUS TRADITIONS; AGING AND THE AGED, *article on* LIFE EXPECTANCY AND LIFE SPAN; BIOLOGY, PHILOSOPHY OF; DEATH AND DYING: EUTHANASIA AND

SUSTAINING LIFE, *article on* HISTORICAL ASPECTS; ENVIRONMENTAL ETHICS, *the* OVERVIEW; EVOLUTION; FOOD POLICY; FUTURE GENERATIONS, OBLIGATIONS TO; MEDICAL ETHICS, HISTORY OF, *section on* EUROPE, *subsection on* ANCIENT AND MEDIEVAL, *and article on* RENAISSANCE AND ENLIGHTENMENT. *Other relevant material may be found under the entries* INTERNATIONAL HEALTH; SEXUAL ETHICS; *and* SUSTAINABLE DEVELOPMENT.

Bibliography

BESEMERES, JOHN F. 1980. *Socialist Population Politics: The Political Implications of Demographic Trends in the USSR and Eastern Europe.* White Plains, N.Y.: M. E. Sharpe.

BOURKE, VERNON J. 1967. "Thomas Aquinas, St." In *Encyclopedia of Philosophy*, vol. 8, pp. 105–116. New York: Macmillan.

CALDWELL, JOHN. 1982. *Theory of Fertility Decline.* New York: Academic Press.

CARR-SAUNDERS, ALEXANDER MORRIS. 1922. *The Population Problem: A Study in Human Evolution.* Oxford: At the Clarendon Press.

CHESNAIS, JEAN-CLAUDE. 1986. *La transition démographique: Étapes, formes, implications économiques: Étude de séries temporelles (1720–1984) relative à 67 pays.* Institut national d'études démographiques travaux et documents, cahier no. 113. Paris: Presses universitaires de France.

CONQUEST, ROBERT. 1990. *The Great Terror: A Reassessment.* New York: Oxford University Press.

DASGUPTA, PARTHA. 1987. "The Ethical Foundations of Population Policy." In *Population Growth and Economic Development: Issues and Evidence*, pp. 631–659. Edited by D. Gale Johnson and Ronald D. Lee. Madison: University of Wisconsin Press.

GLASS, DAVID V. 1973. *Numbering the People: The Eighteenth-Century Population Controversy and the Development of Census and Vital Statistics in Britain.* Farnborough, U.K.: Saxon House.

HEER, DAVID M. 1966. "Economic Development and Fertility." *Demography* 3:423–444.

HILBERG, RAUL. 1973. *The Destruction of the European Jews.* New York: New Viewpoints.

HUTCHINSON, EDWARD PRINCE. 1967. *The Population Debate: The Development of Conflicting Theories up to 1900.* New York: Houghton Mifflin.

LANDRY, ADOLPHE. 1934. *La révolution démographique: Études et essais sur les problèmes de la population.* Paris: Librairie du Recueil Sirey.

NOONAN, JOHN THOMAS, JR. 1965. *Contraception: A History of Its Treatment by the Catholic Theologians and Canonists.* Cambridge, Mass.: Belknap Press.

PETERSEN, WILLIAM. 1979. *Malthus.* Cambridge, Mass.: Harvard University Press.

———. 1988. "Marxism and the Population Question: Theory and Practice." *Population and Development Review* 14 (supp.): 77–101. Edited by Michael S. Teitelbaum and Jay M. Winter. Also published under the title *Population in Western Intellectual Traditions.* Cambridge: At the University Press, 1989.

SAUVY, ALFRED. 1952. *Théorie générale de la population.* 2 vols. Paris: Presses universitaires de France.

STANGELAND, CHARLES EMIL. 1904. *Pre-Malthusian Doctrines of Population: A Study in the History of Economic Theory.* New York: Columbia University Press.

II. NORMATIVE APPROACHES

Population policies raise profound questions of ethics. Is China justified in using coercion to enforce its policy of one child per couple? Is it legitimate for government officials and community peers in Indonesia to apply strong pressure to promote birth control? Should U.S. judges be free to require the insertion of Norplant, a long-lasting, subdermal contraceptive, when sentencing women they consider unfit to be mothers (Feringa et al., 1992)? Do the wealthiest nations of the world have a moral obligation to accept refugees from poor countries?

Answers to such questions require ethical principles applicable to population policies across all countries and cultures. Principles that reflect the standards of only one country or region, such as the United States or Europe, may not persuade leaders and peoples of other countries.

Three schools of thought have guided debates on these principles. The first argues that government programs of any kind must respect human rights as stated in the Universal Declaration of Human Rights adopted by the United Nations in 1948; the International Covenant on Economic, Social, and Cultural Rights (1976); the International Covenant on Civil and Political Rights (1976); and many related U.N. statements (Nickel, 1987; Claude and Weston, 1989). A second school holds that the morality of population interventions must be determined by the country that carries them out, for it has the problem and best understands how to deal with it. This school accepts no universal standards of human rights. It considers attempts by others to impose such standards to be infringements on national sovereignty. The third school recognizes some or all of the human rights affirmed by the United Nations, but claims that when population growth or density create desperate economic or social problems for a country, its government has the right to limit individual reproductive freedom for the common good.

This article develops a framework of ethical principles based on the Universal Declaration of Human Rights, later U.N. statements on human rights, and regional declarations on the same subject, particularly the European Convention on Human Rights. It then applies those principles to population policies. It concludes by contrasting this approach with another ethical framework known as "stepladder ethics."

Five key principles

Ethical evaluation of population policies requires five principles to guide decisions as well as criteria for determining when one principle can be sacrificed for another.

Life heads the list, for without it people cannot benefit from the other four principles. Article 3 of the Universal Declaration of Human Rights states: "Everyone has the right to life, liberty and security of person." The International Covenant on Civil and Political Rights is more specific: "Every human being has the inherent right to life. This right shall be protected by law. No one shall be arbitrarily deprived of his life" (Part III, Article 6).

Life means not only being alive, but enjoying good health and having reasonable security against the actions of others that cause death, illness, severe pain, or disability. Policies on fertility control, migration, and refugees threaten this principle when they take no action to assist people facing starvation or slaughter and when they create incentives for female infanticide (Aird, 1990; Brown and Shue, 1981). Policies endanger health when they promote methods of fertility control, such as sterilizations, oral contraceptives, the intrauterine device (IUD), or injections, that can pose grave risks to physical well-being. Among such risks are cardiovascular diseases, tubal infertility, pelvic inflammatory disease, and septic abortion (National Research Council, 1989; Schearer, 1983). Fertility-control programs may also damage the health of users when they overlook sexually transmitted diseases, such as gonorrhea, or other reproductive-tract infections, including genital herpes, chancroid, genital warts, vaginal infections, and infections of the upper reproductive tract (Dixon-Mueller and Wasserheit, 1991).

Freedom is the capacity and opportunity to make reflective choices and to act on those choices. Freedom requires knowledge about the choices available, such as options for fertility control or migration; a chance to make choices without coercion or strong pressure from others; awareness that one is making choices and of the issues at stake in each; and the possibility of taking action to carry out the choices made (Warwick, 1982, 1990; Veatch, 1977). Restrictions on any of these conditions, such as ignorance of options, decisions made while an individual is being tortured, or barriers to acting on choices made, void or limit freedom.

U.N. statements strongly endorse freedom. According to the Universal Declaration, everyone has the right to freedom of thought, conscience, and religion (Article 18); freedom of opinion and expression (Article 19);

freedom of peaceful assembly and association (Article 20); freedom from slavery and servitude (Article 4); and freedom from arbitrary interference with privacy, family, home, or correspondence (Article 12). Both the International Covenant on Economic, Social, and Cultural Rights and the International Covenant on Civil and Political Rights open with this statement: "All peoples have the right of self-determination. By virtue of that right they freely determine their political status and freely pursue their economic, social, and cultural development" (Part I, Article 1, in both covenants). In the World Population Plan of Action developed at the World Population Conference in 1974, delegates agreed to the following statement on reproductive freedom: "All couples and individuals have the basic right to decide freely and responsibly the number and spacing of their children and to have the information, education, and means to do so . . ." (World Population Conference, 1975, p. 7).

Welfare means a standard of living adequate to provide food, clothing, housing, health care, and education. Affirmed in Articles 25 and 26 of the Universal Declaration, this standard was both repeated and broadened in the International Covenant on Economic, Social, and Cultural Rights. That statement spoke specifically about the right to continuous improvement in living conditions; the steps needed to protect the right to be free from hunger; the right of everyone to the highest attainable standard of physical and mental health; the widest possible protection and assistance for the family; special protection for mothers before and after childbirth; and protection of children and young persons from social and economic exploitation, including work that threatens their lives or is harmful to their morals and health. The World Population Plan of Action of 1974 also explicitly tied population policies to human welfare: "The principal aim of social, economic, and cultural development, of which population goals and policies are integral parts, is to improve levels of living and the quality of life of the people" (World Population Conference, 1975, p. 7). Population programs, therefore, should not aim only to raise or lower fertility, reduce mortality, or control migration, but to be instruments for promoting human welfare.

Fairness refers to an equitable distribution of the benefits and harms from population policies. It does not require an equal distribution of benefits and harms, but it does demand that one individual or group should not receive disproportionate advantages or disadvantages from a given policy. The Universal Declaration strongly endorses fairness in Article 1: "All human beings are born free and equal in dignity and rights." Article 2 continues: "Everyone is entitled to all the rights and freedoms set forth in this Declaration, without distinction of any kind, such as race, colour, sex, language, religion, political or other opinion, national or social origin, property, birth, or other status." The 1967 U.N. Protocol Relating to the Status of Refugees established principles for determining fairness in refugee and immigration policies.

In 1972, Ugandan President Idi Amin Dada ordered the expulsion of between 40,000 and 50,000 Asians living in Uganda. His action is an extreme example of the unfairness seen when the costs of population policy are borne by a single ethnic group. India's use of coercion to promote sterilization among beggars and other poor people between 1975 and 1977 was another case of unfair policy implementation (Gwatkin, 1979). Other examples include the testing only in low-income areas of contraceptives designed for all women (Holmes et al., 1980), and failing to tell uneducated candidates for sterilization how this operation is carried out, what it means for fertility, and what medical risks and side effects accompany it. In each of these cases the political, economic, social, and medical harms of population interventions fall more heavily on one group than another.

Truth-telling requires accurate information about population policies and avoiding lies, misrepresentations, distortions, and evasions about their content, implementation, and consequences. Though truth-telling is not explicitly stated in U.N. declarations of human rights, it is a prerequisite for the other four principles cited. Lies about policies of fertility control, migration, and refugees can jeopardize human life when they involve fatal risks, such as death from infections or from being shot in enemy territory. They limit freedom by depriving individuals of the knowledge necessary to make an informed choice, such as information about the side effects of sterilization. Lies harm welfare when they cause risk to one's income, education, or job prospects, and they violate fairness when they are more likely to be told to one group, such as the poor or an ethnic minority, than to others.

Life, freedom, welfare, fairness, and truth-telling can conflict with each other. Faced with what they see as excessive population growth, government officials may claim that the common welfare demands restrictions on reproductive freedom and allows distortions of the truth, such as not disclosing the medical risks of contraceptives, in order to make birth control seem attractive. Also citing the national interest, political leaders may decide to exterminate members of a specific religion, such as Jews in German territory during World War II; expel an entire ethnic group from the country, as happened in Uganda; or put severe limits on the entry of immigrants they define as hostile to the national interest, as happened when the U.S. government used

ships to block the entry of Haitian refugees in the early 1990s. All three policies subordinate fairness toward religious and ethnic groups to local definitions of the common welfare. Are such policies justified, or are there some principles that cannot be sacrificed to promote others?

The Universal Declaration puts no relative weights on the many rights it endorses. However, later agreements do set priorities among rights. In Article 15, the European Convention on Human Rights states that even in national emergencies, governments cannot use murder, torture, degrading punishments, slavery, or servitude. These rights thus hold the highest rank. Nothing, including government concerns about the damage due to population growth, can override them. The International Covenant on Civil and Political Rights, drafted after the European Convention, accepts all the rights that the Convention declares immune to being overridden and adds others, particularly freedom of thought, conscience, and religion. Henry Shue (1980) and James Nickel (1987) suggest comparable criteria for weighing human rights while Sissela Bok (1978) discusses the value of truth-telling and the conditions under which it may be suspended.

Application to population interventions

The viability of any framework of population ethics depends on its ability to illuminate right and wrong in specific policies, strategies, and sets of actions. Policies set the directions for population interventions, strategies show the broad plans for following those directions, and actions indicate what happens in the field, whether intended or not. The ethics of the three are not necessarily the same. Policies may be stated in humane terms and yet be accompanied by strategies that are coercive. Strategies can be expressed in benign language but, through deliberate initiatives or neglect, lead to field actions that compromise truth, limit freedom, damage human welfare, and in extreme cases, threaten life. Ethical analysis must pay close attention not only to official statements of policies and strategies, but also to how the programs they generate are carried out.

The five ethical principles will now be applied to three examples of interventions begun by population policies. In each case the aim will be to lay out the key principle or principles involved and to indicate how apparent tensions among principles might be resolved.

The "population problem." Population policies usually begin with some notion of a problem. For strong advocates of fertility control, such as Paul Ehrlich and Anne Ehrlich (1990), the problem is captured in phrases such as "the population bomb" or "the population explosion." According to others, particularly Julian Simon

(1981), population growth brings many benefits to society, including the stimulation of human creativity. And for some, fertility, migration, and refugees are complex phenomena that must be carefully studied and that may produce no catchwords that draw public attention.

Any definition of a population problem, or a statement that there is none, must be governed by the principle of truth-telling. Those claiming a problem exists should indicate the good promoted or the evil created by fertility, migration, and refugees. What, precisely, has population done to make it qualify as a problem or a nonproblem?

Statements of a problem should also give a fair summary of the evidence bearing on the subject and its limitations. If the findings are drawn from simulations, or cover a small sample of the countries in the world, those points should be disclosed. Scholars violate truth-telling when they say or imply that simulations done through a hypothetical model of reality are equivalent to data on what people or organizations actually do. Further, when scholars who write on population work for or are funded by organizations promoting or trying to prevent action on population, such as the World Bank or a right-to-life committee, can it be determined whether they have remained objective or have taken on the advocacy role of their sponsors? If scholars have merged research and advocacy, do they indicate where research stops and advocacy begins? Truth-telling requires that all relevant information be presented, even when it may harm one's active endorsement of a policy.

Claims that a problem exists must next show the specific connection between research evidence and the good or evil that makes it a problem. That connection often proves elusive. Data showing that the poorest nations of the world have the highest fertility and the wealthiest nations the lowest fertility may seem to establish a link between population growth and economic development. Indeed, such data are commonly used to support claims of a "population bomb." Yet many studies have failed to show that rapid population growth holds back economic development in the industrialized or developing countries, and a few suggest that it may have advantages (Boserup, 1990; National Research Council, 1986). To meet the standard of truth-telling, scholars should not, as often happens, cite only those studies that support the view of a population problem to which they subscribe and omit contrary evidence.

Using coercion.   China has used coercion to force some of its citizens to limit fertility. "Coercion" means using or threatening to use physical force or severe deprivation in order to make people do things they would not normally do. Governments apply physical force when they order armed police or military officers to take citizens against their will to clinics that perform abortion or sterilization, or when they credibly threaten

with torture couples who have more than two children. They use severe deprivation when they require that poor citizens be sterilized before they can obtain a job or receive food supplies necessary for their own and their family's welfare; warn that parents with more than a certain number of children will be put in prison or have their houses demolished; or use other threats that carry serious risks to life, health, and welfare.

China has relied on coercion to carry out its one-child-per-couple policy (Aird, 1990). The Chinese government claims that its policies are voluntary, but its pressure on field workers to meet their targets, particularly in cities, has led to coercive implementation. According to Tyrene White: "Beijing's penetration to the household is awesome. In 1979 mobilization campaigns for 'voluntary' sterilizations, abortions, and adoption of contraceptive measures were widespread, and the fine line between persuasion and coercion was crossed frequently" (1987, p. 315). Two other scholars comment: "During 1979 and in some subsequent years, in some urban areas and provinces, women pregnant with a second or higher order child were required to abort the pregnancies. Instances of mandatory sterilization were also reported" (Hardee-Cleaveland and Banister, 1988, p. 275).

China's use of coercion and heavy pressures to reduce fertility has, from indications, led to female infanticide and adoption (Johansson and Nygren, 1991). In traditional China, men had the basic duty of continuing the descent line of their fathers by having a son. This boy could carry on the family name, support his parents in their old age, and inherit their property. Failure to have a son showed ingratitude to one's ancestors and discredited men in their own communities. This tradition has continued to the present. If a man's only child is a daughter, he and his neighbors may feel that he has not fulfilled one of his most basic duties in life. Yet a successful one-child policy would mean that many males could not have a son. Demographic analysis strongly suggests a clash between a couple's normal desire to keep and raise their daughters and the limits on having sons imposed by the country's policies on fertility control.

Terence Hull (1990) shows that in 1987 the sex ratios in China—the number of males per 100 females—were nearly 111, compared to an earlier reference norm of 106. Using comparable data, Sten Johansson and Ola Nygren (1991) estimate that from 1985 through 1987 the average number of missing girls (those normally expected to be in the population but, in fact, missing from it) was about 500,000 per year or 1,500,000 for those three years alone. These authors and others writing about the many millions of missing girls in China attribute this phenomenon to the one-child-per-couple policy. They offer four possible explanations: infanticide caused by deliberate actions of the parents or neglect leading to fatal illnesses; a higher proportion of abortions for female than male babies; births not properly registered with the authorities, usually because they were beyond the local quota for couples; and the practice of offering female children for adoption. The evidence offered by Johansson and Nygren suggests the presence of excess female infant deaths, whether from infanticide or other reasons; unregistered babies; and female adoption.

China's coercive policies show the severe tensions between limiting population for the common good and life, freedom, and fairness. If, in response to the one-child norm, Chinese couples have used female infanticide to raise their chances of having a son, compulsion clashes with the infant girl's right to life. Government officials may say that they never intended to encourage infanticide, but that statement does not absolve them of responsibility for the deaths that take place. A full ethical analysis of policies must take account not only of official declarations and intentions, but also of the actions to which they lead. If, as seems to be the case, the policy of one child per couple has led to infanticide, by U.N. standards of human rights this sacrifice of life cannot be justified by the argument that China's overpopulation demands stringent control of fertility. In social policies, life holds such a high value that it cannot be traded off for even the most compelling public claims.

Coercive policies also put unjustifiable limits on human freedom. Unlike life, freedom can be and often is restricted for the common good. Laws, tax regulations, and many other policies indicate what individuals and groups must and must not do. But forcing citizens to undergo sterilizations or abortions that they do not want, as has happened in China, violates the principles of liberty and human dignity endorsed in all U.N. declarations of human rights. The moral question is not whether individuals should be totally free to set their family size—which they are not in any country or culture—but whether some limits on reproductive choice violate human rights. Using force to promote small family sizes does violate those rights.

China's population interventions further raise the question of fairness. Policies leading directly or indirectly to female infanticide, the abortion of female children, or female adoption put a far heavier burden on girls than boys. Abortion and infanticide mean that, through the decisions of their parents, girls stand a lower chance than boys of being born or of surviving to be adults. With adoption, young girls survive but do not have the same opportunity as male children to be raised by their parents. All three outcomes violate fairness by providing more benefits to boys than to girls and more harms to girls than to boys.

Inadequate medical support. Fertility control programs in low-income countries sometimes lead to a conflict between efficiency in delivering services and health care for those receiving the services. To raise efficiency, program managers may insist that field workers meet the targets set for them and threaten with severe punishments those who do not comply. During India's birth-control campaign between 1975 and 1977, which relied heavily on forced sterilization, the Chief Secretary of the state of Uttar Pradesh sent this telegraph to his subordinates: ". . . Failure to achieve monthly targets will not only result in the stoppage of salaries but also suspension and severest penalties. Galvanise entire administrative machinery forthwith and continue to report daily progress by . . . wireless to me and secretary to Chief Minister" (Gwatkin, 1979, p. 41).

Managers and staff working under such pressures often provide little or no health support for those receiving their services. In India during the period mentioned, hundreds of men died from infections that developed after hastily performed sterilizations with no medical follow-up (Gwatkin, 1979, p. 47). Other health hazards caused by fertility-control methods include severe, and sometimes fatal, upper reproductive-tract infections among women not properly screened for the intrauterine device; medical complications produced by using the Dalkon shield and high-dose oral contraceptives in developing countries when their risks were well-known in the United States and Europe; reproductive-tract infections among thousands of women in poor countries; and disruptions of the menstrual cycle, heavy bleeding or spotting, weight gain, depression, headaches, dizziness, fatigue, bloating, or loss of libido among women using the injectable contraceptive Depo-Provera (National Research Council, 1989; Schearer, 1983).

Ethical responsibilities of fertility-control programs

Given these risks to life and health, officials responsible for fertility-control programs face three questions of ethics. The first question concerns the amount of information about the hazards of a particular method that should be disclosed by program staff to their clients. With heavy pressure from their superiors to meet their targets, field workers often emphasize the benefits of a method and conceal its risks. This practice violates the principle of freedom, which requires that clients have reasonable information about risks and benefits to make an informed choice about fertility control. Even when clients cannot grasp sophisticated explanations of medical hazards, they can be told what is at stake in language that they understand. When the risks not disclosed are serious, clients may also face threats to their life, their health, or their welfare.

The second ethical question concerns the adequacy of health services to deal with the hazards created by methods of fertility control. Some argue that, given the severity of the population problem, governments are morally justified in operating fertility-control services well ahead of health-support services. Others, particularly groups supporting the rights of women in family-planning programs, claim that this strategy not only violates human rights but produces a backlash against birth control. Clients who have not been told of any possible side effects or complications from the methods offered and who then suffer poor health can retaliate in many ways. They may discontinue the methods they have started, accept a method but not use it, start rumors about the physical dangers of birth control, stay away from family-planning clinics and field workers, enlist religious leaders or political parties to make fertility control a political issue, vote against the government in the next election, or, if they are truly angry, riot against the government in power. Many of these reactions followed India's use of coercion between 1975 and 1977.

The third ethical question is fairness in the distribution of medical harms and benefits among individuals and groups. This issue arises in the testing as well as the distribution of fertility-control methods. Beginning with the contraceptive pill, whose main evaluation was carried out in Puerto Rico, drug companies have often tested new methods of fertility control on poor individuals in developing countries. Government regulations on testing in those countries have been far less strict than in the United States. Moreover, the low-income individuals chosen for the testing asked few questions about what was being done and were unlikely to mount political protests or begin lawsuits to receive compensation for damage to their health. During the distribution of fertility-control methods, poor individuals in many countries likewise have received less adequate explanations and suffered more health hazards than those with higher incomes. As one example, for many years the U.S. government, citing health risks, banned the domestic use of the injectable contraceptive Depo-Provera. But it saw no problem including Depo-Provera as part of the contraceptive services in poor nations supported by U.S. foreign aid.

Four ethical guidelines help to resolve these conflicts. First, no program should knowingly threaten the life of its clients by using methods that can cause death or by failing to provide health services. If, as happened in India, sterilized males apply animal dung to areas of pain, and if that folk remedy proves fatal, fertility-control programs must take all possible steps to prevent its use.

Second, programs must offer health care for all users of methods with serious medical risks. In its villages, Indonesia has developed a simple system of health care often located in the home of the village head or another resident. Should clients show symptoms that cannot be treated there, they are referred to the nearest health clinic or hospital.

Third, clients must be told, in words they understand, about the risks as well as the benefits of fertility-control methods. To deny potential users information about risks unjustifiably limits their freedom of choice. Explanations need not be elaborate to be accurate, but they must be given.

Fourth, the distribution of risks and benefits from fertility-control programs should be fair, though not necessarily equal. Poor persons should not be the main candidates on whom fertility-control methods are tested, nor should some groups of citizens receive adequate health support while others receive little or none.

To promote user freedom and welfare, program designers and field workers can be trained to adopt the standards of quality suggested by Judith Bruce (1990). Quality care requires technical competence that gives accurate information to users in language they understand; informed consent that shows sensitivity to concerns about modesty among women and girls; pain management; and continuous rather than one-time service to clients. Instead of aiming only to avoid violations of human rights, which might attain that goal but result in mediocre care, staff can be taught to seek high client satisfaction with fertility-control services.

Stepladder ethics: A contrast

Ethical principles based on internationally accepted standards of human rights contrast sharply with the stepladder ethics proposed by Bernard Berelson and Jonathan Lieberson (1979). Berelson was president of the Population Council, a visible center of research, training, and advocacy on population policy, and Lieberson was a philosopher who served as adviser to the Population Council and taught at Columbia University. These two authors commanded attention and respect, and their article was the first and last systematic analysis of ethics to appear in *Population and Development Review*, the leading journal on population policy.

Berelson and Lieberson offered this pivotal statement about population ethics: "Employ less severe measures where possible and only ascend to harsher measures if the problem at hand, as a matter of (established) fact, is clearly grave enough to warrant it" (1979, p. 596). They continued: ". . . The degree of coercive policy brought into play should be proportional to the degree of seriousness of the present problem and should be introduced only after less coercive means have been exhausted. Thus overt violence or other potentially injurious coercion is not to be used before noninjurious coercion has been exhausted" (1979, p. 602). Their moral stepladder involves beginning with voluntary policies and, if they fail, moving up the scale of pressure on people to the point justified by the seriousness of the population problem. They do not mention fertility-control measures involving threats to life, but, by their logic, governments facing exceptionally severe problems from population growth would be allowed to use those methods as well.

The authors state that they are writing out of a Western, individualistic mode, and recognize that other countries draw ethical principles from different philosophical and political traditions. They do not mention U.N. declarations on human rights, or the widely varying views of the world's religions on methods of fertility control. They apply their Western code to the strategies adopted by countries whose local standards are very different from their own. Leaders in countries populated by Catholics, Buddhists, and Muslims, for instance, might vigorously challenge the principle of allowing governments to use any form of coercion in limiting fertility. Stepladder ethics provides no means of developing cross-national ethical principles whose morality derives mainly from religion or from assumptions that differ from those of the authors, including human rights.

Stepladder ethics thus differs greatly from principles based on universally accepted human rights. Norms such as life, freedom, fairness, and welfare provide a basis for developing ethical guidelines for population policies that apply to every society. Like all ethical principles, those norms need clear definition and are often violated in practice, but they open the way for discussion among persons from diverse political systems and religious traditions and beliefs.

Conclusions

To be applicable to the hundreds of countries and cultures across the world, population ethics must be based on widely shared norms. Principles drawing on the assumptions of a single society or culture will often be rejected by those from other backgrounds. Moreover, to be viable in helping decisions about population policies, the principles chosen should have priorities assigned to them. They must be able to answer one of the most challenging questions in ethics: Is it morally acceptable to sacrifice one principle, such as life, for another, such as the common welfare?

This article proposes four principles based on international declarations of human rights: life, freedom, welfare, and fairness. It adds truth-telling as a fifth principle valuable in itself and necessary in reaching the other four. When these principles clash, life receives first priority. In contrast to stepladder ethics, which grants no human rights, the ethical framework proposed here bans any method of population control with serious

risks of death or those relying on torture, slavery, servitude, or other degrading punishments.

If adopted, this ethical framework would have the same advantages and limitations as all universal codes of human rights. The main advantage is that it can be used to educate policymakers and field workers on what is and is not morally acceptable in population programs. When a program violates its standards, U.N. organizations, including the Commission on Human Rights, or private groups, such as Amnesty International, could document the abuses of human rights and demand more humane policies or practices. As has already happened, universal codes can also stimulate geographic regions, such as Europe and Latin America, or major religions to examine human rights from other perspectives. S. M. Haider (1978) and his associates, for example, found many parallels and some differences between Islamic teaching and the Universal Declaration of Human Rights.

The key drawback to this framework is that, like other declarations of human rights, it might be viewed as noble in the abstract but unworkable in practice. Critics could say that it embodies foreign rather than national standards and takes no account of the difficulties with population control that face an overcrowded nation. Even so, it would give local and international advocates of human rights criteria that could be used to develop political and moral pressure to end abuses such as forced sterilization and abortion. And it would avoid the charge, leveled against stepladder ethics, that its ethical standards derive from one country or region, such as the West.

A normative framework based on internationally accepted standards of human rights offers no simple answers to the complex ethical difficulties found in population programs. It does, however, provide a foundation for discussing morality among those who hold widely different views about politics, religion, ethics, and culture. Without that foundation there will never be any serious analysis or lasting agreement about what should and should not be done in population policies and programs.

DONALD P. WARWICK

Directly related to this article are the articles in the other sections of this entry. Also directly related are the entries POPULATION POLICIES; *and* ETHICS, *article on* NORMATIVE ETHICAL THEORIES. *For a further discussion of topics mentioned in this article, see the entries* ABORTION; ADOPTION; FERTILITY CONTROL; FIDELITY AND LOYALTY; FOOD POLICY; FREEDOM AND COERCION; HARM; INFANTS, *article on* HISTORY OF INFANTICIDE; INFORMATION DISCLOSURE; INFORMED CONSENT; JUSTICE; LIFE; MEDICAL ETHICS, HISTORY OF, *section on* SOUTH AND EAST ASIA, *article on* INDIA, *and subsection on* CHINA, *article on* CONTEMPORARY CHINA; PAIN AND SUFFERING;

RIGHTS; RISK; SEXISM; *and* UTILITY. *For a discussion of related ideas, see the entries* ABUSE, INTERPERSONAL, *article on* CHILD ABUSE; CHILDREN, *especially the article on* HISTORY OF CHILDHOOD; FAMILY; FUTURE GENERATIONS, OBLIGATIONS TO; NATIONAL SOCIALISM; *and* VALUE AND VALUATION.

Bibliography

AIRD, JOHN S. 1990. *Slaughter of the Innocents: Coercive Birth Control in China.* Washington, D.C.: AEI Press.

BERELSON, BERNARD, and LIEBERSON, JONATHAN. 1979. "Government Efforts to Influence Fertility: The Ethical Issues." *Population and Development Review* 5, no. 4: 581–613.

BOK, SISSELA. 1978. *Lying: Moral Choice in Public and Private Life.* New York: Pantheon Books.

BOSERUP, ESTER. 1990. *Economic and Demographic Relationships in Development.* Baltimore: Johns Hopkins University Press.

BROWN, PETER G., and SHUE, HENRY, eds. 1981. *Boundaries: National Autonomy and Its Limits.* Totowa, N.J.: Rowman & Littlefield.

BRUCE, JUDITH. 1990. "Fundamental Elements of the Quality of Care: A Simple Framework." *Studies in Family Planning* 21, no. 2:61–91.

CLAUDE, RICHARD PIERRE, and WESTON, BURNS H., eds. 1989. *Human Rights in the World Community: Issues and Action.* Philadelphia: University of Pennsylvania Press.

DIXON-MUELLER, RUTH, and WASSERHEIT, JUDITH N. 1991. *The Culture of Silence: Reproductive Tract Infections Among Women in the Third World.* New York: International Women's Health Coalition.

EHRLICH, PAUL R., and EHRLICH, ANNE H. 1990. *The Population Explosion.* New York: Simon & Schuster.

FERINGA, BARBARA; IDEN, SARA; and ROSENFIELD, ALLAN. 1992. "NORPLANT: Potential for Coercion." In *Norplant and Poor Women,* pp. 57–63. Edited by Sarah-Ellen Samuels and Mark P. Smith. Menlo Park, Calif.: Henry J. Kaiser Family Foundation.

GWATKIN, DAVIDSON R. 1979. "Political Will and Family Planning: The Implications of India's Emergency Experience." *Population and Development Review* 5, no. 1:29–59.

HAIDER, S. M. 1978. *Islamic Concept of Human Rights.* Lahore, Pakistan: Book House.

HARDEE-CLEAVELAND, KAREN, and BANISTER, JUDITH. 1988. "Fertility Policy and Implementation in China, 1986–1988." *Population and Development Review* 14, no. 2: 245–286.

HOLMES, HELEN B.; HOSKINS, BETTY B.; and GROSS, MICHAEL, eds. 1980. *Birth Control and Controlling Birth: Women-Centered Perspectives.* Clifton, N.J.: Humana Press.

HULL, TERENCE H. 1990. "Recent Trends in Sex Ratios at Birth in China." *Population and Development Review* 16, no. 1:63–83.

JOHANSSON, STEN, and NYGREN, OLA. 1991. "The Missing Girls of China: A New Demographic Account." *Population and Development Review* 17, no. 1:35–51.

NATIONAL RESEARCH COUNCIL (U.S.). WORKING GROUP ON THE HEALTH CONSEQUENCES OF CONTRACEPTIVE USE AND CONTROLLED FERTILITY. 1989. *Contraception and Reproduction: Health Consequences for Women and Children in the Developing World.* Washington, D.C.: National Academy Press.

———. WORKING GROUP ON POPULATION GROWTH AND ECONOMIC DEVELOPMENT. 1986. *Population Growth and Economic Development: Policy Questions.* Washington, D.C.: National Academy Press.

NICKEL, JAMES W. 1987. *Making Sense of Human Rights: Philosophical Reflections on the Universal Declaration of Human Rights.* Berkeley: University of California Press.

SCHEARER, S. BRUCE. 1983. "Monetary and Health Costs of Contraception." In *Fertility Regulation and Institutional Influences,* pp. 103–122. Vol. 2 of *Determinants of Fertility in Developing Countries.* Edited by Rodolfo A. Bulatao and Ronald D. Lee. New York: Academic Press.

SHUE, HENRY. 1980. *Basic Rights: Substance, Affluence, and U.S. Foreign Policy.* Princeton, N.J.: Princeton University Press.

SIMON, JULIAN L. 1981. *The Ultimate Resource.* Princeton, N.J.: Princeton University Press.

VEATCH, ROBERT M., ed. 1977. *Population Policy and Ethics: The American Experience.* New York: Irvington Publishers.

WARWICK, DONALD P. 1982. *Bitter Pills: Population Policies and Their Implementation in Eight Developing Countries.* New York: Cambridge University Press.

———. 1990. "The Ethics of Population Control." In *Population Policy: Contemporary Issues,* pp. 21–37. Edited by Godfrey Roberts. New York: Praeger.

WHITE, TYRENE. 1987. "Implementing the 'One-Child-per-Couple' Population Program in Rural China: National Goals and Local Politics." In *Policy Implementation in Post-Mao China,* pp. 284–317. Edited by David M. Lampton. Berkeley: University of California Press.

WORLD POPULATION CONFERENCE. 1975. *Report of the United Nations World Population Conference, 1974, Bucharest, 19–30 August, 1974.* E/CONF.60/19. New York: United Nations.

III. RELIGIOUS TRADITIONS

A. INTRODUCTION

How and to what extent religion influences population policies and the practices of individuals, couples, and larger groups is a very complex question. Although specific religious teachings about marriage, ideal family size, and the permissibility of birth control or abortion would seem to bear on reproductive decision making, the actual effects of these religious beliefs and teachings are not easily traced. Explicitly pronatalist doctrines that espouse the value of having many children and oppose birth limitation sometimes have little effect on reproductive behaviors or policies, while other aspects of religion, seemingly remote from reproductive decision making, can have powerful demographic effects.

Until recently, most major religions stressed marriage as a religiously sanctified state and were pronatalist in outlook; such teachings reflected the perilous demographic circumstances in which these religions were formed. Although Eastern Orthodox Christianity and most Protestant denominations have come to accept the use of contraception for family planning, some other major traditions have concretized traditional religious pronatalism in specific beliefs that discourage the use of birth control. Roman Catholicism continues to prohibit contraception and sterilization; Orthodox Judaism forbids use of the condom or any male methods that prevent insemination. Classical Islam, Hinduism, and Confucianism, while more permissive regarding use of birth control, share the traditional religious bias in favor of marriage and large families. Although abortion has played an important role in societies that have undergone population stabilization, no historical religious tradition favors the use of abortion for purposes of limiting the size of the family.

Other features of religious practice and teaching would seem to have a strong pronatalist effect. Many traditions stress the importance of offspring, especially sons, in carrying out vital religious rituals and in maintaining family continuity. The *Rigveda* (VI.61.1), Hinduism's foundational sacred text, terms a son a *rnachyuta*, one who removes the moral debts of a father and spares him from hell. In Judaism, key rituals emphasize the importance of children, especially male offspring: a son's *bris*, or circumcision ceremony, is a major source of religious joy; children play an important part in the Passover service; and the kaddish right for the dead is ideally performed by a surviving son.

In African tribal societies, veneration of the ancestors is a central religious activity. Whatever immortality awaits the individual after death depends on survivors' continued performance of family rites. Individuals without progeny are viewed as pitiful figures who may become marauding spirits after death (Molnos, 1968). Since ancestors profoundly affect the circumstances of the living, family prosperity and health require the existence of an ample number of descendants to maintain the family cult. In contrast to Euro-American views, popular opinion in some African societies favors providing a scarce, lifesaving medical therapy to a bachelor over a family man (Kilner, 1990). This reflects the belief that an individual's religious and social significance is not established until he or she founds a family.

Popular religious beliefs, as opposed to formal teaching, must also be factored into thinking about reproductive behavior. Orthodox Islam, for example, does not actively prohibit the use of birth control, and most Muslims live under governments with official family-planning programs (Omran, 1992). But popular attitudes about kismet, or fate, and the idea that Allah appoints each couple the children they are to have contribute to a widespread reluctance to adopt family-planning methods (Fagley, 1967). In Africa and elsewhere, popular beliefs about reincarnation or the existence of "souls in heaven" awaiting birth contribute to a reluctance to employ birth control.

Teachings and practices regarding women are another significant aspect of religion that contributes to high birthrates. Hinduism regards women as of lower karmic status and able to effect spiritual ascent by having children and fulfilling family duties. In different ways, most other traditional religions echo these beliefs, removing women from the central sphere of political and religious life and locating whatever spiritual fulfillment that is available to them in the home (Ruether, 1974; Carmody, 1989).

Multiple demographic consequences follow from this history of marginalization of women and treatment of them as "second-class" religious citizens. Early marriage is associated with larger completed family size. Religious values that encourage child marriage, as in India, or that discourage women's education and career preparation before marriage are therefore major contributors to higher birthrates. The existence of highly differentiated social roles for men and women also may lead to larger completed family size, since sons and daughters are less "interchangeable" in terms of their ability to fulfill parental needs (Johnson and Burton, 1989). When religiously influenced values consign women to the home, their social, economic, and spiritual value comes to depend on their reproductive success. In polygynous African tribal societies, a woman's standing among her co-wives depends on the number of her children. Her material well-being also depends on the number of progeny she has to help her with home-based economic tasks and agriculture (Molnos, 1968). Although the consequences of religious teachings and institutional practices about gender have not been measured, they may be among the most important and persistent religious influences on fertility.

These beliefs and practices affect fertility through the behavior of individuals and couples. At the institutional and policy levels, religion affects population through its impact on national and international family-planning programs. During the early 1970s, the Roman Catholic church's opposition to contraception made it difficult for the governments of some Latin American nations to mount family-planning programs (McCoy, 1974). During the 1980s, opposition to abortion by evangelical Christian groups in the United States, among others, led the U.S. government to cease support for international family-planning programs that offered abortion services or counseling. In contrast, some religious pronouncements on behalf of responsible parenthood by religious leaders in Islamic countries may have contributed to the success of family-planning programs. On balance, it is not clear how much difference religious involvement in population policy or programs makes. For example, official Roman Catholic opposition to birth control and abortion has had little or no effect on altering the very low birthrates in Catholic countries such as Austria, Ireland, or Italy.

Whatever the influence of religion at the level of national policies, there is considerable evidence that religious teachings about birth control or family size play a relatively insignificant role in couples' reproductive decision making. Decades ago, sociologists noted that socioeconomic modernization is normally accompanied by a "demographic" transition—from the high birthrates of agricultural and traditional societies to the lower birthrates and family-planning practices of urbanized societies (United Nations, 1977). Once economic and social modernization begins, this demographic transition occurs regardless of the religious basis of the society, casting doubt on the importance of the "religious factor" in reproductive behavior.

More recently, demographers and social scientists have tried to determine the precise role played by religious, economic, or social factors in reproductive decision making. While these studies have not settled all questions, some broad conclusions are widely accepted. Social and economic modernization are held to play a powerful role in reproductive behavior, usually eclipsing specific religious teachings about family size. For example, Joseph Chamie's (1981) study of fertility and religion in Lebanon shows that whatever their traditions teach, educated, urban, middle-class Catholic or Muslim couples make similar decisions about family size and reproduction; and lower-income, agricultural families have higher birthrates, regardless of their creed. In both cases, social and economic circumstances are determinative. The impact of purely religious doctrine on fertility appears significant only while a society is going through economic and social transition, when such doctrine may delay acceptance of birth control.

If a religious group is a minority and holds strong pronatalist views that are heightened by opportunities for group reinforcement, there may be some independent impact of religious teachings on fertility (Kennedy, 1973; Day, 1984; Williams and Zimmer, 1990). Studies of Mormons in the United States, for example, suggest that a pronatalism deeply rooted in Mormon theology and family values, and heightened by intragroup reinforcements, contributes to birthrates among Mormons higher than would be expected among groups of similar social and economic standing (Heaton and Calkins, 1983; Heaton, 1986).

Religious teachings and doctrines, then, may influence reproductive behavior and population growth rates, but probably far less so than the amount of attention given inside and outside religious communities to specific teachings on marriage, birth control, or abortion would suggest. Among religious teachings, those less directly related to reproductive decision making, especially the religiously sanctioned subordination of women, may have the most powerful impact on fertility.

RONALD M. GREEN

While all the articles in the other sections of this entry are relevant, see especially the other articles in this section: ISLAMIC PERSPECTIVES, PROTESTANT PERSPECTIVES, ROMAN CATHOLIC PERSPECTIVES, JEWISH PERSPECTIVES, EASTERN ORTHODOX CHRISTIAN PERSPECTIVES, HINDU PERSPECTIVES, *and* BUDDHIST PERSPECTIVES. *Directly related to this article is the entry* POPULATION POLICIES, *section on* STRATEGIES OF FERTILITY CONTROL. *For a further discussion of topics mentioned in this article, see the entries* ABORTION, *especially the section on* RELIGIOUS TRADITIONS; AFRICAN RELIGION; BUDDHISM; CHILDREN, *articles on* HISTORY OF CHILDHOOD, *and* RIGHTS OF CHILDREN; CONFUCIANISM; EASTERN ORTHODOX CHRISTIANITY; FAMILY; FERTILITY CONTROL; HINDUISM; ISLAM; JUDAISM; MARRIAGE AND OTHER DOMESTIC PARTNERSHIPS; PROTESTANTISM; ROMAN CATHOLICISM; SEXISM; SEXUAL ETHICS; *and* WOMEN, *article on* HISTORICAL AND CROSS-CULTURAL PERSPECTIVES. *For a discussion of related ideas, see the entries* CIRCUMCISION; FEMINISM; FETUS; FUTURE GENERATIONS, OBLIGATIONS TO; INFANTS; JAINISM; LIFE; NATIVE AMERICAN RELIGIONS; RACE AND RACISM; SIKHISM; *and* TAOISM. *Other relevant material may be found under the entries* ENVIRONMENT AND RELIGION; HOMOSEXUALITY; *and* REPRODUCTIVE TECHNOLOGIES.

Bibliography

CARMODY, DENISE L. 1989. *Women and World Religions.* Englewood Cliffs, N.J.: Prentice-Hall.

CHAMIE, JOSEPH. 1981. *Religion and Fertility: Arab Christian–Muslim Differentials.* Cambridge: At the University Press.

DAY, LINCOLN H. 1984. "Minority-Group Status and Fertility: A More Detailed Test of the Hypothesis." *Sociological Quarterly* 25, no. 4:456–472.

FAGLEY, RICHARD M. 1967. "Doctrines and Attitudes of Major Religions in Regard to Fertility." In *Proceedings of the World Population Conference: Belgrade, 30 August–10 September, 1965,* vol. 2, *Selected Papers and Summaries: Fertility; Family Planning; Mortality,* pp. 78–84. E/CONF. 41/ 3. New York: United Nations, Department of Economic and Social Affairs.

HEATON, TIM B. 1986. "How Does Religion Influence Fertility? The Case of the Mormons." *Journal for the Scientific Study of Religion* 25, no. 2:248–258.

HEATON, TIM B., and CALKINS, SANDRA. 1983. "Family Size and Contraceptive Use Among Mormons: 1965–76." *Review of Religious Research* 25, no. 2:102–113.

JOHNSON, NAN E., and BURTON, LINDA M. 1989. "Religion and Reproduction in Philippine Society: A New Test of the Minority-Groups Status Hypothesis." *Women in International Development.* Working Paper #178. East Lansing: Michigan State University.

KENNEDY, ROBERT E., JR. 1973. "Minority-Group Status and Fertility: The Irish." *American Sociological Review* 38, no. 1:85–96.

KILNER, JOHN F. 1990. *Who Lives? Who Dies? Ethical Criteria in Patient Selection.* New Haven, Conn.: Yale University Press.

McCOY, TERRY L., ed. 1974. *The Dynamics of Population Policy in Latin America.* Cambridge, Mass.: Ballinger.

MOLNOS, ANGELA. 1968. *Attitudes Toward Family Planning in East Africa.* Munich: Weltforum Verlag.

OMRAN, ABDEL RAHIM. 1992. *Family Planning in the Legacy of Islam.* London: Routledge.

RUETHER, ROSEMARY RADFORD, ed. 1974. *Religion and Sexism: Images of Woman in the Jewish and Christian Traditions.* New York: Simon and Schuster.

UNITED NATIONS/UNFPA EXPERT GROUP. 1979. *Demographic Transition and Socio-Economic Development.* New York: Author.

WILLIAMS, LINDA B., and ZIMMER, BASIL G. 1990. "The Changing Influence of Religion on U.S. Fertility: The Evidence from Rhode Island." *Demography* 27, no. 3: 475–481.

B. ISLAMIC PERSPECTIVES

Population issues in Islam are the product of the interplay of faith and experience, Muslim belief and local social realities. Like Islam itself, in which unity of faith has been expressed by a diversity of practice, so the application of Islam to population issues has been conditioned by local circumstances and customs as well as personal piety. Understanding the issue of population control in Islam requires an appreciation both of the history of Islamic thought and practice and of its implementation in Muslim countries today.

The impact of Islam on population policies reflects the continuous interaction of religious teaching, local cultural traditions, and national politics. The diverse results of that interaction lead to great variation in the population policies of Muslim countries. Thus the government's approach to fertility control in Indonesia and Egypt differs greatly from that in Saudi Arabia and Iran. The first two have long had active fertility-control programs supported by senior Islamic officials. Saudi Arabia has no active family-planning program. Iran, for religious and political reasons, discontinued its family-plan-

ning program after the country's revolution in 1979 (Ross, 1991). However, in 1992, responding to severe economic and social conditions, including a rapid population growth, Iran reinstated its program with the approval of the religious leaders (*ulama*).

Muslim attitudes toward population control are influenced by beliefs and values concerning the nature and purpose of society, the family, marriage, procreation, and child rearing; they also reflect responses to several centuries of Western influence and dominance. The locus of Muslim norms and ethical standards is the Shari'a, Islamic law, which constitutes the blueprint for the ideal Islamic society. Shari'a consists of those rules and institutions that God has revealed in the Qur'an. In the early centuries of Islam, pious scholars in various Muslim capitals attempted to delineate God's law for the community. They produced a body of law that combined God's word with human interpretation and application of that word. The difference between the divine component of the law and human interpretations or applications of it has provided the rationale for legal change.

Islamic law is based upon four sources: the Qur'an, which Muslims believe is the literal and perfect word of God; the Sunnah, or example of the Prophet Muhammad; analogical reasoning; and the consensus of the community. Islamic law constitutes a comprehensive ideal that provides guidelines for personal and social life, a Muslim's duties to God (worship), and duties to society (social transactions). Jurists also recognized a number of subsidiary sources. Among the most relevant utilized for social and legal reform is public welfare. Sunni and Shiite Islam, the two major groups or traditions within the Islamic community, have a number of law schools, or schools of legal thought. Their laws, while in general agreement, nevertheless include a diversity of orientations, rules, and methods.

Muslim family law, covering marriage, divorce, and inheritance, has long been considered the heart of the Shari'a, an especially sacrosanct component of Islamic law. Historically, the family has been regarded as the basis of Muslim society. As the nucleus of the Islamic community, it is where the next generation receives its religious, social, and cultural training. In modern times, Muslim families, like those in much of the world, have undergone significant change. This is especially clear in the shift from extended to nuclear families as well as in greater educational and employment opportunities for women. These changes have been the subject of continued debate and legal reform.

Reforms in family or gender issues, from family law to population policies, have been widespread and the subject of controversy. During the latter part of the twentieth century, after Muslim nations had gained their independence from European colonial powers, many continued to look to the West for their models or paradigms of development. Political, economic, legal, and social changes were Western-inspired or -oriented, as were modern Muslim elites. As a result, social change, like political and legal reform, has often been judged both in terms of its relationship to the Islamic tradition and its law and within the context of reactions to Western influence, if not hegemony, in the Muslim world.

Marriage and the family

Marriage in Islam is a sacred contract, though not a sacrament, between two individuals and also between their families (Esposito, 1980). Sexuality in Islam is centered on marriage and the family. The married state is the norm—indeed, the ideal—for all Muslims, prescribed by Islamic law and embodied in the life of Muhammad, the exemplar of Muslim life. Celibacy, while permitted if necessary, is not regarded as an ideal. Though procreation and the formation of the family are among the primary purposes of marriage, Muslim jurists from early in Islamic history permitted contraception to limit the size of a family.

Islamic teachings on methods of fertility control depend on the method used. While open to the use of coitus interruptus and methods of contraception such as the pill, many Muslim scholars oppose any form of abortion; others accept it only to save the life of the mother during the first 120 days of pregnancy. Though some Islamic jurists accept sterilization to avoid having more children, most oppose this method unless it is a medical treatment.

Contraception

In contrast to the Christian and Jewish traditions, from earliest times the Islamic tradition showed acceptance of family planning and contraception. From the tenth to the twentieth centuries, the vast majority of legal scholars and all the major schools of law accepted coitus interruptus between a husband and wife. Early acceptance of birth control was built on a combination of sacred texts, biological knowledge, and reason (Musallam, 1978). The Qur'an contains no clear or explicit text regarding birth control. However, the traditions (*hadith*) of the Prophet do. Though some *hadith* forbid birth control, the majority permit it. Muslim jurists were able to construct an argument based on *hadith* and the biological knowledge of the times to declare birth control by means of coitus interruptus as licit. They argued that such means do not limit or counter God's power because they are not foolproof. Thus, if God wanted a woman to become pregnant, his will could and would prevail despite the practice of coitus interruptus.

The prominent religious scholar al-Ghazālī (d. 1111) is representative of the majority of Sunni Muslim jurists who accepted the use of contraception through coitus interruptus. For Ghazālī, coitus interruptus was not only licit but also permissible, regardless of the need to practice it, because there was no explicit text in the Qur'an or Sunnah against it, nor was there clear judicial precedent based on an explicit text:

> We have ruled out its [coitus interruptus] . . . prohibition because, to establish prohibition, one has to have a text [from the Qur'an or Sunnah] or resort to analogous reasoning based on a precedence for which a text is available. In this case . . . there is neither a text nor a precedent for analogical reasoning. (Omran, 1992, p. 80)

The vast majority of Sunni and Shiite jurists believed that birth control through the use of coitus interruptus was permissible. However, because it deprived a woman of her right to children and to sexual satisfaction, her consent was required.

Despite the historical record of jurists regarding the permissibility of contraception, some scholars, such as Ibn Hazm (d. 1064), and local religious leaders viewed contraception as prohibited by Islam because they regarded increase in the number of Muslims as a Prophetic (Muhammad's) command. Though the Qur'an has no text that forbids contraception, critics of contraception interpret it to construct and legitimate their case. Among the major arguments offered are that it (1) constitutes infanticide, which is expressly forbidden by the Qur'an; (2) is contrary to belief in God's power and in divine providence, articulated in the Qur'an's teaching that God is the all-powerful creator and ruler or overseer of the world, and that he determines and controls the destiny of all (81:29 and 11:6); (3) ignores the Qur'anic mandate to trust or rely on God; and (4) ignores the necessary connection between marriage and procreation, the primary purpose of marriage.

In modern times, many Muslims, reacting to the impact of Western colonialism and imperialism, have argued that by diminishing the number of Muslims, contraception undermines the power of the Muslim community. More specifically, they charge that birth-control campaigns and programs are part of a Western conspiracy to limit development in the Muslim world and thus subdue Islam.

Modern Islamic thought

The adoption of Western-inspired legal systems in many Muslim countries in the nineteenth and twentieth centuries limited the scope of Islamic law and the prestige and authority of religious scholars. However, because of the centrality of the family in Muslim society, in most countries family-law and family-planning issues continued to be strongly influenced by Islamic law and ethics. Consciousness of and concern over the implications of a population explosion in areas with limited and shrinking resources, the battle against poverty and illiteracy, urbanization, education and changing expectations, and the development of modern methods of contraception have made the issues of fertility control more prominent and contentious in Muslim societies. Government-sponsored family-planning programs and policies have become common in Muslim countries such as Indonesia, Egypt, Iran, and Bangladesh. Government intervention and implementation of such programs have met with mixed success. In many Muslim countries, when governments introduced fertility-control programs, they often looked to Islamic religious leaders to legitimate their programs and to mobilize popular support. Even when they did not support fertility control, Islamic scholars, viewing it as subject to Islamic law and as a critical area of social intervention, felt it was necessary for them to give moral guidance to Muslim believers.

Legal scholars have generally provided an Islamic rationale for various modern methods to control population growth. Modern Sunni and Shiite jurists, such as Lebanon's Sheikh Muhammad M. Shamsuddin, employing the legal principle of reasoning by analogy, have argued that since birth control in the form of coitus interruptus has been accepted for so long in Islam, then by analogy other, more modern forms of birth control that achieve the same effect are acceptable (Omran, 1992). Both individual jurists and assemblies of religious scholars have issued *fatwas* (formal legal opinions) that have endorsed contraception and in turn not only have informed the consciences of individual Muslims but also have been employed by governments from Egypt to Indonesia to support their birth-control policies and programs.

On the basis of the clear legal precedent of the acceptance of contraception in the form of coitus interruptus, modern jurists have argued for the permissibility of modern chemical and mechanical forms of birth control, such as the diaphragm, the contraceptive pill, and IUDs. Egypt's Sheikh M. S. Madkour, for example, citing the opinions of early jurists, wrote:

> We may say that the first mechanical method known as coitus interruptus, *al-azl* in Arabic, used by our ancestors to prevent pregnancy, corresponds to the device used these days by women and known as the diaphragm or ring to block the uterine aperture, or to another device used by men, the condom. Both are designed to prevent the semen from reaching the ovum and fertilizing it. The second method . . . for temporary contraception [is] . . . the contraceptive pill. Under this heading may also be included the injectables much advertised and supposed to be effective for several months . . . [and] every other beneficial drug which may be discovered by the medical profession for this purpose.
> The third . . . is the [IUD], . . . which . . . prevents the fertilized egg from attaching itself to the uterine wall, and the uterus expels it instead. (Omran, 1992, p. 81)

Sheikh Tantawi, the mufti of Egypt, senior official consultant on Islamic law, in his 1988 *fatwa* recognized several reasons for practicing contraception. Couples may wish to postpone or space the birth of children for financial reasons; others may wish to do so in order to provide a separate room for a son and daughter; even those who are well off but already have three children may wish to avoid another birth because they live in an overpopulated country (Omran, 1992).

Jurists have found many licit reasons for couples to practice contraception: to avoid pregnancy due to health risks to the wife or children resulting from repeated pregnancies, transmission of hereditary or infectious diseases, or genetic risks of inbreeding; economic hardship; to better provide for children's education; and even to preserve a wife's beauty (Omran, 1992).

Muslim jurists have addressed infertility within the context of family planning. They have tended to show the same openness and flexibility in their treatment of infertility. Thus, chemical and surgical treatment, as well as artificial insemination between a husband and wife, are permitted. Insemination of a wife with her husband's sperm or in vitro fertilization is allowed. However, procedures that involve someone other than a spouse, such as inseminating a woman with sperm from a man who is not her husband, are forbidden. Children who result from such procedures are regarded as illegitimate.

Sterilization and abortion

As is the case with contraception, there is no clear text of the Qur'an or Sunnah that forbids sterilization. Although some diversity of opinion exists, the majority of jurists have maintained that sterilization for purposes of contraception, as opposed to its use for medical treatment, is forbidden. Whatever the debate among scholars, local Islamic leaders have tended to oppose sterilization. In recent years, a number of Sunni and Shiite jurists have called for a reconsideration of the legality of sterilization (Omran, 1992).

Abortion is a far more complex and contentious matter. There is a consensus among religious authorities that abortion after 120 days, when the fetus becomes "ensouled" and thus is a person, is absolutely prohibited except to save the mother's life. While many if not most jurists allow abortion as a means of contraception within

120 days of conception, this scholarly and theoretical position stands in sharp contrast with actual practice—abortion is condemned by most religious leaders and omitted from public-sector programs.

Religion, government, and population issues

During the post–World War II period, governments in the Muslim world, faced with rapid population growth, cited religious, demographic, and nationalist reasons for instituting family-planning programs. Some utilized the prestige and authority of the religious establishment to legitimate family-planning policies. In Egypt, the government has often looked to the leadership and scholars of Cairo's al-Azhar University, a historic and authoritative international center of Islamic learning, for support. Fatwas obtained from experts (muftis) in Islamic law have played a prominent role in legitimating population policies throughout the Muslim world. However, differences often exist between official religious decrees and the more conservative responses of local religious leaders and popular beliefs. Since there is no organized church or hierarchy in Islam, and no clear text from revelation or consensus of scholars exists, local religious leaders and their followers are free to hold a variety of opinions.

Islam has legitimated and reinforced traditional pronatalist beliefs and practices in areas where social conditions have made large families desirable. Agricultural and pastoral societies have regarded large families as providing a source of labor, insurance against the loss of help due to high mortality or marriage, and social security in old age. Poverty, illiteracy, lack of educational and employment opportunities, and high mortality often foster and promote a belief in the necessity of a large family. Thus, many Muslims have been raised in a social context in which a primary emphasis on procreation in marriage and large families has been the traditional ideal and norm, a custom reinforced by the preaching and teaching of local religious leaders.

Local beliefs, attitudes, and values have reinforced high fertility rates. Values such as early marriage for women and emphasis on fertility and large families, in particular the importance of having a male child, pressure a young wife to gain the status of motherhood to "prove herself." Women also want to avoid the stigma of infertility and with it the possibility of divorce or of the husband taking a second wife. The importance of motherhood is reflected in the common practice in many Arab countries, once a woman has given birth to a male child, to call her by the name of that firstborn male child, that is, "mother of. . . ."

Government-sponsored programs have varied considerably in their impact and effectiveness. Moderate-to-high contraceptive prevalence rates were indicated in 1994 for Turkey (63 percent), Tunisia (50 percent), Indonesia (50 percent), Algeria (36 percent), and Egypt (47 percent). Muslim countries with low rates reported in 1990 include Somalia (0 percent), Saudi Arabia (1 percent), Afghanistan (2 percent), and Yemen (2 percent) (Ross et al., 1992). Bangladesh's poor performance has been attributed to a "population control battlefield" between contending religious and social forces (Hartmann, 1987); Indonesia, on the other hand, has been identified as a family-planning success story. Since the 1970s, Indonesia has used a carrot-and-stick approach of incentives and state pressure. This policy, combined with socioeconomic changes such as reduced infant mortality, increased educational levels, and rural-to-urban migration, has led to a significant decline in fertility (Hartmann, 1987). Initially, many local religious leaders opposed family-planning programs on moral grounds and because they believed that growth in population was necessary in order to spread Islam. Efforts by the government, early in the program, to consult with religious leaders, and the government's decision to exclude sterilization and abortion from the program, helped counter the opposition.

The role and influence of religious leaders has varied and can often prove significant. The influence of Islam on people's acceptance or rejection of government-sponsored fertility-control programs depends not only on moral teachings of a religious tradition but also on how those teachings are interpreted to local people by religious leaders. If, as in Indonesia, many of those leaders support the program and use occasions such as marriage ceremonies to suggest the value of family planning, acceptance will typically be greater than if those leaders tell believers that using contraceptives to limit birth violates Islamic teaching. Postrevolution Shiite Iran provides a unique example of religious leaders, the ulama, functioning as both the executors and the formulators or legislators of new fatwas on family planning.

The Egyptian government has addressed the population question since the beginning of the rule of Gamal Abdel Nasser in 1952. Because of religious sensibilities, the government moved slowly, employing only the pill. Religious officials, from the government-appointed mufti of Egypt to the rector of the state-supported al-Azhar University, issued a series of fatwas endorsing the use of contraceptives. However, many think the religious establishment has been co-opted by the government. Thus, while Nasser and his successors could marshal the support of the religious establishment, local religious leaders continued to condemn contraception as immoral as well as contrary to Islam, and reinforced traditional emphasis on procreation and acceptance of the will of God, as did other opinion makers, such as midwives.

Like many other countries, Egypt has utilized a centralized, top-down approach, bypassing or ignoring local and regional realities. In 1953, Nasser was concerned that Egypt's population would leap to 44 million (Warwick, 1982). However, little was done about fertility control until the mid-1960s.

In Lebanon, religious sectarianism and communalism have both determined and limited the success of government policy. Lebanon was created as a confessional state whose delicate balance was based upon a system of proportional representation: Maronite Christians were dominant, followed by Sunni and Shiite Muslims and Druze. However, tensions between Christians and Muslims were exacerbated by the socioeconomic dominance and advancement of the Maronites, who had a lower fertility rate than the Muslims. By the mid-1970s, social realities proved explosive, and civil war broke out. The Shiite community, the poorest and most disenfranchised, had grown, and constituted one-third of Lebanon's population.

Given the precarious balance of power and social tensions, the Lebanese government for more than two decades shied away from any official promotion of family planning. However, while contraceptives remained illegal, the government indirectly supported private family-planning projects (Warwick, 1982).

Conclusion

Islam has a well-established body of teaching on fertility control that is closely linked to its views on marriage and the family. The interpretation of these teachings varies from country to country. The openness of individual Muslims to fertility control depends on many variables, including interpretations by local religious leaders of how it should be regarded by Muslims. Countries differ greatly in the extent to which Islamic religious leaders cooperate with government-sponsored fertility-control programs.

Much of the Muslim world faces rapid population growth in a situation of limited resources. Containment or reversal of this trend remains hampered by widespread poverty, illiteracy, and debates about the morality of birth control. In this struggle, the criticisms of local religious leaders combine with voices of many militant Muslims who attack government-sponsored family-planning programs and Western aid as a conspiracy to limit the size of the Muslim community in order to contain and dominate it more effectively.

JOHN L. ESPOSITO

While all the articles in the other sections of this entry are relevant, see especially the INTRODUCTION *and other articles in this section:* PROTESTANT PERSPECTIVES, ROMAN CATHOLIC PERSPECTIVES, JEWISH PERSPECTIVES, EASTERN ORTHODOX CHRISTIAN PERSPECTIVES, HINDU PERSPECTIVES, *and* BUDDHIST PERSPECTIVES. *Directly related to this article are the entries* POPULATION POLICIES; *and* ISLAM. *For a further discussion of topics mentioned in this article, see the entries* ABORTION; CHILDREN; FAMILY; FERTILITY CONTROL; MARRIAGE AND OTHER DOMESTIC PARTNERSHIPS; MEDICAL ETHICS, HISTORY OF, *section on* NEAR AND MIDDLE EAST, *articles on* IRAN, *and* CONTEMPORARY ARAB WORLD, *and section on* SOUTH AND EAST ASIA; REPRODUCTIVE TECHNOLOGIES; RIGHTS; SEXUAL ETHICS; *and* WOMEN, *article on* HISTORICAL AND CROSS-CULTURAL PERSPECTIVES. *For a discussion of related ideas, see the entries* FUTURE GENERATIONS, OBLIGATIONS TO; INFORMED CONSENT; *and* SEXISM.

Bibliography

COULSON, NOEL JAMES. 1964. *A History of Islamic Law.* Edinburgh: Edinburgh University Press.

ESPOSITO, JOHN L. 1980. *Women in Muslim Family Law.* Syracuse, N.Y.: Syracuse University Press.

HARTMANN, BETSY. 1987. *Reproductive Rights and Wrongs: The Global Politics of Population Control and Contraceptive Choice.* New York: Harper & Row.

MUSALLAM, BASIM F. 1978. "Population Ethics. Religious Traditions: Islamic Perspectives." In *Encyclopedia of Bioethics,* pp. 1264–1269. Edited by Warren T. Reich. New York: Macmillan.

———. 1983. *Sex and Society in Islam: Birth Control Before the Nineteenth Century.* Cambridge: At the University Press.

NAZER, ISAM R.; KARMĪ, ḤASAN S.; and ZAYID, MAHMUD Y., eds. 1974. *Islam and Family Planning.* 2 vols. Beirut: International Planned Parenthood Federation.

OMRAN, ABDEL RAHIM. 1992. *Family Planning in the Legacy of Islam.* London: Routledge.

POPULATION REFERENCE BUREAU. 1994. *1994: World Population Data Sheet.* Washington, D.C.: Author.

ROSS, JOHN A.; MAULDIN, W. PARKER; GREEN, STEVEN R.; and COOKE, E. ROMANA. 1992. *Family Planning and Child Survival Programs as Assessed in 1991.* New York: Population Council.

SCHIEFFELIN, OLIVIA, ed. 1972. *Muslim Attitudes Towards Family Planning.* New York: Population Council.

WARWICK, DONALD P. 1982. *Bitter Pills: Population Policies and Their Implementation in Eight Developing Countries.* Cambridge: At the University Press.

———. 1986. "The Indonesian Family Planning Program: Government Influence and Client Choice." *Population and Development Review* 12, no. 3:453–490.

C. JEWISH PERSPECTIVES

"Pronatalism" is the contemporary word describing the classic Jewish tradition regarding fertility. To begin with the religious component of the Jewish culture, procreation is counted as a positive *mitzvah* (a commandment or virtue), given pride of place at the top of rabbinic formulations of Bible commandments. *P'ru ur'vu* ("Be fruitful and multiply," or better, "Be fruitful and increase"—more arithmetic than geometric) in the first chapter of Genesis is a general blessing to other creatures; for humans, it is a behavioral imperative to reproduce. Bible commentators explain this difference in terms of the human differential: The command mode is needed because humankind, created in the image of God, might seek to devote itself entirely to the spiritual and intellectual, and might neglect the material and physical. Accordingly, Scripture thus negates the anti-procreative or celibate views of some cultures. Alternatively, the commandment addresses the fact that only humans are aware of the consequences of sexual activity; they might seek to avoid the attendant responsibilities of procreation while indulging the sexual drive.

On another level, a rabbinic Bible commentary observes that, throughout the first chapter of Genesis, the seal of approval—the announcement that "the Lord saw that it was good"—is repeated for each element of creation. But after Adam was created, "the Lord said, 'It is not good that man [Adam] should be alone.'" Only that which can endure is good; if humankind does not procreate, it will not endure.

Nor will God himself endure, according to the Talmud, without us to acknowledge him: "Not to engage in procreation," we are told, "is to diminish the Divine image." That is why the verse "for in the image of God has He created man" (Gen. 9:6) is followed immediately by the reaffirmation of Genesis 9:7, "Be fruitful and increase" (Yevamot 63b). More to the point, when the later verse (Gen. 17:7) introduces the Lord who will be "thy God and [that] of thy 'descendants after thee,'" the Talmud asks, "If there are no 'descendants after thee,' upon whom will the Divine Presence rest? Upon sticks and stones?" (Yevamot 64a). Without human progeny and continuity, there is no one to worship God. Without the physical body, there is no soul.

The biblical commandment is, as usual, spelled out in its details in Mishnah and Gemara, the two components of the Talmud, setting forth the halakah, the definitive legal ruling as formulated by the Codes. The halakah of "be fruitful" requires that a couple replace itself, that is, give birth to at least a son and a daughter. Having several sons or several daughters still does not fulfill the commandment. Yet, after the fact, the Talmud counts "grandchildren like children," so that parents with progeny of just one gender can be reassured that their children's children will help them measure up. Actually, even two children of different genders are only the bare minimum; in Maimonides' codification, the effort to procreate must continue. In Tosafot, authoritative critical commentaries from medieval France printed on the margin of the Talmud, the fear is expressed that letting the minimum number suffice could result in ethnic extinction (Bava Batra 60b). Infant mortality, as well as the possibility that the offspring may not live to adulthood or not reproduce, requires that more than one son and one daughter be conceived and born.

The duty to go far beyond the minimum has its rationale in the rabbinic dimension of the procreative mitzvah, where it is called, in brief, la-shevet or la-erev. (Deriving legal teaching from biblical books other than the Pentateuch is termed "rabbinic"; only the Five Books of Moses are the source of law called "biblical.") The biblical support for the first, la-shevet, is Isaiah (45:18): "Not for void did He create the world, but for habitation [la-shevet] did He form it." The second, la-erev, comes from Ecclesiastes (11:6): "In the morning sow thy seed, and in the evening [la-erev] do not withhold thy hand [from sowing], for you know not which will succeed, this or that, or whether they shall both alike be good." These verses strongly suggest a moral imperative to continue beyond the minimum.

The broader dimension of the mitzvah is very much an operative part thereof. To illustrate its legal implications, a Sefer Torah (scroll) belonging to an individual requires special care and may not ordinarily be sold for its proceeds. There are two exceptions: It may be sold (1) to finance tuition for the study of Torah, and (2) to dower a bride and thus enable her to marry and procreate. What if she already has a son and daughter? The power of the rabbinic extension of the mitzvah is now seen in the ruling that a Sefer Torah may be sold to finance the remarriage of that woman, so that she may fulfill la-shevet or la-erev.

The traditional pronatalist stance is vividly evident in modern-day rabbinic rulings with respect to reproductive technology. Just as illness or pathology are the targets of Judaism's mandate to heal, whereby Sabbath and dietary laws—and the rest of the Torah—are to be set aside to allow healing procedures to do their work, so barrenness and infertility are seen as pathological states to be overcome by aggressive therapies that may also supersede ritual laws. This equation of barrenness with illness means that fertility problems are to be overcome by such exigencies as in vitro or in utero fertilization, even artificial insemination or gestation by a host mother, for cases in which usual (or "natural") conception and birth are not possible. The principle of the primacy of fertility as a desideratum in a pronatalist tradition is given concrete form by the contemporary application of these legal provisions.

Another technical detail of Jewish law places the mitzvah (commandment) of procreation on the man rather than on the woman, though of course both are needed for procreation and both share in the mitzvah (virtue). This position may have its basis in the theoretical permissibility of polygamy or polygyny, whereby a man could marry more than one wife, but both paternity and maternity would still be known. The husband has to "worry about" the *mitzvah's* accomplishment. An actual sex-role difference derives from the "Be fruitful and increase" of Genesis, which goes on to say "Fill the earth and conquer it." The male is the conqueror, the aggressive one; the female, as the more passive, should not have to "go seeking in the marketplace" (*Yevamot* 65a). If that observation is rooted in anthropology, an explanation based more on ethics is offered by a Bible commentator of the twentieth century, Rabbi Meir Simcha HaKohen (d. 1921): Both the pain and the risk of childbearing are borne by the woman, not the man. Since the Torah's "ways are ways of pleasantness, and all its paths are peace" (Prov. 3:17), the Torah could not in fairness command a woman to undergo pain and assume risk; this must be her choice and it becomes her virtue. For the man, exposed to neither pain nor risk, there is both the command and the responsibility to heed the command (*Meshekh Hokhmah* to Gen. 1:28).

The discussion of what is and what is not a commandment refers to the formulations of the Sinai Covenant, which did in most cases reaffirm the pre-Sinai imperatives of Genesis, and as such applies only to the covenanted Jewish community. What of the rest of the world? A system called "the Seven Commandments of the Children of Noah" was discerned by the Talmudic sages; it is derived from God's charge to Noah after the flood and applied to his descendants in the world at large. These commandments include basic moral imperatives against murder, incest, cruelty to animals, and a directive to establish general law and order. Hence, the Sinai legislation cannot be imposed on mankind in its specifics. Many Jewish teachers see the thrust of *la-shevet* as generally applicable, for that biblical verse holds forth the *telos*, or ultimate end, of the earth, that it be inhabited and populated.

Attitudes toward procreation among Jews were not, of course, shaped by the law alone. Pronatalism partakes of the personal and cultural: In the face of all God's promises, Abraham protests to God (Gen. 15:2): "What canst Thou give me, seeing that I go childless?" The anguish of the barren woman is a recurrent theme in the Bible and beyond. On the other hand, fecundity is the most cherished blessing, exemplified idyllically in the Psalmist image (Ps. 128) of one "whose wife is a fruitful vine" and whose "children are as olive plants around the table" and whose ultimate satisfaction is the sight of "children [born] to thy children."

The natural impulse was buttressed by a national one. Historical circumstances of frequent massacres and forced conversions, with their resulting decimation of Jewish communities, added the impulse to compensate for losses to an existing instinct to procreate. The yearning for offspring was deepened, addressing positively the need to replenish depleted ranks. This contrasts to the response of despair reflected in an antiprocreative stance

taken by some Christian sects in the face of evil. The Gnostics in the first century, the Manichees in the fifth century, and the Cathars in the twelfth century are among the groups that taught and lived by the belief that procreation is to be avoided in a world of evil unredeemed. Apprehensiveness about the eventual well-being of offspring, the Talmud teaches, should not be a reason for not bearing children. This was King Hezekiah's worry, to which the response of Isaiah (38:1–10) is understood to mean: "The secrets of God are none of your business. You fulfill your duty [of procreation]" (*Berakhot* 10a).

In the post-Holocaust days, both the individual and the Jewish collectivity have been encouraged to make up for the physical losses of that tragic period. Nonetheless, realization of this impulse or teaching has not been evident across the board. In fact, the Jewish birthrate in the United States and other developed nations in recent decades was lower than, or as low as, that of the rest of the population. Upward socioeconomic mobility, and an increased pursuit of secular education and professional opportunity, has kept the birthrate down in assimilated families. Jews have, in fact, been visibly active in the movement for zero population growth, advancing a cause they consider ecologically necessary. Reform and, to a greater extent, Conservative Jews generally answer to the influence of Judaic tradition alongside of social considerations, while Orthodox families register the highest rates of reproduction.

Contraception and abortion

Sentiments toward procreation go hand in hand with views and practices of contraception and abortion. The halakah of contraception includes both the problem of method—whether or not a particular means completes the sexual union, or is not onanistic—and of motive—whether medical reasons or convenience are determinant. Contraception is clearly permitted where medically indicated, with even the less preferable methods. For nonmedical reasons, only methods such as rhythm or the pill may be used, providing the motive is acceptable. The preferable methods, such as the pill or Norplant, are not occlusive and not onanistic because sperm has an unimpeded trajectory. Coitus interruptus and the use of condoms are the least acceptable methods. But where AIDS, for example, is a threat, the condom's prophylactic properties take precedence, on the Talmudic principle that "[avoiding] danger is more serious than [avoiding] transgression" (*Chulin* 10a). This clear, medical permission means, incidentally, that in marital relations contraception is to be preferred over sexual abstinence.

Medical reasons are essentially what govern resort to abortion. The distinction is made between murder and killing of the fetus: If abortion were murder, it could only be considered if the life of the mother were at stake; as killing, or taking of only a potential human life, it can be considered to save her health or well-being, emotional as well as physical. As with contraception and pronatalism, Orthodoxy takes a less liberal position on abortion in theory and in practice than do the Conservative and Reform alignments.

The voluminous Responsa (formal replies to queries by rabbinic authorities) on these subjects are addressed to the individual couples and to their queries in deed. Global questions are also addressed, such as population control for ethical reasons as a concern for humanity and for available resources. The counsel of one rabbinic authority invoked the notion of "lifeboat ethics," whereby the lifeboat in which we all find ourselves, like Noah's Ark according to a Talmudic observation, must be kept from sinking as a result of overpopulation. The solicitude in halakic legislation for the welfare of existing children and their mother, before adding to one's family, was also invoked to argue for ecological responsibility.

Birthrate and the state of Israel

Advocacy of world population limitation is not contradicted by efforts to raise the Jewish birthrate. To the extent that growth globally threatens human well-being and Earth's ecology, it is an imperative concern for us all. But the Jewish people, constituting less than 1 percent of the world's population, would not adversely affect that picture even if their numbers doubled. Replacing Jewish losses would not upset the geophysical numerical balance; it would merely keep Judaism alive. Other minorities should similarly be allowed to maintain their existing numbers. Jewish aspirations, as reflected in synagogue liturgy, are not to become predominant in the world, but merely to "preserve the remnant of Israel."

That liturgical phrase refers, of course, to the People of Israel, but the State of Israel reflects similar concerns. At least one reason for the state's establishment in 1948 was demographic. When Palestine was ruled by British mandate, a "white paper" was issued that severely limited immigration by Jews, even hapless Holocaust survivors and internees of Europe's displaced-person camps. Whatever else sovereignty and independence provide, here they were necessary primarily to remove quotas and barriers to Jewish immigration.

After Israel was founded under the sponsorship of the United Nations and Jewish refugees were admitted, interior population growth was encouraged. The Hebrew word for immigration is *aliyah*, or ascendance to the Land of Israel. Now a new term was coined—*aliyah penimit*, or internal immigration—to refer to new births in Israel, encouraged as a patriotic act to build the nation

and its defenses. Also, since the very raison d'etre of the establishment of the state was as a restored homeland and a haven of refuge, the Law of Return was promulgated. It called for the "ingathering of the exiles," inviting Jews to be rehabilitated in their ancestral home, and granting them automatic citizenship upon their arrival.

The politics of population power have been evident not only in control of the disputed territories of Judea and Samaria (West Bank) but also in Israel proper and in the peace efforts begun in 1993. Nationalists express the concern that a disproportionate increase in the Arab birthrate or Arab immigration could effectively dissipate the Jewish character of the world's only Jewish state. On the other hand, during the early 1990s, massive absorption of Jews from the former Soviet Union and from Ethiopia took place; this influx demonstrated the profound demographic and cultural, as well as political, consequences of population factors.

DAVID M. FELDMAN

While all the articles in the other sections of this entry are relevant, see especially the INTRODUCTION *and other articles in this section:* ISLAMIC PERSPECTIVES, PROTESTANT PERSPECTIVES, ROMAN CATHOLIC PERSPECTIVES, EASTERN ORTHODOX CHRISTIAN PERSPECTIVES, HINDU PERSPECTIVES, *and* BUDDHIST PERSPECTIVES. *Directly related to this article are the entries* POPULATION POLICIES; *and* JUDAISM. *For a further discussion of topics mentioned in this article, see the entries* ABORTION, *especially the section on* RELIGIOUS TRADITIONS, *article on* JEWISH PERSPECTIVES; CHILDREN; ENVIRONMENTAL HEALTH; ETHICS, *article on* RELIGION AND MORALITY; FAMILY; FERTILITY CONTROL; MEDICAL ETHICS, HISTORY OF, *section on* NEAR AND MIDDLE EAST, *articles on* ISRAEL, *and* CONTEMPORARY ARAB WORLD; NATIONAL SOCIALISM; PAIN AND SUFFERING; REPRODUCTIVE TECHNOLOGIES; RISK; *and* VIRTUE AND CHARACTER. *For a discussion of related ideas, see the entries* ENVIRONMENT AND RELIGION; FUTURE GENERATIONS, OBLIGATIONS TO; *and* JUSTICE.

Bibliography

FELDMAN, DAVID M. 1968. *Birth Control in Jewish Law: Marital Relations, Contraception, and Abortion as Set Forth in the Classic Texts of Jewish Law.* New York: New York University Press. Also in paperback as *Marital Relations, Birth Control, and Abortion in Jewish Law.* New York: Schocken Press, 1974.

———. 1986. *Health and Medicine in the Jewish Tradition: L'Hayyim—To Life.* New York: Crossroad.

GOLD, MICHAEL. 1988. *And Hannah Wept: Infertility, Adoption, and the Jewish Couple.* Philadelphia: Jewish Publication Society.

GOLDSTEIN, SIDNEY. 1992. "Contemporary Jewish Demography." In *Frontiers of Jewish Thought,* pp. 157–177. Edited by Stephen T. Katz. Washington, D.C.: B'nai B'rith Books.

ROSENTHAL, GILBERT S. 1969. *Generations in Crisis: Judaism's Answers to the Dilemmas of Our Time.* New York: Bloch.

TOBIN, GARY A., and CHENKIN, ALVIN. 1985. "Recent Jewish Community Population Studies: A Roundup." In *American Jewish Year Book, 1985,* pp. 154–178. Philadelphia: Jewish Publication Society.

D. ROMAN CATHOLIC PERSPECTIVES

Roman Catholic teaching on population is a complex blend of theological beliefs, ethical norms, and empirical judgments. The distinctive characteristic of Roman Catholic doctrine is the sustained and significant place its teaching on contraception has held in its population position. Indeed, the detailed discussion of contraception in Catholic moral theology at times conveys the impression that this one issue constitutes the whole Catholic position on population ethics.

It is necessary, therefore, to distinguish two related but not identical moral questions in Catholic theological ethics: the morality of contraception and the teaching on population policy. John Noonan's classic work on contraception identifies moments in the history of the tradition when demographic trends affected the official teaching of the church, but it points out that these instances do not stand out as major determinants in the development of Catholic doctrine on contraception (Noonan, 1965). Noonan's analysis illustrates the complexity of the Catholic response to falling birthrates in the late Roman Empire, in the medieval period, and again in the nineteenth century. During those periods the Catholic position criticized the idea of restraining population growth but did not assert that procreation of children should be fostered without regard to other values. The balancing factors in the Catholic position are the linking of procreation to education and the high status accorded virginity in Catholic life.

It is possible, therefore, to trace a relationship between contraception and population policy throughout Catholic teaching; yet until the twentieth century, the dominant idea is the prohibition of contraceptive and other birth-limiting practices, with the population issue treated as a minor theme. Even in Pius XI's encyclical *Casti Connubii* (1930), which Noonan describes as "a small summa on Christian marriage" (1965, p. 426), the population issue receives only indirect reference. A systematic treatment of the morality of population policy as a distinct issue in its own right is not evident in Catholic thought until the time of Pius XII (Hollenbach, 1975). Beginning with Pius XII's address to the Italian Association of Catholic Midwives in 1951 and continuing through the teachings of Popes John XXIII and Paul VI, Vatican II, the Synod of Bishops (1971), and John Paul II, one can find an articulated ethical doctrine on population policy. The ethical teaching responds to two dimensions of the contemporary population debate: first, intensification of the debate about the relationship of population and resources; second, the move by governments and international institutions to design policies to affect demographic trends.

It is possible to distinguish in the Catholic teaching two species of moral analysis: One focuses on the context of population policy; the other, on the content of the procreative act. David Hollenbach distinguishes these two dimensions as the public and private aspects of Catholic teaching (Hollenbach, 1975).

Population policy

The public dimension is found generally in the social teaching of the church; the principal documents relating to population policy are *Gaudium et Spes* (1965) (Gremillion, 1976), *Populorum Progressio* (Paul VI, 1967), and the interventions of the Holy See on the occasions of international conferences about population, resources, and the environment. These documents manifest a social, structural analysis of the population issue, seeking to place demographic variables within a broadly defined socioeconomic context. The tenor and style of analysis is exemplified in Paul VI's message for the 1974 U.N. Population Year. The Pope's message argues for a broadly based approach to demographic problems with the category of social justice used as a principal theme (Paul VI, 1974a). This perspective is reaffirmed in the Holy See's intervention at the 1984 U.N. Population Conference (Schotte, 1984).

The main presupposition of all these statements is that the population problem is one strand of a larger fabric involving questions of political, economic, and social structure at the national and international levels. While acknowledging the existence of a population problem, this view asserts that it is morally wrong and practically ineffective to isolate population as a single factor, seeking to reduce population growth without simultaneously making those political and economic changes that will achieve a more equitable distribution of wealth and resources within nations and among nations (Rich, 1973; Paul VI, 1974a, 1974b).

The ethical categories used in analyzing the social aspect of the population problem are drawn from Catholic social teaching developed principally in the papal documents from 1891 to 1991 (Calvez and Perrin, 1961; Gremillion, 1976; Pavan, 1967; O'Brien and Shannon, 1992). The foundation of the argument is that the human person, endowed with the gifts of reason and free will, possesses a unique dignity or status in the world. The person, in Christian thought, is regarded as the pinnacle of God's creative action; the uniqueness of the person is argued in Catholic thought in both philosophical and theological terms. The dignity of the person is the source of a spectrum of rights and duties articulated as claims upon and responsibilities toward other persons and society as a whole. The distinguishing mark of the Catholic theory of rights, setting it apart from a classical, liberal argument, is the assertion of the social nature of the person. Society and state are necessary and natural institutions that are presupposed and required for full human development.

The strong social orientation of Catholic political philosophy holds that the way in which society, state, and subordinate social institutions are designed and structured is a moral question of the first order. Society and state are not self-justifying; they exist for the purpose of achieving the common good, defined as the protection and promotion of the rights and duties of each person in the society (Gremillion, 1976).

The central category used in evaluating the organization of social structures and institutions is social justice. This concept has roots in medieval Catholic teaching, but it has been developed and refined in the social encyclicals *Quadragesimo Anno* (1931) (O'Brien and Shannon, 1992) and *Mater et Magistra* (John XXIII, 1961), as well as in the third synodal document, "Justice in the World" (1971), and in the social teaching of John Paul II (O'Brien and Shannon, 1992). As social justice is used in these documents, it measures the role of key social institutions in procuring a fair distribution of wealth and resources nationally and internationally. In *Pacem in Terris*, the normative framework for assessing social institutions is expanded beyond justice to include truth, freedom, and charity (John XXIII, 1963).

The articulation of these categories in Catholic social teaching manifests two stages of development, both pertinent to a population ethic. The social teaching of the period from 1891 through the 1930s focuses on the nation as the unit of analysis; social justice principally means justice within the nation.

Beginning with Pius XII and continuing through John Paul II, the scope of analysis is broadened to focus on the international community. This move from assessing justice within the nation to justice among nations can be charted in the emergence of key concepts. John XXIII (1961) is the first to discuss the international common good as a standard for measuring national policies. The implication of this idea is that an adequate assessment of a state's policy must be calculated in terms of its impact on other states and peoples as well as upon its own citizens. For transnational questions like population and food policy, such a category of analysis opens a whole new set of questions. A similar expansion of a traditional category is found in "Justice in the World" in its discussion of international social justice (Gremillion, 1976). The concept explicitly addresses the structures through which states relate to each other in political and economic affairs. John Paul II develops the notion of solidarity as the ethical category that can direct the increasing interdependence of world politics and economics (O'Brien and Shannon, 1992).

At both the national and international levels, the categories of common good, social justice, and freedom of choice for individuals and families in society are used to define the population question. Among social institutions, the family, based on the covenant of marriage, holds a unique place in Catholic thought (Hollenbach, 1975). It is regarded as the basic cell or unit of society and the Catholic church. In the social hierarchy, reaching from the person through the state to the international community, no other association, save the Catholic church itself, is accorded such status. The demands of the common good and the requirements of social justice are articulated in terms of providing the family and its members with those conditions of life that satisfy basic human needs, protect personal dignity, and allow human development through the exercise of rights and responsibilities in society.

High on the list of inviolable rights is that of marrying and having a family (Hollenbach, 1975). To protect this right and other such rights for each person, Catholic social teaching establishes two parameters: positively, it calls upon the society to guarantee a basic minimum of material welfare, and negatively, it prohibits the state from any significant interference in the exercise of these rights. To summarize the public dimension of Catholic teaching, it accords primary attention to the context of the population question, focusing on the requirements of social justice that should be met as the first step in dealing with the relationship of resources and people. These requirements in specific form include questions of international trade, development assistance, agricultural reform, foreign-investment policies, consumption patterns, and the structure of social relationships within nations. In addition to these contextual issues in the population debate, Catholic teaching also includes a private dimension as regards the content of the procreative relationship.

The teaching on contraception

In contrast to the public teaching that focuses on societal structures, the tradition concerning private matters focuses upon the nature of the conjugal relationship and specifically upon the morality of the conjugal act. The principal issue involves analyzing permissible means of preventing contraception. The private aspect of the tradition is rooted in the extensive Catholic teaching on contraception, which has developed in very complex and detailed fashion since the second century (Noonan, 1965).

The modern expression of the private issues of the tradition is found in Pius XI's *Casti Connubii* (1930),

Pius XII's Address to the Italian Catholic Union of Midwives (1954), Paul VI's *Humanae Vitae* (1968), and John Paul II's *Familiaris Consortio* (1982). The principal private issues in the tradition include the morality of abortion, contraception, and sterilization; in the official teaching, all are rejected as means of preventing conception of birth. The only sanctioned means of limiting conception is some form of natural family planning, that is, one that excludes contraceptives. In contrast to the discussion among theologians on the public tradition, there is a very significant division between the official teaching on contraception and an analysis of contraception by theologians (Hoyt, 1968; Curran, 1969). While official teaching forbids all forms of contraception, many prominent theologians hold for the legitimacy of contraceptive techniques and the use of sterilization under specified conditions.

Population policy and the teaching on contraception

The private dimension of the tradition on population policy has public implications; it seeks to prevent any public policy that would either constrain or induce individuals to procure an abortion or to use contraceptives or would prevent them from choosing to have children. There are themes of coherence and consistency between the public and private aspects of the Catholic tradition: Both are concerned with the procreative process as a sacred dimension of human relationships; both seek to preserve maximum freedom for the couple to determine when to exercise procreative rights; both stress that society and the state exist to serve their members, and the relationship of the state to citizens is articulated in terms of social justice and personal freedom.

Having acknowledged these elements of continuity, it is equally important to illustrate the tension that prevails between the public and private dimensions of Catholic teaching on population policy. The tension can be analyzed by examining two principal texts: *Populorum Progressio*, representing the public dimension, and *Humanae Vitae*, representing the private one (Paul VI, 1967, 1968). These texts, in turn, must be assessed in light of the teaching of John Paul II on population policy. Paragraph 37 of *Populorum Progressio* is a carefully articulated and expansive statement of Catholic teaching on population policy (Gremillion, 1976). The passage contains the following elements: (1) an acknowledgment that a population problem exists in the world; (2) an affirmation that governments have a right and competency to deal with the problem; (3) a prescription that governmental action must be in accord with the moral law. This specific treatment of population policy is couched in the context of Paul VI's most detailed statement of the need for international reform in the political and economic order. Hence, the para-

graph presupposes that the social justice requirements are being addressed, and in that context the paragraph speaks to the question of measures to restrict population growth.

This passage is the clearest statement in Catholic teaching affirming the right of governments to intervene in the population question; left undefined, however, is the permissible scope of governmental intervention. The phrase that renders the policy ambiguous is that public intervention must be "in conformity with the moral law." In this area of public policy, what measures fall within the moral law? One way to clarify and specify the public tradition is to use *Humanae Vitae* as the guide for interpreting the moral law. The principal argument of the encyclical is that the moral law requires each and every act of intercourse to be open to procreation. A supporting reason offered for this position is that any compromise on this point opens the way to unregulated governmental intrusion into the sacred domain of family life (Gremillion, 1976). Presumably, then, the conjunction of *Humanae Vitae* and *Populorum Progressio* would limit the scope of governmental intervention to supporting and fostering only that means of population restraint approved in *Humanae Vitae*.

This is a restrictive reading of the texts; another view would stress the distinction between public and private dimensions of Catholic moral teaching as the key to interpreting Catholic teaching on population policy. This distinction is crucial in recognizing the different ethical norms used in Catholic thought for personal and social morality. A characteristic feature of Catholic social teaching is its sense of the multiple levels of society (Murray, 1960). The state is distinguished from society, and voluntary associations are distinguished from the state. Each principal part of the societal fabric is regarded as having a specific, limited role to play.

Two corollaries flow from this carefully delineated perspective on society. First, there is the recognition that personal conceptions of morality cannot be directly translated into requirements of social morality or public policy; to attempt to do so ignores the distinct nature of social and institutional relationships in society and thereby "makes wreckage not only of public policy but also of morality itself" (Murray, 1960, p. 286). Second, a recognition of two related but distinct levels of moral discourse—public and private—yields the jurisprudential distinction of moral law and civil law (Murray, 1960). While every human action and all human relationships fall under the moral law, only those that have a demonstrable effect on the public order and are open to state regulation without sacrificing other proportionately significant values are to be included under civil law or public policy. Since Catholic theology recognizes distinctions between public and private morality and between civil and moral law, it is possible for Catholic teaching to oppose an action or policy on moral grounds but not be inevitably committed to seek legal or political means to prevent its implementation.

The use of these distinctions between public and private morality and between civil and moral law could yield a more flexible reading of *Populorum Progressio*. First, such a reading would accent the state's right to intervene in the population question. Second, it would then treat the *Humanae Vitae* argument as being principally applicable in the area of personal morality and not an adequate framework for examining population policy. Third, it would acknowledge the disputed character of *Humanae Vitae* in the Catholic community, even as a norm of personal morality. The purpose of bringing to light the opposing Catholic views on papal teaching regarding contraception (as expressed in *Humanae Vitae*) would simply be to acknowledge that, when such dispute exists within the Catholic community, there is strong reason not to seek to make such a norm a standard of public policy in a pluralistic world. Finally, while not interjecting the specific prescriptions of *Humanae Vitae* into public debate, such a Catholic stance could still speak to the limits of permissible state intervention on population questions. The criteria for setting limits could be drawn from the human-rights standards of the public ethic in the tradition, including a stance against abortion (on human-rights grounds), protection of the person from coercion regarding procreative practice (particularly regarding sterilization), and a respect for religious and moral pluralism as a guide for governmental action.

This broadly designed "public" approach to population policy, one cast in terms of human rights and social justice, is defensible in terms of principles of Catholic moral theology. It is not, however, the direction Pope John Paul II has set for the church's approach to population questions since his election to the papacy in 1978. His approach has been to tie the public and private dimensions of policy more tightly together, thereby raising the visibility and role of the teaching on contraception in the overall direction of policy. The impact of John Paul's leadership can be found in his own teaching and in the positions the Holy See has taken in international conferences on population-related issues.

Teaching of John Paul II

John Paul's influence can be summarized in terms of four contributions. First, in his encyclical on Catholic moral theology *Veritatis Splendor* (1993), the pope reaffirmed the structure of moral argument that sustains traditional Catholic teaching, not only on abortion but also on sterilization and contraception. The encyclical did not break new ground on these issues, but the effect of it has been a call for greater restraint on theological dissent from the teaching on contraception and sterilization. The scope of *Veritatis Splendor* is much broader than spe-

cific issues of sexual morality; its influence on population policy lies in its resistance to an interpretation of Catholic teaching that would treat contraception as an internal issue of church discipline but not a position to be espoused in public policy. Prior to the encyclical, the pope's thinking was made clear in the Holy See's intervention at the 1984 U.N. Conference on Population at Mexico City. The Vatican's statement affirmed "that the Catholic Church has always rejected contraception as being morally illicit. That position has not changed but has been reaffirmed with new vigor" (Schotte, 1984, p. 207).

Second, the weight given to the private dimension of Catholic teaching does not, however, mean that John Paul II has forsaken the broader public dimensions of the teaching on population policy. Indeed, the second dimension of his contribution to population policy in the church has been to expand and develop the social justice theme espoused by Paul VI and the 1971 Synod of Bishops. John Paul's contribution is found in a series of encyclical letters, from *Redemptor Hominis* (1979) through *Centesimus Annus* (1991). In his social teaching, John Paul develops a moral vision rooted in human rights, including both political and economic rights, and shaped by principles of social justice and solidarity. The papal teaching takes the international community as the unit of analysis, and John Paul II argues that a broadly defined notion of human, economic, and social development should be the context for examining population questions. John Paul II substantially extends Paul VI's critique of international institutions and practices in the socioeconomic order. Like his predecessor, John Paul II primarily emphasizes deep and extensive changes in international economic policies as the response to demographic pressures. In *Sollicitudo Rei Socialis*, he argues that "one must denounce the existence of economic, financial and social mechanisms which . . . often function almost automatically, thus accentuating the situation of wealth for some and poverty for the rest" (O'Brien and Shannon, 1992, p. 404). In the same encyclical, John Paul II cites the need "for a solidarity which will take up interdependence and transfer it to the moral plane" (1992, p. 411). In subsequent teaching, he explicates some of the policy demands of solidarity as they affect international distribution, problems of the Third World debt, and protection of human rights within nations and through the work of international institutions.

Third, a dimension of Catholic teaching which holds a prominent place in the pontificate of John Paul II is the relationship of migration and population. The teaching and the practice of the church both testify to a deep concern for the welfare of migrants and refugees. At the level of the Holy See, in the structure of national episcopal conferences, and in the work of dioceses and religious orders, the pastoral care of migrants and refugees holds a substantial place in the ministry of the church.

This ministry is supported by Catholic teaching on migration. The perspective on the right of the person to emigrate and immigrate is based on Catholic teaching on human rights and on the moral structure of the international order. The right of the person to emigrate places upon the international community, and states within it, the responsibility for developing fair policies regarding immigration. Catholic teaching does not assert an unlimited duty to receive migrants and refugees, but it does not specify particular limits either. The emphasis of the teaching falls on a duty of international solidarity that then must find expression in international and national policies regarding migrants and refugees. In John Paul II's teaching, "the state's task is to ensure that immigrant families do not lack what it ordinarily guarantees its own citizens as well as to protect them from any attempt at marginalization, intolerance or racism . . ." (John Paul II, 1994, p. 718).

This expansive conception of the duty of states to be open to the movement of populations when they are driven by war, famine, economic necessity, or human-rights violations provides another social instrumentality, along with the teaching on social justice, to complement the Vatican's restrictive policy regarding the limitation of population.

In summary, there is substantial continuity between Paul VI and John Paul II on the public dimensions of population policy. The public argument about human rights and social justice remains the context in which population policy is addressed. Within that context, however, there is a difference in the way John Paul II relates the public and private dimensions of Catholic teaching.

This is the fourth aspect of his teaching, and it does not point toward more active Catholic engagement concerning population issues. Paul VI had acknowledged the objective dimensions of demographic problems, and the duty of governments to address these; John Paul II places the emphasis in a different direction. He also acknowledges that population growth can create "difficulties for development," but his concern is principally about the abuses public agencies commit in pursuit of population policies (O'Brien and Shannon, 1992). There is undoubtedly a need for the multiple concerns expressed by the pope himself and by the Holy See in its 1984 intervention at Mexico City. The values and principles stressed in the Holy See's intervention at the Mexico City conference and reiterated in 1994 by Pope John Paul II in preparation for the U.N. Population Conference at Cairo—protection of the rights of the person and the family, resistance to conditioning economic assistance on the basis of population targets, restraints on the role of the state—are necessary for an ethically sound population policy. But there is less pos-

itive encouragement or guidance for the state or international agencies to take responsibility for population issues. The principal guidance for public authorities is to reject abortion, sterilization, and contraception in the implementation of population policy. These restrictions are matched with a statement of the duty states have to create conditions within which parents can make responsible choices about family size (e.g., John Paul II, 1994).

Clearly, any Catholic policy will oppose abortion because of the deeply held conviction that a human life is at stake, and it will be deeply suspicious of state intervention in any decisions and choices about procreation that are basic to the dignity and freedom of married couples. The question of whether all forms of contraception would have to be explicitly opposed, save that described in Catholic thought as "natural family planning," is what lay implicit in Paul VI's statement of 1967. John Paul's response is decisively in the direction of treating abortion, sterilization, and contraception in similar fashion; although different in nature, all three are to be opposed in population policy.

The basic lines of Catholic policy, in both its public and private dimensions, have been firmly set for centuries. The policy combines a powerful vision of economic justice and human rights with a comprehensive resistance to most specific measures of population limitation. At the level of implementation, does the policy framework allow for or manifest any differentiation? Two possibilities exist: at the level of pastoral care and the level of principles and rules of conduct.

The pastoral level involves the advice, counsel, and direction provided by the ministers of the church to Catholics as guidance for conscience. The pastoral level also involves the degree of activism that marks Catholic life on population issues at national and local levels of the church. The other possibility for differentiation would involve an attempt to change the basic principles of Catholic teaching in its public or private dimensions.

In his history of the teaching on contraception, John Noonan illustrates the fact that some difference has often marked the church's life between what has been prohibited at the level of principle and how distinctions were made to accommodate the specific conditions in the lives of individuals. In the years since *Humanae Vitae* (1968) was issued, substantial differences have existed between the principles of the encyclical and the choices individuals have made, often with advice from theologians or pastors. John Paul II has been vigorous in his attempt to close this gap. While pastoral practice undoubtedly affects the population issue, its primary impact is felt not at the level of church policy or involvement in the public debate on population issues but in the lives of individuals.

In terms of the principles of Catholic population policy, it is useful to compare the universal teaching and the role of the church within nations. It is clear that the church ministers in nations with very different approaches to population policy, some close to Catholic principles and others in direct opposition to either the public or private dimensions of Catholic teaching. It is also clear that in the period since the Second Vatican Council, there has been greater possibility in Catholic polity for national episcopal conferences to take initiatives in applying the church's teaching to specific local circumstances. Examples of this include Latin American hierarchies addressing human rights and economic justice, and the hierarchy of the United States engaging the issues of nuclear deterrence and economic policy.

Population policy, however, is not an area where much latitude exists for national or local voices. The Holy See, through its teaching office and its diplomatic engagement, is clearly the primary and predominant voice on population issues. National hierarchies may coexist with governmental programs that differ from Catholic teaching, but they seldom seek to challenge or change the principles of Catholic teaching to meet their local situations. Examples of national teaching that do seem to press for some change in the understanding or application of the teaching (particularly in its private dimensions) are recognized as rare exceptions. Such is the case of the Indonesian bishops who issued a statement in 1968 and then were required to provide clarification of their position in 1972 (Indonesian Bishops, 1972). The normal practice for episcopal conferences is to take the Holy See's principles as the premise of their position and then try to relate these principles to the broader policy debate in their own countries; this has been the policy followed by the U.S. bishops in their 1973 and 1994 statements on the population question (National Conference, 1973; U.S. Cardinals, 1994).

In the 1984 U.N. Conference on Population in Mexico City and in the preparatory debate leading to the 1994 Cairo conference, John Paul II has forcefully reasserted the papal role as the decisive voice on population issues. His position of tightly integrating the public and private dimensions of the teaching, and seeking to shape global policy in both areas, sets the standard for any other voice in the Catholic church. No Catholic policy would forsake either the socioeconomic principles of justice or its opposition to abortion as a method of population limitation. The effect of John Paul II's leadership is to reaffirm these dimensions and to diminish the likelihood that any distinction will be made in the policy debate between the public and private dimensions of Catholic teaching (John Paul II, 1994).

J. BRYAN HEHIR

While all the articles in the other sections of this entry are relevant, see especially the INTRODUCTION *and other articles in this section:* ISLAMIC PERSPECTIVES, PROTESTANT PERSPECTIVES, JEWISH PERSPECTIVES, EASTERN ORTHODOX CHRISTIAN PERSPECTIVES, HINDU PERSPECTIVES, *and* BUDDHIST PERSPECTIVES. *Directly related to this article are the entries* POPULATION POLICIES; *and* ROMAN CATHOLICISM. *For a further discussion of topics mentioned in this article, see the entries* ABORTION, *especially the section on* RELIGIOUS TRADITIONS, *article on* ROMAN CATHOLIC PERSPECTIVES; FAMILY; FERTILITY CONTROL; FOOD POLICY; JUSTICE; MARRIAGE AND OTHER DOMESTIC PARTNERSHIPS; MEDICAL ETHICS, HISTORY OF, *section on* EUROPE, *subsections on* ANCIENT AND MEDIEVAL *and* NINETEENTH CENTURY; PASTORAL CARE; RACE AND RACISM; *and* RIGHTS. *For a discussion of related ideas, see the entries* AUTHORITY; AUTONOMY; BEHAVIOR CONTROL; DOUBLE EFFECT; ENVIRONMENTAL POLICY AND LAW; ETHICS, *article on* SOCIAL AND POLITICAL THEORIES; FETUS; FREEDOM AND COERCION; HUMAN NATURE; NATURAL LAW; *and* SEXISM. *Other relevant material may be found under the entries* EASTERN ORTHODOX CHRISTIANITY; *and* PROTESTANTISM.

Bibliography

CALVEZ, JEAN-YVES, and PERRIN, JACQUES. 1961. *The Church and Social Justice: The Social Teaching of the Popes from Leo XIII to Pius XII (1878–1958)*. Translated by J. R. Kirwan. Chicago: Henry Regnery.

CURRAN, CHARLES E., ed. 1969. *Contraception: Authority and Dissent*. New York: Herder & Herder.

FERREE, WILLIAM. 1948. *Introduction to Social Justice*. New York: Paulist Press.

GREMILLION, JOSEPH, ed. 1976. *The Gospel of Peace and Justice: Catholic Social Teaching Since Pope John*. Maryknoll, N.Y.: Orbis Books. Cites many of the papal messages mentioned in this article.

HOLLENBACH, DAVID. 1975. "The Right to Procreate and Its Social Limitations: A Systematic Study of Value Conflict in Roman Catholic Ethics." Ph.D. dissertation, Yale University.

HOYT, ROBERT G., ed. 1968. *The Birth Control Debate*. Kansas City, Mo.: National Catholic Reporter.

INDONESIAN BISHOPS. 1973. [1972]. "Population: Indonesian Bishops Statement." *Origins* 3, no. 16:250-251.

JOHN XXIII. 1961. "*Mater et Magistra*: Christianity and Social Progress (May 15, 1961)." In *The Gospel of Peace and Justice: Catholic Social Teaching Since Pope John*, pp. 143–200. Edited by Joseph Gremillion. Maryknoll, N.Y.: Orbis Books.

———. 1963. "*Pacem in Terris*: Peace on Earth (April 11, 1963)." In *The Gospel of Peace and Justice: Catholic Social Teaching Since Pope John*, pp. 201–241. Edited by Joseph Gremillion. Maryknoll, N.Y.: Orbis Books.

JOHN PAUL II. 1979. *Redemptor Hominis: Redeemer of Man*. Washington, D.C.: U.S. Catholic Conference.

———. 1982. *Familiaris Consortio: The Role of the Christian Family in the Modern World*. Washington, D.C.: U.S. Catholic Conference.

———. 1993. "*Veritatis Splendor:* The Splendor of the Truth." *Origins* 23, no. 18:298–334.

———. 1994. "Population Conference Draft Document Criticized." *Origins* 23, no. 41:716–719.

MURRAY, JOHN COURTNEY. 1960. *We Hold These Truths: Catholic Reflections on the American Proposition.* New York: Sheed & Ward.

NATIONAL CONFERENCE OF CATHOLIC BISHOPS. 1973. "Statement on Population." In *Pastoral Letters of the United States Catholic Bishops,* pp. 380–383. Edited by Hugh J. Nolan. Washington, D.C.: U.S. Catholic Conference.

NOONAN, JOHN THOMAS, JR. 1965. *Contraception: A History of Its Treatment by the Catholic Theologians and Canonists.* Cambridge, Mass.: Harvard University Press.

O'BRIEN, DAVID J., and SHANNON, THOMAS A. 1992. *Catholic Social Thought: The Documentary Heritage.* Maryknoll, N.Y.: Orbis Books.

PAUL VI. 1967. "*Populorum Progressio:* On the Development of Peoples (March 26, 1967)." In *The Gospel of Peace and Justice: Catholic Social Teaching Since Pope John,* pp. 387–415. Edited by Joseph Gremillion. Maryknoll, N.Y.: Orbis Books.

———. 1968. "*Humanae Vitae:* On the Regulation of Birth (July 25, 1968)." In *The Gospel of Peace and Justice: Catholic Social Teaching Since Pope John,* pp. 427–444. Edited by Joseph Gremillion. Maryknoll, N.Y.: Orbis Books.

———. 1974a. "Paul VI/Population Year: The Common Future of the Human Race." *Origins* 3, no. 43:670–672. Message on the U.N. Population Year.

———. 1974b. "Address of His Holiness Pope Paul VI to the Participants of the World Food Conference, Rome (November 9, 1974)." In *The Gospel of Peace and Justice: Catholic Social Teaching Since Pope John,* pp. 599–606. Edited by Joseph Gremillion. Maryknoll, N.Y.: Orbis Books.

PAVAN, PIETRO P. 1967. "Social Thought, Papal." In *New Catholic Encyclopedia,* vol. 13, pp. 352–361. New York: McGraw-Hill.

PIUS XI. 1930. "*Casti Connubii.*" *Acta Apostolicae Sedis* 22, no. 13:539–592.

PIUS XII. 1954. "His Holiness Pope Pius XII's Discourse to Members of the Congress of the Italian Association of Catholic Midwives" (October 29, 1951). In *Catholic Documents: Containing Recent Pronouncements and Decisions of His Holiness Pope Pius XII.* London: Pontifical Court Club by the Salesian Press.

RICH, WILLIAM. 1973. *Smaller Families Through Social and Economic Progress.* Washington: Overseas Development Council.

SCHOTTE, JAN. 1984. "Perspectives on Population Policy." *Origins* 14, no. 13:205–208. Intervention of the Holy See at the U.N. International Conference on Population at Mexico City.

SYNOD OF BISHOPS. SECOND GENERAL ASSEMBLY. 1971. "Justice in the World (November 30, 1971)." In *The Gospel of Peace and Justice: Catholic Social Teaching Since Pope John,* pp. 513–529. Edited by Joseph Gremillion. Maryknoll, N.Y.: Orbis Books.

U.S. CARDINALS and PRESIDENT OF THE NATIONAL CONFERENCE OF CATHOLIC BISHOPS. 1994. "Letter to President Clinton." *Origins* 24:58–59.

E. EASTERN ORTHODOX CHRISTIAN PERSPECTIVES

Population questions have not received a great deal of treatment in Orthodox theology or ethics. What little has been written comes out of other, related interests. Even in patristic times, population concerns usually appeared within the framework of discussion on Christian marriage and attendant issues, the most important of which was the place of procreation as a purpose, or even as *the* purpose, of marriage. The fourth-century writings of Saint John Chrysostom, for example, suggest that the purpose of marriage is in part determined by population considerations.

Recent literature

The relevant Eastern Orthodox literature on the contemporary situation may be divided into two periods.

First period: 1933–1969. During this time, Orthodox thinking discounted the threat of overpopulation, which was either ignored or seen as a dubious argument to support birth control. If it was taken seriously, it was perceived to be a false issue, unsupported by the evidence. This position aimed to undercut support for conception control, especially in regard to maintaining the strength of ethnic groups. Many traditionally Orthodox countries (e.g., Greece, Bulgaria, Romania, Serbia) were experiencing a reduced birthrate, which was often perceived as putting them at a political and military disadvantage in relation to neighboring countries. Hence, their interest was in increasing rather than decreasing their populations.

The first important work of this period appeared in 1933: Seraphim G. Papakostas's *To zetema tes teknogonias: To demographihon problema apo Christianikes apopseos* (The Question of the Procreation of Children: The Demographic Problem from a Christian Viewpoint), which places birth control and population concerns within family ethics. The population issue appears under the rubric "The Arguments of the Supporters [of birth control]," where the author holds that arguments drawn from the threat of overpopulation, financial considerations, the improvement of conditions of life for both individual and nation, and other such positions are inadequate to justify the practice of birth control. After discussing the relationship between population and cultivated land, Papakostas concludes that "the means of support are increasing faster than the population" (p. 53). Numerous factors contribute to overpopulation, he argues, and all must be functioning in order for it to occur. His conclusion is that "the danger of overpopulation is non-existent" (p. 57).

In 1937 the Holy Synod of the Church of Greece, its highest governing body, issued an encyclical against the practice of birth control that reflected Papakostas's views. (Papakostas was very likely the author of the encyclical.) Although the document treats birth control almost without reference to the population issue, the encyclical does characterize birth control as an agent of "permanent harm to the Greek Nation because of the reduction of the population."

A similar treatment of the subject, written by the *hegoumenos* (abbot) of one of the monasteries of Athos, Gabriel Dionysiatou, was published in 1957. In this work, *Malthousianismos: To englema tes genoktonias* (Malthusianism: The Crime of Genocide), concern with overpopulation is believed to be unwarranted. The author, however, does not foresee the progress of technology and the resulting increase of agricultural productivity and distribution. The study is based on the view that the primary purpose of marriage is the procreation of children.

Second period: 1970 to the present.   The second period of the treatment of the population issue, beginning in 1970, continues to deal with its relationship to birth control. A significant number of writers now feel that birth control is not the unmitigated evil described in the previous period. Most have adopted their view not because of population issues but through a rejection of Augustinian understandings of sin and "concupiscence" and a more Eastern patristic understanding of the purposes of marriage. While the Western patristic approach drew moral teaching primarily from natural law, the Eastern view was based on a Trinitarian approach that emphasized the interpersonal dimensions of marriage.

Of great importance is Alexander Stavropoulos's *He ekklesia tes Hellados enanti tou problematos tes technogonias* (The Church of Greece and the Question of the Procreation of Children), published in 1977. Using textual analysis, Stavropoulos shows that both Papkostas's work and the encyclical of 1937 were based not on patristic sources but on Western prototypes. As a result of Stavropoulos's work, the encyclical ceased to be considered an authoritative text for Orthodox theological and ethical reflection. Efforts were made to include the issue of conception control in the themes of a forthcoming Great and Holy Council of the Orthodox church, but eventually it was dropped.

Some Orthodox writers treat the issue on the basis of theological grounds without reference to population concerns (Meyendorff, 1975; Constantelos, 1975; Zapheiris, 1974, 1991; Harakas, 1982). During this period a revival of patristic thought and method in theology, emphasizing the importance of the interpersonal dimensions of Eastern Orthodox Christianity, has been instrumental in changing the attitude toward ethical issues as well. These theological developments focus on the human dimensions of Orthodox Trinitarian theological perspectives, since the doctrine of the Holy Trinity as "three persons in unity" is seen as paradigmatic for human beings, in that the goal of human life is growth toward Godlikeness.

Several new treatments of birth control in relation to population issues have appeared in this period. The debate now focuses on the actual (or the mistakenly perceived) danger of overpopulation. In *The Sacrament of Love,* Paul Evdokimov (1985) makes explicit reference to the danger of overpopulation as an argument for the use of birth control.

Similarly, Nicon Patrinacos (1975) deals with ethnic demographic implications, placing the population issue in historical perspective. Explaining the traditional emphasis on the procreative dimension of marriage, he notes: "As with all societies and nations of [the Byzantine] era, numbers were extremely important to the survival of the country and nation" (p. 3). He comments that many factors explain Orthodox emphasis on population increase: high infant mortality; population depletion resulting from frequent wars; and lack of adequate sanitary conditions, medical care, and food. Unlike the writers of the pre-1970 period, Patrinacos is convinced of the reality and dangers of the population explosion. Rather than discounting it, he takes it as one of the chief elements of his moral reasoning. He condemns as evasive and morally irresponsible those positions that ignore the issues created by overpopulation. He is convinced that "unlimited reproduction of our own kind has reached the point of impoverishing rather than enriching humanity" (p. 46).

Patrinacos holds that the command God gave to Adam and Eve to multiply and populate the Earth has been realized. The church must now provide new guidance: "Birth control is, in more than half of today's world, as important and as urgent as feeding the millions of starving. More births would mean more hunger, more pain, more deaths" (p. 48).

The revival of the patristic mind-set in Orthodox theology, with its emphasis on both divine and human relationality, makes untenable the older argument that the only or primary purpose of marriage is procreation. The theology of marriage has come to focus on the interpersonal unity and relationship of spouses. Studies by Megas Farantos (1983), Paul Evdokimov (1985), Haralambos Hatzopoulos (1990), Chrysostom Zapheiris (1991), W. Basil Zion (1992), and Stanley Harakas (1992), among others, reject the previous approach as not reflective of authentic Eastern Orthodox perspectives, and approve conception control within marriage. Some of these writers connect conception control to population issues.

Nicholas Bougatsos's 1994 work, *He rhythmise tes teknogonias: Orthodoxos kai Hellenike apopse* (The Regulation of Childbearing: Orthodox and Hellenic View), discounts the issue of overpopulation for Greece and Europe in general (it does not deal with population issues in the Third World). Nevertheless, Bougatsos argues that for theological reasons, different approaches to the issue of conception control are ethically possible. These may include the practice of birth control by spouses for a number of reasons, among them the enhancement of interpersonal relations and growth in the unity of Christian marriage.

A population agenda for Orthodox Christian ethics

The crucial differences between the earlier and later aspects of this discussion are traceable both to theological outlooks and to concern with issues of population. The foundations now exist for the development of an Orthodox population ethic, which might include a number of elements.

Theological appropriateness of population concerns. It is true that "the Fathers of the Church were . . . uninterested in the economic implications of population growth . . . and early Christian writers can, indeed, hardly be considered to have had a population policy" (Callahan, 1970, p. 187). However, contemporary Orthodox ethics is concerned with population as both an imperative of present existential realities and a demand of the implications of the faith. Orthodox ethics cannot ignore the implications of the fact that there has been an enormous increase in the rate of world population growth, especially in the Third World. It cannot limit its teachings on conception control to the geographical areas where its members reside. Humanity must "maintain some balance between [its] numbers and the finite dimensions of this planet" (Freedman, 1964, p. 18).

Theology of human dominion over the earth. Theological anthropology has ecological and population implications. Traditionally, political implications have been discerned in humanity's creation in the image of God by finding parallels between the kingship of God and that of political leaders. The same doctrine requires human responsibility for creation, including ecological and population dimensions. Further, the dominion of humanity over the environment is an appropriate aspect of the Orthodox doctrine of divine providence in conjunction with the doctrine of "synergy," which calls for the cooperation of the human with the divine. Orthodox ethicists (e.g., Demetropoulos, 1970) have expressed some renewed interest in this approach.

Ethical doctrine of philanthropy. One of the chief theological and ethical categories of Eastern Christianity is *philanthropia,* a concept that transcends mere charity and includes the heartfelt identification of God, the church, and the individual Christian with all of humanity. *Philanthropia,* long a fruitful concept for Eastern

Orthodox thought and life (Constantelos, 1968), has implications for population issues.

Fertility guidelines. Orthodox personal ethics and the ethics of marriage and family have not adequately elucidated the implications of population realities. Both church leaders and scholars tend to leave such issues to "private conscience" or the "guidance of father confessors," although public teaching on the matter is now more widespread than it was earlier (Harakas 1982; Meyendorff, 1975).

Justice and distribution policies. The Orthodox churches tend to focus on national cultures and heritages. This is a result of their strong "incarnational" emphasis, based on the theological teaching in regard to the second person of the Holy Trinity, the Son, who took on full human nature and lived on Earth. The divine, as fully present in the created human reality of the one person Jesus Christ, becomes a model for all creation and relationships. Sacraments, icons, and church architecture are religious examples of this modeling in that in and through them the divine is made significant. Relationships, both formal and informal, are also imbued with the divine. Among these, marriage and marital relationships are thus understood incarnationally.

Global perspectives focusing on structural injustices, especially as they relate to population concerns, are equally incarnational concerns. The Orthodox Christian conscience has always had a universal dimension. Orthodox anthropology does not permit the view that equitable food distribution policies are utopian, nor that population concerns are limited to a single nation or region (Patrinacos, 1975).

An ecumenical approach. Concern for population problems must be a shared endeavor. This may come closest to the original intent of Orthodox involvement in the ecumenical movement, the original justification of which was based on interchurch cooperation toward the solution of social problems. The ecumenical approach, however, must go beyond church cooperation and include collaboration with local and international agencies concerned with hunger and population problems.

Policy and practice. The recent direction in Orthodox thought has been to become more deeply involved in social issues. If this increased social involvement is to be put into practice seriously, Orthodox leaders will seek practical policy changes. For example, if birth control is to be considered by the Orthodox to be "one of the more effective means by which a balancing between eaters and food to be eaten, consumers and goods, and services and labor" can occur (Patrinacos, p. 48), this implies a commitment to a positive emphasis on conception control, coupled with sex education founded on a deeply considered theology of marriage. In addition, the Orthodox church must develop acceptable practices to influence national and international policymaking, legislation, corporate decision making, and public opinion. Serious concern with population issues necessarily requires what has been called "eco-tactics" (De Bell, 1970)—what used to be called in Orthodox history "whispering in the ear of the Emperor in the name of Christ."

In conclusion, both the imperatives and the potentials for involvement by the Orthodox church in population concerns are found within its tradition.

STANLEY S. HARAKAS

While all the articles in the other sections of this entry are relevant, see especially the INTRODUCTION *and other articles in this section:* ISLAMIC PERSPECTIVES, PROTESTANT PERSPECTIVES, ROMAN CATHOLIC PERSPECTIVES, JEWISH PERSPECTIVES, HINDU PERSPECTIVES, *and* BUDDHIST PERSPECTIVES. *Directly related to this article are the entries* POPULATION POLICIES; *and* EASTERN ORTHODOX CHRISTIANITY. *For a discussion of topics mentioned in this article, see the entries* CHILDREN; ENVIRONMENTAL ETHICS; ENVIRONMENT AND RELIGION; FAMILY; FERTILITY CONTROL; *and* MARRIAGE AND OTHER DOMESTIC PARTNERSHIPS. *For a discussion of related ideas, see the entries* ABORTION, *especially the section on* RELIGIOUS TRADITIONS; FOOD POLICY; *and* FUTURE GENERATIONS, OBLIGATIONS TO.

Bibliography

BOUGATSOS, NICHOLAS. 1994. *He rhythmise tes teknogonias: Orthodoxos kai Hellenike apopse.* "Apostolike Diakonia" of the Church of Greece.

CALLAHAN, DANIEL, ed. 1970. *The American Population Debate.* Garden City, N.Y.: Doubleday.

CONSTANTELOS, DEMETRIOS J. 1968. *Byzantine Philanthropy and Social Welfare.* Rutgers Byzantine Series. New Brunswick, N.J.: Rutgers University Press.

———. 1975. *Marriage, Sexuality and Celibacy: A Greek Orthodox Perspective.* Minneapolis: Light and Life.

DE BELL, GARRETT, ed. 1970. *The Environmental Handbook.* New York: Ballantine Books.

DEMETROPOULOS, PANAGIOTES C. 1970. *Orthodoxos Christianike ethike.* Athens: Author.

EVDOKIMOV [EVDOKIMOFF], PAUL. 1985. *Sacrement de l'amour.* Translated by Anthony P. Gythiel and Victoria Steadman under the title *The Sacrament of Love: The Nuptial Mystery in Light of the Orthodox Tradition.* Crestwood, N.Y.: St. Vladimir's Seminary Press.

FARANTOS, MEGAS. 1983. "Ta antisylliptika kai ethike." In part 4 of *Dogmatika kai ethika,* pp. 337–344. Athens: Author.

FREEDMAN, RONALD, ed. 1964. *Population: The Vital Revolution.* VOA Forum Series. Garden City, N.Y.: Doubleday/Anchor.

GABRIEL, DIONYSIATOU. 1957. *Malthousianismos: To englema tes genoktonias.* Volos, Greece: Holy Mountain Library.

HARAKAS, STANLEY. 1982. *Contemporary Moral Issues Facing the Orthodox Christian.* Newly rev. & exp. ed. Minneapolis: Light and Life.

———. 1992. *Living the Faith: The Praxis of Eastern Orthodox Ethics.* Minneapolis: Light and Life.

HATZOPOULOS, HARALAMBOS. 1990. *To hiero mysterion tou gamou: Oi miktoi gamoi.* Athens: Author.

MEYENDORFF, JOHN. 1975. *Marriage: An Orthodox Perspective.* 2d ed. Crestwood, N.Y.: St. Vladimir's Seminary Press.

PAPKOSTAS, SERAPHIM. 1947. [1933]. *To zetema tes teknogonias: To demographihon problema apo Christianikes apopseos.* Athens: Brotherhood of Theologians "Zoe."

PATRINACOS, NICON D. 1975. *The Orthodox Church on Birth Control.* Garwood, N.J.: Graphic Arts Press.

STAVROPOULOS, ALEXANDER. 1977. *He ekklesia tes Hellados enanti tou problematos tes tachnogonias.* Athens: Author.

ZAPHEIRIS, CHRYSOSTOM. 1974. "The Morality of Contraception: An Eastern Orthodox Opinion." *Journal of Ecumenical Studies* 11, no. 4:677–690.

———. 1991. *Ai ambloseis kai e Orthodoxos ekklesia: Theseis kai antitheseis.* Athens: Author.

ZION, WILLIAM BASIL. 1992. *Eros and Transformation: Sexuality and Marriage: An Eastern Orthodox Perspective.* Lanham, Md.: University Press of America.

F. PROTESTANT PERSPECTIVES

Protestantism generally includes all Christian movements, denominations, and sects whose histories can be traced to or related to the sixteenth-century Reformers, especially Martin Luther and John Calvin. Hundreds of such Christian bodies exist worldwide. They represent very diverse theological orientations and forms of church discipline. It is possible to characterize a "mainstream" position on many theological and ethical issues held by major denominational families associated with the World Council of Churches (WCC), including Anglicanism (or Episcopalianism), Lutheranism, Presbyterianism, Methodism, Congregationalism, and various national united churches, such as the United Church of Canada and the Church of North India. Many other Protestant bodies, such as the Assemblies of God, Southern Baptists, and Jehovah's Witnesses are outside such a consensus. Even within the so-called mainline churches sharp differences exist. On many issues, some Protestants take positions completely at odds with others even within their own denominations while finding themselves in agreement with persons in other denominations or even with non-Christians. In recent years, there has been a sharp increase in numbers of Protestants in traditionally Roman Catholic Latin America, in Africa, and in parts of Asia. At the same time, there has been a marked falling off of active participation in the churches in such traditionally Protestant countries as Sweden and the United Kingdom.

It is therefore difficult to generalize about any one Protestant position on population ethics. This article focuses primarily on the mainstream churches and theologians for three reasons. First, these bodies represent the main currents of Protestant Christian history. Second, these bodies have taken the most explicit positions on population issues. Third, theologians representing these bodies present us with the clearest connections between distinctively Protestant theological emphases and ethical applications.

Early Protestant thought on population

The Reformers did not have theories about population as such, although their views on human sexual relations and procreation are relevant to discussions about methods of limiting population growth. Both Luther and Calvin understood sexual relations within marriage as a morally acceptable outlet for sexual drives quite apart from the purpose of procreation. Both, especially Calvin, also viewed sexual relations within marriage as an expression of loving companionship between a husband and wife (Fagley, 1960). Early Protestantism coincided in time with the decimation of Europe's population through the plague and the Hundred Years' War, so discussions of population during that period—which were mostly by secular writers—emphasized the need for population growth, not limitation. In contrast, Robert Malthus, whose demographic theories, published in 1798, first expressed alarm over excessive population growth rates, was a Protestant clergyman. His views derived more from economic thought than from Protestant theology, but the laissez-faire economic theories that exerted primary influence upon him may themselves have been encouraged by individualistic aspects of Protestant thought, especially the heightened importance of the "calling" each person has from God and the demand that each person respond, through faith, to God's grace (Weber, 1950).

Population issues were not intrinsically important to nineteenth-century Protestant thought except at three points. First, Malthus's pessimistic views of population growth were countered by various Protestant divines who considered them an impious reflection on the goodness of God's providence (Hutchinson, 1967). Second, in Anglo-Saxon countries, attitudes toward sexual relations during the Victorian era were often repressive. This gave rise to some rejection of contraceptive methods of birth control early in the twentieth century. Third, the nativist movement in North America, which sought to inhibit immigration from Roman Catholic countries, arose almost exclusively among Protestants. That movement exerted influence on subsequent anti-immigration legislation until the mid-twentieth century.

Theological support for family planning

Protestant support for planned parenthood dates from early in the twentieth century. The early American movement in support of family planning and use of artificial methods of birth control, exemplified especially by Margaret Sanger (1883–1966, founder of Planned Parenthood), was more secular and humanist than Protestant, but it began to attract a serious following among Protestant thinkers and churches. The Lambeth Council of worldwide Anglicanism declared in 1930 that contraceptive methods could be justified when there is "a clearly felt moral obligation to limit or avoid parenthood and where there is a morally sound reason for avoiding complete abstinence." (Noonan, 1986, p. 125). During the thirty years thereafter, a strong consensus developed among mainline denominations and theologians in support of that position.

The preeminent Protestant theologian of that period, Karl Barth, wrote, "There is agreement to-day among all serious Christian moralists . . . that although the choice for or against generation and conception is not a matter for human caprice, it should not be left to chance and therefore lack the character of true decision, but must always be a matter of free obedience and therefore free consideration and decision" (Barth, 1968, p. 273). Artificial means of contraception must not, he wrote, be considered evil "just because they are so manifestly artificial" (Barth, 1968, p. 275). Dietrich Bonhoeffer, another European theologian of the midcentury, wrote, "It would not be right for blind impulse simply to run its course as it pleases and then to go on to claim to be particularly pleasing in the eyes of God; responsible reason must have a share in this decision" (Bonhoeffer, 1955, p. 177). While Bonhoeffer strongly opposed abortion, on the grounds that in the pregnancy "God certainly intended to create a human being" (Bonhoeffer, 1955, p. 176), he explicitly related support for planned parenthood to rapid population growth rates, which concerned him.

Barth's and Bonhoeffer's views are ultimately grounded in their respective views of creation. God's purposes for human life can be supported or obstructed by events in the natural order, including human interventions. When couples have children for which they are not prepared, this falls outside God's life-giving intentions. The same can be said of whole societies or of the world in general: Too rapid population growth can diminish the possibilities for humanity to find its God-intended fulfillment in the created order. Barth, therefore, did not limit his ethical perspective on family planning to decisions by individual couples about what is right for them. There was also the question of what was best for society as a whole. Humankind, in his view, is no longer under the divine command of Genesis 1, "Be fruitful, and multiply."

A leading American liberal theologian, Albert C. Knudson, expressed typical American Protestant thought in insisting (1) that procreation is not the only purpose of sexual intercourse; (2) that "there is nothing in the use of contraceptives that is inconsistent with a sincere faith in Divine Providence," since there is no religious duty to let nature run its own course; and (3) that the general improvement in the standard of living requires lowering the rate of population growth (Knudson, 1943, pp. 209–210).

The first two of these points have been so generally characteristic of mainline Protestant thought and official denominational statements that one is hard pressed to find exceptions. The third has been in some dispute.

The evolution of Protestant views in the twentieth century

We may broadly characterize three main periods in the middle to later twentieth-century Protestant church teaching on population matters.

The first period, roughly from the Lambeth statement of 1930 to the late 1960s, emphasized the companionate, love-enhancing possibilities of sexual intercourse within the bonds of marriage while deemphasizing the moral obligation of married couples to have children. Contraception was generally accepted as a morally legitimate means toward the end of expressing love within marriage for its own sake. Birth control, or "planned parenthood," was, however, considered mainly within the family unit. Couples should be able to have as many children as they wish: no more, no less. Since the real issue was whether people could decide to limit their family size by conscious decision and employing contraceptive means, the net effect of such teaching was to encourage a diminishing birth rate. But during this period comparatively little attention was given to the world population growth rate.

The second period, coinciding with the emergence of the environmental movement in the late 1960s and 1970s and the publication of neo-Malthusian literature on the "population explosion," found Protestant teaching focusing primarily on the dangers of population growth and a corresponding moral responsibility by societies to find ways to limit it. Many of the mainline church declarations date from this period, with revisions added in subsequent years.

The third period, beginning in the late 1970s and corresponding to the growth of the liberation theology movement (the movement that began in the 1960s and

that emphasizes freedom from external oppression as a central theme of Christian faith), witnessed greater criticism of neo-Malthusianism as a way to avoid social justice issues in the distribution of the world's resources. There was less inclination to treat population growth rates themselves as the primary problem. During this period, the mainline denominations continued to affirm the importance of family planning and to recognize the morality of the use of contraceptive measures of birth control. But there was a growing tendency to consider population limitation as a by-product of increased social justice and economic prosperity rather than the reverse.

In the United States, this period also witnessed the rise of evangelical Christian movements critical of mainline denominations and of what was taken to be their laxness in sexual morality and family values. Evangelicals often deemphasized the population issue while reemphasizing the restriction of sexual intercourse to marriage and strongly opposing abortion. Evangelicals, as a force in U.S. politics, played a role in the decision by the administration of President Ronald Reagan to oppose the United Nations Fund for Population Activities at the Second World Conference on Population (Mexico City, 1984) and to withdraw funding from the International Planned Parenthood Federation.

Official positions of mainline Protestant churches

Official statements by mainline denominations illustrate the continuing importance of views developed in each of these three periods.

Among the mainline denominations, the United Methodist Church developed what may be the most systematic position on population ethics. The principal outlines of its position were adopted in 1972 as part of a broader declaration of social principles. Subsequent revisions did not substantially modify this position, although various resolutions adopted by the denomination's General Conference show the influence of the third period of Protestant thinking. In its 1992 form the United Methodist statement cites the strains on food, mineral, and water supplies by growing populations and asserts, "People have the duty to consider the impact on the total world community of their decisions regarding childbearing, and should have access to information and appropriate means to limit their fertility, including voluntary sterilization" (United Methodist Church, 1992, p. 40). A 1980 resolution by that denomination adds a theological rationale: "Our goal in history is that everyone may have the conditions of existence necessary for the fulfillment of God's intentions for humanity. Our context in history is the preciousness of life and the love of God and all creation" (United Methodist Church, 1992, p. 345).

The United Methodists have also dealt at length with questions related to the migration of populations. While stopping short of supporting unlimited movement across national borders, the Methodist statement reminds its readers of biblical support for strangers and sojourners, and calls upon the leaders of all nations "to welcome generous numbers of persons and families dislocated by natural disasters, war, political turmoil, repression, persecution, discrimination, or economic hardship" (United Methodist Church, 1992, p. 510). This document also calls upon governments "to alleviate conditions and change internal politics that create a momentum for the migration of people over the world" while seeking "protection of the basic human rights of immigrants . . . for both documented and undocumented, permanent or transient refugees or immigrants" (United Methodist Church, 1992, pp. 509–510).

Another mainline denomination, the Presbyterian Church in the U.S.A. (and its predecessor denominations), advocated voluntary planned parenthood and population limitation as early as 1965. In that year, the General Assembly of the United Presbyterian Church in the United States of America (UPCUSA) (one of the predecessor communions) called upon the United States to "assist countries who request help in the development of programs of voluntary planned parenthood as a practical and humane means of controlling fertility and population growth" (Presbyterian Church in the U.S.A., 1991). In 1971, that body came to "recognize that reliance on individual desires and private decisions to effect voluntary [birth] control, however well supported by information and means, will not be sufficient to provide the necessary limitation of population growth unless there is a radical and rapid change in the attitudes and desires" (Presbyterian Church in the U.S.A., 1991). This document challenged "the assumption that couples have the freedom to have as many children as they can support," asserting that "we can no longer justify bringing into existence as many children as we desire" (Presbyterian Church in the U.S.A., 1991). In 1984, the Presbyterian General Assembly again voiced its awareness "of the increasing size of the world's population and conscious[ness] of the potential consequences of unlimited growth, of resource limitations, of insufficient public responses, and of unmet population needs" (Presbyterian Church in the U.S.A., 1991). It called "upon the U.S. government to participate fully in the International Conference [on population] and to give generous and continuing financial and logistical support to United Nations programs designed to address specific population needs" (Presbyterian Church in the U.S.A., 1991).

The American Baptist Churches adopted a policy statement in 1976 supporting "efforts to develop programs which encourage family planning in an environ-ment of free individual choice" (American Baptist Churches, 1976). Subsequent declarations emphasized social and economic justice without much specific application to population questions. A 1988 resolution indicated the denomination's internal divisions on the abortion question while opposing abortion "as a means of avoiding responsibility for conception" or "as a primary means of birth control" (American Baptist Churches in the U.S.A., 1988, p. 9).

The Friends Committee on National Legislation (FCNL) has long supported family planning, but that position receives comparatively little emphasis in statements adopted during what I have characterized as the third period in the evolution of Protestant views on population. A lengthy 1987 statement on a variety of social-political-economic issues, for instance, merely repeats the FCNL's "support for safe and non-coercive family planning as one element of an effective national population policy" (FCNL, 1988, p. 5).

The same 1987 statement does, however, contain a much lengthier section dealing with immigration and refugees. That section expresses the belief that "the world should evolve toward a global community whose people can choose freely where they wish to live and work" (FCNL, 1988, p. 6). The FCNL's "long-range ideal" is, therefore, "a world of open borders that ensures both asylum for refugees escaping oppression and freedom to migrate for those who hope to improve their living conditions" (FCNL, 1988, p. 6). Such a world would require "a more equitable distribution of the world's wealth, more respect for human rights, and greater tolerance of differences than exist at present (FCNL, 1988, p. 6).

The Unitarian Universalist Association continues to support family planning as a response to "the crush of overpopulation" that "is frequently associated with increasing the pollution of the water, air, soil, and ozone shield, and further depleting the earth's finite resources" as well as being a factor in "aggressive and destructive behavior." This denomination, like the other mainline churches, supports full access to contraception while going further than most in its direct support for "the right to choose abortion" (Unitarian Universalist Association, 1990, p. 56).

This sampling of denominational statements on population-related issues in the latter third of the twentieth century suggests no diminution of commitment to planned parenthood and the full rights of access to contraceptive technologies. At the same time, churches devoted less attention to population issues during the 1980s and 1990s and seemed more reluctant to grant full moral legitimation to abortion.

Protestant denominational statements do not generally enjoy the authoritative status of Roman Catholic papal encyclicals, though they do reflect deliberation by official bodies. When the official statements are seriously inconsistent with the deeper convictions of members, mechanisms are usually present to enact changes. That fact itself reflects a deep historic theme in most Protestant theology: God has immediate access to every believer. Consequently, the views of every church member, when expressed in good faith, must be taken seriously. Not surprisingly, therefore, Protestant viewpoints on population policy and other issues can change without threat to the basic body of shared doctrine. It is more difficult to ascertain the extent to which denominational statements on such issues reflect nontheological sociocultural influences. But the deliberative process of decision making in Protestant churches generally affords ample opportunity, over time, for purely secular influences to be criticized on the basis of shared faith traditions.

Protestant positions into the twenty-first century

Projecting the future of Protestant views on population, there seems little prospect that the basic commitments to planned parenthood will change during the period ahead. The amount of emphasis given to the issue may well vary, however, with perceptions of the effects of population growth rates and patterns of migration. Protestant churches worldwide will doubtless continue to reflect a wide variety of views on these and other subjects. Historically, however, Protestant views on such issues have tended to be framed in response to empirical problems and opportunities. Evidence mounts that the churches will increasingly have to respond to global environmental problems, and the continuing growth of world population will remain a significant factor in that (Nash, 1991). The churches' response to population migration may be even more interesting as the world moves into the twenty-first century. Toward the end of the twentieth century, ethnic nationalism was felt as a major political force in some parts of the world, such as the Middle East, the former Yugoslavia, and the former Soviet Union. Nevertheless, the growing integration of global economics, increased facilities for communication and transportation, and the conclusion of the Cold War between the United States and the Soviet Union all point toward greater pressure on the increasing irrelevance of national boundaries. While addressing problems related to population growth, religious bodies may find it equally necessary to respond to archaic restrictions of movement.

J. PHILIP WOGAMAN

While all the articles in the other sections of this entry are relevant, see especially the INTRODUCTION *and other articles in this section:* ISLAMIC PERSPECTIVES, ROMAN CATHOLIC PERSPECTIVES, JEWISH PERSPECTIVES, EASTERN ORTHODOX CHRISTIAN PERSPECTIVES, HINDU PERSPECTIVES, *and* BUDDHIST PERSPECTIVES. *Directly related to this article are the entries* POPULATION POLICIES; *and* PROTESTANTISM. *For a further discussion of topics mentioned in this article, see the entries* ENVIRONMENTAL ETHICS, *especially the* OVERVIEW; ENVIRONMENT AND RELIGION; ETHICS, *article on* RELIGION AND MORALITY; FERTILITY CONTROL, *article on* SOCIAL ISSUES; JUSTICE; MARRIAGE AND OTHER DOMESTIC PARTNERSHIPS; SEXUAL ETHICS; *and* SEXUALITY IN SOCIETY, *article on* SOCIAL CONTROL OF SEXUAL BEHAVIOR. *For a discussion of related ideas, see the entries* ABORTION, *especially the section on* RELIGIOUS TRADITIONS, *article on* PROTESTANT PERSPECTIVES; FOOD POLICY; FREEDOM AND COERCION; HOMOSEXUALITY; LOVE; MEDICAL ETHICS, HISTORY OF, *section on* EUROPE, *subsections on* RENAISSANCE AND ENLIGHTENMENT, *and* NINETEENTH CENTURY; ROMAN CATHOLICISM; *and* WARFARE, *article on* PUBLIC HEALTH AND WAR. *Other relevant material may be found under the entries* FEMINISM; INTERNATIONAL HEALTH; SEXISM; *and* WOMEN, *article on* HISTORICAL AND CROSS-CULTURAL PERSPECTIVES.

Bibliography

AMERICAN BAPTIST CHURCHES IN THE U.S.A. 1976. Policy statement on hunger, Valley Forge, Pa.
———. 1988. Resolution concerning abortion and ministry in the local church, Valley Forge, Pa.
BAINTON, ROLAND H. 1962. *Sex, Love and Marriage: A Christian Survey.* London: Collins.
BARTH, KARL. 1968. *Church Dogmatics.* Translated by Geoffrey W. Bromiley and Thomas F. Torrance. Edinburgh: T. & T. Clark.
BONHOEFFER, DIETRICH. 1955. *Ethics.* Translated by Neville Horton Smith. New York: Macmillan.
FAGLEY, RICHARD M. 1960. *The Population Explosion and Christian Responsibility.* New York: Oxford University Press.
FRIENDS COMMITTEE ON NATIONAL LEGISLATION (FCNL). 1988. *FCNL Washington Newsletter,* January.
HUTCHINSON, EDWARD P. 1967. *The Population Debate: The Development of Conflicting Theories up to 1900.* Boston: Houghton Mifflin.
KNUDSON, ALBERT C. 1943. *The Principles of Christian Ethics.* New York: Abingdon-Cokesbury Press.
LUCAS, GEORGE R., JR., and OGLETREE, THOMAS W., eds. 1976. *Lifeboat Ethics: The Moral Dilemmas of World Hunger.* San Francisco: Harper & Row.
NASH, JAMES A. 1991. *Loving Nature: Ecological Integrity and Christian Responsibility.* Nashville, Tenn.: Abingdon Press.
NOONAN, JOHN T., JR. 1986. "Contraception." In *The Westminster Dictionary of Christian Ethics,* pp. 124–126. Edited by James F. Childress and John Macquarrie. Philadelphia: Westminster Press.
PRESBYTERIAN CHURCH IN THE U.S.A. 1991. *Social Policy Compilation.* Louisville, Ky.: Author.

UNITARIAN UNIVERSALIST ASSOCIATION. 1990. *Resolutions of the Unitarian Universalist Association.* Boston: Author.

UNITED METHODIST CHURCH. 1992. *The Book of Resolutions of the United Methodist Church.* Edited by Neil M. Alexander. Nashville, Tenn.: United Methodist Publishing House.

WEBER, MAX. 1950. [1904–1905]. *The Protestant Ethic and the Spirit of Capitalism.* Translated by Talcott Parsons. New York: Scribner.

WOGAMAN, J. PHILIP, ed. 1973. *The Population Crisis and Moral Responsibility.* Washington, D.C.: Public Affairs Press.

[Note: *Official declarations on population-related issues by Protestant and ecumenical church bodies are rarely available in libraries or in trade publication form. They generally can be obtained from denominational or ecumenical offices.*]

G. HINDU PERSPECTIVES

Hinduism includes a complex array of teachings related directly and indirectly to population dynamics (fertility, mortality, and migration) and to the ethics of population-related behavior. Its rich heritage spans millennia and embraces diverse populations. Hindus are found in many world regions, both within and beyond South Asia, its area of origin. Hinduism is the predominant religious tradition of India (for a general overview, see Hiltebeitel, 1987). It is practiced in one form or another by about 80 percent of the approximately 800 million people living there. Another 20 million Hindus live in nations other than India, including Fiji, Indonesia, Singapore, Guyana, Trinidad, Canada, the United States, and the United Kingdom. Diaspora Hindu communities increased in number and prominence in the United States beginning in the late 1960s, when the law was changed to allow immigration of educated professionals. The construction of major Hindu temples in such cities as Pittsburgh, Chicago, New York, and Washington, D.C., demonstrates the vitality of this international growth.

Basic Hindu teachings on population-related ethics and behavior will have different impacts depending on the context in which Hinduism is practiced. Within a particular locality, socioeconomic class, caste, and ethnicity are associated with differences in awareness of and adherence to Hindu religious teachings. Moreover, social resistance to certain aspects of orthodox Hindu religious teachings is being voiced around the world, particularly by ethnic minorities and women's groups.

This article first considers key aspects of Hindu religious teachings. It then focuses on Hindu values in India and how they contribute to demographic practices and outcomes. Last, it offers some observations on how members of Hindu communities in the United States are revising Hindu values related to population.

Hindu teachings related to population

Several key teachings of Hinduism relate to population dynamics and have implications for how governments might formulate policy. A primary value is on *ahimsa* (this word combines the prefix *a,* non, with *himsa,* harm, thus meaning nonviolence or nonkilling). A well-known source of Hindu teachings on proper behavior, *The Laws of Manu* (Doniger and Smith, 1991), describes the model of four life stages (*ashramas*): student, householder, celibate, forest dweller. Manu's guidelines about marriage stipulate that the best form involves the father giving a virgin daughter, implying that the marriage is arranged by the parents of the bride and groom. Repeated statements in *The Laws of Manu* emphasize the importance for a woman of bearing offspring, especially sons. Other popular classical Hindu myths, such as in the epic *Mahabharata,* contain messages relevant to population. One is that the world is overpopulated, and that renunciation of the world is a valid means for release from personal, familial, and other worldly attachments. Celibacy is honored as reflecting a high level of self-control and spiritual attainment. Teachings about celibacy are linked with a strongly enunciated value on premarital chastity for females.

It is likely that these general teachings are known to Hindus throughout India and across most social divisions. It is also likely that links between people's knowledge of Hinduism and their population practices vary markedly across regions because India's demography differs dramatically by region and class (see Miller, 1981). Fertility is much higher in the northern plains than in the south and east. Mortality is more gender-differentiated in the northern plains, with excess female mortality, and is less severely skewed by gender in the south and east.

Thus we are confronted with a puzzle: Basic Hindu teachings are espoused by India's Hindu population more or less equally, but Hindu demography does not present a smooth pattern. We must therefore assume a loose linkage between Hindu teachings and demographic outcomes such as fertility rates and child survival by gender. In other words, as an explanatory variable affecting population dynamics, Hindu teachings are partial at most.

Population issues in India

Fertility.   Reproduction should, according to Hindu cultural norms, take place only within marriage. Stigma is attached to a premarital pregnancy, a situation that may bring serious consequences to the persons involved. A high premium is placed on marriage as a universal life stage through which, ideally, everyone should pass. As a householder, one marries, has children, and raises them. Reproduction is the primary goal of marriage. For Hindu women, the key to auspiciousness (a highly desired status for women that implies the opposite of stigma) involves being married, being devoted to one's husband, and bearing sons. All these values are clearly pronatal.

Hindu values support the bearing of children within marriage, and they emphasize the bearing of sons. Sons provide social security for their aged parents. The social security function of sons is especially marked in the northern Indian kinship system, which is followed strictly by Hindus and Jains. North Indian kinship rules stipulate that a daughter must marry a man from outside her natal village while a married son remains with his parents and brings a bride into his family. Another primary value of Hindus is to have a son light one's funeral pyre; a daughter cannot perform this task. The Sanskrit word for "hell" is *put*; the word for son, *putra*, means "the one who saves his ancestors from hell" (May and Heer, 1968, p. 200). Given mortality rates of the mid-1960s, demographers estimated that in order for a man to have a son who would be alive when he was sixty-five years old, his wife would have to bear seven children. Preference for male children operates to promote fertility and also plays a role in excess female mortality and indirect fertility reduction as discussed below. Desire for sons prompts families to keep trying until they have one, and then to have a second or third son as well.

The pervasiveness of the Hindu teachings on the value of having sons may be regionally variable in terms of intensity. Social surveys across the nation reveal that a stated preference for sons is stronger in the northern region than in the south and east (Dyson and Moore, 1983). This difference arises because socioeconomic factors such as the gender division of labor, marriage and kinship patterns, and the costs of marriage operate to affect the level of son preference (Miller, 1981; Dyson and Moore, 1983).

Other important fertility-reducing factors related to Hindu beliefs include ritually determined rules for sexual abstinence that limit the frequency of intercourse. One study found a total of 120 days mentioned for abstention (Nag, 1972). Such rules may be linked to a lower frequency of intercourse among Hindus than among Muslims, since the latter do not have such ritually proscribed days. Also important are the positive value placed on male self-control, including control of sexuality, and male anxiety about semen loss (Bottero, 1991). No one knows how much of an effect these conditions might have on the frequency of intercourse or actual reproductive rates, but one could posit at least some impact on both compared with non-Hindu populations.

Hindu views concerning widowhood may also lower fertility, since widows should not remarry and therefore should not reproduce (Mandelbaum, 1974). Restrictions on widow remarriage most significantly decreases fertil-ity when women are widowed at a young age, as they often are in India.

Direct methods of fertility control, such as condoms, birth-control pills, or sterilization, are not antithetical to Hindu teaching since sexual intercourse is not seen solely as a means to achieve pregnancy. In contrast with this fairly liberal understanding, the famous leader of the independence movement and national hero, Mohandas Gandhi, supported abstinence as the only appropriate contraceptive.

Abortion for sociomedical reasons has long been legally allowed in India, except in the predominantly Muslim state of Kashmir (Chandrasekhar, 1974). In spite of legal provisions for abortion, safe services are lacking (Dixon-Mueller, 1990). This situation reflects the political priorities of the central and state governments more than religious doctrine.

Sex-selective abortion, a practice begun in the 1980s, is done almost exclusively to abort female fetuses. One study of a large number of hospital births in the Ludhiana area of the state of Punjab in northwestern India found that after 1983, when sex-selection became possible through amniocentesis, the sex ratio at birth rose from a normal of 105 boys per 100 girls to 117 boys per 100 girls in 1989 (Sachar et al., 1990). Many feminist activists in India wish to maintain a woman's right to seek an abortion while striving to ban sex-selective abortion. The debate on prenatal sex selection in the public media in India has been largely secular.

Mortality. India is well known for its gender bias in survival of males and females. Hindu teachings that favor males provide the ideological justification for better treatment of males than females. But it is not possible to explain the scarcity of females relative to males in the Indian population solely on Hinduism. North India and neighboring Pakistan, which is predominantly Muslim, have similar gender patterns in mortality. Recent demographic data on China reveal substantial differences in mortality rates between males and females there as well. Economic, political, and social factors are important in explaining this phenomenon.

In the northern plains of India, son preference is linked with behavior termed "daughter neglect" (Miller 1981, 1987). This neglect, which takes the form of biased allocations of food, medical care, and psychological attention, can be fatal. It skews the sex ratio among children as well as in the general population. In northern India, census data from the first part of the twentieth century indicated that unbalanced juvenile sex ratios favoring boys characterized all major religious groups in the area: Sikhs, Hindus, Muslims, and Jains. Son preference interacts with daughter neglect to create excess female child mortality. The indirect fertility-reducing effect of excess female child mortality is clear:

If daughters experience higher mortality than sons, then the number of future childbearers is reduced in comparison with what would be the case without excess female child mortality. In such a demographic regime, the ratio of living sons to daughters is maintained over time, as brides are brought in from other villages and regions to marry sons; thus, no "shortage" of brides to produce future sons is perceived or experienced.

Hindu beliefs seem implicated in the high mortality rates of widows, which are caused by general neglect and nutritional deprivation (Chen and Drèze, 1992). More extremely, the low value placed on a woman once her husband has died relates to the uncommon practice of *sati*, the suicide of a Hindu widow on the funeral pyre of her husband. In general, the value of female self-sacrifice is long-standing in Hinduism, and it supports socialization patterns of girls that train them in self-denial of food and other resources.

Migration.   According to traditional Hindu teaching, migration beyond the boundaries of India was grounds for outcasting. Since the late nineteenth century, however, the rate of migration of Hindus outside of India has increased substantially (Madhavan, 1985), and anxiety about "outcasting" appears to be nonexistent among migrants. With international migration, Hindu traditions are being reshaped in local contexts.

The United States

In the United States, most Hindus are middle or upper class (Helweg and Helweg, 1990), although large populations, especially in New York City and New Jersey, are less well off. Among this employed and generally well-educated population, fertility rates are low, infant and child mortality rates are low, and longevity is high.

The value placed on having a son among the Hindu population of the United States is an important but unresearched question. Undocumented sources indicate numerous cases of demand for prenatal sex determination, in order to keep male fetuses, by South Asian immigrants in the United States and Canada. As of 1994, U.S. law prohibits abortion based on the sex of the fetus, but people circumvent this rule. They may have a test done ostensibly to reveal genetic abnormalities in the fetus and, in the process, find out its sex. If the fetus is female, they go to another doctor and present a story about genetic abnormalities in their family that cannot be proved or disproved because the relatives who are claimed to have the genetic problems are in South Asia. On this basis, the couple requests an abortion.

Within the teachings of Hinduism, nothing specifically argues against sex-selective abortion per se, since traditional teachings do not address the topic of abortion from a gender-specific perspective. This issue will pose a challenge for contemporary theologians and ethicists working within the Hindu tradition.

Another issue being quietly contested in the everyday lives of Hindus and Jains in the United States is premarital chastity. In opposition to the more liberal sexual mores among the general population, many Hindu and Jain parents apply pressures on their children, especially daughters, to maintain their virginity before marriage. Depending on how conservative the family is, more or less intergenerational conflict ensues.

Many Hindu and Jain communities have started Sunday schools (never a tradition in India) and summer camps where religious values are instilled in young children and teenagers. Such values include premarital chastity. At the same time, marked liberalizing changes are being made in some Hindu rituals in the United States, as a response to lowered fertility rates (many Hindu families have only one child) and an interest in treating daughters the same as sons. In the early 1990s, the Hindu-Jain temple of Pittsburgh held its first *upanayana* (sacred thread) ceremony for girls. Several liberal-minded leaders promoted this reform of Hindu tradition, which restricts the *upanayana* ceremony to boys of the upper castes.

The challenge of change

Neither Hinduism nor population dynamics is static. Contemporary movements in Hinduism range from conservative trends that could be termed fundamentalist to more liberal tendencies among some migrant communities. The greatest challenges to the study of the relationship between Hindu teachings and population lie in the following directions: the links that individuals make in their thinking between Hindu tenets and their own demographic practices; the reactions of Hindu theologians to new questions such as sex-selective abortion; and governments' policies in dealing with such problems as population growth and excess female mortality within a moral framework that would be acceptable to Hindu constituents.

BARBARA D. MILLER

While all the articles in the other sections of this entry are relevant, see especially the INTRODUCTION *and other articles in this section:* ISLAMIC PERSPECTIVES, PROTESTANT PERSPECTIVES, ROMAN CATHOLIC PERSPECTIVES, JEWISH PERSPECTIVES, EASTERN ORTHODOX CHRISTIAN PERSPECTIVES, *and* BUDDHIST PERSPECTIVES. *Directly related to this article are the entries* POPULATION POLICIES; *and* HINDUISM. *For a further discussion of topics mentioned in this article, see the entries* ABUSE, INTERPERSONAL, *articles on* CHILD ABUSE, *and* ABUSE BETWEEN DOMESTIC PARTNERS; DEATH; FERTILITY CONTROL, *article on* SOCIAL ISSUES;

Marriage and Other Domestic Partnerships; Public Health, *article on* determinants of public health; *and* Reproductive Technologies, *article on* sex selection. *For a discussion of related ideas, see the entries* Abortion; Environment and Religion; Environmental Ethics, *especially the* overview; Genetic Testing and Screening, *article on* prenatal diagnosis; Islam; Jainism; Medical Ethics, History of, *section on* south and east asia, *article on* india; *and* Sikhism. *Other relevant material may be found under the entries* Feminism; Food Policy; Maternal–Fetal Relationship; Sexism; *and* Women, *article on* historical and cross-cultural perspectives.

Bibliography

Bottero, Alain. 1991. "Consumption by Semen Loss in India and Elsewhere." *Culture, Medicine, Psychiatry* 15, no. 3:303–320.

Chandrasekhar, Sripati. 1974. *Abortion in a Crowded World: The Problem of Abortion with Special Reference to India.* Seattle: University of Washington Press.

Chen, Marty, and Drèze, Jean. 1992. "Widows and Health in Rural North India." *Economic and Political Weekly of India* 27, nos. 43–44:W5-81–W5-92.

Dixon-Mueller, Ruth. 1990. "Abortion Policy and Women's Health in Developing Countries." *International Journal of Health Services* 20, no. 2:297–314.

Doniger, Wendy, and Smith, Brian K., trans. 1991. *The Laws of Manu.* New York: Penguin.

Dyson, Tim, and Moore, Mick. 1983. "On Kinship Structure, Female Autonomy, and Demographic Behavior in India." *Population and Development Review* 9, no. 1: 35–60.

Helweg, Arthur W., and Helweg, Usha M. 1990. *An Immigrant Success Story: East Indians in America.* Philadelphia: University of Pennsylvania Press.

Hiltebeitel, Alf. 1987. "Hinduism." In vol. 6 of *The Encyclopedia of Religion*, pp. 336–360. Edited by Mircea Eliade. New York: Macmillan.

Madhavan, M. C. 1985. "Indian Emigrants, Numbers, Characteristics, and Economic Impact." *Population and Development Review* 11, no. 3:457–481.

Mandelbaum, David G. 1974. *Human Fertility in India: Social Components and Policy Perspectives.* Berkeley: University of California Press.

May, David A., and Heer, David M. 1968. "Son Survivorship Motivation and Family Size in India: A Computer Simulation." *Population Studies* 22, no. 2:199–210.

Miller, Barbara D. 1981. *The Endangered Sex: Neglect of Female Children in Rural North India.* Ithaca, N.Y.: Cornell University Press.

———. 1987. "Female Infanticide and Child Neglect in Rural North India." In *Child Survival: Anthropological Perspectives on the Treatment and Maltreatment of Children*, pp. 95–112. Edited by Nancy Scheper-Hughes. Dordrecht, Netherlands: D. Reidel.

Nag, Moni. 1972. "Sex, Culture, and Human Fertility: India and the United States." *Current Anthropology* 13, no. 2:231–237.

Sachar, R. K.; Verma, J.; Prakash, V.; Chopra, A.; Adhlaka, R.; and Sofat, R. 1990. "The Unwelcome Sex: Female Feticide in India." *World Health Forum* 11, no. 3:309–310.

H. BUDDHIST PERSPECTIVES

Buddhism is a dominant cultural force in most parts of Asia. Theravada Buddhism, also known under the name of Hinayana or "Small Vehicle," prevails in such Southeast Asian countries as Sri Lanka, Thailand, Burma, Cambodia, and Laos; its sister sect, Mahayana Buddhism, or "Great Vehicle," is currently found in Tibet, Japan, Taiwan, and Korea. This article focuses on Theravada Buddhism, especially as practiced in Thailand.

Though Therevadins have their own sacred literature that distinguishes them from the rest of Buddhism, they do share certain central beliefs with other Buddhists. Among these beliefs are those concerned with *samsara, karma,* and *nirvana,* which are the key concepts of all forms of Buddhism. *Samsara* refers to the round of existence, or the cycle of rebirth, in which all beings revolve according to their *karma.* This perpetual cycle comprises three realms of rebirth, namely, the realm of desire (*kamaloka*), the realm of forms (*rupaloka*), and the formless realm (*arupaloka*). These realms have thirty-one subspheres containing different forms of life, such as humans (*manussa*); animals (*tirachan*); ghosts or unhappy departed beings with deformed bodies (*peta*); spirits or wandering ghostly beings (*bhuta*); hell-beings or tortured beings (*niraya*); titans (*asura*); and gods (*deva*). The realm of desire consists of the higher spheres of gods; the middle spheres, of sentient beings, humans, and animals; and the lower spheres, of ghosts, spirits, and hell-beings. The celestial realm of forms and the formless realm are the abodes of the most refined and subtle beings (*brahman*). Despite differences in life span, beings in all realms are subject to death and rebirth.

Karma means intentional, mental, verbal, or physical action and its result (*vipaka*). The sequence of actions, or deeds, and their effects, known as the law of *karma,* act both as the natural law of cause and effect (operating in the physical realm) and as the moral law (governing the moral sphere that regulates the movement of beings between rebirths). Rebirths of all beings are the natural results of their own deeds, good or bad, and not "rewards" or "punishment" imposed by a supernatural, omniscient ruling power. All beings reap what they sowed in the past, and all will be reborn according to the nature of their present deeds—they are "heirs" to their actions. When a being dies, the karmic result, acting as the individual life-force, passes to other lives, endlessly exalting or degrading successive rebirths. This life-force will become completely inactivated only with the cessation of craving (*tanha*), the inherent force of karmic action. Such cessation is referred to as *nirvana* and can be achieved through following the Middle Path (*Majima Patipada*) consisting of wisdom (*panna*), morality (*sila*), and concentration (*samadhi*).

Buddhist concepts in population growth and control

There is no fixed number for population in *samsara* existence. It is in a state of flux, with continual migration of beings from one realm to the others regulated by the law of *karma* and continuously readjusted to the nature and the quality of *samsara* dwellers. An increase of population in one realm means a decrease of population in others, and vice versa. Human rebirth is considered incomparably precious because the human realm is the only place where there is enough suffering to motivate humans to seek ways to transcend misery and enough freedom to act on their aspirations. In the higher and lower spheres, by contrast, beings are fully reaping the karmic results, good and bad: The gods are too absorbed in the blissful state to find ways out of *samsara* existence while animals, ghosts, spirits, and hell-beings are in irremediable misery and have little freedom to do either good or evil. These suffering beings will gain the precious human rebirth only when the results of bad *karma* that led to their lower rebirths are exhausted. When this happens, the results of their previous good actions performed when they were human will lead them to better rebirths and, sooner or later, to the human level again.

From this view, an increase in the human population is desirable for it means more beings will have the rare human opportunity to transcend suffering. In theory, then, Buddhists should welcome population growth. But the fact that increasing numbers of Buddhists use contraceptives in countries such as Thailand, where 98 percent of the population is Buddhist, seems to indicate a different position. Family planning has been quite successful in both urban and rural areas of Thailand. Apart from the contributing factors of the economy, social change, and education, there are some Buddhist tenets that may account for the low fertility rate. The most important one is the emphasis on the quality of human life concomitant with the high value it gives to human rebirth.

In the Buddhist perspective, the rare human rebirth is meaningless if there is no quality in it. The value of life does not depend on its duration but on its quality. For life to be worth living, it should be lived with the ultimate purpose of attaining *nirvana,* the final emanci-

pation. This goal, however, like all spiritual progress, cannot be achieved without a certain degree of material and economic security. Below the level of subsistence, human life lacks real meaning because it consists only of hunger, illness, and unrelieved misery. This emphasis on material necessities was made by the Buddha as a necessary condition for a truly enlightened, meaningful life. The Buddha himself once refused to preach to a starving man until his hunger had first been appeased. He also recommended that monks who lead the life of renunciation depend on the lay community for food, shelter, and clothing.

This emphasis on life's material necessities is an important part of the Buddhist perspectives on population control and thus needs to be considered together with the Buddhist endorsement of human rebirth. That is, human rebirth, though desirable, needs adequate supporting conditions (*upatthambhaka*) to enable it to be worthwhile. Since famine is one of the most powerful forces (*upapilaka*) working against spiritual development, Buddhism does not approve of population growth disproportionate to a society's available resources of food. Because of this, Buddhists in Thailand and other countries do not attribute large family size to good *karma.* Unlike the Hindu householder, who believes he must have sons to perform the prescribed rituals for him after his death, Buddhist parents are not anxious to have sons to be ordained as monks. Although ordination is considered a meritorious act that will ensure good rebirth after death, many other means of receiving merit are also available, including offering food to monks, listening to sermons, and building or repairing temples.

The lack of anxiety for sons or large families supports the practice of family planning among Thai Buddhists. Unlike abortion, which is still socially unacceptable in Thailand and not as widely practiced as it is in Japan, birth control is believed by Thai Buddhists to be in line with Buddhist teachings concerning marriage and family life. Though the Buddha considered celibate life superior to married life, he did not advise it for all his followers. Realizing that all humans were at different stages of spiritual evolution, he did not commend the same codes of conduct to all. To his lay followers who could not lead the austere life of monks and nuns, he recommended marriage but stressed spiritual progress, and not procreation, as its main goal. For those with children he devised a code of discipline, emphasizing responsible childbearing and child rearing.

For Thai Buddhists birth control, unlike abortion, does not transgress the Buddhist precept of nonkilling, nor does it interfere with the working of the law of *karma.* In Buddhist understanding, conception begins only when three factors merge: the coitus of the parents, the woman's generative capability, and the presence of the *gandhabba*, the karmic life force of one who has died. By preventing pregnancy, birth control makes human rebirth more difficult but it does not interfere with the operation of the law of *karma*.

From the Buddhist viewpoint, the fruition of good or bad karma requires the right supporting conditions; without them the karmic life-force cannot express itself. Only beings who are fully qualified for human rebirth can be reborn in the human realm. Under unfavorable physical conditions a being, though possessing the good *karma* to be reborn as a human being, must dwell in his or her sphere waiting until the opportune moment. Buddhism does not oblige parents to open the gate of human rebirth to all beings with good *karma* by having as many children as they can. The Buddhist concept of *karma* assigns to each person sole responsibility for his or her own life. According to the Buddhist analysis of human nature, one's sexual life is the outcome of the urge to satisfy one's sexual craving. Whether sexual activity produces children or not is a matter to be decided by the couples themselves. The autonomy of individuals to choose their own destiny and to be responsible for their own actions is a crucial element in Buddhist population ethics.

Self-restraint and the control of the senses and passions are recommended as important forms of population control and to prevent the sexual indulgence that widespread use of artificial means of birth control may lead to. Following this teaching, many Buddhists in Thailand, Sri Lanka, and Burma have contributed to population control by practicing sexual continence, leading celibate lives as monks or nuns, and using contraceptives.

PINIT RATANAKUL

While all the articles in the other sections of this entry are relevant, see especially the INTRODUCTION *and other articles in this section:* ISLAMIC PERSPECTIVES, PROTESTANT PERSPECTIVES, ROMAN CATHOLIC PERSPECTIVES, JEWISH PERSPECTIVES, EASTERN ORTHODOX CHRISTIAN PERSPECTIVES, *and* HINDU PERSPECTIVES. *Directly related to this article are the entries* POPULATION POLICIES; *and* FERTILITY CONTROL. *For a further discussion of Buddhist religious traditions, see the entries* BUDDHISM; MEDICAL ETHICS, HISTORY OF, *section on* SOUTH AND EAST ASIA; DEATH, *article on* EASTERN THOUGHT; *and* EUGENICS AND RELIGIOUS LAW, *article on* HINDUISM AND BUDDHISM. *Other relevant material may be found under the entries* CONFUCIANISM; ENVIRONMENTAL ETHICS, *especially the* OVERVIEW; ENVIRONMENT AND RELIGION; REPRODUCTIVE TECHNOLOGIES; *and* TAOISM.

Bibliography

CHOPRA, PRAN NATH. 1983. *Contribution of Buddhism to World Civilization and Culture.* New Delhi: S. Chand & Company.

CHULALONGKORN UNIVERSITY. INSTITUTE OF POPULATION STUDIES. 1991. *Population in Thailand in 25 Years (1965–1990).* Bangkok: Chulalongkorn University Press.

GOMBRICH, RICHARD, and OBEYESEKERE, GANANATH. 1988. *Buddhism Transformed: Religious Change in Sri Lanka.* Princeton, N.J.: Princeton University Press.

HARVEY, PETER. 1990. *An Introduction to Buddhism: Teachings, History and Practices.* Cambridge: At the University Press.

LAFLEUR, WILLIAM R. 1992. *Liquid Life: Abortion and Buddhism in Japan.* Princeton, N.J.: Princeton University Press.

SMITH, BARDWELL. 1992. "Buddhism and Abortion in Contemporary Japan: Mizuko Kuyo and the Confrontation with Death." In *Buddhism, Sexuality, and Gender,* pp. 65–90. Edited by José Ignacio Cabezon. Albany: State University of New York Press.

POPULATION POLICIES

I. STRATEGIES OF FERTILITY CONTROL

A. CHANGES IN ATTITUDE AND CULTURE

Demographic transition theory posits that the Western fertility transition (the reduction in family size that began in France in the late eighteenth century and more generally in northwestern and central Europe and the English-speaking countries of overseas European settlement in the second half of the nineteenth century) was the product of changing attitudes, culture, and social structures, as well as of material conditions. It follows that one way of accelerating fertility decline in contemporary Third World countries might be to change attitudes and society by means of educational and motivational campaigns aimed at altering attitudes on family size, or the prime desirability of children, or altering behavior with regard to age at marriage, or the practice of birth control.

Such campaigns inevitably raise questions both about whether they constitute an assault on cultures and whether that can be justified, and about whether they are actually presenting proven facts about the advantages to be derived from controlling family size. The justification for the attempt to change cultures is usually either that people will benefit in a range of ways from liberation from restrictive traditions, or that the advantages likely to result from decreasing rates of population growth outweigh any damage done to societies by changing the society or fertility behavior at an earlier time than economic development and social change would have spontaneously brought about. The ethical issues involved are sharpened by the fact that the encouragement for such campaigns usually originates in the West and through international organizations.

At individual level, motivational campaigns are deemed necessary by many advocates of family-planning programs on the grounds that contraception is innovational behavior in the society, requiring support and leadership. Indeed, they argue, the adoption of family planning in a society with low levels of contraceptive use involves substantial psychic costs. Such motivational efforts to change individual behavior, and inevitably the nature of societies that favor large families, constitute only a modest part of contemporary Third World population programs, probably more because they have proved to be relatively difficult and unrewarding than because of misgivings about attacks on culture. Most national family-planning programs have found it easier to provide plentiful cheap or free contraceptives, to inform potential clients where they are to be obtained, to offer incentives or disincentives, or, in some programs, to employ directly coercive measures.

Justifying changing attitudes and culture

From the time of Thomas Malthus's publication of the first version of An Essay on the Principle of Population (1798), his followers were able to claim that the danger presented by population growth outstripping subsistence was so great as to justify quite extreme measures. Those measures included long-delayed marriage and strict abstention from sexual relations while single. Because such

behavior was in accordance with middle-class morality of the time, and because he argued that expenditure on assisting the poor in accordance with the Poor Laws was pointless since any resultant reduction in mortality would result in additional population growth and ultimately just as much misery, the English establishment was largely convinced by the analysis.

It was the socialists, especially Karl Marx, who accused Malthus of preaching a political message—less taxation for the rich and less help for the poor—in the guise of a social analysis. This debate led to opposition to organized birth control by many socialists that still continues, with the claim that the advocates of birth control aim to postpone the appearance of capitalism's contradictions. From about the 1870s, the new birth-control movement stressed the situation of women and the range of disabilities they suffered from continuous childbearing. This movement certainly aimed at changing society, but the most accurate historical judgment is that the movement was the outgrowth of the culture itself.

Most sensitivity to induced cultural change arises when the stimuli are external and the debate really centers on international efforts to curb Third World population growth. No social scientists have had more influence on these programs than the group of demographers associated during the 1940s and 1950s with Princeton University's Office of Population Research and its director, Frank Notestein. They focused their interest first on the historic fertility transition in the West, then on European colonies in Asia and Africa, and finally on all developing countries, arguing that social-science knowledge should be employed to accelerate a global transition to low levels of fertility and slow population growth.

Notestein's attitudes and interpretations influenced a generation of demographers and the new Third World family-planning programs. He concluded that the human race had survived only because cultural props, such as the idealization and religious sanctification of high female fertility and the mandating of early female marriage, had kept birth rates "artificially high" in order to overcome the ravages of high levels of mortality. As mortality declined (as evidenced by a widening gap between birth and death rates and accelerating population growth), the props became not only outdated but even dangerous, and efforts to make them wither at a faster rate could hardly be condemned. Notestein believed that fertility decline would be enhanced by the replacement of extended families by nuclear families, which he regarded as freeing individuals from the control of their relatives and, in agreement with Wilbert Moore, as being necessary to produce societies more attuned to the modern economy. He wrote of producing "a population increasingly freed from its old taboos" through "the development of a rational and secular point of view" (Notestein, 1945, 1953). Donald Warwick (1982) identified views of this type in a 1969 report justifying the development of a family-planning program in Kenya. Notestein was not a cultural relativist and certainly believed that people were better off when they were freed from their ancient taboos and had ready access to contraception. In the 1940s he thought that this would come only from evolutionary historical change, but by the 1960s he was happy to see this process hastened by national family-planning programs and their "educational" efforts.

The belief that family-planning programs were ethically justified in attempting to change societies because they liberated individuals and raised living standards can hardly be treated alone, for the programs were just one part of massive post–World War II international efforts to accelerate economic development, efforts that were also characterized by the belief that people would benefit from a loosening of the bonds of traditional society and traditional families, as well as from being richer. Family-planning programs drew attention to more sensitive issues because they dealt with very intimate personal behavior that was often the central concern of traditional culture and religion. Agencies providing international aid claimed that Third World governments represented their people and cultures, and hence that programs those governments requested usually were ethically correct. The problem with this stance was similar to that encountered with building dams or clearing tropical rain forests: Governments tended to represent the educated, modernizing elites with international viewpoints and economic interests, while the resistance came from remoter populations with older traditions still more intact.

In the 1950s and 1960s, the international family-planning movement suspected that most people in developing countries did not favor fertility control and that a great deal of persuasion would be needed to change that situation. The moral basis for attempting this change was at first very largely the Malthusian one: that future catastrophe threatened and individuals might be required to make sacrifices or to moderate their behavior for the eventual common good. The threat of exponential population growth was demonstrated by a virtual demographic industry devoted to producing ever more sophisticated projections of population growth and centering on the United Nations Population Division's series beginning in 1951. This apparently threatening growth was contrasted with the likely limited availability of resources, especially food. In a 1968 paper, "The Tragedy of the Commons," Garrett Hardin argued that "the population problem has no technical solution; it requires a fundamental extension in morality" (p. 1243).

His conclusion was that "freedom to breed is intolerable," and his direction for population programs was "Mutual coercion mutually agreed upon." His argument has two obvious weaknesses. First, there was no proof that there was no technical solution. Many demographers believed that population growth could be halted within the bounds set by agriculturalists for the ceiling on food production while continuing to allow reproductive free choice. Second, mutual agreement was always improbable; at best it was likely to be majority coercion of the minority. Proponents of views similar to Hardin's were William and Paul Paddock (1967) and Paul Ehrlich (1968).

Limitations advocated by environmentalists

About 1966, when Kenneth Boulding coined the phrase "Spaceship Earth," a greater emphasis began to emerge on the limitations imposed on human growth by all resources, the need to save the environment, the fragility of Earth, and the need for a long-term strategy of sustainable growth. These concerns culminated in a debate in the late 1960s, mostly in the pages of *Science,* where Kingsley Davis (1967) argued that it was irresponsible to rely on family-planning programs alone for the containment of population growth and that more positive governmental initiatives would be needed to change the nature of the family. Bernard Berelson (1969) replied that the record of family-planning programs did provide evidence that they could halt population growth in time, that they were acceptable to individuals and morally tolerable to providers, in that coercion or direct attempts to change society's basic units were not required. The issue here, conspicuous since Malthus, was whether all humankind and all cultures would have to concede some independence in order to ensure the survival of the human race on the planet.

Fertility control as a concern of women

Different ethical issues had begun to emerge in the West in the nineteenth century, issues associated with names like Marie Stopes and Margaret Sanger. The family-planning associations and clinics were mostly run by women for women, on the grounds that reproduction and its containment was predominantly a female concern because, at the individual level, women had more to lose or gain than did men. In the United States there was persistent legal prosecution of doctors and others who gave contraceptive advice or distributed or mailed information on the subject. Some doctors were sent to jail for years, and in 1917 Sanger spent a month in prison. The opposition to family planning was partly religious, especially among Catholics, on the grounds that contraception was against the divine law, but mostly moral, on the grounds that contraceptive knowledge would encourage premarital sexual relations and that such intimate discussion of the psychology of sex was "obscene, lewd and lascivious." These were the words of the 1873 Comstock Law, which forbade the use of the mail for distributing contraceptive information. The main thrust of the law was against the mailing of erotic postcards, which had become common, but sections were added to curb the propagation of birth-control advice.

Twentieth-century feminist scholars have tended to argue that traditional culture, far from deserving to be hallowed as a social consensus, usually takes the form of a patriarchy dominated by men who exploit women. Sandra Tangri argued in the first volume of *Signs* (1976) that women should have control over their own bodies, and that family-planning programs were commendable if they supported that achievement; however, population control was a secondary issue, and "the concrete needs of individuals should take precedence over some abstract notion of what is good for society" (p. 899). Judith Bruce (1987) argued that everyone needs to feel some unease about the fact that women's bodies are the main vehicle for achieving population control—indeed, family-planning programs appear to blame women for the world's difficulties. Bruce also felt that secrecy might in many circumstances be unethical, yet, given the patriarchal traditions of societies in many developing nations, there might well be a moral good in family-planning programs in such societies providing contraception that was female-controlled and undetectable, thus investing women with reproductive decision-making power. International agencies, while having a commitment to the self-determination of societies, also became at least as dedicated to furthering the rights of women and their children, with little reference to culture or stage of history.

Economics and other issues

The ethical value of the case for employing more forcible family-planning programs depends on the strength of the proof of the cases put forward by those advocating such measures, and also on an estimate of what is lost to the individual and to society in implementing the programs. In spite of very plausible theoretical models, there is surprisingly little empirical evidence that countries with more slowly growing populations have benefited economically in contrast with comparable societies having high rates of population growth (although Ansley Coale [1967] has pointed out that in all countries where fertility is low, over 90 percent of children attend primary school and at least half of the population lives in urban areas). Colin Clark (1967) and Julian Simon (1981) have argued that there is every reason why eco-

nomic gains have not accrued from slowing population growth. They argue that the real price of most raw materials has been falling persistently and that they are either in virtually limitless supply or easily substitutable. Less convincingly, they argue that past rises in food production were as rapid as population growth and that this would probably continue to be the case even if special efforts were not made to control population growth. Simon (1981, p. 67) becomes more agnostic on the issue: "It is not necessary or useful to discuss whether there is an 'ultimate' limit to the supply of any natural resource including food. . . . We know for sure that the world can produce vastly more food than it now does." Simon also argues that people are the important resource and that large populations have more taxpayers and more geniuses. The latter argument is very different from the conclusion that might be drawn from the experience of Athens in the fifth century B.C.E.: that the right conditions and circumstances, rather than sheer numbers, are more likely to produce geniuses.

Huge international survey programs, including the KAP (knowledge, attitudes, and practices with regard to family planning) surveys of the 1960s–1970s, the World Fertility Surveys of the 1970s–1980s, and the Demographic and Health Surveys of the 1980s–1990s, have been employed to show that there is a KAP gap: Many Third World women have more children than they desire, because they have insufficient access to contraception, are troubled about employing it, or are overruled by husbands and other relatives. The exact size of the gap is difficult to estimate, as Charles Westoff showed in a revision of some of his earlier conclusions (Westoff and Pebley, 1981). Donald Warwick (1982) has argued that the surveys came to these conclusions by employing international questionnaires, little modified for different societies, and addressed themselves only to women of reproductive age.

The Catholic church argues that the ethical case against promoting national family-planning programs offering artificial contraception rests not on a denial that rapid population growth threatens living standards but on the fact that the use of artificial contraception is in conflict with natural law, and that too much concentration on population control denies the high value that should be placed on human life and ignores the cooperation that fecundity displays with the creative activity of God. There are elements of these views in all the major religions. Marxists have argued that each economic system has its own laws and that the creation of national family-planning programs assumes a wrong priority: First, socialist societies should be created that will have very different relations to employment, resource utilization, and even population growth. Some critics, especially in the United States, see problems not in family-planning programs as such but in those that advocate or facilitate abortion, or provide information or services to adolescents. Family-planning programs have been regularly attacked in Africa, by men arguing with politicians or writing to the press, for putting the idea of risk-free, nonmarital sexual activities before unmarried young women or wives, and in both Africa and Asia for using the media or billboards to present messages about delicate matters in a way that is an affront to the cultures.

Family-planning programs in practice

The attempt to increase fertility control by changing attitudes and culture is close to what W. Parker Mauldin and colleagues have called "program effort," the factor that they have determined to be one of the main components in determining family-planning success (Mauldin and Ross, 1991). The organized influences on individual women, families, or communities usually come from three sources: family-planning workers or visitors, usually women, who take their message from door to door; messages in the media; and political leadership in the form of exhortations from national or local leaders. Very little research has been reported on the content of their messages—especially those of the all-important family-planning workers—so the content cannot be assessed. It is clear that these messages promise a better future if family size is restricted, less commonly offer women better health, and provide reassurance about the safety of contraception and the lack of serious side effects.

Family-planning workers are regarded as successful if they receive more clients and keep them practicing family planning by means of these assurances rather than according to the extent to which they involve themselves in a dialogue with clients, trying to assess whether economic gains are likely or if the side effects make the use of contraception more unpleasant than it is worth. In the better programs, family-planning workers arrange for clients to secure medical advice or to change contraception, and frequently they provide some forms of contraception. Sometimes their jobs, their promotion, or part of their income—and always their self-respect and the esteem in which the program holds them—depend on how persuasive they can be. The program at Matlab, Bangladesh, run by the International Centre for Diarrhoeal Disease Research, recruited as family-planning workers only educated young women, practicing family planning and married into the leading and most powerful families of the district, so that they could provide leadership and change models (Caldwell and Caldwell, 1992).

In rural south India, John Caldwell and his colleagues (Caldwell et al., 1988) found that the decision of women to be sterilized depended to a great degree on the firm conviction of the family-planning worker that this was the proper and moral thing to do, and that economic benefits would flow to the family from this action. They also found that the workers regarded such certainty as evidence of just how professional they were, even though off duty most were much less certain that contraception was safe and that family limitation was certain to bring economic benefits to individuals and families. The greater material success attained by those who had restricted fertility could not be proved by the social-science research. In both Matlab and south India, the success of the workers depended on the frequency of their visits and on a reluctance of women and families continually to disappoint them.

Kim Streatfield (1986) reports that the Indonesian family-planning program in Bali achieved much of its success through meetings of the *banjar*, a subvillage unit. The headman presented the government policy in monthly meetings and stated that subsequent decisions were supposed to be by consensus, with behavior conforming to these decisions. Certainly there was at least moral pressure on individuals: In the case of couples who did not appear to be complying with the family-planning guidelines, the husbands were regularly questioned. There was also pressure on the headman, who had to make quarterly reports to a government official on the use of family planning by each married person in his *banjar*.

In south India, where a woman's parents-in-law have traditionally dominated most of the couple's decision making, family-planning workers, who represent official government policy, approach the wife directly. As a result, parents now tend to regard family planning as the business of the young. More direct efforts to change family structures aim at increasing female autonomy, often by providing women with work or an income, as has occurred in an experimental project in Vellore, south India, and as is planned by the nongovernmental development organization BRAC (Bangladesh Rural Advancement Committee) in Matlab.

Research on every Third World continent shows that radio has more impact on family-planning practice than any other segment of the media. It is widely accessible, heard by women even when they are in another room, and understood even by illiterates. The message is of better economic circumstances and health, of the safety of contraception and where it can be obtained. Television has been less successful, although experimental programs, such as one shown in three Nigerian cities, have increased levels of family planning. Newspaper articles have had less impact than might have been anticipated, possibly because more men than women read newspapers. In some societies, women's magazines have been more successful. Firm, moral statements by national leaders have been widely found to be effective.

One example is the repeated statement by President Ibrahim Babangida of Nigeria, "Four is enough." Most women in the country know the slogan, which appears to have been successful at least in part because of the legitimation thereby given by the state for women to make reproductive decisions without consulting their husbands or husbands' relatives.

Some family-planning programs have, under the leadership of the government, employed group pressures to encourage family planning. For example, successive regimes from the Dutch colonizers onward have re-molded Indonesia's community organization to the government's purposes. In a society where few people wish to be outsiders, the present government has employed the village structure to propagate the family-planning message powerfully. Annual campaigns, run mostly in rural areas by retired army officers, arouse enthusiasm for practicing family planning. The government has changed the community, and the community has changed the family. In China the government has used workplace and residential groups to argue the case for family planning with all defaulters from the program. This can also happen more spontaneously: In Matlab, Bangladesh, more couples practice contraception in those villages where the leader has been convinced by the program's arguments (Caldwell and Caldwell, 1992). In south India, during the 1975–1977 emergency, the period when Prime Minister Indira Gandhi ruled by decree and forcefully accelerated various development programs, including national family planning, local elites backed the government and insisted to their employees and potential employees that fertility control was in the national economic interest (Caldwell et al., 1988). China has attempted to limit fertility not only by strongly encouraging small families but also by exhorting later marriage.

Asian national family-planning programs from India to Korea have raised levels of contraceptive use and reduced fertility through a kind of moral leadership in which national political leaders and the programs themselves argue that they know what is good for the country and its citizens. This success is understandable in Confucian and Hindu societies, where there is a long history of elite and religious moral leadership, but more surprising in Southeast Asia, although in some countries in that region armies have assumed a not dissimilar role. Opposition in India has come from the Muslim community, who charge that Hindus have always worshiped government, while the Muslims have a book and a prophet. Asian programs may have received their original ideologies from the West and some of their program ideas from international agencies, but their governments have long been indigenous driving forces, with a commitment to changing society and culture in regard to reproduction and many other things.

In Singapore and Malaysia, the governments have changed their messages with regard to family values and marriage in order to attempt to halt or reverse the fertility decline. In sub-Saharan Africa, many politicians and bureaucrats avoid identifying themselves too closely with the family-planning programs or their messages so as not to be accused of deserting African culture.

The ethical issues

Most family-planning workers and media campaigns, with the support and at the direction of programs, provide potential clients with messages about the economic benefits likely to accrue to them from smaller families, and about the safety of contraception and the unimportance of side effects—messages that are more assured, optimistic, and unilateral than the proven facts will sustain. They do this with a feeling that it is their professional duty rather than that they are presenting a dubious case. Neither they nor the programs indicate that these overly optimistic messages are unethical because they identify the overriding good as being on another plane: saving the planet, delaying famine, raising living standards, or freeing women from the burden of large families. It might be argued that research has not demonstrated any certainties in these areas either. But it is probable that it will eventually be shown that slower population growth will bring individual and community benefits, and that policymakers should support what is probably true rather than cause damage by procrastinating until there is certainty. As Ruth Macklin wrote, "In a world of scarce resources, it surely seems immoral to pour money and personnel into ineffective or minimally effective programs in the interest of preserving freedom of contraceptive choice. These funds and workers could contribute to more effective efforts elsewhere, or in some other field" (1981, p. 356). Dennis Hodgson (1983) charged that not only family planners but also demographers have been activists, attempting to promote the programs rather than being social-scientifically objective.

Family-planning programs, like all modernizing and technical-aid–driven programs, have little interest in preserving indigenous cultures from change. They will bow to national governments, which they regard as preserving the national interest, but not to minorities, or even majorities who prefer the old ways. It might be argued, but rarely is, that family-planning programs are different from other aid programs in that they attempt to change sexuality, reproduction, and fertility, as well as the family and marriage—matters that lie at the heart of most cultures. The question could also be raised, as Paul Demeny (1988) has: Since the West achieved small families without external encouragement or help, why should the contemporary Third World be treated differently? Most actors in the programs would argue that it is unethical to hinder development and not to attempt to close the gap between the West and the rest of the world. Interestingly, for a considerable period two of the most aggressive family-planning programs adopted the view that there were cultural minorities who should be shielded from the full force of the national family planning program: in China with regard to the non-Han minorities and in Indonesia in terms of the outer islands.

International programs and national governments have made value-laden decisions in other areas of population behavior with even fewer hesitations about ethical issues than in the family planning field. In the health field, they have mandated compulsory vaccination and a range of other public-health measures; in terms of marriage, they have set minimum ages and sometimes demanded health tests; with regard to migration, they have limited international migration and, more rarely, rural–urban migration. In all these areas they have followed George Bernard Shaw's admonition against governments allowing so much freedom that they refuse to legislate about which side of the road to drive on.

The West and international organizations took the initiative in urging Third World family-planning programs because they increasingly believed that rapid population growth was hampering economic development in poor countries and that too large a global population would eventually impoverish everyone. By the 1980s they also felt that even a population that could still be adequately fed might be too high for the preservation of the world's environment and of its indigenous fauna and flora and their habitats. Some groups also felt that all women of the world had a moral right to gain access to the knowledge and facilities needed to control family size. Many Westerners assumed that the West would provide leadership because of its greater capacity for research and training and the provision of expertise and funds, but perhaps also because postdemographic-transition societies were felt to have a better perspective on the situation. There is little evidence that fear of being swamped by huge Third World populations was a major motivation; rather, there was a fear that these populations might come to inhabit the world's slums because of the deleterious economic effects arising from their inability to control the growth of their numbers.

JOHN C. CALDWELL

While all the articles in the other sections of this entry are relevant, see especially the other articles in this section: INCENTIVES AND DISINCENTIVES, STRONG PERSUASION, *and* COMPULSION. *Also directly related are the entries* POPULATION ETHICS; *and* FERTILITY CONTROL. *For a further discussion of topics mentioned in this article, see the entries*

AUTONOMY; BEHAVIOR CONTROL; COMMUNICATION, BIOMEDICAL, *article on* MEDIA AND MEDICINE; FAMILY; FEMINISM; FREEDOM AND COERCION; SUSTAINABLE DEVELOPMENT; UTILITY; *and* WOMEN, *article on* HISTORICAL AND CROSS-CULTURAL PERSPECTIVES. *For a discussion of related ideas, see the entries* ABORTION; AGING AND THE AGED, *article on* SOCIETAL AGING; CONFUCIANISM; FOOD POLICY; FUTURE GENERATIONS, OBLIGATIONS TO; HEALTH OFFICIALS AND THEIR RESPONSIBILITIES; HEALTH PROMOTION AND HEALTH EDUCATION; HINDUISM; MARRIAGE AND OTHER DOMESTIC PARTNERSHIPS; NATURAL LAW; RACE AND RACISM; ROMAN CATHOLICISM; *and* SEXISM.

Bibliography

BERELSON, BERNARD. 1969. "Beyond Family Planning." *Science* 163, no. 3867:533–543.

BOULDING, KENNETH E. 1966. "The Economics of the Coming Spaceship Earth." In *Environmental Quality in a Growing Economy: Essays from the Sixth RFF Forum,* pp. 3–14. Edited by Henry Jarrett and Kenneth E. Boulding. Baltimore: Johns Hopkins University Press.

BRUCE, JUDITH. 1987. "Users' Perspectives on Contraceptive Technology and Delivery Systems: Highlighting Some Feminist Issues." *Technology in Society* 9, nos. 3–4: 359–383.

CALDWELL, JOHN C. 1982. *Theory of Fertility Decline.* London: Academic Press.

———. 1991. "The Soft Underbelly of Development: Demographic Transition in Conditions of Limited Economic Change." In *Proceedings of the World Bank: Annual Conference on Development Economics 1990,* pp. 207–253. Edited by Stanley Fischer, Dennis de Tray, and Shekhar Shah. Washington, D.C.: World Bank.

CALDWELL, JOHN C., and CALDWELL, PAT. 1986. *Limiting Population Growth and the Ford Foundation Contribution.* London: Frances Pinter.

———. 1987. "The Cultural Context of High Fertility in Sub-Saharan Africa." *Population and Development Review* 13, no. 3:409–437.

———. 1992. "What Does the Matlab Fertility Experience Really Show?" *Studies in Family Planning* 23, no. 5: 292–310.

CALDWELL, JOHN C.; ORUBULOYE, I. O.; and CALDWELL, PAT. 1992. "Fertility Decline in Africa: A New Type of Transition?" *Population and Development Review* 18, no. 2: 211–242.

CALDWELL, JOHN C.; REDDY, P. H.; and CALDWELL, PAT. 1988. *The Causes of Demographic Change: Experimental Research in South India.* Madison: University of Wisconsin Press.

CLARK, COLIN. 1967. *Population Growth and Land Use.* New York: St. Martin's Press.

COALE, ANSLEY J. 1967. "Factors Associated with the Development of Low Fertility: An Historic Summary." In vol. 2 of *Proceedings of the World Population Conference, 1965,* pp. 205–209. New York: United Nations.

DAVIS, KINGSLEY. 1967. "Population Policy: Will Current Programs Succeed?" *Science* 158, no. 3802:730–739.

DEMENY, PAUL. 1988. "Social Science and Population Policy." *Population and Development Review* 14, no. 3:451–479.

EHRLICH, PAUL R. 1968. *The Population Bomb*. New York: Ballantine.

GREEN, RONALD M. 1976. *Population Growth and Justice: An Examination of Moral Issues Raised by Rapid Population Growth*. Missoula, Mont.: Scholars Press.

HARDIN, GARRETT. 1968. "The Tragedy of the Commons." *Science* 162, no. 3859:1243–1248.

———. 1974. "Living on a Lifeboat." *Bioscience* 24, no. 10:561–568.

HODGSON, DENNIS. 1983. "Demography as Social Science and Policy Science." *Population and Development Review* 9, no. 1:1–34.

LAPHAM, ROBERT J., and MAULDIN, W. PARKER. 1985. "Contraceptive Prevalence: The Influence of Organized Family Planning Programs." *Studies in Family Planning* 16, no. 3:117–137.

LIEBERSON, JONATHAN. 1987. "Ethics of Family Planning." *Technology in Society* 9, nos. 3–4:481–495.

MACKLIN, RUTH. 1981. "Ethics, Effectiveness and Efficiency in Population Programs." In *Ethical Issues of Population Aid: Culture, Economics, and International Assistance*, pp. 333–360. Edited by Daniel Callahan and Philip G. Clark. New York: Irvington.

MALTHUS, THOMAS R. 1993. [1798]. *An Essay on the Principle of Population*. Edited by Geoffrey Gilbert. Oxford: Oxford University Press.

MAULDIN, W. PARKER, and ROSS, JOHN A. 1991. "Family Planning Programs: Efforts and Results, 1982–1989." *Studies in Family Planning* 22, no. 6:350–367.

NOTESTEIN, FRANK W. 1945. "Population—The Long View." In *Food for the World*, pp. 36–57. Edited by Theodore W. Schultz. Chicago: University of Chicago Press.

———. 1953. "Economic Problems of Population Change." In *Proceedings of the 8th International Conference of Agricultural Economists*, pp. 13–31. London: Oxford University Press.

PADDOCK, WILLIAM, and PADDOCK, PAUL. 1967. *Famine, 1975: America's Decision: Who Will Survive?* Boston: Little, Brown.

REINING, PRISCILLA, and TINKER, IRENE, eds. 1975. *Population: Dynamics, Ethics, and Policy*. Washington, D.C.: American Association for the Advancement of Science.

SIMON, JULIAN L. 1981. *The Ultimate Resource*. Princeton: Princeton University Press.

STREATFIELD, KIM. 1986. *Fertility Decline in a Traditional Society: The Case of Bali*. Canberra: Department of Demography, Australian National University.

TANGRI, SANDRA S. 1976. "A Feminist Perspective on Some Ethical Issues in Population Programs." *Signs* 1, no. 4:895–904.

WARWICK, DONALD P. 1982. *Bitter Pills: Population Policies and Their Implementation in Eight Developing Countries*. Cambridge: At the University Press.

WESTOFF, CHARLES F., and PEBLEY, ANNE R. 1981. "Alternative Measures of Unmet Need for Family Planning in Developing Countries." *International Family Planning Perspectives* 7, no. 4:126–136.

B. INCENTIVES AND DISINCENTIVES

The following is a revision and update of the first-edition article "Population Policy Proposals: Governmental Incentives" by the same author.

Incentives designed to modify population-related behavior are among the alternatives considered by governments in planning systematic population policies. Many countries have experimented with antinatalist incentives in some form. Other countries have attempted pronatalist incentives. In one sense any governmental policy that influences population-related behavior could be labeled an "incentive." This article is limited to conscious governmental efforts to produce demographically related behavior by offering economic inducements or related material goods and services. It does not treat educational, health, and other programs designed for demographic impact; programs that depend on legal or physical coercion; and government-subsidized or free distribution of contraceptives and other population-related materials and services.

Types of governmental population incentives

The range of governmental incentives designed to affect population-related behavior is so great that in order to analyze critically the ethical implications of various incentive schemes, it is first necessary to classify the existing plans.

(1) The *incentive* offered can be monetary or material. Pronatalist monetary inducements such as family allowances have sometimes been offered to affect fertility-related behavior, sometimes simply to provide for the welfare of the offspring. Japan offers a "reward" of 5000 yen (about $38 U.S.) per month for each preschool-age child and twice that for a third child (Weisman, 1991). India is a major example of experiments with a wide range of antinatalist incentives. The Ammanpettai Family Welfare Program, which began in 1985 in India, offered women small cash incentives to come to a clinic where they learned about and were provided with the pill, condoms, or the intrauterine device (IUD) (Stevens, 1992). The Bangladesh government pays individuals who undergo sterilization (Cleland and Mauldin, 1991). The payment is about the equivalent of a week's earnings for an unskilled rural laborer. The individuals are also provided with clothing. In China couples may sign a contract with the state agreeing to have only one child. They receive a reward of a yearly cash bonus that may be as much as one third the average worker's monthly pay, larger food subsidies, longer maternity leave, more farmland, improved housing opportunities, and special priority for admission to school, medical service, employment, and housing (Gregory, 1992; Office of the Education, Science, Culture and Public Health Committee of the National People's Congress and the

General Office of the State Family Planning Commission, the People's Republic of China, 1984).

The first formal governmental antinatalist incentive scheme was in Madras State (now Tamil Nadu) in India. In 1956, ten rupees (about $1.33 at then-current exchange rates) was offered for "diffusers" (i.e., those who recruit candidates) and thirty rupees ($4.00) to "acceptors" of vasectomies (Repetto, 1968). Proposals to offer bonds, tax rebates, tax penalties, and social security bonuses are variants on monetary schemes. The significant ethical differences that may arise among these types of monetary incentives will be discussed below.

While incentive schemes have been developed primarily in less developed countries, at least two state legislatures of the United States have considered proposals that would offer financial incentives to women on welfare who receive Norplant contraceptive implants (Scott, 1992).

(2) Incentives may also be classified on the basis of *who receives the incentive*. While individuals whose fertility is to be affected are the most obvious recipients, field workers, local political leaders, and communities may also be the target (as is seen in the Indian example in which those who diffuse the contraceptive techniques as well as those who accept them are rewarded).

Government-offered goods and services that target a variety of recipients have included medical services, maternity leaves, educational opportunities, food, jobs, clothes, transistor radios, wedding costs, and even governmental favors. Iran has adopted a plan that excludes families with fourth-born children from a plan to provide coupons permitting them to buy basic foods at subsidized prices (Murphy, 1992). China has offered "single child certificates" that entitle couples to preferential medical and schooling benefits (United Nations Fund for Population Activities [UNFPA], 1985; Farrell, 1984). Nepal has endorsed a 20 percent increment on earned pension for all government employees with two living children or fewer at the time of retirement (UNFPA, 1991).

Community incentives are designed to generate community pressures to achieve fertility-related behaviors (Wolfson, 1987). In China and Indonesia, communities are given prizes based on aggregate fertility statistics (Ross and Isaacs, 1988). In Thailand a village tied loans from a revolving loan fund to whether the applicant used family planning (Ross and Isaacs, 1988). Incentives may pass from the central government of a nation to individual states or towns. In India the central government has paid the states Rs. 30 (30 Indian rupees, the equivalent of about $3.33 U.S.) for each woman and Rs. 40 for each man who accepts sterilization. Some of this money is, in turn, used to provide small cash incentives to family planning motivators and awards to government functionaries and public servants who achieve high acceptance levels in their communities (Satia and Maru, 1986).

(3) The *behavior to be induced* is another important variable with both practical and moral implications. Probably the most common objective of incentive plans has been sterilization. Such programs have been attempted in India (Kabra and Narayanan, 1990; Farrell, 1984); Bangladesh, Korea, Nepal, Pakistan, Vietnam, and Sri Lanka also pay for sterilizations (Ross and Isaacs, 1988; UNFPA, 1991). Other less permanent but less easily monitored behaviors have included incentive proposals for the use of condoms, diaphragms, oral contraceptives, and IUDs. Bangladesh and India both pay for IUDs (Ross and Isaacs, 1988). Bangladesh also pays incentives to receive implants of the contraceptive Norplant (Ubinig, 1991). While these objectives are less permanent and thus more attractive because they permit a couple to keep options open, they are also inefficient and extremely difficult to monitor. Policy planners have tended to opt for advocating the more efficient, less reversible methods of conception control as the object of incentives.

Another approach, considered for Pakistan (Sirageldin and Hopkins, 1972), is simply to offer incentives for family size or for periods of nonpregnancy, leaving the choice of method to the couple. Gujarat state in India rewards couples without sons (UNFPA, 1991). Governmental incentives have been used to induce increases in the birthrate as well as decreases (Pohlman, 1971). As many as fifty-nine countries have had family allowances, and eighty-one countries maternity benefits. In some cases these are supported for health and welfare purposes, in others (e.g., France and Mongolia) for explicit demographic purposes. While incentives to lower birthrates have been much more controversial and are the main focus of this article, most of the ethical issues raised—the conflict of individual and group rights, the limits of freedom, and the problems of justice—apply to pronatalist incentives as well.

(4) The *timing of the incentive* is important in determining the nature of its impact. One of the moral problems with any incentive scheme is that it often has its impact on the offspring, who are not responsible for the population-related behavior of their parents. If disincentives penalize parents financially for higher fertility, the children may be the ones affected. In order to overcome this problem, some have advocated giving a bond to parents that will mature after the female parent reaches menopause. The couple would gain the proceeds if their completed family size remained small enough. Since one of the motivating forces for bearing children is the need for financial support in old age, some have proposed the delayed incentive of social security bonuses for couples with few children. Such delayed incentives might lessen the impact on the offspring.

In India, for example, three tea estates developed a deferred bonus scheme that provides each woman worker an extra day's bonus credit for each month she is not pregnant (World Bank, 1984). One township in China developed a deferred scheme that would pay for the high-school education of children of two-child families (World Bank, 1984).

(5) Incentives may also be classified by their rates. The *rate of the incentive* may be the same for all acceptors (flat rate) or it may vary. A program may pay more for sterilization after three or fewer children than after four or five. In some cases higher incentives are offered for younger acceptors. One of the serious moral issues in incentives is the problem of differential impact. A flat-rate incentive will have very different impacts on different individuals. Questions of justice arise if a small economic incentive has virtually coercive force over a poverty-level family but no significant impact on a wealthy family. If the goal is to reduce the society's fertility efficiently, then flat-rate incentives may work. They will reduce overall fertility, but do so by changing behavior of those most susceptible to small incentives. Often these will be the poorest members of the society. If the moral objective is to distribute justly the burden for changing population size or growth rates, then variable rates may be necessary. These issues will be discussed below when considering the problem of justice.

(6) A final way to classify incentives is by their psychological impact. The *psychological impact of the incentive* may vary substantially, depending upon whether the incentive is positive or negative. Positive efforts to induce desired behavior are often believed to be more acceptable than negative fees or penalties. Negative incentives differ substantially, however, in their psychological impact. If the negative incentive is called a "penalty" or a "fine," the impression is given that the penalized behavior is wrong in itself. A "charge" or a "fee," however, does not have the same connotation. Fees are charged to pay actual costs, or for services such as parking permits, to discourage a behavior that is not in itself bad but creates a social problem when too many engage in the behavior too often. In fact, the distinction between positive and negative incentive is dependent upon what is taken to be the normal baseline. If one normally expected to get a service for one's children and had it taken away if too many children were born, it would be seen as a penalty. But if a new service were offered to children and limited to those in small families, it might be seen as a positive incentive.

Governmental incentive schemes can incorporate any combination of these incentive variables, rewarding and discouraging a wide range of behaviors by different people at different times by offering different goods and services. Disincentives include limitations on income tax deductions, child allowances, and maternity benefits beyond a few births. These are reported to occur in Ghana, Malaysia, Pakistan, and the Philippines (World Bank, 1984). Tanzania limits maternity leave to once every three years. In the early 1980s, Singapore limited income tax relief to the first three children and restricted paid maternity leave. It also gave children from smaller families priority for school admission (World Bank, 1984). Examples of integrated incentive proposals have been discussed in the literature (Kangas, 1970; Enke and Hickman, 1973).

Ethical dimensions of population incentives

Relatively little explicit ethical analysis of population incentive plans is available (Veatch, 1977; Berelson and Lieberson, 1979). Most of the discussion of criteria for incentive programs has been oriented to efficiency, that is, the amount of change in population-related behavior per unit of expenditure. TEMPO, a division of General Electric Company, did work on population-incentive schemes for the United States Agency for International Development. It listed five criteria for a good incentive program: it must have wide appeal and should be economically efficient, administratively feasible, "cheat-proof," and politically acceptable (Hickman, 1972).

Efficiency and political acceptability are generally presumed to be good characteristics, but they are more central to some ethical theories than others. The issues raised by different ethical theories can be analyzed in terms of the conflict between the social good and individual rights and benefits, the problems of freedom and coercion, and problems of distributive justice.

The social good and individual rights and benefits. Often governmental incentives schemes are evaluated in terms of the economic value to the national economy of preventing a birth in comparison with the economic cost of preventing that birth (Enke and Hickman, 1973; Enke and Brown, 1972). If the cost of preventing the birth is less than the cost of raising the child, then, according to this approach, the cost is justified. The ethical theory that most clearly supports this conclusion is the economic utilitarianism of Jeremy Bentham and John Stuart Mill. That act is right, according to this theory, which provides the greatest good for the greatest number. While the good is not necessarily reduced to social and economic considerations, this simplification is often made, especially when computerized cost–benefit analyses require quantifiable data. Many of those working extensively on governmental incentives to affect population-related behavior are trained in economics and are perhaps unconsciously socialized into this particular ethical principle of maximization of the social good and to a quantitative approach to measuring it.

Western ethical theories have never completely accepted the principle that that policy is right that produces the greatest good for the greatest number. The tradition of John Locke, Thomas Hobbes, and Jean-Jacques Rousseau recognizes the moral significance of individual rights that may conflict with the social good. The Kantian tradition, a major root of Western deontological ethics, holds that actions or policies are right or wrong because of their inherent moral characteristics rather than because of their consequences. In evaluating governmental population incentives, individual rights and inherent right-making characteristics are critical for those standing in these ethical traditions.

One moral problem with incentives is the risk of harm to innocent individuals, particularly the children born to couples who do not follow the desired behavior patterns. If hospital care, food, or the right to education at government expense is denied to families with more than the approved number of children, it is the children rather than (or in addition to) the parents who are going to suffer.

However procreational behavior is interpreted, it cannot be that children are responsible for their own births. Even if such incentives may serve the greatest good of the society in the long run, it is still very much an open question whether they are ethically acceptable, according to ethical stances that give weight to the rights of innocent parties. Even positive incentives may indirectly have harmful consequences for innocent parties. This problem has been discussed in conjunction with the Taiwan plan, which offers educational opportunities to children of couples who limit their family size (Finnigan and Sun, 1972). If bearing no more than n children will entitle the couple to a social security benefit, the child born after the nth may be blamed by the parents. It may also be blamed by its siblings for burdening them with support of the parents in old age. If the psychological interpretation of the incentive is such that it places the blame on innocent parties or deprives them of goods received by other innocent parties who are morally identical, then moral problems arise for those who hold ethical theories recognizing such individual rights and the correlative responsibility of others.

Freedom and coercion.   A second major moral issue arising from the governmental population incentives is the extent to which they interfere with free choice in the fundamental area of procreation. Many claim there is a right, even an inalienable right, to bear children. If freedom is a good valued over and above its ability to serve the general welfare, then we must come to terms with the charge that incentives modify and limit the choice options, thus limiting individual freedom.

Incentives fall on a continuum between a completely free choice and decisions that are totally coerced. The matter becomes more complex, however, when one realizes that all procreative choices are influenced by ex-

isting social structures, income levels, and opportunities for child nurture and education. Some incentives approach coercion. Offers of money many times the couple's annual income or penalties of withholding food from a starving family or nation may come close to coercion. In fact, they may be more potent than physical force. On the other hand, some incentives that provide for life's necessities or counter existing cultural pressures may actually increase the choice options.

Increasing sophistication in planning incentives has heightened the potential for manipulation of fertility behavior. Early incentive schemes were initiated as pragmatic means of speeding the diffusion and adoption of contraceptive ideas, but research is increasing knowledge of the impact of incentives. This gives policy planners the capacity for increased efficiency, but at the same time runs the risk that they will be accused of manipulating or coercing patterns of social behavior (Rogers, 1973; Aird, 1990).

Some freedoms in the procreation area may also be more fundamental than others. The freedom to bear a child may not be equated to the freedom to bear as many children as one wants. Presumably plans that offer incentives only after two or three children have been born or that pay larger amounts for sterilization early in the procreative history of the recipient implicitly hold this view. The negative right not to be interfered with in one's decisions about procreation may also differ from the positive right to have government assist one socially and economically in exercising the right to procreate. Governmental incentives to influence procreative behavior are, by definition, conscious efforts to modify the choice structure of the couple. Whether the incentives always reduce freedom, and whether they reduce it in ethically objectionable ways, will depend on the ethical theory one brings to bear in the evaluation, the weight that is given to various individual and group rights at stake, and the empirical circumstances.

Justice.   A third group of moral issues raised by governmental incentives focuses on the problems of justice. Incentive proposals have often been criticized because they are specifically targeted at the poor or have their greatest impact on the behaviors of the poor (Scott, 1992). If carried out, every population policy, including every incentive plan, will redistribute goods, money, and children in the society.

Different theories of justice will evaluate incentives in radically different ways. In order to evaluate incentive proposals, we must know more precisely what the objective is. We can presume that any governmental incentive will have as its immediate objective a change in population size or growth rate. But the question must be asked why this objective is sought and what other ordering principles are at stake. Assuming the goal is to lower the size of the next cohort, is this to be done in a manner that will produce the maximum social benefits, as the utilitarians hold? Is it to provide every couple with a certain equal number (n) of children? Is it to provide psychologically equal incentive offers to each couple? Or is it to distribute the burden of lowering societal fertility equally?

Each goal will probably lead to a different incentive policy. If, for instance, the goal is to minimize the dollar costs of positive incentives, then small incentives will be tried. These might be raised gradually until the desired population effect is produced. Those affected will be those most influenced by relatively small amounts of money. This will target incentive programs for two groups: those for whom another child is marginal, and the poor, for whom even a small incentive is relatively coercive. Distributing the same (flat rate) incentive to everyone may be efficient in dollar terms but still grossly discriminatory.

Another objective might be to serve the societal good, even if the dollar amounts of the incentives are not equal. If, for instance, it were determined that some social group was of superior social worth, they might be exempt from a negative incentive scheme, even though their fertility would be lowered if the incentive were applied to them. Of course, serious problems of social justice arise when interpersonal social worth comparisons are made. Many would find such a scheme ethically unjustified even if it hypothetically served the general welfare.

Still another objective might be to distribute children (or the right to children) equally among all couples in society. Such a goal might give rise to the n-child proposals where positive incentives are offered only to couples who have n children or fewer and negative incentives are brought to bear on those who have more than n children. Several moral problems arise from such proposals, however. In effect, they place the perceived burden of lowering population on couples who value children relatively highly. They place no such burden (and in fact may increase the financial means) of those who do not value children, but who highly value material goods. If the population problem arises because of a combination of population size and growth rate with consumption and pollution problems, it is not clear why it is morally right to place the obligation for problem resolution only on those who value children. Justice might require distributing the burden to the consumption-oriented as well.

There are other problems with the n-child proposals. They create the impression of making the n-child family the norm, creating a burden for children born after the nth. Psychological burdens may be inflicted upon the parents even if they were not responsible for their family size. The n-child norm may suggest that that family size is socially preferable when there is little evidence for that conclusion. It may be that a mix with some smaller and some larger families would be both better and fairer.

Another theory of justice would take as the goal of governmental incentives the even distribution of the burden for bringing about the socially desirable population characteristics. According to this understanding of justice it would be unacceptable to have "free-riders," that is, those who reap the benefits without paying their share of the costs, benefiting from the induced behavior of others. Everyone should share equally in the sacrifice. A flat rate incentive scheme or an n-child incentive scheme would probably be ruled out according to this view (although in a society where the vast majority had similar family-size desires or had similar incomes this might not be the case). A sliding scale incentive scheme has been advocated as a way of spreading the burden more fairly. A positive incentive scheme providing a higher payment (and thus a similar psychological force) for those with greater income, however, would appear unacceptable. It would require higher payments to the rich in order to induce them to give up future children in numbers comparable with the poor. A negative, graduated, sliding-scale fee or tax on childbearing has been advocated as a policy that would distribute burdens more evenly to the rich and the poor and to those who want few and many children (Veatch, 1977). It would require a proportionally higher fee for childbearing for the wealthy than the poor. Complex graduation schemes, including some linked to property ownership, annual income, or annual income tax have been proposed. Whether such a scheme is feasible would depend upon local conditions. Also fairness might be bought at the expense of efficiency. At that point the moral problem is one of harmonizing competing ethical claims. Holders of differing ethical theories will resolve these conflicts in differing ways. It is important to realize, however, that an incentive plan cannot be justified on moral grounds simply because it is efficient in reducing fertility—unless one constructs the moral argument linking efficiency to moral rightness.

In the ideal world probably no one would favor governmental incentive schemes. Incentive schemes are proposed by those who are convinced that if a society relies on voluntary procreation decisions it will be contrary to the social good and by those looking for some means of governmental intervention short of outright coercion. The number of such possibilities is limited. Educational campaigns, the structuring of society to induce acceptable and apparently free choice, campaigns of persuasion, and basic social structural changes that will have a demographic impact are the main alternatives to governmental incentives. The explicit ethical evaluation of governmental incentive proposals must take place in the context of a particular country, culture, or cultural milieu and in contrast with other possible policies for that country or culture. It is beyond the scope of this article to do the country-by-country comparative analysis necessary to apply the general framework for analysis outlined here. If, however, one concludes that alternative policy options will not work or will raise even more serious moral problems, then governmental incentives become a candidate for population policy. Besides efficiency, other moral principles including individual rights, freedom, and justice must be used in evaluating such incentive plans.

ROBERT M. VEATCH

While all the articles in the other sections of this entry are relevant, see especially the other articles in this section: CHANGES IN ATTITUDE AND CULTURE, STRONG PERSUASION, *and* COMPULSION. *Directly related to this article are the entries* POPULATION ETHICS; *and* FERTILITY CONTROL. *For further discussion of topics mentioned in this article, see the entries* CHILDREN, *articles on* HISTORY OF CHILDHOOD, *and* RIGHTS OF CHILDREN; FAMILY; FREEDOM AND COERCION; HARM; JUSTICE; RIGHTS; *and* UTILITY. *For further discussion of related ideas, see the entries* CONFLICT OF INTEREST; ENVIRONMENTAL ETHICS; FUTURE GENERATIONS, OBLIGATIONS TO; INTERNATIONAL HEALTH; RACE AND RACISM; SEXISM; *and* WOMEN, *articles on* HISTORICAL AND CROSS-CULTURAL PERSPECTIVES, *and* HEALTH-CARE ISSUES. *Other relevant material may be found under the entries* REPRODUCTIVE TECHNOLOGIES; *and* RESPONSIBILITY.

Bibliography

AIRD, JOHN S. 1990. *Slaughter of the Innocents: Coercive Birth Control in China.* Washington, D.C.: AEI Press.

BERELSON, BERNARD. 1969. "Beyond Family Planning." *Studies in Family Planning* no. 38:1–16.

BERELSON, BERNARD, and LIEBERSON, JONATHAN. 1979. "Government Efforts to Influence Fertility: The Ethical Issues." *Population and Development Review* 5, no. 4: 581–613.

CLELAND, JOHN, and MAULDIN, W. PARKER. 1991. "The Promotion of Family Planning by Financial Payments: The Case of Bangladesh." *Studies in Family Planning* 22, no. 1:1–18.

ENKE, STEPHEN, and BROWN, RICHARD A. 1972. "Economic Worth of Preventing Death at Different Ages in Developing Countries." *Journal of Biosocial Science* 4, no. 3: 299–306.

ENKE, STEPHEN, and HICKMAN, BRYAN D. 1973. "Offering Bonuses for Reduced Fertility." *Journal of Biosocial Science* 5, no. 3:329–346.

FARRELL, LAURA E. 1984. "Population Policies and Proposals: When Big Brother Becomes Big Daddy." *Brooklyn Journal of International Law* 10, no. 1:83–114.

FINNIGAN, OLIVER D., III, and SUN, T. H. 1972. "Planning, Starting, and Operating an Educational Incentives Project." *Studies in Family Planning* 3, no. 1:1–7.

GREGORY, LISA B. 1992. "Examining the Economic Component of China's One Child Family Policy Under International Law: Your Money or Your Life." *Journal of Chinese Law* 6, no. 1:45–88.

HICKMAN, BRYAN D. 1972. *Economic Incentives: A Strategy for Family Planning Programs.* Technical Report no. 72, TMP–33. Santa Barbara, Calif.: General Electric Co., TEMPO Center for Advanced Studies.

INTERNATIONAL PLANNED PARENTHOOD FEDERATION. 1969. *Incentive Payments in Family Planning Programmes.* Working Paper no. 4. London: Author.

ISAACS, STEPHEN L. 1981. "Incentives and Disincentives: Socio-Economic Laws and Policies." In his *Population Law and Policy: Source Materials and Issues,* pp. 307–347. New York: Human Sciences Press.

KABRA, S. G., and NARAYANAN, RAMJI. 1990. "Sterilisation Camps in India." *Lancet* 335, no. 8683:224–225.

KANGAS, LENNI W. 1970. "Integrated Incentives for Fertility Control." *Science* 169, no. 3952:1278–1283.

MURPHY, CARYLE. 1992. "Iran Promoting Birth Control in Policy Switch." *Washington Post,* May 8, A17, A20.

OFFICE OF THE EDUCATION, SCIENCE, CULTURE AND PUBLIC HEALTH COMMITTEE OF THE NATIONAL PEOPLE'S CONGRESS AND THE GENERAL OFFICE OF THE STATE FAMILY PLANNING COMMISSION. THE PEOPLE'S REPUBLIC OF CHINA, ed. 1984. "Family Planning." In *China: Population and Development,* pp. 7–8. Beijing: Foreign Languages Printing House.

POHLMAN, EDWARD. 1971. *Incentives and Compensations in Birth Planning.* Carolina Population Center Monograph no. 11. Chapel Hill: Carolina Population Center, University of North Carolina.

RABIN, EDWARD H. 1972. "Population Control Through Financial Incentives." *Hastings Law Journal* 23, no. 5:1353–1399.

REPETTO, ROBERT. 1968. "India: A Case Study of the Madras Vasectomy Program." *Studies in Family Planning* 31:8–16.

ROGERS, EVERETT M. 1973. "Incentives in the Diffusion of Family Planning Innovations." In his *Communication Strategies for Family Planning,* pp. 152–224. New York: Free Press.

ROSS, JOHN A., and ISAACS, STEPHEN L. 1988. "Costs, Payments, and Incentives in Family Planning Programs: A Review for Developing Countries." *Studies in Family Planning* 19, no. 6:270–283.

SATIA, J. K., and MARU, RUSHIKESH M. 1986. "Incentives and Disincentives in the Indian Family Welfare Program." *Studies in Family Planning* 17, no. 3:136–145.

SCOTT, JULIA R. 1992. "Norplant and Women of Color." In *Norplant and Poor Women: Dimensions of New Contraceptives,* pp. 39–52. Edited by Sarah Samuels and Mark D. Smith. Menlo Park, Calif.: Henry J. Kaiser Family Foundation.

SIRAGELDIN, ISMAIL, and HOPKINS, SAMUEL. 1972. "Family Planning Programs: An Economic Approach." *Studies in Family Planning* 3, no. 2:17–28.

STEVENS, JANICE. 1992. "Introductory Small Cash Incentives to Promote Child Spacing in India." *Studies in Family Planning* 23, no. 3:171–186.

UBINIG. 1991. "'The Price of Norplant is TK.2000! You Cannot Remove It.' Clients Are Refused Removal in Norplant Trial in Bangladesh." *Issues in Reproductive and Genetic Engineering: Journal of International Feminist Analysis* 4, no. 1:45–46.

UNITED NATIONS FUND FOR POPULATION ACTIVITIES (UNFPA). 1985. *Annual Review of Population Law, 1983.* New York: Author.

———. 1991. *Annual Review of Population Law, 1988.* New York: Author.

VEATCH, ROBERT M. 1977. "Governmental Population Incentives: Ethical Issues at Stake." *Studies in Family Planning* 8, no. 4:100–108.

WEISMAN, STEVEN R. 1991. "In Crowded Japan, a Bonus for Babies Angers Women." *New York Times*, February 17, 1, 14.

WISHIK, SAMUEL M. 1978. "The Use of Incentives for Fertility Reduction." *American Journal of Public Health* 68, no. 2: 113–114.

WOLFSON, MARGARET. 1987. *Community Action for Family Planning: A Comparison of Six Project Experiences.* Paris: Development Centre of the Organisation for Economic Co-operation and Development.

WORLD BANK. 1984. "Slowing Population Growth." In *World Development Report: 1984*, pp. 106–126. New York: Oxford University Press.

C. STRONG PERSUASION

As a category of fertility control measures, "strong persuasion" lies at an intermediate level of severity. Fertility change brought about by manipulation of economic incentives can often be considered ethically innocuous, while change enforced by stringent physical sanction or threat is widely viewed as ethically inadmissible. Strong persuasion, roughly situated between incentives and compulsion, encompasses social and administrative pressures or economic penalties that lessen but do not extinguish a person's perceived freedom to act contrary to the approved behavior. This approach has characterized particular phases of antinatalist (fertility-reducing) strategies in a number of societies, and it characterizes many policies proposed for countries where rapid population growth is seen as harmful and has resisted milder measures. Some pronatalist (fertility-raising) strategies also entail strong persuasion.

The scope of reproductive freedom

Ethical assessment of strategies employing persuasion would typically start from the premise that individuals are autonomous actors with well-established preferences concerning fertility. If choice is not constrained by ignorance or extreme poverty, reproductive freedom exists when fertility decisions are based on those preferences. Fertility decisions are of course influenced by the effect that family size has on family economic well-being. Incentive strategies can make use of this effect without seriously curtailing reproductive freedom. Strong persuasion, by definition, does seriously curtail it.

The ethical position that would accord individuals full reproductive freedom in this sense derives from the concept of "negative" liberty or freedom in Western liberal thought. Negative freedom is immunity from interference by others. The scope of a person's activities to which that freedom applies sets the bounds of a private sphere of behavior. Political philosophies differ in views of how extensive the private sphere should be. Its bounds might depend, for example, on the supposed minimum degree of interference needed to ensure social harmony or, more relevant here, on the extent to which particular activities of a person are seen as potentially harming others (Berlin, 1969; Patterson, 1991). If it were not for the possibility of causing harm, reproductive behavior would have a compelling claim to be considered private.

International declarations and conventions bear out this position with respect to the responsibilities of national governments. The Universal Declaration of Human Rights asserts a general protection of privacy, which signatory states have undertaken to recognize. Subsequent international declarations, although carrying less weight, have identified numerous more specific human rights, among them one that confers on individuals the freedom to choose the number of their children (United Nations, 1990).

The ethical problem is not so simply resolved, however. No society countenances complete reproductive freedom. In most contemporary societies, for example, monogamy is enforced, as is a minimum age of marriage; there are rules against incest. By and large, such restrictions do not occasion protest as infringements on individual choice. In some societies, abortion is limited or prohibited—a measure that may "compel" a pregnant woman to give birth. In this case, protest is more common, but the issues extend well beyond those of privacy. Other pressures on fertility are so long-standing that they are barely recognized as such, being built into the society's institutions. American society, Judith Blake has argued, is "pervaded by time-honored pronatalist constraints" (Blake, 1972, p. 105). Thus, there is some arbitrariness in declaring that numbers of children should be an inviolable object of choice. Bernard Berelson and Jonathan Lieberson make this point when they write, "We see no fundamental ethical or philosophical difference between sanctions on monogamy or vaccination on the one hand, and sanctions on fertility on the other— only sociological and historical differences" (Berelson and Lieberson, 1979, p. 604).

Exclusion of all stringent fertility-control measures from ethical admissibility therefore cannot be drawn from abstract libertarian principle. Support for such a standpoint appears to derive from convention—one that emerged in historical situations where societal welfare was not drastically affected by the aggregate demographic result of individual free choice. As Paul Demeny has remarked, James Madison wrote nothing about fertility, but if the United States in his time had had a population of one billion instead of four million, and could foresee a near-term doubling of that size, "the Federalist Papers would probably have given the question of population growth, and the question of what Americans might do about it, a great deal of attention" (Demeny, 1986, p. 483).

If reproductive freedom is less than absolute, ethical assessment of fertility-control strategies must involve a weighing of individual interests against some broader set of interests—typically, those of a community or larger society of which the individual is a member. This group whose interests are to be considered is often called the "moral community." There is a range of ethically defensible positions on the scope of the moral community. What, for example, should be the significance of national borders in delimiting it? Should moral consideration be extended to nonhuman sentient creatures (a case that is increasingly being argued)? Moreover, if the familiar practice of time-discounting is permitted, reducing the weight of future members of the group in the calculation, can some analogous discounting be applied to geographical distance or to remoteness in kinship or level of sentience (Bayles, 1980; Feinberg, 1980)?

Taking just the case of the "society" (most often identified with nation), the potential existence of a societal interest in decisions bearing on family size or composition is clear: The size no less than the socialization of the next generation has implications for a society's identity and well-being, and thus may properly be a concern of its members as a whole. The case is analogous to that of admitting new members through immigration. How social interests are determined—in particular, the degree of participation and consent entailed and the protection granted to dissent—is a critical issue, but it is no different here than in any other policy domain. There are circumstances in which the societal interest in modifying reproductive behavior may be very strong: for example, where fertility is at a level that causes population size to double in a generation or to fall by one-third. A canvassing of policy preferences in such societies might well endorse vigorous efforts to moderate the pace of change.

Cases of strong persuasion

To give empirical content to the discussion of the ethics of such efforts, consider some cases of fertility control where the term "strong persuasion" appears to be applicable.

1. India's family-planning program has long favored sterilization (mainly of men) over reversible contraceptive methods, with financial incentives offered to clients and to the officials and private "motivators" who recruit them. Except during the nineteenth-month period in 1975–1977 when civil liberties were suspended under a declaration of national emergency and press-gang methods of recruitment were reportedly widespread, India has stressed the voluntary nature of its program. Nominal voluntarism, however, has been compatible with active recruitment efforts, encouraged by the incentives offered the recruiters and in some regions—especially during the campaigns associated with the "vasectomy camps" that were an important constituent of the program—by pressures on program officials to achieve target numbers of clients. In a highly stratified society, clients came disproportionately from the most disadvantaged groups, where effects of incentives were strongest, susceptibility to browbeating greatest, and assurance of informed consent weakest (Gwatkin, 1979; Vicziany, 1982).

2. In Indonesia, the government's family-planning program, begun around 1970, has sought to mobilize regional and local government officials from provincial down to village level to generate administrative pressures in support of its efforts to increase use of modern contraception—chiefly, pills and intrauterine devices (IUDs). With reversible methods dominant, initial acceptance is a less serious decision for a couple than in the case of sterilization. However, antinatalist effect then requires long-term contraceptive use: Continuation rates are as important as acceptance rates. As in India, special drives—here, "safaris"—have sometimes been associated with reports of strong-arm recruitment tactics. A distinctive additional feature of the Indonesian program has been its use of program clients as a pressure group within each local community, informally backed by village leaders, in gaining new recruits and monitoring continuation. Especially in rural areas, nonacceptance of program services may have called for some degree of defiance of authority. In Bali, where a person's cultural ties to his or her hamlet were particularly strong, the community pressures invoked by the program were formalized at the hamlet level—for example, by making the contraceptive use or nonuse of each couple a matter of public record and, more generally, by bringing contraceptive practice into the arena of socially pressured conformity. At such closeness of range, persuasion is necessarily strong (Warwick, 1986; Streatfield, 1986).

3. China experienced a 50 percent decline in fertility during the 1970s. A vigorous antinatalist campaign—"later-longer [birth intervals]-fewer"—instituted in 1971, combined provision of contraception and abortion services with close surveillance of couples' demographic behavior and imposition of political penalties for noncompliance. The campaign worked through the dense network of Communist party–controlled intermediate institutions: production teams and brigades, communes,

study groups, and party cells. This political pressure modified the existing parental benefit–cost calculus on the value of children, tipping the balance sharply toward low fertility. Pressure reportedly shaded into compulsion in some regions, depending on local interpretations of central policy dictates—although less commonly than during the initial years of the subsequent "one child per family" campaign begun in 1979 (Banister, 1987; Greenhalgh, 1990).

4. Although not in any sense reflecting an intentional fertility policy, in some European societies before industrialization the leadership of local communities exercised fairly stringent oversight within their boundaries of marriage or establishment of a household—factors then directly if incompletely governing fertility. In English parishes of the seventeenth and eighteenth centuries, for example, there was a community responsibility to support indigent members, creating a collective incentive to limit their numbers. Together, the parish system, property requirements for marriage, and the Poor Laws constituted a devolved institutional framework through which community interests could influence fertility. The framework was later dissolved by the changes in labor relations and mobility wrought by the industrial revolution. Analogous community-level systems of demographic control could be found in many other parts of Europe and in Japan (McNicoll, 1975).

A common feature of these cases is that fertility, or behavior bearing on fertility, is the subject of close-at-hand social or administrative pressure on individuals or couples. Often there is some intimation of political or economic sanctions for noncompliance, but social sanctions such as shaming or ostracism may be perceived to be just as severe. There are ethically relevant differences in the overall degree of pressure imposed, in the justice or fairness of its application across the population, and in the intrusiveness of the methods of fertility control employed.

Criteria for ethical acceptability

In their review of the ethics of fertility control programs, Berelson and Lieberson (1979) argue that there is a hierarchy of permissible interventions paralleling the degree of gravity of the fertility problem: "The degree of coercive policy brought into play should be proportional to the degree of seriousness of the present problem and should be introduced only after less coercive means have been exhausted" (p. 602). As a practical political proposition, this may be regarded as common sense: use the minimum pressure to attain a given objective, assuming that the objective is legitimately set. Strong persuasion would be defensible for a middle range of fertility predicaments, plausibly including the cases of India, Indonesia, and China cited above. However, as an ethical

maxim, what Berelson and Lieberson call "the stepladder approach" is quite vague. It reflects the authors' denial that there can be a set of agreed ethical principles applicable to all demographic situations. Donald Warwick criticizes them for this stance: Their framework, he writes, "is politically expedient, lacking in solid ethical foundations, and easily becomes a rationalization for suppressing civil liberties" (Warwick, 1990, p. 33).

An alternative way of assessing the ethical standing of fertility control measures is to judge each against a set of value criteria. Daniel Callahan (1971) selected three: freedom, justice, and security/survival. Warwick (1990) added two more: truth-telling and welfare. Strategies using strong persuasion would barely pass the test of freedom and, in many cases, would fail one or more of the other criteria. For example, adverse side effects of proffered contraceptive methods may not be explained, violating "truth-telling" and, if damage to health follows, security/survival. This approach identifies a subset of control strategies that pass muster on all counts. However, it does not rank them; more important, it does not distinguish among strategies that fail one or more of the tests. Thus it may be of little help in determining a best course of action in the more serious demographic predicaments in which strong persuasion is likely to be contemplated. In both approaches, assessment of a proposed strategy employing strong persuasion requires combining judgments on factors that are strictly incommensurable—deciding, for example, whether a reduction in freedom can be offset by a gain in welfare. The chief difference between the two approaches lies not so much in the choice of which criteria, beyond freedom, are to be applied as in how serious the fertility problem has to be for some departure from voluntarism to be acceptable.

Gauging how much reproductive freedom has been sacrificed in a particular fertility control strategy is complicated by the fact that fertility preferences may shift. Preferences change in fairly predictable ways over the course of economic and social development. For example, urbanization and industrialization create conditions that powerfully favor smaller families. When accompanied or soon followed by rapid economic development, strong antinatalist persuasion, where it is adopted, is thus likely to be operative in influencing behavior only for a limited period: individual demand for fertility control soon takes over as the driving force of demographic change. By the end of the 1980s, this shift had probably occurred in Indonesia and in parts of China. At the same time, economic development brings greater population mobility and freer information flows, making tight political or administrative control of fertility less feasible.

To some extent, preferences can also be manipulated. All governments attempt this in some policy domains. At its worst, the result is an insidious extension of direct pressures on behavior. In relatively open societies, however, such efforts are often better seen as part of the give-and-take of politics—analogous in the public domain to commercial advertising—than as a deliberate undermining of consumer sovereignty. The Indonesian government, for example, has used a barrage of publicity measures to instill in the population the ideal of a small family. The behavioral effect is uncertain but is likely to have been small in comparison to the government's wielding of village-level peer pressures. Subsequently, both efforts would have been dwarfed in their effect by the rapid social and economic changes that have made children much more costly to parents.

Policy fairness

The justice or fairness of a strategy of strong persuasion is clearly central to an ethical assessment, but the application of such a criterion is not straightforward. One interpretation of distributional equity might favorably regard China's efforts to limit fertility to one or two children per couple. The policy seeks to impose a radical equality of fertility outcome across the population: "Fairness" is achieved. Equality of outcome would, of course, disguise substantial inequalities in perceptions of pressure: persons with strong preferences for large families suffer greatly, some others with different preferences not at all. This is a familiar problem with any rationing scheme: The half-serious proposal of Kenneth Boulding (1964) to establish a market in childbearing rights was aimed at alleviating that objection. Directing antinatalist persuasive efforts at disfavored minority groups or at those with least political access, such as the groups lowest in socioeconomic status, would be deemed ethically objectionable on equity grounds. It may be objectionable even if their fertility were higher than average. Such groups are often poorly placed to resist strong persuasion by program officials and in consequence, as the Indian case might suggest, would tend to become prime program targets.

Other dimensions of justice or fairness are also raised by persuasion-based fertility policy. Three deserving particular attention are equity between men and women, equity across generations, and equity between societies. The common assumption that the two members of a couple have similar family-size desires is often invalid. The fallback position that whatever differences do exist are private matters to be negotiated between them is undercut where there are institutionalized power differences between husband and wife affecting whose preferences dominate. The traditional patriarchal family, still common in South Asia and Africa, embodies such differences. Another example is the institution of *purdah,* which severely constrains the life choices avail-

able to women in some Muslim societies. Persuasion that in effect seeks to modify behavior in the direction of the preferences of the weaker party may contribute to equity.

The extent to which culturally entrenched gender inequality warrants ethical respect is contentious. Acceptance of universal criteria of gender equality is clearly gaining in the modern world. Most present-day governments give at least nominal recognition to equal rights for women and support international instruments containing strong endorsements of equality, suggesting their recognition of ethical judgments made from that premise. Equalizing responsibility for and risks of fertility control between men and women would be an immediate corollary.

An analogous problem of equity arises between generations. Children have interests in the number of siblings they have. Those interests, however, are often ignored when a couple is deciding on family size. Moreover, any particular couple, even if it did take account of those interests, has no influence over the fertility decisions of other couples and thus over the size and per-capita inheritance of the next generation as a whole. This predicament, in which an outcome recognized to be unfavorable can result from the separate, rational decisions of individuals, is familiar in many social contexts and is known in game theory as "the prisoner's dilemma." In the field of population, it is one of the standard justifications for strong state action to restrain rapid growth (Hardin, 1968). The many philosophical intricacies of intergenerational equity in fertility policy are discussed by Richard Sikora and Brian Barry (1978). Broader custodial claims by government—for example, claims to stewardship of environmental stability or of biodiversity—can be grounds for sterner policy interventions, although the fertility connection in such arguments is often fairly tenuous.

Finally, there are equity-based ethical issues in efforts to persuade another society to adopt measures to alter its demographic behavior, paralleling the situation of families within a society. The persuasion contained in international instruments like the 1984 Mexico City Declaration on Population and Development is vanishingly weak, in deference to national sovereignty. Overt pressure from international agencies like the World Bank to introduce antinatalist measures would probably be resisted by most governments, even though far-reaching policy realignment is frequently demanded and obtained in other spheres. Behind the scenes, however, pressure to adopt or strengthen antinatalist programs is probably fairly common in international dialogues on foreign assistance. Formally, the bargaining situation vis-à-vis population policy is quite similar to other circumstances where effects of activities in one country spill over its frontiers—for example, the case of "greenhouse gas" emissions—although fertility control may evoke sharper national sensibilities. Of course, nominal accession to such pressure, if lacking domestic political support, is unlikely to translate into effective fertility-control measures.

Fertility-control methods

Ethical justification of strong persuasion in a given fertility situation can never be carte blanche, since ethical assessment of the specifics of the control measures proposed is also needed. A given amount of pressure judged in terms of the fertility outcome may entail varying degrees of intrusiveness into individual or family behavior, depending on the details of the measures employed. Protection of privacy, an ethical value bound up with freedom, calls for minimizing that intrusiveness. This principle does not give a simple ranking of fertility-control methods but would, for example, prefer social pressure to adopt safe, reversible contraceptive practice over comparable pressure for sterilization. Browbeating a woman to have an abortion, a practice reported in some studies of China's antinatalist program, would of course be found highly objectionable. Outcome-based persuasion directed at reducing, say, fourth or higher-order births but leaving choice of means open and providing a range of safe and convenient contraceptive options for both men and women might appear less intrusive than persuasion directed at, say, acceptance of IUDs or contraceptive implants.

Cultural acceptability is a consideration in such rankings of specific measures. The more acceptable the measure, the less the perceived pressure submitted to in adopting it. Among the cultural factors that affect whether a measure is deemed objectionable are notions of privacy, shame, and personal autonomy; beliefs about health and therapeutics; and the expected level of communication between sexual partners. Cultural acceptability may also be influenced by the kinds of pressures routinely applied elsewhere in the society in efforts to change other behaviors or those that are exercised in social life generally. If daily life is minutely regulated, whether by an intrusive government or by neighborly meddlesomeness, pressures on fertility may be a comparatively small additional invasion of privacy. Practices such as neighborhood surveillance of pregnancies in urban China or the month-by-month listing of couples' contraceptive status in village registers in Bali should be judged not alone but along with the polities they manifest.

Some religious beliefs and moral codes make distinctions among birth-control methods. Particular methods—abortion most frequently—may be prohibited outright. For believers, the sanctions for violating such a prohibition, possibly extending into afterlife, can clearly warrant the term "strong persuasion." The position of the Roman Catholic church on contraception, as set out in Pope Paul VI's 1968 encyclical *Humanae Vitae*, entails discriminating between "natural" and "artificial" methods. The church opposes all forms of artificial birth control. In this case, however, the perceived strength of the sanctions has been vitiated, at least in the United States and other affluent countries, by shifts in Catholics' attitudes toward church authority in that domain. Contraceptive behavior in these countries has shown an increasing departure from the church's teaching on the subject, and differences between the family size of Catholics and non-Catholics have largely vanished.

Pronatalist strategies

Most of the above discussion has been concerned with antinatalist strategies, the principal arena of ethical debate on population policy matters. Looking ahead, it is likely that situations of very low fertility and rapid natural decrease of population will become increasingly common. Immigration is at best a partial substitute for births: with very low fertility, the scale of immigration needed to maintain a nation's population size and limit the rise in its average age may be incompatible with maintenance of its cultural identity. Assuming a compelling social interest in demographic continuity, fertility policy would then reemerge on the public agenda, directed at pronatalist objectives.

Pronatalist strategies based on incentives have a long history but have shown at best modest results for quite large public expenditures. Strong pronatalist persuasion, a more recent phenomenon, has perhaps even less to show (David, 1982). Two contrasting instances where such policies did have significant demographic effects were in Romania and Iran. In 1966, Romania outlawed abortion, previously widely practiced, resulting in an estimated 40 percent more births over 1966–1976 than would have been expected in the absence of the policy shift, albeit with the excess concentrated in the initial years. In Iran, the enforcement of traditional sex roles and dismantling of the family-planning program after establishment of the Islamic Republic in 1979 were accompanied by a substantial rise in fertility.

In most respects, the ethical issues raised by pronatalist strategies mirror those of antinatalist strategies. Economic incentives can be designed to be ethically inoffensive, but the scale of transfers needed to make them effective may be too large a burden on public revenue. Strong persuasion, as before, is ethically problematic, even well short of Romanian- or Iranian-style restrictions. A nation facing rapid demographic decline might well arrive at a collective decision to try to raise fertility by means formally analogous to the community-level peer pressure discussed earlier and involving the same array of ethical considerations. The Romanian and Iranian measures could call on no such demographic rationale or implied social consensus; in revoking options and opportunities formerly available, both were ethically retrogressive.

The chief objection to complete reproductive freedom is that societies have legitimate interests in their demographic futures. The proposition is readily assented to when the society is a nation-state and the policy issue is the number of immigrants to be admitted. Fertility policy, concerned with the other source of new members, entails balancing the interests of individuals as parents or members of a family against their interests as citizens. Traditions of Western liberalism, taken over and elaborated in international covenants on human rights, emphasize freedom from interference by government as a salient value. Where social interests, properly determined, are seriously threatened by existing levels of fertility, there is an ethically defensible case for abridging that freedom. Ethical assessment of particular fertility-control strategies requires weighing that abridgment against the perceived threat. It also requires testing the strategies against additional standards—especially that of fairness. This procedure, however, does not yield a cut-and-dried ranking or decision on admissibility. A problem of judgment remains, in which cultural features of the society and perhaps the political predilections of the assessor will play a part.

GEOFFREY MCNICOLL

While all the articles in the other sections of this entry are relevant, see especially the other articles in this section: CHANGES IN ATTITUDE AND CULTURE, INCENTIVES AND DISINCENTIVES, *and* COMPULSION. *Directly related to this article are the entries* POPULATION ETHICS; *and* FERTILITY CONTROL. *For a further discussion of topics mentioned in this article, see the entries* ABORTION; BEHAVIOR CONTROL; ETHICS, *articles on* NORMATIVE ETHICAL THEORIES, *and* RELIGION AND MORALITY; FAMILY; FREEDOM AND COERCION; HARM; JUSTICE; MARRIAGE AND OTHER DOMESTIC PARTNERSHIPS; MEDICAL ETHICS, HISTORY OF, *section on* SOUTH AND EAST ASIA, *articles on* INDIA, *and* SOUTHEAST ASIAN COUNTRIES, *and section on* CHINA, *article on* CONTEMPORARY CHINA; NATURE; RIGHTS; *and* ROMAN CATHOLICISM. *For a discussion of related ideas, see the entries* AGING AND THE AGED, *article on* SOCIETAL AGING; AUTHORITY; CHILDREN, *article on* RIGHTS OF CHILDREN; FUTURE GENERATIONS, OBLIGATIONS TO; PRIVACY IN HEALTH CARE; SEXISM; *and* WOMEN, *article on* HISTORICAL AND CROSS-CULTURAL PERSPECTIVES.

Bibliography

BANISTER, JUDITH. 1987. *China's Changing Population.* Stanford, Calif.: Stanford University Press.

BAYLES, MICHAEL D. 1980. *Morality and Population Policy.* Tuscaloosa: University of Alabama Press.

BERELSON, BERNARD, and LIEBERSON, JONATHAN. 1979. "Government Efforts to Influence Fertility: The Ethical Issues." *Population and Development Review* 5:581–613.

BERLIN, ISAIAH. 1969. "Two Concepts of Liberty." In his *Four Essays on Liberty.* Oxford: Oxford University Press.

BLAKE, JUDITH. 1972. "Coercive Pronatalism and American Population Policy." In *Aspects of Population Growth Policy.* Edited by Robert Parke, Jr., and Charles F. Westoff. Commission on Population Growth and the American Future, Research Reports, vol. 6, pp. 81–109. Washington, D.C.: Government Printing Office.

BOULDING, KENNETH E. 1964. *The Meaning of the Twentieth Century.* New York: Harper & Row.

CALLAHAN, DANIEL. 1971. *Ethics and Population Limitation.* New York: The Population Council.

DAVID, HENRY P. 1982. "Eastern Europe: Pronatalist Policies and Private Behavior." *Population Bulletin* 36, no. 6:1–48.

DEMENY, PAUL. 1986. "Population and the Invisible Hand." *Demography* 23:473–487.

FEINBERG, JOEL. 1980. *Rights, Justice, and the Bounds of Liberty.* Princeton, N.J.: Princeton University Press.

GREENHALGH, SUSAN. 1990. "The Evolution of the One-Child Policy in Shaanxi Province, 1979–88." *China Quarterly* 122:191–229.

GWATKIN, DAVIDSON R. 1979. "Political Will and Family Planning: The Implications of India's Emergency Experience." *Population and Development Review* 5:29–59.

HARDIN, GARRETT. 1968. "The Tragedy of the Commons." *Science* 162:1243–1248.

MCNICOLL, GEOFFREY. 1975. "Community-Level Population Policy: An Exploration." *Population and Development Review* 1:1–21.

PATTERSON, ORLANDO. 1991. *Freedom in the Making of Western Culture.* New York: Basic Books.

SIKORA, RICHARD I., and BARRY, BRIAN, eds. 1978. *Obligations to Future Generations.* Philadelphia: Temple University Press.

STREATFIELD, KIM. 1986. *Fertility Decline in a Traditional Society: The Case of Bali.* Canberra: Department of Demography, Australian National University.

UNITED NATIONS. SECRETARIAT. 1990. "Relationship Between Human Rights and Population Issues: Standard-Setting Activities of the United Nations Organization, 1980–1988." In *Population and Human Rights,* pp. 54–74. New York: Author.

VICZIANY, MARIKA. 1982. "Coercion in a Soft State: The Family Planning Program of India." *Pacific Affairs* 55:373–402, 557–592.

WARWICK, DONALD P. 1986. "The Indonesian Family Planning Program: Government Influence and Client Choice." *Population and Development Review* 12:453–490.

———. 1990. "The Ethics of Population Control." In *Population Policy: Contemporary Issues,* pp. 21–37. Edited by Godfrey Roberts. New York: Praeger.

D. COMPULSION

Compulsion in fertility control goes far beyond persuasion. To compel (or coerce; the terms are often used interchangeably), a fertility-control measure must employ force, the threat of force, or extreme penalties and pressures that leave people no choice but to comply. Compulsion need not be absolute—some people may be able to withstand pressures that overwhelm others—but it must be powerful enough to compel many people to act in ways contrary to their wishes. When individuals use contraception against their will, abort wanted pregnancies, or are forced to undergo sterilization, they are evidently experiencing compulsion, even if the inducements employed to achieve these results are only psychological.

Some family-planning advocates limit the term "coercion" to the use of physical force. For ethical purposes, that definition is too narrow. Incentive and disincentive measures may, in some circumstances, result in compulsion. People who practice family planning out of fear of public humiliation; strong peer pressures; such penalties as loss of food, housing, employment, possessions, or essential services; or simply because of threats and intimidation are acting under compulsion even if no overt force is in evidence.

Incentives for couples who accept contraception or abide by family size limits are usually not coercive unless they involve services essential to life or health (e.g., food or medical care) that are not readily available to those who do not comply. Disincentives are not coercive for those who can disregard them and have the children they want, but they may be coercive for people whose subsistence or general welfare is seriously threatened by them. Threats are not coercive if there is no follow-up and no one takes them seriously. However, when people comply with family-planning demands out of fear, they are clearly acting under compulsion.

National fertility policies

National fertility policies may be either pronatalist (fertility-raising) or antinatalist (fertility-reducing). Pronatalist policies are sometimes, as in the case of Germany in the 1930s, prompted by concern that low fertility or negative population growth rates threaten national political or economic well-being, or the belief, as in the People's Republic of China in the early 1950s, that a large population is a source of economic, political, and military power. The leadership of a country whose population is not growing may fear aggression by more populous or faster-growing neighbors or an overwhelming influx of immigrants differing in language, culture, or ethnicity. Pronatalist policies may also reflect religious values that treat procreation as a fulfillment of natural law or divine commandment.

Antinatalist policies are usually inspired by the view that current fertility levels constitute an impossible or undesirable burden on the government because of the costs of providing health care, education, employment, housing, and other essential services, or the belief that population growth threatens prospects for economic development, improved living standards, nutrition, the supply of natural resources, the environment, and the survival of humankind and other species. This view is often taken as received wisdom that requires no further investigation and needs only to be asserted to be proven. For example, since 1974 the government of China has justified its family-planning program on the grounds that population growth threatens economic development and living standards in general, including education, employment, housing, and even food supply.

However, these arguments, like the pronatalist arguments they superseded, consist largely of categorical assertions never put to an empirical test and sometimes contain contradictions. Although the Chinese government claims that population growth prevents it from investing in consumer needs, it has been spending heavily for armaments since the late 1980s. In 1993, the government insisted that China's then modest natural increase rate threatened economic growth at the same time that it worried publicly about "overheating" in an economy growing at about 14 percent per year, faster than any other in the world! Such incongruities suggest that official explanations do not necessarily reveal the actual reasons for national policies. China is not the only country to which this caveat applies.

National fertility policies can be completely voluntary, but some use compulsion and go to great lengths to conceal and deny the fact. Denial helps avoid domestic and international criticism on humanitarian grounds and obviates the necessity of justifying coercion. The Chinese government has consistently maintained, in spite of abundant contrary evidence, that its program is voluntary; foreign supporters of the Chinese program, including the United Nations Population Fund and the International Planned Parenthood Federation, ostensibly accept and reiterate the Chinese claims.

Pronatalist compulsion

The most common forms of pronatalist compulsion are government policies that deny access to contraception or abortion. In the early 1950s the Chinese government denounced birth control as a foreign plot to "kill off the Chinese people without shedding blood," banned imports of contraceptives, and prohibited abortion. Restrictions on abortion are also found throughout Latin America except Cuba. Until the collapse of Communist governments in 1990 and 1991, liberal abortion laws prevailed in eastern Europe except in Romania, but in 1991 and 1992 Poland, Czechoslovakia, and Hungary adopted measures that increasingly restricted the practice. Legislation adopted in Poland tripled the cost of contraceptives, making them less accessible to many people (Boland, 1992). Prohibiting particular contraceptive measures may constitute compulsion in the absence of effective alternatives, but only if the prohibition is enforced. Brazil, for example, has a law against sterilization that is generally ignored; an estimated 40 percent of Brazilian women have been sterilized.

Some people have applied the term "coercive" to traditional pronatalist values emphasizing the need to bear children to ensure family prosperity, provide support in old age, carry on the family line, or demonstrate virility or fecundity—attitudes common in many developing countries, especially among rural people. These values are often reinforced by religious institutions favoring large families or condemning specific birth-control practices. Cultural factors are indeed coercive when they compel couples (or women) to have children against their will, specifically in situations in which the desires of women to limit childbearing are overridden by prevailing norms and institutions in a male-dominated society (but not in cases in which both husband and wife accept the cultural imperatives and comply willingly).

Pronatalist compulsion is usually not as coercive as antinatalist compulsion. Even the most coercive pronatalist policies have been relatively ineffectual except for brief periods (Demeny, 1986b), probably because government strategies for compelling pregnancy are more easily and inconspicuously evaded than are those for preventing or terminating pregnancy. Antinatalist compulsion leaves couples no choice but to have fewer children than they might want. Pronatalist compulsion may narrow the range of contraceptive options but can seldom stop couples from limiting fertility if they are resolved to do so. Voluntary fertility control was practiced quite effectively in several European countries long before modern contraceptive techniques had been devised and without recourse to abortion.

Antinatalist compulsion

Antinatalist compulsion has been brought to public attention in recent years by the conspicuously coercive family-planning measures employed in India and China. A sterilization program promoted by the Indian government in the mid-1970s generated compulsion because of demands from the top that assigned targets be achieved by whatever means necessary. In April 1976 the government issued a national policy statement authorizing state legislatures to adopt legislation for compulsory sterilization. One state, Maharashtra, did so, but instances of forced sterilization were widely reported in other areas as well. Local officials used control over permits, licenses, employment, and school admissions, and denial of food rations, salary forfeitures, threats, and physical force to compel people to submit. One analyst attributed the coercion to intense central government pressure on local authorities to carry out large numbers of sterilizations immediately, with no excuses accepted and no questions asked (Gwatkin, 1979). Between July and December 1976, six million people were sterilized. The Indian experience provoked a public reaction that helped to bring down the government.

The Chinese family-planning program has used compulsion more extensively than has any other national program. The compulsion began early in the 1970s, with an attempt to impose a two-to-four-child limit by requiring women to use intrauterine devices (IUDs) to prevent further pregnancies. Chinese sources do not reveal exactly how this policy was implemented, but the media openly advocated publicizing individual "birth plans," setting target figures for contraceptive use, and conducting "mass mobilizations." Those who resisted were to be declared "class enemies" and subjected to "political struggle" (Aird, 1981).

Pressures for compliance escalated during the rest of the decade, except for a brief remission in 1978, and culminated in the adoption of the one-child policy in 1979. Another remission occurred in 1980, but by 1981 the pressures were resumed and reached a peak in 1983, when Chinese government policy, adopted by the State Family Planning Commission with prior approval of the Communist Party Central Committee and the State Council, demanded IUD insertion for women with one child, sterilization for couples with two or more children, and abortion for pregnancies without official approval. Mobile birth-control surgery teams ranged over the countryside, apprehending those to whom the policy applied and carrying out the operations on the spot; many of these operations had complications because some of the teams were inadequately trained. Nearly twenty-one million sterilizations were performed in 1983 alone, three-quarters of them on women. Most of them were undoubtedly involuntary, as was implied by Chinese sources at the time. One source revealed that the purpose of the sterilization requirement was not just to eliminate third and higher-order births but also to make couples with one child avoid further pregnancies. This explanation implies that sterilization was compulsory and was meant to be intimidating.

Strong adverse public reaction obliged the regime to moderate its policies in 1984. Sterilization quotas were abandoned, family-planning workers were advised to be "fair and reasonable" and avoid coercion, and the categories of special circumstances under which some couples could be allowed a second child were increased; thereupon enforcement of policy requirements promptly lapsed. For a few years most provinces allowed rural couples whose first child was a girl to have a second child, and several provinces allowed all rural couples to have two children. These measures were intended to enlist public support for the elimination of higher-order pregnancies, but they did not work. Alarmed by rising birthrates, the central authorities attempted to tighten up again, and by the end of the decade, policy enforcement had become very strict.

In April 1991, the central authorities ordered a further major escalation, with startling results. For the first time, fertility in China dropped below the replacement level in 1992, and coercion increased sharply. The authorities demanded that the crackdown continue without change to the end of the century. New population targets were established, and efforts to penalize officials who failed to fulfill them were intensified. Provincial family-planning regulations were stiffened, and new laws were adopted to control fertility among migrants, to limit adoptive families to one child, and to eliminate childbearing by those deemed unfit for "eugenic" reasons. The 1983 rules for IUD insertion, sterilization, and abortion were reinstated. The one-child limit is rigidly maintained in most urban areas, and the number of exceptions permitted in rural areas is being reduced. Since the 1950s most ethnic minorities had been subjected to somewhat less stringent rules (e.g., a two-child limit) to avoid charges of "Han chauvinism," but in the early 1990s steps were taken to narrow their options as well (Banister, 1987; Aird, 1990).

Forms of compulsion

Physical compulsion is the most direct and extreme form of compulsion used in fertility control. In includes such measures as rounding up women pregnant without government permission and transporting them to clinics for forced abortions—sometimes in handcuffs, bound with ropes, or in hog cages, practices reported from time to time in China and in Tibet. Physical compulsion is also involved when urban doctors in China, threatened with loss of their jobs if they permit unauthorized newborns to leave the hospital alive, destroy them during delivery by injecting lethal substances into their fontanels or crushing their heads with forceps, as was reported by several sources in the 1980s (Aird, 1990). It is implicit in the mass "mobilizations" for abortion, sterilization, and IUD insertion, from which people reportedly sometimes flee their homes and go into hiding because, once apprehended, they have no choice but to submit.

Physical compulsion occurs without overt force when women in China who ask for removal of IUDs or reversal of sterilizations are refused, and when women in Bangladesh suffering serious side effects from Norplant implants (subcutaneous devices that release fertility-inhibiting hormones for five years or more) are told they cannot be removed (Ubinig, 1991). Fertility-control techniques that are effective for long periods or permanently, such as long-lasting injections or implants, are more susceptible to compulsory applications than are contraceptives that depend upon user initiative and sustained efforts. This is especially true for measures that can be implemented without the consent or knowledge of the recipient while other medical services are being provided, such as injections of chemical abortifacients, abortions, and sterilizations.

Threats and commands issued by officials are often coercive in societies in which the authorities exercise such power that people dare not defy them. Intimidation is clearly the intent of the "heart-to-heart talks" with family-planning cadres that Chinese women reluctant to practice family planning are obliged to endure until they succumb to the pressure. The same applies to the "study classes" for nonconforming women, who are forced to attend and are not allowed to return home until they promise to comply (Aird, 1990; Mosher, 1983). A threat of legal action against nonconformists is implicit in the provision in the Chinese Constitution making family planning a citizen's "duty" and in provincial regulations mandating family-planning requirements, as well as in the requirement that an official permission slip be obtained from local authorities before starting a pregnancy. In the 1980s, Balinese Hindus who resisted birth-control demands were threatened with expulsion from their villages or with refusal to allow them to cremate deceased relatives in the village graveyards, both awesome threats in the context of their culture (Warwick, 1990). In India, government officials used their status to bully beggars into submitting to sterilization (Warwick, 1990).

Peer pressure can sometimes be made coercive in the service of family-planning programs. In China such pressures are deliberately instigated by imposing collective punishments for individual noncompliance. In several Chinese provinces in the late 1980s, rural couples eligible under official policies to have a second child were refused permission until all unauthorized pregnancies in their village were terminated. In some factories, bonuses and expansion plans were denied to the entire work force if a single employee had an unauthorized child (Aird, 1990). Under these circumstances, offending couples in essentially closed communities can be ostracized and subjected to reprisals by local officials and by neighbors or coworkers until the stress reaches unbearable levels.

Some of the disincentives imposed on violators of family-planning rules in China are so severe that they are obviously meant to be coercive, and often are. Provincial family-planning regulations may require a couple that has an unauthorized child to forfeit 20, 30, or 40 percent of their total income for up to fourteen years (Aird, 1992). One-time penalties may be several times the family's total annual income (Barnett, 1992). Other penalties include cutting off electricity, water, and food allotments; confiscating household possessions, livestock and farm implements; expelling people from their homes; and even tearing down the houses (Aird, 1992). In 1993, for the first time there were reports of family-planning violators being beaten with electric batons. In India some couples were told that their children could not attend school until one of the parents was sterilized. Unemployed workers were required to show sterilization certificates before they could be hired. Some villages were allowed irrigation water at subsidized prices only if they had the requisite number of sterilizations (Warwick, 1982).

Incentives that include vital necessities can amount to compulsion for the indigent. In Bangladesh, a destitute woman seeking free food was told she must first be sterilized (Warwick, 1990), and other women were required to undergo sterilization to qualify for health care (Hartmann, 1990). In Egypt in the early 1970s, some women were forced to buy contraceptive pills if they wanted other medical treatment (Warwick, 1990). In general, incentives are more compelling for poor families than for the rest of the community.

Penalties and incentives applied to local officials to make sure they attain their family-planning targets often cause them to resort to compulsory measures. Target numbers of acceptors of IUDs, sterilization, implants, and other contraceptive methods are generally intended to pressure local authorities to obtain compliance from their people. In China, national targets for population size and rate of growth are allocated to the provinces, which are expected to set lower-level targets accordingly. Other targets are designed to increase the percentages of women using contraception or accepting one-child certificates, and to reduce the percentages of third and higher-order births. Chinese provinces are ranked according to their success in meeting their targets, and laggard provinces are ordered to catch up with the rest.

The pressures are transmitted mainly through a nationwide system of signed contracts called the "responsibility system." Provincial and lower-level leaders in China who fail to meet their targets may lose bonuses, promotions, and even their jobs (Aird, 1990). When such systems are instituted without effective safeguards against coercion, local leaders naturally assume that the higher levels are not deeply concerned about preventing it. Even targets not intended to be compulsory can lead to coercion at the grass-roots level, as has happened in India, Bangladesh, the Philippines, Indonesia, and Vietnam (Warwick, 1982; Cohen, 1991; Hafidz et al., 1992; Banister, 1989, 1991). Organizations such as the World Bank and the U.S. Agency for International Development have sometimes made target attainment a prerequisite for continued assistance to client countries, thus creating conditions in which local authorities may feel obliged to resort to compulsory measures (Hartmann, 1991–1992).

Ethical considerations

Granted that most of the measures described above are either compulsory or tend to lead to compulsion in implementation, are compulsory family-planning measures unethical? Certainly they violate the right of reproductive freedom embraced by the world population conferences at Bucharest in 1974 and at Mexico City in 1984, and in other international declarations on human rights. All international agencies promoting family planning and most professionals in the field at least nominally subscribe to the Mexico City declaration that all individuals and couples have the right to "decide freely and responsibly the number and spacing of their children," and that parents should be allowed to fulfill their responsibilities "freely and without coercion" (International Conference on Population, 1984). The rationale for including reproductive freedom among the basic human rights is that decisions about childbearing are so personal and so important for the happiness of parents that they should be protected against encroachments by state authority.

However, the consensus about the inviolability of reproductive freedom is not as solid as public declarations make it seem. Many family-planning advocates, demographers, economists, and environmentalists have accepted the view that world population growth constitutes a serious threat to human welfare and even to the survival of the planet. In one form or another, this view has become the received wisdom in intellectual circles throughout much of the Western world. Although few of its adherents have openly advocated compulsory family planning, many have privately accepted the idea. In 1978 a survey taken of members of the Population Association of America found that 56 percent of the respondents believed that compulsory measures must be taken in the future to avoid catastrophe, and 34 percent felt that some countries needed to adopt such measures immediately (Population Association of America, 1978). Some people of this persuasion urge consideration of measures that go "beyond family planning" and openly express admiration for the aggressive tactics used in China.

Presumably those who express guarded approval of compulsory family planning consider it a lesser evil from a humanitarian standpoint than the consequences of continued population growth, and hence a legitimate exercise of authority by the state in its role as protector of the public welfare. But is this perception valid? On this question there is sharp disagreement among demographers and economists. The broad consensus about the dangers of population growth that existed through the 1960s has seriously eroded in subsequent years (Menken, 1986; Demeny 1986a; Warwick, 1990). The idea of an imminent "population crisis" has not been sustained either by relevant statistical evidence assembled during the 1970s and 1980s or by actual experience in developing countries.

In the late 1960s, Simon Kuznets and Richard Easterlin warned that the effects of population growth on economic development were not well understood and that there was no correlation between population growth and per capita income in developing countries (Kuznets, 1967; Easterlin, 1967). In 1971, a study by the National Academy of Sciences concluded, on the basis of evidence from India and Mexico, that rapid population growth had serious negative consequences. However, in 1973, Julian Simon and Avery Guest challenged the notion of overpopulation (in Pohlman, 1973), and in 1977, Simon cited evidence that moderate population growth stimulates economic development, rapid and slow growth are slight deterrents, and no growth or a decline in population seems to be a strong deterrent (Simon, 1977).

In 1986, a second National Academy of Sciences study, drawing on extensive international statistical data, found that population growth plays a relatively minor role in economic development, insufficient to justify extreme fertility-control measures. One participant in the study, Samuel Preston, noted that "so much of the [doomsday] rhetoric is simple-minded and incorrect, casually attributing any human problem to there being too many humans" (1985, p. 10). Meanwhile, some of the more sensational doomsday predictions, notably Paul Ehrlich's warning of an inescapable worldwide famine in the 1970s (Ehrlich, 1968), failed to come true. In many heavily populated developing countries, per capita food availability rose instead.

Obviously the last word has not been written on this issue. The debate among demographers and economists will undoubtedly continue, and the final outcome is uncertain. Still, it seems unlikely that the notion of a "population crisis," in the world as a whole or in particular countries, can be demonstrated beyond reasonable doubt. If the relationship between population growth and human welfare were as direct, preponderant, and negative as the "crisis" view assumes, at least a modest correlation should have appeared by now in international statistics. Instead, as Preston observed, the relation appears "about as random and unstructured as any . . . in the social sciences" (1985, p. 11). Moreover, demographic projections are not meant to be predictions, and in the long term often turn out to be wide of the mark; economic forecasts are generally much more inaccurate and often contradictory. Prognostications that combine both surely compound the probability of error. There is therefore no justification for the certainty with which conclusions about the effects of population growth on human welfare are usually advanced.

In view of the lack of definitive knowledge about the consequences of population growth, there seems to be no empirically sound basis for antinatalist encroachments on reproductive freedom. If the case for compulsion can ever be made, it must be based on evidence that is systematic, substantial, and conclusive. The interpretation of the evidence must not be entrusted to persons and institutions with a vested interest in the outcome, which would exclude most family-planning advocates and agencies, at least some demographic and economic research institutions, the agencies that fund their activities, and other organizations and individuals that have an ax to grind on the questions at issue. Despite much public rhetoric from interested quarters, no such case has yet been made. Until an unequivocal verdict has been reached under circumstances with proper safeguards, compulsory fertility-control measures must be regarded as unethical.

JOHN S. AIRD

While all the articles in the other sections of this entry are relevant, see especially the other articles in this section: CHANGES IN ATTITUDE AND CULTURE; INCENTIVES AND DISINCENTIVES; *and* STRONG PERSUASION. *Directly related are the entries* POPULATION ETHICS; FERTILITY CONTROL; *and* FREEDOM AND COERCION. *For a further discussion of topics mentioned in this article, see the entries* ABORTION; AUTONOMY; BEHAVIOR CONTROL; ENVIRONMENTAL POLICY AND LAW; EUGENICS; FOOD POLICY; HARM; NATURAL LAW; *and* WOMEN, *article on* HISTORICAL AND CROSS-CULTURAL PERSPECTIVES. *For a discussion of related ideas, see the entries* AGING AND THE AGED, *article on* SOCIETAL AGING; AGRICULTURE; CHILDREN; ENVIRONMENTAL HEALTH; FUTURE GENERATIONS, OBLIGATIONS TO; LIFE; PUBLIC HEALTH, *articles on* DETERMINANTS OF PUBLIC HEALTH, *and* PHILOSOPHY OF PUBLIC HEALTH; RACE AND RACISM; ROMAN CATHOLICISM; SEXISM; *and* UTILITY. *Other relevant material may be found under the entry* MEDICAL ETHICS, HISTORY OF, *section on* SOUTH AND EAST ASIA, *articles on* INDIA, *and* SOUTHEAST ASIAN COUNTRIES, *and subsection on* CHINA, *article on* CONTEMPORARY CHINA; *section on* EUROPE, *subsection on* CONTEMPORARY PERIOD, *article on* GERMAN-SPEAKING COUNTRIES AND SWITZERLAND; *and section on* THE AMERICAS, *article on* LATIN AMERICA.

Bibliography

AIRD, JOHN S. 1981. "Fertility Decline in China." In *Fertility Decline in the Less Developed Countries*, pp. 119–227. Edited by Nick Eberstadt. New York: Praeger.

————. 1990. *Slaughter of the Innocents: Coercive Birth Control in China*. Washington, D.C.: American Enterprise Institute.

————. 1992. "Foreign Assistance to Coercive Family Planning in China." Canberra: Australian Senate.

BANISTER, JUDITH. 1987. *China's Changing Population*. Stanford, Calif.: Stanford University Press.

————. 1989. "Vietnam's Evolving Population Policies." In *International Conference on Population, New Delhi, 1989, September 20–27*. Liège, Belgium: International Union for the Scientific Study of Population.

————. 1991. "Vietnam: Population Dynamics and Prospects." Washington, D.C.: U.S. Bureau of the Census, Center for International Research.

BARNETT, ROBERT. 1992. "Documents Give Tibetan Birth Control Regulations." *South China Morning Post* (Hong Kong), October 7, p. 11.

BOLAND, REED. 1992. "Selected Legal Developments in Reproductive Health in 1991." *Family Planning Perspectives* 24, no. 4:178–185.

COHEN, MARGOT. 1991. "Success Brings New Problems." *Far Eastern Economic Review* (Hong Kong) 151, no. 16 (April 18):48–49.

DEMENY, PAUL G. 1986a. *Population and the Invisible Hand*. Working Paper no. 123. New York: Population Council, Center for Policy Studies.

————. 1986b. *Pronatalist Policies in Low Fertility Countries: Patterns, Performance, and Prospects*. Working Paper no. 129. New York: Population Council, Center for Policy Studies.

EASTERLIN, RICHARD A. 1967. "Effects of Population Growth on the Economic Development of Developing Countries." *Annals of the American Academy of Political and Social Science* 369:98–108.

EHRLICH, PAUL R. 1968. *The Population Bomb*. New York: Ballantine.

GWATKIN, DAVIDSON R. 1979. "Political Will and Family Planning: The Implications of India's Emergency Experience." *Population and Development Review* 5, no. 1:29–59.

HAFIDZ, WARDAH; TASLIM, ADRINA; and ARIPURNAMI, SITA. 1992. "Family Planning in Indonesia: The Case for Policy Reorientation." *Inside Indonesia* (March):19–20, 22.

HARTMANN, BETSY. 1990. "Bankers, Babies, and Bangladesh." *Progressive* 54, no. 9:18–21.

————. 1991–1992. "Population Control as Foreign Policy." *CovertAction Information Bulletin* 39 (Winter):26–30.

INTERNATIONAL CONFERENCE ON POPULATION. 1984. *Report of the International Conference on Population, 1984*. New York: United Nations.

KUZNETS, SIMON. 1967. "Population and Economic Growth." *Proceedings of the American Philosophical Society* 111, no. 3:170–193.

MENKEN, JANE A. 1986. "Introduction and Overview." In *World Population and U.S. Policy: The Choices Ahead*, pp. 6–26. Edited by Jane A. Menken. New York: W. W. Norton.

MOSHER, STEVEN W. 1983. *Broken Earth: The Rural Chinese*. New York: Free Press.

NATIONAL ACADEMY OF SCIENCES. 1986. *Population Growth and Economic Development: Policy Questions*. Washington, D.C.: National Academy Press.

POHLMAN, EDWARD, comp. 1973. *Population: A Clash of Prophets*. New York: New American Library.

POPULATION ASSOCIATION OF AMERICA. 1978. *P. A. A. Affairs* (Fall):p. 2.

PRESTON, SAMUEL H. 1985. Paper in *Are World Population Trends a Problem?* Edited by Ben J. Wattenberg and Karl Zinsmeister. Washington, D.C.: American Enterprise Institute.

SIMON, JULIAN L. 1977. *The Economics of Population Growth*. Princeton, N.J.: Princeton University Press.

Ubinig. 1991. "'The Price of Norplant is TK.2000! You Cannot Remove It.' Clients Are Refused Removal in Norplant Trial in Bangladesh." *Issues in Reproductive and Genetic Engineering* 4, no. 1:45–46.

WARWICK, DONALD P. 1982. *Bitter Pills: Population Policies and Their Implementation in Eight Developing Countries*. Cambridge: At the University Press.

————. 1990. "The Ethics of Population Control." In *Population Policy: Contemporary Issues*. Edited by Godfrey Roberts. New York: Praeger.

II. HEALTH EFFECTS OF FERTILITY CONTROL

Concern about possible side effects of contraceptives is the most common reason women in the United States at risk of unintended pregnancy give for not using them (Silverman et al., 1987). Because many people do not consider the beneficial effects of contraceptive use on women's current and future health, there may be unbalanced perceptions of their real health effects.

Sexually transmitted diseases (STDs), including human immunodeficiency virus (HIV) infection, continue to spread in the United States and worldwide. As the incidence of STD rises, so does the incidence of upper genital tract infections and ectopic (tubal) pregnancy, potential consequences of STD infection that can lead to infertility. Also, because more and more women are postponing childbearing until the middle or later years of their reproductive life, preventing infertility has become an important companion goal of postponing pregnancy.

To choose an appropriate method of contraception, individuals need to know whether they have a medical condition (e.g., high blood pressure) that might rule out the use of certain methods; whether their own behavior (e.g., having multiple sexual partners or smoking) contraindicates the use of a method; or whether the method itself could threaten their health.

To assess the health consequences of contraceptive choices among sexually active, fecund women who do not want to become pregnant, investigators compare the risks of pregnancy, infertility, heart disease, cancer, and death faced by women using various methods with those faced by women using no method. Because of the paucity of information from other countries, the assessment that follows is based on data primarily from the United

States and the conclusions also pertain to the United States.

Preventing pregnancy

Pregnancy rates among women who use no contraceptive method are at least four times as high as the rate among those using any method (Trussell et al., 1990). Failure rates vary widely. The highest rates occur among typical users of periodic abstinence, withdrawal, or barrier and spermicide methods (10 to 22 percent become pregnant in the first twelve months of use), followed by users of the pill and the intrauterine device (IUD) (3 to 4 percent), and by women who rely on implants, injectables, or sterilization (less than 1 percent) (Harlap et al., 1991).

Women who use no method during their entire reproductive life span and who never have an induced abortion have far more births than women who use any of the contraceptive methods and have a birth every time they become accidentally pregnant (eighteen vs. five, respectively, or fewer) (Harlap et al., 1991). Likewise, among women who terminate all their pregnancies by induced abortion, those using no method of contraception have far more abortions than contraceptive users, including women who use the least effective methods (thirty-five vs. six, respectively, or fewer). Among women using the least effective methods—periodic abstinence, withdrawal, condoms, or spermicides—those who have an abortion every time they become pregnant have more pregnancies than those who give birth every time they become pregnant, because they would be exposed to the risk of a subsequent pregnancy much sooner than women who carry every pregnancy to term. However, regardless of how women resolve their pregnancies, use of even the least effective contraceptive results in many fewer pregnancies than use of no method.

Preserving fertility

Most women and men in the United States have more than one sexual partner during their lifetime. Two-thirds of all U.S. women who have ever had intercourse have had more than one partner. Many of them, especially young women, have more than one partner within a short time (Kost and Forrest, 1992). With each new sexual partner, a woman faces the risk of becoming infected with an STD.

Some STDs can cause upper genital tract infections—such as pelvic inflammatory disease (PID) or infections following pregnancy (whether it ends in spontaneous abortion, induced abortion, or birth)—that can damage a woman's reproductive organs and lead to ectopic pregnancy or tubal infertility. The more episodes of upper genital tract infection a woman has, the more

likely it is that a subsequent pregnancy will be ectopic. Moreover, once a woman has experienced an ectopic pregnancy, it is more likely that subsequent pregnancies will be ectopic. Women who have had an ectopic pregnancy are likely to become infertile, and the risk of infertility rises quickly with increasing numbers of ectopic pregnancies.

Among women at low risk of STD infection, estimated rates of tubal infertility for those using any contraceptive method are lower than rates for women using no method (who have a high risk of pregnancy-related upper genital tract infections because of their large numbers of pregnancies). Among women at high risk of STDs, the contraceptive method used can have a significant effect on the risk of developing tubal infertility. For these women, rates of tubal infertility are lowest among users of barrier and spermicide methods and highest among those using the IUD, periodic abstinence, or no method (Harlap et al., 1991).

Protecting health

Pregnancy and childbirth, once major causes of mortality among women in the United States, are now much safer; however, they still account for 1 to 2 percent of all deaths each year among women aged fifteen to forty-four (National Center for Health Statistics, 1990). Ectopic pregnancy is the outcome with the greatest risk of death, and induced abortion the one with the least. Other pregnancy-related deaths are from giving birth, upper genital tract infections, and rare cancers associated with abnormal embryonic development (e.g., trophoblastic disease). By preventing pregnancy, contraceptives reduce the risk of such deaths. In many parts of the world where pregnancy and childbirth are still major causes of death, contraceptive use can have an even greater impact on the risk of maternal mortality.

Mortality rates among users of various methods differ according to the failure rate of each method; that is, methods with the highest failure rates have higher risks of death than those with lower failure rates. Women who have a contraceptive failure and choose to have an abortion face a lower risk of death than those who choose to give birth. Using no contraception carries the greatest risk of death, although choosing abortion rather than childbirth greatly reduces the risk.

In the United States, only a few deaths can be directly attributable to the contraceptive method (about one or fewer per 100,000 users; see Kost et al., 1991). Methods that carry such risks are oral contraceptives, long-acting hormonal methods, tubal sterilization, and vasectomy. The risk of death from a sterilization operation is a one-time risk to the person being sterilized (male or female). The method-related deaths for users of oral contraceptives and long-acting hormonal methods result from cardiovascular disease.

Cardiovascular disease.   Researchers have found that women who took oral contraceptives in the 1970s had an increased risk of cardiovascular disease (Sartwell and Stolley, 1982; Stadel, 1981a, 1981b). However, since the discovery of this association, use of the pill has become safer. The doses of estrogen and progestin have been markedly reduced, and available evidence suggests that compared with the earlier formulations, current preparations are associated with a lower risk of cardiovascular disease among users relative to that of earlier preparations (Croft and Hannaford, 1989; Porter et al., 1985; Vessey et al., 1989).

Oral contraceptive use has been shown to affect only certain cardiovascular diseases, such as myocardial infarction (heart attack), venous thrombosis and embolism (blood clots), and two kinds of strokes—those resulting from subarachnoid hemorrhage and those caused by thrombosis or embolism (nonhemorrhagic strokes). The risk of cardiovascular disease increases with age, partly because the prevalence of predisposing risk factors (e.g., high blood pressure, diabetes, and physical inactivity) increases with age. Smoking also increases the risk among all women, whether or not they use oral contraceptives.

The overall added risk of cardiovascular disease for users of oral contraceptives is very low in young women and nonsmokers who are healthy and who have no predisposing factors for the disease. It is now possible to identify many women who are at high risk for cardiovascular disease prior to their using the pill. For example, women older than age thirty-five who smoke and younger women who smoke heavily (25 or more cigarettes a day) are contraindicated for pill use because, for some cardiovascular diseases, oral contraceptive use adds to the already increased risk from smoking. Thus, such women can either choose another method or quit smoking (the latter option is likely to have other health benefits, as well). Women without such contraindications can be reassured that the likelihood of their developing a cardiovascular illness due to oral contraceptive use is extremely small.

Minipills, injectables, and implants contain no estrogen, and their daily doses of progestin are considerably lower than those found in combined oral contraceptives. For this reason, such progestin-only methods may have little effect on a user's risk of cardiovascular disease (Harlap et al., 1991). However, conclusive data on these effects are not yet available.

Cancers.   In the United States, cancers of the reproductive system—those affecting the cervix, ovaries, endometrium, or breasts—make up about 40 percent of all cancers diagnosed in women. Media reports of an association between oral contraceptive use and breast cancer have left millions of women wondering if their past or current use of the pill has endangered their health, or even their lives. Of all women aged fifteen to forty-four

who have had intercourse, 79 percent have used oral contraceptives; about 25 percent of those women are current users (Forrest, 1990).

Cervical cancer is thought to be related, at least in part, to infection by certain strains of human papilloma virus, an STD. The risk of this cancer is related to the number of sexual partners a woman, or her partner, has had. Cervical cancer is more likely to be diagnosed among women older than thirty than among those who are younger; and in every age group, women who have never used barrier and spermicide methods are almost twice as likely as even occasional users of those methods to develop this cancer.

The risks of ovarian and endometrial cancer rise steadily with age, but the likelihood of being diagnosed with either of these cancers among women who have ever used the pill is about 30 to 80 percent less than the incidence among those who have never used it, depending on length of use; the risk is lowered by longer duration of pill use. In addition, the protective effect continues for many years after pill use ends (Harlap et al., 1991; Booth et al., 1989; La Vecchia et al., 1984; Schlesselman, 1989).

The full relationship between oral contraceptive use and breast cancer is still unclear. Among all women aged fifteen to fifty-four, the risk of a breast cancer diagnosis is the same among "ever-users" and "never-users." Furthermore, studies have shown that women who first use the pill at age twenty-five or older have the same rate of breast cancer diagnosis as women who never use it (Prentice and Thomas, 1987). Some studies have suggested that women who begin use of the pill in their adolescence or early twenties are more likely than those who begin use later to be diagnosed with breast cancer in their thirties and early forties. However, the evidence also suggests that at older ages, these women have lower rates of breast cancer than women who never used the pill (Paul et al., 1986; United Kingdom National Case-Control Study Group, 1989; Wingo et al., 1990).

Several explanations have been suggested for the apparent increase in the risk of breast cancer diagnosis among oral contraceptive users in the middle reproductive ages (25–34) and for the possible decrease in risk at older ages. Because pill users are screened for breast cancer more frequently than nonusers (Skegg, 1988), their breast cancers may be detected earlier. Another hypothesis is that the hormones in oral contraceptives accelerate the growth of an undiagnosed breast cancer (or of certain types of breast cancer) but do not cause its initial development. This effect would be consistent with the way pregnancy temporarily increases the risk of breast cancer (Bruzzi et al., 1988).

To put into perspective the pill's overall effect on the risk of cancers—ovarian, endometrial, and breast cancers combined—ever-users of the pill in each age group can expect fewer cancer diagnoses than never-users except at ages twenty-five to thirty-four, when women who have ever used oral contraceptives will experience nearly the same overall incidence of cancer as women who have never used the pill.

Overall, any pill-related increases in the risk of breast cancer are more than offset by corresponding decreases in ovarian and endometrial cancers, so women who have used oral contraceptives develop fewer cancers than women who have never used them. The difference between the two groups widens in the middle to late reproductive years as the incidence of ovarian and endometrial cancers rises.

Conclusion

As women pass through different stages of their reproductive life, each contraceptive method offers a somewhat different combination of risks and benefits, not only to their current well-being but also to their chances of being able to bear children and remain in good health in the future. As their needs, options, and preferences change over time, women must reevaluate their choice of contraceptive.

Physicians and other medical providers should take a more active role in helping both their female and male patients make contraceptive choices by initiating discussion of their childbearing aspirations, their sexual behavior, their individual and family health history, their health habits, and perhaps most important of all, their willingness and ability to use a particular method consistently and correctly. In addition, medical providers should encourage discussion of ongoing experience with a method in the event that it is no longer meeting the patient's needs. Individuals who have been educated about how current or future behavior might affect their health and influence the effects of a contraceptive method can make better-informed choices about their behavior and select methods that are better tailored to their own concerns and goals.

Three factors—multiple sexual relationships, smoking, and irregular or incorrect method use—have particularly strong effects on whether a woman will be able to reach her reproductive and health goals. A sexually active woman who does not want to become pregnant greatly increases her chances of maintaining good health if she and her partner use contraceptives consistently and follow some general guidelines for the selection of a method. Couples should use barrier and spermicide methods when their relationship is not mutually monogamous or when one of them has an STD (for protection against infection, infertility, and cervical cancer); use oral contraceptives at some time during the woman's reproductive years (for protection against ovarian and endometrial cancer); stay informed and aware of health conditions (such as high blood pressure) and behavior (such as smoking) that may contraindicate their use of

particular methods; and rely on an extremely effective method once childbearing is completed.

Because pregnancy can affect women's health in numerous ways, the prevention of pregnancy has a significantly beneficial effect on women's health. Yet the virtual elimination of pregnancy-related complications by the most effective contraceptive methods—the pill, the IUD, long-acting hormonal methods, and sterilization—is a benefit often overlooked when the health effects of methods are considered.

KATHRYN KOST

While all the articles in the other sections in this entry are relevant, see especially the section on STRATEGIES OF FERTILITY CONTROL. *Directly related to this article are the entries* POPULATION ETHICS, FERTILITY CONTROL, *especially the article on* MEDICAL ASPECTS; *and* WOMEN, *article on* HEALTH-CARE ISSUES. *For a discussion of topics mentioned in this article, see the entries* ABORTION, *especially the article on* MEDICAL PERSPECTIVES; AIDS; CHILDREN; EUGENICS, *article on* ETHICAL ISSUES; FAMILY; FEMINISM; FETUS, *article on* HUMAN DEVELOPMENT FROM FERTILIZATION TO BIRTH; FREEDOM AND COERCION; INTERNATIONAL HEALTH; REPRODUCTIVE TECHNOLOGIES; SEXISM; *and* SUBSTANCE ABUSE, *article on* SMOKING. *For a discussion of related ideas, see the entries* ADOLESCENTS; LIFESTYLES AND PUBLIC HEALTH; MATERNAL–FETAL RELATIONSHIPS; *and* ROMAN CATHOLICISM.

Bibliography

BOOTH, M.; BERAL, V.; and SMITH, P. 1989. "Risk Factors for Ovarian Cancer: A Case Control Study." *British Journal of Cancer* 60, no. 4:592–598.

BRUZZI, PAOLO; NEGRI, EVA; LA VECCHIA, CARLO; DECARLI, ADRIANO; PALLI, DOMENICO; PARAZZINI, FABIO; and DEL TURCO, MARCO R. 1988. "Short Term Increase in Risk of Breast Cancer After Full Term Pregnancy." *British Journal of Medicine* 297, no. 6656:1096–1098.

CENTERS FOR DISEASE CONTROL (U.S.). 1989. *Division of STD/HIV Prevention: Annual Report.* Atlanta, Ga.: Author.

CROFT, PETER, and HANNAFORD, PHILIP C. 1989. "Risk Factors for Acute Myocardial Infarction in Women: Evidence from the Royal College of General Practitioners' Oral Contraceptive Study." *British Medical Journal* 298, no. 6667:165–168.

FORREST, JACQUELINE DARROCH. 1990. "The Demographics of Oral Contraceptive Use." Report prepared for the Institute of Medicine and National Academy of Sciences. New York: Alan Guttmacher Institute.

HARLAP, SUSAN; KOST, KATHRYN; and FORREST, JACQUELINE DARROCH. 1991. *Preventing Pregnancy, Protecting Health: A New Look at Birth Control Choices in the United States.* New York: Alan Guttmacher Institute.

KOST, KATHRYN, and FORREST, JACQUELINE DARROCH. 1992. "American Women's Sexual Behavior and Exposure to Risk of Sexually Transmitted Diseases." *Family Planning Perspectives* 24, no. 6:244–255.

KOST, KATHRYN; FORREST, JACQUELINE DARROCH; and HARLAP, SUSAN. 1991. "Comparing the Health Risks and Benefits of Contraceptive Choices." *Family Planning Perspectives* 23, no.2:54–61.

LA VECCHIA, CARLO; FRANCESCHI, S.; and DECARLI, ADRIANO. 1984. "Oral Contraceptive Use and the Risk of Epithelial Ovarian Cancer." *British Journal of Cancer* 50, no. 1:31–34.

NATIONAL CENTER FOR HEALTH STATISTICS (U.S.). 1990. *Vital Statistics of the United States, 1987.* Vol. 2, *Mortality,* Part A. Washington, D.C.: U.S. Government Printing Office.

PAUL, CHARLOTTE; SKEGG, DAVID C. G.; SPEARS, G. F. S.; and KALDOR, J. M. 1986. "Oral Contraceptives and Breast Cancer: A National Study. *British Medical Journal* 293, no. 6549:723–726.

PORTER, JANE B.; HUNTER, J. R.; JICK, HERSHEL; and STERGACHIS, A. 1985. "Oral Contraceptives and Nonfatal Vascular Disease." *Obstetrics and Gynecology* 66, no. 1: 1–4.

PRENTICE, ROSS L., and THOMAS, DAVID B. 1987. "On the Epidemiology of Oral Contraceptives and Disease." *Advances in Cancer Research* 49:285–401.

SARTWELL, PHILIP E., and STOLLEY, PAUL D. 1982. "Oral Contraceptives and Vascular Disease." *Epidemiologic Reviews* 4:95–109.

SCHLESSELMAN, JAMES J. 1989. "Cancers of the Breast and Reproductive Tract in Relation to Use of Oral Contraceptives." *Contraception* 40, no. 1:1–38.

SILVERMAN, JANE; TORRES, AIDA; and FORREST, JACQUELINE DARROCH. 1987. "Barriers to Contraceptive Services. *Family Planning Perspectives* 19, no. 3:94–97, 101–102.

SKEGG, DAVID C. G. 1988. "Potential for Bias in Case-Control Studies of Oral Contraception and Breast Cancer." *American Journal of Epidemiology* 127, no. 2: 205–212.

STADEL, BRUCE B. 1981a. "Oral Contraceptives and Cardiovascular Disease" (first of two parts). *New England Journal of Medicine* 305, no. 11:612–618.

———. 1981b. "Oral Contraceptives and Cardiovascular Disease" (second of two parts). *New England Journal of Medicine* 305, no. 12:672–677.

TRUSSELL, JAMES; HATCHER, ROBERT A.; CATES, WILLARD, JR.; STEWART, FELICIA HANCE; and KOST, KATHRYN. 1990. "Contraceptive Failure in the United States: An Update." *Studies in Family Planning* 21, no. 1:51–54.

UNITED KINGDOM NATIONAL CASE-CONTROL STUDY GROUP. 1989. "Oral Contraceptive Use and Breast Cancer Risk in Young Women." *Lancet* 1, no. 8645:973–982.

VESSEY, MARTIN P.; VILLARD-MACKINTOSH, L.; MCPHERSON, KIM; and YEATES, D. 1989. "Mortality Among Oral Contraceptive Users: 20 Year Follow-Up of Women in a Cohort Study." *British Medical Journal* 229, no. 6714: 1487–1491.

WINGO, PATRICIA; LEE, NANCY C.; ORY, HOWARD W.; BERAL, VALERIE; and PETERSON, HERBERT B. 1990. "Age-Specific Differences in the Relationship Between Oral Contraceptive Use and Breast Cancer." Paper presented at the Conference on Oral Contraceptive Use and Breast Cancer, Irvine, Calif., May 30.

III. MIGRATION AND REFUGEES

Global migration is as old as history, but its significance has waxed and waned over the centuries. In the late twentieth century, political, economic, and social factors have brought it once more to prominence; a 1993 United Nations Population Fund report asserted that migration "could become the human crisis of our age."

What accounts for the contemporary significance of global migration? For one thing, the world no longer contains politically unincorporated territories, so that every instance of migration is not only a move *from* some nation or other; it is a move *to* some nation or other. Nations are sovereign states whose recognized rights include the right to control their borders—the right, therefore, to decide who may enter their territory. Thus a decision to migrate *to* some place is a decision that, politically if not morally, is not for an individual alone to make; it requires the consent of the receiving country. In some cases, even the decision to migrate *from* a place has been taken out of the hands of the individual; some nations, that is, have claimed the authority to decide who may leave as well as who may enter.

There are further reasons for the increased significance and magnitude of international migration: explosive, uneven population growth in different nations; large disparities in economic wealth and economic development between countries; special interdependencies between particular countries; and advances in transportation and communications systems. Not surprisingly, people tend to move from crowded, poor countries to less crowded, richer ones where economic and other opportunities are better. The desire to migrate may be fostered by television and other mass media, which arouse awareness of opportunities in faraway places; the ability to migrate may be aided by transportation systems that make relocation easier. It has been said that the question is not why people migrate but why they do not migrate more often, given conditions in many "sending" countries and the basic economic principle that resources flow to optimal locations. Migration always involves both "push" factors that give people reason to want to leave a place and "pull" factors that attract them to someplace else.

International migration raises fundamental ethical questions about the moral significance of national boundaries and social communities, the nature and extent of human rights, and the circumstances in which people have moral obligations to aid others or to accept them into their communities. It also raises a host of empirical questions about the effects of migration on both sending and receiving countries and about the extent to which migration can be controlled. On the basis of our current knowledge, it cannot be said that the empirical questions are any more tractable than the ethical ones. Both the facts about migration, and the relevant moral principles, are highly controversial.

A framework for migration issues

It seems a safe assumption that, other things being equal, most people would rather remain in their native countries than begin anew in a strange land. But other things are not always equal. The contemporary world is organized into nation-states possessing very different characteristics, a situation creating disequilibrium. Countries that are relatively rich, safe, or politically free tend to attract people—either as permanent residents or as temporary workers—from countries not possessing these features. Not only do individuals in such circumstances have reason to migrate, but the countries from which they come may view emigration as a way to relieve political or economic pressures. Moreover, receiving countries often have powerful economic interests in acquiring foreign labor. Disentangling the various interests at stake—between sending and receiving countries, and between different groups and classes within each—is a complex task.

The pressure point in contemporary discussions of migration centers primarily on its effects on receiving countries. It is perhaps a truism that if too many people come to those countries, they will eventually cease to be attractive either to their original inhabitants or to anyone else. But the question is how many are too many, and why? How should a receiving country decide which of those seeking entry ought to be admitted?

These questions are misleading if they suggest that an immigration policy is simply a way of implementing charity or beneficence. Immigrants, legal and illegal, serve important interests of receiving countries, or of significant groups within them. We can organize the issues at stake by elaborating four considerations appropriate to formulating an immigration policy—leaving aside, for the moment, the perspective of sending countries. First, what is at stake for those seeking entry? Second, is immigration the only way their needs can be met? Third, what costs and benefits—economic, social, cultural—are at stake for the receiving country as a whole and for particular groups within it? Should these costs and benefits be weighed differently depending on who bears them? Fourth, do receiving countries sometimes have moral obligations to accept potential immigrants—on the basis of past actions, a special

relationship with the sending country, or general humanitarian grounds? We can begin to address this fourth question only after the first three have been explored.

Refugees, immigrants, and migrants

The first two considerations—what is at stake for those seeking entry, and the extent to which migration is the only way their needs can be met—are captured in the way different categories of people who migrate are usually described. The basic distinction is between refugees and immigrants.

According to the 1951 Convention Relating to the Status of Refugees and the 1967 Protocol Relating to the Status of Refugees, the definition accepted by the United Nations says a refugee is a person who, "owing to well-founded fear of being persecuted for reasons of race, religion, nationality, membership of a particular social group or political opinion, is outside the country of his nationality and is unable or, owing to such fear, is unwilling to avail himself of the protection of that country; or who, not having a nationality and being outside the country of his former habitual residence as a result of such events, is unable or, owing to such fear, is unwilling to return to it" (Article 1.A.2, in Goodwin-Gill, 1983, p. 253). Essentially this definition has been in force since shortly after World War II, in response to the upheavals surrounding that conflict.

The meaning of "immigrant" or "migrant" has traditionally been understood by contrast to refugees: Those who migrate are not fleeing political persecution. The difference between migrants and immigrants, furthermore, is not a formal one; but based on common usage, we may say that migrants relocate temporarily, or travel back and forth between their home country and another, while immigrants relocate permanently.

The suggestion is typically that immigrants move for economic betterment, with the implication that they are "pulled" rather than "pushed." But this implication, although often reasonable, is sometimes highly misleading. Even to speak of economic betterment misleadingly suggests an acceptable baseline from which one aims to improve; but many who migrate for economic reasons find themselves in desperate circumstances—as desperate, sometimes, as those of political refugees. The causes of migration may be natural disaster, external aggression, civil war, or internal oppression, all of which can severely affect even those who do not suffer direct political persecution. Furthermore, it may be that those who wish to migrate cannot be helped where they are. Recognizing these problems and the possible bias in the U.N. definition, the Organization of African Unity (OAU) in its 1969 Convention added the following to the definition of a refugee: "every person who, owing to external aggression, occupation, foreign domination or events seriously disturbing public order in either part or the whole of his country of origin or nationality, is compelled to leave his place of habitual residence in order to seek refuge in another place outside his country of origin or nationality" (Article I, Section 2). Thus, for example, "environmental refugees" may be forced to flee their homeland because of deforestation resulting from trading practices and the import strategies of rich countries or international institutions. The OAU definition accommodates the truth that in today's world—as Aristide Zolberg, Astri Suhrke, and Sergio Aguayo argue—"The causes of life-threatening conditions in the developing world stem from an interpenetration of national and transnational, or global, processes" (Zolberg et al., 1989, p. 33).

Why does it matter how we define "refugee"? The reason is that the term has special legal, moral, and emotional force; to be counted a refugee is to be treated as having a compelling claim to admission, whereas potential immigrants have a much weaker claim, in part because of the assumption that their needs can be met without relocation. Many countries are bound by international agreements forbidding *refoulement,* the forcible return of a refugee to his or her country. To exclude from the definition extremely pressing claims that do not result directly from persecution has a powerful influence on the lives and well-being of millions of people.

The definition of a refugee can be manipulated in other ways. Thus, although the United States helped draft the 1951 Convention Relating to the Status of Refugees, it did not ratify it, and adopted the U.N. definition only in the Refugee Act of 1980. Until that time, ideological considerations played a large part in U.S. policy; priority was given to those fleeing "Communist or Communist-dominated" societies. Even since 1980, ideological considerations have continued to influence U.S. refugee admissions.

Of course, many of those seeking to migrate—for example, Mexicans to the United States, Turks to Germany—are not in desperate straits. They are poor compared to most people in the receiving countries, but they do not usually come from the poorest stratum of their own society; the poorest lack the physical, emotional, and economic resources to uproot themselves from their homes and begin again. What is at stake for these potential immigrants? A better life, a decent life—a life that most of those in the receiving countries would consider much superior to what is available in the sending countries, but one that it is in no way inappropriate to aim for. The life left behind, then, is not desperate, but it may not be acceptable either.

Costs and benefits to receiving countries

No one would oppose immigration unless he or she believed it presented significant drawbacks or costs. Those who favor stricter limits on the number of immigrants, or stricter conditions of entry, typically argue that at certain levels (often current levels), immigration carries significant economic, social, or cultural costs. Sometimes the concern is primarily with those who enter illegally, either because it is believed that the flow of illegal immigrants inflates the number of outsiders to unacceptable limits, or because *as* illegal immigrants they pose special problems not posed by those admitted through legal channels.

A central debate concerns the effects of immigrant labor on jobs for natives. In the United States, the debate takes the following form: Some who wish to restrict immigration believe that immigrant labor displaces the worst-off native citizen groups and depresses wages (Briggs, 1992). Immigrants, it is said, will work for wages that citizens, possessing the elevated standards prevalent in more developed societies, find unacceptable. Illegal immigrants make things even worse, these critics argue, because they are fearful and thus willing to accept whatever they can get. Proponents of immigration argue, on the other hand, that immigrants do work that citizens consider too menial, such as domestic work and hard agricultural labor. In addition, they say, because the labor market is not a zero-sum game and because immigrants are also consumers, they often stimulate the economy, thereby creating new jobs (Simon, 1989).

It is extremely difficult to sort out the various issues implicit in these claims and to derive conclusions with any degree of certainty. Immigration has multiple effects, and unequivocal conclusions about these effects lack plausibility. Most economists seem to agree that immigration increases aggregate national wealth, but that some displacement of low-skilled workers and depression of their wages do occur. For obvious reasons, the welfare of low-income citizens should be of special concern: Policies that make the worst-off even worse off are difficult to justify. But economists disagree about the magnitude of these problems, and many argue that in some occupations, immigrants and citizens do not compete.

In any case, it is easy to see how foreign labor serves business interests. This is especially true in industries dominated by undocumented migrant labor—those that are part of the "informal economy"—where workers' docility and fear are easy to exploit. In some industries, like the garment industry in the United States, women, who sometimes do "homework," are particularly at risk (Fernandez-Kelly and Garcia, 1989).

Another issue that is partly economic and partly social concerns the extent to which immigrants burden a society's social services and, particularly because of language deficiencies and cultural differences, its educational institutions. Even if new immigrants do utilize such services disproportionately—and this remains a point of controversy—they also contribute significantly to a nation's tax base. Some argue, furthermore, that countries with low population growth, like the United States and the nations of western Europe, will need immigrants to help pay for programs such as Medicare and Social Security for older citizens. In the United States, these costs and benefits cannot be easily weighed against each other, since for the most part social services are funded locally, and local jurisdictions are not reimbursed proportionately for the services they render. The countries of western Europe may face different and greater problems because of their more comprehensive social-support systems.

Perhaps the most complex "costs" that immigration is said to impose are social and cultural. Several issues are relevant. For one thing, immigration sometimes produces conflict among ethnic groups. In part, this can arise because low-income native-born groups regard the newcomers—accurately or inaccurately—as competing for jobs and resources. But it may also occur when immigrants constitute "middleman minorities," a role played historically in many countries by Jews, Asian Indians, and Chinese (Portes and Rumbaut, 1990). Conflict of this kind exists today in the United States, for example, between African-Americans and the Korean merchants who own shops in their communities.

Some critics argue that too many immigrants may threaten a society's distinctive way of life, diluting or destroying its identity and its institutions. This is a difficult criticism to assess, in part because the values said to be at stake are elusive and vague. Historically, immigrants have often been viewed with suspicion and fear (Higham, 1963), and sometimes the concern about culture amounts to no more than veiled xenophobia or racism. The immigration policies of many countries, such as the United States and Australia, have during extended periods excluded or severely limited the entry of non–northern European or nonwhite immigrants (Jones, 1992). When immigrant groups consist partly or largely of nonwhite peoples, as they often do today, it is difficult to avoid the suspicion that claims of cultural integrity contain a racial component.

Let us suppose that these attitudes do not exhaust the concern about cultural integrity. Then we are faced with difficult questions about what a culture is and how immigrant groups mix or assimilate into it, or do not (Gordon, 1964). It may be argued that the worry about cultural integrity rests on a misconception about culture. A culture is not an unchanging entity that is threatened by, and too inflexible to accommodate, influences from without or within. Especially in the contemporary world, cultures change. We can imagine radical, unacceptable changes that render the old culture unrecognizable; but the burden of proof is on the critic to show that immigrant groups cause such transformations.

In the United States, immigrant groups have shown a remarkable capacity to assimilate into the dominant culture. Historically, the nations of western Europe have had less experience with immigration than the United States; partly for that reason, the citizens of such a nation do not see themselves as part of a "melting pot," a "salad," or a "nation of immigrants," as Americans often do. Apart from this matter of self-conception, these societies are ethnically less heterogeneous than the United States. But one cannot conclude from this alone that they have more to fear from immigration.

Costs and benefits to sending countries

Just as costs and benefits to receiving countries are controversial, so are those to sending countries. "Out-migration" serves to reduce economic and population pressures, but it can also cause "brain drain"—loss of some of the most productive members of a society—and it can reduce the pressure for needed social, economic, and political reforms. On the other hand, some countries, such as the Philippines and El Salvador, now earn more from remittances sent home by migrants than from any export. Thus migration can produce important benefits to sending countries and to families within them.

But as important as these issues are, the central point of controversy today concerns the impact of migration on receiving countries. This is not unconnected with the fact that the moral and legal right to leave a place is generally accepted; debate centers on the right to enter. Thus, even if overall a decline in emigration benefited a sending country, few would endorse prohibitions against leaving. Thus the hard core of the argument—about what people or nations have the *right* to do or to prevent, about what strictures on mobility ought to be implemented—concerns the point of entry, not the point of exit.

If immigration today is more imminently pressing than emigration, then the problems it poses—that is, problems in receiving countries—will be the engine that drives new approaches and policies. At the same time, as the world becomes increasingly interdependent economically, as well as in every other way, it is clear that there can be no "solution" to immigration that is not at the same time a solution to emigration. If people are to stop coming to the developed countries, conditions in their home countries will have to become more attractive. Policies are needed to weaken both the pulls and the pushes of migration.

Migration and morality

Uncertainties about the effects of migration on sending and receiving countries and on particular groups within them; a sense that to a large extent these phenomena exemplify forces beyond our control; the legacy of political realism, according to which ethical considerations do not and should not operate in international relations—all of these may contribute to the view that moral questions have no place at all in discussions of migration.

But such questions cannot be avoided. In the case of refugees and others not officially designated as such but who are equally desperate, migration confronts us with clashes between the claims of some individuals both to survive and to attain basic levels of health and well-being, on the one hand, and the claims of nations, or individuals within them, to exclude these people from such basic goods by refusing them entry, on the other hand. Even when the needs of those seeking entry are not quite so stark, migration poses difficult questions about the relationship between rich and poor—both individuals and countries—and the nature of the moral ties between them. Do rich countries have an obligation to aid poor countries, either by accepting immigrants or by some other means? On what basis could such a moral obligation stand? And how far does it extend?

According to a commonly held view, nations have the right to prevent the entry of whomever they wish. But this claim needs further analysis. It may be uncontroversial that nations have the *legal* right to refuse entry to noncitizens and thus may use whatever criteria they like to decide admissions. Even this claim is somewhat misleading, however, because nations bound by agreements forbidding *refoulement* may not ordinarily expel refugees even if they have entered illegally. But refusing admission to those who have not yet entered does not constitute a violation of international law.

Yet a legal right is not a moral right, nor is it equivalent to what is morally right. Consider the well-known case of the *St. Louis*. In June 1939, the United States turned away a German vessel carrying more than 900 Jews fleeing Nazi Germany. They had been promised, then denied, visas by Cuba; proceeding up the U.S. coast, they requested refuge from the American government. These "boat people" were not inside U.S. territorial waters, and in any case, international agreements regarding refugees had not yet been established; thus there is no doubt that the United States was within its legal rights in refusing the refugees' appeal. But did it have a moral right to refuse their request? Or did it, on the contrary, have a moral obligation to provide at least a temporary haven?

Some people may shy away from speaking in terms of rights and obligations in this context. But few today would deny that the United States ought to have taken in the refugees, or that it was wrong and reprehensible for it to have refused. The moral principle underlying such a judgment might be expressed thus: If a person or a nation can prevent a great harm at little or no cost to itself, it is wrong not to do so.

This principle fits the case under discussion because taking in the *St. Louis* passengers, whose lives hung in the balance, would have had no adverse effects on the United States. The issues confronting us today, however, raise two kinds of questions not raised by this example. First, in most cases, those seeking entry are not as desperate as were the refugees from Nazi Germany. It might be argued that what is at issue in such cases is not preventing a great harm but providing a good, and that people are not obviously worthy of blame if they choose not to provide that good.

In any case, it is the second question raised by contemporary migration that more seriously challenges the relevance of the principle that one ought to act if one can do so with little or no cost to oneself. The great number of people who might be inclined to migrate—and who might be encouraged to do so if they were aware that others have been admitted—calls into question the assumption that migration imposes no costs on countries that open their doors, or on particular groups or individuals within them.

Debate continues about the economic, social, and cultural costs of migration. Some hold that the costs of migration at current levels are not significant, while others claim that it has adverse effects on the well-being of groups in the resident population. Thus, two critical empirical questions are at what point migration brings harm to groups in the receiving country, and which groups there are affected. The crucial moral question is whether and to what extent people in receiving countries should bear the costs of accommodating immigrants.

Haves and have-nots

Why, morally, should people in receiving countries bear any costs to promote immigration? Two kinds of reasons can be offered. First, it might be argued that it is wrong or indecent for some to have so much while others have so little, even if the haves are in no way responsible for the plight of the have-nots. Second, it can be argued that the haves owe something because they bear some responsibility for the situation of the have-nots, perhaps in virtue of some prior or current relationship between them. Let us consider these two kinds of reasons in turn.

From a moral point of view, the global distribution of wealth and poverty as it affects individuals is largely arbitrary. Whether one happens to be born in Sweden or Pakistan, Australia or Somalia, is a matter of chance, but it makes all the difference to a person's life prospects. What follows morally from this fact? There is little consensus. To some, it seems obvious that radical inequalities are unfair or otherwise unacceptable to the extent that they are undeserved. On this view, since people in rich countries are lucky to have been born there and those in poor countries are unlucky, and since these chance occurrences have much to do with how people fare in the world, something ought to be done to redistribute wealth from rich to poor. The same conclusion regarding the need for redistribution might be based not on the arbitrariness of birthplace but on a principle of humanitarianism or benevolence: Those who can help people in dire need ought to do so.

Migration is one way to achieve redistribution. Whether and in what circumstances it is preferable to other approaches, such as humanitarian or development assistance to poor countries, will depend on a variety of factors.

But others draw no such conclusion from the moral arbitrariness of nationality. In part, their refusal may flow from the conviction that this line of thinking "proves too much": Not only does one not deserve to be born in a rich country, but one does not deserve to be born to rich parents, or to be endowed with superior genes. Taken to its logical conclusion, the critics say, this argument removes the grounds for all systems of rewards and punishments, and would mark the end of a free society. For this or other reasons, such critics insist that although it might be decent or nice or admirable for rich countries to share their wealth, the fact that birthplace is arbitrary implies no moral obligation to do so; and poor people or poor countries who do not receive such benefits have no cause for complaint.

Disagreement about what follows from the moral arbitrariness of nationality goes to the deepest questions about moral responsibility and social justice. Progress toward resolving these questions, if it can be achieved at all, is impossible without extensive and detailed argument. But there is another rationale for the conclusion that rich countries ought to make some sacrifices for the well-being of immigrants from poor countries—a rationale that does not depend on the moral arbitrariness of birthplace or on simple humanitarianism. This is the view that rich countries owe something to poor countries on the basis of past or present actions and relationships. For example, in 1974 the U.N. General Assembly's Declaration on the Establishment of a New International Economic Order argued that rich countries have "underdeveloped" poor countries: that it is because of colonialism and exploitation, at least in part, that there are now radical disparities in wealth and well-being among nations, and that poor countries are poorer than they would have been had there been no interaction. If this is true, then poor countries are owed something by way of reparations or compensation, not simply in virtue of benevolence.

There are several problems with such claims. Even if one agrees that rich countries did mistreat poor countries in various ways, it is difficult to know what the victims of such exploitation and harm would be like today in the absence of these actions. Without knowledge of this kind, it is almost impossible to decide what reparations or compensation are owed. Moreover, it is possible that in the absence of colonialism, some developing countries would not exist and would be even worse off than they are today. And some, such as Singapore, have fared well despite a colonial legacy.

An obligation may rest more specifically on a particular relationship between countries. For example, acceptance by the United States of large numbers of refugees and immigrants from Vietnam can be viewed as acknowledgment of the moral import of U.S. involvement in Vietnam and the U.S. debt to the Vietnamese people. American relations with Mexico fit this principle as well, although in a less extreme form. Mexican labor was crucial to the growth of many American industries, and recruitment of Mexican labor by U.S. mining and railroad companies and by agricultural growers dates to the middle of the nineteenth century. European countries' use of "guest workers" can be understood similarly to generate obligations: Having brought workers to one's country when they were deemed necessary, one is not free to sever the relationship after the "guests" have set down roots.

Beyond "us" and "them"

Whether on grounds of the moral arbitrariness of nationality, general humanitarianism, or compensatory justice, it seems clear that developed countries, which tend to be the recipients of immigrants and refugees, have moral obligations to developing countries. To what extent such obligations are best fulfilled through migration requires further investigation: In some cases it will make more sense to move resources to people than to move people to resources.

More fundamental questions remain, however. How extensive are these moral obligations? How much ought people in rich countries to sacrifice, if that is necessary, to raise the welfare of poor and oppressed people to tolerable levels? It is clear that no general answers can be given to these questions. In part, the answers depend on how obligations to those outside one's country are to be weighed against obligations to those within. Does one not, it may be asked, owe more to the poor within one's own society than to those elsewhere? And is it not likely that serious commitment to fulfilling obligations to our fellow nationals will strain our resources and therefore our virtue as it is?

Perhaps we can find part of an answer to this question by addressing the concerns of those who view claims about the moral obligations of rich countries to poor countries as misplaced or pointless, because they believe that national policies are not based on such considerations, or even that they should not be. Obviously the foregoing discussion rejects this view. Nevertheless, it is important to see—both because it is true and because it may motivate those unmoved by considerations of morality—that "self-interest rightly understood," in Alexis de Tocqueville's phrase, may also serve to support policies that reduce global inequalities.

In what ways? With international economic interdependence ever increasing—and telecommunications and transportation systems rendering the world of the haves more accessible both psychologically and physically to the have-nots—in the long run, rich countries will be unable to keep their privileges to themselves without employing methods that are repellent, and perhaps ineffective. One might go further and say that the same factors that render the world more interdependent and the North more visible and immediate to the South also render the South more visible and immediate to the North. And so it will become more difficult for those in the North to maintain their humanity while denying their connections with distant strangers of whose suffering they are aware. The reasons that we have duties to those within our community, and that our well-being depends on the well-being of other members of our community, still stand. But the boundaries of our community now may have to be enlarged.

JUDITH LICHTENBERG

While all the articles in the other sections of this entry are relevant, see especially the section on DONOR AGENCIES, *article on* MIGRATION AND REFUGEES. *Directly related to this article is the entry* POPULATION ETHICS. *For a further discussion of topics mentioned in this article, see the entries* BENEFICENCE; ENVIRONMENTAL HEALTH; ENVIRONMENTAL POLICY AND LAW; FREEDOM AND COERCION; HARM; JUSTICE; LIFE; OBLIGATION AND SUPEREROGATION; RACE AND RACISM; RIGHTS; SEXISM; UTILITY; WARFARE, *especially the article on* PUBLIC HEALTH AND WAR; *and* WOMEN, *article on* HISTORICAL AND CROSS-CULTURAL PERSPECTIVES. *For a discussion of related ideas, see the entries* AUTONOMY; CONFLICT OF INTEREST; FOOD POLICY; *and* TRAGEDY.

Bibliography

BRIGGS, VERNON M., JR. 1992. *Mass Immigration and the National Interest.* Armonk, N.Y.: M. E. Sharpe.

BROWN, PETER G., and SHUE, HENRY, eds. 1981. *Boundaries: National Autonomy and Its Limits.* Totowa, N.J.: Rowman and Littlefield.

————. 1983. *The Border That Joins: Mexican Migrants and U.S. Responsibility.* Totowa, N.J.: Rowman and Allanheld.

Convention Relating to the Status of Refugees. 1951. Reprinted in *The Refugee in International Law,* by Guy S. Goodwin-Gill. Oxford: At the Clarendon Press, 1983.

FERNANDEZ-KELLY, M. PATRICIA, and GARCIA, ANNA M. 1989. "Informalization at the Core: Hispanic Women, Homework, and the Advanced Capitalist State." In *The Informal Economy: Studies in Advanced and Less Developed Countries,* pp. 247–264. Edited by Alejandro Portes, Manuel Castells, and Lauren A. Benton. Baltimore: Johns Hopkins University Press.

GALBRAITH, JOHN KENNETH. 1979. *The Nature of Mass Poverty.* Cambridge, Mass.: Harvard University Press.

GOODWIN-GILL, GUY S. 1983. *The Refugee in International Law.* Oxford: At the Clarendon Press.

GORDON, MILTON. 1964. *Assimilation in American Life: The Role of Race, Religion, and National Origins.* New York: Oxford University Press.

HIGHAM, JOHN. 1963. *Strangers in the Land: Patterns of American Nativism, 1860–1925.* New York: Atheneum.

JONES, MALDWYN ALLEN. 1992. *American Immigration.* 2d ed. Chicago: University of Chicago Press.

LOESCHER, GILBURT D., and SCANLAN, JOHN. 1986. *Calculated Kindness: Refugees and America's Half-Open Door, 1945 to the Present.* New York: Free Press.

MAZUR, LAURIE ANN, ed. 1994. *Beyond the Numbers: A Reader on Population, Consumption, and the Environment.* Washington, D.C.: Island Press.

MULLER, THOMAS. 1993. *Immigrants and the American City.* New York: New York University Press.

ORGANIZATION OF AFRICAN UNITY. 1969. Convention on Refugee Problems in Africa. Reprinted in *The Refugee in International Law,* by Guy S. Goodwin-Gill. Oxford: At the Clarendon Press, 1983.

PORTES, ALEJANDRO, and RUMBAUT, RUBEN G. 1990. *Immigrant America: A Portrait.* Berkeley: University of California Press.

Protocol Relating to the Status of Refugees. 1967. Reprinted in *The Refugee in International Law,* by Guy S. Goodwin-Gill. Oxford: At the Clarendon Press.

ROTHSTEIN, RICHARD. 1993. "Immigration Dilemmas." *Dissent* 40:455–462.

SCHUCK, PETER. 1993. "The New Immigration and the Old Civil Rights." *American Prospect* 15, no. 3:102–111.

SIMON, JULIAN L. 1989. *The Economic Consequences of Immigration.* Oxford: Basil Blackwell.

TOMASI, LYDIO, ed. Annual. *In Defense of the Alien: Proceedings of the Annual National Legal Conference on Immigration and Refugee Policy.* New York: Center for Migration Studies.

ZOLBERG, ARISTIDE R.; SUHRKE, ASTRI; and AGUAYO, SERGIO. 1989. *Escape from Violence: Conflict and the Refugee Crisis in the Developing World.* New York: Oxford University Press.

IV. DONOR AGENCIES

A. FERTILITY CONTROL

Donor organizations and the fertility-control programs they support often face ethical dilemmas arising from donor assistance. In some countries donor representatives pressure program managers to increase their commitment to family planning, expand the size of their programs, and use fertility-control methods local managers consider medically unsafe or unsuitable to national conditions. In other countries, such as China, donors and potential donors lobby program officials not to use forced sterilization and abortion or other strong measures.

Ethical dilemmas created by donor assistance can arise in any fertility-control program, but they are most acute in developing countries. Many of those countries do not have the health facilities necessary to deal with the medical side effects of family planning. Some also have autocratic governments with few or no procedures for protecting human rights. Hence, when the government begins a fertility-control program, it often does so in conditions that can pose serious threats to the freedom, health, and welfare of clients.

The following discussion considers the extent to which donors fund fertility-control programs in developing countries; reasons why they use their resources for that purpose; the main agencies involved; and ethical issues raised by their assistance.

Donors and funding

In 1990, grants for international population activities reached a high of $801.8 million (United Nations Population Fund, 1993). Ten donor countries, led by the United States, contributed 96 percent of that total. Other sources of funds included the World Bank, which spent over $169 million on population assistance in 1990; U.N. agencies, which committed about $86 million; and private sources, which provided $48 million.

Why do national governments, international agencies, and private organizations contribute funds for population assistance? Each donor has its own reasons, but almost all claim that controlling rapid population growth helps a poor country to reach and sustain economic development. Most also believe that swelling populations limit the possibilities for educating children, create hazards for public health, damage the environment, and threaten a country's ability to feed its citizens. Many donors likewise see family planning as a way of giving a country's citizens greater reproductive freedom. Critics have challenged the links claimed between population control and economic development and the harmful effects attributed to population density (Simon, 1990; National Research Council, 1986; Kasun, 1988). But their views have had no impact on the statements made by donors about why they offer population assistance.

Two main groups make decisions about how to use international population funds: donor agencies and national authorities. Ethical difficulties are most severe when national authorities who accept donor funding adopt policies directly threatening human rights. These policies include any use of coercion; putting strong political and social pressure on community members to adopt fertility control; distributing medically risky contraceptives without adequate monitoring for their suit-

ability to clients and their side effects; failure to provide health facilities to deal with those side effects; and refusing to remove contraceptives, such as the intrauterine device, at the client's request.

The most influential donors in fertility control are the U.S. Agency for International Development (AID), the main organization responsible for U.S. foreign assistance; the U.N. Population Fund (UNFPA); and the World Bank. All three promote fertility control, but in different ways.

As the best-funded donor organization, AID supports population programs in about fifty countries. Its Office of Population has over forty grant agreements and contracts with U.S. government and private agencies to advise those programs, provide them with contraceptives, conduct population research, and carry out other activities (U.S. Bureau for Research and Development, Office of Population, 1993). In assisting a single country, AID seeks to "(1) strengthen government commitment to voluntary family planning; (2) develop effective public and private family planning programs; (3) increase the utilization of those programs; and (4) decrease dependence on external donors for program support" (U.S. Bureau for Research and Development, Office of Population, 1993, p. 4).

UNFPA assists national population programs and funds population work by other U.N. agencies, such as the World Health Organization, the International Labor Organization, and UNICEF (Sadik, 1990). It also gives grants to private organizations such as the Population Council and Worldwatch. The World Bank actively promotes fertility control through loans for family-planning programs in developing countries as well as through its research and publications (Sai and Chester, 1990). Also working in developing nations are private organizations such as the International Planned Parenthood Federation, the Population Council, the Pathfinder Fund, and the Association for Voluntary Surgical Contraception. These organizations receive funding from AID, UNFPA, private foundations, and other sources.

The ethics of donor interventions

Donor agencies face moral dilemmas when their own activities and those of the programs they fund clash with five ethical principles: a respect for life; reproductive freedom; the welfare of clients; fairness in the distribution of benefits and harms from population programs; and truth-telling.

Donors violate respect for life when, as a direct or indirect result of their activities, participants in fertility-control programs die. This happens when a method of birth control provided by the donor, such as a procedure for sterilization, leads to the death of clients. Donors help to limit reproductive freedom if national managers of the fertility-control programs they support coerce or strongly pressure clients to adopt contraceptives, sterilization, or abortion. They can harm the welfare of clients when, in the programs that they fund, they do not object if national authorities provide no facilities to deal with the health problems caused by medically risky methods of fertility control. Donors may violate fairness when programs they assist create more health risks for poor than for rich clients. And they can reduce truth-telling when they initiate, encourage, or tolerate information campaigns claiming more benefits or fewer harms from fertility control than actually exist.

Three cases will give a more detailed sense of the ethical conflicts caused by donor interventions in fertility control.

Defining the population problem

The first challenge for donors when they enter a country is to provide clear evidence that the country has a population problem. Limiting fertility will be much easier if citizens feel that population growth is causing damage to them and the country than if they think that large families are net assets.

Donors, often working closely with officials in collaborating countries, have used several devices to create the sense of a problem. The most common, no longer used, was Knowledge-Attitude-Practice (KAP) surveys to assess what fertile women knew, felt, and were doing about birth control. Such surveys not only provided that information but also had value in convincing national elites that there was a market for family planning. According to Bernard Berelson of the Population Council, "Such a survey should probably be done at the outset of any national program—partly for its evaluational use, but also for its political use, in demonstrating to the elite that the people themselves strongly support the program and in demonstrating to the society at large that family planning is generally approved" (1964, p. 11). Donors sponsored hundreds of KAP studies and used their results as Berelson suggested.

KAP surveys illustrate the tensions between the mission of fertility control and the principle of truth-telling. Donors often saw this research as an invaluable means of showing popular demand for birth control. But to make that case they often violated professional norms for conducting household surveys. They chose samples that were not representative of the population about which conclusions were drawn; assumed that those interviewed had thought enough about fertility to have an opinion about family size and would tell it to a stranger who arrived unannounced and stayed just a short time; used questions that led individuals to approve family planning; overlooked errors caused by the interviewers; and overinterpreted the findings (Warwick, 1982, 1993).

A few surveys followed the procedures necessary to portray the situation as it actually was, but many of them sought any finding that would make a strong case for birth control.

In the 1980s and 1990s donor-sponsored studies, such as Demographic and Health Surveys, have paid more attention to the methodological procedures necessary to obtain valid data. There is still some pressure to bend the evidence, but the methods followed show less bias than those in most KAP surveys.

Tensions between the mission of fertility control and truth-telling likewise arise in discussions of the relationships between population growth and economic development. In its *World Development Report 1984*, a forcefully argued and widely read statement on population, the World Bank concluded that "population growth at the rapid rates common in most of the developing world slows development" (1984, p. 105). Among its many effects, high fertility makes it harder to provide health, education, and other services for poor people, and more difficult for governments to finance the investments in education and infrastructure needed for economic growth.

Two specialists on population claim that the World Bank's statements about the consequences of population growth come more from simulations, projections, and hypotheses than from empirical evidence (Leibenstein, 1985; Lee, 1985). Its conclusions also receive little support from a scholarly analysis of the relationships between population growth and economic development (National Research Council, 1986).

These examples show how donors advocating fertility control have collected and presented evidence favoring their case and have left out or misrepresented findings that weaken their arguments. Scholars opposed to family planning have done much the same by presenting research indicating that population growth brings benefits and poses few threats to individuals and society (Simon, 1990; Kasun, 1988).

Strategies of fertility control

Once countries believe that they have a problem of rapid population growth, donors can recommend strategies for reducing fertility. They usually suggest meeting existing user interest through voluntary means and stimulating demand for family planning through national publicity campaigns and other forms of education. Some donors, including the World Bank, also have endorsed financial incentives to individuals, couples, or communities for adopting fertility control and to field workers for recruiting new acceptors. Donors may also give open or tacit support to programs, such as that in Indonesia, using strong community and peer pressure to bring in new clients.

Donors face acute moral and political dilemmas when governments they assist use coercion and tight monitoring to ensure that citizens comply with national policies on fertility control. Agencies providing population assistance often wish to help programs taking measures likely to be effective in reducing birth rates. But they are also sensitive to criticism that, in supporting such measures, they are encouraging violations of human rights. For example, since 1978 China has had a policy of one child per couple. To enforce that policy, the Chinese government has relied heavily on compulsory sterilization and abortion, fines, and other heavy pressures on clients. It has, for instance, required women using the intrauterine device to be X-rayed to see if that device is still in place (Aird, 1990).

In response to China's use of coercion, many donors refused to provide any funding for its fertility-control program. But some, led by UNFPA, continued to assist China. UNFPA believed that it was not the responsibility of international agencies to supervise the policies of national governments. In the words of its executive director,

> UNFPA does not support abortion programs in any country; neither of course does it support coercion. It also does not intervene in the "management" of any national program, which is the exclusive prerogative of the recipient government. (Sadik, 1990, p. 204)

However, U.S. critics, including members of Congress, claimed that even if it was not involved in program management, by assisting China's program UNFPA was condoning its violations of human rights (Crane and Finkle, 1989). To show that it was serious about its criticisms, the U.S. government withdrew its contribution to UNFPA between 1985 and 1993.

Methods of fertility control

Once governments have chosen their program strategies, donor agencies can help them to select and distribute methods of fertility control and related services, such as health care. In choosing methods and program services, both governments and donor agencies make decisions affecting life, reproductive freedom, human welfare, fairness, and truth-telling.

A critical moral question concerns the bases for selecting methods of fertility control. Donor representatives and national providers of family-planning services usually prefer methods that are effective in reducing fertility and have little risk of failure. Their frame of reference centers on fertility control. Other groups consider fertility regulation too narrow a perspective for selecting methods. For example, the International Women's Health Coalition views fertility regulation as only one aspect of reproductive health and rights. A more holistic view, its vice president has argued, leads women's health advocates "to seek methods that not only regulate fertility, but also protect against sexually transmitted diseases and their consequences, such as infertility" (Germain, 1993, p. 4). Still others, including many advocates of economic development, argue that programs of fertility control will be both more fair and more effective when they work in tandem with national efforts to increase education, employment, and income. Education, for instance, makes potential clients of fertility control better able to understand the range of methods available, their benefits, and the risks and complications of each method.

Donors also make moral choices in deciding how to deal with countries that accept their funds for programs to limit fertility. Some, such as UNFPA in China, take the position that they have no obligation to interfere in the implementation of national family-planning programs. In UNFPA's view, because program management falls entirely under the jurisdiction of the government, donors should not press for changes in how fertility control is carried out. Even when a program uses coercion and imposes severe penalties on those who disobey its rules, as has happened in China, funding organizations should not complain to the government or others about violations of human rights, in this view.

A massive campaign for birth control in Bangladesh showed how donor agencies can both support and challenge government activities. In 1983, according to Betsy Hartmann (1987), AID, the World Bank, and UNFPA circulated a position paper recommending a drastic reduction in population growth; a National Population Control Board with emergency powers; and frequent visits by high-level government and army officials to promote family planning in villages. It also urged the government to increase the financial incentives for sterilization.

With heavy funding from donor agencies, particularly AID, Bangladesh set up a sterilization program providing incentives to those receiving the operation as well as to doctors and clinic staff, government health and family-planning workers, and village midwives. Those responsible for carrying out the sterilizations paid little attention to requirements for informed consent and worked in conditions of very poor hygiene. A Western health adviser gave this blunt assessment of the campaign: "If people die during the operation or there is a complication, their records will be torn up" (Hartmann, 1987, p. 216).

In 1983 the Bangladesh Army joined this effort with a campaign of compulsory sterilization. Working in one of the country's northern districts, military staff rounded up villagers reported to have more than three children, forced them to sign statements giving their informed consent, and had them sterilized. In a few weeks this campaign led to the sterilization of over five hundred people, mostly poor women from a minority tribal community (Hartmann, 1987, p. 217).

Donor agencies varied in their reaction to this effort. The Swedish International Development Agency (SIDA) claimed that the use of incentives could lead to the indirect coercion of poor clients and make it difficult to honor the principle of free choice endorsed in the U.N. World Population Plan of Action. SIDA, Dutch and Norwegian development agencies, and UNICEF also argued that incentives for sterilization worked against basic health care for the citizens of Bangladesh. Faced with a choice between recruiting for sterilization, which brought a bonus, and providing health care, which brought no bonus, poorly paid government employees would often opt for sterilization. AID, which had pressured the government to increase its efforts at fertility control and had provided much of the funds for incentives and referral fees, also became concerned about a political backlash in Bangladesh when it learned about the army campaign. It asked the government to stop that campaign.

The fertility-control program in Bangladesh illustrates the conflicts that can occur between government initiatives and key ethical principles. Donor agencies become involved in these conflicts to the extent that the programs described are the result of their pressures and operate with their financing.

The most severe ethical conflict takes place when clients die as a result of the sterilization operation. In that case fertility control poses a direct threat to life. The use of financial incentives for clients raises questions about the economic fairness of the sterilization campaign. If those incentives are more appealing to destitute than to affluent citizens, they disregard fairness by making a long-term method of fertility control more attractive to the poor. By using coercion on clients, as happened in the army campaign, and by often disregarding the government's own procedures for informed consent, the sterilization program also violated reproductive freedom.

The Bangladesh program would also threaten human welfare if, as appears to have happened, it led to a reduction in government health services. By using financial incentives to press health workers to focus on sterilization rather than on their other duties, the government would in effect be reducing the priority it put on health care. Finally, the program would not respect truth-telling if the motivators for sterilization failed to explain the exact nature of the operation and did not disclose its medical risks. More broadly, truth-telling requires family planning clinics to ensure that clients know about other methods of fertility control and do not believe that sterilization is the only option available.

Donor responsibilities

In conclusion, what are the ethical obligations of donor agencies when they provide assistance to fertility-control programs? Do they have the right to pressure government and other organizations to be more active in fertility control? Once they have chosen the programs they will support, should they try to influence the ways in which those programs are carried out? Or should they claim that program design and management are not their responsibility?

In principle, donors have the right to provide funds to government and private organizations for initiatives those organizations wish to undertake. While one might debate the need for programs and their content, if a government wishes to set up a fertility-control program and accepts donor assistance for that purpose, the relationship between the government and the donor is on solid moral ground. If, on the other hand, a government decides not to become involved in fertility control and a donor tells national officials that, as a result, it will cut its assistance in areas where the government does want aid, the donor could be pressuring a country to set up a program it does not want. The government might well feel that the donor is making unfair use of its funding power.

Once a donor has provided funds to a recipient organization, it has responsibility for what happens in the program receiving its aid. While donors must respect national sovereignty, they also have an obligation to monitor the programs they support for violations of human rights. If they find that fertility-control programs are causing threats to human life and other harms to clients, they can urge the recipient to remove the sources of those difficulties. In the recipient refuses to deal with the issues raised, the donor can scale back or end its funding of that effort.

DONALD P. WARWICK

While all the articles in the other sections of this entry are relevant, see especially the companion article in this section: MIGRATION AND REFUGEES. *Directly related are the entries* POPULATION ETHICS; *and* FERTILITY CONTROL. *For a further discussion of topics mentioned in this article, see the entries* AUTONOMY; ENVIRONMENTAL HEALTH; ENVIRONMENTAL POLICY AND LAW; FIDELITY AND LOYALTY; FOOD POLICY; FREEDOM AND COERCION; JUSTICE; RIGHTS; *and* UTILITY. *For a discussion of related ideas, see the entries* ABORTION; BENEFICENCE; HARM; HEALTH POLICY, *article on* HEALTH POLICY IN INTERNATIONAL PERSPECTIVE; HEALTH PROMOTION AND HEALTH EDUCATION; MEDICAL ETHICS, HISTORY OF, *section on* SOUTH AND EAST ASIA, *subsection on* CHINA, *article on* CONTEMPORARY CHINA; *and* SEXISM.

Bibliography

AIRD, JOHN S. 1990. *Slaughter of the Innocents: Coercive Birth Control in China.* Washington, D.C.: AEI Press.

BERELSON, BERNARD. 1964. "National Family Planning Programs: A Guide." *Studies in Family Planning* 1, no. 5(suppl.):1–12.

CRANE, BARBARA B., and FINKLE, JASON L. 1989. "The United States, China, and the United Nations Population Fund: Dynamics of U.S. Policymaking." *Population and Development Review* 15, no. 1:23–59.

GERMAIN, ADRIENNE. 1993. "Are We Speaking the Same Language? Women's Health Advocates and Scientists Talk About Contraceptive Technology." In *Four Essays on Birth Control Needs and Risks*, pp. 3–6. By Ruth Dixon-Mueller and Adrienne Germain. New York: International Women's Health Coalition.

HARTMANN, BETSY. 1987. *Reproductive Rights and Wrongs: The Global Politics of Population Control and Contraceptive Choice.* New York: Harper & Row.

KASUN, JACQUELINE R. 1988. *The War Against Population: The Economics and Ideology of World Population Control.* San Francisco: Ignatius.

LEE, RONALD. 1985. Review of *World Development Report 1984. Population and Development Review* 11, no. 1: 127–130.

LEIBENSTEIN, HARVEY. 1985. Comment on *World Development Report 1984. Population and Development Review* 11, no. 1:135–137.

NATIONAL RESEARCH COUNCIL. WORKING GROUP ON POPULATION GROWTH AND ECONOMIC DEVELOPMENT. 1986. *Population Growth and Economic Development: Policy Questions.* Washington, D.C.: National Academy Press.

SADIK, NAFIS. 1990. "The Role of the United Nations—From Conflict to Consensus." In *Population Policy: Contemporary Issues*, pp. 193–206. Edited by Godfrey Roberts. New York: Praeger.

SAI, FRED T., and CHESTER, LAUREN A. 1990. "The Role of the World Bank in Shaping Third World Population Policy." In *Population Policy: Contemporary Issues*, pp. 179–191. Edited by Godfrey Roberts. New York: Praeger.

SIMON, JULIAN L. 1990. *Population Matters: People, Resources, Environment, and Immigration.* New Brunswick, N.J.: Transaction.

UNITED NATIONS POPULATION FUND. 1993. *Global Population Assistance Report 1982–1991.* New York: Author.

U.S. BUREAU FOR RESEARCH AND DEVELOPMENT. OFFICE OF POPULATION. 1993. *User's Guide to the Office of Population: January, 1993.* Washington, D.C.: U.S. Agency for International Development.

WARWICK, DONALD P. 1982. *Bitter Pills: Population Policies and Their Implementation in Eight Developing Countries.* Cambridge: At the University Press.

———. 1993. "The KAP Survey: Dictates of Mission vs. Demands of Science." In *Social Research in Developing Countries: Surveys and Censuses in the Third World*, pp. 349–363. Edited by Martin Bulmer and Donald P. Warwick. London: UCL Press.

WORLD BANK. 1984. *World Development Report 1984.* New York: Oxford University Press.

B. MIGRATION AND REFUGEES

Central to any understanding of the ethical dilemmas facing those who provide aid to migrants, refugees, displaced persons, and other victims of disasters and emergencies is an appreciation of the fundamental structure of the international order in which such aid is provided. The most important actors in the humanitarian assistance network are ultimately governments, since they create and direct the international agencies, provide the lion's share of the resources, and determine when and how aid to distressed populations will be dispensed. Governments alone retain the characteristics of sovereignty. Intergovernmental organizations, such as the United Nations High Commissioner for Refugees (UNHCR) and the World Food Program (WFP), derive their authority from the agreement of governments and pursue their mandates under governmental supervision. Nongovernmental organizations (NGOs), such as CARE, Oxfam, Catholic Relief Services (CRS), and the International Committee of the Red Cross (ICRC), though not created by governments, cannot provide overseas humanitarian aid without the permission of the host governments; in many cases, NGOs also derive a substantial portion of their revenues from the donor governments.

Governments as source of conflict and relief

One of the realities of international humanitarian aid, then, is that it is constrained by the political interactions of governments. Governmental persecution frequently is directly responsible for the creation of refugee flows. Governmental incapacity to provide security often indirectly causes such flows. Disputes over the control of governments can deteriorate into civil wars that displace people from their homes and homelands. Policies of foreign governments toward these conflicts can either exacerbate or mitigate them. They mitigate such situations by providing humanitarian aid and opportunities for refugee resettlement, promoting resolution of the conflicts, encouraging local settlement of refugees until such resolutions occur, and assisting repatriation when people decide to return home (Gorman, 1993a).

Governments sometimes undertake these tasks bilaterally, through their own diplomatic activity and assistance organizations. The United States, for instance, provides small amounts of bilateral refugee aid through its Bureau for Refugee Programs, and larger amounts of longer-term bilateral development aid through its Agency for International Development. It also provides large amounts of refugee aid through multilateral channels, to such international agencies as the UNHCR, the ICRC, the United Nations Relief and Works Agency for Palestine (UNRWA), and the International Organization for Migration (IOM), as well as emergency food aid and development resources through such agencies as WFP, the United Nations Development Program (UNDP), and the United Nations Children's Fund (UNICEF). Many donor governments give aid through multilateral channels in order to avoid entangling humanitarian aid too directly with political considerations, and to ensure that aid will be available to cope more efficiently with emergencies that arise throughout the globe. The structure of multilateral assistance that has been created by governments is based on the ethical principle of depoliticizing humanitarian aid.

In addition to providing aid, governments often find it necessary to resettle large numbers of refugees, particularly when repatriation is not possible and when the countries in which refugees first seek haven are unwilling to permit long-term settlement or permanent integration. Although governments and aid agencies consider third-country resettlement less desirable than repatriation (the preferred solution) or local settlement (considered the second-best solution), it is often a necessary step to ensure the protection of refugees and a viable and durable solution to their predicament. Despite its lowly place in the hierarchy of preferred solutions for refugees, third-country resettlement often enjoys preferred treatment in terms of the amounts of revenue spent on it. Although this solution addresses the needs of only a small percentage, usually no more than 1 or 2 percent of the global refugee population in any given year, some governments spend as much as half of their refugee assistance allocation on it.

Third-country resettlement, then, is very expensive and reaches only a small fraction of refugees. Do the numbers justify the expenditure? Many refugee advocates believe that they do, and that even more refugees ought to be resettled (Singer and Singer, 1988; Stein, 1991). Indeed, the political activity of refugee advocacy groups helps to sustain high levels of resettlement quotas and expenditures. Nevertheless, many government officials and some scholars have questioned whether the emphasis on resettlement may be commanding resources more urgently needed for drought prevention, development infrastructure, rehabilitation programs, and the like in refugee-affected areas of the globe, especially in the Third World (Gorman, 1993b; Gorman, 1991). Third-country resettlement was a major feature of refugee programs during the early years of the Cold War in Europe. However, the vast majority of refugees, mostly women and children, now flee from violence in poor countries of the Third World, raising the question of whether development-related humanitarian aid should now receive higher priority.

Nongovernment and intergovernment aid

Governments, the chief actors in providing humanitarian aid, are joined by a range of intergovernmental agencies and NGOs. Within the United Nations system alone, more than a dozen agencies participate in one way or another in the provision of aid to migrants or refugees. In 1991, the United Nations consolidated its humanitarian activities under the Department of Humanitarian Affairs (DHA), which assumed the role previously performed by the United Nations Disaster Relief Organization. Facing an increasing number of difficult humanitarian emergencies with the passing of the Cold War, governments decided that the United Nations should have a stronger and more centralized coordination mechanism for humanitarian assistance. DHA was given this authority. It is charged with coordination of an interagency standing committee, with administering the $50 million Central Emergency Revolving Fund, and, when the latter is inadequate, with the coordination of consolidated appeals for assistance in responding to disasters, to refugee situations, and to other emergencies.

Other U.N. agencies continue their specific mandates. UNHCR is principally responsible for protecting and assisting refugees, and UNRWA provides health programs and education to Palestinian refugees in the Middle East. WFP provides emergency food aid and food-for-work programs in all sorts of emergencies, including those involving refugees. IOM handles transportation arrangements for refugees resettling to third countries, supports research on migration, and operates the Return of Talent program to help reverse the brain drain that has seen many of the most talented individuals from poor countries seek professional employment in the developed world. UNICEF operates oral rehydration (through administration of electrolyte solutions), sanitation, health, and education programs for children. UNDP promotes coordination of technical assistance intended to enhance development and ease the impact of emergencies. The World Health Organization (WHO) provides emergency medical assistance. The World Bank indirectly finances infrastructural development programs in areas heavily affected by refugees, as well as employment opportunities for refugees and host country people. The International Labour Office (ILO) supports income-generation projects. The U.N. Population Fund conducts research on the effects of migration on local economies, and the U.N. Environment Program (UNEP) devises programs to remedy the effects of large-scale refugee movements, which often result in deforestation and degradation of the environment in the vicinity of refugee settlements.

While more than a dozen U.N. agencies provide some form of assistance to refugees or migrants, hundreds of NGOs provide programs in almost every country of the globe. Most U.N. agencies do not consider themselves to be operational agencies, directly responsible for the implementation of assistance programs in the field. This is usually left to the host country's governmental agencies or to indigenous or expatriate-based NGOs. UN agencies coordinate and monitor refugee and emergency assistance, while governments and NGOs provide for the staffing of implementation.

NGOs are very diverse in their countries of origin and nationality. The United States leads the list with the largest number of NGOs; Australia, Canada, and the countries of western Europe have large numbers of such agencies as well. Virtually every nation on the globe has indigenous voluntary groups that are engaged in some sort of humanitarian aid. The Red Cross, headquartered in Switzerland, for instance, has national affiliates in about 150 countries. Some NGOs are sponsored by specific churches or religious organizations. CRS, Lutheran World Relief, World Vision, and the World Council of Churches (WCC) fit into this category. Other agencies, such as the British agency Oxfam, and the American agency CARE, are strictly secular. Some NGOs—such as CRS and CARE—are very large and serve as a conduit for substantial governmental humanitarian aid. Others, such as the Mennonite Central Committee and the American Friends Service Committee, are quite small and refuse to accept any governmental resources.

Some NGOs focus on refugee and emergency aid; others, on resettlement of refugees; and still others, on long-term development assistance. Other NGOs, such as Church World Service, WCC, Amnesty International, the U.S. Committee for Refugees, the British Refugee Council, AUSTCARE, and the Lawyers Committee for Human Rights, are engaged in political advocacy for refugee and emergency assistance. NGOs are ideologically diverse, ranging across the continuum from conservative to liberal. This diversity ensures that U.N. agencies and governments will have no lack of interested agencies and volunteers wherever humanitarian emergencies arise across the globe (Gorman, 1985; Lissner, 1977; Nicols, 1988).

NGOs have been subjected to numerous criticisms. Some religious agencies are accused of being overly concerned with proselytization. Others are criticized for using too many foreigners and not enough indigenous personnel in implementing programs. Some adopt questionable advertising campaigns to raise money, such as running film footage of emergencies to gain public sympathy long after those emergencies have passed. Although such ethical concerns clearly face NGOs as they provide overseas relief, there can be little doubt that they are an indispensable feature of contemporary humanitarian programs (Gorman, 1985).

Ethical issues facing governments and aid agencies

Several ethical questions face the donor community. What kinds of assistance should be given priority by governments and donor agencies? How should one determine where aid is to be allocated and why? Should need be the determining criterion, or should political factors control the decision? Should the international donors ignore the sovereign prerogatives of governments responsible for massive human suffering among their own citizens, and intervene to provide humanitarian aid? How should the agencies deal with corrupt host governments and with large-scale diversion of humanitarian aid for private commercial gain? How should agencies cope with the potentially adverse effects of emergency assistance on the local economies? How quickly should agencies respond to potential emergencies?

International practice suggests that the two varieties of assistance that command the highest priority for funding are refugee resettlement programs and emergency aid. The areas of funding receiving the least attention are those that address longer-term, development-oriented programs on behalf of host countries and their populations even though these programs, if aggressively pursued, could mitigate future disasters, reduce the loss of life during famines and emergencies, and ease the provision of future emergency assistance. Lack of funding for these programs reflects the tendency for the United Nations, governments, and NGOs to separate their refugee and humanitarian emergency aid programming from their long-term development programming, and the tendency, when resources are scarce, to allot them for immediate needs and the saving of life during emergencies rather than to focus on the less dramatic and less compelling long-term preventive assistance measures. U.N. agencies are also limited by their original mandates in how and where they provide aid. UNHCR, for instance, is not usually given lead responsibility for aid to persons displaced inside their own states. This responsibility lies with DHA, UNDP, and other U.N. development agencies, as well as with ICRC on the NGO side. On the other hand, flexible application of U.N. agency mandates does occur. UNHCR assisted refugees and famine victims in eastern Sudan in the mid-1980s, and has been designated the lead agency for humanitarian assistance to the Balkans for both refugees and displaced persons.

Matching need. One of the principal concerns of U.N. aid agencies is to match the need for assistance with programs that address those needs. Generally U.N. agencies such as the UNHCR allocate budgets in rough proportion to the needs for refugee programs in various regions (Pitterman, 1985). However, the nature of refugee programs in some regions (Indochina and Central America) made them more expensive, on a per capita basis, than those in South Asia and Africa. In part, these discrepancies result from the principle that the refugees in a particular region should be given aid that will permit them to live at a standard comparable with the surrounding host population. Not placing refugees in a privileged position helps mitigate resentment among the host population. Because regional and local standards of living vary substantially, so does the level of refugee assistance. In addition, if refugee resettlement programs are crucial to the protection of refugees, as was the case in Indochina, per capita costs of refugee programs rise because resettlement is expensive. In Africa, by contrast, local settlement in relatively poor areas can be achieved at considerably less expense. Programs, in short, are devised by aid agencies to cope with the special circumstances surrounding each refugee situation, and it is almost axiomatic (with very rare exceptions, such as aid to the Kurds inside Iraq) that aid is not provided unless the government that controls the territory in which the humanitarian emergency exists, requests international involvement.

An increasingly difficult ethical question for governments and aid agencies is how and whether they should provide assistance to needy peoples who have become victims of their own government and have been unable to flee across borders. This is most common in civil war situations. The ICRC, for instance, operated a land-bridge operation from eastern Sudan into Ethiopia in the months preceding the deepening of the Ethiopian famine in 1984–1985, to ensure that some food reached people trapped in rebel-held areas of Ethiopia (Gorman, 1993a). U.N. agencies could not have provided such aid without the explicit approval of Ethiopia. Later, when the famine spread, agreements between donor governments, U.N. agencies, and the Ethiopian government enabled food aid to reach areas the government did not control. On occasion, however, U.N. agencies have undertaken assistance to people in opposition-held territory, as they did in Kurdish areas of northern Iraq that were placed under international protection after concerted attempts by the Iraqi military to suppress Kurdish rebellion. This represented a substantial departure from the normal concessions to national sovereignty, and an indication that compelling humanitarian need might give rise to international intervention. Legally, such intervention is on shaky ground, although compelling ethical and moral arguments support it in some situations (Macalister-Smith, 1985; Adelman, 1992).

Aid agencies often must deal with inefficient or corrupt host country governments. In such cases, food diversion is not uncommon. Some food diversion in poor countries can be and is tolerated as a necessary price of delivering humanitarian aid. If 10 or 15 percent of food aid is lost to diversion, overall operations are not badly inhibited, and usually such food finds its way into the mouths of hungry local people, even if they are not the target population. However, rampant food diversion debilitates the overall relief effort and must be corrected. Aid agencies do this by insisting on accurate censuses of beneficiary populations; gaining control over the offloading of food shipments at ports, along transportation lines, and at storage areas; and through ration card systems at the points of distribution. CARE is one NGO that specializes in food distribution logistics.

In addition, the provision of too much external food aid can ruin the local food market by glutting it and lowering prices that indigenous producers can get for their produce. Thus, aid agencies try first to purchase relief supplies from locally available stocks before seeking external food shipments. Over the long run, the ratio of external food supplies to local production must be carefully managed to ensure that international emergency aid does not induce disincentives to local production and self-reliance.

Determining when to supply aid. When should agencies respond to emergencies? Ideally, they should do so at the first evidence that a refugee flow or famine is imminent, thus prepositioning food supplies and avoiding substantial loss of life. Through early warning mechanisms, donors and agencies can ensure that enough aid is present to save lives. However, humanitarian aid typically must await the request of governments, which may be reluctant to preposition emergency food stocks for fear of precipitating refugee flows into their own territories. This political obstacle frequently prevents the international community from responding to emergencies early enough to prevent them entirely or to reduce their negative effects substantially.

Other obstacles also can retard the response. In Somalia, the lack of a government and the existence of widespread violence caused U.N. aid agencies to pull out. They did not return until a modicum of security was afforded to relief personnel. In the meantime, hundreds of thousands of Somalis starved. The balance of security for aid workers versus the gravity of the humanitarian emergency remains a difficult political and ethical question. Similarly, in the Balkans, questions have been raised about whether relief agencies should deal with governments that exploit humanitarian aid for their own political ends.

Apart from the assistance questions involved in refugee affairs, a set of ethical concerns surround when and whether countries have an obligation to accept asylum seekers or resettled refugees permanently. From a legal standpoint, most governments do not consider themselves obligated to accept claims of asylum, although most recognize the right of individuals to *seek* asylum. On the moral and ethical side, however, questions remain concerning whether a country may preserve its security, cultural character, or economic prosperity by limiting the acceptance of migrants, refugees, and asylum seekers. Some ethicists, using the "equal consideration of interests" principle, believe that wealthy countries have a duty to accept large numbers of such migrants, up to the point that the discomfort their citizens experience as a consequence of the immigration begins to match that of the refugees or immigrants seeking entry (Singer and Singer, 1988). Others, while recognizing the validity of extending aid, believe that limitations regarding cultural issues and security permit a more restrictive approach to immigration (Walzer, 1983). Still others find that the countries that generate refugee flows have a responsibility to avoid behavior that produces refugees, while other governments, including those of first asylum and potential resettlement, have a range of responsibilities to ensure that refugees are adequately protected, assisted, and provided meaningful, durable solutions (Shacknove, 1988).

The international community as a whole, in this view, has a duty to provide aid to refugees and other emergency victims. Each country involved has particular obligations depending on its capacity to provide material aid or resettlement opportunities, its proximity to the refugee situation, its past involvement in the conflict that eventually produced refugees, and other factors such as cultural compatibility and existing population pressures. The one certain obligation that governments accept is that they may not involuntarily repatriate genuine refugees to the country from which they fled, fearing persecution. Beyond this, the debates in legal and ethical circles have yet to reach a clear consensus (Gibney, 1988; Ellis, 1986).

ROBERT F. GORMAN

While all the articles in the other sections of this entry are relevant, see especially the companion article in this section: FERTILITY CONTROL. *Directly related to this article is the entry* POPULATION ETHICS. *For a further discussion of topics mentioned in this article, see the entries* CHILDREN, *article on* RIGHTS OF CHILDREN; FOOD POLICY; INTERNATIONAL HEALTH; WARFARE, *article on* PUBLIC HEALTH AND WAR; *and* WOMEN, *article on* HISTORICAL AND CROSS-CULTURAL PERSPECTIVES. *For a discussion of*

related ideas, see the entries LIFE; PUBLIC HEALTH, *article on* DETERMINANTS OF PUBLIC HEALTH; RACE AND RACISM; RIGHTS; TRAGEDY; *and* UTILITY. *Other relevant material may be found under the entries* AGRICULTURE; AUTONOMY; BENEFICENCE; EVOLUTION; FUTURE GENERATIONS, OBLIGATIONS TO; *and* WARFARE, *article on* INTERNATIONAL WEAPONS TRADE.

Bibliography

ADELMAN, HOWARD. 1992. "Humanitarian Intervention: The Case of the Kurds." *International Journal of Refugee Law* 4, no. 1:5–38.

ELLIS, ANTHONY, ed. 1986. *Ethics and International Relations.* Manchester, U.K.: Manchester University Press.

GIBNEY, MARK, ed. 1988. *Open Borders? Closed Societies? The Ethical and Political Issues.* New York: Greenwood Press.

GORMAN, ROBERT F. 1985. "Private Voluntary Organizations and Refugee Relief." In *Refugees and World Politics,* pp. 82–104. Edited by Elizabeth G. Ferris. New York: Praeger.

———. 1991. "U.S. Overseas Refugee Policy." In *Refugee Policy: Canada and the United States,* pp. 118–142. Edited by Howard Adelman. Toronto: Center for Refugee Studies, York University, Center for Migration Studies of New York.

———. 1993a. *Mitigating Misery: An Inquiry into the Political and Humanitarian Aspects of U.S. and Global Refugee Policy.* Lanham, Md.: University Press of America.

———, ed. 1993b. *Refugee Aid and Development: Theory and Practice.* Westport, Conn.: Greenwood Press.

KENT, RANDOLPH C. 1987. *The Anatomy of Disaster Relief: The International Network in Action.* London: Pinter.

LISSNER, JORGEN. 1977. *The Politics of Altruism: A Study of the Political Behaviour of Voluntary Development Agencies.* Geneva: Lutheran World Federation.

MACALISTER-SMITH, PETER. 1985. *International Humanitarian Assistance: Disaster Relief Actions in International Law and Organization.* Dordrecht, Netherlands: Martinus Nijhoff.

NICHOLS, J. BRUCE. 1988. *The Uneasy Alliance: Religion, Refugee Work, and U.S. Foreign Policy.* Oxford: Oxford University Press.

PITTERMAN, SHELLY. 1985. "International Responses to Refugee Situations: The United Nations High Commissioner for Refugees." In *Refugees and World Politics,* pp. 43–81. Edited by Elizabeth G. Ferris. New York: Praeger.

SHACKNOVE, ANDREW E. 1988. "American Duties to Refugees: Their Scope and Limits." In *Open Borders? Closed Societies?,* pp. 131–149. Edited by Mark Gibney. New York: Greenwood Press.

SINGER, PETER, and SINGER, RENATA. 1988. "The Ethics of Refugee Policy." In *Open Borders? Closed Societies?,* pp. 111–130. Edited by Mark Gibney. New York: Greenwood Press.

STEIN, BARRY N. 1991. "Refugee Aid and Development: Slow Progress Since ICARA II." In *Refugee Policy: Canada and the United States,* pp. 143–170. Edited by Howard Adelman. Toronto: Center for Refugee Studies, York University, Center for Migration Studies of New York.

WALZER, MICHAEL. 1983. *Spheres of Justice: A Defense of Pluralism and Equality.* New York: Basic Books.

PORTUGAL

See MEDICAL ETHICS, HISTORY OF, *section on* EUROPE, *subsection on* CONTEMPORARY PERIOD, *article on* SOUTHERN EUROPE.

POWER OF ATTORNEY FOR HEALTH-CARE DECISIONS

See DEATH AND DYING: EUTHANASIA AND SUSTAINING LIFE, *article on* ADVANCE DIRECTIVES.

PRENATAL DIAGNOSIS

See GENETIC TESTING AND SCREENING, *article on* PRENATAL DIAGNOSIS.

PRENATAL INJURIES

See MATERNAL–FETAL RELATIONSHIP.

PRESCRIPTION DRUGS

See PHARMACEUTICS.

PREVENTIVE MEDICINE

See HEALTH PROMOTION AND HEALTH EDUCATION; PUBLIC HEALTH; *and* SOCIAL MEDICINE. See also HEALTH SCREENING AND TESTING IN THE PUBLIC-HEALTH CONTEXT; *and* OCCUPATIONAL SAFETY AND HEALTH.

PRINCIPLES OF BIOETHICS

See AUTONOMY; BENEFICENCE; BIOETHICS; ETHICS, *article on* NORMATIVE ETHICAL THEORIES; *and* JUSTICE.

PRISONERS

I. Health-Care Issues
  Nancy Neveloff Dubler
II. Torture and the Health Professional
  Elena O. Nightingale
  Julia C. Chill
III. Research Issues
  Roy Branson

I. HEALTH-CARE ISSUES

The goal of medical care is to diagnose, comfort, and cure; the goal of a prison or jail is to confine and punish. The inevitable tension between these two goals underlies much of the substandard or abusive care provided for many incarcerated persons in the United States and throughout the world. Health-care providers must see their patients as equals in the tasks of examining health-care options and choosing the most individually appropriate care plan; correctional officers, on the other hand, must see their charges as inferior beings in order to enforce the punishments of society.

Most correctional facilities are not pleasant places to work in either for security staff or for other professionals; locked doors confine inmates and staff together in spaces filled with deprivation and anger. Facilities, especially in the United States, are increasingly inadequate and overcrowded as the number of inmates continues to expand from 644,000 in 1983 to 1,217,000 in 1990 (U.S. Department of Justice, 1990, 1992). "Prison Doc," a term of opprobrium until quite recently, accurately reflected the inadequate quality of medical staff generally willing to work behind bars.

Until the early 1970s the correctional system in the United States was largely protected from public exposure and from judicial review. Historically, correctional facilities were built away from centers of population and were shielded from scrutiny. Furthermore (until 1974), the "hands-off doctrine," then a guide for judicial opinions, held that the problems of prisons and jails were so complex and intractable, and so ill-suited to resolution by juridical decree, that administrative decisions should be given such discretion as to be largely unreviewable (*Procunier v. Martinez*, 1974). And yet, commentators from Fyodor Dostoyevsky to John Rawls have asserted that one gauge of a society's humanity is how it treats its least well-positioned. In its treatment of prisoners, the United States has become more humane, but only with the constant efforts of prisoners' rights attorneys and the consistent supervision of the federal courts.

Systemic abuses

In the 1960s, spurred by the developing civil-rights movements, a new class of publicly funded attorneys emerged who were not dependent on clients' funds for their fees and were, therefore, able to represent prisoners who were generally penniless. These lawyers were also reacting to the more frequent prison exposés in the press and to the particularly horrifying reports of the Attica (New York) prison rebellion in 1971.

Federal courts, in analyzing petitions and evidence, struggled to fashion a constitutional standard that would protect inmates from a deprivation of rights without creating a rule that was so broad that the federal courts could be asked to supervise all correctional medical-care interactions (Neisser, 1977). Early cases reasoned that a denial of medical care or the provision of "grossly inadequate" or "callously indifferent" care was unconstitutional. The Eighth Amendment's prohibition of "cruel and unusual" punishment provided the legal basis for this new expansion of constitutional protection. These new perspectives were grounded in contemporary notions of Eighth Amendment jurisprudence that described a changing understanding of permissible punishments: "The term [cruel and unusual punishment] cannot be defined with specificity. It is flexible and tends to broaden as society tends to pay more regard to human decency and dignity and becomes, or likes to think that it becomes, more humane" (*Holt* v. *Sarver*, 1970).

The facts of the prisoner cases that were litigated revealed horrendous and torturous medical interactions. One case described the plight of an inmate following leg surgery whose doctor's orders were ignored by the prison supervisor and corrections officers: He was forced to stand and walk, and was denied his pain medications (*Martinez* v. *Mancusi*, 1970). In another case, an inmate was brought to the physician along with a portion of his right ear that had been severed in a fight with another inmate. The physician told him that he did not need his ear, threw it away, and sewed up the stump with ten stitches (*Williams* v. *Vincent*, 1974). In *Newman* v. *State of Alabama* (1974), attorneys challenged the conditions in an entire state prison system. When analyzing the adequacy of medical-care services, the court found corroborated allegations that unsupervised prisoners without formal training regularly pulled teeth, screened sick-call patients, dispensed as well as administered medication (including dangerous drugs), gave injections, took X rays, sutured, and performed minor surgery. The court also cited several dramatic instances of abuse in which patients died neglected, covered in maggots, and lying in their own filth. These conditions, said the U.S. Federal Court of Appeals for the Fifth Circuit, were consti-

tutionally impermissible (*Newman* v. *State of Alabama*, 1974).

The debate on the constitutional standard was resolved in 1976, when the U.S. Supreme Court decided the case of *Estelle* v. *Gamble*, holding that: "Deliberate indifference to the serious medical needs of prisoners constitutes the 'unnecessary and wanton infliction of pain' . . . proscribed by the Eighth Amendment. This is true whether the indifference is manifested by prison doctors in their response to the prisoner's needs or by prison guards in intentionally denying or delaying access to medical care or intentionally interfering with the treatment once prescribed" (*Estelle* v. *Gambler*, 1976, p. 104).

Health-care rights of prisoners

Because of legal precedents set during the 1960s and 1970s, inmates in U.S. prisons and jails have a right to physical and mental health care that is protected by the Eighth Amendment. Since 1976, numerous cases in the federal courts have determined the precise scope of this right by defining the minimum constitutional standard of acceptable care. These cases established three basic health rights of inmates: the right to access to care; the right to care that is ordered; and the right to a professional medical judgment (Boney et al., 1991).

Access to care must be provided for any condition, whether medical, dental, or psychological, if the denial of care might result in pain, suffering, deterioration, or degeneration. The second component—care that is ordered—is violated when needed prescribed care of any category is denied to any inmate. Finally, the right to a professional medical judgment assures that: "decisions concerning the nature and timing of medical care are made by medical personnel, using equipment designed for medical use, in locations conducive to medical functions, and for reasons that are purely medical" (Boney et al., 1991, p. 36). This last right is obviously the key to ensuring the independence of health-care practitioners in the correctional environment, where security concerns are always paramount. It is never comfortable or convenient for correctional officers to accommodate inmate movement at nonprescribed times even if care regimens demand. If guards can regulate behavior, they will; that is the nature of punitive administration. In contrast, medical care is based on an assessment of individual need, a process antithetical to correctional practice.

In addition to prescribing an inmate's right to care, the federal courts have also required a constitutional system of care. Courts have held that the state's obligation is threefold, reflecting the three dimensions of the inmate's right. "First, prisoners must be able to make their medical problems known. . . . Second, the medical staff must be competent to examine inmates and to diagnose their illnesses. And, third, the staff must be able to treat the inmate's medical problems or to refer inmates to outside medical sources who can" (Boney et al., 1991, p. 37).

Legal issues

In the process of stipulating constitutional guarantees and supervising health-care reform, the courts have identified several problems that have both legal and ethical dimensions. In general, the standard of review in effect in the 1990s provides that administrative regulations and decisions that are "reasonably related to legitimate penological interests" (*Turner v. Safley*, 1987, p. 482) will be upheld by the court. This standard permits a greater infringement of inmate freedoms than tolerated by the federal courts in the 1970s and 1980s. While this is not a reestablishment of the "hands-off" doctrine, it does present prison administrators with greater latitude than prison advocates deem appropriate, given the continued abuses within the system.

Despite this retreat from a prior policy of aggressive judicial supervision of patterns of prison administration, inmates retain enforceable rights within the health-care system. There is some right to confidentiality for medical records and information, although the right is not absolute, and confidentiality may be breached for issues of public health that, in a prison context, include order. The acquired immunodeficiency syndrome (AIDS) epidemic also has limited confidentiality. Some prison systems require HIV testing and provide separate housing for those who test positive. The special care needed by persons with AIDS makes them visible within the facility. Inmates also have the right to consent to care, while not possessing a coequal right to refuse care. A Massachusetts case regarding an inmate's refusal of dialysis held that life-sustaining care could be imposed. The court balanced the inmate's right to refuse care against the state's interest in upholding orderly prison administration and permitted the prison to impose care (*Commissioner of Corrections v. Myers*, 1979).

The U.S. Supreme Court in 1990 upheld a policy of allowing forced administration of antipsychotic drugs over a prisoner's objection if an administrative hearing conducted by prison officials (the prisoner was seeking an independent judicial hearing) supported the finding of the facility's physician and found that the prisoner suffered from a "mental disorder" and was "gravely disabled" or "posed a likelihood of serious harm to self or others" (*Washington v. Harper*, 1990). A disturbing aspect of the case was that the court relied on the rule upholding the validity of administrative process and permitted the care decision to be based on an admin-

istrative assessment of the inmate's medical interest. Previously this sort of case would have received independent judicial review rather than administrative—nonindependent—review. Administrative review is far more likely to reflect institutional bias and correctional needs than a medical or judicial review conducted by independent physicians or judges.

Federal court cases since 1976 have further delineated the parameters of required care: The increasingly common practice of contracting with private health-care corporations to provide correctional health-care services does not shield the correctional agency from fulfilling the constitutionally required dimensions of health care (*West v. Atkins*, 1989); an inmate cannot be held responsible for the costs of an otherwise legal abortion—such costs must be borne by the correctional facility (*Monmouth County Correctional Institute Inmates v. Lanzaro*, 1987); and conditions of confinement that expose inmates to communicable disease and other identifiable health threats violate the Eighth Amendment (*Jones v. Diamond*, 1981). The federal courts have also confronted many aspects of the treatment of prisoners with AIDS, including mandatory screening, segregation, standards for treatment, and access to clinical trials (Boney et al., 1991). The results vary, but in general the federal courts favor the particular medical policy proposed by the states or by the Federal Bureau of Prisons. The U.S. Supreme Court, however, has not ruled on any of these issues regarding AIDS.

Ethical dilemmas

In addition to constitutional mandates and the range of medical/ethical problems complicated by the prison context, there is a series of ethical dilemmas peculiar to correctional settings. Health-care providers in correctional settings are bound by the same guidelines as their colleagues who work in more conventional medical spaces: They must promote the welfare of patients, advocate their medical needs, inform them about their diagnoses and prognoses, and protect their privacy. However, providers in correctional settings also face ethical challenges for which there are no parallels in the outside world. The prison setting exerts a continual pressure on professional judgment. Seasoned care providers report that they must be consciously and continuously vigilant to avoid becoming co-opted by correctional assumptions regarding moral culpability and characterological deficits and goals of restricting liberty and personal choice, and by patterns of officer–inmate interactions (Dubler and Anno, 1991).

Often providers are asked to act as impartial arbiters of potentially explosive or violent situations. Thus they are asked to witness forced transfers or to supervise punishment. It is assumed that their presence will prevent violence or that their skill and special status will render searches less painful and intrusive and the punishment less destructive. Acquiescing to these requests, however, may destroy the provider's ability to act independently as the patient's advocate. Such participation violates the particular provider–patient relationship, and by extension, relationships with other inmates (Dubler, 1986; Dubler and Anno, 1991).

Other assignments that tend to undermine the provider–patient relationship include collecting forensic information for prosecutors, using restraints for nonmedical purposes, agreeing to endorse a "special diet" that is actually a nutritionally adequate yet inedible punishment, permitting a medical note about an inmate's noncompliance with a care plan or follow-up appointment to be used to trigger disciplinary action, agreeing to monitor a hunger strike, certifying that a prisoner has been successfully executed, or helping to determine whether an inmate is "competent"—sufficiently mentally intact and aware—for execution. Deciding how to respond to requests for such assistance is a difficult and complex task. The institutional pressures for provider participation may be enormous, yet many scholars and commentators have argued, consistent with comprehensive standards published by the National Commission on Correctional Health Care and by the American Public Health Association, that if professional ethics would prohibit an action in a community setting, they prohibit it in a correctional setting as well (National Commission, 1992a, 1992b; Dubler, 1986).

Inmates are not passive in the process. Not surprisingly, as the prison erects barriers to communication with the outside world, inmates focus more on self. "Everything hurts more in prison" (Dubler, 1983, p. 20). The uncertain prison work ethic, the need for a medical note to avoid assignment, and the lack of available over-the-counter medications all encourage heavy use of the medical service. Prisoners, who are largely poor and did not have adequate access to medical and dental care before incarceration, tend to have more significant medical problems than a matched age cohort. Finally, prisoners may view medical-service personnel as more humane and caring than the rest of the prison staff and for this reason seek to spend inordinate amounts of time in their presence. Such use of the medical service to meet "nonmedical" needs, although perhaps a rational coping strategy in a dehumanizing environment, may elicit hostility from the medical staff (Dubler, 1983).

Care-provider ethics in the larger world are based on mutual respect and patient trust. The doctrine of informed consent is premised on the respect for patient autonomy that grounds the individual's right to make personal choices about care. This model clashes with the correctional model, which is not based on mutual respect. By definition, the inmate is of lesser moral worth and possesses fewer rights and privileges than the staff. In this setting, confidentiality, the right to consent to and refuse care, and the very essence of the provider–patient relationship come daily under attack.

The administration and management of prisons and jails is a growth industry. This means that increasing numbers of health-care providers will be faced with the challenge of practicing their profession in alien surroundings that perpetually challenge professional skill, personal commitment, and notions of fairness and justice.

NANCY NEVELOFF DUBLER

Directly related to this article are the other articles in this entry: TORTURE AND THE HEALTH PROFESSIONAL, *and* RESEARCH ISSUES. *Also directly related are the entries* DIVIDED LOYALTIES IN MENTAL-HEALTH CARE; AUTONOMY; FREEDOM AND COERCION; AUTHORITY; DEATH PENALTY; RIGHTS; PATIENT RIGHTS; *and* CONFLICT OF INTEREST. *For a further discussion of topics mentioned in this article, see the entries* BEHAVIOR CONTROL; BENEFICENCE; CIVIL DISOBEDIENCE AND HEALTH CARE; CONSCIENCE; HARM; HEALTH-CARE RESOURCES, ALLOCATION OF, *article on* MACROALLOCATION; *and* RESEARCH POLICY, *article on* RISK AND VULNERABLE GROUPS.

Bibliography

BONEY, JACQUELINE M.; DUBLER, NANCY N.; and ROLD, WILLIAM J. 1991. "The Legal Right to Health Care in Correctional Institutions." In *Prison Health Care: Guidelines for the Management of an Adequate Delivery System.* Edited by B. Jaye Anno. Washington, D.C.: U.S. Department of Justice, National Institute of Corrections.

Commissioner of Corrections v. Myers. 1979. 399 N.E.2d 452 (Mass.).

DUBLER, NANCY NEVELOFF. 1983. "Prison Health Care: Difficulties in Meeting the Legal Standard." In *Health Care in Prisons, Jails and Detention Centers: Some Legal and Ethical Dilemmas.* Edited by Margaret D. Wishart and Nancy N. Dubler. Bronx, N.Y.: Montefiore Medical Center.

———, ed. 1986. *Standards for Health Services in Correctional Institutions.* 2d ed. Washington, D.C.: American Public Health Association.

DUBLER, NANCY NEVELOFF, and ANNO, B. JAYE. 1991. "Ethical Considerations and the Interface with Custody." In *Prison Health Care: Guidelines for the Management of an Adequate Delivery System.* Edited by B. Jaye Anno. Washington, D.C.: U.S. Department of Justice, National Institute of Corrections.

Estelle v. Gamble. 1976. 429 U.S. 97, 104–105, 97 S. Ct. 285, 290.

Holt v. Sarver. 1970. 309 F. Supp. 362, 380.

Jones v. Diamond 1981. 636 F.2d 1364 (5th Cir.).

Martinez v. Mancusi. 1970. 443 F.2d 921 (2d Cir.).

Monmouth County Correctional Institute Inmates v. Lanzaro. 1987. 834 F.2d 326 (3rd Cir.).

National Commission on Correctional Health Care. 1992a. *Standards for Health Services in Jails.* Chicago: Author.

———. 1992b. *Standards for Health Services in Prisons.* Chicago: Author.

Neisser, Eric. 1977. " 'Is There a Doctor in the Joint?' The Search for Constitutional Standards for Prison Health Care." *Virginia Law Review* 63:921–973.

Newman v. State of Alabama. 1974. 503 F.2d 1320 (5th Cir.).

Procunier v. Martinez. 1974. 416 U.S. 405, 416.

Turner v. Safley. 1987. 482 U.S. 78, 89, 107 S.Ct. 2254, 2261.

U.S. Department of Justice. Bureau of Justice Statistics. 1990. *Sourcebook of Criminal Justice Statistics.* Washington, D.C.: U.S. Government Printing Office.

———. 1992. *Sourcebook of Criminal Justice Statistics.* Washington, D.C.: U.S. Government Printing Office.

Washington v. Harper. 1990. 494 U.S. 210, 221, 110 S.Ct. 1028, 1036.

West v. Atkins. 1989. 487 U.S. 42.

Williams v. Vincent. 1974. 508 F.2d 241 (2d Cir.).

II. TORTURE AND THE HEALTH PROFESSIONAL

Definition and history

As a consequence of the brutalities perpetrated by the Axis countries (Germany, Italy, and Japan) during World War II, many nations in the world community agreed that human rights should be an international concern. In 1948, the United Nations adopted the Universal Declaration of Human Rights, which set forth the fundamental rights to which all human beings are entitled (U.N. General Assembly, 1949). Since then, the United Nations and many of its member countries have adopted additional binding covenants and declarations, including the Declaration on the Protection of All Persons from Being Subjected to Torture and Other Cruel, Inhuman or Degrading Treatment or Punishment (1975), and the Convention Against Torture and Other Cruel, Inhuman or Degrading Treatment or Punishment, adopted in 1984 (United Nations, 1985).

The purpose of torture is to destroy the dignity, self-respect, and will of the victim. The torturer has complete control over every aspect of the victim's being, thus negating any sense of freedom the victim might have felt previously. Torture may take many forms: physical, such as beatings, electrical shock, prolonged exposure to extremes of temperature, rape, and other sexual abuse; psychiatric, such as intimidation, sham executions, and incarceration in psychiatric prisons and hospitals; pharmacological, in which the victim is drugged with mind-altering and pain-causing substances; as well as deprivations of the basic necessities of life— food, clothing, or adequate sanitary facilities. Torture also exists as individual acts, such as child and spouse abuse. This article is limited to a discussion of torture as a state-sanctioned human-rights violation.

In the Convention Against Torture and Other Cruel, Inhuman or Degrading Treatment or Punishment, the United Nations defines torture as

> any act by which severe pain or suffering, whether physical or mental, is intentionally inflicted on a person for such purposes as obtaining from him or a third person information or a confession, punishing him for an act he or a third person has committed or is suspected of having committed, or intimidating or coercing him or a third person, or for any reason based on discrimination of any kind, when such pain or suffering is inflicted by or at the instigation of or with the consent or acquiescence of a public official or other person acting in an official capacity. (United Nations, 1985)

In its Declaration of Tokyo, the World Medical Association similarly defines torture as "the deliberate, systematic or wanton infliction of physical or mental suffering by one or more personas acting alone or on the orders of any authority, to force another to yield information, to make a confession, or for any other reason" (World Medical Association, 1975).

According to Amnesty International, torture is currently practiced or condoned by more than one-third of the nations of the world, many of which are signatories of the various declarations and conventions prohibiting torture. A number of countries use torture as the legal punishment for objectionable behavior. For example, in Iran, convicted thieves face amputation of fingers and women who violate the dress code face flogging. In Singapore, caning is a mandatory punishment for offenses including illegal immigration, robbery, murder, and rape. For certain offenses, legal requirements in many countries mandate capital punishment that, at least in the United States, can be overseen by a physician. Participation in these activities, however, is contrary to the oaths taken by physicians. Contradictions sometimes exist between a culture's civil laws and its medical code of ethics. The Islamic Shari'a law, for example, calls for the amputation of the right hand for theft, while the Islamic Code of Medical Ethics, adopted by the International Conference on Islamic Medicine in 1981, charges physicians, "by God, the Great" to "protect human life in all stages and under all circumstances, doing my utmost to rescue it from death, malady, pain and anxiety; to keep people's dignity, cover their privacies and lock up their secrets" (see Appendix, Volume 5). Often, if a physician does not participate in state-sanctioned punishments, he or she may jeopardize his or her own safety and perhaps further endanger prisoners. The dilemma posed by such a situation was addressed by the Commonwealth Medical Association with the following guideline:

Individual physicians opposed to such activities should be supported and encouraged, and those who participate in them should be sensitized to the implications of their participation, in the international quest for the elimination of degrading punishment and coercive forms of control as defined in the International Convention against Torture and other Cruel, Inhuman or Degrading Treatment or Punishment. (Commonwealth Medical Association, 1993, p. 11)

Torturing human beings to obtain information such as confessions, evidence against family members and friends, and lists of participants in antigovernment groups seldom has been shown to be effective. Although governments justify torture as a means to ensure the security of the state and the protection of its citizens, in reality torture is a political tool. Governments silence dissent by humiliating and physically injuring victims until they do not wish to, or physically cannot, continue their alleged rebellious behavior. The victim becomes an object lesson for others in the community who might wish to speak or act in dissent, and coerced statements renouncing certain ideals become propaganda for the state. The dissident's family or friends may also be apprehended and tortured to convince the dissident to cease the behavior perceived by the government as threatening.

Torture occurs most often in secret while victims are in the custody of police officials before charge or trial. During this time, detainees remain anonymous—they are not listed as prisoners because they have not been charged with crimes. Their anonymity allows police officials to torture them without fear of discovery. A victim's death is noted as merely a "disappearance."

Health-care professionals as violators of human rights

Although the practice of torture can be traced to ancient Greece and the Roman Empire, documented proof of physician involvement in torture dates back to the sixteenth century, when physicians were called upon by Holy Roman Emperor Charles V to determine whether defendants could withstand torture (Stover and Nightingale, 1985). Although torture was almost eliminated by the end of the nineteenth century in Europe, the unification of pseudoscientific theories with the political ideology of the Nazi party greatly increased its use. During World War II, physicians were involved in every step of the Nazi plan to create a racially "pure" state. Physicians progressed from forcibly sterilizing those who were thought to be genetically inferior, to killing the mentally ill and handicapped in hospitals, and finally to assisting in mass exterminations in concentration camps. Physicians not only sanctioned and assisted in killings but also helped develop effective means for mass murder under

the guise of scientific inquiry. Some, such as Joseph Mengele, used concentration camp inmates for cruel human experiments (Lifton, 1986).

Torture and medical ethics

Professional guidelines for physicians' conduct have existed in most societies for many centuries. The basis for many of today's medical codes can be traced to the fifth century B.C.E. and the Hippocratic oath, in which a doctor states, among other things, his or her intention to guard the sick from harm and injustice. The modern version of the Hippocratic oath, the Declaration of Geneva adopted by the World Medical Association in 1948, emphasizes that the health of a patient is the physician's first concern. The Declaration of Tokyo, which deals specifically with torture, states:

> The doctor shall not countenance, condone or participate in the practice of torture or other forms of cruel, inhuman or degrading procedures, whatever the offence of which the victim of such procedures is suspected, accused or guilty, and whatever the victim's beliefs or motives, and in all situations, including armed conflict and civil strife. (World Medical Association, 1975)

The Declaration of Tokyo led to the Principles of Medical Ethics, adopted by the United Nations in 1982, which defines the role of all health professionals regarding the treatment of prisoners and asserts:

> It is a gross contravention of medical ethics, as well as an offense under applicable international instruments, for health personnel, in particular physicians, to engage actively or passively in acts which constitute participation in, complicity in, incitement to or attempts to commit torture or other cruel, inhuman or degrading treatment or punishment. (U.N. General Assembly, 1983)

Many other groups, such as the World Psychiatric Association, the International Council of Nurses, and the International Conference on Islamic Medicine have developed ethical codes or passed resolutions on ethical standards.

Physicians may participate as both perpetrators and enablers of torture. As perpetrators, physicians examine the victim for those who plan torture, design torture for the individual victim, or monitor torture to ensure that the torturer does not accidentally kill the victim. In some instances, physicians treat victims in order to improve their condition enough to allow torture to continue. In other instances, physicians ignore injured or sick victims and fail to provide any type of medical care. In the latter case, medical conditions that are easy to treat, such as dehydration, may progress to a point where the victim dies.

Physicians may also perform the torture themselves. In the former Soviet Union, dissidents were incarcerated in special prisons for those whose ideologically incorrect beliefs were held to be a form of mental illness; doctors administered drugs like sulfizine, which caused "intense fever, excruciating pain, convulsions, and disorientation" but had absolutely no therapeutic effect (Klose, 1985, p. 168). Physicians also participated in torture during Augusto Pinochet's regime in Chile. Chilean law stated that prisoners had to be examined both on entering and leaving prison. However, many physicians examined prisoners merely to determine their fitness for torture. Physicians also advised the military on specific torture methods and on ways to keep prisoners alive during torture (Stover, 1987).

In order to support governments' denials regarding the occurrence of torture, physicians may also falsify medical records, death certificates, and autopsy reports. In 1977, South African police detained and tortured Steven Biko, an activist working to end apartheid. When Biko became unresponsive to questioning, police summoned a district surgeon, that is, a general practitioner employed by the Department of Health, to determine whether Biko had a stroke. During a series of examinations, this physician failed to perform rudimentary medical tests (blood and urine analysis and temperature), ignored obvious signs of serious injury (head contusions, bloodstained cerebrospinal fluid, and extensor plantar reflex), and failed to treat Biko, who died. During the inquest, the district surgeon and other physicians admitted that they misstated the facts in the medical records and on the death certificate, and that the patient's interests "were subordinated to the interest of security" (Rayner, 1987, p. 30). Despite these admissions, the Medical and Dental Council found no evidence of improper conduct by the physicians. Only after seven years of legal wrangling did the council take disciplinary action against Biko's physicians, who were found guilty of improper and disgraceful conduct (Rayner, 1987).

Physicians participate in torture for many reasons. Some fear that they will lose their jobs or that they or their families will be detained and tortured. Others participate voluntarily for power and gain, or because they share the politics or ideology of the state that recruits them.

Health-care professionals as protectors of human rights

By virtue of their oaths as health-care professionals, physicians and other health professionals have a special responsibility to fight against torture and other human-rights abuses. In countries where human rights are not respected, physicians are often the only outsiders who have access to detainees. Consequently, they have a unique opportunity to examine the detainees, document incidences of torture, and ensure that medical records and death certificates are accurate. They can bear witness to the world community that torture is taking place. In addition, health-care professionals are ethically obligated to report members of their profession who violate human rights. Failure to protest abuse allows abusers to justify their actions, while protest may cause abusers to rethink and stop the abuse. Health-care professionals can also offer their skills to treat and help survivors of torture.

Health-care professionals may advocate for human rights by urging their medical societies and professional organizations to form human-rights committees to help conduct fact-finding missions, research human-rights abuses, and pressure abusers and countries that sponsor abuse to cease this practice. Because of their international and internal networks, these groups, much more than individuals, are able to mobilize and support colleagues who are under pressure to collaborate or who are already in detention for not complying. Organizations of health professionals can act on behalf of individuals, as well as alert governments that human-rights abuses will not be tolerated by the world medical community.

A number of professional organizations have established committees to oppose human-rights abuses worldwide. These include the American Association for the Advancement of Science Committee on Scientific Freedom and Responsibility; the National Academy of Sciences Committee on Human Rights; the American College of Physicians; the American Academy of Pediatrics; and the American Psychological Association. Physicians for Human Rights, an organization of health professionals, uses the skills of member physicians and scientists to "expose violations through documentary and physical evidence." The evidence is then used to "hold governments which violate human rights accountable for their actions" (Physicians for Human Rights, 1993, p. 2). In addition, a number of centers, including the Rehabilitation and Research Center for Torture Victims (Copenhagen, Denmark); the Canadian Centre for Victims of Torture (Toronto); and the Center for Victims of Torture (Minneapolis, Minnesota) specialize in the treatment of torture survivors (Gruschow and Hannibal, 1990).

In countries such as the United States, as the refugee population becomes larger, physicians face the increased chance that they will treat someone who has been tortured. Physicians and other health-care professionals must be able to recognize such a patient, acknowledge that a physician may have been involved in the torture, and recommend a treatment that will not cause further trauma. Little is known about the long-term consequences of torture for survivors or about effective treatment, and research in this area is needed.

ELENA O. NIGHTINGALE
JULIA C. CHILL

Directly related to this article are the other articles in this entry: HEALTH-CARE ISSUES, *and* RESEARCH ISSUES. *Also directly related are the entries* NATIONAL SOCIALISM; EUGENICS, *article on* HISTORICAL ASPECTS; HARM; FREEDOM AND COERCION; PAIN AND SUFFERING; DIVIDED LOYALTIES IN MENTAL-HEALTH CARE; *and* CONFLICT OF INTEREST. *For a further discussion of topics mentioned in this article, see the entries* BEHAVIOR CONTROL; DEATH PENALTY; RIGHTS; *and* WARFARE, *article on* MEDICINE AND WAR. *See also the* APPENDIX (CODES, OATHS, AND DIRECTIVES RELATED TO BIOETHICS), SECTION II: ETHICAL DIRECTIVES FOR THE PRACTICE OF MEDICINE, DECLARATION OF GENEVA *of the* WORLD MEDICAL ASSOCIATION.

Bibliography

AMNESTY INTERNATIONAL. 1984. *Torture in the Eighties.* London: Author.

AMNESTY INTERNATIONAL and MARANGE, VALÉRIE. 1991. *Doctors and Torture: Resistance or Collaboration?* London: Bellew.

BRITISH MEDICAL ASSOCIATION. 1992. *Medicine Betrayed: The Participation of Doctors in Human Rights Abuses.* London: Zed.

COHN, JORGEN, ed. 1991. "Proceedings of the International Symposium on Torture and the Medical Profession, June 5–7, 1990." *Journal of Medical Ethics* 17, no. 4 (suppl.). Special issue.

COMMONWEALTH MEDICAL ASSOCIATION. 1993. *Medical Ethics and Human Rights: The Commonwealth Medical Association Project on the Role of Medical Ethics in the Protection of Human Rights.* London: Author.

GRUSCHOW, JANET, and HANNIBAL, KARI. 1990. *Health Services for the Treatment of Torture and Trauma Survivors.* Washington, D.C.: American Association for the Advancement of Science.

Human Rights Quarterly. 1981–. Baltimore: Johns Hopkins University Press.

INTERNATIONAL CONFERENCE ON ISLAMIC MEDICINE. 1981. *Islamic Code of Medical Ethics: Kuwait Document.* Kuwait: Author.

KLOSE, KEVIN. 1985. "A Question of Conscience: The Cases of Alexei Nikitin and Anatoly Koryagin." In *The Breaking of Bodies and Minds: Torture, Psychiatric Abuse, and the Health Professions,* pp. 164–182. Edited by Eric Stover and Elena O. Nightingale. New York: Freeman.

LAWSON, EDWARD. 1991. "Convention Against Torture and Other Cruel, Inhuman or Degrading Treatment or Punishment." In *Encyclopedia of Human Rights,* p. 245. Bristol, Pa.: Taylor and Francis.

LIFTON, ROBERT JAY. 1986. *The Nazi Doctors: Medical Killing and the Psychology of Genocide.* New York: Basic Books.

NIGHTINGALE, ELENA O. 1990. "The Role of Physicians in Human Rights." *Law, Medicine and Health Care* 18, nos. 1–2:132–139.

PETERS, EDWARD. 1985. *Torture.* New York: Basil Blackwell.

PHYSICIANS FOR HUMAN RIGHTS. 1993. *Annual Report.* Boston: Author.

RANDALL, GLENN, and LUTZ, ELLEN L. 1991. *Serving Survivors of Torture: A Practical Manual for Health Professionals and Other Service Providers.* Washington, D.C.: American Association for the Advancement of Science.

RAYNER, MARY. 1987. *Turning a Blind Eye? Medical Accountability and the Prevention of Torture in South Africa.* Washington, D.C.: American Association for the Advancement of Science.

SCARRY, ELAINE. 1985. *The Body in Pain: The Making and Unmaking of the World.* New York: Oxford University Press.

STOVER, ERIC. 1987. *The Open Secret: Torture and the Medical Profession in Chile.* Washington, D.C.: American Association for the Advancement of Science.

STOVER, ERIC, and NIGHTINGALE, ELENA O., eds. 1985. *The Breaking of Bodies and Minds: Torture, Psychiatric Abuse, and the Health Professions.* New York: Freeman.

UNITED NATIONS. 1985. *Convention Against Torture and Other Cruel, Inhuman or Degrading Treatment or Punishment.* London: HMSO.

———. GENERAL ASSEMBLY. 1949. *Universal Declaration of Human Rights.* Lake Success: U.N. Department of Public Information.

———. 1983. "Principles of Medical Ethics." In *Principles of Medical Ethics Relevant to the Protection of Prisoners Against Torture.* Geneva: Council for International Organizations of Medical Sciences.

WORLD MEDICAL ASSOCIATION. 1970. [1948]. "Declaration of Geneva." In *Declaration of Geneva; Declaration of Helsinki; Declaration of Sydney; Declaration of Oslo.* New York: Author.

———. 1975. *Guidelines for Medical Doctors Concerning Torture and Other Cruel, Inhuman or Degrading Treatment or Punishment in Relation to Detention and Imprisonment.* [Declaration of Tokyo]. Ferney-Voltaire, France: Author. Reprinted in *Medicine Betrayed,* by Clare Anthony, pp. 210–211.

III. RESEARCH ISSUES

Since the 1980s, virtually no prisoners in the United States have been used in biomedical experimentation that does not benefit prisoners as individuals or as a class. A principal reason is that ethical reflection on this topic in the 1970s not only decisively affected public policy but also shaped an enduring moral consensus in society.

A crucial year in that process was 1976. The Federal Bureau of Prisons announced an indefinite moratorium on nontherapeutic biomedical experimentation conducted in any federal prison. That same year, the board of directors of the American Correctional Association—the professional organization of U.S. prison officials at all levels of government—officially adopted a statement urging responsible bodies at federal, state, and local levels to eliminate the use of prisoners as subjects of medical pharmacological experimentation.

Most important, the U.S. National Commission for the Protection of Human Subjects of Biomedical and Behavioral Research (National Commission) recommended to the secretary of the Department of Health, Education and Welfare (now the Department of Health and Human Services, DHHS) that a moratorium on approving and funding prisoner experimentation be declared until certain specified minimum standards had been met by any prison allowing experimentation on inmates. The work of the National Commission deserves special attention because it was pivotal, at a critical moment in the 1970s, in articulating connections between moral principles and public policies concerning prisoner experimentation (U.S. National Commission, 1976a, 1976b).

Some debate continued over government regulations implementing the National Commission's recommendations, but by the 1980s, experimentation that was not therapeutic for the individual prisoner or prisoners as a class had virtually come to an end. With the crucial help of the National Commission, American society had reached a moral consensus already achieved by the rest of the world.

Practices

Such a consensus did not always exist. Rulers in ancient Persia permitted physicians to use prisoners as experimental subjects. Rome tested poisons on prisoners. European physicians in the eighteenth century used prisoners in experiments, exposing them—sometimes through injections—to venereal disease, cancers, typhoid, and scarlet fever.

In the United States, prisoners were used for experimentation from at least 1914, when white male convicts in Mississippi were used in pellagra experiments. During World War II, prisoner experimentation assumed a morally favorable aura when prisoners, to show their patriotism, signed up in large numbers for experimental studies. After reviewing this experimentation, several state commissions encouraged the use of prisoners (Beecher, 1970).

The American Medical Association underscored the degree to which participation in medical experimenta-

tion was viewed as morally admirable. It adopted a resolution disapproving of the practice of permitting prisoners convicted of murder, rape, arson, kidnapping, treason, or other heinous crimes to participate in medical experimentation. They were not considered sufficiently virtuous to be part of such a noble enterprise (Katz, 1972).

After World War II, when it became known that Nazi physicians had used concentration camp prisoners in medical experiments that mutilated and killed their subjects—innocent Jewish citizens of all ages—Europe found the use of any incarcerated persons in experimentation morally repugnant. An early draft of the Declaration of Helsinki included the following provision: "Persons retained in prisons, penitentiaries, or reformatories—being 'captive groups'—should not be used as subjects of experiment; nor persons incapable of giving consent because of age, mental incapacity, or being in a position in which they are incapable of exercising the power of free choice" (U.S. National Commission, 1976a, essay 16, p. 4).

However, the provision was deleted from the final version of the 1964 Declaration, reportedly because of pressure from the United States. Not only did the United States have an extended history of approving prisoner experimentation, but during the post–World War II years there was a substantial increase in biomedical experiments, including those using prisoners.

The federal government funded a wide variety of biomedical and behavioral experiments using prisoners, including numerous studies on infectious diseases, and the Atomic Energy Commission (later absorbed by the Department of Energy) conducted experiments involving radiation of male prisoners' genitals. From 1970 to 1975, five of the six government agencies that supported experimentation—all within the Public Health Service of the Department of Health, Education and Welfare—used prisoners in 125 biomedical studies and 19 behavioral research projects (U.S. National Commission, 1976b).

The greatest use of prisoners was in initial tests of drugs, performed primarily by private drug companies. In 1962, following the thalidomide tragedy, the U.S. Congress passed legislation requiring that before drugs were released for therapeutic use, their safety and efficacy must be tested on humans. To ensure an increased and steady supply of experimental subjects, pharmaceutical companies built facilities within prisons.

Prisoners became the principal subjects in the United States for testing new drugs. By 1975, according to a survey conducted by the Pharmaceutical Manufacturers Association (whose members develop most of the prescription drugs in the United States), at least 3,600 U.S. prisoners were the first humans on whom the safety of new drugs was tested. Prisoners in the United States were even being used to test drugs for researchers in other countries (Pharmaceutical Manufacturers Association, 1976).

Principles

When the National Commission conducted its deliberations on prisoners, the Department of Health, Education and Welfare was already on record as being enthusiastic about the advantage of using prisoners in research. The president of the Pharmaceutical Manufacturers Association testified before the National Commission that his organization believed there were few alternatives to using prisoners in drug tests. Given that factual assumption, the moral argument was made that the good of society required the use of prisoners.

In its *Report and Recommendations* the National Commission moved beyond the moral appeal to the good of society by challenging the factual assumption that prisoners were necessary for at least initial drug trials. The commission found several drug-testing programs in the United States that successfully used healthy, nonincarcerated volunteers (U.S. National Commission, 1976b). Thus prisoners were not essential for biomedical experimentation. Having established that empirical fact, the National Commission then devoted considerable attention to two of the three ethical principles it said should govern experimentation with human subjects.

Respect for persons. According to the National Commission, the fundamental moral principle of respect for persons includes respect for their dignity and autonomy. Experimentation with autonomous persons demands obtaining their consent to participate. The basic principle of respect for persons thus justifies the bioethical guideline of informed consent. Debates arising from the moral principle of respect for persons revolve around whether prisoners can provide a sufficiently voluntary consent to participate in experimentation.

One line of reasoning argues that prisoners obviously are competent to volunteer for experiments. After all, conviction for a crime presupposes that the citizen has been found sufficiently competent to be held accountable for his or her acts. Also, the citizen who enters prison has had certain rights legally recognized, such as the right to sue for freedom of worship and even to obtain compensation for injuries sustained in prison jobs (McDonald, 1967).

According to this line of thinking, prison inmates participate in remunerated occupations that put them at some risk. No one challenges the capacity of prisoners to volunteer for these tasks—for example, stamping license plates in prison factories. Why should there be

moral outrage at prisoners' *choosing* (they are permitted to refuse) to participate in medical experiments that admittedly provide financial inducements but also may do less physical harm?

Those who oppose prisoner experimentation argue that the relationship of persons to their bodies is very different from their relationship to their productive goods; the former comprises their relationship to themselves. There is a distinction between activities in which impinging on a person's body is accidental or unavoidable, as in a job, and those in which it is the very purpose of the activity, as in experimentation (Fried, 1974). The argument runs that since consent to a job is different from consent to experimentation, prisoners may be sufficiently free to consent to prison jobs but not sufficiently free to consent to experimentation.

Among those who cite the principle of free and informed consent as part of their opposition to the use of prisoners in experimentation, some argue that prisoners cannot in principle give a sufficiently free consent (American Civil Liberties Union, 1974). Others who oppose the use of prisoners in experimentation admit that in principle it might be possible for an inmate in some ideal correctional institution to give a sufficiently free and informed consent. However, they argue that in fact either the structure or the administration of the penal system in the Unted States makes it impossible for prisoners to give a sufficiently free consent to experimentation.

This argument relies on analyses of the basic structure of American prisons made by historians and sociologists. According to historians, the coercive structure of the American prison and its powerful impact on the attitudes of prisoners are not accidental. After the 1820s, foreign officials came to the United States to observe the unique lengths to which the country went in creating new institutions called *penitentiaries*. They were designed not only to incarcerate criminals but also to shape their behavior and their character (Rothman, 1971).

Those opposed to prisoner participation in experimentation argue that medical experiments cannot remain unaffected by the social environment of what sociologist Erving Goffman calls a "total institution," such as a penitentiary. In a total institution a single authority tightly controls the entire space and time of each person within it, including a series of abasements, degradations, and humiliations designed to convince inmates to accept the single authority's view of them. In such institutions the entire social environment is designed to elicit cooperation with the central authority. It is argued that in total institutions even the attractive and beneficial features of an activity such as experimentation can overcome the inmates' ability to give a sufficiently free consent (Goffman, 1961).

The National Commission's investigations revealed that in U.S. prisons there appeared to be limited alternatives to experimentation among available prison activities. Other activities were not conducted in comparably secure surroundings, and there appeared to be a paucity of meaningful, alternative ways for prisoners to express any altruism they might have. Most importantly, no other prison activity paid comparably. The National Commission learned of differences in payment between experimentation and other prison activities that ranged to well over ten to one. Not surprisingly, surveys showed that 70 percent of prisoner research subjects volunteered primarily for the money (Arnold et al., 1970).

Ethicists who served on the National Commission, or as staff and consultants, have subsequently emphasized that the commission believed prisoners were able to consent to experimentation under some conceivable conditions. However, the actual and likely conditions of American prisons raised genuine questions concerning prisoners' being able to give sufficiently free and informed consent. A distinction between coercion and manipulation of a prisoner's consent may be useful, although even a manipulated consent to participation in experimentation may be impermissible (Beauchamp and Childress, 1989; Faden et al., 1986).

Justice.   A significant contribution of the National Commission was making not only respect for persons but also justice central to ethical considerations of prisoner experimentation. A few voices defended the use of prisoners as a form of reparative justice. Prisoners, they said, have committed crimes against society, and it is inherently appropriate, as an act of reparation for those crimes, for prisoners to serve society by being used in research. Opponents of prisoner experimentation responded that society, through its legal system, had already pronounced sentence on prisoners for whatever crime they committed, and medical experimentation should not be considered a form of punishment.

The National Commission brushed past discussions of reparation to questions raised by comparative justice. The essence of comparative justice is that like cases or classes are to be treated alike, and different cases or classes are to be treated differently (Feinberg, 1973). Problems of remuneration immediately came to the fore. Considerations of justice would require paying prisoners participating in experiments the same as free volunteers. However, the amounts would be so much greater than remuneration otherwise available in prison that the payments could become so irresistible as to be coercive. Thus, in its final report, the National Commission included suggestions that researchers pay the same rate for prisoners to participate in experiments as they did for nonincarcerated volunteers; however, individual prisoners would receive the same amount they received for other prison jobs. The excess would go into a fund for

the general benefit of prisoners, or into escrow accounts paid to each participant at the time of his or her release from prison (Branson, 1976).

Comparative justice leads in biomedical ethics to considerations of the selection of subjects for experimentation. With respect to nontherapeutic experimentation in particular, risks and benefits should be distributed equitably among classes and groups of experimental subjects. The implications of comparative justice specifically for the gender and race of prisoners selected for experimentation received some attention from the National Commission. It heard testimony from black prisoners that they did not have equal opportunity to participate in experiments. Better-educated whites were disproportionately enrolled in prisoner experimentation. In its report the National Commission also noted that less research was conducted in women's prisons than in men's.

More fundamental were concerns about the justice of selecting prisoners at all for research benefiting society generally. A principal moral concern was that prisoners bore a disproportionate share of the burdens of research benefiting society as a whole—for example, initial drug trials on humans.

Comparative justice refers not only to similarities but also to differences between groups. Unequal treatment—for example, permitting free subjects, but not prisoners, to participate in experimentation—can be justified when individuals or groups are different in relevant respects. Prison populations are significantly different from the free society. Prisoners live in an institutional environment that is more coercive than that of free-living volunteers, and prisoners are less likely to receive equivalent health care. They also receive a minuscule percentage of the financial benefits given to free research subjects.

That prisoners are considered to be in so many relevant respects different from, and unequal to, the rest of society is a principal reason they are considered to be treated justly if they do not participate in research that does not benefit them directly.

Policies

In 1976, the National Commission recommended that research involving prisoners that posed more than minimal risk, that was not studying the process of incarceration, and that did not directly improve the health or well-being of individual prisoners should not be conducted unless the reasons for the research were compelling and "a high degree of voluntariness on the part of the prospective participants and openness on the part of the institution(s) to be involved would characterize the conduct of the research." The National Commission included a long list of acceptable prison conditions. Showing its concern for justice, the commission also said that research would have to satisfy "conditions of equity" (U.S. National Commission, 1976b, p. 16).

In 1978, the DHHS published final regulations on research involving prisoners that were more restrictive than the recommendations of the National Commission. The department threw up its hands at trying to find prisons that met the commission's conditions of openness, and prohibited research on prisoners that did not benefit them as individuals or as a class ("Additional DHHS Protections," 1993).

DHHS limited research involving prisoners to (1) studies, involving no more than minimal risk or inconvenience, of the possible causes, effects, and processes of incarceration and criminal behavior; (2) studies of prisons as institutional structures, or of prisoners as incarcerated persons; (3) research on particular conditions affecting prisoners as a class; and (4) research involving a therapy likely to benefit the prisoner subject. Minimal risk was defined as risk normally encountered by non-prisoners ("Additional DHHS Protections," 1993).

The Federal Bureau of Prisons has maintained a policy that is even more restrictive. It prohibits biomedical research and drug testing on its inmates unless an individual, sick federal prisoner could benefit directly from an experimental therapy. Even then, a federal prisoner can be enrolled in a relevant clinical trial only if the responsible physician recommends it, the experiment has been approved by the DHHS, the prisoner consents, and the medical director of the Federal Bureau of Prisons approves the individual case (Federal Bureau of Prisons, 1990).

The U.S. Food and Drug Administration (FDA), which has authority over private drug companies, announced regulations in 1980 that were essentially the same as those of DHHS. But in 1981 the FDA "stayed indefinitely" its proposed regulations concerning use of prisoners. As a result, as of 1993, no regulations were in place that would prevent private drug companies from arranging with somewhat less than half the state prisons of the United States to resume using prisoners as subjects of initial drug trials (Penslar, 1993).

However, drug companies have evidently taken to heart the view expressed in the FDA's proposed regulations that sponsors of research could never establish a compelling need to use prisoners ("Protection of Human Subjects," 1981). Ethical discussion, most notably that of the National Commission, not only affected public policy. It also created a persistent moral consensus in society that prisoners should not be used in experimentation that does not specifically benefit them as individuals or as a class.

ROY BRANSON

Directly related to this article are the other articles in the entry: HEALTH-CARE ISSUES, *and* TORTURE AND THE HEALTH PROFESSIONAL. *Also directly related are the entries* RESEARCH, HUMAN: HISTORICAL ASPECTS; RESEARCH, UNETHICAL; *and* RESEARCH POLICY, *article on* RISK AND VULNERABLE GROUPS. *For a further discussion of topics mentioned in this article, see the entries* AUTONOMY; EUGENICS, *article on* HISTORICAL ASPECTS; FREEDOM AND COERCION; INFORMED CONSENT, *article on* CONSENT ISSUES IN HUMAN RESEARCH; JUSTICE; NATIONAL SOCIALISM; *and* RISK. *Other relevant material may be found under the entries* MINORITIES AS RESEARCH SUBJECTS; *and* RESEARCH BIAS. *See also the* APPENDIX (CODES, OATHS, AND DIRECTIVES RELATED TO BIOETHICS), SECTION IV: ETHICAL DIRECTIVES FOR HUMAN RESEARCH.

Bibliography

"Additional DHHS Protections Pertaining to Biomedical and Behavioral Research Involving Prisoners as Subjects." 1993. 45 *Code of Federal Regulations* 46, subpart C.

AMERICAN CIVIL LIBERTIES UNION. NATIONAL PRISON PROJECT. 1974. *Complaint before United States District Court of Maryland.* See also *Bailey v. Lally,* 481 F. Supp. 203 (D. Md. 1979).

ARNOLD, JOHN D.; MARTIN, DANIEL C.; and BOYER, SARAH E. 1970. "A Study of One Prison Population and Its Response to Medical Research." *Annals of the New York Academy of Sciences* 169, art. 2:463–470.

BEAUCHAMP, TOM L., and CHILDRESS, JAMES F. 1989. *Principles of Biomedical Ethics.* 3d ed. New York: Oxford University Press.

BEECHER, HENRY K. 1970. "The Subject: Prisoners." In his *Research and the Individual: Human Studies,* pp. 69–78. Boston: Little, Brown.

BRANSON, ROY. 1976. "Philosophical Perspectives on Experimentation with Prisoners." In *Research Involving Prisoners: Appendix to Report and Recommendations.* DHEW Publication no. (OS) 76-132. Bethesda, Md.: U.S. National Commission for the Protection of Human Subjects of Biomedical and Behavioral Research.

FADEN, RUTH R.; BEAUCHAMP, TOM L.; and KING, NANCY M. P. 1986. *A History and Theory of Informed Consent.* New York: Oxford University Press.

FEDERAL BUREAU OF PRISONS. 1990. *Health Services Manual,* Program statement 6000.3, pp. 6800–6818. Washington, D.C.: Federal Bureau of Prisons.

FEINBERG, JOEL. 1973. *Social Philosophy.* Englewood Cliffs, N.J.: Prentice-Hall.

FRIED, CHARLES. 1974. *Medical Experimentation: Personal Integrity and Social Policy.* Amsterdam: North-Holland.

GOFFMAN, ERVING. 1961. *Asylums: Essays on the Social Situation of Mental Patients and Other Inmates.* Chicago: Aldine.

KATZ, JAY, ed. 1972. *Experimentation with Human Beings: The Authority of the Investigator, Subject, Professions, and State in the Human Experimentation Process.* New York: Russell Sage.

LEVINE, ROBERT J. 1986. *Ethics and Regulation of Clinical Research.* 2d ed. New Haven, Conn.: Yale University Press.

MCCARTHY, COLLEEN M. 1989. "Experimentation on Prisoners: The Inadequacy of Voluntary Consent." *New England Journal on Criminal and Civil Confinement* 15, no. 1:55–80.

MCDONALD, JOHN C. 1967. "Why Prisoners Volunteer to Be Experimental Subjects." *Journal of the American Medical Association* 202, no. 6:511–512.

PENSLAR, ROBIN LEVIN. 1993. *Protecting Human Research Subjects: Institutional Review Board Guidebook.* 2d ed. Bethesda, Md.: National Institutes of Health, Office for Protection from Research Risks, Office of Extramural Research.

PHARMACEUTICAL MANUFACTURERS ASSOCIATION. 1976. "Survey: Use of Prisoners in Drug Testing." In *Research Involving Prisoners: Appendix to Report and Recommendations,* doc. no. 11, pp. 1–9. DHEW publication no. (OS) 76-132. Bethesda, Md.: U.S. National Commission for the Protection of Human Subjects of Biomedical and Behavioral Research.

"Protection of Human Subjects: Prisoners Used as Research Subjects: Reproposal of Regulations." 1981. *Federal Register* 46, no. 245 (December 18): 61666–61671.

ROTHMAN, DAVID J. 1971. *The Discovery of the Asylum: Social Order and Disorder in the New Republic.* Boston: Little, Brown.

U.S. NATIONAL COMMISSION FOR THE PROTECTION OF HUMAN SUBJECTS OF BIOMEDICAL AND BEHAVIORAL RESEARCH. 1976a. *Research Involving Prisoners: Appendix to Report and Recommendations.* DHEW publication no. (OS) 76-132. Bethesda, Md.: Author.

———. 1976b. *Research Involving Prisoners: Report and Recommendations.* DHEW publication no. (OS) 76-132. Bethesda, Md.: Author.

PRIVACY AND CONFIDENTIALITY IN RESEARCH

When people seek the help of health-care providers, and thus become patients, they exchange some of their privacy for the chance to be healed, diagnosed, and protected from illness. Health-care providers in turn promise to keep patients' private information confidential by sharing it only with those whose knowledge stands to benefit the patient, unless overwhelming necessity requires that the promise be broken, or the patient has consented to other uses of the information. When private information is shared not for treatment purposes but in research, the exchange is necessarily different: Research subjects are not the same as patients and researchers are not the same as persons offering treatment. The research context may alter not only what information individuals consider private and the

extent to which they are willing to share it, but also the potential harms and wrongs that may result from breaches of privacy and confidentiality.

Issues of privacy and confidentiality in human-subjects research can arise in three contexts. First, patient care can give rise to research questions, as when researchers wish to use data from patients' medical records or contact health providers for the names of patients with specific health problems to ask them to participate in research projects. Second, human subjects of biomedical, behavioral, or social-science research can be harmed or wronged in a variety of ways by the gathering or the use of information. Finally, what has been called therapeutic research or experimental treatment has its own particular risks to privacy and confidentiality, as when the media and the public claim a special interest in the first patients to receive a novel therapy. In all of these circumstances we must examine the disclosure, sharing, and publication of information, and the interests of both researcher and subject, as well as the legal, policy, and practical protections that are available to preserve subjects' privacy and the confidentiality of their private information.

Privacy, as a right belonging to persons, and confidentiality, as an attribute of data that arises from a promise made by researchers, can readily be seen as intimately related to the principles of autonomy, respect for persons, and beneficence, and to the requirement of informed consent. In the United States, federally funded research is governed by consolidated regulations for the protection of human subjects, which require that all research collecting identifiable private information about living individuals be reviewed by an institutional review board. This review must minimize the risks that research poses to subjects, determine that the risks are reasonable in relation to anticipated benefits, ensure that informed consent is obtained, and require "adequate provision to protect the privacy of subjects and to maintain the confidentiality of data." The required informed consent includes "a statement describing the extent, if any, to which confidentiality of records identifying the subject will be maintained" ("Federal Policy for the Protection of Human Subjects," 1991).

According to these regulations, if confidentiality is promised by researchers, they must be able to provide it; but confidentiality need not be promised, so long as subjects are informed that confidentiality is not offered and can freely choose to participate based on that knowledge. The "ethical baseline" thus provided by the regulations must then be supplemented by professional codes and other guidelines, as well as by existing federal, state, or local privacy laws.

Many professional codes discuss the ethics of research and scholarly publication; the attention each gives to privacy and confidentiality necessarily varies, with each such code generally combining an aspirational morality with a particularized professional focus. For example, the Council for International Organizations of Medical Sciences' (1991) "International Guidelines for Ethical Review of Epidemiological Studies" contains an extensive discussion of confidentiality protection in large data sets; the World Medical Association's "Declaration of Helsinki" (1990) includes only a statement of the importance of respecting the subject's privacy; and the Nuremberg Code (Germany [Territory Under Allied Occupation . . .], 1949), devoted to the subject's right to consent, does not mention privacy or confidentiality at all.

Becoming a research subject

Usually, research subjects are enrolled in a study after giving their informed consent to participation. However, subjects in studies in which obtaining individual consent is considered impracticable and in studies that examine information about which there is considered to be a lesser expectation of privacy (e.g., large-scale record abstraction that collects no identifying information, or studies observing public behavior) may never know that they have been the subjects of research. Violations of privacy may occur in such studies. For example, some subjects may not want researchers to read their records even though only aggregate data are recorded; and some subjects may feel wronged if they know their behavior is being observed for research purposes, even though many strangers who are not researchers observe the same behavior. However, the balance of benefits and harms is generally considered to warrant exempting such studies from the informed-consent requirements that would alert subjects to participation ("Federal Policy for Protection of Human Subjects," 1991; Capron, 1991).

The fact of study participation is generally treated as confidential information, especially when the category of subjects or the purpose of the research carries potential social stigma (e.g., studies of AIDS patients, familial mental illness, genetic disease, or drug abuse). Inclusion in the subject pool may be enough to warrant confidentiality protection for potential subjects who decline to participate. Persons approached to participate in some studies may not want others to know that they fall into a category appropriate for inclusion. Others may be concerned that their participation may signal the existence of desirable information about them to employers, insurers, treating health professionals, or other authorities, placing the confidentiality of collected data at particular risk (Melton and Gray, 1988).

Privacy and the researcher–subject relationship

Once enrolled, the subject is asked to disclose private information to a researcher. Such disclosure can take place in a variety of ways, from giving up tissue samples to answering extensive questions about personal history and psychology. The subject's judgment regarding the privacy of such information is highly dependent upon the circumstances. Someone enrolled in an addiction-control program may have little difficulty discussing alcohol consumption with health professionals in that program, but may have some hesitation about discussing it with a researcher collecting epidemiological information on the health of the person's county of residence, and even more when it is requested as part of a survey about the effects of television on perceptions about violence.

Sometimes the revealing of personal information (e.g., giving a blood sample, disclosing personal habits, recounting a past experience, or discussing physical limitations) can cause psychological or physical distress. According to federal regulations, subjects must be informed when the research may be painful or address sensitive topics. Subjects must also be informed of their rights to refuse to answer individual questions and to terminate participation in the research at any time ("Federal Policy for the Protection of Human Subjects," 1991).

Interview studies raise an additional privacy concern when the information sought concerns persons other than the subject. For example, much survey research asks questions about the habits and activities of the subject's family, household, and associates. Some questions may concern sensitive topics or disfavored or illegal conduct. Although persons other than the subject are not named, they may be identifiable through naming of the relationship to the subject. Even if they are not identifiable, they may be wronged, simply because information about them is revealed without their consent or knowledge (Capron, 1991).

A similar concern can arise when others are asked to provide information about study subjects. In long-term studies, some subjects may become decisionally incapacitated, and investigators may turn to others, perhaps family members or institutional caregivers, to provide needed data. This violation of subjects' privacy can be avoided by dropping these subjects from the study, or ameliorated by anticipating the problem and discussing with all subjects the designation of appropriate proxies should that become necessary.

The promise of confidentiality

The promise of confidentiality given by researchers to subjects extends not only to the information actually collected but also to whatever information the researcher encounters in the course of the data collection, regardless of whether that information is recorded. Thus, for example, when medical records are abstracted, information read by researchers as part of the abstraction process must be kept confidential, and information conveyed but not used in interviews similarly must not be divulged. Research projects that make use of record abstractors or interviewers generally require them to sign pledges of confidentiality promising that they will discuss no information outside the research project.

The information collected in human-subjects research needs protection not only from careless disclosure but also from intentional disclosure to those with a particular interest in the data. For example, study results may be offered as evidence in civil or criminal litigation, and both plaintiffs and defendants may seek to challenge the research by reexamining the data used or even by reinterviewing subjects. Criminal or social services authorities may seek access to study data that could inform them of ongoing violations. Health insurers may want to know whether those they insure have been tested for HIV or genetic disorders (Holder, 1986; Lansing, 1984; Yolles et al., 1986).

In order to protect subjects from court-ordered disclosure of information that puts them at risk of civil or criminal prosecution, federal certificates of confidentiality are available for human-subjects research that addresses criminal-justice questions or touches on alcohol and drug use and mental health. Certificates of confidentiality must be applied for by the investigator, and do not cover all situations in which they might be desired, but they can offer considerable protection. They preclude only the release of information that would identify specific individual research subjects and connect their identities with their data (Reatig, 1979). The concept of a researcher–subject privilege is not well established in the law, but courts that have considered requests for research data have generally required a strong showing of necessity and the deletion of all information that could lead to identification of subjects, even when the subjects' identities are a critical part of the request. Commentators have called for further attention to this problem, and for expanding the applicability of certificates of confidentiality to protect identifying information in sensitive research for which certificates are not currently available (Bayer et al., 1984; Holder, 1986; Lansing, 1984; Tribe, 1988, §15-14).

Confidential or anonymous?

One way to ensure that confidentiality is not breached is to ensure that the information collected in research is anonymous—that is, that no information is recorded that could identify subjects. Confidentiality in research is often accomplished by stripping collected data of identifying information, substituting a subject identification code, and creating a secured "linkage file" that contains information connecting the subject's name and/or other identifying information to the code. The complexities of confidentiality protection can be considerable, espe-

cially in large projects, conducted at multiple sites, that collect data on hard copy that must then be computer-encoded. Many different means of protecting confidentiality for different types of data have been devised (Schiedermayer, 1991).

Anonymous research virtually eliminates the risk of breaching confidentiality. However, anonymity may not be practicable. Researchers may wish to recontact subjects for a follow-up study, or may be conducting a long-term study that requires multiple contacts. Studies may collect health information, such as blood pressure or blood cholesterol levels, that subjects have been promised as an inducement to participation, or investigators may feel the need to inform subjects of potentially dangerous health situations that data collection may uncover. Anonymity may also be seen as a justification for not seeking participants' consent in studies that can be conducted without their knowledge (Bok, 1992).

Giving up anonymity in order to protect subjects' other interests can be highly problematic. AIDS research provides an excellent example. Because of the stigma associated with even the possibility of membership in an at-risk population and the difficulty in obtaining consents in sufficient numbers, epidemiological researchers in the United States have conducted anonymous studies of the percentage of persons testing HIV-positive in large populations in order to obtain basic information about the spread of the disease. This makes it impossible to identify persons found to test positive, so that they can be counseled and treated. In effect, it precludes offering research subjects the opportunity to become patients.

Some European researchers resist the idea of anonymous HIV studies out of a felt obligation to offer counseling and treatment to those who test positive, as well as out of concern that testing without consent is a violation of subjects' rights even when it is anonymous. As the need for full epidemiological study of the AIDS epidemic grows and the prospects for effective early therapeutic intervention also increase, the tension between public-health goals and the ethical imperatives of notification and clinical intervention is likely to increase, and to require new solutions (Bayer et al., 1990).

New uses for old data

Data-sharing problems arise when researchers seek access to previously collected information. Researchers may seek to abstract information from the medical records of both currently and formerly hospitalized patients, or to perform additional tests on samples of blood or tissue obtained for diagnostic purposes. Study subjects may be approached by other researchers, or the data collected about them may be sought for new research uses. Stored research data may even yield information that is thought to be of therapeutic usefulness, as when information collected in the course of research could identify tissue matches for a patient in need of transplantation (Benbassat and Levy, 1988; Medical Research Council, 1985; Tribe, 1988, §15-16).

Each of these cases raises one or more of several recurring problems: Is the new use one that was contemplated in the original consent? Is it one that the person would or would not be likely to find objectionable? Can the person be contacted for a new consent? If not, is proceeding without consent appropriate? If contact is necessary or desirable, does such a contact in itself constitute an unacceptable breach of confidentiality? The use of medical records for research has been addressed by asking patients at the time of hospital admission to give blanket consent to confidential or anonymous use of record data; by permitting researchers to contact patients for consent to specific uses; and by using the treating physician to screen researchers' requests. Each of these solutions provides a different balance between the burden on researchers and the wrongs, harms, and benefits to subjects (Appelbaum et al., 1984).

Where stored data have a potential therapeutic use, the situation is even more sensitive. A subject who participates in blood and tissue studies does not thereby consent to be contacted with a request to become a bone marrow donor for a specific patient. Such a contact could easily place extreme pressure on some subjects; others may want to have the opportunity to make such a donation, and may feel guilt at not having been afforded it. The temptation to compromise on privacy and confidentiality may be quite strong here. However, like the use of treatment information for research purposes, this situation can be addressed by asking research subjects whether they agree to be contacted later should a specific therapeutic need arise. The argument that the needs of the patient should outweigh the privacy interests of a potential donor has not been embraced by the courts that have heard such cases (Davis, 1983; Lansing, 1984).

Publicity, privacy, and voice in research

Publicity is most notably a problem for participants in therapeutic research and experimental treatment, such as the first recipients of organ transplants, the first patients to receive a novel treatment for AIDS, or the first patients to receive somatic-cell gene therapy. The invasions of privacy threatened by the public interest in the lives of persons suffering from exotic diseases and undergoing unprecedented treatments may constitute civil wrongs if the media cannot claim First Amendment protection (Tribe, 1988, §§12-14, 15-16). The civil right to privacy is encompassed by several distinct courses of action, including the rights of private persons to be free from intrusion upon their solitude, to keep private information from being made public, and to prevent the publication of true information that places them in a "false light" (Warren and Brandeis, 1890).

A related threat to privacy and confidentiality is posed by the growing emphasis on narrative in research and teaching. Publication of research results is permitted, in professional and international codes and regulations, either when the subject has consented or when identifying information has been deleted or altered so as to preclude identification of the subject by readers and audiences, so long as the data are not misrepresented thereby (International Committee of Medical Journal Editors, 1991).

In many circumstances, such as in ethnographic research and increasingly in medical ethics generally, it may not be possible to disguise stories adequately and still use them pedagogically (Davis, 1991). Very well-known cases cannot be disguised at all. The scholarly community and the public have learned much from widespread discussion of Baby Fae, Barney Clark, and many others, but not without costs to them and their families. And in less famous cases, even when a stripping of details is sufficient to disguise a patient-subject for a scholarly audience without misrepresenting the data, it may not be sufficient to disguise that person from family, associates, and treating health professionals who may chance to read a publication.

Finally, recognition of the patient-subject by others may not constitute the only or the greatest wrong. Recognizing oneself in a public depiction can produce shame even when no one else knows and regardless of whether the depiction is perceived to be accurate or distorted and whether the patient-subject has consented to the publication.

Some researchers address this complex problem by developing long-term collaborative relationships with subjects. Collaboration can reduce the exclusive control the researcher has over the story by including the subject's voice, but such a solution is unlikely to be helpful in many cases. As the importance of "thick description" makes the ethics of telling stories a primary issue for bioethics itself (Davis, 1991), it may be important to consider whether some stories should be learned from but be kept in confidence, so that not the stories themselves, but only their lessons, are retold.

NANCY M. P. KING

Directly related to this entry is the entry CONFIDENTIALITY. *For a further discussion of topics mentioned in this entry, see the entries* AIDS, *article on* HEALTH-CARE AND RESEARCH ISSUES; LAW AND BIOETHICS; PRIVACY IN HEALTH CARE; *and* PRIVILEGED COMMUNICATIONS. *This entry will find application in the entries* AGING AND

THE AGED, *article on* HEALTH-CARE AND RESEARCH ISSUES; CHILDREN, *article on* HEALTH-CARE AND RESEARCH ISSUES; GENETICS AND HUMAN BEHAVIOR, *article on* SCIENTIFIC AND RESEARCH ISSUES; FETUS, *article on* FETAL RESEARCH; MILITARY PERSONNEL AS RESEARCH SUBJECTS; MINORITIES AS RESEARCH SUBJECTS; MULTINATIONAL RESEARCH; PRISONERS, *article on* RESEARCH ISSUES; SEX THERAPY AND SEX RESEARCH; *and* STUDENTS AS RESEARCH SUBJECTS. *For a discussion of related ideas, see the entries on* AUTONOMY; INFORMED CONSENT, *article on* CONSENT ISSUES IN HUMAN RESEARCH; *and* TRUST. *Other relevant material may be found under the entries* RESEARCH, UNETHICAL; RESEARCH ETHICS COMMITTEES; RESEARCH METHODOLOGY; *and* RESEARCH POLICY. *See also the* APPENDIX (CODES, OATHS, AND DIRECTIVES RELATED TO BIOETHICS), SECTION IV: ETHICAL DIRECTIVES FOR HUMAN RESEARCH.

Bibliography

APPELBAUM, PAUL S.; ROTH, LOREN H.; and DETRE, THOMAS. 1984. "Researchers' Access to Patient Records: An Analysis of the Ethical Problems." *Clinical Research* 32, no. 4:399–403.

BAYER, RONALD; LEVINE, CAROL; and MURRAY, THOMAS H. 1984. "Guidelines for Confidentiality in Research on AIDS." *IRB* 6, no. 6:1–7.

BAYER, RONALD; LUMEY, L. H.; and WAN, LOURDES. 1990. "The American, British and Dutch Responses to Unlinked Anonymous HIV Seroprevalence Studies: An International Comparison." *AIDS* 4, no. 4:283–290.

BENBASSAT, JOCHANAN, and LEVY, MICHA. 1988. "Researchers' Access to Stored Medical Data: The Israeli Experience." *IRB* 10, no. 3:1–3.

BOK, SISSELA. 1992. "Informed Consent in Tests of Patient Reliability." *Journal of the American Medical Association* 267, no. 8:1118–1119.

CAPRON, ALEXANDER M. 1991. "Protection of Research Subjects: Do Special Rules Apply in Epidemiology?" *Journal of Clinical Epidemiology* 44 (suppl. 1): 81S–89S.

COUNCIL FOR INTERNATIONAL ORGANIZATIONS OF MEDICAL SCIENCES. 1991. "International Guidelines for Ethical Review of Epidemiological Studies." *Law, Medicine & Health Care* 19, nos. 3–4:247–258.

DAVIS, DENA S. 1983. "Case Study: 'Dear Mrs. X. . . .'" *IRB* 5, no. 6:6–9.

———. 1991. "Rich Cases: The Ethics of Thick Description." *Hastings Center Report* 21, no. 4:12–17.

"Federal Policy for the Protection of Human Subjects: Notices and Rules." 1991. *Federal Register* 56:117 (June 18); pp. 28001–28132. See pp. 28012–28018 for the text of the common rule adopted.

GERMANY (TERRITORY UNDER ALLIED OCCUPATION, 1945–1955: U.S. ZONE). MILITARY TRIBUNALS. 1949. "Permissible Medical Experiments." In vol. 2 of *Trials of War Criminals Before the Nuremberg Military Tribunals Under Control Council Law no. 10: Nuremberg, October 1946–1949,* pp. 181–184. Washington, D.C.: U.S. Government Printing Office.

HOLDER, ANGELA R. 1986. "The Biomedical Researcher and Subpoenas: Judicial Protection of Confidential Medical Data." *American Journal of Law and Medicine* 12:405–421.

INTERNATIONAL COMMITTEE OF MEDICAL JOURNAL EDITORS. 1991. "Statements from the International Committee of Medical Journal Editors." *Journal of the American Medical Association* 265, no. 20:2697–2698. Includes "Guidelines for the Protection of Patients' Right to Anonymity."

LANSING, PAUL. 1984. "The Conflict of Patient Privacy and the Freedom of Information Act." *Journal of Health Politics, Policy and Law* 9, no. 2:315–324.

MEDICAL RESEARCH COUNCIL. 1985. "Responsibility in the Use of Personal Medical Information for Research: Principles and Guide to Practice." *British Medical Journal* 290:1120–1124.

MELTON, GARY B., and GRAY, JONI N. 1988. "Ethical Dilemmas in AIDS Research: Individual Privacy and Public Health." *American Psychologist,* January, pp. 60–64.

REATIG, NATALIE. 1979. "Confidentiality Certificates: A Measure of Privacy Protection." *IRB* 1, no. 3:1–4, 12.

SCHIEDERMAYER, DAVID L. 1991. "Guarding Secrets and Keeping Counsel in the Computer Age," *Journal of Clinical Ethics* 2, no. 1:33–34.

TRIBE, LAURENCE H. 1988. *American Constitutional Law.* 2d ed. Mineola, N.Y.: Foundation Press.

WARREN, SAMUEL D., and BRANDEIS, LOUIS D. 1890. "The Right to Privacy." *Harvard Law Review* 4:193–220.

WORLD MEDICAL ASSOCIATION. 1990. "Declaration of Helsinki: Recommendations Guiding Physicians in Biomedical Research Involving Human Subjects." *Bulletin of the Pan American Health Organization* 24, no. 4:606–609.

YOLLES, BRYAN J.; CONNORS, JOSEPH C.; and GRUFFERMAN, SEYMOUR. 1986. "Obtaining Access to Data from Government-Sponsored Medical Research." *New England Journal of Medicine* 315, no. 26:1669–1672.

PRIVACY IN HEALTH CARE

Privacy is a complex concept with a major role in the assessment of health-care practices, policies, and law. It has become increasingly commonplace to ascribe important health-related privacy interests to individuals, families, and institutions, and then to criticize public and private sector failures to protect those interests. The word "privacy" has three major usages, corresponding to what some scholars regard as three distinct forms or conceptions of privacy: physical privacy, informational privacy, and decisional privacy. Issues relating to all three pervade health care.

Privacy and health services

Physical privacy. Under one popular usage of the term, "privacy" denotes freedom from contact with other people. The desire for limited physical accessibility—for seclusion and solitude conducive to peace of mind and intimacy—is a desire for privacy in this first sense. Members of the general public regard many social, business, and governmental contacts as privacy intrusions. These include door-to-door, street corner, telephone, and mail solicitation; some forms of sexual harassment; beeper and cordless telephone monitoring; and employers' performance, polygraph, drug, and alcohol testing. Traditional governmental practices are controversial for their threats to physical privacy, especially the use in foreign intelligence gathering and domestic surveillance of high-powered binoculars, concealed tape recorders, cameras, wiretaps, and pen registers. The loss of physical privacy is sometimes a concern when criminal-justice officials rely on body-cavity searches, prison-cell searches, and electronic monitoring of probationers; or when the police operate "checkpoints" to detect violations of curfew, seat-belt, and drunk-driving laws.

Complete physical privacy is inconsistent with the demands of modern health care. The modern delivery of health services presupposes that patients and medical professionals mutually accept nudity, touching, and observation as unavoidable aspects of examination, treatment, surgery, and hospitalization. Typical patients willingly sacrifice the desire for bodily concealment and seclusion for a chance at better health. Yet patients often expect their physicians, nurses, and other caretakers to guard assiduously against unnecessary bodily exposure or contact. The examination gowns and pajamas worn by patients respond to the expectation of privacy, as well the need for warmth.

Hospital patients—and their lawyers—have sometimes characterized unauthorized medical treatments as invasions of privacy, along with the bedside presence of inessential medical attendants, spectators, or cameras. The desire for physical privacy may lead patients who have a choice to choose single over shared hospital rooms. Because for many Americans bodily exposure to persons of the opposite sex is a more significant loss of privacy than same-sex exposures, the desire for physical privacy has led some patients to prefer physicians of their own sex. Norms of quietude surrounding hospitals reflect the sentiment that patients have heightened physical and psychological needs for solitude and peace of mind.

Informational privacy.   Under a second popular usage, "privacy" is synonymous with secrecy, confidentiality, or anonymity. It requires limits on the accessibility of personal information. The expectations of privacy surrounding health information are especially high, but not unique. Significant expectations of privacy exist also for information related to employment, education, Social Security numbers, criminal arrest, library use, video

rentals, motor vehicle registration, taxes, consumer credit, and banking.

Informational privacy concerns in the health-care setting have traditionally focused on the confidentiality of the physician–patient relationship and on limiting access to medical and insurance records (Bruce, 1988). But proposals for governmentally or institutionally mandated testing, reporting, and identification raise other informational privacy concerns. The public-health community recognizes the potential threat to privacy and other important interests posed by nonanonymous AIDS testing or reporting and mandatory medical insurance identification cards.

Informational privacy in health care is not solely a matter of safeguarding information about individuals. By virtue of genetic ties, family members may share health conditions or predispositions. Progress by researchers toward the goal of mapping and sequencing the human genome has heightened ethical concerns about possible family, as opposed to individual, privacy interests in the information coded in a person's genetic materials (Powers, 1994).

Informational privacy requires appropriate forms of secrecy, sometimes defined as intentional concealment of fact (Bok, 1981); and confidentiality, defined as selective disclosure of fact to authorized persons (Allen, 1988). In institutional settings security requires mechanisms capable of limiting access to information, such as locked office doors and file cabinets. The security of health data shared on computers may require user identification passwords and encoding. In addition to security, concern about privacy of information overlaps with concern about what are sometimes called "fair information" practices. These include maintaining accurate information in confidence. The accuracy of information contained in health, insurance, adoption, and gene-research records potentially bears on the quality of health care, and therefore holds special importance.

Decisional privacy.   Individuals, families, and domestic partners typically define some decisions as personal decisions and certain conduct as intimate conduct. Under its third usage, "privacy" denotes autonomous choices about the personal and intimate matters that constitute private lives. Decisional "privacy" signifies the ability to make one's own decisions and to act on those decisions, free from governmental or other unwanted interference. Decisional privacy concerns in the health context relate to responsibility for important decisions about treatment, the termination of treatment, and the allocation of scarce medical resources. Legal and ethical disagreements about who has the "right to decide" or the "right to choose" sometimes have turned collaborating patients, physicians, nurses, hospitals, families, researchers, and lawmakers into competitors and litigants.

In the United States, conceptions of decisional privacy have come to dominate discussions of government regulation of abortion and the treatment of patients who are severely disabled, terminally ill, or in a persistent vegetative state. In the context of so-called surrogate motherhood, privacy for infertile couples has meant the freedom to make legally enforceable agreements to procreate with the assistance of third parties. Gay men and lesbians invoke the ideal of privacy in their quest for the freedom to engage in consensual adult sexual relationships and marriage, free from the fear of criminal prosecution and legally sanctioned discrimination. Parents sometimes invoke "family privacy" to mean the freedom of heads of households to decide how those for whom they are responsible will be reared, educated, and medically assisted. Invocations to respect privacy accompany defenses of limited government and autonomous decision making respecting heterosexual sex, contraception, midwifery, women's prenatal conduct, use of experimental medical remedies, psychotropic drug therapy, organ sales and transplants, hunger striking, prostitution, and pornography.

Theories about privacy

Definitions of privacy. Privacy was once a neglected subject. However, theorists have begun to debate how precisely to define, value, and protect privacy (Schoeman, 1992; Inness, 1992; Wacks, 1989; Allen, 1988). Although many acknowledge that privacy is used in distinguishable physical, informational, and decisional senses, no single definition of privacy in any of its senses has gained universal acceptance. Nor has any theory of the value of privacy gained universal acceptance.

Scholars disagree about how to approach defining privacy (Allen, 1988). Some say privacy should be defined as a value or moral claim (Inness, 1992), others as a fact or a legal right (Gavison, 1980). Some say definitions of privacy should prescribe ideal uses of the term (Gavison, 1980), others that definitions should describe actual usage (Allen, 1988). Debates over the definition of privacy may seem arcane. Yet, the outcome of the debates bears importantly on the framing of ethical and legal issues raised by health care. For example, some theorists contend that the popular privacy arguments for abortion rights are unsound because they confuse privacy with liberty, autonomy, or freedom.

Proposed definitions of privacy range from the very expansive "being let alone," popularized by Samuel Warren and Louis Brandeis (1890), to Alan F. Westin's more specific "claim of individuals, groups or institutions to determine for themselves when, how, and to what extent information about them is communicated to others" (Westin, 1967, p. 7). Many definitions characterize privacy in its physical and informational senses as denoting conditions of restricted access to persons, their mental

states, or information about them (Allen, 1988). According to Ruth Gavison, "[i]n perfect privacy no one has information about X, no one pays attention to X, and no one has physical access to X" (Gavison, 1980, p. 428). So conceived, privacy functions as an umbrella concept, encompassing a family of concepts each of which denotes a form of limited access to others. There is disagreement about the composition of the privacy family's membership list. However, the list arguably includes seclusion, solitude, anonymity, confidentiality, modesty, intimacy, reserve, and secrecy.

The debate over the relationship between the concepts of privacy and secrecy exemplifies the bewildering extent of disagreement about how to define privacy and related concepts. Although some scholars view secrecy as a form of privacy, others view privacy as a form of secrecy (Friedrich, 1971). Still others view them as distinct concepts. Sissela Bok (1984) urges that privacy and secrecy are wholly distinct concepts—the former referring to limited physical and information access, the latter to intentional concealment of information.

A number of definitions of privacy instead emphasize control, whether control over information or control over avenues of observation and physical contact (Fried, 1968; Westin, 1967). In our media-saturated and government bureaucracy-dependent society, it is perhaps unsurprising that one scholar has suggested we think of privacy as the possession of undocumented information (Parent, 1983a, 1983b). Other legal and moral theorists stress privacy as a social practice with normative functions (Inness, 1992). Jeffrey Reiman links privacy to the formation of individuality and personhood: "Privacy is a social ritual by means of which an individual's moral title to his own existence is conferred" (Reiman, 1976, p. 39).

The decisional privacy controversy. Perhaps the greatest source of definitional disagreement surrounding the concept of privacy has related to the decisional usage of privacy. Decisional privacy has been defined as control over intimate aspects of personal identity. In our society, aspects of the human body, sex, reproduction, marriage, and family are generally considered as numbering among the intimacies of personal identity. The U.S. Supreme Court popularized the decisional usage of privacy in the 1960s and 1970s by characterizing laws restricting birth control, abortion, marriage, and parental authority as burdening the right to privacy. Decisional privacy rights in the law presuppose a private sphere of conduct immune from state or federal regulation. Some scholars emphasize the ideal of privacy as the ideal of limited government (Rubenfeld, 1989).

Many theorists insist that privacy in the decisional sense is not properly understood as a sense of privacy at all (Gavison, 1980; Parent, 1983; McCloskey, 1980; Ely, 1973). They raise several arguments. First, they argue, as an aspect of liberty, freedom, or autonomy, decisional privacy stands apart from paradigmatic forms of privacy, such as seclusion, solitude, and anonymity. Second, we lose our ability to treat privacy and liberty as distinct concepts if we speak of "decisional" privacy. Confused, ambiguous uses of the concept of privacy in the U.S. Supreme Court's first contraception and abortion cases helped to raise this widespread objection.

Defenders of the decisional usage of the term "privacy" counter that decisional privacy is worthy of the name (DeCew, 1987). They emphasize that although decisional privacy denotes aspects of liberty, freedom, and autonomy, it denotes aspects of these that pertain to deeply felt conceptions of a private life beyond legitimate social involvement. Controversial or not, using "privacy" to denote a domain outside of legitimate social concern is now an entrenched practice in the United States.

The public and the private in political thought.   Linkage with the Graeco-Roman heritage of Western law and political theory may provide a degree of historic and etymological validity to the controversial practice of referring to freedom from interference with personal life as "privacy." The decisional usage of "privacy" has origins in classical antiquity's distinction between private and public spheres.

The Greeks distinguished the "public" sphere of the polis, or city-state, from the "private" sphere of the *oikos*, or household. The Romans similarly distinguished *res publicae*, concerns of the community, from *res privatae*, concerns of individuals and families. The ancients celebrated the public sphere as the sphere of political freedom for citizens. The public realm was the sector in which select men—free men with property whose economic virtue had earned them citizenship and the right to participate in collective governance—could truly flourish. By contrast, the private realm was the sector of mundane economic and biologic necessity. Wives, children, and slaves populated the private economic sphere, living as subordinates and ancillaries to autonomous male caretakers.

The post-Enlightenment Western liberal tradition inherited the premise that social life ought to be organized into public and private spheres (Arendt, 1958; Habermas, 1989). It also inherited the premise that the private sphere is properly constituted by the home, the family, and intimate association. However, while ancient thought tolerated the private and celebrated the public, modern liberal thought often reflects an opposing tendency: It tolerates the public as pervasive and necessary for collective welfare, but celebrates the private as an essential expression of personal identity, freedom, and responsibility.

The political concept of a limited, tolerant government—elaborated by John Locke and Thomas Jefferson as a requirement of natural rights, and by John Stuart Mill and Adam Smith as a requirement of utility—entails a nongovernmental, private sphere of autonomous individuals, families, and voluntary associations. Mill emphasized the importance of government tolerance, arguing that government is not well situated to assess the utility of "self-regarding" acts that potentially harm only the actors themselves. Self-regarding conduct "neither violates any specific duty to the public, nor occasions any perceptible hurt to any assignable individual except himself" (Mill, 1978, p. 80). It is, in other words, conduct that is restricted to an individual's own body and property and that may offend others but imposes no risk of significant harm on others. The contractarian political tradition of American democratic liberalism requires tolerance for religious minorities, political dissenters, and unpopular lifestyles. The ideal of tolerance is arguably the ultimate foundation of the case for sexual privacy for homosexuals and women seeking abortions (Richards, 1986).

The ideal of a private sphere free of government and other outside interference has currency, despite the reality that in the United States and other Western democracies, virtually every aspect of nominally private life is a focus of direct or indirect government regulation. Marriage is considered a private relationship, yet governments require licenses and medical tests, impose age limits, and prohibit polygamous, incestuous, and same-sex marriages. Procreation and childrearing are considered private, but government child-abuse and neglect laws regulate, if at times inadequately, how parents, and possibly even pregnant women, must exercise their responsibilities. The ideal of a private sphere can be no more than an ideal of the ability of ordinary citizens to make choices that are relatively free of the most direct forms of governmental interference and constraint.

The worthiness of this ideal has been called to question in the United States, where problems of domestic violence suggest a need for more rather than less involvement in the traditionally "private" spheres of home and family life (MacKinnon, 1991). In addition, the ideal of a private sphere has been the ideal of a sphere of negative as opposed to positive freedom. The right to privacy in the context of contraception and abortion has meant a negative right against government decision making respecting procreation, not a positive right to governmental programs designed to make contraception and abortion services available to those who cannot afford to pay. Critics blame the emphasis on privacy and negative freedom for the failure of legal efforts to secure government funding of abortions for women who are poor.

Ethical values.   Physical and informational privacy practices serve to limit observation and disclosure deemed inimical to well-being. Psychologists have long emphasized the unhealthful effects of depriving individuals of opportunities for socially defined modes of privacy (Schneider, 1977). Many philosophers maintain that respecting physical, informational, and decisional privacy is paramount for respect for human dignity and personhood, moral autonomy, and workable community life (Schoeman, 1992; Allen, 1988; Kupfer, 1987; DeCew, 1986; Feinberg, 1983; Benn, 1971). Lawyers view the moral value of privacy as the basis of moral rights deserving legal protection (Greenawalt, 1974; Fried, 1970; Westin, 1967).

Scholarly disagreement about how best to characterize the ethical value of privacy is fundamental (Inness, 1992). One axis of disagreement concerns whether "privacy" denotes a value or a state of affairs. A second axis of disagreement concerns whether "privacy," presumed to denote a state of affairs, refers to a state of affairs with necessary moral legitimacy or merely contingent moral legitimacy. A third axis of disagreement concerns whether the value of privacy, presumed to denote a state of affairs with only contingent moral legitimacy, should be measured against relevant consequentialist criteria, such as promoting aggregate happiness or efficiency; or deontological criteria, such as respect for personhood, personal identity, or humanity.

From the consequentialist perspective, privacy has value to the extent that it is useful in promoting, for example, aggregate happiness or the diverse interests of individuals, groups, or government. In this vein, scholars commonly argue that privacy has value because it functions to create or enhance human personhood in ways that promote liberal social and political institutions. Privacy practices promote individuality and the formation of self-concept presupposed by democratic self-government. Some accounts stress the utilitarian value to society of restraining government power in the spheres of what John Stuart Mill called "self-regarding" actions (Mill, 1978, p. 80).

Scholars also argue that privacy has instrumental value relative to its role in creating and enhancing relationships. The traditional argument is that only in isolation from others can desirable forms of intimacy and friendship flourish; only if individuals and families can seclude themselves from others, can the potentially stifling and emotionally explosive social demands of group life be abated. In reply, it is argued that privacy practices have facilitated both the mistreatment of women and children, and the disregard for the ideal of aggregate as opposed to individual responsibility. The ethical challenge posed by these criticisms is to describe social arrangements that vigorously protect states of physical and informational privacy in the name of individuality, creativity, family, and free association, but that avoid the subordination and alienation often associated with modern Western liberal societies.

Scholars sometimes explain what they regard as the value of privacy by reference to the importance of personhood and personal dignity to individuals. These arguments draw connections between limited physical and informational access and/or the ability to make important decisions for oneself and the very idea of rational moral autonomy. Stanley Benn argued, for example, that the principle of respect for persons provides a moral reason for not interfering with personal privacy (Benn, 1971). David A. J. Richards argued by appeal to the "social contract" metaphor, for legal privacy protections, stressing the fundamental value of government toleration of the choices individuals make for themselves pertaining to procreation, sexuality, and religion (Richards, 1986).

Privacy in the United States

Cultural and historical dimensions. Focusing on physical and informational privacy, anthropologist Barrington Moore observed that both the desire for privacy and the ability to satisfy it are unequally distributed among and within human societies (Moore, 1984). Although some cultures do not emphasize privacy at all, privacy protection practices are found in virtually every human culture (Moore, 1984; Altman, 1977; Westin, 1967). Strikingly, what is treated as private can vary significantly from society to society (Pennock and Chapman, 1971). In one culture, defecation and sexual intercourse may be performed openly without embarrassment or shame; in another they are deeply private. One culture shields religious rites in secrecy, while another performs them on the commons. Female breasts and breast feeding require concealment for modesty's sake in one place, but not another. Nuclear family problems are personal information in one society, but are freely shared with leaders of one's tribe or village elsewhere.

The protection of personal privacy is among the most important public issues in the Western nations of the world (Flaherty, 1989). These nations have in common large, well-developed bureaucracies and advanced information technologies (Bennett, 1992). Categories of data western Europeans and North Americans deem personal include health information, criminal convictions, disciplinary measures, religious beliefs, political opinions, racial origin, trade union membership, sexual life, and intimate private life (Nugter, 1990).

U.S. culture is dominated by widely shared aspirations for lifestyles that afford frequent opportunities for privacy and intimacy. Although the "taste" for privacy is strong in the United States, it competes with the principle of a "public right to know" reflected in the practices of government and the media. Commercial, professional, and personal relationships of many kinds presuppose a high degree of self-disclosure and physical contact. As a consequence, the United States is not a country in which expectations of physical or informational privacy are easily satisfied.

American culture was not always dominated by articulated concern for privacy. Nor have deeply private lifestyles often been the norm. The Colonial lifestyle "left little room for privacy or nonconformity even among the free and the affluent" (Flaherty, 1972, p. 172). Concerns for physical and informational privacy achieved prominence as public issues for the first time in the nineteenth century, when a sharp increase in technology and industrialization had begun to transform the agrarian and mercantile culture to one of urban capitalism, and when the courts and legislatures began expressly to regulate marriage and family life (Garrow, 1994).

According to Alan Westin, nuclear family lifestyles, mobility in work and residence, and the decline of religious authority meant "greater situations of physical and psychological privacy" for mid- and late-nineteenth-century Americans (Westin, 1967, p. 21). However, at about the same time that some middle-class and wealthy Americans were enjoying more privacy than ever before, a number of factors appear to have increased Americans' privacy-related anxieties. The simultaneous growth of crowded cities, the closing of the western frontier, the invention of commercial photography, and the rise of mass circulation newspapers may explain the emergence during the late nineteenth century of public concern about lost privacy (Allen and Mack, 1990; Copple, 1989).

The development in the early twentieth century of a social welfare bureaucracy and surveillance technologies may have further increased concerns about privacy. Indeed, the Supreme Court's first pronouncement about the right to privacy came in a dissenting opinion in *Olmstead* v. *United States* (1928), a case that validated telephonic eavesdropping by government. But the development of powerful computers capable of storing personal data appears to have spawned another, larger wave of concern about privacy in the 1960s and 1970s, the decades of origin for many of the major federal privacy laws currently on the books (Miller, 1971; Turkington et al., 1992). Finally, the rhetorical success of legal claims based on the "right to privacy" after 1965 in Supreme Court contraception and abortion cases spawned additional interest in fending off interference with choices people make respecting their bodies, health care, families, and lifestyles.

Legal dimensions.   Near ubiquitous recognition of the importance of privacy is suggested by the language of key international human-rights documents. Privacy is mentioned, for example, in the Universal Declaration of Human Rights, adopted by the United Nations General Assembly in 1948. Article 12 provides that "No one shall be subjected to arbitrary interference with his pri-

vacy, family, home, or correspondence, nor to attacks upon his honor and reputation" and that "Everyone has the right to the protection of the law against such interference or attacks" (Henkin et al., 1987, p. 144). In fact, the law of most modern legal systems prohibits, at least officially, physical privacy invasions and assaults on honor of the sort identified by Article 12. Western nations typically regulate several forms of physical, informational, and decisional privacy. Access to health-related information is limited by statute in most industrialized nations and the European Economic Community (Nugter, 1990).

Great Britain and the United States share a common legal heritage and protect many of the same forms of privacy. Yet courts and legislatures in the United States have been more willing than their English counterparts to multiply the number of express privacy protections. The reasons for this difference are unclear, although one explanation may be greater concerns in Britain about creating rights of uncertain application (Wacks, 1989). In the United States privacy interests are protected, often expressly, by tort law, the Constitution, and numerous federal and state statutes.

Tort law.   The first privacy rights to be recognized expressly in United States law were rights of physical and informational privacy. The express right to privacy first came into existence through the common-law process of judicial recognition. Endorsed by Samuel Warren and Louis Brandeis in a famous 1890 *Harvard Law Review* article stressing the importance of freedom from unwanted publicity, the invasion of privacy tort was officially adopted by the Georgia Supreme Court in *Pavesich* v. *New England Life Insurance Company* (1905). Many other state courts eventually followed suit.

By 1960, William Prosser could identify, not one, but four common-law privacy rights recognized by courts in the United States (Prosser, 1960). Today, most states have adopted one or more of Prosser's four privacy rights through their courts or legislatures. The influential *Restatement of the Law Second: Torts 2d* (American Law Institute, 1986), a summary and exposition of developments in personal injury law, embraced Prosser's analysis. In states that have adopted Prosser's analysis, a person may bring a privacy-invasion lawsuit claiming highly offensive conduct consisting of either (1) interference with seclusion, solitude, and anonymity; (2) publication of embarrassing private facts; (3) publicity placing a person in a false light; or (4) appropriation of name, likeness, or identity. In addition, most states permit privacy-invasion-related claims involving unauthorized publicity; breach of confidence or secrecy; and unfair business practices involving misappropriation, trade secret, trade name, and copyright violations. Plaintiffs have alleged invasion of privacy in cases related to health services. An Oregon physician was sued for disclosing the identity of an adult adoptee's birth mother. A New Yorker whose photograph appeared in a newspaper accompanying a story about an AIDS treatment facility sued the publisher.

Constitutional law.   Although the Constitution makes no express mention of the term "privacy" itself, the constitutional law of the United States protects physical, informational, and decisional privacy interests. The First Amendment, the guarantor of freedom of speech and association, protects the physical and informational privacy concerns of exclusive clubs or political groups. In effect, the Supreme Court has held that the Fourth Amendment guarantees a right of physical privacy when it limits warrantless search and seizure, and that the Fifth Amendment guarantees a right of informational privacy when it limits compulsory disclosure and self-incrimination. Although the Supreme Court has never held as much, some judges and lawyers maintain that the Ninth Amendment, which provides that the "enumeration in the Constitution, of certain rights, shall not be construed to deny or disparage others retained by the people," implies decisional privacy rights. The Supreme Court has established First and Fourteenth Amendment limits on government recordkeeping and access to personal information. In *Whalen* v. *Roe* (1977), a major Supreme Court case involving a data bank of prescription drug users maintained by New York officials, the Court held that the First and Fourteenth Amendments require states seeking to deter drug abuse to implement confidentiality safeguards.

The U.S. Supreme Court and many lower courts have held that the Constitution protects decisional privacy respecting aspects of health, reproduction, sex, and family life, deriving this brand of privacy from the "penumbra" of the Bill of Rights and the Fourteenth Amendment. The Fourteenth Amendment, which provides that no state may deprive a person of liberty without due process, is the most frequently cited basis of the decisional privacy right protecting autonomous decision making respecting contraception, abortion, and the termination of medical treatment. *Griswold* v. *Connecticut* (1965) and *Roe* v. *Wade* (1973) established the right to contraception and abortion. The privacy doctrine that originated in the *Griswold* and *Roe* cases has come under repeated attack from critics who stress the absence of a textual basis for reproductive privacy rights. Some critics have urged that gender equality and equal protection of the laws, rather than privacy and liberty, are the core values served by reproductive rights.

In *Planned Parenthood* v. *Casey* (1992), the Supreme Court affirmed the essential holding of *Roe* v. *Wade*, reiterating the Fourteenth Amendment as protection for reproductive privacy. However, the Court backed away from *Griswold*'s and *Roe*'s characterization of the right to privacy as a "fundamental" right that cannot be breached except where there is a truly "compelling" governmental interest. *Cruzan* v. *Missouri Dept. of Public Health* (1990) recognized an adult patient's privacy right—not her parents'—to terminate life-sustaining medical treatment. Yet *Cruzan* and *Casey* applied weaker standards of review than *Roe* v. *Wade*. Abortion restrictions "rationally related" to a "legitimate state interest" that do not "unduly burden" the woman's constitutional right to privacy are valid. And restrictions on the right to refuse treatment that reasonably relate to a legitimate state interest are also valid.

Statutory law.   The U.S. Congress enacted a number of federal statutes after 1970 to protect informational and physical privacy interests. The Privacy Act (1974), the Freedom of Information Act (1974), the Family and Educational Privacy Act (1974), the Right to Financial Privacy Act (1978), and the Electronic Communications Privacy Act (1986) protect information privacy by limiting access to personal information held in government, school, and bank records. The federal Employee Polygraph Protection Act protects workers from potentially incriminating self-disclosure in the workplace by limiting use of the "lie-detector" test. Other federal statutes protect against intrusive searches utilizing electronic surveillance, wiretapping, and other unauthorized access to telephones or computers. A proposed federal Human Genome Privacy Act limits access to genetic information about individuals. A proposed Fair Health Information Practices Act of 1994 requires the maintenance of confidentiality and security of health-related information.

State statutes in virtually every state address concerns about the privacy of information related to medical care, criminal histories, and adoption. Newer state statutory regulations include the decisional privacy protections of Virginia's Natural Death Act, and Pennsylvania's Confidentiality of HIV-Related Information statute. Recently, state constitutions in Montana, California, and Florida have been amended or interpreted to require physical, informational, and decisional privacy protections. For example, in a pre-*Casey* decision, the Florida high court held that the state constitution protects decisional privacy to the same degree as *Roe* v. *Wade*.

Patients' privacy rights.   One of the most important areas of health law is the broad field of patients' rights. Discussions of patients' rights include the physical, informational, and decisional privacy rights recognized under tort, constitutional, and statutory law.

The oldest American legal case decided by reference to rights of privacy, *DeMay* v. *Roberts* (1881), vindicated interests in physical privacy and modesty. A Michigan husband and wife successfully sued a physician who permitted an "unprofessional young, unmarried man" to enter their home and help deliver their baby. A century later a married couple in Maine brought *Knight* v. *Penobscot Bay Medical Center* (1980), a similar, though unsuccessful, lawsuit claiming that a hospital violated their privacy by permitting a layperson, the spouse of a nurse, to observe delivery of their child through a glass partition from a distance of twelve feet. The issue of whether women should be able to choose who is present at the birth of their children—including whether delivery is undertaken with the aid of a midwife, nurse practitioner, or physician—is clearly both a physical and a decisional privacy issue.

All patients generally may share the obstetrical patient's sense that adequate privacy is lacking in hospitals where well-intentioned medical, administrative, and support staff move freely in and out of (even nominally "private") in-patient wards. The feeling that one's privacy has been invaded may be especially acute in busy, crowded public hospitals serving low-income patients, or in any hospital where groups of several physicians, interns, and medical students simultaneously conduct physical examinations and discussions at one's bedside. Some men and women report feeling their privacy invaded by having to share a room in an intensive-care unit with a person of the opposite sex. The law is unclear about the extent to which medical resources or the general written consent to treatment patients give upon admission to hospitals eliminates legitimate expectations of physical and informational privacy. Specific waivers of legal privacy claims may give patients clear notice of the privacy losses associated with treatment in teaching and research hospitals, but arguably do not eliminate hospitals' ethical obligations to respect privacy to the extent possible.

Moral outrage over the discovery that health-care providers have recorded, filmed, or photographed a patient for scholarly or research purposes sometimes, though infrequently, results in litigation. Respect for privacy would appear to dictate obtaining prior consent to the publication of graphic images of a person, particularly if the person is identifiable in an image or is named in connection with its publication.

The legal importance of obtaining prior informed consent was underscored by the holding of the California court in the highly publicized case, *Moore* v. *Regents of University of California* (1990). John Moore brought a multimillion dollar lawsuit when he discovered that University of California medical researchers who treated him for hairy-cell leukemia had failed to disclose that "certain blood products and blood components were of great value in a number of commercial and scientific efforts." Moore's right to privacy claims were based on the notion that exploitation of his blood for commercial purposes was a highly offensive appropriation of a person's name, likeness, or identity compensable as an invasion of privacy under state tort law.

The court threw out Moore's privacy claims on the ground that the researchers did not appropriate Moore's likeness or identity in a sense recognized by law. Typical cases of the sort Moore cited as precedents involved appropriation of photographic images of a person's face or the use of a person's distinctive name or voice in product advertising. Although Moore lost his privacy battle, the court held he could validly assert claims of breach of fiduciary duty and lack of informed consent. According to the California court, a patient has a right to know the medical purpose of treatment and the treating physician's personal economic stake; otherwise treatment is battery, presumably no better than sterilizing a fertile woman or performing a cesarean section on a cancer patient without her consent.

As noted earlier, abortion and euthanasia are approached in the United States as patient privacy issues. Opponents of laws prohibiting abortions say that state and federal regulations should not prevent women from acting on their own decisions about whether to terminate pregnancy through medical abortion. On the other hand, it is also argued on privacy grounds that women should not be forced or counseled to abort for any reason, including where they are seropositive for the virus that causes AIDS. "Privacy" can signify freedom to choose the circumstances of death for oneself, a family member, or an intimate friend. It means the absence of criminal laws and bureaucratic procedures that constrain the choice to accelerate the death of a person who is terminally ill or to refuse artificial nutrition and hydration to preserve life in a person in a persistent vegetative state. The right to privacy may also prove to be the ethical refuge of supporters of physician-assisted suicide of nonterminally ill, fully competent adults.

The privacy implications of nonvoluntary and routine AIDS testing of obstetrical patients, surgical patients, and newborns have been of great interest to public authorities and private health-care providers for two reasons. First, nonconsensual testing is a prima facie denial of decisional privacy or autonomy. Some individuals prefer not to be tested and forced to confront the specter of terminal illness. And while this precise concern has never applied to newborns, newborn testing can reveal the HIV status of birth mothers. Second, where the confidentiality of an HIV- or AIDS-infected person is breached by medical or insurance providers, far-ranging implications for private lives and employment can follow due to prejudice and discrimination. In this context, policy analysts often assert that the individual interest in privacy is outweighed by societal interests, including the societal interest in controlling the spread of deadly disease through inappropriate handling of contaminated blood and other tissues. But societal interests do not always outweigh individual privacy rights.

The federal courts have upheld the mandatory AIDS-testing policies of the United States military and the nation's prisons. However, in *Glover* v. *Eastern Nebraska Community Office of Retardation* (1989), a federal court struck down a state requirement that all persons working closely with mentally retarded clients disclose their HIV and hepatitis B status, and undergo periodic HIV and hepatitis B blood testing. Against the argument that persons working in highly regulated state agencies have lower expectations of privacy, the court stressed that constitutional values do not permit mandatory testing where the risk of disease transmission is extremely low. A similar weighing of the costs of testing against its benefits in view of the low risk of transmission may explain government reluctance to mandate AIDS testing for all dentists, physicians, and other health-care providers who come in close contact with patients.

Conclusion

Privacy is likely to have an important role in bioethical discussions for some time. The English political philosopher James Fitzjames Stephens wrote in 1873 that "conduct which can be described as indecent is always in one way or another a violation of privacy" (Stephens, 1873, p. 160). These words capture a truth about the broad usage the term "privacy" enjoys in the health field. Patients and those who care about them consider a diverse spectrum of "indecencies," ranging from maltreatment and breach of confidentiality to interference with decision making, as "invasions of privacy." Accordingly, the ethics, law, and politics of privacy have made what may be an indelible mark on the future of health care and health research.

ANITA L. ALLEN

Directly related to this entry are the entries CONFIDENTIALITY; PRIVACY AND CONFIDENTIALITY IN RESEARCH; PRIVILEGED COMMUNICATIONS; RIGHTS, *article on* RIGHTS IN BIOETHICS; *and* PROFESSIONAL–PATIENT RELATIONSHIP, *article on* ETHICAL ISSUES. *For a further discussion of topics mentioned in this entry, see the entries* ABORTION, *section on* CONTEMPORARY AND LEGAL ASPECTS; AIDS; AUTONOMY; BIOETHICS AND LAW; DEATH AND DYING: EUTHANASIA AND SUSTAINING LIFE; ETHICS, *article on* NORMATIVE ETHICAL THEORIES; FIDELITY AND LOYALTY; MORALITY AND LAW; REPRODUCTIVE TECHNOLOGY, *articles on* ETHICAL ISSUES, *and* LEGAL AND REGULATORY ISSUES; *and* TRUST. *This entry will find application in the entries* FERTILITY CONTROL, *article on* ETHICAL ISSUES; GENETIC COUNSELING; HEALTH SCREENING AND TESTING IN THE PUBLIC-HEALTH CONTEXT; LIFESTYLES AND PUBLIC HEALTH; *and* MEDICAL INFORMATION SYSTEMS. *Other relevant material may be found under the entries* CLINICAL ETHICS, *article on* ELEMENTS AND METHODOLOGIES; HEALTH OFFICIALS AND THEIR RESPONSIBILITIES; *and* MEDICAL CODES AND OATHS. *See also the* APPENDIX (CODES, OATHS, AND DIRECTIVES RELATED TO BIOETHICS), SECTION II: ETHICAL DIRECTIVES FOR THE PRACTICE OF MEDICINE, *and* SECTION III: ETHICAL DIRECTIVES FOR OTHER HEALTH-CARE PROFESSIONS.

Bibliography

ALLEN, ANITA L. 1988. *Uneasy Access: Privacy for Women in a Free Society.* Totowa, N.J.: Rowman and Littlefield.

ALLEN, ANITA L., and MACK, ERIN. 1990. "How Privacy Got Its Gender." *Northern Illinois University Law Review* 10, no. 3:441–478.

ALTMAN, IRWIN. 1977. "Privacy Regulation: Culturally Universal or Culturally Specific?" *Journal of Social Issues* 33, no. 3:66–74.

AMERICAN LAW INSTITUTE. 1986. *Restatement of the Law Second: Torts 2d.* Chap. 28 A, sections 652 B, C, D, & E. St. Paul, Minn.: Author.

ARENDT, HANNAH. 1958. *The Human Condition.* Chicago: University of Chicago Press.

BENN, STANLEY I. 1971. "Privacy, Freedom and Respect for Persons." In *Privacy: Nomos XIII*, pp. 1–26. Edited by J. Roland Pennock and John W. Chapman. New York: Atherton Press.

BENNETT, COLIN, J. 1992. *Regulating Privacy: Data Protection and Public Policy in Europe and the United States.* Ithaca, N.Y.: Cornell University Press.

BLOUSTEIN, EDWARD J. 1978. *Individual and Group Privacy.* New Brunswick, N.J.: Transaction Books.

BOK, SISSELA. 1984. *Secrets: On the Ethics of Concealment and Revelation.* Oxford: Oxford University Press.

BOONE, C. KEITH. 1983. "Privacy and Community." *Social Theory and Practice* 9, no. 1:1–30.

BRANDEIS, LOUIS, and WARREN, SAMUEL. 1890. "The Right to Privacy." *Harvard Law Review* 4:193–220.

BRUCE, JO ANNE CZECOWSKI. 1988. *Privacy and Confidentiality of Health Care Information.* 2d ed. Chicago: American Hospital Publishing.

COPPLE, ROBERT F. 1989. "Privacy and the Frontier Thesis: An American Intersection of Self and Society." *American Journal of Jurisprudence* 34:87–131.

Cruzan v. *Missouri Dept. of Public Health.* 1990. 497 U.S. 261.

DECEW, JUDITH WAGNER. 1986. "The Scope of Privacy in Law and Ethics." *Law and Philosophy* 5:145–173.

———. 1987. "Defending the 'Private' in Constitutional Privacy." *Journal of Value Inquiry* 21:171–184.

DeMay v. *Roberts.* 1881. 46 Mich. 160, 9 N.W. 146.

ELY, JOHN HART. 1973. "The Wages of Crying Wolf: A Comment on *Roe* v. *Wade*." *Yale Law Journal* 89:920–949.

FEINBERG, JOEL. 1983. "Autonomy, Sovereignty, and Privacy: Moral Ideals and the Constitution?" *Notre Dame Law Review* 58:445–492.

FLAHERTY, DAVID H. 1972. *Privacy in Colonial New England.* Charlottesville: University Press of Virginia.

———. 1989. *Protecting Privacy in Surveillance Societies: The Federal Republic of Germany, Sweden, France, Canada, and the United States.* Chapel Hill: University of North Carolina Press.

FRIED, CHARLES. 1968. "Privacy." *Yale Law Journal* 77:475–493.

FRIEDRICH, CARL. 1971. "Secrecy Versus Privacy: The Democratic Dilemma." In *Privacy: Nomos XIII*, pp. 105–120. Edited by J. Roland Pennock and John W. Chapman. New York: Atherton.

GARROW, DAVID J. 1994. *Liberty and Sexuality: The Right to Privacy and the Making of Roe v. Wade*. New York: Macmillan.

GAVISON, RUTH. 1980. "Privacy and the Limits of Law." *Yale Law Journal* 89, no. 3:421–471.

GERSTEIN, ROBERT S. 1978. "Intimacy and Privacy." *Ethics* 89:76–81.

Glover v. Eastern Nebraska Community Office of Retardation. 1989. 867 F. 2d 461.

GREENAWALT, KENT. 1974. "Privacy and Its Legal Protection." *Hastings Center Studies* 2, no. 3:45–68.

Griswold v. Connecticut. 1965. 381 U.S. 479. 85 S.Ct. 1678.

HABERMAS, JURGEN. 1989. *The Structural Transformation of the Public Sphere: An Inquiry into a Category of Bourgeois Society*. Translated by Thomas Burger. Cambridge, Mass.: MIT Press.

HENKIN, LOUIS; PUGH, RICHARD; SCHACHTER, OSCAR; and SMIT, HANS. 1987. *Basic Documents Supplement to International Law: Cases and Materials*, p. 383. St. Paul: Minn.: West Publishing.

INNESS, JULIE C. 1992. *Privacy, Intimacy and Isolation*. New York: Oxford University Press.

Knight v. Penobscot Bay Medical Center. 1980. 420 A.2d 915.

KUPFER, JOSEPH. 1987. "Privacy, Autonomy, and Self-Concept." *American Philosophical Quarterly* 24, no. 1:81–89.

MACKINNON, CATHERINE A. 1991. "Reflections on Sex Equality Under the Law." *Yale Law Journal* 100, no. 5:1281–1328.

MCCLOSKEY, H. J. 1980. "Privacy and the Right to Privacy." *Philosophy* 55:17–38.

MILL, JOHN STUART. 1978. *On Liberty*. Edited by Elizabeth Rapaport. Indianapolis: Hackett.

MILLER, ARTHUR R. 1971. *The Assault on Privacy: Computers, Data Banks and Dossiers*. Ann Arbor: University of Michigan Press.

MOORE, BARRINGTON. 1984. *Privacy: Studies in Social and Cultural History*. Armonk, N.Y.: M. E. Sharpe.

Moore v. Regents of University of California. 1990. 51 Cal.3d 120, 271 Cal. Rpt. 146, 793 P.2d 479.

NUGTER, A. C. M. 1990. *Transborder Flow of Personal Data Within the EC: A Comparative Analysis of the Privacy Statutes of the Federal Republic of Germany, France, the United Kingdom, and the Netherlands and Their Impact on the Private Sector*. Boston: Kluwer Law and Taxation Publishers.

Olmstead v. United States. 1928. 277 U.S. 438.

PARENT, WILLIAM A. 1983a. "A New Definition of Privacy for the Law." *Law and Philosophy* 2, no. 3:305–338.

———. 1983b. "Recent Work on the Concept of Privacy." *American Philosophical Quarterly* 20, no. 4:341–355.

Pavesich v. New England Life Insurance Co. 1905. 122 Ga. 190, 50 S.E. 68.

PENNOCK, J. ROLAND, and CHAPMAN, JOHN W., eds. 1971. *Privacy: Nomos XIII*. New York: Atherton Press.

Planned Parenthood of Southeast Pennsylvania v. Casey. 1992. 112 S.Ct. 2791.

POWERS, MADISON. 1994. "Privacy and the Control of Genetic Information." In *The Genetic Frontier: Ethics, Law and Policy*, pp. 78–100. Edited by Mark S. Frankel and Albert Teich. Washington: D.C.: American Association for the Advancement of Science.

PROSSER, WILLIAM. 1960. "Privacy." *California Law Review* 48, no. 3:383–423.

RACHELS, JAMES. 1975. "Why Privacy Is Important." *Philosophy and Public Affairs* 4, no. 4:323–333.

REIMAN, JEFFREY H. 1976. "Privacy, Intimacy and Personhood." *Philosophy and Public Affairs* 6, no. 1:26–44.

RICHARDS, DAVID A. J. 1986. *Toleration and the Constitution*. Oxford: Oxford University Press.

Roe v. Wade. 1973. 410 U.S. 113. 35 L.Ed.2d 147. 93 S.Ct. 705.

RUBENFELD, JED. 1989. "The Right to Privacy." *Harvard Law Review* 102:737–806.

SCHEPPELE, KIM L. 1988. *Legal Secrets: Equality and Efficiency in the Common Law*. Chicago: University of Chicago Press.

SCHNEIDER, CARL D. 1977. *Shame, Exposure and Privacy*. Boston: Beacon.

SCHOEMAN, FERDINAND DAVID. 1992. *Privacy and Social Freedom*. Cambridge: At the University Press.

———, ed. 1984. *Philosophical Dimensions of Privacy: An Anthology*. Cambridge: At the University Press.

STEPHENS, JAMES FITZJAMES. 1967. [1873]. *Liberty, Equality and Fraternity*, p. 160. Cambridge: At the University Press.

STORR, ANTHONY. 1988. *Solitude: A Return to the Self*. New York: Free Press.

TEFFT, STANTON K., ed. 1980. *Secrecy: A Cross Cultural Perspective*. New York: Human Sciences Press.

TURKINGTON, RICHARD C.; TRUBOW, GEORGE; and ALLEN, ANITA. 1992. *Privacy, Cases and Materials*. Houston: John Marshall.

UNITED NATIONS. GENERAL ASSEMBLY. 1948. *Universal Declaration of Human Rights: Adopted the 10th December 1948 in Plenary Session by the General Assembly of the United Nations*. S.I.: UNESCO.

WACKS, RAYMOND. 1989. *Personal Information: Privacy and the Law*. Oxford: At the Clarendon Press.

WESTIN, ALAN F. 1967. *Privacy and Freedom*. New York: Atheneum.

Whalen v. Roe. 1977. 429 U.S. 589. 97 S.Ct. 869.

YOUNG, JOHN, ed. 1978. *Privacy*. Chichester, N.Y.: Wiley.

PRIVILEGED COMMUNICATIONS

When a person tells a secret to another, it is ordinarily assumed and hoped that the secret will not be divulged to others unless the person whose secret it is authorizes it. Secrets are a classic example of confidential communications. In some relationships it is also expected that the person who knows the secret will ordinarily not be required to tell others about it. This idea is formalized in the legal doctrine of privileged communications.

Privileged communications are certain confidential communications between persons in a special relationship that may be exempt from disclosure in judicial or administrative proceedings. In general, confidentiality refers to an ethical and sometimes a legal duty to protect certain information from disclosure to unauthorized third parties. Privileged communications are those confidential communications that certain persons may refuse to disclose in legal proceedings. This entry explores reasons for and against the legal protection of privileged communications, some specific aspects of the doctrine, and some typical situations in which a privilege not to disclose information is asserted or restricted.

Legal origins of privileged communications

In general, a court of law may inquire into all relevant facts to pursue the goals of truth and justice. Ordinarily, witnesses must testify truthfully in response to relevant questions. But in some circumstances a witness has the right to remain silent to protect confidential information even if it is relevant (Weiner and Wettstein, 1993). For example, an attorney is not required to disclose information obtained from a client in preparation for a trial. A psychotherapist may withhold sensitive personal information about a client revealed in the context of therapy. Spouses are exempt, in most cases, from testifying against each other. Priests are permitted to protect the confessions of penitents by promising and preserving confidentiality.

Each of these examples concerns communications between persons in a special, intimate relationship where both an expectation and a need for confidentiality exist. Attorney–client privilege has been established for several centuries in the common law, but other professional–client privileges are more recent legislative creations. The physician–patient privilege was first enacted in the nineteenth century and the psychotherapist–patient privilege laws were passed in the twentieth century. They attest to the growing influence of the professions as a political force. Although society may have an interest in the information exchanged, most states have passed statutes that insulate from required disclosure certain communications made in special relationships.

Ethical justifications

Two different ethical rationales support the doctrine of privileged communications. Utilitarians stress collective benefits to society; they argue that the social benefits of fostering certain special relationships outweigh the costs of excluding relevant evidence in legal proceedings. The potential injury to special relationships from lack of confidentiality is greater than the benefits to fact-finders if disclosure is required (Domb, 1990–1991). Deontologists emphasize individual rights; they believe that the doctrine of privileged communications shows respect for the dignity of the individual and the integrity of special relationships in which individuals reveal secrets—private, personal, and often sensitive information—to professionals or intimates such as spouses or priests (Shuman and Weiner, 1987). The right of individuals to protection from intrusion by government or other third parties is derived from concepts of human dignity that preclude disclosure regardless of any social costs or benefits. A clear example is the privilege against self-incrimination; to require individuals to testify against themselves undermines their personal dignity, privacy, and autonomy. Protection of privileged communications in special relationships can be seen as an extension of this reasoning.

Critics of the doctrine of privileged communication argue, however, that the supposed social benefits of fostering special relationships by these means are unproven and unnecessary (Slovenko and Grossman, 1991). It is also sometimes argued that privileged communications are shields from public scrutiny held up by professionals to protect their own interests more than those of clients or patients (Domb, 1990–1991). Others claim that the societal interest in truth and justice should override individual interests in privacy or confidentiality. Although about two-thirds of the legislatures in the United States have sided with the proponents of privileged communications, about one-third have no privilege statutes.

Privileged communications in practice

When one person reveals a secret to another person the communication is not privileged unless certain conditions are met. The communication must be of a type recognized by state law as privileged. A legally recognized special relationship must exist, such as attorney–client, physician–patient, or husband–wife. Telling a secret to a friend, for example, that you lied about your age, does not create a legally privileged communication; it does, however, if you told your lawyer or your psychotherapist in the context of their provision of professional services. A further requirement is that the communication must not be subject to exceptions typically specified by statute, as explained below.

The right to refuse to disclose privileged communications belongs solely to the individual who revealed the information. This person, or the professional on behalf of this person, may assert the right to preclude privileged communications from being introduced as evidence in a judicial or administrative proceeding. But the person who holds the privilege may consent to a disclosure or may waive the privilege and require the professional to testify about otherwise confidential communications. Some professionals feel that they, rather than (or in addition to) the person who revealed information in a confidential relationship, should have a privilege not to disclose such information. But common law courts and nearly all state statutes in the United States specify that the privilege belongs only to the person who communicated confidential information (*Lifshutz*, 1970).

As a practical matter, the law of privileged communication often causes confusion and consternation in the health-care community. When a patient consults a health-care professional, both usually prefer that communications from client to professional be kept confidential. In addition, when a client consults a health professional, neither the professional nor the client usually anticipates that the client will be a party to litigation. For example, a man who seeks psychiatric care for depression or sexual dysfunction is unlikely to think about the possibility of becoming a plaintiff in a personal injury lawsuit.

Information disclosed in the course of mental-health care may, however, be relevant to the judicial process. Suppose, for example, that the man mentioned above sues the driver of a car that crashed into his car. The patient/plaintiff files a claim for damages to the car and for physical and emotional damages. The defendant, in the course of the discovery process, seeks access to the plaintiff's medical and psychiatric records. The defendant argues that such records are relevant to the claim that the plaintiff suffered physical or emotional damage. The otherwise confidential information disclosed to the psychiatrist would then be subject to discovery by the defendant to the extent that it is relevant to the specific issues being litigated. This scenario sketches what is commonly known as the patient/litigant exception to the legal doctrine of privileged communication. The example illustrates a tension in the legal process between the need for access to relevant evidence to promote truth and fairness to one litigant, on the one hand, and the protection of confidential information of the other litigant, even at the expense of truth, on the other.

At this point the plaintiff has several options. He can drop the lawsuit or limit his claim to damages to the car. The defendant then has no right to review any of the plaintiff's medical or psychiatric records. Suppose, however, that the plaintiff drops only the claim of emotional damages from the lawsuit. The defendant clearly has a right to review medical records; it may be argued both ways that the psychiatric records are relevant to the alleged physical injuries. A judge may be asked to rule specifically what information must be disclosed and what remains privileged.

The tension within the legal system created by the individual's entitlement to privileged communication is dynamic; this tension is reflected in restrictions on and exceptions to the legal doctrine of privileged communications. It has already been mentioned that individuals themselves may consent, typically in writing, to the disclosure of otherwise confidential information. They may also lose the privilege if, for example, they have revealed the confidential information publicly, outside the confines of a special relationship. Or the privilege may be lost if an individual fails to claim it in a legal proceeding. The privilege is a right that must be respected by others as well as asserted by an individual who possesses the right.

In addition to the patient/litigant exception discussed previously, numerous standard exceptions to the right of individuals to claim a privilege are established in the law. In general, these exceptions pertain to issues concerning an individual's mental state, payments of services, or protection of another's welfare. For example, when a question arises about a person's emotional stability, sanity, emotional damage, competence to stand trial, make a will, or raise a child, otherwise confidential information is not privileged. In such cases, it is so essential to a fair and reasonable legal process that the value of confidentiality is overridden. Economic considerations also weigh heavily against privileged communications. Not only when litigants seek monetary damages but also when a claim for payment for medical services is at stake are such exceptions made.

Finally, many exceptions arise in connection with protection of others. If a patient sues a physician for malpractice or if a physician is under investigation for disciplinary or criminal charges, the patient's privilege is subordinated. If the patient is a defendant—or sometimes even a witness or a victim—in a criminal proceeding, disclosure of privileged communications may be required. For example, in alleged instances of child abuse, psychotherapists are required to report it and may be required to testify in a trial. Similarly, in rape cases the mental state of victims is subject to investigation and subsequent disclosure, sometimes including revelations to their physicians or therapists. In child abuse, rape, homicide, and other criminal cases, controversy exists about who should be required to testify and how much disclosure should be mandated. Some argue that information relevant to criminal prosecution should be obtained by means other than those that undermine the trust provided by confidentiality. Others argue that confidentiality should not be protected at the expense of persons faced with possible criminal punishment. It should be noted, however, that confidentiality may not require complete protection and that the legal process may not need total disclosure of privileged information. The conflicts can sometimes be mediated by discretionary judicial rulings, compromises among the parties to the litigation, or specific limitations on the scope of confidentiality or an investigation.

Individuals and professionals sometimes fear that exceptions to privileged communications may overwhelm or dilute it; persons who desire access to confidential information sometimes feel that maintaining the privilege shields fraud or crime. Despite these worries, there is still a consensus among interested parties that the conceptual, practical, and professional issues raised by this doctrine are important; they require a delicate balancing of interests in order to protect individual rights as well as society's need for sensitive information.

WILLIAM J. WINSLADE

Directly related to this entry are the entries CONFIDENTIALITY; *and* PRIVACY IN HEALTH CARE. *For a further discussion of topics mentioned in this entry, see the entries* LAW AND BIOETHICS; PROFESSIONAL–PATIENT RELATIONSHIP; *and* PROFESSION AND PROFESSIONAL ETHICS. *This entry will find application in the entry* PRIVACY AND CONFIDENTIALITY IN RESEARCH. *For a discussion of related ideas, see the entries* FIDELITY AND LOYALTY; *and* INFORMATION DISCLOSURE. *Other relevant material may be found under the entries* CONFLICT OF INTEREST; *and* ETHICS, *article on* TASK OF ETHICS.

Bibliography

CHURGIN, MICHAEL J. 1986. "Psychotherapist–Patient Privilege: A Search for Identity." In vol. 2 of *Law and Mental Health: International Perspectives*, pp. 215–264. Edited by David N. Weisstub. New York: Pergamon Press.

"Developments in the Law: Privileged Communications." 1985. *Harvard Law Review* 98, no. 7:1450–1666.

DOMB, BRIAN. 1990–1991. "I Shot the Sheriff, but Only My Analyst Knows: Shrinking the Psychotherapist–Patient Privilege." *Journal of Law and Health* 5, no. 2:209–236.

KNAPP, S., and VANDECREEK, L. 1987. *Privileged Communications in the Mental Health Professions*. New York: Van Nostrand Reinhold.

Lifshutz, In re. 1970. 466 P. 2d 557 (Cal.).

SHUMAN, DANIEL W., and WEINER, MYRON F. 1987. *Psychotherapist–Patient Privilege: A Critical Examination*. Springfield, Ill.: Charles C. Thomas.

SLOVENKO, RALPH, and GROSSMAN, MAURICE. 1991. "Confidentiality and Testimonial Privilege." In vol. 3 of *Psychiatry*, pp. 1–18. Edited by Robert Michels. Philadelphia: Lippincott.

SMITH, STEVEN R. 1986–1987. "Medical and Psychotherapy Privileges and Confidentiality: On Giving with One Hand and Removing with the Other." *Kentucky Law Journal* 75, no. 3:473–557.

SMITH-BELL, MICHELE, and WINSLADE, WILLIAM J. 1994. "Privacy, Confidentiality, and Privilege in Psychother-

apeutic Relationships." *American Journal of Orthopsychiatry* 64, no. 2:180–193.

WEINER, BARBARA A., and WETTSTEIN, ROBERT M. 1993. *Legal Issues in Mental Health Care*. New York: Plenum Press.

WINSLADE, WILLIAM J., and ROSS, JUDITH WILSON. 1985. "Privacy, Confidentiality, and Autonomy in Psychiatry." *Nebraska Law Review* 64:578–636.

PROFESSIONAL–PATIENT RELATIONSHIP

I. Historical Perspectives
   Pedro Laín Entralgo
II. Sociological Perspectives
   Samuel W. Bloom
III. Ethical Issues
   Ruth B. Purtilo

I. HISTORICAL PERSPECTIVES

The following article is a reprint of the first-edition article "Therapeutic Relationship: History of the Relationship" by the same author, with only minor changes.

We give the name "therapeutic relationship" to the link established between an individual (the patient) and another individual or group (the healers), with the aim of curing or relieving the disease suffered by the former. Our problem is to describe as exactly as possible the various forms this relationship has assumed throughout history.

The empirico-magical stage

Ever since records have existed concerning the treatment of the sick, we may distinguish the following four chief forms: (1) the spontaneous or instinctive, (2) the empirical, (3) the magico-religious, and (4) the scientific. In all periods of history, all of these forms have had their practitioners. The mother who holds her feverish child on her lap, embracing it to protect it from the cold air, illustrates the first form, *spontaneous* or *instinctive* help. The second form, *empirical* help, consists in using a remedy because it has provided some relief in similar cases—that is, without asking why the remedy has those particular healing qualities. Medicine owes some very important discoveries to therapeutic empiricism. The treatment of wounds from firearms, discovered by chance by Ambrosio Paré (c. 1510–1590); the introduction of quinine into the Western world; and Edward Jenner's vaccination against smallpox are three superb examples. Generically speaking, in *magico-religious* treatment both healer and patient believe that the cure is due to the action of "supernatural" or "divine" powers available for the purpose. In some cases the curative effectiveness of these powers depends on "who" uses them (medicine man, shaman, witch doctor, etc.); in others, on "how" they are applied (magic ritual); and in others, upon "where" the cure takes place (in localities "singled out" or "favored" for their healing powers—some shrine, island, or spring).

Since scientific treatment in the strict sense began in Greece in the fifth century B.C., we can definitely state that from the origin of the human race and for many thousand years thereafter, the therapeutic relationship was empirico-magical in character, with either the "empirical" or the "magical" element of the healing process dominant, according to circumstances. It is known that in the most highly developed pre-Hellenic cultures of ancient Egypt, China, and India, a form of medicine existed in which strictly "magical" or magico-religious elements were minor compared with the empirical and theoretical. However, a careful study of these three methods of understanding and practicing the care of the sick would reveal to some extent attitudes of the doctor that can only be called "magical" and that, above all, show a lack of principles capable of initiating a way toward purely "scientific" medicine.

The ancient scientific stage

As Aristotle taught, treatment of the sick is scientific ("technical") in the strictest sense when it depends on the knowledge of why it is being done, what is being done, and by what means it takes effect (in other words, what is the disease, what remedy is being used, and by what therapeutic procedure is it administered). Thus the healer's ability to cure does not depend on the agent who applies the remedy, nor on the ceremony accompanying its application, nor on the privileged place where the cure takes place—that is, not on a magical "who," "how," or "where," but on a series of "whats" concerning the illness and its remedy.

Taking as their starting point the most important cosmological idea of the pre-Socratic philosophers—the idea of physis, or "nature"—the group of physicians, the Aesclepiades, known as Hippocratics, originated the technical concept of illness a century before Aristotle formulated the conceptual definitions just mentioned. Consequently, a doctor would try to cure a patient or to alleviate the patient's pain in the rational or scientifically definitive knowledge of the "nature" of humans, of illness in general, of the special disease he was treating, and of the remedy being used—while at the same time having the knowledge and skill to perform everything required by the treatment. This is not to say that Hip-

pocratic medicine—apart from its inevitable deficiencies—was free from some serious errors and superstitious practice but to affirm that it already contained various principles: the notion of physis as the basis of all technical knowledge, the concept of medicine as téchne iatriké, the idea of a method of knowing whose first rule is the attentive sensory examination of the patient's body—as a result of which defects and errors would be gradually corrected.

From Hippocrates to Galen (A.D. 130?–200?)—while the ancient view of technical medicine remained in force—the therapeutic relationship can be described under four heads.

Basis of the therapeutic relationship. Ideally considered, this basis is philanthropia, the "love of man," because, according to a famous saying, "Where there is love of man, philanthropia, there is love of the art [of healing], philotechnia" (Hippocrates, Praeceptiones, L.IX, 258). Of course, this saying belongs to a later, post-Stoic period; but the study of much earlier medical texts, such as the Epidemias, gives grounds for the belief that the Hippocratics, as they were called, practiced philanthropia before the word was invented. In any case, the "love of man" of ancient Greece was the same as "love of nature," of the divine physis, as is specifically and individually realized in the name given to the subject in question: physiophilia. It is not necessary to add that less noble interests, such as love of money and thirst for fame, in practice often obscured this ethical and technical ideal of "physiological philanthropy" as the basis of the therapeutic relationship.

Diagnostic aspect of the relationship. As scientific and effective "knowledge" was the first premise of the technical concept of medicine, the therapeutic relationship required—as it has of doctors since—that the Greek physician should reach a diagnosis by rational means. During the period in the history of medicine here called "ancient scientific," this diagnostic activity appears to have consisted of (1) a fourfold desire to discover whether the illness is determined by an insuperable and necessary cause (kat'ananken) or by some controllable contingency (katà tychen); to identify the typical form (tropos, eidos) of the suffering; to determine its causes, both remote and immediate (aitia, prophasis); and to establish a well-founded prognosis; (2) a series of exploratory maneuvers (anamnesis, study of the surroundings, examination of the patient's body by means of sight, touch, hearing, smell, and taste); and (3) adequate inductive reasoning (logismos).

Curative aspect of the relationship. After some deliberation, the therapeutic activity of the Greek doctor was subjected to the following rules: (1) to help the patient, or at least to do no harm to the patient (Hippocrates, Epidemias, I, L.II, 634); (2) to refrain from interfering if the illness were incurable and inevitably mortal, because in that case the doctor, by intervening, would commit the sin of *hybris*, or rebellion against an edict of the divine and sovereign *physis*; and (3) insofar as possible, to attack the cause of the disease therapeutically. Diet, drugs, surgery, and to a lesser degree "psychotherapy" were the four great healing methods of ancient medicine.

Ethical and social aspects of the therapeutic relationship. One must avoid the common error of seeing the oath contained in the *Corpus Hippocraticum* as the ethical code of Greek medicine; in all probability it was not in force outside the Pythagorean order (Edelstein, 1967). However, it is possible to trace the outline of the medical ethics and social medicine of the ancient Greeks:

1. The doctor's duties to the patient: to help or not to harm, to abstain from the impossible, to adjust the fees to the patient's income.
2. Duties toward other doctors: The ideal principle of regarding colleagues as brothers (Hippocrates, *Praeceptiones*, 4, IX, 258) was very infrequently infringed by the competitiveness of which doctors of antiquity are so often accused (Edelstein, 1967).
3. Duties toward self: A doctor should give attention to personal appearance and behave in a manner that would be called "beautiful and good" (Hippocrates, *Medicus*, L, IX, 204). To serve nature through the application of professional skill (Hippocrates, *Epidemias*, I, L.11, 636) should be the physician's paramount principle.
4. Duties to society: Though clearly stated by Plato (*Republic, Laws*), these are given much less importance in strictly medical writings; in any case (Plato, the Hippocratic treatise *On Diet*), it is certain that there was "medicine for the rich" and "medicine for the poor" in the ancient world.

Christianity and the therapeutic relationship

The propagation of Christianity was not motivated by the need to reform the conduct of doctor toward patient, insofar as this conduct could be held as technical, but because the medical technique prevailing at the time had been created by pagans. Because the Christian concept of love was relatively new, Christ's religious message influenced both the problem and the form taken by the therapeutic relationship in various ways.

Could the pagan medical technique have been accepted without more ado by Christians? Out of excessively vehement opposition to paganism, some of them—Tatian the Assyrian and Tertullian, for instance—gave a negative answer to this question. But the good sense of others prevailed in the end; and thus, from the fourth century to the increasingly strong anti-Ga-

lenism of the sixteenth and seventeenth centuries, the medicine of Christian peoples (e.g., in Byzantium and medieval Europe) showed a progressive intellectual effort to relate the art of healing, inherited from ancient Greece and culminating in the work of Galen, to the Christian worldview.

One can note the novelty of the Christian concept of love and its decisive effect on the form taken by the therapeutic relationship. When this was the direct, pure expression of the evangelical message—in other words, before Constantine's edict led to the primitive Christian communities' becoming involved with the civil power—there were two chief features of its structure.

Ideal basis of the therapeutic relationship. We are no longer facing love of *physis* or universal "nature," as individualized in the sick person; rather, we are confronting his or her unique persona as a "neighbor" (parable of the good Samaritan). Moreover, in helping an ailing neighbor, one is helping Christ (Matt. 25: 39–40).

The therapeutic relationship as help. Herein lie the most significant new developments in primitive or pre-Constantinian Christianity.

1. In the assistance given to the sick person there should be no "natural limits," thus putting an end to the Hellenic imperative to refrain from therapy in cases of "necessarily" mortal or incurable disease. Here, although there is no place for therapeutic technique, the patient can always be helped by spiritual advice.
2. The egalitarian nature of treatment: No difference should be made between Greeks and barbarians, free people and slaves, friends and enemies.
3. The necessity of giving free help: Within a community governed by the principle that possessions are shared (see the texts of Acts of the Apostles), the basic motive of help for the sick was charity, not only on the part of the doctor but also on the part of other people (widows acting as nurses and, later, "deaconesses"). The Greek doctor would give free treatment in exchange for some favor received or to acquire prestige in the town (Hippocrates, *Praeceptiones*, L.IX, 258); the Christian doctor should give help free, on principle.
4. Such practices of the Christian religion as prayer and extreme unction were incorporated into the care of the sick.

The medieval scientific stage

After Constantine's Edict of Milan (C.E. 312), the links between Christianity and the civil power became increasingly strong, and this gave rise to public awareness that the Christian life, such as was led outside the new conventual communities, was losing at least some of its original purity. This is shown by a brief examination of the two main politicosocial forms of Christianity, during the historical period that we call the Middle Ages, in the Byzantine Empire and medieval Europe. Exigencies of space allow no more than a mention of the third great cultural ambit of the Middle Ages: the world of Islam.

Therapeutic relationship in Byzantium. The theocratic fusion between the Christian religion and civil power has never been stronger than in the Byzantine Empire; never has religious error or heresy been more methodically and sternly treated as "political crime." From this are derived the two main characteristics of the therapeutic relationship in Byzantine society: its doctrinal basis and its importance as help. The doctrinal basis of the therapeutic relationship in the Byzantine world was essentially the result of a juxtaposition that never turned out well. On the ethical plane, Byzantine medicine went on accepting and proclaiming the Christian concept of helping the sick; on the technical plane it accepted in principle everything described by the Greeks as "practical," and refused to acknowledge (as pagan and evil) the basic "theoretic" concepts of Hippocratic-Galenic medicine—for example, the notion of *physis* as "divine" and the denial or negation of a personal, spiritual God, creator of the world and transcending it. The doctors of Byzantium did not succeed in connecting the dogmas of their Christian faith with the scientific and philosophic basis of Hellenic *téchne iatriké*.

The most important contribution made by Byzantine Christianity to medical care was the creation of hospitals to treat poor invalids; among them was the famous "hospital city" of Caesarea, founded about the year 370. (Earlier institutions did not strictly deserve the name "hospitals.") In those institutions there were specialists, male and female nurses, surgeons, assistant doctors (*parabalani*), and servants. Charity was the ruling principle in their activity, but that did not prevent the distinction between "medicine for the rich" and "medicine for the poor" from being clearly observed in Byzantium. And finally, we must mention the magical and pseudo-religious cures, which particularly attracted poorer patients.

The therapeutic relationship in medieval Europe. The historical period we call the Middle Ages covers the millennium between the invasion of Rome by the Germanic races and the conquest of Constantinople by the Turks in 1453, and is far from uniform in character—suffice it to compare the life in a feudal castle in the ninth century with that of a Flemish or Italian town in the fifteenth. It is shown also by the gradual changes in the therapeutic relationship throughout this period.

Doctrinal basis of the therapeutic relationship. Two chief aspects must be distinguished—the technical and the ethical. Until the School of Salerno became famous (in the eleventh and twelfth centuries) and the Scholastic medicine of the thirteenth to fifteenth centuries was flourishing, medieval medicine hardly deserves the term "technical" or "scientific" in the strict sense. Mainly practiced by monks ("monastic medicine") either inside or outside monasteries, it was based solely on a certain amount of experience and the extremely scanty remains of ancient learning that had survived the destruction of the Roman Empire.

There was a marked change at the beginning of the twelfth century: Secular doctors with professional degrees became more common; from the time of Roger of Sicily in 1140, Graeco-Arab learning began to spread from Salerno, or from Toledo, and became truly "technical" medicine, an authentic *ars medica*. By means of the intellectual resources provided by the theology and philosophy of the period, the Scholastic European doctors of the thirteenth and fourteenth centuries achieved something not attained by Byzantine medicine; they systematically adapted Hippocratic and Galenic thought to the needs of the Christian faith.

From the ethical point of view, medieval medicine continued to base itself ideally on the Christian concept of aid for the needy and sick—ideally because in practice the pressure of economic interest was not uncommon, nor, sometimes, free from corruption.

Diagnostic aspect of the therapeutic relationship. Though it had become impoverished and schematized in comparison with that of ancient Greece, the diagnostic relationship between doctor and patient—examination and establishment of "genus" and "species" of the affliction observed—remained much the same. Two techniques gained prominence and were gradually perfected: examination of the urine (*uroscopia*) and taking of the pulse. There were also two doctrinal guidelines to help the doctor pass from clinical experience to reasoning, treatises that systematically described the different species of disease (*de passionibus, de affectionibus*) and the didactic descriptions of individual cases of disease (*consilia*).

Curative aspect of the therapeutic relationship. From a technical standpoint the Middle Ages added little that was new to the treatment of the sick as taught by Greek and Arab doctors. Diet, the use of drugs, surgery, and "psychotherapy"—with a Christian orientation—remained the principal methods of treatment. As to theory, the chief concept of Galenic therapy, the "symptom" (*endeixis*), became latinized and scholasticized under the name of *insinuatio agendi*. On the other hand, the problem arose of how to harmonize "technical" requirements derived from the Galenic concept of symptoms with the "moral" rules imposed by the Christian idea of the person: the bond between *ars* and *caritas*. However, medieval physicians did not succeed in solving this delicate human problem coherently or systematically.

Ethical and social aspects of the therapeutic relationship. As to principles and ideals, medieval medical ethics are as faithfully Christian as the society to which they belong; but individual and social realization of this sincere Christianity was very different from that prevailing in pre-Constantine communities. Four reasons contribute to this:

1. The avarice of many clerical and secular doctors: "Doctor, do not be afraid of asking good fees from the rich," wrote Lanfranc in the eleventh century.
2. The growing interference of the civil power in regulating doctors' duties by means of ordinances—relating not only to the healer's technical behavior but also sometimes to his religious conduct—infringement of which was punished.
3. The frequent critico-burlesque attitude of society toward the doctor's greed for gain or lack of skill (John of Salisbury's *Metalogicus* and Petrarch's *Invectivae*).
4. The marked difference between "medicine for the rich" and "medicine for the poor"—in monasteries, the distance separating the *infirmarium* from the *hospitale pauperum*; in cities, the even greater gap between the treatment of those in power—politicians or churchmen, nearly all of whom had their own private doctors—and the almost purely religious treatment given to the unfortunates in hospital beds. Not everything in the Christian Middle Ages was in fact Christian.

Modern scientific stage: Christian modernity

It is a platitude to say that the "modern world" began with the Renaissance or even in the fifteenth century. However, a thorough study of the various characteristics of this modernity—greater knowledge of classical antiquity, importance of worldly matters, new conceptions of science, rationalization of life, awareness of historical progress—clearly shows the roots of all these developments to be present in the transition from the thirteenth to the fourteenth century, when the voluntarism and nominalism of Franciscan thought (e.g., William of Occam, 1285?–1349?) began to influence European culture. When human freedom (and hence human creative ability) was seen as a person's chief similarity to God, the idea of "natural" and "necessary" limitations to human scientific and technical capacity with regard to the cosmos disappeared in principle, and the human mind began to entertain the idea of "indefinite progress." Science and modern techniques took their first steps, in the belief that knowledge of the sensible world consisted in creating abstract symbols—they would soon be called mathematical symbols—by means of which the external world could be understood and dominated. Many years

had to pass, however, for these germinal concepts to be converted into strong, widespread social customs. Only in the secularized society of the eighteenth through the twentieth century would a great tree grow from the tiny seed of the fourteenth century.

Two periods must be distinguished in the history of the modern Euro-American world: In the first, from the fifteenth to the second half of the eighteenth century, by far the largest proportion of society was still nominally Christian, although the form of religion, whether Catholic or Protestant, was growing away from that of the Middle Ages; in the second, the nineteenth and twentieth centuries, society was becoming secularized.

Basis of the therapeutic relationship. Whether Catholic or Protestant, modern Christian doctors still saw the injunction to give charitable help to those in need as the basic ideal of healing activity: They thought of Theophrastus Paracelsus, they remembered the ritual oath taken by newly graduated French doctors in front of the altar of Nôtre Dame. But the diversity of religions in Europe and America, and the growing esteem both for the reality of worldly values and for increasing civil power, led to two new features in this ideal: (1) greater respect for the personal religious life of the patient and (2) an increasing and sharper separation between the spiritual and material worlds, the latter being known and governed by the beginnings of modern science and the technology founded upon it. Two examples of this spiritual–material separation will suffice: Hermann Boerhaave's teaching of the distinction between the mind and the body (*De distinctione mentis a corpore*) and Friedrich Hoffmann's significant anthropological contrast between the physical (*cor corporale*) and the spiritual (*cor spirituale*).

Diagnostic aspect of the therapeutic relationship. The principle of understanding nature in order to master it (Francis Bacon, René Descartes) gained strength in modern society and led to the physician's concern to make diagnoses that were objectively correct. Very briefly, the following are the chief characteristics of the diagnostic aspect of the therapeutic relationship during this period:

1. Understanding of the disease being treated became more individualized, as was very clear in the form taken by case histories (Giovanni Battista Montanus, Boerhaave, etc.).
2. Numerical measurement gradually began to figure in examinations, leading to the first use of instruments such as watches and thermometers.
3. Diagnosis was increasingly used to guess at the existence of an anatomic lesion, which could be proved by an autopsy (Giovanni Maria Lancisi and Hippolyte Albertini, Hermann Boerhaave, Giovanni Battista Morgagni).

4. A more lively and objective interest was evinced in the influence of the social environment on the disease (Paracelsus, Bernardino Ramazzini, Johann Peter Frank).

Curative aspect of the relationship. The spread and strength of the modern scientific mentality required a doctor who wished to keep up with the times to validate by experimentation the efficacy of the available remedies. On the other hand, awareness of human power over natural phenomena demanded a constant increase in the number and curative scope of those remedies. Paracelsus thought that every natural substance could be an efficacious medicament, if convenient means of using it could be discovered; God had disposed the world thus when it was created, and this the inquiring and inventive intelligence of the doctor should be able to make plain. Consequently, doctors no longer saw themselves as "servants of nature by means of their skill," as in ancient Greece but also during the Middle Ages in a Christian interpretation of the words as the true "collaborators of God." Whether Paracelsists or not, the most eminent doctors of the fifteenth to eighteenth centuries made use more or less consciously of this concept of therapeutic activity. But at the same time there was increasing distrust of the healing qualities assumed to belong to many of the remedies traditional practice had recommended.

The main therapeutic methods were still the four employed in Hippocratic medicine: diet (adapted to new ways of life), cure by drugs (enriched by various new medicines), surgery (whose technique had advanced considerably, from Ambrosio Paré to William Cheselden, Percival Pott, and Hunter), and, on a distinctly lower plane, psychotherapy, whose later triumph was unconsciously heralded by Franz Anton Mesmer at the end of the eighteenth century. The separation of healers into "doctors" (or "physicians") and "surgeons" was daily becoming more clear.

Ethical and social aspects of the professional–patient relationship. Since both doctor and patient were Christians, it was natural for doctors to find their ethical principles in those of the Christian life; but at the same time, since the creation and rational order of the world had gained greater stature as explanations of the world, it was also natural for the form in which these principles were individually and socially realized to change to some extent. There should have been, and indeed there was, a relationship between religion and medicine that was both theoretical and practical. As religion was concerned with the life of the spirit and medicine with the life of the body (or what human knowledge tells us about the cosmos), the scientist and the physician did their best to discover and establish points of direct communication between those two worlds. In regard to theory, such communication was guaranteed by the "harmony" between Holy Writ and science, for example, in Francisco Valles's *Sacra philosophia* (sixteenth century) and Friedrich Hoffmann's *Dissertatio theologico-medica* (eighteenth century). Naturally, such communication and the bridge establishing it had to take a different form on the practical level. There the communication gave rise to "medical deontology," a collection of ethical precepts that were to be respected in the healer's technical activity. Examples of both early and mature forms of them are found in certain parts of the *Quaestiones medico-legales* of Paulo Zacchia (1621–1635) and the *Embriologia sacra* of Francesco Emmanuel Cangiamilla (1758).

Between the fifteenth and the seventeenth centuries, and therefore during the ancien régime, the bourgeois structure of society in Europe and America was being developed, and three distinct strata began to emerge: the "upper classes" (aristocrats, magnates of church and state, rich merchants), the "middle classes" (artisans, officials, and members of various professions), and the "lower classes" (laborers, the poor). Parallel strata could be observed in medical care. Ill persons of the upper classes were looked after in their luxurious homes and had a monopoly on more expensive treatments (one need only think of the distribution of quinine in the seventeenth century). The lower classes still went to hospitals for the poor, although during the eighteenth century those were altered or completely rebuilt on a larger scale. But the care of the sick inside those hospitals was far from acceptable (as to dirt, parasites, smell), as can be seen from denunciations by some socially and philanthropically sensitive doctors, like James René Tenon in 1788 and Howard in 1789. Nor was the medical care of the middle classes entirely satisfactory.

Modern scientific stage: Secularized modernity

The process of secularizing society advanced at progressive speed during the nineteenth and twentieth centuries. Certainly there were still many Christians in the cities of Europe and America, but their individual and social style of living, their habits, were affected by this secularization; and it was in the eighteenth century that distinct groups came to be known as "intellectuals" and "aristocrats," and later (from the second half of the nineteenth century) a class came to be known as "proletarian."

Combined with this increasing secularization of behavior, we find that in the nineteenth century life was becoming more technical, and in consequence of the industrial revolution an urban proletariat made its appearance. Submissive at first, the proletariat afterward organized itself as the "workers' movement" and asserted its rights more effectively, so that in one way or another it has decisively contributed to shaping the social scene of the twentieth century. How was the therapeutic relationship to be interpreted in this secularized world, part bourgeois, part proletarian?

Doctrinal basis of the relationship. As had been the case ever since Hippocratic medicine, the doctrinal basis of this relationship had two essential aspects, one ethical, the other scientific or technical. First, from an ethical standpoint, the ideal motive of medical care of the sick was "philanthropy," the feelings and the rules of conduct in which Christian charity was secularized. But modern philanthropy was radically different from the Hippocratic form (which had as its ultimate goal the divine *physis*, or universal nature), in that it was concerned with the "individual persona" of the patient—although the doctor's theory of humanity might not be formally "personalist." During the nineteenth and twentieth centuries many doctors have been "naturalist" in theory (in their scientific concept of human nature) and "personalist" in practice (in their therapeutic relation with the patient). Not until Marxist socialism did there appear a philanthropy based on the notions of "social or civil nature" and "state of nature." Second, from a scientific point of view, the ideal basis of medical care was the concept of medicine as the application of pure natural science. "Medicine should be natural science—in other words, what the second half of the nineteenth century understood as natural science—or it will be nothing" was the oracular saying of Hermann Helmholtz. The sick person was *scientifically* considered as a fragment of the cosmos, acted on by biological evolution and governed by the laws of physics and chemistry. Scientifically, because in practice nearly all doctors obeyed the rule of Joseph Frédéric Bérard and Gluber: *Guérir parfois, soulager souvent, consoler toujours* (heal sometimes, relieve often, always console). This does not, of course, preclude the usual corruption of the medical profession—desire for gain, thirst for social prestige—often contaminating that philanthropic and scientific ideal.

Diagnostic aspect of the relationship. The diagnostic relationship with the patient now conformed to the following principles:

1. The patient was seen, above all, as an individual, capable of being rationally understood.
2. This understanding was increased by means of the instrumental aids to clinical examination (stethoscope, sphygmograph, ophthalmoscope, chemical analysis, X rays, etc.).
3. The disease was scientifically understood by applying rules that were anatomoclinical (diagnosis of anatomical lesions), physiopathological (diagnosis of disorders typical of the functional and material processes of life), or etiopathological (diagnosis of external causes, microbes, poison, etc., of the disease

process); or the doctor could try to coordinate these three approaches.
4. Neurosis, whose frequency increased from the second half of the nineteenth century as a result of industrial civilization, was understood by natural scientific medicine by reference to anatomoclinical (Jean-Martin Charcot) or physiopathological rules (German practice since Friedrich Frerichs and Ludwig Traube).
5. To sum up, the diagnosis was, or tried to be, *at the same time* natural-scientific and individualist.

Curative aspect of the relationship. When medicine was considered as applied natural science, the doctor's powers of healing (by experimental pharmacology, surgery enhanced by the development of anesthesia and antisepsis, synthesis of new drugs, serum therapy, vaccination, etc.) were progressively and wonderfully increased. Moreover, giving broad social expression to what was merely a slight and theoretical germ at the end of the thirteenth century and the beginning of the fourteenth, doctors freed themselves from the Hellenic concept of "natural force" (*ananke physeos*) and began to think of humans as not being, in principle, subject to diseases that were mortal or incurable "of necessity." What could not be cured today might well be curable tomorrow. In fact, the doctor ceased being "the servant of nature by means of skill" and became instead nature's "guardian, master, and sculptor."

Alongside dietetics, now scientifically regulated, increasingly rich therapy by drugs, and increasingly effective surgery, the psychotherapeutic element in treatment was acquiring more importance through several different methods and interpretations. In the history of this renewed importance of psychotherapy, the most distinguished names are those of the Englishmen Daniel Tuke, Alfred John Carpenter, and Hughes Bennet; the Frenchmen Jean-Martin Charcot and Bernheim; and, above all, Sigmund Freud, whose work had already reached maturity at the start of World War I in 1914.

Ethical and social aspects of the relationship. Something has already been said about medical ethics in the society of the nineteenth and twentieth centuries. Like the society to which it belonged, this ethics became more secular, as is shown by the attempts to codify it, beginning with Percival's in 1803. From an ethical and social point of view, medical care was a service purchased at different prices or given free to the poor in hospitals supported by charity and inspired by the new philanthropy. The poor received medical care as a gift.

The sick were cared for in three different ambits.

1. *Hospitals* were supported by charity, the state, the municipality, or the church. Here the patient was one of two things in relation to the doctor: either an object that could be scientifically understood and modified, combined with a human being who was

unknown and indifferent (if the doctor was a cold and matter-of-fact person), or an object that could be scientifically understood and modified, combined with a person suffering and in need of compassion (if the doctor was a person of feeling and carried out the rule of Bérard and Gluber).

2. *The patient's own home.* The patient visited at home was an object that could be scientifically understood and modified, combined with a well-known person—a friend.

3. *The doctor's private consulting room.* Here the patient was, according to circumstances, an object that could be scientifically understood and modified, combined with a person to whom the therapist was indifferent (purely "scientific" doctors); an object that could be understood and modified, combined with a person who paid the fee asked (doctors dominated by desire for gain); or an object that could be understood and modified, combined with a friend in need of compassion (generous, sympathetic doctors).

These three ambits, with certain exceptions, correspond to the three strata into which the bourgeois and proletarian society of the age are divided, and to the three socioeconomic methods of providing medical care: "medicine for the rich" (private consulting rooms for specialists), "medicine for the middle classes" (attendance in their homes), and "medicine for the poor and proletarians" (charitable hospitals). The injustice of this social organization of medicine becomes flagrant and untenable when the proletariat becomes conscious of its right to health and proper medical care, and when, one may add, medical treatment is both efficient and expensive.

Since the second half of the nineteenth century there has been a visible rebellion against this injustice with its politicosocial and clinical aspects. Since Turner Thackrah in 1831, Sir Edwin Chadwick in 1842, and Louis René Villermé in 1840, some doctors have denounced the terrible effects of industrial poverty on health; and workers' movements have included the right to put an end to this painful and unjustifiable situation in their programs for social reform. The great vogue of Friendly Societies in the United Kingdom between 1800 and 1875, the institution of the *zemstvo* system in tsarist Russia in 1867 after the liberation of the serfs, and the creation of *Krankenkassen* in Germany by Otto von Bismarck (1882–1884) are examples of the first medical results of the proletarian rebellion.

Among the clinical results of this rebellion may be counted the increase in neurotic forms of illness, which in some cases were direct consequences of social injustice and maladjustment. The "introduction of the subject in medicine" (von Weizsäcker's term), that is, the methodical study of the patient as an individual, both

in diagnosis and treatment (penetration of hospitals by Freudian psychoanalysis and psychosomatic medicine) and in social pathology and medical sociology (Grotjahn and various English authors), constitutes the response of scientific medicine to the clinical rebellion of the sick against the medical care of the nineteenth century.

To the layperson as well as to the doctor of today, the present period begins with World War I. From that point on, the historian of yesterday must defer to the chronicler of the present day.

PEDRO LAÍN ENTRALGO
[TRANSLATED BY FRANCES PARTRIDGE]

Directly related to this article are the other articles in this entry: SOCIOLOGICAL PERSPECTIVES, *and* ETHICAL ISSUES. *Also directly related are the entries* BENEFICENCE; PATERNALISM; CONFIDENTIALITY; TRUST; INFORMATION DISCLOSURE, *article on* ATTITUDES TOWARD TRUTH-TELLING; INFORMED CONSENT, *article on* HISTORY OF INFORMED CONSENT; HEALING; HOSPITAL, *article on* MEDIEVAL AND RENAISSANCE HISTORY; MEDICAL ETHICS, HISTORY OF, *section on* EUROPE; *and* SURGERY. *For a discussion of related ideas, see the entries* HEALTH OFFICIALS AND THEIR RESPONSIBILITIES; MEDICAL CODES AND OATHS, *article on* HISTORY; MEDICINE, ANTHROPOLOGY OF; MEDICINE, ART OF; MEDICINE, PHILOSOPHY OF; MEDICINE, SOCIOLOGY OF; MEDICINE AS A PROFESSION; *and* NURSING AS A PROFESSION. *Other relevant material may be found under the entries* CARE, *especially the article on* HISTORICAL DIMENSIONS OF AN ETHICS OF CARE IN HEALTH CARE; COMPASSION; FIDELITY AND LOYALTY; HEALTH AND DISEASE, *article on* HISTORY OF THE CONCEPTS; PROFESSION AND PROFESSIONAL ETHICS; PUBLIC HEALTH, *article on* HISTORY OF PUBLIC HEALTH; ROMAN CATHOLICISM; SOCIAL MEDICINE; *and* VIRTUE AND CHARACTER. *See also the* APPENDIX (CODES, OATHS, AND DIRECTIVES RELATED TO BIOETHICS), SECTION II: ETHICAL DIRECTIVES FOR THE PRACTICE OF MEDICINE.

Bibliography

BAAS, KARL. 1915. "Uranfänge und Frühgeschichte der Krankenpflege." *Sudhoffs Archiv für Geschichte der Medizin* 8:146–164.

BALINT, MICHAEL. 1964. *The Doctor, His Patient, and the Illness.* 2d ed. New York: International Universities Press. First published 1957.

BLUM, RICHARD H. 1960. *The Management of the Doctor–Patient Relationship.* Foreword by Joseph Sadusk and Rollen Waterson. New York: McGraw-Hill/Blakiston.

CHRISTIAN, PAUL. 1952. *Das Personverständnis im modernen medizinischen Denken.* Schriften der Studiengemeinschaft der Evangelischen Akademien, no. 1. Tübingen: J.C.B. Mohr.

DUFFY, JOHN. 1979. *Healers: A History of American Medicine.* Urbana: University of Illinois Press.

EDELSTEIN, LUDWIG. 1943. *The Hippocratic Oath: Text, Translation, and Interpretation.* Supplements to the *Bulletin of the History of Medicine* no. 1. Baltimore: Johns Hopkins University Press. Reprinted in *Ancient Medicine: Selected Papers of Ludwig Edelstein,* pp. 3–63. Edited by Owsei Temkin and C. Lilian Temkin. Translated by C. Lilian Temkin. Baltimore: Johns Hopkins University Press, 1967.

FIELD, MARK G. 1957. *Doctor and Patient in Soviet Russia.* Russian Research Center Studies, no. 29. Cambridge, Mass.: Harvard University Press.

FLEURY, MAI L. 1984. *The Healing Bond: Human Relations Skills for Nurses and Other Health-Care Professionals.* Englewood Cliffs, N.J.: Prentice-Hall.

GRACIA, DIEGO. 1989a. "Los cambios en la relación médico-enfermo." *Medicina clínica* (Barcelona) 93:100–102.

———. 1989b. *Fundamentos de bioética.* Madrid: Eudema.

———. 1991. *Procedimiento de decisión en ética clínica.* Madrid: Eudema.

HIPPOCRATES. *Epidemias* I, L.II, 634 and 636. In Littré, *Oeuvres complètes d'Hippocrate,* vol. 2, pp. 634–637. Also in Jones, trans., *Hippocrates,* vol. 1, second constitution, par. 11, 11.10–12 and 13–14, pp. 164–165.

———. *Medicus.* L. IX, 204. In Littré, *Oeuvres complètes d'Hippocrate,* vol. 9, pp. 204–207. Also in Jones, trans., *Hippocrates,* vol. 2, chap. 1, pp. 310–313.

———. *Praeceptiones.* L. IX, 258. In Littré, *Oeuvres complètes d'Hippocrate,* vol. 9, pp. 258–263. Also in Jones, trans., *Hippocrates,* vol. 1, par. 6–7, pp. 318–323.

———. *Regimen.* L. VI, 466. In Littré, *Oeuvres complètes d'Hippocrate,* vol. 6, pp. 466–663. Also in Jones, trans., *Hippocrates,* vol. 4, pp. 224–447.

JONES, WILLIAM HENRY SAMUEL, trans. 1923–1931. *Hippocrates.* 4 vols. Loeb Classical Library. Edited by E. Capps, T. E. Page, and W. H. D. Rouse. London: William Heinemann; New York: G. P. Putnam's Sons. Greek and English.

LAÍN ENTRALGO, PEDRO. 1958. *La curación por la palabra en la antigüedad clásica.* Madrid: Revista de Occidente. Edited and translated by L. J. Rather and John M. Sharp as *The Therapy of the Word in Classical Antiquity.* New Haven, Conn.: Yale University Press, 1970.

———. 1961. *Enfermedad y pecado.* Medicina de hoy. Barcelona: Ediciones Toray.

———. 1962. "La asistencia médica en la obra de Platón." In his *Marañón y el enfermo,* pp. 90–135. Madrid: Revista de Occidente.

———. 1964. *La relación médico-enfermo: Historia y teoría.* Madrid: Revista de Occidente.

———. 1969. *Doctor and Patient.* Translated by Frances Partridge. World University Library. London: Weidenfeld and Nicholson; New York: McGraw-Hill.

———. 1970. *La medicina hipocrática.* Madrid: Revista de Occidente.

———. 1972a. "El cristianismo primitivo y la medicina." In his *Historia universal de la medicina,* vol. 3, pp. 1–7. Barcelona: Salvat.

———. 1972b. *Sobre la amistad.* Colección Selecta, no. 41. Madrid: Revista de Occidente.

LITTRÉ, EMILE, ed. and trans. 1839–1861. *Oeuvres complètes d'Hippocrate. Traduction nouvelle avec le texte grec en regard, collationné sur les manuscrits et toutes les éditions, accompagnée d'une introduction, de commentaires médicaux, de variantes et de notes philologiques; suivie d'une table générale des matières.* 10 vols. Paris: J. B. Baillière. Reprinted Amsterdam: Adolf M. Hakkert, 1961.

MAJNO, GUIDO. 1975. *Healing Hand: Man and Wound in the Ancient World.* Cambridge, Mass.: Harvard University Press.

NUTTING, MARY ADELAIDE, and DOCK, LAVINIA L. 1907–1912. *A History of Nursing: The Evolution of Nursing Systems from the Earliest Times to the Foundation of the First English and American Training School for Nurses.* 4 vols. New York: G. P. Putnam. Translated by Agnes Karll as *Geschichte der Krankenpflege: Die Entwicklung der Krankenpflege—Systeme von Urzeiten bis zur Gründung der ersten englischen und amerikanischen Pflegerinnenschulen.* 3 vols. Berlin: D. Reimer, 1910–1913.

ORR, DOUGLAS W. 1954. "Transference and Countertransference: A Historical Survey." *Journal of the American Psychoanalytic Association* 2, no. 4:621–670.

PARSONS, TALCOTT. 1951. "Illness and the Role of the Physician: A Sociological Perspective." *American Journal of Orthopsychiatry* 21:452–460.

PITTENGER, ROBERT E.; HACKETT, CHARLES F.; and DANEHY, JOHN J. 1960. *The First Five Minutes: A Sample of Microscopic Interview Analysis.* Ithaca, N.Y.: Paul Martineau.

PORTER, ROY, ed. 1986. *Patients and Practitioners: Lay Perceptions of Medicine in Pre-Industrial Society.* New York: Cambridge University Press.

REISER, STANLEY J., and ANBAR, MICHAEL, eds. 1984. *The Machine at the Bedside: Strategies for Using Technology in Patient Care.* New York: Cambridge University Press.

RITTER-RÖHR, DOROTHEA, ed. 1975. *Der Arzt, sein Patient, und die Gesellschaft.* Edition Suhrkamp, no. 746. Frankfurt am Main: Suhrkamp.

ROF CARBALLO, JUAN. 1961. *Urdimbre afectiva y enfermedad: Introducción a una medicina dialógica.* Colección Hombre y Mundo. Barcelona: Editorial Labor.

SIGERIST, HENRY E. 1987. *History of Medicine.* 2 vols. New York: Oxford University Press.

SNYDER, WILLIAM U., and SNYDER, B. JUNE. 1961. *The Psychotherapy Relationship.* New York: Macmillan.

SZASZ, THOMAS S. 1958. "Scientific Method and Social Role in Medicine and Psychiatry." *Archives of Internal Medicine* 101:228–238.

VALABREGA, JEAN-PAUL. 1962. *La Relation thérapeutique: Malade et médecin.* Nouvelle Bibliotheque Scientifique. Paris: Flammarion.

WEISS, GEORG. 1910. "Die ethischen Anschauungen im Corpus Hippokraticum." *Sudhoffs Archiv für Geschichte der Medizin* 4:235–262.

ZBOROWSKI, MARK. 1952. "Cultural Components in Responses to Pain." *Journal of Social Issues* 8, no. 4:16–30

II. SOCIOLOGICAL PERSPECTIVES

The purposes of this article are to provide a sociological perspective of the doctor–patient relationship by sketching the models of it as they have been developed by sociology, and to summarize contemporary sociological analysis. Both are essential for understanding the issues surrounding the therapeutic relationship today.

No other aspect of medicine has attracted more sociological analysis than the medical professional–patient relationship. From a classic view of the relation between doctor and patient "as a pure person-to-person relation" (Sigerist, 1960), the full range of psychosocial and sociocultural influences has been studied. Many of the most distinguished sociologists have used this particular problem to illustrate theories of the field. At the same time, the changing facts of technology, organization, and cost were charted as the necessary context for understanding the changes in professional–patient encounters.

There are also distinctive regional-cultural interpretations of the therapeutic relationship. European sociologists consistently have emphasized the significance of power (Foucault, 1978). This perspective makes the human body, and hence the patient, the passive recipient of pathology, and sees the professional as an agent of the state (Rosen, 1974). David Armstrong, a British medical sociologist, has pointed out that in Britain, not until about 1970 was the importance of the "inherently problematic . . . [aspects of the] . . . doctor–patient relationship" recognized (Armstrong, 1982; Interdepartmental Committee on Medical Schools, 1944). Not until the Todd Report was history taking described as "a great deal more . . . than simply asking a series of prescribed questions and checking the accuracy of the answers" (Great Britain, 1968). Essentially, Foucault viewed the clinical examination as a technique of surveillance. Beginning in the eighteenth century, such surveillance invoked a disciplinary power and required that the body (and hence the patient) be a discrete (passive) object. The change signaled by the Todd Report suggests "the beginnings of the fabrication of patient subjectivity" or, more simply, the activation of the patient (Armstrong, 1982).

Americans, on the other hand, have been preoccupied largely with the analysis of medicine as a profession, placing emphasis upon the role of the physician as a professional with resultant claims to autonomy and dominance (Freidson, 1970b). Initially, this perspective placed the patient in a primarily passive role. The American approach, however, has been to construct models that separate each role according to its structure—its reciprocal privileges and obligations—and its function for the society, defining the doctor as the legitimizer of illness and thereby the agent of social control, and the patient as an involuntary deviant who is allowed temporary exemptions from normal social expectations but is required to resume his or her place as soon as possible. Americans have assumed that within the framework of cultural expectations, behavior in these roles is volun-

tary. Europeans have directed their concern mainly to questions about how the rights and obligations of doctor and patient are inherent and controlled by the state.

These distinctive frames of reference for the analysis of medical relationships are reflected in very different systems for the delivery of health care. European nations, in both financing and service organization, have constructed systems that provide universal access to health care. Whether by a government-run national health service (the British model) or by national health insurance (the government guarantees the payment of fees for service by an essentially independent profession), the goal is to provide health care as a fundamental right for all citizens. The United States, virtually alone among modern industrialized nations—South Africa is its only companion state—has not guaranteed this right for the sick nor established the obligations of the caregiver, choosing instead to rely primarily on an implicit contract between the medical profession and the society. The latter arrangement, on the premises of individualism, claims that the doctor–patient relationship is sacred, based on the privileges of the professional to autonomy and the patient's right to choose his or her doctor. The alternative approach is based on the premise that in the therapeutic relationship, the behavior of the individuals—and their rights—depends upon social controls vested in the state. "Models," the Americans choose to call their explanations, signifying the fullness and reciprocity of the interaction between doctor and patient.

However, the intellectual distance between the continents has steadily grown smaller. When one traces the full history, the American and European interpretations can be seen gradually to converge. The starting point is in the 1930s, with all the major theories of sociological thought applied to the therapeutic relationship. Although the healing art is older than—and practiced by others than—the physician, the doctor's role has been the centerpiece. Other helping roles—the nurse, social worker, and various "allied health professionals"—have received attention (Aiken, 1983), but historically it is the therapist as a professional in modern society who has most interested the sociologist, and medicine is seen as the archetypal profession.

The result has been a changing portrait of both doctor and patient—from a dominantly psychological perspective to a sharp turn when Talcott Parsons introduced the social-system frame of reference (Parsons, 1951), shifting the analysis to the social roles of therapist and client, instilled in each individual by agents of socialization like the family and schools. The idea was that the qualities of patienthood were part of social development. We learn what to expect of physicians and how to behave as patients. Such roles were interpreted as "functional" components fashioned to maintain the society. Within this framework, the doctor's achieved high level of expertise is described as essential to modern scientific health care, and as a consequence, medical education is spotlighted. The medical school is seen as the principal source of attitudes and values as well as of training in skills and knowledge. That approach enhances the physician's image of awesome technological accomplishment and heroic personal attributes, while the patient is relegated to a subordinate, fragile state in which the only requirements are to be motivated to get well and to consult the physician toward that end.

The reaction to this approach, beginning in the 1960s, changed the role images dramatically: Complex bureaucratic forces were elevated to predominance over the voluntaristic choices of individuals (Starr, 1982). The "monopoly of dominance" replaced "technological achievement" as the more popular view of the doctor; the patient came to be viewed as "exploited" by the physician as much as or more than he or she was victimized by the primarily organic forces of illness. The doctor and patient became antagonists, each from a separate world, and their adversarial relationship was described as a "clash of perspectives" instead of a balanced, interdependent system.

In this changing approach, sociological thought has run parallel to the public's attitude toward the medical profession. The sociologists' picture of the physician, at first cautious and respectful, reflected the peak of public prestige and trust that allocated to doctors the privilege of virtually complete autonomy as "high priests in the temples of science" (Churchill, 1949). That pedestal was not an easy resting place, however. Physicians became the objects of public exhortation, government regulation, and legal attack.

The implications of the ethical standards by which physicians are judged are profound. After centuries of struggle to win the right to take risks, under conditions of uncertainty (Sigerist, 1960; Fox, 1957), in the "best interests of their patients," doctors now find themselves confronted by a fresh demand for accountability. The responsibility that was once assumed in trust is increasingly subject to the formal controls either of state-run systems or of various forms of peer review and medical audit. The added pressure of changing definitions of both the onset of life and its termination, stimulated by new technologies, has intensified the challenge to social values (Fox, 1979).

The therapeutic relationship is also responding to changes in the age profile, particularly of the populations of the United States and other modern industrial nations, and altered patterns of illness and disability. The challenge for physicians increasingly has become less a matter of cure and more of maintaining function (Mechanic, 1985).

At the same time, the sciences basic to medical practice—represented by modern molecular biology, ge-

netics, and the neurosciences, together with computer-related technologies—have produced what has been called a "paradigmatic leap" that must profoundly affect the basic human relations of medical practice (Marston and Jones, 1992). As medical knowledge and technology have expanded, public expectations of physicians' expertise and caring have become higher than ever before, complicated by patient needs for a more active, sharing role in therapy.

The development of sociological interpretation of the therapeutic relationship must be viewed as an expansion rather than a linear growth. It is not possible to say that the models have emerged successively, each more valid than its predecessor. The theories represented are still hypothetical. We present them in historical order.

The system model

Functionalism.   As applied to both biology and sociology, functional theory proposes that the relationships between the basic elements, whether chemical and physiological or social roles and institutions, are arranged in systems rather than as sums of their parts. Also basic in this conception is that the system is inherently driven toward equilibrium, a homeostatic balance that is reasserted whenever an intervention or change occurs. This dynamic toward balance and stability is the source of the term "functionalism." It is assumed that living processes, including but not limited to the social, are dominated by relationships that function to maintain or reassert stability to the whole. Thus the terms "system," "function," and "equilibrium" are often used interchangeably: Functionalist theory is system theory.

Although not the first functionalist in social thought, Lawrence J. Henderson pioneered the application of an equilibrium model to the doctor–patient relationship (Henderson, 1935). This he did only in midcareer, after having established himself as an outstanding biological scientist by translating Willard Gibbs's model of physicochemical systems for use in the study of blood physiology. Known as the formulator of the acid–base equilibrium, he applied his functional model with simultaneous equations to explain the quantitative relationship of eight variables of the blood.

Functionalism in physics, chemistry, and biology replaced the linear, cause-and-effect positivism dominant in the nineteenth century. The introduction of this theoretical framework and its mathematical proofs had produced revolutionary effects in biology, and Henderson believed they would be duplicated in social science. The essence of his reasoning was expressed as follows:

> Because every factor interacts in a social system, because everything, every property, every relation, is

therefore in a state of mutual dependence with everything else, ordinary cause-and-effect analysis of events is rarely possible. In fact, it must be regarded as one of the two great sources of error in sociological work. (Henderson, 1970, p. 29)

Henderson's application of the functionalist model to social systems produced a limited conception, and his model was mechanical and simplistic. As a result, his achievement in social science was mainly that of the seminal teacher: to inspire and challenge colleagues and students to take his model further.

Henderson's was soon followed by other interpretations of the social-system model. Illustrations and applications of the theory were drawn from all the major social institutions, especially the industrial and educa-

tional, but the doctor–patient relationship remained important. The major functional analysts of the therapeutic relationship, their illustrative examples, and their special contributions to knowledge are listed in Table 1.

Talcott Parsons, more than any other, carried forward the discussion of the doctor–patient relationship as a social system, giving it full expression as part of sociological theory (Parsons, 1951). He argued that human social relationships can be described as patterns rooted in cultural expectation about the social roles of group members; that the fundamental process of behavior is communication; and that the integrity of the system is maintained by homeostasis, defined as a dynamic force that reacts to any change or intervention by reasserting a balance in the system that enables it to perform its intended function.

TABLE 1.   Functional Models of the Doctor–Patient Relationship, Illustrative Cases, and Effects on the Field, 1930–1965

Models	Illustrative Examples	Effects on the Field
Lawrence J. Henderson 1935	Cancer patient: socioemotional determinants of system process	Established legitimacy of medical relationship as a subject of scientific inquiry
Talcott Parsons 1951	Institutional case: the profession a social system	Contributed to general theory of social behavior
Florence Kluckhohn, John Spiegel 1954	Psychiatric patients, studied according to cultural value orientation	Contributed to general theory of behavior, combining sociological with psychoanalytic concepts: transactional theory
William Caudill 1958	The hospitalized mental patient	Applied social-system theory to analysis of mental hospital; conceived hospital as a functional social system
Thomas Szasz, Marc Hollender 1956	Acute, ambulatory, and chronic diseases, to illustrate behavioral implication of biological symptoms	Operationalized role theory in medical terms; articulated system theory for education of physicians and to improve clinical practice
Michael Balint 1957	Ambulatory patient of general practitioner	Expanded biomedical model (in Great Britain) to include socioemotional; broke down mind–body dualism.
Samuel W. Bloom 1963	Diabetes, mental illness, and multiproblem patient to illustrate sociocultural determinants	Applied functional theory to health care in historical/ developmental terms
Kenneth Arrow 1963	The medical-care market	Adapted Pareto to general economic theory by conceptualizing optimum equilibrium as a theorem of competitive systems
Edward Suchman 1965	A population of "seriously ill" patients: a survey	Operationalized social-system explanation of health-services utilization

Adapted from Bloom and Speedling, 1989, p. 115.

Parsons conceived of the doctor–patient relationship as a social-role interaction in which the sick role is voluntary; for instance, a person can be ill—say, with a cold—but choose not to be "sick," a status that invokes privileges and obligations determined by the cultural expectations of the society. The sick role is a form of social deviance that must be controlled to prevent the abuse of the dependency of illness. The professional role combines healing the patient and social control as the agent of the society. Accordingly, the sick role is temporary, undesirable, and socially disruptive. The professional is a technical expert who legitimizes the claim to illness and is responsible for returning the sick person to his or her normal role in society.

Criticisms of Parsons's views are of two distinct types. One is intellectual, challenging his theoretical premises and argument (Freidson, 1970a). The other is political, interpreting the work of both Henderson and Parsons as a conservative political response to the historical events of the early 1930s, particularly the Great Depression and the rise of communism (Gouldner, 1970).

The theoretical criticism of the model focuses on Parsons's emphasis on the asymmetry of the therapeutic situation—that is, the professional dominance versus the client's dependence—and in the distancing effect of that asymmetry. Parsons is interpreted as a defender of the technical elitism of the modern physician. His patients must be "controlled," lest they take advantage of the privileges of the sick role to prolong dependency; his physicians must be "protected" from emotional overinvolvement with their patients. The consequences, the criticism asserts, are not just to explain a role asymmetry based upon the achieved technical expertise of the professional, but also to categorize and label the roles so that the passive, dependent patient and the expert doctor become hardened stereotypes.

The continuous development of functionalist interpretations of the therapeutic relationship was broken abruptly in the 1960s with the appearance of studies that emphasized the structural, situational determinants and directly challenged the validity of the functional.

Structural conflict theory. Eliot Freidson is the major spokesman for the application of the structural conflict theory to the professional–patient relationship. The therapeutic interaction, he argued, is most effectively analyzed as a clash of perspectives. "The professional expects patients to accept what he recommends on his terms; patients seek services in their own terms. In that each seeks to gain his own terms, there is conflict" (Freidson, 1961, p. 171). The patient, in this formulation, is assumed to be governed by an interpersonal order equal in complexity to that of the professional. The asymmetry of Parsons's model underscoring the physician's technical expertise is discarded. The patient

responds largely on the basis of current experience and sources of influence, not as a result of deeply embedded beliefs and expectation derived from long-term cultural socialization. Between doctor and patient, negotiation, not persuasion, occurs. The critical factor is structure, not function—the structural social positions based on the separate statuses and interests of the client and the professional. The deviance of the sick role, within this framework, becomes more central and more complex than in Parsons. A distinctive influence is assigned to stigma. For example, mental illness and sexually transmitted diseases, Freidson argues, are perceived by society on a variable scale of deviance and stigmatized accordingly; they are not lumped together as diseases that are beyond the control of the patient.

Freidson's critique of Parsons was very specific. First, the Parsons model sees the doctor–patient relationship from too limited a perspective, most essentially that of the physician; it does not pay attention to the varying expectations of all members of the "role-set," including the patients (or, more inclusively, their lay associates as well) and the nurses and other persons involved in the process of treatment. Second, expectations are presented by Parsons as though they are the primary influence on actual behavior; they are only an ideal standard against which actual behavior is judged. Third, influence does not inhere in the expectation but in the position of the person holding it; only from the structure of the situation and the limits imposed by it can one weigh the possibility of an expectation's being met. Fourth and most important, the functional model ignores the necessity of conflict in human relationships. Insofar as each person, the professional and the patient, seeks to gain his or her own terms from the other, there is conflict.

This approach spawned a succession of studies about the therapeutic situation. The major examples are listed in Table 2. Through these studies, the view of the patient was transformed. Fully equal to the physician, the patient might behave passively, influenced either by personality or by the structure of the situation. Nevertheless, the patient role was no longer inherently subordinate by virtue of the physician's technical expertise or of the patient's lack of adequate knowledge.

Neo-Marxism, bureaucracy, and the politics of health

The high point of structural conflict theory occurred with the 1970 publication by Freidson of the second of his two books about the medical profession. Marxist critiques followed by Howard Waitzkin and Barbara Waterman in 1974 and by Vicente Navarro in 1975.

The new Marxism built its argument on the classic conception that social behavior is essentially organized

TABLE 2. Models of the Doctor–Patient Relationship, Their Illustrative Cases, and Effects on the Field: Structuralism (Conflict Theory, Labeling), 1960–1975

Models	Illustrative Examples	Effects on the Field
Erwin Goffman 1961	Hospitalized mental patients	General theory of structured deviance; labeling; social stigma. Concepts: total institution, moral career of patients
Eliot Freidson 1961, 1970b	Health-care institutions; HMOs; the medical profession	General theory of conflict behavior determined by situational factors; clash of perspectives mediated by negotiation; professional autonomy and monopoly; patient networks
David Mechanic 1962	Illness behavior in various contexts	A multivariate theory: synthesized social psychological with situational variables; designed to operationalize for research; problem-oriented. Based on Volkart and W. I. Thomas. Health behavior as coping
Julius A. Roth 1963	Hospitalized tuberculosis patients	General theory: management of illness by normative timetables; institutional organization of illness response
Thomas Szasz 1964	Disabled patients, mental and physical	Critique of functionalism; contribution to deviance and labeling theory
Thomas Scheff 1966	Hospitalized mental patients	General theory of social deviance; labeling

Adapted from Bloom and Speedling, 1989, pp. 122–123.

according to principles of social stratification or social class, based on materialistic determinants, and inevitably dominated by one class, leading to monopolistic control of resources and markets by the dominant class and to the exploitation of subordinate groups for profit or gain of the more powerful class. Waitzkin illustrated what he called the "micropolitics" of the doctor–patient relationship, using the following types of cases: (1) a young worker with occupationally caused sterility; (2) neonatal death attributable to neglect caused by poverty and racial discrimination; (3) an elderly man burdened by costs of technically oriented medicine. Waitzkin analyzed more than 300 taped doctor–patient interviews in an effort to demonstrate that medicine, like other social institutions, functions as part of the "ideologic state apparatus," with the doctor as the agent of ideology and social control. The micropolitics of the doctor–patient relationship, he argued, revealed contradictions that no current political system resolves (Waitzkin, 1991).

The boundaries between this view and that of the earlier structuralists were not as sharp as the demarcations with functionalism. Nevertheless, there are important differences. In Freidson, for example, there is no hint of patient exploitation. Nor does the drive among doctors for "professional autonomy and dominance," as described by the structuralists, mean anything similar to the Marxist description of the physician as a self-interested manager of health resources. What neo-Marxists like Waitzkin added to forecast subsequent trends was the analysis of how both doctor and patient have become captives of monopolistic trends in the health-care industries.

The focus of the 1980s was on the same monopolistic big business, but with a different interpretation. Paul Starr (1982), for example, argued that rational behavior leads to large-scale privatization and the absorption of health care into the marketplace. He described the corporatization of the health-care system of the United States in five dimensions:

1. Change in the type of ownership and control, shifting from nonprofit and governmental service organizations, especially hospitals, to for-profit health-care companies.
2. Horizontal integration, the decline of freestanding institutions and the consequent shift in the locus of

control from community boards to regional and national health-care corporations.

3. Diversification and corporate restructuring, the shift from single-unit organizations operating in one market to conglomerates involved in a variety of health-care markets.

4. Vertical integration, the shift from a single level of care organizations, like acute-care hospitals, to organizations that embrace the various phases and levels of care, such as health maintenance organizations (HMOs).

5. Industry concentration, the increasing concentration of control of health services in regional markets and the nation as a whole.

The implications of these trends, it was argued, are to depersonalize the therapeutic relationship and to change the nature of the social roles. The doctor, increasingly a salaried employee instead of an individual entrepreneur, is losing autonomy and, in effect, is becoming proletarianized. The patient, as a result of pressures to join large health-care organizations, cannot freely choose a doctor or join with the doctor in certain decisions because cost control by the organization intervenes.

Such interpretations were buttressed by the increase in large-scale organizations for the delivery of health care, but the interest of scholars in psychosocial factors in therapeutic encounters continued to be strong. Compliance, the extent to which patients follow the recommendations of their therapists, for example, remained an important problem independent of the organizational framework for health care. Marshall Becker and Lois Maimon (1982) described a "health belief model" that made individual motivations and beliefs about the validity of treatment methods the central factors of health behavior. Attempts to quantify the sociobehavioral determinants of compliance preoccupied many researchers during the next two decades. The physician, at the same time, has been scrutinized in comparable empirical and quantitative detail as a "decision-maker" (Elstein et al., 1978).

This quantitative trend is reflected in the training and assessment of medical students and residents. With the increasing orientation toward the use of measurements of clinical reasoning and behavior, didactic teaching and memorization are being replaced by problem-based learning and experiential learning situations such as simulations of clinical cases, called standardized patient (SP) methods (Woodward and Gerard, 1985). The goal of these efforts to change how physicians are trained is to create a more patient-oriented approach and, at the same time, influence doctors to become active, lifelong learners in order to maintain effectiveness

under conditions of rapidly advancing basic medical sciences (Marston and Jones, 1992).

The nonmedical healing professions

The history of the healing professions has been dominated by medicine. Although nurses, public-health workers, dentists, and social workers have been major contributors to the health of individuals and communities, their professional status and power have always been less than those of physicians. However, dramatic changes have expanded the need for the care of health and disease, challenging the monopoly of doctors. Constantly advancing technology applied to diagnosis and treatment, the increase in life expectancy and consequent growth of the elderly population, and changed patterns of illness and disability have forced physicians to depend on partnerships with members of other healing professions.

Nursing is the outstanding case in point. Nurses, although much more numerous than physicians (four nurses for every doctor), increasingly professionalized (over 100,000 have master's or doctorate degrees), and performing tasks in health settings previously restricted to physicians, continue to struggle for release from the view, argued by Freidson, that, following precedents established by Florence Nightingale more than a century ago, "All nursing work flowed from the doctor's orders . . . [so that] nursing became a formal part of the doctor's work, a technical trade. . . . Nursing thus was defined as a subordinate part of the technical division of labor surrounding medicine" (Freidson, 1970b, p. 61). There is some evidence that success in this struggle is at last being achieved.

Advanced-practice nurses, for example, are registered nurses with specialty training, usually at the master's degree level, in primary care (i.e., nurse practitioners and nurse–midwives) or acute care of in-patients (i.e., clinical nurse specialists). Mary Mundinger writes:

> The practice of nurse practitioners has been evaluated since 1965 when the role was developed by Henry Silver, M.D., and Loretta Ford, R.N. When measures of diagnostic certainty, management competence, or comprehensiveness, quality, and cost are used, virtually every study indicates that the primary care provided by nurse practitioners is equivalent or superior to that provided by physicians. . . .
>
> Over the past few years, state legislatures have broadened the authority of nurse practitioners to receive direct payment and write prescriptions, and the barriers to independence have fallen. As a result, nurse practitioners can establish independent practices that parallel those of primary care physicians (either solo or health maintenance organizations), or they can establish col-

laborative practices in which doctors and nurses care for patients together. (Mundinger, 1994, p. 211)

Initiatives from private foundations and the government have encouraged the professionalization of nursing and the other healing occupations, rewarding the creation of both educational and health-care reforms that foster the creation of teams working together as equals. Nevertheless, these other professions remain in the shadow of medicine. As a consequence, nurses, probably the highest-status members of the paramedicals, earn an average of less than a third of physicians' incomes; their training, except for the 5 percent who have earned higher degrees, is considerably shorter and less rigorous; and nursing is almost totally a women's profession, a fact that, regrettable though it is, remains a classic indicator of low occupational status.

However, as indicated by the testimony of Mary Mundinger above, the status of nursing as a profession has changed. Increasingly, nurses are both trained in and responsible for the complex knowledge and technical aspects of patient care. In 1960, 83 percent of new graduates were trained in hospitals, the rest in colleges and universities. By 1980, those figures had reversed.

We are witnessing, therefore, a historical development in nursing reminiscent of the changes that occurred in medicine in the 1910s. Like medicine in the post-Flexner era (1910 and following), nursing is seeking to increase its professionalism by extending its training in close association with the university. Included is new emphasis on biomedical science and research.

The value implications of these changes are of particular concern. Professionalism for nurses tends to emphasize intellectual and technical skills in an occupation whose major function has been as much the ministering of nurturant and humane care as technical prowess.

For the patient, the options seem to narrow as knowledge and technical skill increase. Whereas once it seemed reasonable to expect physicians to combine technical expertise with emotional sensitivity and skill, and nurses to complement them in both, now the patient gains equality and independence but with increasing emotional distance from caregivers.

Under the current conditions of health care, social workers would seem to have a strategic role. They are, after all, uniquely trained in the skills of interpersonal relations, and professionally are intended to function as the patient's advocate for well-being, both within the period of illness and in preparation for the recovery period. Yet, here, too, the pressures for professional status take an ironic toll. A trend toward private practice with fee-for-service financial rewards attracts social workers toward professional status on the medical model and away from the team model in which their function is to balance the technical with the social.

The same value dilemma confronts all the healing professions. A polarization has developed between two orientations, one centered on the *what* of health care and the other on the *how*. The former has been called a reductionistic approach, emphasizing biomedical knowledge and technology; the latter is the "social ecology" or "humanistic" approach.

The values of these two approaches are significantly different. The more traditional, reductionistic approach is dominated by faith that all problems of health and illness have rational solutions, and by a dedication to competence in practice and to a community of science that transcends personal interest. Patient, societal, and ethical issues are seen as matters of opinion not susceptible to rational discourse (Pellegrino, 1978; Fox, 1979).

The approach of social ecology, on the other hand, rests on a very different set of values. The social and behavioral sciences and even the humanities are here as pertinent as the biological sciences; students are selected on the basis of social concern and interest in people and their problems; emphasis is on caring as much as on curing. The community, not the university hospital, is the proper locus for the education of health professionals.

Although one can say that neither of these approaches has sought or gained exclusive dominance, their differences are important enough to generate partisan claims from each about the failures of the past, the needs of the future, and the implications for patients and society. Both the value of modern science and the critical need for enlightened social and ethical orientations can be found in the way national commissions are addressing the problems of today's healing professions (Marston and Jones, 1992).

Summary and conclusions

The definition of the professions is the foundation of sociological analysis of the professional–patient relationship. Uniquely among modern occupations, a profession has been seen as an activity that requires extensive training based upon a continuously developing knowledge base coupled with the application of such knowledge for the general welfare of society. Therefore, although the rewards of professional life have been substantial, it is assumed that the professional is not free to exploit such skills and knowledge for personal gain alone, as other entrepreneurs may—the so-called principle of *caveat emptor* (let the buyer beware). On the contrary, the professional is granted unusual privileges involving access especially to the personal and biological privacy of patients, but only on an implicit contractual premise that such professional rights will conform to general rules of the welfare of society.

Medicine has been the primary subject of such analysis because it is seen as the archetype of professions.

Virtually every person needs the help of healing occupations; the other classic professions, the law and the clergy, are not so ubiquitous. Therefore, a large sociological literature grew out of the study of medicine as a profession. However, the practice of medicine has changed radically in modern times and continues to change. Research in the biomedical sciences is usually considered the major driving force of this transformation, but changes in the social organization of the delivery of health services, the application side of the medical profession, have been no less dramatic.

In the wake of both the bioetchnological and application developments, new ethical issues have appeared and earlier ones have deepened. Bioethics as a separate discipline has grown significantly, very likely as a direct consequence of these changes. Sociology, meanwhile, has spawned its own forms of interest in medical ethics. In part, sociologists have followed the tradition of individualism, which interprets behavior as a social psychological process determined by the values individuals learn and carry with them into social encounters. A different perspective emphasizes the material technologies and organizational constraints that dominate the therapeutic relationship. For example, the bureaucratization of medicine has advanced, creating a situation in which both doctor and patient meet less as individuals than as members of groups. The resulting formalization has altered the emotional quality of the exchange and the nature of responsibility and accountability for those involved therein.

Conventional wisdom has suggested that the ethical problems of current therapeutic relationships are driven mainly by technical imperatives. Sociologists, in the main, however, have argued that bioethics is determined by the value context in which medical technology must be managed, not by the intrinsic qualities of the technology. The dilemmas—the extension of life at the sacrifice of quality of life, the increased efficiency of neonatology at the cost of disability—are seen as only part of the current medicoethical challenge. Equally important is the unequal access to the benefits of technological advancement for populations that are disadvantaged by poverty, by race, or by other sources of discrimination.

Pressures are increasing for comprehensive entitlement to medical care but, as in the past, the chances for such change remain in doubt. As analysts have noted, the proportion of national income that will be invested in health care is both a value judgment and a product of the political process. As a result, David Mechanic writes:

> When faced with competing claims on national resources, government finds it easier to restrain growth in programs affecting the poor and disabled, who constitute relatively weak constituencies, than to reduce sub-

sidies shared by large, articulate, and sophisticated segments of the larger American public. . . . The imminent risk we face is not a deterioration in medical care overall, but more a continuing erosion of access and appropriate care for our most unfortunate populations. . . . Between 1976 and 1984 the proportion of poor and near poor covered by the Medicaid program decreased from 65 to 52 percent. (Mechanic, 1985, p. 454)

In the pluralistic society that America epitomizes, attitudes have become polarized. At one extreme are those who view the system as basically sound and strongly support the conventional structure of medicine. At the other extreme are those "who view the delivery system as so flawed in its structure and priorities and so dominated by special interests that only major reorganization offers any promise of an equitable and effective delivery system in the future" (Mechanic, 1985, p. 190).

The struggle between these polar opposites will be strongly affected by the values that are basic to American thinking and that inevitably must be reconciled in the policy decisions that will be made. The trend at this time appears to be toward universal health insurance. The methods reinforce organizational development that fosters large corporate structures. Those who cling to the right to choose one's personal doctor, and believe that no health-care system can function effectively otherwise, feel they have been put on the defensive against pressures for cost-effectiveness, even rationing, but nevertheless persevere in a time-honored American belief in individualism.

The contributions of sociologists, if they follow the patterns of the period since the 1940s, will continue to focus on the microrelations of medicine, especially the doctor–patient relationship (Stacey, 1985). They will also explore the ethics of human research, and issues of public policy such as equality of access to care and the role of the professions in determining the availability of medical and health-care services (Sorenson and Swazey, 1989).

Renée Fox lists the primary values of American society as follows: individualism, contractual relations, veracity, the fair allocation of scarce resources, and the principle of benevolence. Individualism, for Fox, is "the primary value-complex on which the intellectual and moral edifice of bioethics rests" (Fox and Swazey, 1984, p. 352). It starts with a belief in the importance, uniqueness, dignity, and sovereignty of the individual. From this flows the assumption that every person has certain individual rights. Autonomy, self-determination, and privacy are fundamental. In addition, individuals are entitled to the opportunity to find, develop, and realize themselves and their self-interests. They are entitled to be and do as they see fit, so long as they do not violate the comparable rights of others.

Can these values be reconciled with the changes in modern American society, especially those that foster large organizational structures? Sociologists will certainly devote themselves to such questions, and include the fate of microrelations such as the professional–patient relationship.

SAMUEL W. BLOOM

Directly related to this article are the other articles in the entry: HISTORICAL PERSPECTIVES, *and* ETHICAL ISSUES. *Also directly related are the entries* ALLIED HEALTH PROFESSIONS; HEALTH AND DISEASE, *article on* SOCIOLOGICAL PERSPECTIVES; MEDICINE, SOCIOLOGY OF; MEDICINE AS A PROFESSION; NURSING AS A PROFESSION; *and* PROFESSION AND PROFESSIONAL ETHICS. *For a further discussion of topics mentioned in this article, see the entries* CONFIDENTIALITY; FIDELITY AND LOYALTY; INFORMATION DISCLOSURE; INFORMED CONSENT; PRIVACY IN HEALTH CARE; *and* PRIVILEGED COMMUNICATIONS. *For a discussion of related ideas, see the entries* AUTHORITY; AUTONOMY; BENEFICENCE; COMPASSION; COMPETENCE; DEATH, *article on* DEATH IN THE WESTERN WORLD (*with its* POSTSCRIPT); HEALING; PATERNALISM; *and* RESPONSIBILITY. *See also the* APPENDIX (CODES, OATHS, AND DIRECTIVES RELATED TO BIOETHICS), SECTION II: ETHICAL DIRECTIVES FOR THE PRACTICE OF MEDICINE, *and* SECTION III: ETHICAL DIRECTIVES FOR OTHER HEALTHCARE PROFESSIONS.

Bibliography

AIKEN, LINDA H. 1983. "Nurses." In *The Handbook of Health, Health Care, and the Health Professions*, pp. 407–431. Edited by David Mechanic. New York: Free Press.

ARMSTRONG, DAVID. 1982. "The Doctor–Patient Relationship: 1930–80." In *The Problem of Medical Knowledge: Examining the Social Construction of Medicine*, pp. 109–122. Edited by Peter Wright and Andrew Treacher. Edinburgh: Edinburgh University Press.

ARROW, KENNETH J. 1963. "Uncertainty and the Welfare Economics of Medical Care." *American Economic Review* 53, no. 5:941–973.

BALINT, MICHAEL. 1964. *The Doctor, His Patient and the Illness.* 2d ed., rev. and enl. London: Pitman Medical.

BECKER, MARSHALL H., and MAIMON, LOIS A. 1983. "Models of Health-Related Behavior." In *The Handbook of Health, Health Care, and the Health Professions*, pp. 539–568. Edited by David Mechanic. New York: Free Press.

BLOOM, SAMUEL W. 1963. *The Doctor and His Patient: A Sociological Analysis.* New York: Russell Sage Foundation.

BLOOM, SAMUEL W., and SPEEDLING, EDWARD J. 1989. "The Education of Physicians: Training for What?" In *Medizin für die Medizin: Arzt und Ärztin zwischen Wissenschaft und Praxis. Festschrift für Hannes G. Pauli*, pp. 107–129. Edited by Peter Saladin, Hans Jurg Schaufelberger, and Peter Schlappi. Basel: Halbing & Lichtenhahn.

CAUDILL, WILLIAM A. 1958. *The Psychiatric Hospital as a Small Society.* Cambridge, Mass.: Harvard University Press.

CHURCHILL, EDWARD D. 1949. "The Development of the Hospital." In *The Hospital in Contemporary Life.* Edited by Nathaniel W. Faxon. Cambridge, Mass.: Harvard University Press.

ELSTEIN, ARTHUR S.; SHULMAN, LEE S.; and SPRAFKA, SARAH A. 1978. *Medical Problem Solving: An Analysis of Clinical Reasoning.* Cambridge, Mass.: Harvard University Press.

FOUCAULT, MICHEL. 1978. *The History of Sexuality.* Translated by Robert Hurley. York: Pantheon.

FOX, RENÉE C. 1957. "Training for Uncertainty." In *The Student-Physician: Introductory Studies in the Sociology of Medical Education*, pp. 207–241. Edited by Robert K. Merton, George G. Reader, and Patricia L. Kendall. Cambridge, Mass.: Harvard University Press.

———. 1979. "Advanced Medical Technology—Social and Ethical Implications." In her *Essays in Medical Sociology: Journeys into the Field*, pp. 413–461. New York: Wiley.

FOX, RENÉE C., and SWAZEY, JUDITH P. 1984. "Medical Morality Is Not Bioethics—Medical Ethics in China and the United States." *Perspectives in Biology and Medicine* 27, no. 3:336–360.

FREIDSON, ELIOT. 1961. *Patients' Views of Medical Practice: A Study of Subscribers to a Prepaid Medical Plan in the Bronx.* New York: Russell Sage Foundation.

———. 1970a. *Professional Dominance: The Social Structure of Medical Care.* New York: Aldine.

———. 1970b. *Profession of Medicine: A Study of the Sociology of Applied Knowledge.* New York: Dodd, Mead.

GOFFMAN, ERVING. 1961. *Asylums.* New York: Doubleday-Anchor.

GOULDNER, ALVIN W. 1970. *The Coming Crisis of Western Sociology: Essays on the Social Situation of Mental Patients and Other Inmates.* New York: Basic Books.

GREAT BRITAIN. ROYAL COMMISSION ON MEDICAL EDUCATION. 1968. *Royal Commission on Medical Education, 1965–1968: Report.* [Todd Report]. London: HMSO.

HENDERSON, LAWRENCE J. 1935. *Pareto's General Sociology: A Physiologist's Interpretation.* Cambridge, Mass.: Harvard University Press.

———. 1970. *On the Social System: Selected Writings.* Edited by Bernard Barber. Chicago: University of Chicago Press.

INTERDEPARTMENTAL COMMITTEE ON MEDICAL SCHOOLS (GREAT BRITAIN AND SCOTLAND). 1944. *Report of the Interdepartmental Committee on Medical Schools.* [Goodenough Report]. London: HMSO.

KLUCKHOHN, FLORENCE R., and SPIEGEL, JOHN P. 1954. *Integration and Conflict in Family Behavior.* Topeka, Kan.: Group for Advancement of Psychiatry.

MARSTON, ROBERT Q., and JONES, ROSEANN M., eds. 1992. *Medical Education in Transition.* Princeton, N.J.: Robert Wood Johnson Foundation.

MECHANIC, DAVID. 1962. "The Concept of Illness Behavior." *Journal of Chronic Diseases* 15, no. 2:189–194.

———. 1968. *Medical Sociology: A Selective View.* New York: Free Press.

———. 1985. "Cost Containment and the Quality of Medical Care: Rationing Strategies in an Era of Constrained Resources." *Milbank Memorial Fund Quarterly/Health and Society* 63, no. 3:453–475.

MUNDINGER, MARY O. 1994. "Sounding Board: Advanced-Practice Nursing—Good Medicine for Physicians?" *New England Journal of Medicine* 330, no. 3:211–214.

NAVARRO, VICENTE. 1975. "Social Policy Issues: An Explanation of the Composition, Nature, and Functions of the Present Health Sector of the United States." *Bulletin of the New York Academy of Medicine* 51, no. 1:199–234.

PARSONS, TALCOTT. 1951. *The Social System.* New York: Free Press.

PELLEGRINO, EDMUND D. 1978. "Medical Education." In vol. 2 of *Encyclopedia of Bioethics,* pp. 863–870. New York: Free Press.

ROSEN, GEORGE, ed. 1974. *From Medical Police to Social Medicine: Essays on the History of Health Care.* New York: Science History Publications.

ROTH, JULIUS A. 1963. *Timetables: Structuring the Passage of Time in Hospital Treatment and Other Careers.* Indianapolis, Ind.: Bobbs-Merrill.

SCHEFF, THOMAS J. 1966. *Being Mentally Ill: A Sociological Theory.* Chicago: Aldine.

SIGERIST, HENRY ERNEST. 1960. "The Physician's Profession Through the Ages." In his *On the History of Medicine,* pp. 3–15. Edited by Felix Marti-Ibanez. New York: MD Publications.

SORENSON, JAMES R., and SWAZEY, JUDITH. 1989. "Sociological Perspectives on Ethical Issues in Medical and Health Care." In *Handbook of Medical Sociology,* 4th ed., pp. 492–507. Edited by Howard E. Freeman and Sol Levine. Englewood Cliffs, N.J.: Prentice-Hall.

STACEY, MARGARET. 1985. "Medical Ethics and Medical Practice: A Social Science View." *Journal of Medical Ethics* 11, no. 1:14–18.

STARR, PAUL. 1982. *The Social Transformation of American Medicine.* New York: Basic Books.

SUCHMAN, EDWARD A. 1965. "Stages of Illness and Medical Care." *Journal of Health and Social Behavior* 6, no. 3: 114–128.

SZASZ, THOMAS S. 1964. *The Myth of Mental Illness: Foundations of a Theory of Personal Conduct.* New York: Harper & Row.

SZASZ, THOMAS, and HOLLENDER, MARC H. 1956. "A Contribution to the Philosophy of Medicine: The Basic Models of the Doctor-Patient Relationship." AMA *Archives of Internal Medicine* 97:585–592.

WAITZKIN, HOWARD. 1991. *The Politics of Medical Encounters: How Patients and Doctors Deal with Social Problems.* New Haven, Conn.: Yale University Press.

WAITZKIN, HOWARD, and WATERMAN, BARBARA. 1974. *The Exploitation of Illness in Capitalist Society.* Indianapolis, Ind.: Bobbs-Merrill.

WOODWARD, C., and GERRARD, B. 1985. "Evaluation of the Doctor–Patient Relationship." In *Assessing Clinical Competence.* Edited by Vic Neufeld and Geoffrey R. Norman. New York: Springer.

III. ETHICAL ISSUES

Writing about and reflection on the ethical issues in the health professional–patient relationship have focused principally on the mutual interactions and expectations of two individuals: a professional (traditionally, a physician) and a patient. Several important basic ethical values, principles, and virtues continue to be relevant to the relationship between a patient and the wide range of health professionals with whom he or she interacts. This article addresses those enduring ethical aspects of the professional–patient relationship. It also discusses issues that have become relevant because of changes in the character and understanding of the relationship. The focus is on the health professional's position in the relationship, though at times the patient's role is highlighted.

As the companion articles in this entry aptly show, the sources of philosophical and moral knowledge on the topic of the physician–patient relationship are rich and varied. Historical knowledge, rational approaches from theological and philosophical ethics, sociological perspectives, and narrative approaches that emphasize story, image, and vision combine to create the major components. The following pages contain themes that are especially instrumental in creating our understanding of the ethical issues inherent in this unique relationship today, with reference to some major sources of each position.

Conduct, virtue, and context in the professional–patient relationship

There are two broad general ethical issues that can be evaluated in a relationship. The first is whether right conduct is exhibited by the parties toward each other and the second is whether praiseworthy character traits and attitudes (virtues) that ought to manifest themselves within the relationship are present. The context in which the relationship takes place also is relevant.

Conduct-related issues. Morally right conduct in relationships is understood through an examination of the principles (moral obligations and rights) in the relationship. The specific principles that ought to be present in the professional–patient relationship are described at length later in this article. Furthermore, judgments about the type of conduct parties ought to display toward each other in a relationship require attention to basic values those parties hold. It follows that the fundamental values of professionals, patients, and society must be taken into account in evaluating that relationship (Brody, 1981).

There are at least three levels of discourse in which we may engage when faced with a judgment about right or wrong conduct in general. Many of our evaluations are at the level strictly of feeling or emotion ("I hate," "I would like"), without any conscious reference to our assessments of right or wrong. At a second level we bring to mind certain moral rules that we believe should be followed, and enunciate those rules as a guide to conduct. At the third level (Henry Aiken's "Level of Ethical Principles") we engage in discourse that reflects a reasoning process about right and wrong, so that we can make a considered judgment about the situation (Aiken, 1962). All three levels are important in relationships as well: Feeling and emotion, as well as the recognition of relevant moral rules, are sources of information, but ultimately the ethical aspect of a judgment requires a readiness to engage in the reasoning process (Callahan, 1988). Complete consensus at the first and second levels still requires the rigor of examining the underlying ethical principles to assure that the rules themselves are appropriate as guides in a given situation.

Virtue-related issues.   A second area of ethical issues regarding a relationship is understood through an examination of virtues: the good or praiseworthy habits and dispositions of the parties. The focus is less on the things people *do* and more on the types of people they *are*. Just as we can engage in reflection about ethical principles that help to elucidate right from wrong conduct, so we can make reasoned judgments about the character traits and attitudes that people ought to exhibit in a relationship. We expect a person who develops and regularly exercises virtuous character traits to be more disposed to honor another's values and to create a better community than would a person who lacks them. In many relationships (such as the professional–patient relationship) one person's deeply held values can be either protected or compromised by the other. On this basis alone it is justifiable to place expectations of virtue on certain relationships. Some basic professional virtues that have bearing on the professional–patient relationship are discussed later in this article.

Contextual considerations.   The specific ethical elements needed for evaluating a relationship—moral obligations, rights, and virtues—will vary according to the context in which the relationship takes place. One needs to assess, for example, the special peculiarities of the way in which the relationship was formed, the basis for explicit or implicit expectations of the parties, the utility and function of the relationship, and the role of society's expectations.

Attempts to characterize the context and essence of the professional–patient relationship have been drawn primarily from the physician's relationship with patients, though important additional voices from nursing and other professions are emerging.

Moral models of the relationship

Assessments of right conduct and good moral habits and dispositions in the professional–patient relationship depend on the way in which the relationship itself is understood from a moral perspective. Several proposals have been made regarding the dominant models that characterize this relationship; a consideration of these

models will influence the understanding of the ethical issues discussed in this article.

Robert Veatch offers four models of the physician–patient relationship: the "engineering model," in which the physician acts as a scientist dealing with facts, divorced from questions of value; the "priestly model," an explicitly paternalistic and value-laden approach in which the physician assumes competence not only for medical facts but also for naming and interpreting value dimensions of health-care decisions on the patient's behalf; the "collegial model," in which physician and patient become "pals" assuming equality through mutual trust, loyalty, and roles; and the "contractual model," which entails a mutual understanding of benefits and responsibilities incumbent on each person involved (Veatch, 1972).

From a nursing perspective, Sheri Smith distinguishes three models of the nurse–patient relationship: In the "surrogate mother" model the nurse is morally obliged to assume ultimate responsibility for the well-being and care of an essentially passive patient; the "technician" model characterizes the nurse's responsibility as being limited to competently applying technical knowledge and skills to meet the patient's needs; and the "contracted clinician" model defines the nurse's responsibility by the values and rights of the patient and assumes that the patient is capable of determining her or his own best interests (Smith, 1980).

Many view a form of the contractual model with considerable favor today, some arguing that informed consent is at the heart of it while others emphasize the patient's interests as the key. But serious reservations have been raised about this model. For example, William F. May proposes that the concept of "covenant" rather than "contract" provides a morally richer basis for conceptualizing this relationship. In his theologically informed approach he argues that a covenant model includes contractual elements of mutual expectations and agreement but goes further. Covenantal ethics places the professional within a context in which he or she not only provides a good but acknowledges being a recipient of goods as well. The professional has received societal support for education and permission to practice as well as continuing to receive many benefits from health-care practice and from the patients themselves. Therefore, this model carries an element of professional gratitude that pushes the health professional to go beyond the bare minimum of what may be agreed upon in a contract-based relationship. In addition, covenant is a less individualized image than that of colleague, priest, or contracting agent, reminding the professional that his or her accountability may go beyond assuring that an individual patient is treated competently (May, 1975).

Paul Ramsey, who also proposes a covenant model, adds that certain moral attitudes and actions owed to each other are inherent in a covenantal context. His emphasis is on covenantal responsibilities (or "canons of loyalty") that we assume when we voluntarily undertake institutional relationships and roles. He names informed consent as a primary "canon of loyalty" in the relationship, but stretches the idea beyond the contract mode to specify that through this doctrine the professional and patient acknowledge full partnership as humans and promise fidelity to each other. "Consent expresses or establishes this relationship, and the requirement of consent sustains it" (Ramsey, 1970, pp. 5–6).

U.S. law places the professional–patient relationship in the class of "fiduciary relationships." In fiduciary relationships "each [person] must repose trust and confidence in the other and must exercise a corresponding degree of fairness and good faith," because the two persons cannot expect to have all of the usual facts that would allow them to contract as equals (Blackwell, 1968). This law is used by the legal profession to help hold physicians (and, to varying degrees, other health professionals) accountable for the fact that they have more power within the relationship and may not be able to equalize that power on the basis of disclosing relevant information to patients. Trust is the bridge to the relationship, and the burden is on the professional not only to expect the patient's trust but also to build a solid foundation upon which the patient can place his or her trust.

These few examples illustrate different models of the professional–patient relationship, each of which features different visions and goals. Each suggests its own list of important values and virtues. The following pages turn from the differences and provide the reader with some basic components of ethical thought common to all of the models.

Ethical principles in the professional–patient relationship

Several ethical principles are relevant in the professional–patient relationship and provide insight into its ethical foundations. Among the most important are respect for persons, nonmaleficence, beneficence, veracity, autonomy, and justice.

Respect for persons.   Respect for persons, highlighting the dignity of the patient as a person, is found in the preambles of most professional codes of ethics, mission statements of health-care organizations, and patient-rights documents, as well as many other ethics writings. The principle assumes that persons have inherent or essential worth simply because they are human beings. Diverse philosophical, religious, and scientific understandings of the nature of humaneness have created a wide base upon which the health professions can ground this ideal (Lammers and Verhey, 1987). But the principle also presents challenges to health professionals: One is to discern categories of beings that are per-

sons; another is to discern practical direction from such a general ideal. For example, two health professionals may agree on the Judaeo-Christian interpretation that all persons have worth or dignity because they are equally children of God or follow the common philosophy attributed to the philosopher Immanuel Kant that "persons must be treated as ends and not as means to ends"; yet the two may differ in their positions regarding the status of the fetus and come to different conclusions about which treatments to provide or withhold from, say, a patient suffering from acute alcohol syndrome. In spite of its difficulties, however, this principle makes a signal contribution to the relationship because it pushes health professionals in the direction of always showing respect for patients qua persons.

Nonmaleficence.   The maxim to do no harm, *primum non nocere*, often is cited as the first ethical principle of medical practice. Curiously, its source as a maxim in health care is unknown. However, its meaning and usefulness can be gleaned from the serious thought given to the concept in deontological (duty-oriented) approaches to moral philosophy. W. D. Ross argues that it is our stringent duty to inflict no harm intentionally, because to live in any other type of society would make each of us too vulnerable. This duty, he adds, is not covered by the duty to prevent or remove harm, or to do good (Ross, 1930). Albert Jonsen suggests that the principle is appropriate in health care because health care is a moral enterprise itself with an inherent understanding that harm should not result from voluntarily placing oneself in the professional–patient relationship. Patients interact with health-care professionals with the reasonable expectation that appropriate care—not careless or negligent or other harmful care—will be provided to the extent that it is within the power of the professional to do so (Jonsen, 1977).

The duty of nonmaleficence also places the professional on alert that society reasonably can expect that he or she will not be an agent of harm. The debates about physician-assisted dying, euthanasia, and abortion often focus on the interpretation of harm and the physician's role in participating in activities that cause harm. Discussion of maleficence must take into account that some types of harm are necessary in the name of that patient's greater good: For example, the patient undergoes the harm of the surgical knife in the name of removing the pathology.

Beneficence.   The principle of beneficence delineates conduct directed to the welfare of others and is pivotal in the understanding of the professional–patient relationship. Since its inception the relationship has had its grounding in the ideal that the professional's ethical priority is to further the welfare of a patient. Today that ideal is interpreted to have the stringency of a special moral obligation on the part of the professional to seek a patient's well-being, guided by that person's health-related concerns and needs. Any other worthy goal, such as furthering the knowledge about disease and its cure, or earning a just wage, or maintaining the efficiency or financial solvency of the institution, is not an appropriate beacon to guide the professional in this relationship.

Taken in combination with the principle of respect for persons, the principle of beneficence highlights the fact that health professionals have a moral obligation to treat all kinds of patients with whom they establish a relationship, assuming that the patient's problem lends itself to health-care intervention and the professional is competent to treat the patient's type of condition. Therefore, the principle is put to the test when the professional is prejudiced against people of color, or the Irish (or another ethnic group), or old people, or any other group, and therefore finds it difficult to treat members of such groups with respect. A health professional also may judge an individual patient "undesirable," "difficult," "disgusting," or even "hateful" on the basis of personal characteristics such as poor personal hygiene, effects of drug or alcohol dependency, irritating personality traits, or lifestyle choices (Groves, 1978). In each case, the health professional must regard the patient in the relationship as worthy of treatment however great a gulf exists between their respective values. If the differences are so disabling as to prevent the professional from providing good care, he or she must attempt to assure that the patient receives it from someone else.

In short, one foundational principle of the relationship is the professional's moral obligation to minister competently to the patient, using all of his or her skills to accomplish the goal of helping the patient. To meet this end, the health professional must focus on the person's needs whether the patient be model citizen or thief, old or young, man or woman, likable or not.

Veracity. Philosophers often treat the principle of truth-telling as a separate principle, but some argue that it is derivative, embedded in respect for persons, promise-keeping, or utility (Beauchamp and Childress, 1989). Robert Weir suggests that its stringency as a moral obligation means, in terms of the professional–patient relationship, that the professional intends to build this relationship on confidence and trust (Weir, 1980).

Given the moral stringency of truth-telling, an interesting ethical quandary arises when it falls to the professional to convey bad news to patients and families. Health professionals long have believed that patients want professionals to help them maintain hope in the face of catastrophe. For centuries this was interpreted as requiring the professional to protect patients from the truth at times, engaging, if necessary, in a "benevolent lie" and bearing responsibility for having breached the patient's moral expectation that veracity would be honored (Hartmann, 1932).

But this belief has shifted, at least in North America, where even in the face of catastrophe hope is believed to be enhanced by the patient's ability to take control of important life events; and this in turn depends on knowing the truth about his or her clinical condition. In other words, hope is not dependent solely on whether or not the truth is shared with the patient, but also on the role of veracity in maintaining a patient's exercise of autonomy.

Autonomy and self-determination. Patient autonomy in the professional–patient relationship honors not only the idea that the patient should have access to "the truth" but also the idea that all conditions required for remaining in control are met.

The principle of autonomy applied to the patient's situation has evolved from being viewed as the patient's prerogative to refuse treatment to the right to refuse it, and finally to the right to play a central role in determining the course of treatment. For example, the increased emphasis on informed consent as the brokering chip in the professional–patient relationship places a major focus on the patient's role as an active agent in care decisions. In 1990 the passage by the U.S. Congress of the Patient Self-Determination Act took patient autonomy further out of the realm of ethics and into the legal arena by making it a legislative mandate that patients have an opportunity to express their wishes about potential treatments in critical situations.

Discussions regarding the appropriate moral limits of patient autonomy range from those that place autonomy at the ethical core of the relationship to others that conceptualize it as important but not governing. For example, H. Tristram Engelhardt sees the relationship through libertarian lenses. He argues that individual autonomy must remain central in a pluralistic society, because no one theology or philosophy exists to mediate deep differences in values (Engelhardt, 1986). Others maintain that the major emphasis on individual autonomy has created (or can create) a situation in which physicians and other health professionals no longer are able to exercise the level of independent judgment required for acting beneficently toward the patient.

Tension sometimes develops between the patient's right to self-determination or autonomy and the professional's obligation to be beneficent. This often is expressed as the issue of paternalism or parentalism: Under what conditions should the physician or other professional usurp the patient's informed preferences so as to pursue the patient's medical well-being? How does the health professional know when the patient's wishes are fundamentally at odds with the patient's welfare? This important topic is discussed elsewhere in this encyclopedia and is not developed further here.

In the tradition of medical ethics, discussion regarding autonomy did not focus on patient autonomy at all, but on the professional's autonomy. Freedom from others' impingement on his or her clinical judgment and practice has been considered one of the prerogatives and desirable attributes of professional practice. This position is based on an assumption about the nature of the profession: Health professionals, the bearers of esoteric knowledge and skills, need to be free from outside pressures to accomplish their professional goal of benefiting patients. However, there are numerous government regulations and other impingements within health care today that restrict professional autonomy, causing thoughtful health professionals sometimes to worry whether they will be able to honor basic professional ideals of service.

One important factor altering the character of professional autonomy has been the patient's active partnership as decision maker. Most health professionals have welcomed this change as being of benefit to everyone involved.

Justice. The principle of justice, stated simply, is that each should get his or her due. At the level of the professional–patient relationship, this has several implications. First, the patient can expect to be treated fairly. Others should not be given any advantage on the basis of arbitrary favoritism. The rules will be applied consistently, taking into account legitimate departures from the norm. For instance, a procedural rule of first come, first served will be applied except in cases where greater need morally requires that the rule be flexible enough to allow for valid exceptions.

The principle of justice also raises perplexing ethical issues related to scarce resources. Health professionals abide by a duty of beneficence, but it is not an absolute duty. Because some resources are scarce, the professional also has a duty to allocate resources according to moral criteria when allocation decisions are in his or her power. The resulting allocation may have a deleterious effect on one or more patients because their benefits are compromised. For example, a nursing shortage on a unit may require the nurses to make difficult (though not arbitrary) decisions about patient-care priorities.

Compensation for harms also derives from our understanding of what justice requires. A patient who is harmed in the relationship has a right to know that the harm has occurred and may wish to seek compensation for the harm.

Serious barriers to justice often arise outside of the relationship. Societal discrimination against patients on the basis of race, ethnicity, religion, sex, and age are well documented, and continue to flourish in spite of legislation designed to prevent it. Other barriers are imposed by today's bureaucratic context of health care: institutional mechanisms and societal arrangements designed to foster efficiency, profit, or other goals, but not the patient's well-being. The relationship does not stand in isolation from these influences, all of which have profound effects on whether the high ideals of the relationship can be upheld.

The health professional who is committed to upholding professional ideals must work not only to preserve justice within the relationship directly but also to remove barriers to it on a broader scale so that the appropriate ends of health care can be realized.

Conflicts among principles

As illustrated by the issue of paternalism in truth-telling situations and the compromise of beneficence in situations of scarce resources, conflicts among principles inevitably arise in everyday professional–patient relationship situations. From an ethical theory point of view, the principles themselves, then, cannot be considered absolute. They can be thought of as prima facie principles, binding when all things are equal. That is, in actual situations the principles must be weighed to ascertain which is the most binding. Institutional mechanisms exist to help resolve difficulties that arise due to conflicting ethical principles in actual decisions. Some of these mechanisms are discussed in the last section of this article.

Virtue in the professional–patient relationship

In recent years the study of ethics in the health professions has included a lively reexamination of the virtues that should be expressed by health professionals. Edmund Pellegrino and David Thomasma conclude that "The contemporary reappraisal is not an abnegation of rights-and-duty-based ethics, but a recognition that rights and duties notwithstanding, their moral effectiveness still turns on dispositions and character traits of our fellow men and women" (Pellegrino and Thomasma, 1988, p. 112).

Within philosophy there are numerous theories of virtue and of the character traits and dispositions that combine to create "a virtuous person." Medical ethics writings about virtue in the professional–patient relationship often draw on major elements of Aristotle's general description of virtue in the *Nichomachean Ethics*. Basically, he said that a life of moral virtue is characterized by dispositions and attitudes that can be cultivated into habits of preparedness that enable a person to act in ways that further the good of a relationship or community. He also underscored the importance of the person's desire to become a good person, which in turn requires knowledge of ultimate goods and ends. Aristotle did not divorce virtue from the realm of feelings and emotions, suggesting instead that acts arising out of various dispositions will give pleasure and that, at the same time, ethical action resulting from a virtuous disposition requires the exercise of reason.

A challenge throughout the ages has been to identify dispositions that the professional should cultivate so as to further the good and proper ends of health care. Many virtues have been proposed, among them benevolence and kindliness, compassion, integrity, honesty, fairness, conscientiousness, fidelity beyond duty, and humility.

These virtues are as appropriate in today's professional–patient relationship as they have always been. However, some things about the relationship are understood differently today than in the past, and our understanding of human relationships in general continues to undergo new evaluation. It is not surprising that our understanding of the virtues also continues to evolve. The following two illustrations of this evolution by no means exhaust the important work that is being conducted in this area.

Benevolence and considerations of trust. The traditional professional virtue of benevolence or kindness has enjoyed a long history in the writing on the professional–patient relationship. This character trait evokes a picture of a physician sitting quietly at the bedside, reassuring a patient, an image consistent with a period in which the professional was viewed as a kindly person who ministered to the medical needs of a trusting, mostly passive patient. Today the notion of benevolence must be refined to adapt to a relationship in which patients are active participants in the interaction, suggesting that simple kindness and blind trust are not adequate ingredients for the mutual tasks to be accomplished.

One step toward an adequate notion of benevolence today is taking place through an examination of how trustworthiness figures ever more prominently as a component of benevolence in the professional–patient relationship.

Erik Erikson is among the school of psychologists who view psychosocial development as entailing a number of stages. He and others have shown that trust plays a central role in our basic developmental tasks of achieving intimacy and individuation (Erikson, 1950). Trust helps one to know not only when to depend on others, but also when and how to take the initiative and responsibility for one's own actions. We assume today that patients who are competent to be active partners in their health-care decisions should take the initiative and responsibility for doing so. It follows that the health professional who is disposed to be benevolent must develop attitudes and conduct that provide a psychologically convincing basis for the patient's trust. Only when the professional is truly trustworthy can the patient's security and, importantly, freedom to act flourish within the complex intermingling of dependence and independence that characterizes today's relationship. The professional cannot rely on patients' blind faith as a sub-stitute for his or her own commitment to treating patients as partners.

Confidentiality, an ethical issue inherent in the professional–patient relationship, illustrates the importance of trustworthiness as a component of benevolence. Confidentiality always has assumed the professional's willingness to keep a professional secret because he or she acknowledges that the patient may have to provide intimate personal details that have the potential to be harmful, shameful, or embarrassing. Still, traditionally the whole way of understanding confidentiality was to focus on the physician's duty. To the extent that the physician had cultivated a benevolent attitude toward the patient, the duty would come more naturally. Today the moral focus has shifted to the patient, particularly to his or her right to confidentiality. Only trustworthiness based on the professional's authentic commitment to respecting patients' rights and dignity assures the patient that he or she is in the hands of a benevolent professional.

A similar idea is advanced and broadened by Edmund Pellegrino and David Thomasma, who suggest that the concept of "beneficence-in-trust" should guide the professional–patient relationship. Trustworthiness, rather than the virtue of traditionally understood benevolence alone, helps to assure that the patient's welfare will be furthered in the relationship (Pellegrino and Thomasma, 1988).

Compassion and considerations of caring. Compassion long has been included in discussions of virtues that should characterize the professional–patient relationship. Compassion often has been interpreted according to its etymological root, "to suffer with." Theories vary about what, exactly, this means in the health-care context, but one central theme is that healing is enabled when professionals exhibit a disposition and ability to sympathize deeply with the patient's plight. The cultivation of this disposition means that the professional may recognize the key issue to be not only Have I done my duty? (e.g., truth-telling) but also Have I been sensitive to the effect my approach will have? (e.g., how, when, by whom, and where this information should be disclosed). To this end William F. May observes, "The moral question for professionals is not simply a question of telling truths, but being true to his [sic] promises regarding the implications of that information" (May, 1975, p. 37). Baruch Brody places the emphasis on the disposition to sympathize with the patient's deeper losses, not only his or her obvious suffering, since compassion may be a virtuous disposition even in the absence of this kind of suffering (Brody, 1988a).

The notion of "caring," which has received vigorous attention as a pivotal value in the professional–patient relationship, sheds light on important ways in which the virtue of compassion might manifest itself in the everyday work of professionals. Warren Reich makes a signal contribution to the understanding of compassion by relating different modes of compassion to different phases of a patient's suffering (Reich, 1989). Care in the relationship between health professional and patient often has been seen as that activity which reflects an attitude of sensitivity to the patient's deepest values and concerns, and constructively addresses them. In other words, a caring person seems to be motivated by a compassionate disposition. Paul Ramsey (1970) associates the idea of care with the sacredness of the human, suggesting that by their expressions of care, professionals pay the deepest respect to the patient as a person.

The language of care and casual caring behaviors may be easier for girls and women to express since they usually place *care within relationships* at the center of their assumptions about the requirements for leading a morally good life (Gilligan, 1982). Comfort with such language and behavior is not gender-specific, though Carol Gilligan's studies show them to be gender-related. Placing care at the center of a relationship may be crucial to healing when human suffering and deep loss are involved. Eric Cassell treats caring as a salve to the type of human suffering brought about by the vicissitudes of illness, injury, and disease, and views it as a powerful tool in the healing of such sufferers (Cassell, 1976). As such, genuine caring is an activity that should be expressed and valued in health-care relationships (Noddings, 1992). The disposition of compassion, which helps give rise to caring behaviors, also should be valued and fostered.

Esther Condon and Hilde Nelson raise worries about care voiced by many nurses and other professionals who are aware of problems created by a sexist society. Caring for others is a trait associated with women, and so is the caregiving role. In a society where traits associated with women often are devalued, both caring and the caregiving role may be devalued in the health-care environment (Nelson, 1992). Therefore, when a health professional expresses care, he or she may also appear to condone injustices that derive from being in a society that devalues women (Condon, 1991).

Existential dimensions of the patient's experience: Implications for the professional–patient relationship

The existential dimensions of the patient's experience are an important area of inquiry that is emerging but has been neglected or incompletely examined in many discussions of professional–patient relationship. ("Existential," as it is used here, refers to the human quest for meaning in the face of our limitations, among them illness and death.) Especially significant are new insights regarding the health professional's role in exploring the existential meaning of illness for a patient. The focus on

the existential meaning of the patient's condition helps to signal how the patient is a partner in the search for the best course to take because the point of reference is the quality of his or her own life, not just freedom from illness.

These insights on the patient's existential situation also highlight the potential for miscommunication and harm resulting from failure to take the patient's perspective fully into account. For example, Richard Baron describes the differences of perception about the patient's situation as "a great gulf" that exists between the professional's perspective and the patient's. His article "I Can't Hear You While I'm Listening" (his response to a patient who asked a question while Baron was listening with his stethoscope to the patient's heart) illustrates the difficulty. The professional's perspective on the problem is that a pathology (disease) is present that must be treated through his or her technologic capability to diagnose it and to prescribe a remedy directed at the body systems. At the same time, the experience for the patient is one of illness in which the world is in a state of disorder, "a loss of the familiar that pervades the way things are for someone" (Baron, 1985, 607).

William F. May bases the dilemma of differing perceptions not only in the differing traditions that professional and patient bring to the therapeutic encounter, but much more deeply in the role that the patient's embodiment plays in his or her experience of the situation:

> The body serves as the medium through which the self discloses itself to others. One does not need to be an existentialist to know that a person not only *has* a body; in a sense, she *is* her body. . . . Catastrophic illness disorients the self in its complicated veiling and unveiling through the medium of the body. . . . What the self shows no longer seems itself, and yet the self must own it. (May, 1991, pp. 10–12)

May's emphasis on the intimate connection of the body to the self gives final shape to the contours of the mold within which all of the ethical issues in the professional–patient relationship ultimately must be cast. The patient's "story," then, goes beyond the clinical dimensions to the meaning of the illness or injury for the patient's life (Hunter, 1991). Failure to take into full account the existential disorientation that a patient experiences due to bodily changes can lead to disastrous results, among them a patient's distrust, a belief that the health professional doesn't care, and even a patient's inability to engage in his or her own healing process (Baron, 1985).

Howard Brody, who also convincingly addresses the necessity of listening for the patient's story, notes that the challenge does not lie only in the professional's desire and willingness to hear the story. Even those who are so disposed may be prevented because both professional and patient believe that the professional holds the key to knowing the "real problem" (i.e., the medical problem). The power differential built into the structure of the relationship means that the professional is believed to be empowered to impute the meaning of the patient's story. A concentrated effort must be made to overcome such a barrier (Brody, 1987).

Other investigators are exploring additional effects of the professional's focus on disease rather than on the patient's perspective regarding his or her own illness. Some observe that a focus on disease is more likely to lead to a professional attitude that is cognitively and logically dominant, distant, and impersonal. The beliefs that objectivity depends on reason and that feeling or emotion clouds reason inform these attitudes. But they show that feelings and an appropriate degree of personal involvement can foster a professional–patient relationship characterized by clear thinking. Professionals may express their feelings much in the way that a mother or friend might be objective but not be completely impartial about what ought to be done (Ruddick, 1989; Callahan, 1988). When the professional shows a self to the patient as a personality with emotions, likes and dislikes, fears and dreams, hopes and faults, the patient understands that there is a *person* in the professional role, not just a bundle of competencies and technical skills. The patient becomes more trusting that his or her own personality has a chance of being taken seriously (Purtilo, 1990).

Emerging from such thinking are new materials for refining the professional–patient relationship, new ethical dimensions to build on the traditional foundations of moral obligations, rights, and virtues. The healing quest will be for the discovery of the patient's lost or changed self, not just for removal of a disease that resides in that person.

In summary, the contributions of those reflecting on the existential aspects of the patient's situation are many. They are helping health professionals and patients to think more substantively about real communication and partnership in the relationship. They show that this orientation opens health professional and patient alike to the awareness that much healing occurs outside the relationship and focuses the goal of the relationship on those ends that the relationship itself is capable of pursuing.

Mechanisms for resolving ethical conflict in the professional–patient relationship

Ethical issues in the professional–patient relationship are receiving more attention in the everyday environments of health care. Inevitably, differences in judgment, even deeply held differences, arise between professional and patient (or the patient's family). "Conflict" does not always denote a feeling of animosity.

Often it signals a frustration shared by all alike in not knowing the best way to proceed.

There are several mechanisms designed to assist patients in such situations. First, the patient representative or patient ombudsperson is an employee of the institution who is charged with being available to patients and their families when dissatisfaction or questions arise. This advocate may learn that a patient or family believes the patient is being harmed by receiving substandard treatment. While not all such situations involve ethical issues, many do. The advocate may act as a direct liaison between the parties or may refer the issue to one of the other mechanisms designed to provide assistance.

Second, ethics consultants are being hired by many major hospitals. Their charge is to deal with ethical issues regarding patient-care decisions. Procedures vary somewhat. Depending on the institution, the ethics consultation service may be accessed by the physician, the nurse or other professional, the patient, or the patient's family. Usually the consultant meets with all the relevant parties to help them identify the ethical issues involved, reason about the issues, and make recommendations for how to weigh conflicting principles in light of the situation. The consultant does not make the final decision, which is correctly left to the professional–patient relationship.

Third, clinical ethics committees are present in many health-care environments. Usually multidisciplinary, they function in a manner similar to the ethics consultant. Sometimes an ethics consultant will be called first, and if he or she thinks that the issue merits further deliberation by several different disciplines and personalities, may call the ethics committee together.

Dispute resolution is a relatively new approach to addressing conflict in the health-care setting. The emphasis is on mediation and facilitation techniques. Specific steps for an institution include orientation and training for all management staff in how to deal with misunderstandings and disagreements, and establishment of an in-house mediation team.

Everyone would agree that whenever possible, prevention is the best approach to moral conflict in a professional or institutional setting. The professional's diligence in communication, technical competence, and caring are keys to conflict prevention, as well as powerful instruments for resolution of conflict when it does occur in the professional–patient relationship.

RUTH B. PURTILO

Directly related to this article are the other articles in the entry: HISTORICAL PERSPECTIVES, *and* SOCIOLOGICAL PERSPECTIVES. *Also directly related are the entries* AUTHORITY; AUTONOMY; BENEFICENCE; JUSTICE; PATERNALISM; RIGHTS; TRUST; VIRTUE AND CHARACTER; *and* MEDICAL CODES AND OATHS, *article on* ETHICAL

ANALYSIS. *This article will find application in the entries* CONFIDENTIALITY; DEATH AND DYING: EUTHANASIA AND SUSTAINING LIFE; INFORMATION DISCLOSURE; INFORMED CONSENT; *and* MEDICINE, ART OF. *For a discussion of related ideas, see the entries* CARE, *articles on* HISTORICAL DIMENSIONS OF AN ETHIC OF CARE IN HEALTH CARE, *and* CONTEMPORARY ETHICS OF CARE; CASUISTRY; ETHICS, *article on* NORMATIVE ETHICAL THEORIES; HEALTH AND DISEASE, *article on* THE EXPERIENCE OF HEALTH AND ILLNESS; NARRATIVE; *and* RESPONSIBILITY. *Other relevant material may be found under the entries* ALLIED HEALTH PROFESSIONS; BIOETHICS EDUCATION, *the* INTRODUCTION *and articles on* MEDICINE, *and* NURSING; CLINICAL ETHICS, *article on* ELEMENTS AND METHODOLOGIES; FEMINISM; HEALTH OFFICIALS AND THEIR RESPONSIBILITIES; MEDICINE AS A PROFESSION; NURSING ETHICS; NURSING AS A PROFESSION; *and* PROFESSION AND PROFESSIONAL ETHICS. *See also the* APPENDIX (CODES, OATHS, AND DIRECTIVES RELATED TO BIOETHICS), SECTION II: ETHICAL DIRECTIVES FOR THE PRACTICE OF MEDICINE, *and* SECTION III: ETHICAL DIRECTIVES FOR OTHER HEALTH-CARE PROFESSIONS.

Bibliography

AIKEN, HENRY. 1962. *Reason and Conduct: New Bearings in Moral Philosophy.* New York: Knopf.

ARRAS, JOHN, and HUNT, ROBERT. 1983. "Part One: Health Professionals, Patients and Society." In their *Ethical Issues in Modern Medicine,* 2d ed., pp. 34–138. Palo Alto, Calif.: Mayfield.

BAIER, ANNETTE C. 1986. "Trust and Antitrust." *Ethics* 96, no. 2:231–260.

BARON, RICHARD J. 1985. "An Introduction to Medical Phenomenology: I Can't Hear You While I'm Listening." *Annals of Internal Medicine* 103, no. 4:606–611.

BEAUCHAMP, TOM L., and CHILDRESS, JAMES F. 1989a. "Ideals, Virtues, and Conscientiousness." In their *Principles of Biomedical Ethics,* 3d ed., pp. 366–399. New York: Oxford University Press.

———. 1989b. "Professional–Patient Relationships." In their *Principles of Biomedical Ethics,* 3d ed., pp. 307–365. New York: Oxford University Press.

BENJAMIN, MARTIN, and CURTIS, JOY. 1981. *Ethics in Nursing.* New York: Oxford University Press.

BLACKWELL, HENRY CAMPBELL. 1968. *Black's Law Dictionary.* 4th ed. St. Paul, Minn.: West.

BRODY, BARUCH A. 1988a. "A New Model for the Patient–Physician Relationship." In his *Life and Death Decision Making,* chap. 4. New York: Oxford University Press.

———. 1988b. "The Virtues in a Pluralistic Society." In his *Life and Death Decision Making,* chap. 1.3. New York: Oxford University Press.

BRODY, HOWARD. 1981. *Ethical Decisions in Medicine.* 2d ed. Boston: Little, Brown.

———. 1987. *Stories of Sickness.* New Haven, Conn.: Yale University Press.

———. 1989. "The Physician/Patient Relationship." In *Med-*

ical Ethics, pp. 65–92. Edited by Robert M. Veatch. Boston: Jones and Bartlett.

CALLAHAN, SIDNEY. 1988. "The Role of Emotion in Ethical Decisionmaking." *Hastings Center Report* 18, no. 3:9–14.

CASSELL, ERIC J. 1976. *The Healer's Art: A New Approach to the Doctor-Patient Relationship.* Philadelphia: J. B. Lippincott.

CONDON, ESTHER H. 1991. "Nursing and the Caring Metaphor: Gender and Political Influences on an Ethics of Care." *Nursing Outlook* 40, no. 1:14–19.

DRANE, JAMES F. 1988. *Becoming a Good Doctor: The Place of Virtue and Character in Medical Ethics.* Kansas City, Mo.: Sheed & Ward.

ENGLEHARDT, H. TRISTRAM, JR. 1986. *The Foundations of Bioethics.* New York: Oxford University Press.

ERIKSON, ERIK H. 1950. *Childhood and Society.* New York: W. W. Norton.

FITZPATRICK, JOYCE J., and WHALL, ANN L., eds. *Conceptual Models of Nursing: Analysis and Application.* Bowie, Md.: Robert J. Brady.

GILLIGAN, CAROL. 1982. *In a Different Voice: Psychological Theory and Women's Development.* Cambridge, Mass.: Harvard University Press.

GROVES, JAMES E. 1978. "Taking Care of the Hateful Patient." *New England Journal of Medicine* 289, no. 16:883–887.

HARTMANN, NICOLAI. 1932. "Truthfulness and Uprightness." In vol. 2 of his *Ethics,* pp. 281–285. Translated by Stanton Coit. New York: Humanities Press.

HUNTER, KATHRYN MONTGOMERY. 1991. *Doctors' Stories: The Narrative Structure of Medical Knowledge.* Princeton, N.J.: Princeton University Press.

JONSEN, ALBERT R. 1977. "Do No Harm: Axiom of Medical Ethics." In *Philosophical Medical Ethics: Its Nature and Significance,* pp. 27–41. Edited by Stuart F. Spicker and H. Tristram Engelhardt, Jr. Dordrecht, Netherlands: D. Reidel.

———. 1990. *The New Medicine and the Old Ethics.* Cambridge, Mass.: Harvard University Press.

LAMMERS, STEPHEN E., and VERHEY, ALLEN, eds. 1987. *On Moral Medicine: Theological Perspectives in Medical Ethics.* Grand Rapids, Mich.: William B. Eerdmans.

MAPPES, THOMAS A., and ZEMBATY, JANE S. 1981a. "Patients' Rights and Professionals' Obligations." In their *Biomedical Ethics.* New York: McGraw-Hill.

———. 1981b. "The Physician–Patient Relationship: Paternalism, Truth-Telling, and Informed Consent." In their *Biomedical Ethics.* New York: McGraw-Hill.

MAY, WILLIAM F. 1975. "Code, Covenant, Contracts, or Philanthropy: Various Models for Professional Ethics Are Available to Medicine." *Hastings Center Report* 5, no. 6:29–38.

———. 1983. *The Physician's Covenant: Images of the Healer in Medical Ethics.* Philadelphia: Westminster.

———. 1991. *The Patient's Ordeal.* Bloomington: Indiana University Press.

NELSON, HILDE LINDEMANN. 1992. "Against Caring." *Journal of Clinical Ethics* 3, no. 1:8–15.

NODDINGS, NEL. 1992. "In Defense of Caring." *Journal of Clinical Ethics* 3, no. 1:15–18.

PELLEGRINO, EDMUND D. 1979. *Humanism and the Physician.* Knoxville: University of Tennessee Press.

Pellegrino, Edmund D., and Thomasma, David C. 1988. *For the Patient's Good: The Restoration of Beneficence in Health Care.* New York: Oxford University Press.

———. 1993. *The Virtues in Medical Practice.* New York: Oxford University Press.

Percival, Thomas. 1849. *Medical Ethics; Or, A Code of Institutions and Precepts Adapted to the Professional Conduct of Physicians and Surgeons.* Oxford: John Henry Parker.

Purtilo, Ruth B. 1990. *Health Professionals and Patient Interaction.* 4th ed. Philadelphia: W. B. Saunders.

Purtilo, Ruth B., and Cassel, Christine K. 1993. *Ethical Dimensions in the Health Professions.* 2d ed. Philadelphia: W. B. Saunders.

Ramsey, Paul. 1970. *The Patient as Person: Explorations in Medical Ethics.* New Haven, Conn.: Yale University Press.

Reich, Warren T. 1989. "Spreading of Suffering: A Moral Account of Compassion." *Soundings* 72:83–108.

Ross, W. D. 1930. *The Right and the Good.* Oxford: At the Clarendon Press.

Rothman, David J. 1991. *Strangers at the Bedside: A History of How Law and Bioethics Transformed Medical Decision Making.* New York: Basic Books.

Ruddick, Sara. 1989. *Maternal Thinking: Toward a Politics of Peace.* Boston: Beacon Press.

Smith, Sheri. 1980. "Three Models of the Nurse–Patient Relationship." In *Nursing: Images and Ideals: Opening Dialogue with the Humanities,* pp. 14–19. Edited by Stuart Spicker and Sally Gadow. New York: Springer.

Spicker, Stuart, and Gadow, Sally, eds. 1980. *Nursing: Images and Ideals: Opening Dialogue with the Humanities.* New York: Springer.

U.S. President's Commission for the Study of Ethical Problems in Medicine and Biomedical and Behavioral Research. 1982. *Making Health Care Decisions: A Report on the Ethical and Legal Implications of Informed Consent on the Patient–Practitioner Relationship.* Washington, D.C.: U.S. Government Printing Office.

Veatch, Robert M. 1972. "Models for Ethical Medicine in a Revolutionary Age." *Hastings Center Report* 2, no. 3:5–7.

Walsh, Diana Chapman. 1987. *Corporate Physicians: Between Medicine and Management.* New Haven, Conn.: Yale University Press.

Weir, Robert. 1980. *Perspectives in Biology and Medicine.* Chicago: University of Chicago Press.

PROFESSION AND PROFESSIONAL ETHICS

Among any society's most important institutions are the social structures by which the society controls the use of specialized knowledge and skills. This fact is particularly true when highly valued aspects of human life depend on such expertise, and all the more so if acquiring such expertise requires lengthy theoretical education and intensive training in its practical application under the supervision of those already expert, thus rendering the valuable knowledge and skills unavoidably exclusive.

Social control over the use of such knowledge and skills is important because the members of the expert group could use their exclusive expertise solely for their own benefit or even hold society hostage to their expertise. But those who might exert such control, if they are outside the expert group, cannot depend on their understanding of this expertise because they lack precisely the relevant knowledge and practical training. How, then, can a society control the use of important, specialized expertise and render those outside the expert group secure that they will be able to enjoy the values that depend on it? One of the most important social structures developed to this end is the institution of profession.

A few social philosophers and a large number of sociologists, following Emile Durkheim and Talcott Parsons, have studied the institution of profession in depth and have attempted to identify its essential elements. This task is not a simple one because so many groups have been eager to appropriate the title of profession in order to enjoy the social rewards that go with it. In addition, the terms "profession" and "professional" have both normative and descriptive uses in ordinary discourse. Nevertheless, by looking for common features among the most obvious examples of this institution, such as medicine, law, and dentistry, a useful listing of characteristic features of the institution of profession is available.

The key features of a profession

Important and exclusive expertise. For an occupational group to be a profession, it must provide its clients with something the larger community judges extremely valuable, either because of its intrinsic value or because it is a necessary precondition of any person's achievement of valued goals, or both. Health and the preservation of life, to take two commonly identified goals of the health professions, are held by almost everyone to be values of the highest order, either as intrinsic values or as necessary preconditions of people's achievement of whatever else they value. In a similar way, security of one's property and person against the errors of others and against the adverse workings of government and the legal system, as one defensible description of the goal of the legal profession, is also widely valued as a precondition of achieving whatever other goals one has.

The expertise of a profession has both cognitive (theoretical and factual) and practical (the fruits of experiential learning) components that are of sufficient subtlety and complexity that only persons who have been specifically and extensively educated in them, by persons already expert, can be depended upon to bring about the relevant benefits for the occupation's clients.

In the practical division of a society's labors, this makes possession of such expertise exclusive to a relatively small group.

Moreover, for the same reason, only persons fully educated in both knowledge and practice of a profession's expertise can be relied on to judge correctly the need for expert intervention in a given situation, or to judge the quality of such an intervention as it is being carried out. Judgments of need and judgments of the quality of the expert's performance by those not so trained are not dependable. Because of the importance of what is at stake, it is not sufficient to judge the performance solely on the basis of its long-term outcomes, even when the nonexpert can accomplish such a judgment unaided. Long-term outcomes will not be known for some time, and the risk of negative consequences in the meantime, in a matter of great importance, means that delayed judgments are simply not enough.

The expertise of a profession involves not only specialized and complex knowledge, both theoretical and practical, but also the application of this knowledge. This is the reason that mastery of a profession's expertise requires experiential as well as cognitive education. This is also why the members of a profession are said to "practice" its expertise. A profession is not made up simply of experts; it is made up of practitioners of a body of expertise.

Internal and external recognition.   A profession, as an occupational group made exclusive by reason of its particular body of expertise, is also characterized by a set of internal relationships of which the most important is a mutual recognition of expertise on the part of its members. These internal relationships may be quite informal or may become quite formal, as when a community of experts who mutually recognize each others' expertise establishes a formal organization. The expression "the profession of medicine" thus refers most properly to all those expert in the practice of medicine, mutually recognized as such by one another, within whatever geographic limits are relevant. This same expression is also used, however, to refer either to the chief national organization of such persons, the American Medical Association (AMA), or to some larger set of associations, including the AMA, to which physicians would be likely to belong. However, it is not the formal character of association among experts, but the fact of their mutual recognition of expertise, that is most important here. Other expressions—for example, "organized medicine"—are available to refer to formally constituted groups.

The expertise of a profession is not only mutually recognized by those who possess it; it is also recognized by the members of the larger community. Because of the exclusive nature of professional expertise and the importance of its application, such external recognition is most often expressed in formal actions of the larger community, such as certification, licensure, and so on, that confer formal authority over the profession's expertise. A profession may receive, for example, exclusive authority both to determine the degree of expertise needed by those who intend to practice it and to test the expertise of those who claim to do so. Since students of the profession must undertake lengthy and specialized training in order to master its expertise, the larger community's authorization is likely to include a grant of exclusive authority to train and certify new members of the profession. But, as with internal recognition, it is not the formal character but the reality of external recognition that is essential to the character of a profession.

Autonomy in practice.   Because the activity of a profession is so valued by its clients, and because proper performance and dependable judgments about performance depend upon expertise that is unavoidably exclusive and therefore not available to the ordinary person, a profession's clients routinely grant its members extensive autonomy in the actual performance of the profession's practice. The term "autonomy" has a number of important uses in moral discourse and often appears when issues in bioethics are under discussion. Here this term refers specifically to the acceptance by clients of the professional's judgments as determinative on any matter that is within the range of the professional's expertise. Such autonomous judgments by professionals arise in three possible arenas.

The first area, autonomy in practice judgments, depends on the assumption that each member of the expert community possesses the relevant professional expertise and is therefore a dependable provider of its benefits. It includes three elements: first, determination of the specific needs of the client in matters within the range of the professional's expertise; second, determination of the likely outcomes of various courses of action that the client, the professional, or some other party might undertake in response to these needs; and third, judgment of which of the possible courses of action is most likely to best meet the client's needs.

Consider, for example, the encounter between a physician or a dentist and a patient. The patient often accepts without question the doctor's judgments regarding the nature of the patient's present condition and of the patient's need for care, if any; the range of courses of action that might be taken in response; and the likelihood that one of these courses of action will best meet the patient's needs.

A fourth possible element of professional autonomy may consist in judgments about the intermediate, instrumental steps appropriate in carrying out the chosen course of action. Although these judgments are often carried out by the professional as well, they can be and frequently are relegated to another party, such as a technician. Such a person, while capable of making judgments about properly applying instrumental actions already identified as needed, is not necessarily capable of judging dependably regarding the need for these actions.

In some circumstances, the instrumental actions needed to respond to the client's situation may depend, like the original judgment of the need for them, upon exclusive expertise. In such cases, the "prescribing" professional may need to refer the client to another professional to have the needed intervention carried out. In this situation, further judgments of need, identification of outcomes, choice of a best course, and choice of instrumentalities are carried out over a much narrower range of alternatives by the specialist to whom the client is referred.

Although each individual client grants autonomy to the professional, clients do not ordinarily do so simply on the basis of their individual judgments of the expertise of the individual professional. They make their judgments rather on the basis of a more complex set of factors involving the community's (external) recognition of the professional group's expertise and the professional group's (internal) recognition of the expertise of the particular professional. Thus, even though this grant of professional autonomy takes place above all between the individual client and professional, its full meaning can only be understood against the background of the institution of profession.

Second, the professional's ability to serve clients by making dependable judgments is often conditioned in turn by various features of the situation in which the client–professional encounter takes place. In order to assure that professionals' judgments are as dependable as possible, professionals often seek, and the larger community and individual clients often grant them, considerable additional autonomy to determine the immediate circumstances of practice.

The extent of this aspect of professional autonomy depends on answers to two questions. What aspects of the immediate circumstances of practice significantly affect the quality of professional performance? And what additional factors do members of the profession also prefer to control, at least for their convenience and perhaps also out of a conviction, which may be unexamined or even mistaken, that they affect the quality of professional performance?

For example, physicians, not their clients, control the daily routine of medical practice. In the marketplace, this control could easily be explained as the producer's control of the product he or she offers. But physicians ordinarily justify such preferred patterns of practice on the grounds that this is the best way to serve all their patients; patients, in turn, ordinarily change their daily schedules accordingly, though many may be doubtful that the inconveniences they accept really are the only way that physicians can best serve all of their patients.

Third, a professional's ability to serve clients by making dependable judgments is also conditioned by other, broader parameters over which professionals may seek, and the larger community may grant, some measure of control. To an even greater degree than autonomy in making practice judgments and in controlling the immediate circumstances of practice, autonomy of this third kind is ordinarily granted to the members of a profession as a group rather than individually.

Physicians' opposition to health-insurance programs in an earlier day, for example, and their later opposition to federally funded health-care programs for the needy were remarkably effective in preserving the medical community's preferred (at that time) economic structure for health-care distribution, namely, the fee-for-service marketplace. At one time, physicians also exercised almost total control over hospitals in the United States. Their consistent rationale—whether correct or not—was that such economic and institutional arrangements as they preferred were the most likely to produce the best health care for their patients; the larger community generally accepted this rationale as an appropriate reason for physicians to try to control health-care economics and health-care institutions.

Other forms of expertise have since been accepted as much more important than medical expertise to health-care economics and health-care administration. Consequently, physicians' autonomy in these areas has been much curtailed since the 1970s. Of course, physicians' reasons for preferring one economic or institutional arrangement rather than another will almost always deserve consideration when broader social and institutional parameters do impact the quality of care they can provide to patients. But this third category of autonomy does not appear to be central to what a profession is.

Professions' and professionals' obligations. The final and, for present purposes, the most important feature of the institution of profession is that membership in a profession implies the acceptance by its members of a set of norms of professional practice. To make this point clear, contrast what may be termed a "normative" picture of a profession with what may be termed a "commercial" picture.

According to the commercial picture, practicing a profession is no different in principle from selling one's wares in the marketplace. According to those who take this view, the professional has a product to sell and makes the appropriate and needed agreements with interested purchasers. Beyond some fundamental obligation not to coerce, cheat, or defraud others, the professional would have no other obligations to anyone except those voluntarily undertaken with specific individuals or groups. According to the commercial picture, in other words, there are no specifically professional values or obligations in any profession. There is nothing to which a person is obligated precisely because he or she is a professional.

Some commentators consider the commercial picture to be an accurate description of what professions are like, while others maintain that professionals or the community at large would be better off if professions conformed to this view more thoroughly (Sade, 1971; Kuskey, 1973). But recall that all professional groups have a corner on some valuable form of knowledge within a society. Wherever this is the case, there is power—power to control the knowledge itself and, especially, power over the aspects of human life that depend upon this knowledge. Now compare how various powerful groups are dealt with in our society. Contrast professionals with politicians, for example.

Experience has taught us that politicians will be tempted to misuse their power. Consequently, we want to keep a close eye on them. This is arguably one reason why we accept without too much complaint the terribly inefficient system of periodic reelection, to take one example, because we want to keep close watch over those with political power. It is arguably one reason why we tolerate the excesses of a free press as well, because a free press means that it will be that much harder for politicians to misuse their power.

But the professions, though they do face some slight measure of regulation through licensing boards and the like, are subjected to remarkably little oversight in U.S. society. In fact, even when there is regulation, it is generally their own members who regulate them, not the larger community. The community assures itself that the power of the profession will not be misused by means of the institution of profession.

This suggests that the way in which a profession functions within the larger community is inherently normative. When a person enters a profession, he or she undertakes obligations, obligations whose content has been worked out and is continually being affirmed or adjusted through an ongoing dialogue between the expert group and the larger community. In other words, there are conventional obligations, over and above obligations incurred in other human relationships, that both individuals and groups have simply because they are members of a profession. Professions and professionals have obligations, and the content of these obligations for each profession is its "professional ethics."

The chief categories of professional norms

Although most professions have articulated a code of ethics or other statements of the norms of their professional practice, such statements are never complete or fully authoritative. They are, at best, good partial representations of the content of the profession's norms and obligations. The full content of these norms is the fruit of an ongoing dialogue between the expert group and the larger community, on whose recognition of expertise and grant of professional autonomy the expert group depends for its status as a profession. Therefore, the effort to answer such questions as "What professional norms apply to this situation?" and "What is a member of this profession obligated to do in this situation?" must include asking what the larger community understands those norms and obligations to be, rather than looking only at the views of the professional group or some organization(s) within it.

Determining what a profession's norms are is therefore a much subtler enterprise than it might seem. Even the well-known moral categories of autonomy, beneficence, maleficence, and justice are only a useful starting point. Another way to examine a profession's norms is in terms of eight categories of professional obligation that have been identified from studies of numerous professional groups (Ozar and Sokol, 1994). Each of these categories provides a set of questions about a profession's norms, both for personal reflection on one's obligations and for scholarly study and professional ethics education.

Briefly stated, the eight categories of questions about professional obligation are:

1. Who is (are) this profession's chief client(s)?
2. What are the central values of this profession?
3. What is the ideal relationship between a member of this profession and the client?
4. What sacrifices are required of members of this profession and in what respects do the obligations of this profession take priority over other morally relevant considerations affecting its members?
5. What are the norms of competence of this profession?
6. What is the ideal relationship between the members of this profession and coprofessionals?
7. What is the ideal relationship between the members of this profession and the larger community?
8. What are the members of this profession obligated to do to preserve the integrity of their commitment to its values and to educate others about them?

The chief client.   Every profession has a chief client or clients. This is the person or set of persons whose well-being the profession and its members are chiefly committed to serving. For some professions, the identification of the chief client seems quite easy. Surely, we might say, the chief client of a physician and a nurse, for example, is the patient. But who is the chief client of a lawyer? Is it simply the party whose case the lawyer represents or to whom the lawyer gives advice? Lawyers are told and they announce in their self-descriptions and codes of conduct that they have obligations to the whole justice system; therefore, there are things that they as professionals may not ethically do, even if doing them would advance the situation of the party they represent or advise. So it appears that the answer to the question about the chief client of the legal profession is complex, involving not only the persons lawyers represent or advise but the whole justice system and/or perhaps the whole larger community served by that system.

Once this sort of complexity about the chief client is noticed, even those cases that appear to be simple prove more complex. The physician and the nurse must attend not only to the patient before them, for example, but also to those in the waiting room or to the other patients on the hospital unit, and so on. In fact, they have some obligations to all the patients in the institution where they work, or to all their patients of record if they are in private practice. They also have significant obligations to the public as a whole; for example, they are obligated to practice with caution so as not to spread infection from patients they are caring for either to themselves or to other patients.

Who, to take another example, is the chief client of the engineer? Is it the party who will pay the engineer's fee? Or, if the engineer is employed, is it the engineer's employer? Or are the engineer's chief clients possibly the people who will directly use the bridge or the building that the engineer designs, or those whose environment will be affected by whatever the engineer produces?

In any case, this question about the chief client is one of the first questions that must be asked if a particular profession's obligations are to become clear. It must also, therefore, be one of the first questions we must address when we are educating the members of a profession in their professional obligations.

The central values of the profession.   Every profession is focused only on certain aspects of the well-being of its clients. The professions' rhetoric to the contrary, no professional group is expected by the larger community to be expert in their clients' whole well-being or to secure for its clients everything that is of value for them. There is, rather, a certain set of values that are the focus of each profession's expertise and that it is the job and obligation of that profession to work to secure for its clients. These values can be called the profession's central values.

Most professions are committed to pursuing more than one central value for clients. Whatever other values are central for a given profession, for example, the value of clients' autonomy is ordinarily a central value as well. Efficiency in the use of resources may have a similar standing. In any case, if there is more than one central value for a given profession, the question can

then be asked whether these values are all equal in rank, or whether the members of the profession are committed to choosing them in some ranked order when they cannot all be realized at once.

For example, the values proposed as the central values that the dental profession is committed to pursuing for its patients are, in order of importance, life and general health; oral health, understood as appropriate and pain-free oral functioning; the patient's autonomy (i.e. the patient's control), whenever practicable, over what happens to his or her body; preferred patterns of practice on the part of the dentist; aesthetic considerations; and efficiency in the use of resources (Ozar and Sokol, 1994).

For every profession, then, questions need to be asked and answered: What are its central values? What specific aspects of human well-being is it the task of each member of this profession to secure for clients? And if there are more than one, which takes precedence?

The ideal relationship between professional and client.   The point of the relationship between a professional and a client is to bring about certain values for the client that cannot be achieved without the expertise of the professional. To achieve this, the professional and the client must both make a number of judgments and choices about the professional's interventions. This third category of professional norms addresses the proper roles of the professional and the client as they make these judgments and choices.

At least four general models of such relationships can be distinguished: (1) a "commercial model," in which only the minimal morality of the marketplace governs; in other words, neither party has any obligations beyond a general prohibition of coercion and fraud unless and until individuals freely contract together to be obligated toward each other in specific additional ways; (2) a "guild model," in which the emphasis is on the professional's expertise and the client's lack of it, so that the professional alone is the active member in all judgments and choices about professional services for the client; (3) an "agent model," in which the expertise of the professional is simply placed at the service of the values and goals of the client without interference by any competing goals or values, including values to which the profession is committed from the start; and (4) an "interactive model," in which both parties have irreplaceable contributions to make in the decision-making process; the professional offers expertise to help meet the client's needs and has a commitment to the profession's central values, and the client brings his or her own values and priorities as well as the value of his or her self-determination. Ideally, in this last model, the two parties choose together how the professional shall benefit the client.

In addition, since the ideal relationship is described in regard to fully functioning adults, a profession's norms must also include how its members are to interact with clients who are not capable of full participation in decision making about the professional's interventions; such clients might include children, the developmentally disabled, and persons whose capacity to participate is diminished by fear, illness, or other conditions.

Sacrifice and the relative priority of the client's well-being. Most sociologists who study professions mention "commitment to service" or "commitment to the public" as one of the characteristic features of a profession. Similarly, in most professions' codes of ethics and other self-descriptions, clients' best interest or service to the public is given a prominent place. But these expressions admit of many different interpretations, with significantly different implications for actual practice.

Consider, for example, what could be called a "minimalist" interpretation of this general norm. According to this interpretation, a professional would have an obligation to consider the well-being of the client as only one among the professional's most important concerns. This is called a "minimalist" interpretation because, if any less consideration than this were given, the client's well-being could not be said to have any priority for the professional.

On the other hand, according to a "maximalist" interpretation, the professional has an obligation to place the well-being of clients ahead of every other consideration, both the professional's own interests and all other obligations or concerns that the professional might have.

It is doubtful that either of these interpretations accurately represents what the larger community wants or understands in this matter. Professional obligation almost certainly requires that members of a profession accept certain sacrifices of other interests in the interest of their clients. On the other hand, even if it were only to make certain that the community continued to have a supply of professionals to meet its needs in the future, the larger community certainly does not understand the commitment of the professional person to be absolute or to impose the utmost of sacrifices for the sake of one's client in all circumstances.

Each professional group has, as part of the content of its obligations worked out over time in dialogue with the larger community, an obligation to accept certain kinds of sacrifices, certain degrees of risk in certain matters, and so on. The risk may be of infection, if facing it is necessary for the sake of one's clients, for health professionals; or it may be the risk of financial loss, or the risk of social loss or criticism. In any case, it should certainly be part of reflection on a profession's ethics and part of professional ethics education to raise this issue and to discuss and try to identify the kinds and degrees of risk that are part of that profession's obligations.

Competence. Every professional is obligated both to acquire and to maintain the expertise needed to undertake his or her professional tasks, and every professional is obligated to undertake only those tasks that are within his or her competence.

Competence is probably the most obvious category of professional obligation. It is also the easiest to describe in a general way. For if a professional fails to apply his or her expertise, or fails to obtain the expertise for undertaking some task, these failures directly contradict both the point of being an expert and the very foundation of the larger community's award of decision-making power to the professional in the first place.

But determining what counts as competence on the part of a member of a given profession, both in general and in relation to specific kinds of tasks, is a complex matter. In practice, and almost of necessity, detailed judgments about requisite expertise are left to those who are expert—the profession itself. But the larger community usually requires that explanations be given regarding the general reasoning involved. In particular, it should understand the risk–benefit judgments involved in every determination of minimal competence. For as the level of competence identified as the minimum acceptable in some matter is raised, the relative availability of that level of expertise to the profession's clients will fall.

Ideal relationships between coprofessionals. Each profession also has norms, mostly implicit and unexamined, concerning the proper relationship among members of the same profession in various matters and also among members of different professions when they are dealing with the same client. Some elements of the proper relationship between a family practitioner and a renal specialist, for example, are not matters of etiquette, but bear directly on the medical profession's ability to achieve its proper ends. The same is true of relationships between physicians and nurses, dentists and dental hygienists, dentists and physicians, and so on, when they are caring for the same patient.

Some aspects of these relationships are dictated by each professional's obligation not to practice beyond his or her competence and so to seek assistance from other professionals when a particular matter requires expertise that the first professional does not possess. But other aspects of coprofessional relationships are also governed by professional norms, though they are rarely explicit. For example, how should coprofessionals communicate with a patient about their differing recommendations for the patient when these differences derive, not from differing interpretations of the facts, but from differing philosophies of practice within their profession or from their being members of different professions with different central values?

The relationship between the profession and the larger community.   The activities of every profession also involve diverse relationships between the profession as a group, or its individual members, and persons who are neither coprofessionals nor clients. These relationships may involve the larger community as a whole, or various significant subgroups, or specific individuals. It is incumbent on a profession that is permitted to be self-regulating by the larger community, for example, that it carry out this task of self-regulation conscientiously. This includes providing and monitoring educational programs and institutions in which new members of the profession receive their formation as professionals. It includes monitoring the collective activities of members of the profession in their various professional organizations to make sure that these organizations act in ways consistent with the other professional obligations of the members. It also includes such measures as are necessary to monitor and correct incompetent or other professionally inappropriate practice on the part of individual members of the group.

The profession as a group and its individual members are also the principal educators of the community regarding such elements of the profession's expertise as the lay community needs to know to function effectively in ordinary life. Thus, for example, the health professions have obligations regarding public education in matters of ordinary health self-care and hygiene; the engineering and scientific professions have obligations regarding ordinary knowledge of safety practices that the lay community needs to know in daily life.

A more subtle kind of obligation has to do with the content of key value concepts that become part of the public culture and play crucial roles in people's private lives and especially in public policy, but whose content is significantly influenced by the members of a profession or of a group of professions. For example, the health professions are more responsible than any other group for educating the public about what it means to be healthy; the engineering professions have a powerful formative influence on the culturally dominant notions of safety and physical risk; and so on. This is an area of professional obligation to the larger community that has received little attention, but it seems one of continuing ethical significance.

Integrity and education. Finally, there is that very subtle component of conduct by which a person communicates to others what he or she stands for, not only in the person's acts themselves but also in how these acts are chosen and in how the person presents himself or herself to others in carrying them out. The two words that seem to communicate the core of this concern are "integrity" and "education," especially when the two words are paired.

Each profession stands for, or "professes," certain values that it is committed to bringing about both for its clients individually and for the community at large. But a professional's personal priorities may communicate a different set of values, even though the professional's choices of interventions for clients and his or her efforts to secure appropriate relationships with clients all conform to acceptable standards. Concern with this kind of communication to their patients and to the general public, for example, motivates some health professionals to establish in their personal lives patterns of healthy living consonant with what they say to their patients. Failure to attend to this element of professional commitment also makes illegal personal activities on the part of lawyers somehow doubly wrong.

Professionals may be obligated, then, to do some things and to refrain from doing others in order to remain true to the values that their profession stands for and thereby to educate others in these values by their own example.

There are undoubtedly other useful ways of dividing the general topic of professional obligation besides these eight categories. The point is that conceptual tools like the key features of the institution of profession and the principal categories of professional obligation can assist professionals in determining their own obligations in general and in particular cases, and can assist scholars and educators of professional ethics in their work for a clearer understanding of professional practice and of the ethical standards that apply to it.

Alternative views of profession

The account just given explains the institution of profession in terms of its function in society, as a means by which a society secures the benefits of specialized expertise for its members and prevents, or at least limits, its misuse by those who possess it. Like every account of a thing's function, this account is both descriptive and normative. It describes how professions and their members act, at least for the most part, and it identifies sets of standards by which their successes and failures to act in those ways are to be judged.

The principal alternative ways of explaining the institution of profession can be described under four headings: historical, critical functionalist, radical democratic, and personalist. Each of these approaches separates the descriptive and normative elements that are interwoven in a functionalist account, with the first and second stressing the descriptive elements and the third and fourth the normative elements.

Historical explanations of the institution of profession identify, through historical study, a developmental pattern that brings an occupational group to the point of being considered a profession. This pattern is then used normatively to determine which occupational groups qualify at any given point in time and what patterns of conduct by the group conform or do not conform to the pattern. Some historical studies of professions do not purport to explain the institution of profession, of course, but simply tell part of its story without attempting to draw normative conclusions. Historical explanations may depend, at least initially, on some functionalist account of profession or on the selection of certain occupations, in their contemporary form or otherwise, as endpoints or at least markers of the developmental process being studied. But once a developmental explanation has been formulated, it can then be offered to replace functionalist accounts on the grounds that these are excessively idealized and are not adequately descriptive of the actual conduct of relevant individuals and groups. For example, the medical profession in the mid-twentieth century has been described as the product of a process of monopolization, or gradual acquisition of control by an exclusive group over a segment of market activity over the years (Berlant, 1975); the institution of profession generally has been described as a specialized mechanism for maintaining economic power and class-based status and dominance (Larson, 1977).

Some critics of the professions formulate a functionalist account of the institution for themselves, or accept someone else's, and then use its normative content to critique current patterns of conduct of individuals and organizations within a particular profession or across the professions generally (Freidson, 1970b). Other functionalist critics argue that currently accepted functionalist accounts are so idealized—that is, pay so little attention to the gap between what is described as the profession's function and actual conduct—that they foster harm to the community, or at least complacency for its good. Therefore, an alternative account of the function of professions and professionals is proposed and its implications for professional conduct are identified (Kultgen, 1988).

Radical democratic critics of the institution of profession believe that any society that accepts this institution makes a profound mistake. It is central to the institution of profession that the possession of expertise is a basis of power and that one element of that power is a grant of autonomy to those possessed of it. By institutionalizing deep inequalities of power and autonomy in this way, these critics argue, the society makes the achievement of genuine democracy almost impossible. According to the radical democrat, the failures in conduct pointed out by functionalist critics and the developmental patterns leading to monopoly and to other forms of economic and class-based inequality that the historical critics point out are not accidental traits of the institution of profession but the inevitable outcomes of its inherently undemocratic constitution. The solution, on which the well-being of the human community depends, is to do away with this institution, and all other institutions grounded on undemocratic premises (Illich, 1973, 1976).

The personalist explanation of profession identifies the individual professional's act of personal commitment upon entering a profession as the basis of everything morally significant about the institution of profession. As centuries ago a solemn vow initiated a person's membership into a profession—a vestige of which remains, for example, in the ceremony in which new physicians speak the Hippocratic oath—so today the act of personal commitment by each member of a profession is what brings the profession continually into being and gives it its character. The contents of its norms are determined by the contents of these personal acts of commitment; and the professional who falls short in conduct fails above all to honor his or her own commitment to serve others, rather than failing to follow a norm created and sustained by the mutual effort of the profession, including the individual professional, and the community at large (Pellegrino, 1979; Pellegrino and Thomasma, 1988).

Each of these approaches stresses a feature of the institution of profession that standard functionalist accounts are held to overlook or underestimate: the developmental patterns by which professionals are formed; the extent to which professions' and professionals' actual conduct falls short of the functionalist's proposed norms; the undemocratic character of exclusive expertise; and the centrality of the act of commitment by which a person becomes a professional. More complex functionalist accounts could incorporate much that is stressed in these other approaches, as more complex versions of each of them could incorporate emphases and concerns from the others. From the point of view of understanding professions as we know them, in other words, each of these approaches teaches something of central importance.

Changing times, changing standards, changing concepts

It is not only the conduct of individuals and groups, as measured by professional norms, that can fall short of what it ought to be. Professional norms themselves can fall short of what they ought to be, particularly when important characteristics of the society have changed. There was a time, for example, when the general level of education in the United States may well have justified physicians and dentists in judging the ideal patient–practitioner relationship to be a relationship according to the guild model rather than the interactive model, which has become normative for these professions in the years since the late 1960s.

A profession's norms and the institution of profession itself are human constructs and, like all things of human making, they can fall short of their intended goals, and the goals in terms of which they are judged can themselves change with changing times. When norms and institutions are no longer serviceable to do the tasks that a society needs them to do, then the society is justified in trying to change them. But social structures such as professions are inherently conservative, in the root sense of that word; they exist to preserve a mode of acting or of organizing conduct that has proven fruitful, and they preserve it by forming in their participants strong habits of perceiving, judging, and acting in ways that support it.

So when times and expectations change, or people's values or abilities change, or the surrounding social institutions change, then it is important to reexamine the relevant norms and institutions to see if they are still appropriate and to change them if they are not, even if this involves a major transformation of a particular profession's norms across many of the eight categories. One of the weaknesses of functionalist accounts of the institution of profession in the minds of their critics is that such accounts seem to say that what is the case is what ought to be the case. But, like the other four approaches, the functionalist account is simply a conceptual tool whose purpose is to help us understand what we have when we have a particular profession with a particular set of norms so we can then make the judgment whether that is the profession we ought to have.

In an analogous way, the new professional enters a profession whose norms are already in place. This does not mean that they cannot be changed, but they achieve their content by means of an ongoing dialogue between the profession and the larger community, and they change their content in the same way. So the new professional cannot create the contents of his or her professional obligations out of whole cloth. Yet, even in the individual case, the norms of the profession are not the ultimate determiners of right and wrong; if these norms are in conflict with one another or with other important moral considerations, or if they are severely defective in some way, then the professional must form his or her conscience carefully in choosing how to act. Situations will arise in which conscientious disobedience of a professional norm will be what a person's moral judgment requires when all things about a situation are considered.

By what standards should a society judge a profession's norms when their adequacy to the society's needs is in question? By what standard should the institution of profession itself be judged? By what standard should the individual professional form his or her conscience when conflict or severe doubt about the adequacy of a professional norm in a particular case suggests that conscientious disobedience may be the correct path? Surely not by the norms of the profession, for these are precisely what are being challenged when such questions arise. It is to the deeper values and standards of human conduct and social life that we must turn at such times,

for it is upon them that the norms of professions rest for their moral force in the first place.

As is true for many other human institutions, if we do not have the institution of profession, we would need to invent it or something like it in order to live together effectively. For we live in a world where no one person can master all the knowledge and skills on which the achievement of so many important values in human life depend. But, like other human institutions, the institution of profession as a whole, and each individual profession, and each normative feature of each profession, requires regular ethical scrutiny to make sure it continues to fulfill the purposes for which it was made. One of the principal roles of the field of bioethics and its practitioners is to provide the members of the health professions and the larger community with effective conceptual tools to employ in this scrutiny.

DAVID T. OZAR

Directly related to this entry are the entries MEDICINE AS A PROFESSION; NURSING AS A PROFESSION; ALLIED HEALTH PROFESSIONS; TEAMS, HEALTH-CARE; PROFESSIONAL–PATIENT RELATIONSHIP, *articles on* HISTORICAL PERSPECTIVES, SOCIOLOGICAL PERSPECTIVES, *and* ETHICAL ISSUES; HEALTH OFFICIALS AND THEIR RESPONSIBILITIES; *and* LICENSING, DISCIPLINE, AND REGULATION IN THE HEALTH PROFESSIONS. *This entry will find application in the entries* DIVIDED LOYALTIES IN MENTAL-HEALTH CARE; IMPAIRED PROFESSIONALS; PSYCHIATRY, ABUSES OF; *and* SEXUAL ETHICS AND PROFESSIONAL STANDARDS. *For a discussion of related ideas, see the entries* AUTONOMY; COMPETENCE; CONFIDENTIALITY; INFORMATION DISCLOSURE; INFORMED CONSENT; *and* RESPONSIBILITY. *For a discussion of the development of medical ethics within medical professions, see the extensive entry* MEDICAL ETHICS, HISTORY OF. *Other relevant material may be found under the entries* BIOETHICS EDUCATION; GENETIC COUNSELING, *article on* PRACTICE OF GENETIC COUNSELING; *and* MEDICAL CODES AND OATHS. *See also the* APPENDIX (CODES, OATHS, AND DIRECTIVES RELATED TO BIOETHICS), SECTION II: ETHICAL DIRECTIVES FOR THE PRACTICE OF MEDICINE; SECTION III: ETHICAL DIRECTIVES FOR OTHER HEALTH-CARE PROFESSIONS; *and* SECTION IV: ETHICAL DIRECTIVES FOR HUMAN RESEARCH.

Bibliography

ABBOTT, ANDREW. 1988. *The System of Professions: An Essay on the Division of Expert Labor.* Chicago: University of Chicago Press.

BAYLES, MICHAEL D. 1989. *Professional Ethics.* 2d ed. Belmont, Calif.: Wadsworth Publishing Company.

BERLANT, JEFFREY LIONEL. 1975. *Profession and Monopoly: A Study of Medicine in the United States and Great Britain.* Berkeley: University of California Press.

CAMENISCH, PAUL F. 1983. *Grounding Professional Ethics in a Pluralistic Society.* New York: Haven Publications.

DURKHEIM, EMILE. 1960. *The Division of Labor in Society.* Translated by George Simpson. New York: Free Press.

ETZIONI, AMITAI. 1969. *The Semi-Professions and Their Organization: Teachers, Nurses, Social Workers.* New York: Free Press.

FREIDSON, ELIOT. 1970a. *Professional Dominance: The Social Structure of Medical Care.* Chicago: Atherton Press.

———. 1970b. *Profession of Medicine: A Study of the Sociology of Applied Knowledge.* New York: Dodd, Mead.

———. 1986. *Professional Powers: A Study of the Institutionalization of Formal Knowledge.* Chicago: University of Chicago Press.

GOLDMAN, ALAN H. 1980. *The Moral Foundations of Professional Ethics.* Totowa, N.J.: Rowman and Littlefield.

GREENWOOD, ERNEST. 1957. "Attributes of a Profession." *Social Work* 2, no. 3:45–55.

HUGHES, EVERETT C. 1965. "Professions." In *The Professions in America,* pp. 1–14. Edited by Kenneth S. Lynn. Boston: Houghton Mifflin.

ILLICH, IVAN. 1973. *Tools for Conviviality.* New York: Harper & Row.

———. 1976. *Medical Nemesis: The Expropriation of Health.* New York: Pantheon Books.

KULTGEN, JOHN. 1988. *Ethics and Professionalism.* Philadelphia: University of Pennsylvania Press.

KUSKEY, G. 1973. "Health Care, Human Rights, and Government Intervention." *California Dental Association Journal* 1, no. 1:10–13.

LARSON, MAGALI SARFATTI. 1977. *The Rise of Professionalism: A Sociological Analysis.* Berkeley: University of California Press.

LUBAN, DAVID. 1988. *Lawyers and Justice: An Ethical Study.* Princeton, N.J.: Princeton University Press.

MILLERSON, GEOFFREY. 1974. *The Qualifying Associations: A Study in Professionalization.* New York: Humanities Press.

OZAR, DAVID T. 1993. "Building Awareness of Ethical Standards and Conduct." In *Educating Professionals: Responding to New Expectations for Competence and Accountability,* pp. 148–177. Edited by Lynn Curry and Jon F. Wergin. San Francisco: Jossey-Bass.

OZAR, DAVID T., and SOKOL, DAVID J. 1994. *Dental Ethics at Chairside: Professional Principles and Practical Applications.* St. Louis, Mo.: Mosby.

PARSONS, TALCOTT. 1951. *The Social System.* New York: Free Press.

———. 1954. *Essays in Sociological Theory.* Rev. ed. Glencoe, Ill.: Free Press.

PELLEGRINO, EDMUND. 1979. "Toward a Reconstruction of Medical Morality: The Primacy of the Act of Profession and the Fact of Illness." *Journal of Medicine and Philosophy* 4, no. 1:32–56.

PELLEGRINO, EDMUND D., and THOMASMA, DAVID C. 1988. *For the Patient's Good: The Restoration of Beneficence in Health Care.* New York: Oxford University Press.

SADE, ROBERT M. 1971. "Medical Care as a Right: A Refutation." *New England Journal of Medicine* 285, no. 23: 1288–1292.

STARR, PAUL. 1982. *The Social Transformation of American Medicine.* New York: Basic Books.

WILENSKY, HAROLD L. 1964. "The Professionalization of Everyone?" *American Journal of Sociology* 70, no. 2:137–158.

PROLONGATION OF LIFE

See DEATH AND DYING: EUTHANASIA AND SUSTAINING LIFE. *See also* ARTIFICIAL ORGANS AND LIFE-SUPPORT SYSTEMS.

PROSTITUTION

While the term "prostitution" has been applied to various human activities, in contemporary industrialized societies it commonly refers to a practice in which a woman makes herself sexually available to a man for a fee or some form of material compensation. Since indiscriminate, nonamorous sexual activity is considered in many societies to be debasing to women, when women act in this way for material gain their sexual and economic behavior is regarded as a form of prostitution. Commercialized sexual transactions typically are highly stigmatizing for the women, and sometimes the men, who participate in them; the existence of such activities is often treated as a sign of personal, spiritual, and social corruption and decay. As a potent symbol of moral disorder, prostitution is commonly viewed as a threat to social cohesion and individual well-being. In other words, prostitution is seen to corrupt and defile both the social body and the physical human body. This association between prostitution and degeneration or disease informs many legal, political, and intellectual responses to prostitution.

Moral questions

Some moral questions that prostitution poses can be raised, in general, about nonmarital and nonamorous sex. Does sexual activity outside marital and romantic social relationships degrade or harm the participants? Does it create harms for innocent third parties—for example, by contributing to the spread of sexually transmitted diseases, by weakening marital bonds or marriage as an institution, or by demeaning sexual activity? And does extramarital casual sexual activity inevitably conflict either with moral duties to loved ones or with some moral principle or ideal—such as universal human respect, faithfulness, honesty, or fairness?

Prostitution also raises moral questions pertaining to its social origins and consequences. Does prostitution reflect and reinforce the social subordination of women? Is prostitution produced and reproduced, in part, by social privileges based on race, ethnicity, class, and age? If prostitution is a function of the social dynamics of power and privilege, then is the prostitute's behavior determined by pernicious social forces rather than informed choice? Finally, the economic aspects of prostitution pose further ethical issues. Are prostitutes economically coerced and exploited by others? Does an organized practice that commercializes sex create a public danger or nuisance? And is the performance of a sexual act for money, without any other purpose or motive, morally base or reprehensible? Does it represent the encroachment of market forces into inappropriate areas of people's lives, leading to the domination of materialistic values over other values?

The existence of prostitution involving children or adolescents, both male and female, raises some different moral concerns. Since children and adolescents are presumably incapable of fully understanding the significance and consequences of sexual activity, especially paid sexual activity, their participation in prostitution is likely to involve a substantially higher degree of coercion and exploitation than prostitution involving only adults. Sexual activity with preadult prostitutes may involve a nonconsenting partner or the lack of a partner's informed consent. Depending upon the age of the minor prostitute, it may endanger the prostitute's physical and mental health. In addition, child prostitution promotes the moral corruption of children.

A relatively small portion of prostitution involves male prostitutes (adults, children, and adolescents) with female and male customers. Since indiscriminate, nonamorous heterosexual sexual behavior by men typically receives less social disapproval, male prostitutes with female clients—like the male clients of female prostitutes—have received little attention from moralists, social theorists, and the criminal justice system. Male prostitutes who serve a predominantly gay male clientele are more frequently subjects of moral and social analysis. Theorists and social reformers who have considered this latter group typically raise the same moral questions about their behavior as those above concerning the activities of female and child prostitutes. In short, the gender biases that condition the commercial sex industry also condition intellectual and social responses to it.

Prostitution sometimes involves sexual behaviors that are socially stigmatizing even in noncommercial contexts: same-sex sex, interracial sex, sadistic and masochistic sex, group sex, and child–adult sex. Prostitution involving such behaviors raises moral questions that pertain to the origins, consequences, and acceptability of these behaviors. This entry will focus on the most common form of prostitution: heterosexual prostitution involving adult female prostitutes.

Historical perspectives

Women have engaged in materially compensated sexual activities with men with whom they had no ongoing social relationship (unlike mistresses or concubines) in a variety of social, cultural, and historical contexts. In ancient Babylon, for example, women offered sexual services to male temple patrons, and even to the gods, as part of a religious ritual aimed at promoting the fertility of nature (Lerner, 1986; Goldman, 1983). In ancient India, female children were recruited for temple prostitution, and were trained in dancing and music (Bullough and Bullough, 1987). In ancient Greece and China, women prostitutes, or courtesans, provided extramarital companionship, entertainment, and sexual services to men from the highest social classes. Chinese Taoists apparently believed that certain forms of sex could promote a man's health and longevity, and that these personal benefits could be derived from prostitutional sex (Bullough and Bullough, 1987).

Brothel prostitution, publicly sanctioned and regulated, was popular in many medieval European cities. The Christian church condemned prostitution but saw its existence as a necessary evil. Prostitution provided an outlet for sexual desires that, if left unfulfilled, could lead to more sinful sexual behaviors. While celebrating virginity and celibacy and condemning all nonmarital sexual acts, the church fathers nevertheless were sympathetic to the social and economic plight of prostitutes. They were viewed as capable of repentance and potentially worthy of salvation (Rossiaud, 1988; Otis, 1985).

In the contemporary industrialized world, prostitutes are active predominantly in urban centers and ply their trade in a variety of ways. In some Asian cities where tourism is promoted, prostitutes are typically associated with bars and hotels, which offer the prostitute's services to their customers (Truong, 1990). In the contemporary United States and parts of Europe, prostitutes solicit customers on city streets (streetwalkers), through houses of prostitution and massage parlors (brothel workers), and through escort services and private networks (call girls). In colonial Nairobi, Kenya, during the first part of the twentieth century, prostitutes predominantly served an indigenous colonial work force; they typically took customers to their own rooms, where they could sell other domestic comforts such as food and baths (White, 1990).

The existence of labor forms similar to contemporary prostitution in a variety of historical and cultural settings has led many theorists to view prostitution as an inevitable component of human civilization. Some theorists attribute prostitution to a natural male (or human) desire for unlimited sexual gratification in an economy where opportunities for sex are in scarce supply (Ericsson, 1980). Other theorists see prostitution not as an inevitable human practice but as one that is contingent upon forms of social stratification that arose historically in capitalist and patriarchal societies (Overall, 1992; Pateman, 1983). For these theorists, prostitution is an extreme form of the dehumanized social relations that exist in capitalist and patriarchal social orders. However, given the variety of human sexual activities, both religious and economic, to which "prostitution" refers, it is unlikely that a single causal account will explain its existence.

Legal aspects

In many countries across Europe, Asia, and America, prostitution is legally prohibited or heavily regulated. In the contemporary United States, prostitution is illegal everywhere except in certain counties of Nevada. Prostitution in these counties is limited to licensed brothels, and prostitutes are subject to mandatory health exams, curfews, and residence restrictions. In England, following the Wolfenden Report (1957), private acts of prostitution are legal, whereas any public manifestation of prostitution, such as the open solicitation of customers or advertising through public media, is illegal. In some countries, like Germany, prostitution has been decriminalized and, in certain cities, deregulated to some extent. Many groups, ranging from feminist organizations like the National Organization for Women to prostitute collectives like COYOTE (Call Off Your Old Tired Ethics), support removing criminal sanctions from the prostitute's work (Cooper, 1989; Matthews, 1986; Delacoste and Alexander, 1987).

Laws prohibiting prostitution usually aim to protect society against the spread of venereal disease, to prevent the erosion of a shared public moral order, to protect women both from exploitation by others and from self-inflicted harm, and to prevent the creation of a public nuisance. Yet antiprostitution laws may be ineffective in achieving these aims.

Many legal scholars have argued that the criminalization of prostitution neither eliminates nor reduces prostitution, but only increases the difficulty of imposing health safeguards and of monitoring and curtailing the spread of disease through commercial sex. Legalized prostitution would allow the state to introduce measures that might better protect the health of the prostitute and her customer, and thus the health of all citizens.

Others have argued that criminalizing prostitution to preserve a shared public moral order falsely presupposes the existence of homogeneous moral beliefs and attitudes regarding prostitution. For it may not be the case that all social groups or religions regard the sale of sexual services as inherently immoral. At least, it is incumbent upon those who justify the criminalization of prostitution in this way to demonstrate the existence of a shared moral perspective regarding prostitution. If this presupposition is false, then criminalizing prostitution may preserve values that are not widely held. Moreover, even if there were a public consensus regarding the moral status of prostitution, some theorists question whether it is the proper role of the state to attempt either to influence moral values or to inhibit private sexual conduct between consenting adults.

Some feminist theorists have argued that laws prohibiting prostitution do not protect women but, rather, render them more vulnerable to abuse from others. Laws against prostitution often lead to the harassment of poor women, who are frequently subject to the arbitrary and abusive application of such laws by local officials (Walkowitz, 1980; Cooper, 1989; Symanski, 1981). Moreover, such laws diminish the prostitute's ability to seek legal redress for harms she may suffer from clients or her associates. In addition, laws that aim to protect adult women from self-harm and exploitation by others may be overly paternalistic, since they assume that women are incapable of determining what is in their own best interest. Perhaps the only sort of laws that might protect women are those that criminalize the coercive and exploitative behaviors of the prostitute's customers and managers.

Finally, while the prevention of a potential public nuisance may provide a good reason for regulating prostitution, it does not support imposing laws to prohibit it. The nuisance to others that an organized commercial sex industry might pose can be contained by denying it access to noncommercial districts and by imposing normal standards for business operations on the industry.

In sum, unless there are better reasons than those considered here for applying criminal sanctions to people who participate voluntarily in acts of prostitution, outlawing prostitution may be neither feasible nor justifiable. Yet, like other labor forms and commercial operations that create risks for workers, customers, and society at large, prostitution could be regulated by the state. The regulations imposed could seek to protect the prostitute, as well as the customer and society. These regulations could especially seek to prevent large-scale commercial interests from drawing profits in ways that dehumanize or degrade workers (Matthews, 1986).

Prostitution, AIDS, and drugs

The current AIDS epidemic raises both new and old moral questions regarding prostitution. Is prostitution partly responsible for the spread of AIDS? What steps is the state morally obligated or allowed to take toward HIV-positive prostitutes and customers? Are HIV-positive prostitutes and customers who practice safe sex entitled to as much privacy as HIV-positive dentists or surgeons, for example? Do the moral rights of innocent third parties (such as the spouses, partners, and children of prostitutes and customers) outweigh the privacy rights of prostitutes and customers? What steps is the state morally obligated or permitted to take to protect prostitutes from being coerced into performing, or to prevent prostitutes and customers from consensually performing, sexual acts where the risk of HIV exposure is high?

While many prostitutes are HIV-positive, some researchers have argued that prostitutes are more likely to be exposed to HIV through intravenous drug use than through commercial sexual activities, in which they are more likely to take precautions (Delacoste and Alexander, 1987; Decker, 1987). Some have argued that since profits in prostitution depend upon the commercial sex industry's ability to offer services that are relatively safe, tolerating prostitution will promote safer sexual practices, especially those involving condom use. However, the profit motive may encourage some "safe" sexual practices that are highly problematic, such as the use of presumably virginal child prostitutes, or voyeuristic sex in which the voyeur pays to watch a couple engage in unsafe sex, and so on. In these cases, prostitution is safe only for the customer. In order to prevent commercial interests from overriding the rights of prostitutes and children, the state should regulate commercial sexual interactions, and stringently enforce criminal laws pertaining to the sexual violation and commercial exploitation of children.

Many researchers have observed and confirmed a significant correlation between women who work as prostitutes and women who are drug addicts or substance abusers (Goldstein, 1979). Does prostitution lead to drug use, or does drug use lead women to prostitution? What are the moral implications of these possible causal relationships? If prostitution characteristically leads women to substance abuse or drug dependency, then there may be some features of the work that encourage drug use. Theorists have identified a number of possible features of prostitution that may contribute to the prostitute's evolution into a substance abuser: Prostitutes operate in a social milieu where drug abuse is common; the work of a prostitute, or the social stigma it creates, requires mood alteration or mental escape; the commission of the criminal act of prostitution lowers one's inhibitions toward committing other criminal acts; and prostitutes are encouraged to become drug addicts by pimps who wish to control them. The features of prostitution that lead to substance abuse may be alterable, and thus social policies regarding prostitution should be designed to minimize these features.

Where substance abuse leads women to prostitution, the causes appear to be primarily economic.

Women who are drug addicts may find prostitution sufficient or necessary to support an expensive drug habit. However, the fact that drug addiction can lead to prostitution does not seem to illuminate any morally relevant aspect of prostitution.

Prostitution as the subordination of women

Some feminist theorists have argued that prostitution involves not just the exploitation of female bodies or sexuality, but of female persons, because the product purchased or consumed in prostitution cannot be separated from the person who exchanges it—a separation that may be made in other kinds of trade (Pateman, 1983; Barry, 1979). Other feminists have argued that prostitution inevitably involves illegitimate forms of human subordination. On this view, prostitution has a value or purpose only when it is performed for someone socially privileged by gender, race, class, or age, and by someone socially disadvantaged by the same factors; thus when these illegitimate forms of social privilege disappear, so will prostitution (Overall, 1992). Yet there are cases where prostitution is performed by men for women (Karch and Dann, 1981), by working-class people for each other (White, 1990), and by white North Americans and Europeans for Asians (e.g., the "blond geishas" in Japan). Thus, in some cases the customer may be socially privileged by some factors while the prostitute is socially privileged by others. In short, prostitution appears desirable to some participants even when the social power and status of the prostitute and customer are, on balance, seemingly comparable.

In the United States, the commercial sex industry does appear to be organized by, and may ultimately serve to reproduce, cultural ideologies that place women in subordinate social roles (Shrage, 1989). Prostitution in this context reflects the cultural ideology that men have sexual needs that can be met by impersonal sexual encounters, and that while men benefit from heterosexual intercourse in these contexts, women are harmed and defiled. The composition of the prostitute work force also reflects racist and pernicious social myths about the sexuality of women of color (Shrage, 1992). While prostitution may not involve the subordination of women in all societies, in the contemporary United States and many similar industrialized parts of the world, it reflects beliefs that continue to promote the subordination of women.

Yet the commercialization of sex is neither a universal cause nor a symptom of the subordination of women. Rather, the degraded social position of women and the cultural myths that sustain it in a particular society can shape sex commerce into a practice that reflects and reinforces women's subordinate social status (Dominelli, 1986). Therefore, those who oppose the subordination of women should challenge not sex commerce but the cultural ideologies and customs that give it its historically specific form. This should involve devising social policies regarding trafficking in sex that challenge cultural myths regarding proper sexual and social roles for women and men. Moreover, social policies that economically empower women—especially single mothers—and reduce their level of financial dependence on others would also serve more directly to challenge the subordination of women than would the repression of sex commerce.

Some feminist prostitutes have argued that prostitution itself challenges the subordination of women. Since prostitution affirms a woman's right to control her own body, including the right to exploit it for economic gain, it challenges the notion that women are economically dependent on men (Pheterson, 1989). Yet, just as it is unlikely that prostitution inherently supports and reflects the subordination of women, so it is unlikely that prostitution inherently supports and reflects the social empowerment of women. In the United States, for example, prostitution may challenge deeply instilled stereotypes of women as nonproviders, but it reinforces the pernicious notion that it is a woman's primary function to satisfy men sexually.

Conclusion

Most of the moral questions about prostitution, and some of the medical and empirical concerns upon which they rest, can be answered only by studying particular cases of sex commerce. It is possible, then, that the moral status of prostitution in colonial Nairobi or ancient Babylon, for example, may be different from the moral status of an outwardly similar phenomenon in contemporary Asia. Moral theorists need to examine the cultural factors that shape sex into work, that form the provision of sex into an occupation, and that place the sex worker under the moral category of prostitute—a person who alienates from herself a basic human good for material gain. In some cases prostitution may involve illegitimate forms of human subordination and exploitation (for example, where child prostitutes or impoverished women are involved), and thus may approach something akin to rape—that is, coerced sex. In other cases, prostitution may occur between persons of comparable social status and means, as part of a voluntary and mutually satisfying arrangement. Moral theorists need to pay close attention to the social and cultural contexts in which prostitution occurs in order to isolate features that morally distinguish different cases. In this way we can explore and question the conceptualization of sex commerce in terms of the powerful metaphors of disease and degeneration.

LAURIE SHRAGE

For a further discussion of topics mentioned in this entry, see the entries AIDS; FEMINISM; HOMOSEXUALITY; MARRIAGE AND OTHER DOMESTIC PARTNERSHIPS; SEXUAL ETHICS; SEXUALITY IN SOCIETY; SUBSTANCE ABUSE; and WOMEN, especially the article on HISTORICAL AND CROSS-CULTURAL PERSPECTIVES. For a discussion of related ideas, see the entries AUTONOMY; and PATERNALISM. Other relevant material may be found under the entries ABUSE, INTERPERSONAL; HEALTH SCREENING AND TESTING IN THE PUBLIC-HEALTH CONTEXT; PUBLIC HEALTH AND THE LAW, article on LEGAL MORALISM AND PUBLIC HEALTH; and SEXISM.

Bibliography

BARRY, KATHLEEN. 1979. *Female Sexual Slavery*. New York: Avon.

BELL, LAURIE, ed. 1987. *Good Girls/Bad Girls: Feminists and Sex Trade Workers Face to Face*. Seattle: Seal.

BULLOUGH, VERN L., and BULLOUGH, BONNIE. 1987. *Women and Prostitution: A Social History*. Buffalo, N.Y.: Prometheus.

CAMPAGNA, DANIEL S., and POFFENBERGER, DONALD L. 1988. *The Sexual Trafficking in Children: An Investigation of the Child Sex Trade*. Dover, Mass.: Auburn House.

COOPER, BELINDA. 1989. "Prostitution: A Feminist Analysis." *Women's Rights Law Reporter* 11, no. 3:98–119.

DECKER, JOHN F. 1987. "Prostitution as a Public Health Issue." In *AIDS and the Law: A Guide for the Public*, pp. 81–89. Edited by Harlon L. Dalton, Scott Burris, and the Yale AIDS Law Project. New Haven, Conn.: Yale University Press.

DELACOSTE, FREDERIQUE, and ALEXANDER, PRISCILLA, eds. 1987. *Sex Work: Writings by Women in the Industry*. Pittsburgh, Penn.: Cleis.

DOMINELLI, LENA. 1986. "The Power of the Powerless: Prostitution and the Reinforcement of Submissive Femininity." *Sociological Review* 34, no. 1:65–92.

ERICSSON, LARS O. 1980. "Charges Against Prostitution: An Attempt at a Philosophical Assessment." *Ethics* 90, no. 3:335–366.

GOLDMAN, EMMA. 1983. "The Traffic in Women." In *Red Emma Speaks: An Emma Goldman Reader*, pp. 175–189. Edited by Alix Kates Shulman. New York: Schocken.

GOLDSTEIN, PAUL J. 1979. *Prostitution and Drugs*. Lexington, Mass.: Heath.

KARCH, CECILIA A., and DANN, GRAHAM H. S. 1981. "Close Encounters of the Third World." *Human Relations* 34, no. 4:249–268.

LERNER, GERDA. 1986. "The Origin of Prostitution in Ancient Mesopotamia." *Signs: Journal of Women in Culture and Society* 11, no. 2:236–254.

MATTHEWS, ROGER. 1986. "Beyond Wolfenden? Prostitution, Politics and the Law." In *Confronting Crime*, pp. 188–211. Edited by Roger Matthews and Jock Young. London: Sage.

OTIS, LEAH L. 1985. *Prostitution in Medieval Society: The History of an Urban Institution in Languedoc*. Chicago: University of Chicago Press.

OVERALL, CHRISTINE. 1992. "What's Wrong with Prostitution? Evaluating Sex Work." *Signs* 17, no. 2:705–724.

PATEMAN, CAROLE. 1983. "Defending Prostitution: Charges Against Ericsson." *Ethics* 93, no. 3:561–565.

PHETERSON, GAIL. 1989. *A Vindication of the Rights of Whores.* Seattle: Seal.

ROSSIAUD, JACQUES. 1988. *Medieval Prostitution.* Translated by Lydia G. Cochrane. Oxford: Basil Blackwell.

SHRAGE, LAURIE. 1989. "Should Feminists Oppose Prostitution?" *Ethics* 99, no. 2:347–361.

———. 1992. "Is Sexual Desire Raced? The Social Meaning of Interracial Prostitution." *Journal of Social Philosophy* 23, no. 1:42–51.

SMART, CAROL. 1984. "Researching Prostitution: Some Problems for Feminist Research." *Humanity and Society* 8, no. 4:407–413.

STEWARD, SAMUEL M. 1991. *Understanding the Male Hustler.* New York: Haworth.

SYMANSKI, RICHARD. 1981. *The Immoral Landscape: Female Prostitution in Western Societies.* Toronto: Butterworths.

TRUONG, THANH-DAM. 1990. *Sex, Money and Morality: Prostitution and Tourism in South-East Asia.* London: Zed.

WALKOWITZ, JUDITH R. 1980. *Prostitution and Victorian Society: Women, Class, and the State.* Cambridge: At the University Press.

WHITE, LUISE. 1990. *The Comforts of Home: Prostitution in Colonial Nairobi.* Chicago: University of Chicago Press.

PROTESTANTISM

Protestantism began in the sixteenth century as a reform movement within the Roman Catholic church. Soon and sadly, the reformers found themselves outside the Catholic church, forced to establish churches of their own. The movement spread quickly through northern Europe and was transplanted to North America; eventually churches were established all over the world.

As the movement spread, it also splintered. Different visions of the form that a reformed church should take led to a variety of liturgical practices, systems of governance, and creedal statements. This diversity has also characterized Protestant reflection about morality, including medical morality. Protestant reflection about medical ethics defies generalization. Even so, a tradition and efforts to describe it—and the struggles of Protestants to be faithful to it—have contributed to medical ethics.

The origin of Protestantism and its enduring witness

Protestantism was a movement of protest against what were perceived to be the corruptions of discipline and doctrine in the medieval church, but as the Latin word *protestari* ("to give testimony") suggests, it was also a movement of affirmation and of testimony. Some of the things to which Protestantism has consistently given testimony may be discovered in the story of its beginnings.

In 1517 a young German monk and theologian named Martin Luther challenged the medieval church's practice of selling indulgences, or papal grants of forgiveness, and testified to his conviction that God's grace could not be earned or purchased but only received. He had intended only a little debate about indulgences, but he quickly found himself in an enormous struggle with Pope Leo X over fundamental questions of the thought and life of the Church. The breach came in 1520, when Luther wrote three treatises against the papal church that gave enduring shape to the Protestant witness.

The sovereignty of God and the freedom of Christians. Luther's treatises testified to the sovereignty of a gracious God. The sovereignty of God meant at least the freedom of God; it was not an arbitrary or capricious power, but the free and purposeful decision of God to be the righteous and gracious Sovereign made known by Jesus Christ and by the scriptures that witnessed to Christ. That free decision entailed freedom for the Christian, too; it freed sinful human beings to have Christ as lord, to live in the righteousness and grace of God, to be a servant of God and of the neighbor. In Luther's paradoxical but illuminating propositions, "A Christian is a perfectly free lord of all, subject to none. A Christian is a perfectly dutiful servant of all, subject to all" (Luther, 1960, p. 277).

Faith and works: The suspicion of casuistry. Luther also objected to a sacramental system that made it the prerogative of the church or its clerics or its pope to confer or to withhold the grace of God. The grace of God was free. The sacramental system, Luther protested, domesticated the grace of God and diminished the freedom of both God and the Christian.

One of the sacraments was penance, and Luther objected vigorously to the way it was conducted. The priest in the confessional functioned as jurist, identifying sins and determining fit penance. Canon law provided the basis for such adjudication, and confessional manuals were developed to aid the priest in discovering and dealing with a variety of sins, including the sins of physicians. By means of this practice and the casuistic literature that guided it, the Roman Catholic church exercised a remarkable control over every part of life, including medicine. For Luther, however, the root sin was a failure to trust God, and the number and gravity of particular sins was not nearly as significant as the fundamental failure to trust God. He warned against the juridical and casuistic practice of penance as an invitation to self-justification. Ironically, Luther's heightened sense of sin resulted in a diminished attention to individual sins. Luther's testimony to the freedom of God and of the Christian made him suspicious of "legalism," of moralism, and of casuistry and any juridical role for clergy.

The priesthood and worldly vocation of all believers.   Luther also called for a reform of the hierarchical structure of the church. He rejected the authority of the pope, not only because Leo X excommunicated him and resisted reform but also because there was one head of the church, namely, Christ, and the hierarchy misrepresented the way Christ's authority functions in the church and arbitrarily diminished the freedom of the Christian. In relation to Christ, all the distinctions of ecclesiastical hierarchy were relativized.

Each believer, Luther said, was baptized into Christ, had "put on Christ," and was called to represent Christ to the neighbor: "Through baptism all of us are consecrated to the priesthood" (Luther, 1960, p. 14). Each Christian was gifted and called, as priest, to represent the grace of God to the neighbor and to intercede for the neighbor to God. The "priesthood of all believers" underscored both the dignity of the individual believer and the importance and necessity of Christian community. The claim is not that each one is one's own priest but rather that each is priest to the other. Their mutual ministry signals the priesthood and rule of Christ in the church.

Luther also rejected the distinction between the "spiritual estate" and the "temporal estate," the double standard of medieval Christendom that distinguished religious callings from secular callings. Each believer, as priest, had a "calling" or "vocation" to service. The secular or "this-worldly" work of the cobbler and the caregiver were given a dignity no less than the "religious" work of the priest or monk. In the exercise of this vocation, the believer's freedom was not to be arbitrarily diminished by the priest or by canon law.

Consciences taken captive by scripture.   Called before the Diet at Worms in 1521 by Emperor Charles V and ordered to recant, Luther refused, stating that his conscience had been "taken captive" by scripture and that, unless he were convinced by the testimony of scripture or by clear reason, he could not recant. "Here I stand," he said, "I cannot do otherwise."

Eight years later, at the Diet of Speyer, Charles V again attempted to suppress the Lutheran "heresy." Nineteen estates (of the 400 represented at the Diet) registered their "protest," testifying like Luther at Worms to their submission to scripture's authority and to their confidence in the sovereignty of God in spite of the power of the pope and Charles V. These representatives—and soon all members of the movement—were called "Protestants."

The young monk and theologian of Wittenberg was joined by other reformers, such as Philipp Melanchthon in Wittenberg, Ulrich Zwingli in Zurich, John Calvin in Geneva, Menno Simons in the Netherlands, and Thomas Cranmer in England. Sometimes the other voices were more radical; sometimes they were more conservative and conciliatory. The voices did not always sound in unison or even in harmony. As early as the sixteenth century, the movement splintered. Lines were drawn between the followers of Luther and the followers of Calvin (who came to be called Reformed or Presbyterian) and between those groups and both the more radical reformers (e.g., the Mennonites) and the less radical reformation of the Anglicans.

Protestantism and the scientific revolution

The scientific revolution of the sixteenth and seventeenth centuries coincided with the Reformation and flourished in Protestant lands. The causes for the advances of science and medicine during this time are complicated, and the new research was hardly a monopoly of Protestantism. Nevertheless, a number of historians of science have called attention to the contributions of Protestantism (Cohen, 1990; Hooykaas, 1972; Merton, 1970), its affirmation of the sovereignty of God, its suspicion of casuistry, its celebration of a worldly "calling," and its readiness to question the authority of tradition.

That the affirmation of God's sovereignty played an important role is widely recognized, but the Calvinist doctrines of predestination and providence were not, as some historians of science have suggested (Mason, 1962), the theological precursors for the mechanistic determinism of the scientists. The Reformers' denial that things happened by chance was not an affirmation of fate or mechanistic necessity, but an affirmation of God's rule. Order comes from the gracious hand of God no less than extraordinary events, "nature" no less than "miracle." The order of the universe and of the body is simply an example of the way God ordinarily works, and the study of God's work—as by medicine—simply provides evidence of the "wonderful wisdom" of God (Calvin, 1960, I.v.2, p. 53).

The other side of the Reformers' appreciation for God's work in the order of things was their suspicion of extravagant claims made for the miraculous effects of relics and shrines. Not science but Protestantism first challenged the magical account of diseases and cures. Protestants repudiated the popular and magical understanding of the use of relics, the invocation of saints, the pilgrimages to shrines, and the use of holy water (Thomas, 1971). Their moral and theological suspicion of any magical manipulation of a sovereign God fostered the "disenchantment of the world" and prepared the way for medicine to be medicine while God was God.

Protestants were also suspicious of the juridical power of the clergy and of the penitential casuistry by which the medieval church had exercised control over the conduct of people, including physicians. The Protestant affirmation of salvation by grace through faith contributed to the emancipation of artisans, including physicians, from the control of the church. Protestant physicians were free to assert the autonomy of the profession, to look to the scientist rather than the cleric for advice about the practice.

The Protestant notion of the "priesthood of all believers," and its correlative notion of a worldly "calling," not only emancipated physicians, scientists, and hospitals but also gave them a new dignity and their work a new direction. Their "priesthood" made them not only "perfectly free lord of all, subject to none" but also "perfectly dutiful servant of all, subject to all." The science and the practice of medicine were called and ordered toward the relief of humanity. Francis Bacon's call for an "advancement of learning" resonated on Protestant ears and was echoed by many Puritan voices (Cohen, 1990; Hooykaas, 1972; Webster, 1976). Knowledge should not be merely speculative but also practical, tested by experience and experiment, and apt for the restoration of dominion over nature to human hands and so, for progress toward human well-being. The optimistic expectation of great benefit to humanity through science gave many Puritans a positive, indeed religious, motive for scientific inquiry (Webster, 1976). Finally, as Thomas Sprat observed in his 1667 *History of the Royal Society*, there was a certain congruity between the new science and Protestantism, in their common rejection of the authority of tradition and doctrinal authority and in their common appeal to experience (Mason, 1962).

The place and meaning of healing

The "enlightenment" of the eighteenth-century philosophers followed hard on the heels of scientific revolution. The harmony of religion and science remained, but control had shifted to science. If the Puritan had concluded that nature must have an order because God's rule is orderly rather than capricious, the Protestant deist concluded that God must be a designer because the universe is a machine. This different conception of God led inevitably to a certain indifference to the God so conceived. Only a few were prepared to dispense with God altogether, but God was hardly personal and never inconvenient. Human freedom and reason—and gradually also human disease and cure—were understood apart from God. Grace was transformed to virtue and technical competence, and salvation was transferred from divine to human hands.

But the eighteenth century was not only the age of reason; it was also the age of renewal. The revivals of "the Great Awakening" stressed conversions and discipleship and "awakened" Protestantism from the rationalism of Protestant scholasticism and from the

indifference of the deists. The assumption of a harmony between science, especially medical science, and religion remained, revealed not only in the scientific curiosity of Jonathan Edwards, the great Calvinist theologian and preacher, but also in the medical practice and writing of John Wesley, the Anglican who founded the Methodist church.

As a missionary in America, Wesley supplemented his evangelism with opposition to hard liquor and tobacco and with some medical care, but when he returned to England and saw the sickness and suffering of the poor, he undertook a more regular practice. The desire to identify remedies available to the poor led to the publication in 1747 of *Primitive Physick*. Some of the remedies collected by Wesley sound quaint and quackish by today's standards, but two things are worth noting about the collection. First, Wesley drew from the best physicians of the day and selected remedies then regarded as cheap and safe. Second, he defended the tradition of the "empirics," whose remedies could be and had been tested by the trial of experience (Holifield, 1986).

Wesley did not share the conviction of the Reformers that the gift of "spiritual" healing had vanished from the church, and he certainly had no sympathy with the "enlightened" view that the biblical miracles were not only past but naive and mythological accounts of that past. He conducted his medical practice side by side with a growing confidence in and curiosity about spiritual healing. He did not see these healing practices as in conflict; all healing, after all, was finally from God (Holifield, 1986). What Wesley regarded as harmonious, however, was regarded by some of his more "enlightened" Protestant contemporaries as a mixture of "enthusiasm" with proper religion and of "Romish magic" with proper medicine.

During the nineteenth century, medicine developed not only its scientific and technical competence, but also its social authority and cohesiveness. By the end of that century, training requirements and licensing restrictions brought a virtual halt to the tradition of clergy practicing medicine. Mainline Protestantism aligned itself with the developing medical orthodoxy, while sectarian Protestantism favored sectarian medicine. Mormons favored Thomsonian medicine; Seventh-Day Adventism was allied with hydropathy; and Christian Science was indebted to Phineas Quimby's New Thought. Each eventually broke with sectarian medicine. Mormonism and Seventh-Day Adventism adopted strong attachments to conventional medicine while they continued to emphasize abstention from caffeine and nicotine. Christian Science repudiated Quimby's doctrines but continued to avoid conventional medicine as contradictory to its belief that disease and death are illusions.

The Protestant mainstream generally welcomed the professional autonomy of medicine and embraced medical care as a way to express the healing ministry of Christ. At the beginning of the missionary movement of the nineteenth century, there were only a few medically trained professionals involved, and their task was the care of the missionaries. By the end of the century, however, they were an integral part of the missionary movement itself, and not simply a means to win a hearing for the preaching of the missionary. Medicine was seen as a continuation of the healing ministry of Jesus and as a response to his command to preach the gospel and to heal the sick, a necessary expression of faithfulness to the mission of God.

Much conventional Protestantism ensured the harmony of medicine and religion by compartmentalizing life; the body was regarded as the object of the physician's care and skill, and the spirit or soul as the object of the attention of the church and its clergy. The progressive impulse of liberal theology in the nineteenth century celebrated the triumph of Bacon's vision and shared his confidence in knowledge as power over nature to secure human well-being. At the beginning of the twentieth century, therefore, many Protestant physicians and scientists, emancipated from the control of magisterial ecclesiastical authority and canon law and increasingly secularized, could pursue their work with a strong sense of the significance of their "calling" but with little sense of the guidance and limits provided by religion. Many Protestant churches and their members could regard medicine as a good gift of God but none of their business—best left in the hands of competent and compassionate physicians.

Some other Protestants, however, regarded spiritual healings as more apt to express the healing ministry of Jesus. While many Protestants regarded such healings as both bad medicine and bad Protestantism, others—especially in popular rather than in elite and intellectual cultures—regarded healing gifts as evidence of the presence and power of the Spirit and of grace. The Holiness Movement among Methodists in the nineteenth century was hospitable to spiritual healing, while other Methodists like James Buckley, the editor of the *Advocate*, described faith healing as "a kind of quackery of faith" (Holifield, 1986, p. 40).

In the twentieth century, "healing" continued to divide Protestantism. Pentecostalism was born out of the Holiness revivals and camp meetings at the beginning of the twentieth century. In typical Protestant fashion, it called for the renewal of the church according to its early pattern, but it identified that pattern with the gifts of the Spirit, including the gift of healing. It attracted people from a wide variety of Protestant denominations, and an even wider variety of new Pentecostal denomi-

nations (over 1,000 of them) were formed. In the Charismatic movement of mid-century, many more experienced the gifts (the charismata) of the Spirit, including healing, but stayed in their own denominations. These Charismatics are a sizable group in many Protestant churches and in the Roman Catholic church. There has been a phenomenal growth of such Pentecostal and Charismatic groups, especially in South America, Africa, and Asia. Enormous diversity characterizes these groups, but generally they share Wesley's view that all healing—and not just spiritual healing—comes from God.

Buckley's early resistance to faith healing was echoed again and again in Protestant publications through the twentieth century in response to the claims of Pentecostalism: Faith healing was medical quackery and religious superstition, unworthy of human reason and of God's rule. In the midst of his polemic against faith healers, Buckley called for an alternative Protestant piety relative to healing: the building of hospitals. Such a piety was aligned with human reason and with reform; it recognized the harmony of science and religion and it could enable the church to follow Jesus (and Wesley) by caring for the sick poor. The call for construction of hospitals was also echoed again and again in Protestant publications in the late nineteenth and early twentieth centuries and Protestants were often moved by piety to build hospitals, whether public or denominational. Almost from the very beginning, however, it was difficult to distinguish Protestant from secular hospitals. Such was the confidence in a harmony of science and religion.

The Protestant debate about faith healing was frequently, but not always, polemic. Protestant churches with a tradition of spiritual healing learned sometimes to be careful about pride in spiritual gifts and sloth with respect to more conventional therapies, and Protestant churches with a tradition of supporting medical healing listened well enough to acknowledge the danger of dualism, of reducing an embodied patient to manipulable nature. In 1920, for example, an Anglican conference (the Lambeth Conference) issued a report calling for the cooperation of those who cared for the body and those who cared for the soul.

One effect of this call for cooperation was the development of hospital chaplaincy. In 1936 Richard Cabot, a physician at Massachusetts General Hospital, and Russell Dicks, a minister who served as chaplain there, published *The Art of Ministering to the Sick*. In it they called attention to the "whole person" and insisted that healing is not simply a matter of curing the body by scientific medicine. Their model was cooperation in a joint ministry to the whole person, rather than compartmentalization of care for the body and care for the soul. In good Protestant fashion, they appealed to scripture to justify the presence of the minister in the hospital room: "The minister goes to the sickroom because he is the duly recognized representative of Him who said, 'For . . . I was sick and ye visited me'" (Cabot and Dicks, 1936, pp. 12–13; the authors did not notice that the text makes the sick rather than the visitor the representative of Christ). By 1940 the American Protestant Hospital Association (formed in 1921) adopted a set of standards for hospital chaplaincy, and hospital chaplaincy developed quickly thereafter.

Chaplaincy was sometimes co-opted by the therapeutic agenda of medicine, and religion was sometimes valued instrumentally for its contributions to that agenda. Even so, the emphasis on the whole person by chaplains such as Russell Dicks and Seward Hiltner (1943), and by physicians such as Paul Tournier (1954), prepared Protestantism to raise questions of medical ethics.

Protestant perspectives on medical ethics

Although it was not the first book by a Protestant on the theology and ethics of medicine (Jenkins, 1949, and Sperry, 1950, were earlier), Joseph Fletcher's *Morals and Medicine* (1960) was a groundbreaking work, self-consciously set against the tradition of Catholic casuistry. Fletcher's selective retrieval of the Protestant tradition focused on human freedom, the suspicion of "legalism," the Baconian confidence in knowledge as mastery over nature to provide human well-being, and the autonomy of a conscience informed by scripture (whose significance was reduced to the love commandment). In Fletcher's hands, the Protestant tradition was thoroughly "enlightened." It provoked response not only from Catholics but also from another Protestant thinker, Paul Ramsey (1956).

During the next decade, Protestant attention focused on issues of civil rights and just war, but then Ramsey returned to questions of medical ethics, first with essays on genetic control and abortion and then with *The Patient as Person: Explorations in Medical Ethics* (1970). This book, more than any other, marked what LeRoy Walters called the "renaissance of medical ethics" and led to the "flowering" of the discipline (Walters, 1985).

Protestants made substantial contributions to the literature on medical ethics during the next decade. Besides Fletcher and Ramsey, other important Protestant contributors include James F. Childress, Arthur Dyck, John C. Fletcher, James Gustafson, Stanley Hauerwas, Karen Lebacqz, William F. May, J. Robert Nelson, Gene Outka, David H. Smith, Harmon Smith, Kenneth Vaux, Robert Veatch, and LeRoy Walters. There is a characteristic Protestant diversity among these authors, and generalizations are hazardous. They are heirs of a tradition that includes, after all, not only the Reformation of the sixteenth century but also the Puritan adoption of a Baconian vision in the seventeenth century, both the "enlightenment" and the "awakening" of the eighteenth century, and attitudes toward medicine that range from celebration to suspicion. Even so, some of the things to which Protestantism has consistently given testimony since its origin have continued to shape Protestant perspectives on medical ethics.

The sovereignty of God: Idolatry and dualism. Protestants did not invent the notion of the sovereignty of God, but they used it against any and every confusion of the rule of God with lesser authorities, whether pope or king, whether canon law or the dicta of magistrates. God alone is God, and God alone is worthy of absolute trust and confidence, of absolute faith. In this theocentric perspective, the great moral dangers are idolatry and dualism, to treat some relative good as absolute and to treat some relative evil as ultimate.

The rejection of idolatry is a theme to which Protestant medical ethics returns regularly. Karl Barth, for example, while commending the respect due life as the gift and command of God, wrote, "Life is no second God, and therefore the respect due to it cannot rival the reverence owed to God" (Barth, 1961, p. 342). Life is a great good, a gift of God, but the sovereignty of God prohibits both an absolute prohibition against taking life and an absolute requirement to prolong it.

Similarly, health is a great good but no second God, either. The relief of pain is a great good, but in the midst of pain there is a great temptation to idolatry, to curse God or to damn the neighbor, to do or undo anything for the sake only of relieving one's pain. Children are a precious gift from God, but even children can be the object of idolatrous loyalty and expectation. It is a commonplace that children are the hope for the future, but it is nevertheless blasphemous. The sovereign grace of God is the hope for the future, and Protestant sensibilities toward children regard them as a sign of such confidence (Hauerwas, 1986).

Technology may be the most tempting idol in the contemporary pantheon. Protestants trained at the feet of "Baconian Puritans" are partly responsible for the extravagant expectations attached to technology, but more than one Protestant has issued a prophetic protest against idolatrous confidence in and expectations of technology. Of course, many Protestants do continue to reject as "idolatrous" submissiveness to "Mother Nature" and to cultural taboos that interfere with seizing technological opportunities for human well-being.

The rejection of idolatry does not tell the Protestant precisely what ought to be done or left undone, but it has served to keep Protestantism critical and self-critical. Unfortunately, it is a good deal easier to say that a relative value is not ultimate than it is to say precisely how it is relative to the sovereign One. The Protestant task is captured in the theocentric exhortation of James Gustafson to relate to all things in ways appropriate to the relation of all things to God (Gustafson, 1981).

If Protestants have wanted to avoid absolutizing any relative goods, they have also wanted to avoid regarding any relative evil as ultimate. Protestants formed by this testimony to God's sovereignty and constancy can endure pain, sorrow, suffering, and death, remaining content to be human and not God, thankful for the good gifts of God, nonchalant in the face of adversity, confident that nothing can separate them from the love of God. In the face of suffering and death the Protestant is sustained by the readiness to let God be sovereign and by the recognition that the powers of evil are ultimately powerless against God's grace and future.

William F. May, for example, acknowledges the "sacral power of death" in Western culture but affirms the sovereignty of God. Death is powerlessness against the grace of God made known in Jesus. There are not "two Lords." "The lord of the church is not ruler of a surface kingdom. His dominion is nothing if it does not go at least six feet deep" (Lammers and Verhey, 1987, p. 178). May protests against using the machinery of medicine either to conceal or to eliminate death (or suffering). Neither the church nor medicine can deny the reality or the menace of death, or pretend to messianic powers against it. Death threatens to separate people from their bodies, from their communities, and from God. The threat is real and terrible, but in the confidence of God's final victory over death, the church and medicine can minister to the dying by nurturing their relation to their own flesh, by sustaining their relations with community, and by refusing to abandon them. Such words and deeds give "indirect" testimony to the God who rules and will rule.

The sovereignty of God is appealed to in other areas of medicine as well. Paul Ramsey, for example, accused the Nobel Prize–winning geneticist H. J. Muller of describing "the pollution of the gene pool" as an ultimate evil and of entertaining extravagant and idolatrous expectations of genetic control (Lammers and Verhey, 1987). The consequences of the "pollution of the gene pool" could be and were being debated scientifically, but Ramsey insisted that, even if Muller's predictions were right, one who affirmed the sovereignty of God would "need neither fear the problem nor trust the solution of it too much" (Lammers and Verhey, 1987, p. 364). Such nonchalance is neither Pollyanna optimism nor an excuse for doing nothing. Since the future is finally in God's hands, humans may and must attend not only to consequences but also to the rightness of the means to achieve them. One more illustration: Stanley Hauerwas has suggested, in thoroughly Protestant fashion, that the critical question for the debate about abortion is not "When does life begin?" but "Who is its true sovereign?" (Hauerwas, 1981, p. 226).

The freedom of the Christian: The autonomy of patients. The corollary of the sovereignty of God in Martin Luther was human freedom, and much of Protestant moral reflection about medicine has underscored the significance of freedom. Robert Veatch has suggested that "the most important contribution of Protestant thinkers to medical ethics" has been the emphasis on the role of the layperson in their approach to medical ethical problems. The Protestant tradition, he has said, is committed to protecting the freedom of the layperson against the arbitrary dominance of the powerful professional—whether ecclesiastical or medical (Veatch, 1989, p. 15).

Veatch is surely right when he says that the approach of many Protestant commentators on medical ethics has emphasized freedom. So, for example, Joseph Fletcher described his position in his early work as "personalist" (Fletcher, 1960, p. xx), developed the notion of "respect for persons" along the lines of Kant's second maxim that persons ought never to be treated merely as a means to an end, emphasized the moral priority of free and informed consent, and underscored in chapter titles and exposition a number of "rights." Similarly, Ramsey announced the theme of his groundbreaking book in its title, *The Patient as Person* (1970). He used the notion of "person" as a Kantian or deontological check against medicine's devotion to maximizing certain "benefits," whether knowledge or life. He insisted that free and informed consent was critical to respect for "the patient as person" and to "the canon of loyalty," the covenant that linked physician to patient.

Fletcher and Ramsey disagreed fundamentally about a number of points surrounding the issue of freedom and the principle of respect for persons. They disagreed, for example, about who counted as a "person" and about whether "respect for autonomous choices" was a sufficient account of "respect for persons." According to Fletcher, a "person" was one who had "cerebral function," capacities for knowledge and choice. Ramsey regarded such an account of "person" as a reductionistic denial of the embodiment of human beings. Fletcher's account permitted him to regard "respect for persons" as irrelevant to fetuses, newborns, and those in persistent vegetative state, and therefore also permitted him to consider the treatment of these in terms of maximizing the benefit to others. Ramsey's insistence upon embodiment led him not only to include fetuses and newborns in the category "person" but also to insist that human creatures have "a sacredness" not only in their capacities to choose but also "in bodily life" (Ramsey, 1970), "that there are more ways to violate man-womanhood than to violate the *freedom* of the parties; and that something voluntarily adopted can still be wrong" (Lammers and Verhey, 1987, p. 365).

The Protestant tradition provides resources to underscore the significance of freedom. James F. Childress, for example, calls attention to the Quaker tradition of "answering that of God in every person," to the persistence of the "image of God" in the capacities to understand and to choose, and to the persistence of the requirement to respect that image even when, in conditions of finitude and sin, people understand poorly and choose badly (Verhey and Lammers, 1993, pp. 127–156).

The Protestant tradition, however, also provides resources to challenge any reduction of human freedom to individual choices to do whatever one wishes. The "freedom of the Christian," according to Luther and Calvin, was not an arbitrary autonomy; it was joined to the sovereignty of God. Indeed, it was the freedom to have Christ as Lord, to live in the righteousness and grace of God, to be a servant of God and of the neighbor.

Gustafson, in a deliberate (and selective) retrieval of the Protestant tradition of Calvin and Edwards, argues that, while respect for persons surely includes respect for their rational autonomy, the fact that persons are embodied, communal, and finite means that respect for them may not be reduced to respect for autonomy (Gustafson, 1981; Childress and Macquarrie, 1986).

Still more radically, some Protestant moral theologians, most notably Hauerwas, have criticized this "Protestant approach," this single-minded attention to autonomy, as corrupted and corrupting. According to Hauerwas, it is corrupted by the Enlightenment project to "free" people from the chains of historical particularity, to "free" reason from determination by a specific tradition, and to make politics a matter of simply securing cooperation between self-interested individuals (Hauerwas, 1986). From this perspective "the Protestant approach" described and celebrated by Veatch owes more to the "enlightened" variation of the Protestant tradition than to the sixteenth-century movement of protest and testimony (Hauerwas, 1986).

The suspicion of casuistry: Protestant discernment.   Ever since the sixteenth century, the Protestant tradition has been suspicious of "legalism" and casuistry. There is nothing in the Protestant tradition to compare with the Catholic tradition of casuistry that surrounded the confessional, nor to compare with the Jewish tradition of Torah, Talmud, codes, and responsa. (There have been, to be sure, some significant examples of Protestant casuistry over the centuries, notably in the Anglican and Puritan traditions.)

Of course, any significant moral reflection is to some extent casuistic; that is, it must deal with the decisions to be made in particular cases and with the strategies, principles, and perspective appropriate to making them. But Protestants who began to work in medical ethics could not and did not rely on a tradition of casuistry already formed, on a consistent set of past decisions, or even on a coherent framework for making decisions that was utilized by their predecessors—at least not to the extent that Jews and Catholics could and did.

Protestant pastors were not examiners of conscience or judges of conduct in the same way that Catholic priests or Jewish rabbis were. For Protestant clergy the emphasis was more pedagogical than juridical. And with respect to the pedagogical function of pastors, there was nothing to correspond to the Catholic "magisterium." The work of the Protestant theologian was correspondingly different, and the works of moral theologians understandably diverse. The Protestant mode of casuistry was repeatedly reinvented.

Joseph Fletcher attempted to capitalize on the Protestant suspicion of legalism and casuistry to defend "situation ethics." Any appeal to rules or to any principle other than "do the loving thing" was regarded as a form of legalism and as unfaithful to the Protestant witness. While opposing "legalism," however, Fletcher in effect invented a mode of attention to cases that focused on freedom and on the calculation of the consequences of an action, and he did not shrink from calling it "love's casuistry." Fletcher's "casuistry" ended up looking very much like act-utilitarianism, the philosophical moral theory requiring that every act be governed by a calculation of the greatest good for the greatest number.

Other Protestants, notably Ramsey, were opposed to "situation ethics," especially to the utilitarianism of Fletcher but generally to the relativism and the lack of intellectual rigor of Protestant moral analysis. As Ramsey sought to identify those "actions and abstentions" required by "a rational and charitable justice" (Ramsey, 1970, p. xvii), he attempted to articulate and apply the "unexceptionable moral principles" that genuine love would not and could not violate. According to Ramsey "love's casuistry" required not only intellectual rigor but a deontological form.

A third position has refused the alternatives of focusing on the consequences or on the rules as a strategy for thinking about choices. Instead, some Protestants have proposed focusing on the agent, on the historical situation of the agent and his or her choices, on the particular formation of dispositions and possibilities, on the virtues and vision of actors. James Gustafson led the way. In "A Protestant Ethical Approach" to abortion (Lammers and Verhey, 1987, pp. 403–412), Gustafson rejected the position of external judge and stressed instead empathetic identification with the person who must assume responsibility for the decision. Rather than juridically judging whether an action conformed to a rule or not, Gustafson emphasized that the agent was involved in a web of human relationships and faced a concrete choice with limited possibilities. This "wider context of human values, responsibilities, and aspirations" (Lammers and Verhey, 1987, p. 411) must not be eclipsed by the physical aspects of abortion or by the single relation of patient and physician. Attitudes and affections, and the faith which evokes and informs them, have a greater role than is characteristic of rationalistic attention to natural law. Gustafson's approach "subordinates law to virtue as points of reliance in making moral decisions" (Lammers and Verhey, 1987, p. 411).

These diverse strategies for discernment represent different Protestant casuistries. Protestants continually return to questions not only about what to decide, but about how to decide.

Calling and profession.   The notion of a "calling" or "vocation" served in early Protestantism to emancipate physicians from the control of the medieval church and to vest their work with a new dignity and direction. Once physicians had asserted the autonomy of the profession, Protestants continued to invoke the notion of calling, now to resist the tendency to reduce the profession to a marketable technical competence and to direct it in response to grace toward "service."

In 1909, for example, Walter Rauschenbusch, one of the founders of the movement for social reform known as "the social gospel," prayed that doctors and nurses would recognize "that their calling is holy and that they, too, are disciples of the saving Christ" (Lammers and Verhey, 1987, p. 5). A sense of calling was needed to resist the temptation of professionals to "become hirelings who serve only for money." A "sense of a divine mission" should move the professional to be "doubly faithful in the service of the poor."

Gustafson identifies more general implications of invoking the language of calling to describe the professions. He admits that a calling without professional competence would be inept and dangerous, but he insists still more strongly that "a profession without a calling" lacks the resources to keep motivation alive, to keep human sensitivities and sensibilities alert, and to envision the larger ends, the common good, that our individual professional efforts can serve (Gustafson, 1982, p. 514).

When Protestants name medicine a calling, they assert that medicine, too, can serve the cause of God. The same point is sometimes made by using the language of "covenant." The notion of covenant was an important one for Ramsey (and informed consent was the "cardinal *canon of loyalty*" that marked the covenant between physician or researcher and patient) (Ramsey, 1970, p. 5). Ramsey, however, frequently left implicit the theology of covenant that undergirded his emphasis on covenants between persons.

Veatch takes the language of covenant and uses it to refer simply to a contract between autonomous individuals (Veatch, 1981). William F. May, on the other hand, insists that the transcendent reference of covenant not be forgotten, and in describing the professions as covenantal, he describes them as responses to grace, and so orients them toward the care and respect due persons. He criticizes construals of medicine as a technical proficiency, as philanthropy, and as contract. All of them, he says, "are devices for evading ties" with the suffering or dying patient (May, 1983, p. 128). Technique is then used as a shield against patients; philanthropy deteriorates into the condescension of the self-sufficient benefactor; and contractors intentionally limit their commitments to what can be bought and sold. In place of these accounts of medicine, May commends covenant and its attention to God. Then professional service is put "in the context of a primordial act of receiving a gift not wholly deserved" (May, 1983, p. 108). Receipt of such a gift creates bonds with others, and the bonds are expressed in care. Moreover, looking to "a creative, nurturant, and donative" God enables medical professionals to enter the world of the suffering or dying patient "without panicking before it" (May, 1983, p. 127). They do not need to substitute for some absent God.

Scripture.   When sixteenth-century Reformers argued against medieval Catholicism (and then against the direction in which others were taking the movement), they appealed again and again to scripture. And while Protestants refused to submit to popes or kings, they boasted of their submissiveness to scripture. With virtually one voice, contemporary Protestants affirm that scripture is authoritative for medical ethics, but there are many different voices when the question is not whether but how it is relevant to medical ethics.

Some Protestants identify the human words of scripture with the Word of God, and treat it as a revealed medical text and as a timeless moral code. Jehovah's Witnesses, for example, use a set of texts about blood (Gen. 9:4, Lev. 17:13–14, Acts 15:19) to prohibit blood transfusion (Numbers and Amundsen, 1986). John Frame begins his sophisticated book on medical ethics by affirming the "inerrancy" of scripture and construing it as "a *system* of divine law" (Frame, 1988, p. 10). Some other Protestants contrast the human words of scripture with the divine Word and rely on other sources (moral philosophy or experience or "common sense") to identify and select the words of scripture that are judged to be normative, perhaps the love commandment, for example.

Most Protestants find themselves between these two extremes, affirming that scripture is both the Word of God and human words, and struggling to hold that conjunction without either confusing the one with the other or simply contrasting them. Since scripture itself involves a process of tradition, of continuity and change, appeals to it ought also to involve both fidelity and creativity. This broad, middle position includes a number of diverse uses of scripture. Thus, some identify certain moral principles or "guides" in scripture that give direction to the moral life. For example, John Kilner identifies and develops four "guides": life, freedom, truth, and justice (Kilner, 1992). They are not understood as "rationalistic principles," but as elements of the creative and redemptive intention of God made known in scripture (Kilner, 1992, p. 53). In hard cases of medical ethics they can conflict; still, they form the intention of one whose conscience has been taken captive by scripture.

Others have called attention not to biblical principles but to a biblical perspective on the situation; they have appealed to scripture to form the way people see and describe the world. So, for example, it has been used to defend seeing the human self as embodied and to caution against reducing the self either to mere biological organism or to mere capacities for agency. Ramsey's theme of embodiment, of the coinherence of body and soul, is explicitly tied to scripture. Again, scripture has sometimes shaped the way Protestants see the self in community; death and suffering (Hauerwas, 1986), sex and begetting (Lebacqz, 1983), scarcity, and the sharing of resources (Kilner, 1986).

Hauerwas (1981) has suggested that scripture is normative as "narrative," indeed preeminently as the story of Jesus. He refuses to infer from the stories certain moral themes and to identify those themes as the moral message of scripture. To understand scripture is to remember these stories, within the church, as the stories of our life as a Christian community. In these stories we find identity and community and the meaning of otherwise vacuous concepts like "love" and "freedom" and even "God." Of course, different understandings of the "plot" of the narrative will authorize different particular uses of scripture. To focus on the event of the nonviolent and patient endurance of suffering on a cross has a different effect on the use of scripture than to plot the story as creation-fall-redemption-consummation (Kilner, 1986) or as liberation (Lammers and Verhey, 1987, pp. 64–69).

The Protestant conscience is still taken captive by scripture. In the midst of diverse uses, it continues to provide a common story and a common language for Protestants. Identity is formed by it; virtue and vision are shaped by it; and finally choices are tested by whether they are "worthy of the gospel" that is found in scripture.

Protestant contributions to medical ethics have been marked by diversity, but also sometimes by a Protestant passion to bear witness to the sovereignty of God and to the freedom of patients, by a Protestant patience with moral ambiguity, by a powerful sense of vocation, and by appeals to scripture to support and guide people in their suffering and in their care for the suffering.

ALLEN VERHEY

Directly related to this entry are the entries ABORTION, *section on* RELIGIOUS TRADITIONS, *article on* PROTESTANT PERSPECTIVES; *and* ROMAN CATHOLICISM. *For a further discussion of topics mentioned in this entry, see the entries* AUTHORITY; AUTONOMY; CASUISTRY; CONSCIENCE; DEATH; DEATH AND DYING: EUTHANASIA AND SUSTAINING LIFE; FREEDOM AND COERCION; HEALING; LIFE; LOVE; MEDICAL ETHICS, HISTORY OF, *section on* EUROPE, *subsections on* RENAISSANCE AND ENLIGHTENMENT, *and* NINETEENTH CENTURY; NARRATIVE; PAIN AND SUFFERING; PASTORAL CARE; PERSON; *and* PROFESSION AND PROFESSIONAL ETHICS. *For a further discussion of related ideas, see the entries* BODY, *article on* CULTURAL AND RELIGIOUS PERSPECTIVES; JUSTICE; PROFESSIONAL–PATIENT RELATIONSHIP; TECHNOLOGY; TRUST; *and* VIRTUE AND CHARACTER. *Other relevant material may be found under the entries* AFRICAN RELIGION; ALTERNATIVE THERAPIES; BUDDHISM; CONFUCIANISM; EASTERN ORTHODOX CHRISTIANITY; FEMINISM; HINDUISM; ISLAM; JAINISM; JUDAISM; *and* SIKHISM.

Bibliography

BARTH, KARL. 1961. *The Doctrine of Creation.* Vol. 3 of his *Church Dogmatics.* Edited by G. W. Bromiley and T. F. Torrance. Edinburgh: T. & T. Clark.

CABOT, RICHARD C., and DICKS, RUSSELL L. 1936. *The Art of Ministering to the Sick.* New York: Macmillan.

CALVIN, JOHN. 1960. [1559]. *Institutes of the Christian Religion.* Vols. 20 and 21 of *The Library of Christian Classics.* Edited by John T. McNeill. Translated by Ford Lewis Battles. Philadelphia: Westminster.

CHILDRESS, JAMES R., and MACQUARRIE, JOHN, eds. 1986. *The Westminster Dictionary of Christian Ethics.* Philadelphia: Westminster.

COHEN, I. BERNARD, ed. 1990. *Puritanism and the Rise of Modern Science: The Merton Thesis.* New Brunswick, N.J.: Rutgers University Press.

DILLENBERGER, JOHN, and WELCH, CLAUDE. 1954. *Protestant Christianity Interpreted Through Its Development.* New York: Scribner.

FLETCHER, JOSEPH. 1960. [1954]. *Morals and Medicine: The Moral Problems of the Patient's Right to Know the Truth, Contraception, Artificial Insemination, Sterilization, Euthanasia.* Boston: Beacon Press.

FRAME, JOHN M. 1988. *Medical Ethics: Principles, Persons, and Problems.* Phillipsburg, N.J.: Presbyterian and Reformed.

GUSTAFSON, JAMES M. 1981. *Theology and Ethics.* Vol. 1 of his *Ethics from a Theocentric Perspective.* Chicago: University of Chicago Press.

———. 1982. "Professions as 'Callings.'" *Social Service Review* 56, no. 4:501–515.

———. 1987. "A Protestant Ethical Approach." In *On Moral Medicine: Theological Perspectives in Medical Ethics,* pp.

403–412. Edited by Stephen E. Lammers and Allen Verhey. Grand Rapids, Mich.: William B. Eerdmans.

HAUERWAS, STANLEY. 1981. *A Community of Character: Toward a Constructive Christian Social Ethic.* Notre Dame, Ind.: University of Notre Dame Press.

———. 1986. *Suffering Presence: Theological Reflections on Medicine, the Mentally Handicapped, and the Church.* Notre Dame, Ind.: University of Notre Dame Press.

HILTNER, SEWARD. 1943. *Religion and Health.* New York: Macmillan.

HOLIFIELD, E. BROOKS. 1986. *Health and Medicine in the Methodist Tradition: Journey Toward Wholeness.* New York: Crossroad.

HOOYKAAS, REIJER. 1972. *Religion and the Rise of Modern Science.* Grand Rapids, Mich.: William B. Eerdmans.

JENKINS, DANIEL T. 1949. *The Doctor's Profession.* London: SCM.

KILNER, JOHN F. 1986. "A Needy World—A Needed Word: Scarce Medical Resources and the Christian Story." *Asbury Theological Journal* 41, no. 2:23–58.

———. 1992. *Life on the Line: Ethics, Aging, Ending Patients' Lives, and Allocating Vital Resources.* Grand Rapids, Mich.: William B. Eerdmans.

LAMMERS, STEPHEN E., and VERHEY, ALLEN, eds. 1987. *On Moral Medicine: Theological Perspectives in Medical Ethics.* Grand Rapids, Mich.: William B. Eerdmans.

LEBACQZ, KAREN. 1983. *Genetics, Ethics and Parenthood.* New York: Pilgrim.

LUSTIG, B. ANDREW, ed. 1993. *Theological Developments in Bioethics: 1990–1992.* Bioethics Yearbook, vol. 3. Dordrecht, Netherlands: Kluwer.

LUTHER, MARTIN. 1960. [1520]. *Three Treatises.* Translated by C. M. Jacobs, A. T. W. Steinhäuser, and W. A. Lambert. Philadelphia: Fortress.

MARTY, MARTIN E. 1983. *Health and Medicine in the Lutheran Tradition: Being Well.* New York: Crossroad.

MARTY, MARTIN E., and VAUX, KENNETH L., eds. 1982. *Health/Medicine and the Faith Traditions: An Inquiry into Religion and Medicine.* Philadelphia: Fortress.

MASON, STEPHEN F. 1962. *A History of the Sciences.* New rev. ed. New York: Collier.

MAY, WILLIAM F. 1983. *The Physician's Covenant: Images of the Healer in Medical Ethics.* Philadelphia: Westminster.

MERTON, ROBERT K. 1970. *Science, Technology and Society in Seventeenth Century England.* New York: Harper & Row. The classic thesis on the contribution of Puritanism to science; a reprint of Merton's 1938 work.

NUMBERS, RONALD L., and AMUNDSEN, DARREL W., eds. 1986. *Caring and Curing: Health and Medicine in the Western Religious Traditions.* New York: Macmillan.

RAMSEY, PAUL. 1956. "Freedom and Responsibility in Medical and Sex Ethics: A Protestant View." *New York University Law Review* 31 (November):1189–1204.

———. 1970. *The Patient as Person: Explorations in Medical Ethics.* New Haven, Conn.: Yale University Press.

SCHUBERT, HARTWIG VON. 1991. *Evangelische Ethik und Biotechnologie.* Frankfurt: Campus.

SHEILS, W. J., ed. 1982. *The Church and Healing: Papers Read at the Twentieth Summer Meeting and the Twenty-First Winter Meeting of the Ecclesiastical History Society.* Oxford: Basil Blackwell. Historical essays on "spiritual" healing in Christian communities.

SHELP, EARL E., ed. 1985. *Theology and Bioethics: Exploring the Foundations and Frontiers.* Dordrecht, Netherlands: D. Reidel.

SMITH, DAVID H. 1986. *Health and Medicine in the Anglican Tradition: Conscience, Community, and Compromise.* New York: Crossroad.

SPERRY, WILLARD L. 1950. *Ethical Basis of Medical Practice.* New York: Paul B. Hoeber.

THOMAS, KEITH. 1971. *Religion and the Decline of Magic.* New York: Scribner.

TOURNIER, PAUL. 1954. *A Doctor's Casebook in the Light of the Bible.* Translated by Edwin Hudson. London: SCM.

VAUX, KENNETH L. 1984. *Health and Medicine in the Reformed Tradition: Promise, Providence, and Care.* New York: Crossroad.

VEATCH, ROBERT M. 1981. *A Theory of Medical Ethics.* New York: Basic Books.

———, ed. 1989. *Medical Ethics.* Boston: Jones and Bartlett.

VERHEY, ALLEN, and LAMMERS, STEPHEN E., eds. 1993. *Theological Voices in Medical Ethics.* Grand Rapids, Mich.: William B. Eerdmans.

WALTERS, LEROY. 1985. "Religion and the Renaissance of Medical Ethics in the United States: 1965–1975." In *Theology and Bioethics: Exploring the Foundations and Frontiers,* pp. 3–16. Edited by Earl E. Shelp. Dordrecht, Netherlands: D. Reidel.

WEBSTER, CHARLES. 1976. *The Great Instauration: Science, Medicine, and Reform 1626–1660.* New York: Holmes and Meier.

PROXY CONSENT

See DEATH AND DYING: EUTHANASIA AND SUSTAINING LIFE, *article on* ADVANCE DIRECTIVES.

PSYCHIATRY, ABUSES OF

The concept of the abuse of psychiatry conjures up a situation in which a psychiatrist acts improperly, causing a patient to experience some sort of harm. The concept of psychiatric abuse, however, is more complex than it appears to be at first sight. This article examines the notion of abuse in an effort to determine its accurate meaning so that steps can be taken to remedy it when it occurs or prevent it from taking place.

Historical background

In recent decades evidence has emerged of such practices as the abuse of psychiatry for political purposes in the former Soviet Union (Bloch and Reddaway, 1977, 1984), a similar pattern of abuse in Cuba limited to suppression of political dissent (Brown and Lago, 1991), the deployment of psychiatric knowledge and personnel in torture and interrogation in Northern Ireland in 1971 (Bloch, 1990), and pursuit of financial profit as a priority in Japanese private psychiatric hospitals (Harding, 1991). The tragic abuse of psychiatry during the Nazi era, especially the program in which tens of thousands of chronic psychiatric and mentally retarded patients were killed, and similar numbers were sterilized without their consent, is no doubt the grossest instance of abuse of which we have historical records (Lifton, 1986; Mitscherlich and Mielke, 1962).

Commentary on psychiatric abuse not uncommonly refers to its widespread prevalence, particularly in the United States and South Africa. But, as will become evident in the section below on definitions, care must be taken to distinguish between intentional misapplication of psychiatric knowledge, skills, and technology and inadequate or negligent practices. In the South African case, the state policy of apartheid over four decades led to a massive inequity in the provision of mental-health services, with blacks allocated substantially fewer resources compared with whites despite their equivalent medical needs. On the other hand, the allegation of the misuse of psychiatry to suppress black political activism has never had any basis ("Apartheid and Psychiatry," 1984).

In the United States, similar discriminatory practices have occurred, but they have been due more to economic than to explicitly political factors. With millions of Americans unable to afford health insurance and long-standing inadequate budgets for public psychiatric services, the inevitable result has been woefully substandard care in state mental hospitals, particularly for minority groups and the poor (frequently the same population) (Stone, 1984; Robitscher, 1980).

The abuse of psychiatry for political or other purposes in the United States has been sporadic, the examples of the poet Ezra Pound and General Edwin Walker being especially well known. In the case of Pound, psychiatry was recruited to deal with a politically sensitive and complex situation: A celebrated poet, indicted for treason following his pro-Axis broadcasts in Italy during World War II, was facing possible execution. Although the evidence was equivocal, Pound was deemed incompetent to stand trial and transferred to St. Elizabeth's Psychiatric Hospital in Washington, D.C., where he spent thirteen years. The indictment was then dismissed and Pound was released. Whether psychiatry was employed to extricate the U.S. government from an embarrassing quandary or Pound was genuinely deluded, which would account for this wartime behavior, remains a controversial question. Suffice it to say, the case clearly demonstrates the vulnerability of psychiatry to exploitation by political forces.

Similar factors were pertinent in the case of Edwin Walker, a highly decorated major general in the U.S. army who overtly supported the extreme right-wing position during the desegregation movement of the 1950s and the 1960s in the Deep South. His mental competence became a matter of dispute after he had been charged with a number of offenses related to his political activism. Although he was declared competent to stand trial (the case was later dismissed for technical reasons), the available evidence raises the possibility of the government's recourse to psychiatry in order to deal more conveniently with a "troublemaker" (Stone, 1984).

A final comment in this necessarily brief historical background concerns the criticism of psychiatry for its demeaning, patronizing attitude toward women. The dramatic case of Mrs. Packard in 1860 illustrates how prejudice and bias can undermine sound clinical judgment. Upon the insistence of her husband, a fundamentalist clergyman, that she harbored dangerous religious beliefs, Mrs. Packard was involuntarily committed to an Illinois mental hospital, where she remained confined for three years. Upon her release, she launched a campaign against the expression of opinions as a reason for psychiatric commitment (Musto, 1991).

Over a century later, Phyllis Chesler (1972) was among the first critics to argue that psychiatry's view of women was so distorted and blinkered as to influence its diagnostic objectivity. Other feminist perspectives on women and mental health have followed (e.g., Showalter, 1987). According to this view, women not conforming to stereotypic roles have been too readily regarded by a male-dominated profession as at best psychologically suspect and as at worst emotionally disturbed. Sigmund Freud's contribution to gender psychology has no doubt been influential in the maintenance of such attitudes. Rigid views about gender roles emerged clearly in an empirical study by Broverman et al. (1970), published shortly before Chesler's book. Clinicians regarded healthy women and healthy men as having quite different characteristics, the distinguishing features echoing prevailing sex-role stereotypes. What emerged from the inquiry was a distinct double standard of mental health.

Definitions

Psychiatric "abuse" can be defined according to specific criteria and should be differentiated from other undesirable practices, which are best termed "malpractice." "Abuse" refers to the intentional, improper application of the knowledge, skills, and technology of psychiatry for a purpose other than serving the interests of the patient or for the purpose of harming, in diverse ways, persons who do not warrant the status of psychiatric patienthood in the first instance. Abuse is usually perpetrated by psychiatrists (or other mental-health professionals) in collaboration with other persons or agencies, such as a state security service or political authority.

Such institutional abuse always constitutes unethical conduct in that the protagonist intentionally carries out an act in the knowledge that the act is intrinsically wrong (whether or not it turns out to harm the patient), explicitly violating the ethics of the psychiatric profession. A psychiatrist who misuses the profession in this way, claiming that he or she is obliged to follow the orders of superiors and in that sense is not autonomous, is inexcusably rejecting the responsibility to make sure that regulations serve good, not bad, professional goals. In such circumstances, even if psychiatrists covertly ameliorate the welfare of their patients, claiming that this is the only available means to maintain an ethical stance, their behavior, by virtue of their collusion in an abusive practice, is an inherent part of the abuse.

Reference to institutional abuse, on which this article focuses, does not negate the possibility of individual psychiatrists abusing one or more of their own patients. A similar ethical violation takes place in both cases, psychiatrists in the latter exploiting patients to meet their personal needs, on the pretext that the practice applied is clinically indicated and appropriate. The most clear-cut example is sexual involvement, but other forms of abuse of power intrinsic to the psychiatrist–patient relationship, such as financial and religious, are relevant here. This sort of abuse may mar any doctor–patient relationship, but the not uncommon situation in psychiatric treatment of an excessively vulnerable patient seeking comfort and succor from an ostensibly all-caring psychiatrist is arguably more conducive to its occurrence than is the case in other areas of medical practice.

Abuse can also be perpetrated by a psychiatrist in conjunction with or acceding to attempts by laypeople to exploit the discipline for nonmedical purposes. Consider this example: A husband who knows that his wife is not mentally ill persuades a psychiatrist to commit her to a psychiatric hospital. His interests are other than the welfare of his partner; he desires to wield power over her and recruits the psychiatrist as his accessory (Robitscher, 1980).

"Malpractice" can be distinguished from abuse with respect to the psychiatrist's intent. Malpractice is admittedly a term used in diverse ways, but an alternative term is elusive; "inadequate practice" comes closest to the meaning intended here. A psychiatrist who does not set out to use knowledge, skills, or technology improperly but who employs these in an inadequate or unskilled fashion is engaging in malpractice. An example is the not uncommon practice of prescribing tranquilizing drugs for patients upon the request of nursing staff, who insist that they are otherwise unable to manage "behav-

ior," in cases where the patients do not need such medication. The psychiatrist does not pervert his or her science in these circumstances but fails to adhere to a fundamental standard of practice that requires prescription of drugs only when clinically indicated.

Malpractice can be differentiated from "errors in clinical judgment" when that judgment has been made in good faith. Psychiatrists, like any other professionals, err on occasion. Although the consequences may simulate the effects of malpractice, malpractice is not actually committed.

The vulnerability of psychiatry to abuse

Abuse appears to be more common in psychiatry than elsewhere in medicine, probably because psychiatry is inherently more vulnerable to it. This is the case in at least three respects: (1) the boundaries of psychiatry remain exceedingly blurred and ill defined; (2) diagnosis in psychiatry is often conducted in the absence of objective criteria; and (3) the psychiatrist is granted immense power over the fate of other people, even to the extent of detaining them.

Blurred boundaries. The absence of a well-demarcated conceptual boundary in psychiatry leads to a correspondingly ill-defined role for its practitioners. Debate has been ongoing since the 1960s among psychiatrists themselves, and in the wider community, as to what constitutes their legitimate role (Dyer, 1988). Attitudes vary considerably, even to the point of contradiction. The following views, expressed by former presidents of the American Psychiatric Association, reflect this diversity. Ewald Busse (1969) argued for a limited role whereby the psychiatrist restricts his or her focus to the suffering patient, and psychiatric services are accordingly confined to "patient-oriented activities designed to reduce pain and discomfort." His colleague, Raymond Waggoner (1970), had a much wider perspective, calling upon the profession to pursue "fundamental social goals," concerning themselves with "individual liberty and communal responsibility"; psychiatrists should be not only pragmatists but also "dreamers with a vision of the future."

Definitions of health and ill health are pertinent to the above positions. Thus, a "visionary" outlook facilitates psychiatrists' entry into the realm of social policy. Their active involvement in a context beyond hospital and clinic is boundless, offering the potential for professional pronouncements, ostensibly derived from expertise, on such social phenomena as unemployment, racism, poverty, religious cults, child-rearing practices, sexual offenders, and so forth. Psychiatrists may adopt roles, including those of social commentator, political advocate, and lobbyist, that lie well beyond their more traditional role as clinical practitioner.

Whatever the role adopted, the psychiatrist is buffeted by the demands of multiple loyalties. He or she is caught ineluctably between the responsibilities to patients and to society, the latter potentially including a patient's family, an employer, the courts, prison officials, and military authorities. In these circumstances he or she has to weigh the interests of patients against those of social agencies; in so doing, he or she may be subject to such intense pressure as to cause subordination to social forces, with corresponding neglect of the primary obligation to patients.

Returning to the issue of professional boundaries, it seems that psychiatry's role is more clear-cut when it is limited to an exclusively medical function. But this generally depends on the psychiatrist's capacity to make diagnostic assessments that are relatively objective and value-free—for example, in the case of a patient with an organic disorder like dementia. This brings us to the second feature of psychiatry that contributes to its vulnerability to abuse.

Lack of objective criteria in diagnostic assessment. Notwithstanding the evolution of psychiatry as a scientific discipline since the second half of the nineteenth century, and progress in the field of taxonomy (see, e.g., American Psychiatric Association, 1987), the profession still wrestles with the fundamental question of what constitutes mental illness (Fulford, 1989). No satisfactory criteria are available to define precisely most of the conditions with which psychiatry deals. Compared with those in other medical fields, many conventionally labeled psychiatric diagnoses derive from clinical observation only, and lack identifiable pathological or pathophysiological correlates. Objective tests that determine the presence or absence of a psychiatric condition are uncommon.

Moreover, in the diagnostic task the psychiatrist is obliged to rely in uncomfortably large measure on social criteria and value judgments. As the British sociologist Kathleen Jones (1978) reminds us, society would not be able to determine what was normal if it failed to designate certain acts and certain people as abnormal or antisocial.

William Fulford and Walter Reich have contributed handsomely to the question of what constitutes psychiatric disease, and have illuminated the complex procedure whereby psychiatrists determine when a diagnosis is legitimately applied to a particular set of mental or behavioral states. Fulford (1991) stresses the fundamental place of values in medicine generally, contending that all diagnoses involving physical and mental disease are an admixture of the factual and the evaluative. As he puts it, the "ethically contentious concept of mental illness [is put] on an equal logical footing with the relatively uncontentious concept of physical illness" (1991, p. 95).

Reich (1991) makes explicit what has long discomforted psychiatrists—the vulnerability of their diagnostic process to error. The factors are manifold here: reliance on subjective criteria; the intrusion of bias and prejudice; doubtful reliability; and shifting criteria leading to inconsistency and frequent change. Mention of a few illustrative diagnostic controversies buttresses Reich's observations: the deletion of homosexuality as a clinical condition following a poll of members of the American Psychiatric Association in 1973; long-standing debates over whether such concepts as simple schizophrenia and hyperactivity in children are valid; the addition of two new personality disorders (sadistic and self-defeating) in a category labeled "needing further study," in the revision of *DSM-III* (American Psychiatric Association, 1987) as if they had not occurred previously; the dispute over whether sociopathic behavior is due to an unfortunate and serious disorder of personality functioning or to social deviance (and therefore belongs within the sphere of crime and delinquency). Many more examples could readily be added to this list.

The psychiatrist's power. Within the context of an ill-defined professional framework and the vague criteria for diagnosis, the psychiatrist is sanctioned by law to manage the situation in which a person suffers or is suspected of suffering from mental illness that may require enforced hospitalization in order to protect the individual's welfare and/or the welfare of others (Chodoff, 1984; Miller, 1991). This is exceptional authority, inasmuch as the person is deprived of liberty, loses many civil rights, and is subject to a wide range of institutional regulations.

Commitment statutes in many legal jurisdictions, particularly those pertaining to the more accurate determination of the risk of dangerousness to self and/or others, have been subject to rigorous scrutiny and improvement. However, a disconcerting degree of uncertainty remains as to what constitute relevant criteria. Psychiatrists are often caught in the dilemma of having to make a judgment about a person's clinical needs while safeguarding his or her civil rights. The civil libertarian would urge that the individual's inalienable right to liberty be protected above all other considerations, while advocates of a paternalistic view would argue that society, through its sanctioned agents, sometimes has an obligation to take necessary measures, including forcible hospitalization, to protect the patient, society, or both from harm.

Soviet psychiatric abuse

Ill-defined boundaries, the subjective basis of assessment, and the authority to detain and treat a person involuntarily combine to make psychiatry especially vulnerable to abuse. The most clear-cut illustration of this was the use of psychiatry in the former Soviet Union to suppress political, religious, and other forms of dissent. These Soviet practices have been described and analyzed at length by several observers (Bloch and Reddaway, 1977; 1984; see also Bukovsky, 1978; Fireside, 1979; Podrabinek, 1980).

Soviet psychiatry's boundaries were drawn in a way that made the entire profession subject to the pervasive influence, both overt and covert, of the Soviet state and, more particularly, of the Communist party. The pyramidal form of the administrative structure, with power tightly wielded by a small, compliant group of psychiatrists, enabled a political authority to determine the role and function of all Soviet psychiatrists. Even if the boundaries of psychiatry had been clearer, the totalitarian nature of the Soviet state ensured that psychiatrists could not function autonomously. The fact that boundaries were blurred made it all the easier for the state to exert control and mold the profession in accordance with its ideology. The state's avowal that the interests of the social collective were at least as important as those of the individual led to the virtually complete undermining of the principle of respect for autonomy.

The Soviet case is a blatant reminder that psychiatrists may function in a state whose interests do not serve those of the public. The corollary is abundantly clear: Psychiatrists must act autonomously with regard to ethical standards, which are above politics.

The lack of an objective basis of diagnostic practice permitted the evolution of an idiosyncratic scheme in Soviet psychiatry between the 1950s and the 1980s. Professor Andrei Snezhnevsky rapidly ascended to the leadership of the psychiatric establishment during the 1950s, and from that powerful position launched a unique classificatory system of mental illness. A crucial result was the profound shift in the way schizophrenia was conceptualized. Snezhnevsky promoted several claims, among them the notion that since the illness could be present in a person showing only minor symptoms, schizophrenia was substantially more common than previously thought. A particular form of the illness, "sluggish schizophrenia," named thus because of its extremely slow rate of progression, accounted for the wider limits placed on the use of the diagnosis. From the 1960s on, when suppression of dissent by psychiatric means escalated, the diagnosis "sluggish schizophrenia" was comonly applied to political, religious, and other dissidents the state wished to disempower and punish (Reich, 1991).

Although the Soviet diagnostic schema was not originally devised with the purpose of curbing dissent, the vagueness of its concepts facilitated the application of a disease label to people whom psychiatrists elsewhere would have regarded as normal, mildly eccentric, or at worst neurotic.

The inadequacy of explicit criteria to determine the risk of harm to a person and/or to others makes psychiatry vulnerable to improper use of its sanction to detain. As part of the Soviet abuse, the concept of "social danger" was invoked. In a letter to the Western press in 1973 ("The Soviet Psychiatrists Reply," 1973), the Soviet psychiatric establishment, defending itself against Western allegations that psychiatry was being misused, argued that in a certain proportion of patients, their disease could lead to antisocial actions, including "disturbances of public order, dissemination of slander, and manifestations of aggressive intentions." They commented further on the "seeming normality" of such patients in their commission of dangerous acts. Aggression in the mentally ill leading to self-harm or harm to others was conflated with disturbance of public order and slander. Well-documented cases of dissenters in Soviet hospitals pointed to an obvious conclusion: that Soviet psychiatrists had broadened the concept of dangerousness in an ethically unacceptable fashion.

Preventing abuse

Legislation, professional self-regulation, establishment of watchdog committees, and adherence to appropriate codes of ethics are complementary means designed to deal with psychiatric abuse. Legislation can help protect patients' civil rights, hold psychiatrists accountable for their actions, and define their powers and functions as specifically as possible. Mental-health law here is akin to a double-edged sword, on the one hand promoting patients' rights, and thus protecting them from abusive psychiatry, and on the other hand, setting standards of clinical conduct whose neglect by the psychiatrist is tantamount to illegal practice.

Peer review and audit exercises help psychiatrists to prevent or identify ethically dubious judgments or actions. Many national associations of psychiatrists have procedures to discipline members who violate basic principles of clinical care: informal warning, reprimand, suspension, or expulsion (see, e.g., Royal Australian and New Zealand College of Psychiatrists, 1992). The Royal College of Psychiatrists in Britain and the American Psychiatric Association have created influential committees to investigate and campaign against psychiatric abuse.

As a corporate group, psychiatrists, both nationally and internationally, need to be vigilant in the face of attempts by governmental or nongovernmental entities to coerce them to use their discipline for purposes that do not serve the health and well-being of individuals and the public at large. Psychiatrists practicing in totalitarian states may not be in a position to do this without jeopardizing their professional and personal welfare. Ukrainian psychiatrists Semyon Gluzman and Anatoly

Koryagin experienced years of incarceration for openly criticizing the political misuse of psychiatry in the former Soviet Union.

In the context of the ethics of psychiatric practice, psychiatrists are obliged to condemn abuse of their profession wherever it occurs. Such protests, not strictly medical activities, point to the political and social role psychiatrists may be required to play.

Finally, psychiatrists need to be familiar with, and adhere to, relevant ethical codes, from that of Hippocrates, which stipulates that the doctor will "keep [the sick] from harm and injustice," to psychiatrists' own *Declaration of Hawaii* (World Psychiatric Association, 1984), which affirms that they should not use their professional position for the maltreatment of individuals. The ethical code of the Royal Australian and New Zealand College of Psychiatrists (1992) is even more explicit in its reference to abuse; it includes the principle that "Psychiatrists shall not allow the misuse of their professional knowledge and skills." A series of annotations covers such issues as the prohibition of diagnosing persons as mentally ill solely on the basis of their political, religious, ideological, moral, or philosophical beliefs; the impermissibility of using nonconformity with a society's prevailing values as the determining factor in diagnosing mental illness; and the ethical unacceptability of psychiatrists' participation in torture and executions.

Conclusion

The history of psychiatry has been tarnished by the occurrence of gross abuse, the Soviet, Nazi, and Japanese cases being especially prominent. Public attention to such cases has produced a heightened ethical sensitivity within the psychiatric profession. Although this constitutes a pivotal safeguard against abuse now and in the future, both the profession and society need to maintain a rigorous defense against any malignant forces that would exploit psychiatry's vulnerability and thus jeopardize its integrity.

SIDNEY BLOCH

Directly related to this entry are the entries COMMITMENT TO MENTAL INSTITUTIONS; INSTITUTIONALIZATION AND DEINSTITUTIONALIZATION; *and* DIVIDED LOYALTIES IN MENTAL-HEALTH CARE. *For a further discussion of topics mentioned in this entry, see the entries* MEDICAL MALPRACTICE; PATIENTS' RIGHTS, *article on* MENTAL PATIENTS' RIGHTS; PSYCHOANALYSIS AND DYNAMIC THERAPIES; SEXUAL ETHICS AND PROFESSIONAL STANDARDS; *and* WOMEN, *article on* HEALTH-CARE ISSUES. *For a discussion of related ideas, see the entries* AUTONOMY; BEHAVIOR CONTROL; CONFLICT OF INTEREST; FREEDOM AND COERCION; HARM; LICENSING, DISCIPLINE, AND REGULATION IN THE HEALTH PROFESSIONS; PATERNALISM; PROFESSION AND PROFESSIONAL ETHICS; *and* VALUE AND VALUATION. *Other relevant material may be found under the entries* MENTAL HEALTH; MENTAL-HEALTH SERVICES; MENTAL-HEALTH THERAPIES; MENTAL ILLNESS; *and* MENTALLY DISABLED AND MENTALLY ILL PERSONS. *See also the* APPENDIX (CODES, OATHS, AND DIRECTIVES RELATED TO BIOETHICS), SECTION II: ETHICAL DIRECTIVES FOR THE PRACTICE OF MEDICINE, HIPPOCRATIC OATH; *and* SECTION IV: ETHICAL DIRECTIVES FOR HUMAN RESEARCH, ETHICAL PRINCIPLES OF PSYCHOLOGISTS *and* CODE OF CONDUCT *of the* AMERICAN PSYCHOLOGICAL ASSOCIATION.

Bibliography

AMERICAN PSYCHIATRIC ASSOCIATION. 1987. *Diagnostic and Statistical Manual of Mental Disorders: DSM-III-R.* 3d ed. rev. Washington, D.C.: Author.

BLOCH, SIDNEY. 1984. "Apartheid and Psychiatry." *Lancet* 2, no. 8414:1252–1253.

———. 1990. "Interrogation and Torture." In *Principles and Practice of Forensic Psychiatry,* pp. 617–624. Edited by Robert Blugrass and Paul Bowden. Edinburgh: Churchill Livingstone.

BLOCH, SIDNEY, and REDDAWAY, PETER. 1977. *Russia's Political Hospitals: The Abuse of Psychiatry in the Soviet Union.* London: Gollancz.

———. 1984. *Soviet Psychiatric Abuse: The Shadow over World Psychiatry.* London: Gollancz.

BROVERMAN, INGEK; BROVERMAN, DONALD M.; CLARKSON, FRANK E.; ROSENKRANTZ, PAUL S.; and VOGEL, SUSAN R. 1970. "Sex-Role Stereotypes and Clinical Judgements of Mental Health." *Journal of Consulting and Clinical Psychology* 34:1–7.

BROWN, CHARLES, and LAGO, ARMANDO M. 1991. *The Politics of Psychiatry in Revolutionary Cuba.* New Brunswick, N.J.: Transaction.

BUKOVSKY, VLADIMIR KONSTANTINOVICH. 1978. *To Build a Castle: My Life as a Dissenter.* Translated by Michael Scammell. New York: Viking.

BUSSE, EWALD W. 1969. "APA's Role in Influencing the Evolution of a Health Care Delivery System." *American Journal of Psychiatry* 126, no. 5:739–758.

CHESLER, PHYLLIS. 1972. *Women and Madness.* Garden City, N.Y.: Doubleday.

CHODOFF, PAUL. 1984. "Involuntary Hospitalization of the Mentally Ill as a Moral Issue." *American Journal of Psychiatry* 141, no. 3:384–389.

DUNPHY, J. ENGELBERT. 1977. "Malpractice, Medical." In *Dictionary of Medical Ethics,* pp. 195–197. Edited by Archibald S. Duncan, Gordon R. Dunstan, and Richard B. Welbourn. London: Darton, Longman and Todd.

DYER, ALLEN R. 1988. *Ethics and Psychiatry: Toward Professional Definition.* Washington, D.C.: American Psychiatric Press.

FIRESIDE, HARVEY. 1979. *Soviet Psychoprisons.* New York: W. W. Norton.

FULFORD, WILLIAM. 1989. *Moral Theory and Medical Practice.* Cambridge: At the University Press.

———. 1991. "The Concept of Disease." In *Psychiatric Ethics,* 2d ed., pp. 77–99. Edited by Sidney Bloch and Paul Chodoff. Oxford: Oxford University Press.

HARDING, TIMOTHY. 1991. "Ethical Issues in the Delivery of Mental Health Services: Abuses in Japan." In *Psychiatric Ethics,* 2d ed., pp. 473–491. Edited by Sidney Bloch and Paul Chodoff. Oxford: Oxford University Press.

JONES, KATHLEEN. 1978. "Society Looks at the Psychiatrist." *British Journal of Psychiatry* 132 (April):321–332.

LIFTON, ROBERT J. 1986. *The Nazi Doctors: Medical Killing and the Psychology of Genocide.* New York: Basic Books.

MILLER, ROBERT. 1991. "The Ethics of Involuntary Commitment to Mental Health Treatment." In *Psychiatric Ethics,* 2d ed., pp. 265–289. Edited by Sidney Bloch and Paul Chodoff. Oxford: Oxford University Press.

MITSCHERLICH, ALEXANDER, and MIELKE, FRED. 1962. *The Death Doctors.* Translated by James Cleugh. London: Elek.

MUSTO, DAVID. 1991. "A Historical Perspective." In *Psychiatric Ethics,* 2d ed., pp. 15–32. Edited by Sidney Bloch and Paul Chodoff. Oxford: Oxford University Press.

PODRABINEK, ALEKSANDR PINKHOSOVICH. 1980. *Punitive Medicine.* Ann Arbor, Mich.: Karoma.

REICH, WALTER. 1991. "Psychiatric Diagnosis as an Ethical Problem." In *Psychiatric Ethics,* 2d ed., pp. 101–133. Edited by Sidney Bloch and Paul Chodoff. Oxford: Oxford University Press.

ROBITSCHER, JONAS B. 1980. *The Powers of Psychiatry.* Boston: Houghton Mifflin.

ROYAL AUSTRALIAN AND NEW ZEALAND COLLEGE OF PSYCHIATRISTS. 1992. "Code of Ethics." Melbourne, Australia: Author.

SHOWALTER, ELAINE. 1987. *The Female Malady: Women, Madness and English Culture, 1830–1980.* London: Virago.

"Soviet Psychiatry: The Doctors Reply." 1973. *Guardian,* September 29, 1973, p. 10.

STONE, ALAN A. 1984. *Law, Psychiatry, and Morality: Essays and Analysis.* Washington, D.C.: American Psychiatric Press.

WAGGONER, RAYMOND W. 1970. "The Presidential Address: Cultural Dissonance and Psychiatry." *American Journal of Psychiatry* 127, no. 1:1–8.

WORLD PSYCHIATRIC ASSOCIATION. 1984. *Declaration of Hawaii.* Honolulu: Author. Reprinted in *Psychiatric Ethics,* 2d ed., pp. 524–526. Edited by Sidney Bloch and Paul Chodoff. Oxford: Oxford University Press, 1991.

PSYCHOANALYSIS AND DYNAMIC THERAPIES

The term "psychoanalysis," in its narrow sense, refers to a method of psychological therapy originally developed by Sigmund Freud around the turn of the twentieth century and now practiced by analysts trained in the intellectual and clinical tradition that has followed Freud. The earliest psychoanalytic investigations led to revolutionary discoveries about the working of the mind, and therefore the term "psychoanalysis" refers also, in a broader sense, to the accumulated body of findings and theories about human mental functioning that have resulted from clinical psychoanalysis, and that are available to guide psychoanalysts in continuing their work.

Clinical psychoanalysis is used as a treatment for a variety of psychological conditions, including both specific symptoms and more general personality problems. The treatment involves individual meetings with an analyst, several times per week, over a period of several years. The patient usually lies on a couch and is instructed to say whatever comes to mind (a technique called free association), including symptoms, life events, memories, fantasies, dreams, physical sensations, and feelings about the analyst. The analyst listens to this material, and eventually interprets it as revealing conflicts between emotional forces ("dynamic" conflicts) of which the patient had previously been unconscious. Feelings about the analyst, called transference feelings, are particularly important for this purpose, since these feelings are unconsciously transferred onto the analyst from significant persons in the patient's past, and can be used to interpret and rework current conflicts derived from these past relationships.

Psychoanalytic theory has been continually revised and expanded since its inception. Its earliest form was codified in Freud's major work, *The Interpretation of Dreams* (1900). In this volume he presented the topographic theory, which emphasized the division of the mind into conscious and unconscious realms, and explained not only neurotic symptoms but also normal phenomena, such as dreams and slips of the tongue, as the results of unconscious wishes breaking through, in disguised and distorted form, into consciousness. Psychoanalytic techniques, such as free association and the use of the couch, were intended to maximize the possibility of such breakthroughs. In this way, unconscious wishes could be interpreted and made conscious, and the symptoms resulting from those wishes could be relieved.

Dreams, errors, and symptoms remain useful sources of interpretable material for the modern analyst, but topographic theory has been subsumed by later theoretical developments. Freud's "The Ego and the Id" (1923) presented a structural theory, in which the mind includes three agencies: the id, ego, and superego. Each agency has wishes and directions of its own, and they often come into conflict with each other. Neurotic symptoms, as well as character traits, are interpreted as the results of conflicts among these structures, and the goal of analysis is to strengthen the ego, the structure responsible for resolving conflicts within the mind and negotiating compromises between internal wishes and external reality.

Structural theory forms the core of a theoretical tradition known as "ego psychology," one of the dominant schools of thought in modern psychoanalysis, along with object-relations theory and self psychology. Object-relations theory places greater emphasis on the effects of early relationships, most importantly with the mother. It holds that pathological early relationships are internalized and unconsciously repeated, causing problems in later relationships. Self psychology emphasizes the role of early trauma and parental failure in preventing the establishment of a stable and coherent self. Proponents of these theories hold that they are more serviceable than structural theory for the treatment of seriously disturbed patients, those whose pathological early lives prevented the formation of stable mental structures.

The applicability of clinical psychoanalysis is limited by a number of practical and psychological factors. There are many patients for whom psychoanalytic ideas and insights might be useful, but who cannot be treated with clinical psychoanalysis because they cannot afford the time or money required, because they are interested only in more limited treatment for well-circumscribed problems, or because they do not have the necessary psychological resources, such as curiosity about the mind, access to dreams and fantasies, and an ability to tolerate frustration. The term "dynamic therapies" refers to a variety of psychotherapeutic techniques that have evolved for use in these situations.

The dynamic therapies, which are now considered the treatment of choice in some situations, are similar to psychoanalysis in that they involve regular meetings between patient and therapist in which talking is the primary therapeutic activity, an effort is made to understand the unconscious origins of the patient's problems, the patient's relationship to the therapist is used as an important source of information and a vehicle for change, and the practitioner is guided by psychoanalytic ideas about the working of the mind, including the idea that psychological problems are caused by "dynamic" conflict between unconscious forces. The dynamic therapies differ from psychoanalysis in that they are usually less intensive and involve less frequent meetings, the patient usually sits in a chair facing the therapist, the overall duration of the treatment may be shorter, the treatment may be focused on more specific goals, and the therapist is more likely to use techniques that offer emotional support to the patient as well as exploration of the unconscious. To the extent that the dynamic therapies are derivatives of psychoanalysis, similar considerations of ethics and values apply to both. This article will focus on ethical and value-related issues in psycho-

analysis, with the understanding that similar considerations apply to the other dynamic therapies.

Training and practice

Freud was trained as a neurologist, but most medical psychoanalysts have been psychiatrists. Freud believed that a medical background was not necessary for analysts (1926), and in Europe it has been common for nonphysicians to become analysts. In the United States, however, analysis has been seen primarily as a subspecialty of psychiatry, and until recently only a few nonphysicians were admitted to analytic training.

Training in psychoanalysis begins after the completion of professional school and specialty training, and includes classroom education, a personal analysis of the trainee, and the treatment of several analytic cases under the supervision of senior analysts. Becoming a psychoanalyst involves not only mastering theory and technique but also becoming a member of another profession, and accepting the profession's ethical judgments. The psychoanalytic profession's formal organization, the International Psychoanalytical Association, and its component associations, articulate and enforce ethical standards for the profession, as well as standards for training and procedures for certifying the skills of psychoanalysts. However, these bodies have no legal authority and cannot prevent nonmembers from calling themselves psychoanalysts.

The field of psychotherapy is much less organized and regulated. Individuals from many different professional backgrounds are free to call themselves therapists. Those individuals may be answerable to the standards of their own professions, but there is no overarching set of standards for training or ethical practice in psychotherapy.

Clinical theory versus theory of the mind

Over the decades, psychoanalysis has evolved two related but quite different bodies of theory. The first, "clinical theory," is a set of ideas about how the process of psychoanalysis works and a set of principles about how the analyst should behave. The second, comprising ideas about the working of the human mind that have resulted from psychoanalytic investigations in the past, might be broadly termed a psychoanalytic "theory of the mind"; this body of theory includes ideas about normal development, about the nature and origins of psychopathology, and about the structure and functioning of the mind (a branch of theory termed metapsychology). For the purpose of ethical analysis, these two bodies of theory present quite different challenges. Psychoanalytic clinical theory strives to remain value-neutral, while the psychoanalytic theory of the mind embodies a host of value-laden assumptions about normality and deviance, health and sickness, and the relationship of the individual to society, many of which have been challenged by critics of psychoanalysis.

Freud argued strongly that psychoanalysis was a scientific method of investigation, and therefore neutral with respect to values (1927). Clearly this claim cannot apply to the theory of the mind, and its applicability to clinical theory is arguable. The assertion that clinical analysis is value-neutral is related to the tenet in clinical theory that the analyst is guided by the principles of abstinence (Freud, 1915a) and neutrality (Freud, 1919; see also LaPlanche and Pontalis, 1967). The principle of abstinence enjoins the analyst from indulging in any kind of gratification (for patient or analyst) other than the satisfactions of analysis itself; sexual contact between analyst and patient, extra-analytic friendship, and nonanalytic emotional support are all proscribed.

The principle of neutrality dictates, in terms of structural theory, that the analyst should occupy a position equidistant from the competing forces in the mind (Freud, 1946), analyzing the conflict between them but not trying to influence the outcome of that conflict. In lay terms, the principle of neutrality means that the analyst should not try to influence the patient to adopt any particular set of values, or to conduct his or her life in any particular way; the analyst's job is only to analyze conflicts and remove inhibitions. Neurotic inhibitions limit the patient's freedom, and their successful removal liberates the patient to live however he or she chooses.

The limits of neutrality

The attitude of neutrality is not easy to adopt or to maintain. It requires that the analyst first become aware of his or her own values and preferences, unconscious as well as conscious, and then exert a constant and vigilant self-discipline, in order not to let these personal values influence the conduct of analysis. Much of the analyst's lengthy training, especially the personal analysis that he or she must undergo, is directed toward this end. However, it can be argued that absolute neutrality is not possible, even with a thorough personal analysis and a consistent adherence to the principle. The process of psychoanalysis necessarily embodies certain values, both in its selection of patients and in the ideals that inhere in the process itself.

The analyst can adopt the attitude of neutrality only if certain preconditions are met in the patient. Patient and analyst must have a common view of reality, at least in a broad way, for the analyst will probably find it impossible to remain neutral with respect to frankly psychotic ideas. Similarly, if the patient's illness is of the type that produces serious danger to the patient or oth-ers, the analyst may be unable to remain neutral with respect to that danger, and may instead intervene to protect the values of life and health, concluding that these medical and therapeutic values take precedence over analytic goals in this situation. In order to adopt an attitude of neutrality, the analyst must also believe that the patient possesses an adequately sound moral character; if the analyst believes the patient to be an evil person, neutrality will be impossible. It is part of the individual analyst's clinical and ethical responsibility to become aware of the kinds of patients with whom he or she has particular difficulty. Thus, some of the preconditions in the selection of patients for analysis embody value-laden assumptions that limit the scope of the principle of neutrality.

Moreover, the process of analysis itself can be seen to embody certain values that are not universally held and deviate from absolute neutrality (Michels and Oldham, 1983). Psychoanalysis assumes that insight is a goal worth pursuing; that it is always better to know things, especially about oneself, than not to know them; and that greater knowledge will ultimately lead to decreased suffering. This is a common belief, but by no means an unquestionable one; indeed, the Greek drama on which Freud based much of his theory of the mind, Sophocles' *Oedipus Rex*, primarily concerns the question whether knowledge or insight is an unmitigated good.

Clinical analysis also embodies the value of individuality; it is a process in which an individual patient spends a great deal of time, energy, and money exploring his or her individual mind and personal history in order, ultimately, to achieve greater individual happiness. This is not to say that relationships with others are neglected, or that the individual is encouraged to promote his or her welfare at the expense of others. However, to members of other cultures, especially non-Western ones, the idea of devoting so much attention to the individual alone, rather than as a member of the group, would seem strange and inappropriate. Thus the principle of neutrality, while central in clinical theory, is limited in its scope; the process requires that patient and analyst share certain value-laden assumptions about the perception of reality, about morally acceptable behavior, and about the importance of individuality and insight.

Limitations on the analyst's role

The principles of abstinence and neutrality dictate that the analyst may not assume other roles in the patient's life. As noted above, nonprofessional contacts, such as sexual, social, or business relationships, or exchanging gifts with patients, are inconsistent with analytic abstinence. Certain other professional functions, which might well be beneficial, are still proscribed because they are inconsistent with neutrality, and therefore are not analytic. For example, advising the patient on life decisions or on how to manage relationships with important others, as one might do in a supportive psychotherapy, would constitute a deviation from analytic neutrality. Similarly, certain assessment or advocacy functions, such as testifying on a patient's behalf in a legal proceeding, would violate the analytic role. In certain circumstances, such violations are inescapable or necessary; if an analytic patient becomes suicidally depressed, the analyst may have to intervene in a nonabstinent and nonneutral fashion. However, such a situation is best understood not as an exception to the principles of analysis but as a point at which other values, such as preserving life, override the importance of analysis, and the analyst chooses temporarily to suspend analysis in order to serve other goals.

The analyst's obligations

In the broadest sense, the analyst's primary obligation is to give good treatment. In practice, this means ensuring that he or she is well-trained; that his or her skills remain current and consistent with professional standards, by keeping up with the analytic literature and being involved with professional associations; selecting patients for analysis carefully, to be sure that they have the psychological resources necessary for analysis, and that there is no more appropriate treatment for each patient's condition; and conducting the analysis under the guidance of the principles of neutrality and abstinence. By adhering to these guidelines, the analyst will fulfill most of his or her ethical obligations. However, certain obligations deserve particular notice.

Countertransference. Just as the patient in a successful analysis predictably develops intense transference feelings about the analyst, the analyst predictably develops intense feelings about the patient, which are called countertransference. These feelings may be positive or negative, and their specific content will be determined both by the nature of the patient's transference and by the analyst's own history and unconscious dynamics. In any case, countertransference feelings, especially unconscious ones, constitute the most serious challenge to analytic neutrality. The ability to recognize and manage countertransference feelings is both an essential goal of analystic training and supervision, and an ongoing ethical obligation for the practicing analyst.

Sexual misconduct. A very common variety of transference and countertransference involves erotic attraction between patient and analyst. The analyst is under a strict ethical obligation to strive to recognize the transferential origin of this attraction and, in any event, to refrain from acting on it (Freud, 1915a). Sexual con-

tact between doctor and patient is prohibited in general medicine, as stated in the Hippocratic Oath, and in psychiatry, but there are additional reasons for this rule in psychoanalysis. In general medicine and psychiatry, the patient is in a dependent position, and the chance that the patient's needs could be exploited for the doctor's sexual satisfaction is so great that the American Medical Association has seen fit to ban sex between physicians and their current patients (Council on Ethical and Judicial Affairs, 1991). In 1993 the American Psychiatric Association (APA) went further and stated in their *Principles of Medical Ethics with Annotations Especially Applicable to Psychiatry* that "Sexual activity with a current or former patient is unethical" (p. 4).

In psychoanalysis, the same argument about dependency and exploitation applies, but another and more encompassing argument exists as well. The conduct of psychoanalysis rests on the proposition that the treatment is conducted in words only, not in action; the patient is free to say or imagine anything, because no action will ensue. If this principle is violated and the patient and analyst act on their erotic attraction to each other, either during or long after the analysis, the credibility of the treatment itself is seriously damaged, and the interests of those who might benefit from analysis in the future are thus harmed. Accordingly, the American Psychoanalytic Association, recognizing that the unconscious is timeless (Freud, 1915b), absolutely prohibits sexual contact between analyst and patient, with no special exemption for a postanalytic relationship (American Psychoanalytic Association, 1983).

Confidentiality. The analyst's obligation to respect the patient's confidentiality derives not specifically from the principles of clinical psychoanalysis but from the general principle of confidentiality recognized in both physician–patient and therapist–client relationships. However, the principle assumes special importance in psychoanalysis, since the analyst specifically instructs the patient to hold no information back, and thereby acquires the obligation to treat the patient's communications with full respect for privacy.

Psychoanalysis and social values: Common criticisms

Criticisms of the theory of the mind. Many of the value-laden assumptions embodied in the psychoanalytic theory of the mind have been attacked as promoting negative stereotypes and producing destructive social consequences. For example, feminist critics have argued that the psychoanalytic theory of female development and psychology offers a negative view of women as psychologically inferior to men. The argument is based on Freud's early position that women do not experience castration anxiety in the same way men do, and are therefore less likely to develop a rigorous superego. This criticism is generally accurate with respect to Freud's original theory, which was very much a product of the culture in which he lived and his personal predilections. However, psychoanalytic ideas about female psychology and social roles have been extensively revised since that time, with the result that current psychoanalytic theorizing on the subject offers a much fuller, more positive, and more nuanced view of both male and female development and psychology.

Similarly, spokespersons for the gay community have argued that psychoanalysis treats gays unfairly and advances a biased view that homosexuality is invariably a pathological outcome of disturbed development. This criticism is directed at organized psychoanalysis after Freud, since Freud himself argued strongly that homosexuality need not be considered a form of pathology (1905). Debate on this subject is currently very active, and involves such questions as whether homosexuality has significant concurrence with certain forms of psychopathology, especially narcissistic disorders; whether the psychopathology seen in homosexuals can be understood as a result of familial and social condemnation of biologically determined orientation; whether heterosexuality can or should be a goal of analytic treatment; and whether homosexuals are acceptable candidates for training as analysts.

Another important criticism of psychoanalysis, deriving largely from the circumstances of Freud's personality and culture, is that it is hostile to religion. Freud himself made clear his belief that religion was nothing more than a cultural neurosis (1927). For many years, psychoanalysis and religion saw each other as enemies, but in recent decades this situation has changed. Analysts have come to recognize religion as an important domain of human mental activity, not to be lightly dismissed, and theologians have become increasingly interested in the use of psychoanalytic insights in their thinking and pastoral practice.

The concept of "psychic reality" is both a central tenet of psychoanalytic theory and a source of some important criticisms of that theory. The concept appeared when Freud revised his theory about the role of childhood seduction in causing neurosis; at first, he believed his patients' frequent stories of being sexually abused as children were historically accurate, but later he came to appreciate the psychological importance of fantasies and wishes as capable of producing neurosis even in the absence of actual seduction. Critics have argued that psychoanalytic theory went too far in this direction, presenting a view in which all memories of childhood sexual abuse were dismissed as fantasies, and that this development was responsible for long-standing and widespread denial, until recently, of the extent of actual sexual abuse of children.

Finally, psychoanalysis has been criticized by the antipsychiatry movement as a form of mind control. Spokespeople for this movement are opposed to all psychiatric practice as a tool of social control that imposes on patients a view of reality acceptable to the politically powerful. As a particularly influential form of psychiatric treatment, these critics argue, psychoanalysis is very effective in imposing the analyst's view of reality on the unsuspecting patient. Whether this general criticism is valid or not, the behavior it describes is clearly inconsistent with analytic neutrality and good analytic practice.

Criticisms of clinical theory and practice. Various ethical objections have been raised against clinical psychoanalysis, concerning both its status as a form of treatment and the effects it has on individuals and on society.

Critics have argued that it is impossible for a patient to give informed consent to analysis, since the patient cannot possibly appreciate beforehand what an exploration of the unconscious will involve. This situation is analogous to other investigative procedures in medicine, in which neither patient nor doctor can know beforehand what will be found, and the patient can be informed only as to the risks and potential benefits of the procedure itself, with the understanding that the findings cannot be predicted. In clinical analysis, the patient's act of giving consent is ongoing throughout the treatment. Opponents of psychoanalysis, including many prominent psychiatrists, have argued extensively that it is unethical to offer a treatment, like psychoanalytic therapy, the value of which has not been demonstrated in controlled statistical studies, when other treatments are available that have been shown by such studies to be effective (Klerman, 1990). However, the vast majority of treatments and practices in clinical medicine have not yet been proven effective in this rigorous fashion. The fact that psychoanalysis still awaits such proof requires only that the prospective patient be informed of what is known about the treatment's effectiveness, and of other treatments that might be available.

With respect to the effects of analysis, critics have argued that it discourages spontaneity, encourages dependence and self-centeredness, excuses evil or criminal behavior, and medicalizes human relationships. For the most part, these criticisms describe expectable complications and distortions of the analytic process, or inappropriate applications of analytic principles outside of analytic treatment, rather than the process of analysis as it should be conducted.

The idea that analysis discourages spontaneity by requiring that the patient substitute thought for action presents a common and analyzable distortion of the process. While it is true that analysis requires substituting thought for action during the analytic hour, it does not follow that the patient is expected to behave this way outside the hour. In fact, an inhibition of spontaneity outside of analysis would usually be seen as a manifestation of obsessional pathology, in which thought is substituted for action, or as an enactment of the transference—and in any case as an indication for further analytic work. Similarly, the idea that the focus on oneself required in the analytic hour should extend to the rest of life is a miscarriage of analysis, requiring interpretation and correction.

The argument that analysis encourages dependency results from the fact that a dependent transference toward the analyst commonly develops, since the patient's relationship to important others in the past will often have been a dependent one, or that the experience of a dependent time of life is remembered when regression occurs in the analysis. However, analysis itself neither encourages nor discourages dependency; it encourages only the emergence and resolution of the transference, whatever its content may be. If the patient is reluctant to relinquish this dependent posture, that development is an interpretable distortion. Some varieties of dynamic therapy, in contrast, may encourage dependency as the cost of attaining important therapeutic goals.

Debates about the insanity defense in criminal proceedings have often involved a misapplication of the psychoanalytic principle of neutrality. Critics argue that by trying to make all behavior understandable in terms of the interplay of unconscious forces, psychoanalysis has removed the sense of personal responsibility for behavior. However, as described above, the principle of neutrality is employed only in a very specific setting, the psychoanalytic hour, and only with a well-selected population and for a specific limited purpose. Analysts do not encourage society to adopt an attitude of neutrality outside of clinical psychoanalysis (Gaylin, 1982).

The argument that psychoanalysis tends inappropriately to medicalize problems in human life and relationships is based partly on a peculiar historical association between analysis and medicine. Freud was a physician, as were his earliest disciples, but the psychoanalytic movement in Europe rapidly expanded to include nonmedical practitioners. In America, analysis has been dominated by the medical profession, though the 1991 decision of the American Psychoanalytic Association to approve full training for nonmedical candidates presages a significant increase in the proportion and influence of nonmedical analysts in the United States. The distinction between prescribing analysis and conducting analysis may be useful in elucidating the proper relationship between medicine and analysis. The

act of prescribing psychoanalysis as the treatment of choice for a particular patient is a medical act, since it requires diagnosing the patient's problem and knowing the possible alternative treatments; but the act of conducting the analysis, while it requires good clinical judgment, does not require medical knowledge or training.

Public-health issues.   Some criticisms of psychoanalysis contend that it is a luxury for the rich, is suitable only for a tiny minority of the most prosperous and least disturbed members of society, and consumes a vast amount of medical resources that could be put to better use meeting the needs of the poor and the seriously mentally ill. Psychoanalysts offer several rebuttals. First, it is not true that the problems of psychoanalytic patients are trivial; while analysis does require certain particular psychological strengths, patients in analysis can be seriously impaired and genuinely suffering in many ways, and analysis can provide significant relief to them. Second, the benefits of psychoanalysis extend well beyond the patients who are treated with full analysis. Many other forms of treatment, including the dynamic therapies and even pharmacotherapy and general medical treatment, can be rendered more effective if the practitioner understands and makes use of psychoanalytic insights about human motivation. Finally, analysts recognize that few individuals can afford to pay a standard psychiatric fee several times per week over many years, and many analysts are willing to reduce their fees to enable a wider range of people to benefit from psychoanalytic treatment. These financial problems could be mitigated if systems of reimbursement paid for cognitive and interpersonal services fairly in comparison with surgical and invasive procedures. But, such decisions are usually governed by political and economic concerns rather than by ethical imperatives.

Conclusion

Until the 1960s, psychoanalysis was the dominant theory, and psychoanalytically derived therapies were the most common treatment, in the mental professions. Since then the dominance has waned, partly as a result of economic forces leading to the development of briefer treatments, and partly as the result of the rise of biological psychiatry and the development of effective pharmacologic treatments. In recent decades only a small fraction of psychiatrists have chosen to become psychoanalysts, and only a small fraction of patients are treated with full psychoanalysis. However, the influence of analytic theories and findings continues to be felt throughout the fields of psychiatry, psychotherapy, and medicine. It is likely that there will remain a population of patients who have problems of sufficient breadth and depth and who can support its financial costs, who will choose psychoanalysis and its related therapies as their treatments of choice.

KEVIN V. KELLY

For a further discussion of topics mentioned in this entry, see the entries ABUSE, INTERPERSONAL, *article on* CHILD ABUSE; CHILDREN; CONFIDENTIALITY; ETHICS, *article on* RELIGION AND MORALITY; FEMINISM; HOMOSEXUALITY; INFORMED CONSENT; MENTAL-HEALTH SERVICES; MENTAL-HEALTH THERAPIES; NARRATIVE; PSYCHIATRY, ABUSES OF; PSYCHOPHARMACOLOGY; RESPONSIBILITY; SEXISM; SEXUAL ETHICS AND PROFESSIONAL STANDARDS; VALUE AND VALUATION; *and* WOMEN. *For a discussion of related ideas, see the entries* BEHAVIOR MODIFICATION THERAPIES; COMMITMENT TO MENTAL INSTITUTIONS; DIVIDED LOYALTIES IN MENTAL-HEALTH CARE; ELECTROCONVULSIVE THERAPY; HYPNOSIS; MENTAL HEALTH; MENTAL ILLNESS; MENTALLY DISABLED AND MENTALLY ILL PERSONS; PROFESSIONAL–PATIENT RELATIONSHIP; *and* SEXUAL DEVELOPMENT.

Bibliography

AMERICAN PSYCHIATRIC ASSOCIATION (APA). 1993. *Principles of Medical Ethics: With Annotations Especially Applicable to Psychiatry.* Washington, D.C.: Author.

AMERICAN PSYCHOANALYTIC ASSOCIATION. 1983. *Principles of Ethics for Psychoanalysts and Provisions for Implementation of the Principles of Ethics for Psychoanalysts.* New York: Author.

APPELBAUM, PAUL S., and JORGENSON, LINDA. 1991. "Psychotherapist–Patient Sexual Contact After Termination of Treatment: An Analysis and a Proposal." *American Journal of Psychiatry* 148, no. 11:1466–1473.

COUNCIL ON ETHICAL AND JUDICIAL AFFAIRS. AMERICAN MEDICAL ASSOCIATION. 1991. "Sexual Misconduct in the Practice of Medicine." *Journal of the American Medical Association* 266, no. 19:2741–2745.

FREUD, ANNA. 1946. *The Ego and the Mechanisms of Defense.* New York: International Universities Press.

FREUD, SIGMUND. 1953–1974. [1886–1940]. *The Standard Edition of the Complete Psychological Works of Sigmund Freud.* Translated and edited by James Strachey, Anna Freud, Alix Strachey, and Alan Tyson. 24 vols. London: Hogarth. Hereafter SE.

———. 1900. *The Interpretation of Dreams.* In vols. 4 and 5 of SE, pp. 1–625.

———. 1905. "Three Essays on the Theory of Sexuality." In vol. 7 of SE, pp. 123–245.

———. 1915a. "Observations on Transference-Love." In vol. 12 of SE, pp. 157–173.

———. 1915b. "The Unconscious." In vol. 14 of SE, pp. 159–215.

———. 1919. "Lines of Advance in Psychoanalytic Therapy." In vol. 17 of SE, pp. 157–168.

———. 1923. "The Ego and the Id." In vol. 19 of SE, pp. 3–66.

———. 1925. "An Autobiographical Study." In vol. 20 of SE, pp. 1–74.

———. 1926. "The Question of Lay Analysis." In vol. 20 of SE, pp. 177–258.

———. 1927. "The Future of an Illusion." In vol. 21 of SE, pp. 1–56.

GAYLIN, WILLARD. 1982. *The Killing of Bonnie Garland: A Question of Justice.* New York: Simon and Schuster.

KLERMAN, GERALD L. 1990. "The Psychiatric Patient's Right to Effective Treatment: Implications of *Osheroff* v. *Chestnut Lodge.*" *American Journal of Psychiatry* 147, no. 4:409–418.

LAPLANCHE, JEAN, and PONTALIS, J. B. 1967. *Vocabulaire de la psychoanalyse.* Paris: Presses universitaires de France. Translated under the title *The Language of Psychoanalysis* by D. Nicholson-Smith. New York: W. W. Norton, 1973.

MICHELS, ROBERT, and OLDHAM, JOHN M. 1983. "Value Judgements in Psychoanalytic Theory and Practice." *Psychoanalytic Inquiry* 3, no. 4:599–608.

PSYCHOPHARMACOLOGY

Psychopharmacology is the study of drugs used to alter mood, behavior, and mental functioning across a broad range of illnesses and conditions. While many drugs used in general medicine (e.g., antihypertensives, hormonal therapies) produce behavioral or psychological symptoms, psychopharmacologic agents are used specifically for their behavioral or mental effects. These agents have arrived late into the hands of physicians—nearly all since 1955. While serendipitous discovery played a major role in the emergence of many psychopharmacologic compounds, neuroscience has reached a level of sophistication where drugs are now used as probes for complex aspects of brain function. The boundary between the "hard" sciences of neurophysiology and neuropharmacology and the study of the behavioral or social symptoms produced by psychiatric illness is becoming less distinct, often as a result of these drug therapies.

The ethical issues in psychopharmacology focus on the overuse of such agents, including excessive dosage, the use of multiple drugs when not clearly indicated (polypharmacy), and the use of such agents when pharmacological treatment is not indicated or is unnecessary. The issue of informed consent in psychiatric patients, as well as the broad spectrum of adverse effects from psychotropic agents, provide additional ethical dilemmas. The introduction of new drugs has greatly increased the cost of treatment, and the controversy surrounding drug marketing raises further concerns. These individuals often lack the ability to protect their rights as patients because of limited intellect, judgment, or experience. Special populations, including confused, demented, retarded, or pediatric populations, are also likely to receive psychotropic drugs and are incapable of self-protection. This entry will also discuss the ethics of antianxiety drugs and their complications as well as other specific drug classes. Drugs will be referred to by their generic name with the American trade name indicated in parentheses. This entry will focus chiefly on drugs used for therapeutic purposes in a medical setting and will not cover alcohol and drug abuse.

The commercial development of psychopharmacologic agents has grown into a multimillion-dollar industry. The development of a drug in the United States or Canada may take a decade and hundreds of millions of dollars to accomplish. The initial testing of drugs on humans produces unknown risks, first to healthy volunteers and later to patients suffering from the illness in question. In the clinical trials of a new drug, scientific rigor requires that neither patient nor physician know if the patient is on the experimental agent or a placebo, a procedure known as "double blind." It is not unusual for investigators participating in drug trials to act also as consultants for these drug companies, possibly compromising their scientific objectivity. This system depends upon physicians, organizations (e.g., the American Medical Association), and governmental regulatory bodies (e.g., the U.S. Food and Drug Administration) to play an essential role in seeking to balance the pressures of the market with concerns for the public welfare. With each of the agents discussed there is an implicit ethical issue of balancing what is desired (valued) against what is not desired (disvalued). This balance requires of the clinician a sensitivity to the needs, interests, and wants of each patient and a thorough effort to communicate with each patient.

Classes of psychopharmacologic agents

Antipsychotics. Antipsychotic drugs have made possible fundamental changes in the treatment of the most severe psychiatric disorders, enabling many patients to control incapacitating symptoms, such as delusions (falsely held beliefs) and hallucinations (e.g., voices heard by the patient). Prior to the introduction of antipscyhotics in 1952, the treatment of psychosis was largely ineffectual, and lengthy or indefinite hospitalization of questionable value was the principle intervention provided. Schizophrenia was the illness most impacted by these drugs. Schizophrenia affects 1 percent of the population worldwide, and today the majority of these patients are treated with one of the antipsychotics. Antipsychotics are especially useful in treating hallucinations, delusions, and a variety of paranoid symptoms. They greatly reduce the patient's hostility and combative behavior, which can pose a substantial risk to the caregivers or families of schizophrenic patients. The

drugs reduce the need for physical restraint (tying the patient to a bed or chair) by both reducing hostility and producing sedation.

Most schizophrenic patients have the onset of their illness in early adulthood, with relapses of psychotic behavior that can occur for decades to come. Thus, after treatment of the initial episode of psychosis, longer-term or maintenance therapy is usually indicated. In the acute psychotic episode, there are few guides as to how to determine the dosage of these drugs. The measurement of drug levels in blood are for the most part inexact and disappointing in clinical use. Dosing involves assessing the reduction in the patient's psychotic symptoms balanced against the drug's adverse effects (discussed below), but this equation is by no means exact. It is universally agreed that antipsychotic agents speed recovery and enable a more rapid discharge from the hospital. Only a minority of patients can improve without drugs.

Despite their effectiveness, antipsychotics are far from ideal. They produce a number of uncomfortable and sometimes irreversible effects on brain and behavior. Although schizophrenic patients are less psychotic and less dangerous with these drugs, they are not well. Lesser symptoms remain: social withdrawal, loss of motivation, slowed thinking, blunted mood, and bizarre behavior.

Pharmacologically, antipsychotics include chlorpromazine, haloperidol, thioridazine, thiothixene, trifluoperazine, loxapine, and others. Chlorpromazine (Thorazine) was the first antipsychotic introduced. Currently, haloperidol (Haldol) is the most widely used in the United States. Remarkably, until the introduction of atypical antipsychotics in the 1980s, all these other drugs were of equal benefit clinically. The atypical antipsychotics combine novel pharmacologic effects with increased effectiveness on psychosis.

Antipsychotics work by occupying and blocking dopamine receptors in specific areas of the brain that are known to mediate psychotic behavior. Receptors are the receiving terminals of chemical messengers (in this case, dopamine) released from one nerve cell to the next. Other messengers (e.g., serotonin) fulfill specific brain functions at set locations. The receptor is usually specific for each messenger and can also be affected by various drugs. Increased dopamine activity appears to make individuals more psychotic, and blocking dopamine reduces psychosis. In addition to this role in mental functioning, dopamine is also involved in muscular function and in the synthesis of norepinephrine, a chemical messenger important in arousal and attention. Therefore, blocking dopamine produces uncomfortable muscular symptoms (stiffness, rigidity, tremor, restlessness) and a reduction in alertness and attention. In addition to affecting dopamine, these antipsychotics are well known for affecting (usually adversely) receptors of many other brain systems.

A newer family of atypical antipsychotics includes clozapine (Clozaril), risperidone (Risperdal), melperone, and others. These drugs are of greater clinical benefit than other antipsychotics by virtue of their ability to target dopamine receptors important in psychosis, while sparing other dopamine areas (e.g., those involved in involuntary muscular movement). In addition, they block serotonin receptors; this feature is emerging as possibly helpful in schizophrenia, depression, and manic-depressive disorders. While blocking serotonin appears to stabilize mood in psychiatric disorderes, its role is very complex and incompletely understood.

Adverse effects.   Antipsychotic drugs are not popular with patients because of their unpleasant side effects. Many patients who feel sedated, slowed, and uncomfortable become noncompliant with the drug therapy. Most of the adverse effects of antipsychotics are a result of the same dopamine blockade that controls psychosis. Blocking the involuntary movement system produces rigidity, tremor, slowing of movement, and an unpleasant muscular restlessness. Moreover, a significant proportion of patients with long-term therapy develop tardive dyskinesia, a neurological disorder of involuntary mouth, face, neck, and body movement that can become permanent. Each additional year of antipsychotic exposure increases a patient's chance of developing tardive dyskinesia. After three years of therapy (not an unusual length of treatment in schizophrenia), 15 percent of patients will develop tardive dyskinesia. Elderly, hospitalized psychiatric patients have the highest rates of this disorder, with many surveys finding over 50 percent affected (American Psychiatric Association Task Force, 1980).

These alterations in movement may make social interaction more difficult for patients, and many patients also experience reduction or loss of motivation, both of which are also symptoms of schizophrenia. Dry mouth, constipation, and loss of some or all sexual function result in a truly unpleasant experience for many patients. Fatal effects are rare, but they can occur from alterations in heart rhythm and from a loss in white blood cells, an effect seen in about 1 percent of patients taking clozapine (Clozaril).

Antidepressants.   Antidepressants are widely used, reflecting the high prevalence rates of depression in the U.S. population; lifetime prevalence of depression is at least 6 percent (Kaplan and Sadock, 1991). The introduction of these drugs followed closely the discovery of antipsychotics, and created a totally new approach to the treatment of depression. Their effectiveness has increased our understanding of it as a medical disorder analogous to diabetes or hypertension. As with antipsy-

chotics, they have reduced the need for hospitalization and shortened its duration when it becomes necessary. Unlike the antipsychotics, there are multiple mechanisms of action for the antidepressants and some have no known pharmacologic mechanism. The first antidepressants, the tricyclics (so-called because they all possess a 3-cycle ring), act by blocking the reuptake of norepinephrine or serotonin at the junction between nerve cells. Unused neurotransmitter substance is taken back into the cell to be reused, a process known as reuptake. By blocking reuptake, antidepressant agents make more neurotransmitters available to the receptor, thus increasing the firing frequency of the cell. Depression is felt to result from defects in norepinephrine or serotonin pathways, which explains the effectiveness of these agents.

While norepinephrine was the primary target of early antidepressants, newer agents have more prominent effects on serotonin. Reductions in serotonin have been identified in suicidal behavior, obsessive-compulsive disorder, and some behaviors associated with violence or impulsivity. Thus, as these antidepressants block the reuptake of serotonin, more serotonin becomes available to the receptors, alleviating all these symptoms. Other antidepressants block monoamine oxidase, the enzyme that degrades both norepinephrine and serotonin; they are known as monoamine oxidase inhibitors.

Several drugs specific for action on serotonin have been introduced: fluoxetine (Prozac), sertraline (Zoloft), paroxetine (Paxil), and clomipramine (Anafranil). These drugs have taken the medical community by storm and have been extensively prescribed; 7 million Americans receive fluoxetine alone. All are easy to prescribe and are used much more by primary care physicians than by psychiatric specialists. They are also expensive. It should be remembered that because depression can relapse, many patients will require long-term therapy, perhaps for decades or more. Serotonergic agents have also been effectively utilized in the treatment of obsessive-compulsive disorder, an illness of repetitive, ritualistic behavior, which may begin in adolescence.

Lithium is considered an antidepressant, but is much more widely used in manic-depressive illness. Although its mechanism of action is not fully understood, it can block recurrence of manic depression as well as treat acute episodes of both mania and depression.

Psychomotor stimulants have been used to a limited extent in depression, although they are used most frequently in attention deficit disorder in pediatric populations. These drugs, which are chemically related to cocaine, have been prone to abuse. Stimulants include dextramephetamine (Dexedrine), methylphenidate (Ritalin), and pemoline (Cylert). They accentuate the output of both norepinephrine and dopamine in the brain, and will produce agitation or psychotic behavior in high doses. Stimulant psychosis, producing a picture of agitation and paranoid delusions, is a well-recognized syndrome among high-dose drug abusers.

Adverse effects. Adverse effects of antidepressants are mild compared to those of antipsychotics, but they can be problematic. The tricyclic antidepressants produce dry mouth, constipation, and some sedation, but the sedative effect can be used to treat the insomnia that frequently accompanies depression. In cases of overdose, monoamine oxidase inhibitors and tricyclics can produce dangerous cardiac arrythmias. Monoamine oxidase inhibitors can also produce serious blood pressure elevations if they are combined with certain other drugs or foods. Patients must strictly adhere to dietary guidelines to prevent problems.

The newer serotonergic antidepressants produce a different spectrum of adverse effects: nausea, diarrhea, weight loss, and occasional agitation; but they are far safer in cases of overdose. The serotonergic compounds can also cause a sometimes striking reduction in sexual interest along with problems in achieving orgasm. Other antidepressants produce some difficulties in sexual function, but they are less severe. With antidepressants, the balance between therapeutic and adverse effects is straightforward and usually clear to both the physician and the patient. Lithium may also have long-term effects—especially on the kidneys—that are less apparent. Psychomotor stimulants produce a slowing of bone growth (a very important concern in treating children) as well as insomnia, excess arousal, and habituation in some patients.

Antianxiety drugs and their complications

Antianxiety drugs (anxiolytics) are used medically to treat primary anxiety disorders as well as anxiety that surfaces secondary to a number of medical conditions (for example, myocardial infarction). Alcohol is the oldest antianxiety agent. Medical use of anxiolytics began with the barbiturates and propanediols, drugs with sedative and anxiety-reducing effects, which also slowed thinking and alertness. In the late 1960s, the benzodiazepines were developed as drugs that reduced anxiety but preserved cognitive function and physical activity. These drugs include diazepam (Valium), lorazepam (Ativan), and alprazolam (Xanax). Benzodiazepines are believed to stimulate another neurotransmitter, gamma aminobutyric acid, which plays an inhibitory role in brain function, lessening arousal and anxiety. Benzodiazepines were much safer than the earlier antianxiety drugs, which could impair breathing or cause death in high doses and which were also highly liable to abuse and serious withdrawal syndromes. Nevertheless, toler-

ance (the need for higher doses) and withdrawal, the hallmarks of abusable drugs, do occur with the benzodiazepines.

Anxiety and panic disorder, for which these drugs are primarily used, are the most frequently noted of psychiatric disorders. The lifetime prevalence of anxiety disorders is close to 15 percent (Rickels and Schweizer, 1987); and in one extensive community survey, 8.3 percent of the U.S. adult population reported being affected by an anxiety disorder in the prior 6 months (Shapiro et al., 1984). Because of the extensive prevalence of anxiety symptoms, it is not surprising that these drugs are so widely used, even though fewer than one quarter of the people suffering from anxiety ever seek treatment.

Pharmacologists have searched for antianxiety drugs that do not produce tolerance or addiction. One approach has been to develop an agent to stimulate a part of the serotonergic system; Buspirone (Buspar) is the first of a number of drugs in this category. Almost all the antidepressant agents can reduce anxiety, but benzodiazepines appear to be the most effective and to have the most immediate effect, valuable traits in antianxiety agents.

Hypnotic agents. Most hypnotic (sleep-inducing) agents are also benzodiazepines. The hypnotic benzodiazepines include flurazepam (Dalmane), triazolam (Halcion), and temazepam (Restoril). They are structurally similar to the anxiolytics, sharing their advantages and drawbacks. Overdosage of the barbiturates, formerly used as hypnotics, was frequently fatal. Today's sleeping pills are far safer and fatal overdoses are rare. The ideal sleeping pill would have a fast onset of action, would produce a natural sleep, and would not impair wakefulness or alertness the next morning. Like anxiety, insomnia is present in about one fourth of the U.S. population. Hypnotics are used by almost 3 percent of the population (Balter and Uhlenhuth, 1992). Intermittent use is the most common pattern.

Adverse effects. Adverse effects of antianxiety agents are generally extensions of their therapeutic effect: sedation, impaired motor performance or attention, tolerance, and physical dependency (addiction); the sedative effects impair driving and attention to mechanical tasks. However, untreated anxiety or insomnia can produce serious problems in these same functions. Thus, the prescriber must carefully weigh the risks and benefits. The risk of addiction to these drugs is considerably less than with barbiturates and other older sedatives. Nevertheless, physical addiction can occur with tolerance and a withdrawal state can arise, characterized by symptoms opposite to the therapeutic effects of these drugs—that is, increased anxiety, restlessness, nausea, and insomnia. In some cases, seizures may develop from withdrawal of short-acting benzodiazepines (lorazepam, alprazolam, triazolam). How much risk do typical patients face? During short-term, low-dose therapy, the risk is low; however, patients with prior drug abuse or alcoholism are at higher risk for these problems as are patients who take higher doses over longer periods. The short-acting sleeping pills (such as triazolam) may produce a rebound insomnia after use. Here the patient's insomnia is temporarily exacerbated by withdrawal of the hypnotics. Some hypnotic agents can produce confusion or memory loss, especially if combined with alcohol.

Ethical dilemmas in psychopharmacology

Consent to treatment.   A principal ethical dilemma involves the use of psychopharmacologic agents in patients who are in fact impaired by their condition and who are unable to make an informed choice as to their treatment and its risks and benefits. Antipsychotic drugs are prescribed chiefly to psychotic patients, many of whom will be paranoid and suspicious, especially about drugs they may be asked to take. The prescriber faces a dilemma: How reasonable is the patient's option to accept or refuse treatment for an illness that renders him or her unable to process reality, likely to suspect all who hope to help him or her, and even likely to constitute a risk to self or others?

All competent patients have the right to refuse treatment of any kind. Unfortunately, state laws have not clearly defined competency in regard to psychotic conditions. Competency hearings may delay decision making for weeks and are expensive for both patient and treating physician or facility. If a patient's refusal to take medication results in a danger to her- or himself (e.g., refusing to eat) or to others (e.g., attacking feared persecutors), both common sense and state statutes advocate temporarily forcing medication if necessary. Forced medication involves administering these drugs to a patient against his or her will. In less extreme cases, patients are participants in their treatment; but on a locked unit, in a totally controlled environment, how free can this choice truly be? One study demonstrated that the most severely psychotic patients refuse treatment more frequently than patients who are less symptomatic (Marder et al., 1983).

As patients improve from their acute psychotic state, the ethics of deciding to continue drug therapy becomes less clear. As noted above, the adverse effects of antipsychotics are unpleasant and may interfere with patients' social, vocational, or sexual functioning; the specter of tardive dyskinesia, for example, is so clearly understood that patients should be specifically informed about it. Yet the antipsychotics can block the recurrence of psychotic states that might require further hospitalization. Written consents may serve as guides to the informed-consent process, and they are helpful in situations involving antipsychotics. However, there is no substitute for a relationship in which the prescriber supplies information in response to the patient's needs and wishes. This is a dynamic and changing process, and the risks for various adverse effects change from month to month. This is made much more difficult when the physician, or treating facility, changes as is common for indigent, psychotic patients. Ideally, as patients respond to therapy, they become less psychotic and more able to participate with their physicians to make reasoned, informed decisions about their treatment.

Consent by proxy has not been supported by any state in cases of determining the need for forced medication. However, many physicians involve the family in this decision. Because family members are acutely aware of the problems and risks the patient poses, they may become overzealous advocates for drug treatment, especially if violent behavior has occurred or has been threatened by the patient. From the perspective of the paranoid patient, an alliance between doctor and family poses grave risks, as the doctor may carry out the wishes of the family.

Special populations.   Demented and retarded patients are two groups for whom antipsychotics are frequently used and who are likely to encounter drug therapy in institutional settings. These populations also have memory deficits and alterations in thinking that profoundly affect their ability to consent to or understand treatment. Demented patients (most frequently those with Alzheimer's disease) have psychotic symptoms as a result of their profound memory loss and confusion. They may develop hallucinations and delusions that create a perception of threat from family or caregivers. Demented patients may wander out in the cold in search of their home, or attack a spouse who they do not recognize. Antipsychotics have been prescribed indiscriminately to demented patients in nursing-home settings. In these settings, where staffing is minimal, nondrug therapies may be underutilized. The value of antipsychotics in treating dementia is clinically evident to some, but many studies have raised questions about whether their effect is superior to no drug treatment. More research is needed to provide clinicians with information on this neglected area of study.

Psychopharmacologic agents are widely used in patients who are mentally retarded. Retarded patients may exhibit psychotic, aggressive, or impulsive behavior without necessarily being psychotic. The limited awareness of the risks and benefits of antipsychotics in this population requires the participation of the family and/or patient advocates in making treatment decisions. Tardive dyskinesia has been widely reported in retarded populations on whom antipsychotics have been used, suggesting a special vulnerability of these patients. In addition, antipsychotics are known to slow learning and responses to behavioral programming. Most states and many facilities utilize aggressive checks on the extensive or long-term use of antipsychotics and require periodic follow-up and assessment. As with demented nursing-home populations, pharmacologic intervention with the mentally retarded may be used as the simplest or least expensive intervention, although patients might derive more benefit from a more personalized behavioral or social approach.

Drug therapy and resource allocation. The use of clozapine in schizophrenia has presented a model of an ethical interface between the drug manufacturer, physician, and patient. The drug has made a dramatic difference in the lives of many patients who have experienced relief of disabling symptoms ineffectively treated by other antipsychotics. In many patients, this improvement has led to discharge from a hospital or boarding home, and even to gainful employment. However, the drug can produce a dangerous drop in the body's ability to fight infection; this side effect has been fatal in a handful of patients out of the more than 40,000 exposed to the drug in the United States.

In addition, the extremely high cost also limits the use of this drug. When clozapine was first introduced into the United States, its cost of approximately $9,000 per year was unthinkable for the majority of patients who would otherwise have used it: chronic schizophrenics who had already used any resources or insurance in the early phases of their illness. The cost was eventually reduced to about $5,000 annually, and because the drug has greatly reduced hospitalization rates, most states have decided to assume the cost of clozapine prescriptions for their indigent patients. Due to the success of the drug, public-sector expenses and presumably corporate profits have been large in the service of an underprivileged patient population. Clozapine remains among the most expensive drugs used for any medical condition. This inordinate expense is not related to the manufacture of clozapine, but rather to the associated testing and development. Estimates indicate that at the current price it would cost the United States nearly $1.5 billion per year to give the drug to all people for whom it is appropriate. In the United Kingdom, clozapine costs £2000 per patient year, compared to the most expensive antidepressants, which cost £300–400 per patient year. A balance among patient needs, the government's ability to pay, and market forces will provide the optimal solution, so that patients who might benefit from such a drug should not be denied it.

Alternative treatments—diagnostic considerations. Psychopharmacologic agents have been effective in alleviating the symptoms of psychiatric illness: Schizophrenic patients become less psychotic and more accessible, depressed patients are able to work and func-

tion, and sufferers from anxiety find their problem reduced to manageable levels. To the prescriber, these improvements raise the ethical problem of whether to provide nondrug treatments to complement the improvement garnered by drugs. The worldwide movement to reduce or eliminate hospital beds for chronic schizophrenic patients would not have been possible without the benefit of antipsychotics that control disruptive and destructive behavior.

However, development of adequate outpatient services has not kept pace with progress in treating acute psychosis. Thus, patients are well enough to be discharged from the hospital, but not well enough to be able to live independent lives. Patients are left with residual symptoms of schizophrenia: loss of motivation, reduced emotional responsivity, impaired thinking, and social withdrawal. Drugs have been less effective in treating these symptoms. Some psychiatrists argue that the ready availability of antipsychotic drugs has allowed physicians to neglect social and interpersonal aspects of treatment. These partially treated patients leave the hospital in large numbers to return home, where they are unable to work, or to live in board-and-care facilities that may or may not provide ongoing treatment. While better drugs may improve the lot of these patients, it is clear that physicians are faced with patients who need repair and rehabilitation that go beyond the scope of drug therapy alone.

Psychotherapy of various kinds was once the only therapy available for depression. Today antidepressant prescriptions are numbered in the millions, prescribed by physicians who may never bother to take a detailed personal history of the patient. With the advent of the new serotonergic agents, adverse effects have been minimized and patients may not even feel they are on medication. These drugs have also been prescribed for much broader and less severe conditions. Whereas previously antidepressants were given primarily for major depressive disorders, the newer agents may be given to alleviate disappointment, to reduce the pain of daily living for normal individuals, and even to alter character traits. Peter Kramer, in his popular book *Listening to Prozac* (1993), argues that the newer serotonergic agents produce neurochemical changes that alter what was formerly viewed as character. Certain obsessional and compulsive behaviors are uniquely responsive to these drugs. Disorders once felt to be solely within the realm of psychotherapy are now treated pharmacologically.

It could be argued that such drugs are too casually prescribed. Physicians' excitement with these newfound agents, combined with pharmaceutical encouragement and public interest, has created an atmosphere in which the prescriber simply provides a drug to cause patients to feel and function better, without the careful diagnosis, judgment, and supervision that this process requires.

While most patients do well with antidepressants, clinicians have noted a loss of inhibition in some patients given serotonergic antidepressants, with the new appearance of suicidal thoughts or actions (Teicher et al., 1990). In other patients, at least one-third report reductions in sexual interest or functioning.

Another unusual effect from serotonergic antidepressants provides an example of how complex the behavioral effects of these drugs may be. Patients have reported loss of initiative, and negligence, indifference, and apathy, with striking loss of drive. It has been theorized that the complex behavioral effects of these drugs, which give relief to so many patients, may be a problem for others. Clearly, the use of these agents should be accompanied by a careful supervision and assessment by the prescribing physician.

The issue of drug therapy and its effect on other therapies is present with both antidepressants and antianxiety agents. Both drugs relieve painful symptoms that might otherwise motivate patients to seek other psychotherapies. While studies clearly indicate that patients do better with psychotherapy and drug therapy in combination, this often does not occur.

Under ideal circumstances, antianxiety drugs are used for brief periods, from weeks to months, until normal adaptive processes can take over. This pattern holds for most patients. In some patients, however, the drugs are used for longer periods or even indefinitely. Whereas some patients could not function effectively without these drugs, others experience troublesome adverse effects and are exposed to the risk of tolerance and habituation long after therapeutic effects have ceased. In alcoholic patients and those with a history of drug abuse, antianxiety drugs may activate the substance-abuse process. Forty-three percent of patients who take benzodiazepines for a year or longer can expect a clear-cut withdrawal syndrome, and some authors report even higher figures (Rickels and Schweizer, 1987). When patients experience these withdrawal symptoms, they may confuse them with the underlying anxiety state for which the drugs were first prescribed, and assume that they require longer-term treatment. Patients should be informed of these effects throughout drug therapy, and the benefits and risks of treatment should be reassessed on several occasions. Other treatments for anxiety and depression, including psychotherapy, behavioral therapy, and relaxation therapy, should also be offered.

Drugs and women.   Women receive more prescriptions for all psychotropic drugs than do men. This discrepancy is in part explained by the higher incidence of anxiety and depressive disorders in women. However, there is evidence that gender biases the use of drugs, especially antianxiety drugs. Because most physicians are male, it has been assumed in the past that male physicians are more prepared to medicate female patients than other males. In fact, doctors do prescribe drugs (primarily benzodiazepines) more frequently to women than to men. Interestingly, it appears that if the physician is a woman, she is even more likely to prescribe a psychotropic drug to a woman (Morabia et al., 1992). While these data may indicate that women physicians share their male counterparts' prejudice toward drug treatment of women, more complex explanations appear at least as attractive. These include the different epidemiology of psychiatric illness in men versus women, the nature of the doctor–patient contact, and the possibility that benzodiazepines may be underprescribed to men because they underreport emotional symptoms (Morabia et al., 1992).

Pediatric psychopharmacology.   Psychotropic drugs have been clearly beneficial in treating such childhood and adolescent disorders as anxiety, school refusals, and separation anxiety. In childhood psychotic disorders, antipsychotic agents are commonly used with good effect. All the side effects noted in adults can also occur in children. Informed consent here generally involves the parents, who have the responsibility to authorize treatment until the child reaches eighteen.

Attention deficit disorder with hyperactivity (ADDH) is a childhood syndrome of excessive muscular activity, attention problems, restlessness, and impulsivity. Symptoms are generally worse at school and may be accompanied by poor frustration tolerance, poor peer relations, aggressiveness, and deficient academic performance. Antipsychotics and antidepressants have been used to treat this disorder, but psychostimulants, such as methylpenidate (Ritalin), have been the mainstay of treatment. The rate of success with methylphenidate is as high as 90 percent (Gittleman and Kanner, 1984).

While pathological symptoms of ADDH improve with treatment, it is important to note that the performance of normal children also improves on stimulants. There is some dispute as to the role of these drugs in improving academic performance. Some have argued that the drugs improve classroom manageability, not academic skills. In addition, drug treatment does not alter the long-term course of the disorder, according to some studies (Weiss et al., 1975; Klein et al., 1980). Thus the overzealous use of these agents in classrooms may reflect the needs of the school rather than the needs of the student. It is also common for teachers to participate in the administration of these drugs. From a treatment standpoint, drug therapy is continued as long as the hyperactivity persists, although many adults who had ADDH in childhood still benefit from stimulants. The drugs reduce appetite and impair sleep. A complex equation between the child's needs, his school performance, and his social milieu must be solved individually. Parents, teachers, and physicians ideally should share the decision making to initiate and to terminate treatment.

Summary

Psychopharmacologic treatments are becoming more successful, and the use of psychoactive medications is widespread. Our increasing awareness of these drugs' various properties must be balanced by an awareness of their impact on the patient and his or her individual needs. In most cases, an awareness of the ethical dilemmas concerning treatment will lead the clinician to involve patients in decision making and to weigh with patients and their families the risks and benefits of treatment.

WILLIAM M. PETRIE

Directly related to this entry are the entries BEHAVIOR MODIFICATION THERAPIES; *and* MENTAL-HEALTH THERAPIES. *For a further discussion of topics mentioned in this entry, see the entries* CHILDREN, *article on* MENTAL-HEALTH ISSUES; FAMILY; HEALTH-CARE RESOURCES, ALLOCATION OF, *article on* MACROALLOCATION; INFORMED CONSENT, *especially the article on* ISSUES OF CONSENT IN MENTAL-HEALTH CARE; MENTAL HEALTH; MENTAL-HEALTH SERVICES; MENTAL ILLNESS; MENTALLY DISABLED AND MENTALLY ILL PERSONS; PHARMACEUTICS; *and* WOMEN, *articles on* HISTORICAL AND CROSS-CULTURAL PERSPECTIVES, *and* HEALTH-CARE ISSUES. *Other relevant material may be found under the entries* COMMITMENT TO MENTAL INSTITUTIONS; ELECTROCONVULSIVE THERAPY; INSTITUTIONALIZATION AND DEINSTITUTIONALIZATION; LONG-TERM CARE, *article on* NURSING HOMES; PATIENTS' RIGHTS, *article on* MENTAL PATIENTS' RIGHTS; *and* PSYCHOANALYSIS AND DYNAMIC THERAPIES.

Bibliography

AMERICAN PSYCHIATRIC ASSOCIATION TASK FORCE ON LATE NEUROLOGICAL EFFECTS OF ANTIPSYCHOTIC DRUGS. 1980. "Tardive Dyskinesia: A Summary of a Task Force Report." *American Journal of Psychiatry* 137:1163–1172.

BALTER, MITCHELL B., and UHLENHUTH, E. H. 1992. "New Epidemiologic Findings About Insomnia and Its Treatment." *Journal of Clinical Psychiatry* 53, no. 12 (suppl.): 34–39.

GITTLEMAN, RACHEL, and KANNER, ANDRES. 1984. "Overview of Clinical Psychopharmacology in Childhood Disorders." In *Clinical Psychopharmacology*, 2d ed., pp. 189–210. Edited by Jerrold G. Bernstein. Boston: John Wright.

HOHMANN, ANN H. 1989. "Gender Bias in Psychotropic Drug Prescribing in Primary Care." *Medical Care* 27, no. 5: 479–490.

KAPLAN, HAROLD I., and SADOCK, BENJAMIN J. 1991. *Synopsis of Psychiatry.* Baltimore: Williams and Wilkins.

KLEIN, DONALD F.; GITTELMAN, RACHEL; QUITKIN, FREDERICK; and RIFKIN, ARTHUR. 1980. *Diagnosis and Drug Treatment of Psychiatric Disorders: Adults and Children.* 2d ed. Baltimore: Williams and Wilkins.

KRAMER, PETER D. 1993. *Listening to Prozac.* New York: Penguin.

MARDER, STEPHEN R.; MEBANE, ANDREW; CHIEN, CHINGPIAO; WINSLADE, WILLIAM J.; SWANN, ELIZABETH; and VAN PUTTEN, THEODORE. 1983. "A Comparison of Patients Who Refuse and Consent to Neuroleptic Treatment." *American Journal of Psychiatry* 140, no. 4:470–472.

MELLINGER, GLEN D., and BALTER, MITCHELL B. 1973. "Psychotherapeutic Drugs: A Current Assessment of Prevalence and Patterns of Use." In *Society and Medication: Conflicting Signals for Prescribers and Patients*, pp. 137–154. Edited by John P. Morgan and Doreen V. Kagan. Lexington, Mass.: Lexington Books.

MORABIA, ALFREDO; FABRE, JEAN; and DUNAND, JEAN-PHILIPPE. 1992. "The Influence of Patient and Physician Gender on Prescription of Psychotropic Drugs." *Journal of Clinical Epidemiology* 45, no. 2:111–116.

RICKELS, KARL, and SCHWEIZER, EDWARD E. 1987. "Current Pharmacotherapy of Anxiety and Panic." In *Psychopharmacology: The Third Generation of Progress*, pp. 1193–1203. Edited by Herbert Y. Meltzer. New York: Raven Press.

SHAPIRO, SAM; SKINNER, ELIZABETH A.; KESSLER, LARRY G.; VON KORFF, MICHAEL; GERMAN, PEARL S.; TISCHLER, GARY L.; LEAF, PHILIP J.; BENHAM, LEE; COTTLER, LINDA; and REIGER, DARREL A. 1984. "Utilization of Health and Mental Health Services." *Archives of General Psychiatry* 41, no. 10:971–982.

TEICHER, MARTIN H.; GLOD, CAROL C.; and COLE, JONATHAN O. 1990. "Emergence of Intensive Suicidal Preoccupation During Fluoxetine Treatment." *American Journal of Psychiatry* 147:207–210.

UNITED STATES PHARMACOPEIAL CONVENTION. 1993. *United States Pharmacopeic Dispensing Information, Volume I (Drug Information for the Health Care Professional).* 13th ed. Rockville, Md.: Author.

WEIS, GABRIELLE; KRUGER, ELENA; DANIELSON, URSEL; and ELMAN, MERYL. 1975. "Effect of Long Term Treatment of Hyperactive Children with Methylphenidate." *Canadian Medical Association Journal* 112:159–165.

PSYCHOSURGERY

I. Medical and Historical Aspects
   John C. Oakley
II. Ethical Aspects
   Harold Merskey

I. MEDICAL AND HISTORICAL ASPECTS

Psychosurgery is the surgical removal or destruction of brain tissue with the intent of normalizing behavior in otherwise disabling psychiatric disorders. The patients selected for treatment generally have certain types of symptoms rather than being a part of entire nosological groups or diagnostic categories. Examples of such symptoms include phobias, anxieties, depressions, obsessive compulsions, and affective components of schizophrenia—behaviors that include, but are not limited to, incapacitating alterations in mood with loss of interest in usually pleasurable activities; persistent and irrational fear of an object, activity, or situation; or feelings of apprehension or dread about the future. Routine neurosurgical procedures are employed, including cutting, burning, or irradiation of brain tissue. Neurosurgical procedures for psychosurgical purposes are performed in the absence of definable, structural brain changes such as tumors, vascular malformations, or posttraumatic scarring. Surgical intervention in the brain for the purpose of treating a structural lesion, or other definable pathology such as an epileptic focus or tumor, would not be considered psychosurgery even if the procedure resulted in some behavioral alteration. Regarding pain-relieving procedures, some of which employ these techniques, there is no clear consensus. Such procedures clearly are designed to alter the perception of pain, thereby altering the behavioral response to that pain. These procedures have not been included in most discussions of psychosurgery unless they are specifically oriented toward altering an emotional or affective disorder associated with the pain.

Mechanisms

The best results of treating psychiatric disease by neurosurgical interventions follow destruction of some part of the frontal lobes or their connections to other brain structures. The limbic system—that portion of the brain including the white-matter fiber tracts (consisting of nerve fibers covered with myelin and hence white in appearance) of the corpus callosum (connecting the two hemispheres of the brain), the cingulate, the fornicate, and the angulate gyri, and the amygdala and hippocampus of the temporal lobes, as well as the deeper nuclei (consisting of cell bodies or gray matter), the thalamus, and the hypothalamus—is now generally accepted to control behavior and the emotions. While the relationship of these structures to behavior and emotions is accepted, the specific functions of the various segments have not been identified with any certainty. The present state of knowledge about the physiological mechanisms for the control of normal emotions, to say nothing of the mechanisms involved in affective disorders, can only be characterized as rudimentary and empirical. Hence, there is no pathophysiological rationale for selecting targets for psychosurgical procedures. There is no good answer at present to the question of how these treatments work. It is, therefore, of critical importance to prospectively evaluate outcomes of treatment in relation to the initial patient symptoms.

The development of psychosurgery

Psychosurgery began in the 1930s in the Yale University laboratory of neurophysiologist John Fulton. Based on a growing background of knowledge from animal experiments using selective destruction of frontal lobe areas, combined with behavioral training from a number of laboratories, and on a specific observation from Pavlov (1928) concerning the production of neurotic behavior in dogs presented with confusing reinforcement symbols, he and his colleague Carlyle Jacobsen conducted behavioral experiments on two chimpanzees trained to solve complex problems in order to obtain food rewards. When frustrated with attempts to obtain food, they became agitated and aggressive. Fulton and Jacobsen then performed frontal lobectomies, literally cutting out the anterior frontal lobes of the brain, and noted that the animals became immune to frustration, although they performed assigned tests slightly less well.

Fulton and Jacobsen reported their observations at a 1935 London neuroscience meeting (Fulton and Jacobsen, 1935; see also Fulton, 1942, 1951). In attendance was a noted Portuguese neuroscientist, Egas Moniz, who, with his neurosurgical colleague Almeida Lima, performed the first procedures in humans a few months thereafter. The initial operation involved placing two holes through the skull three centimeters from the midline over the frontal area, with injection of alcohol to destroy the brain substance. In subsequent operations a wire loop was used to cut the frontal lobe connections. Thus they modified the Fulton procedure, performing only a frontal lobotomy or, as Moniz termed it, a *leucotomy* (cutting of the white matter) (Moniz, 1936). Moniz was awarded the 1949 Nobel Prize for his discovery of the therapeutic value of prefrontal leucotomy in certain psychoses.

Neuropsychiatrist Walter Freeman of the United States also attended the London conference. He and his neurosurgical colleague James Watts introduced psychosurgery to the United States. They pioneered the *lobotomy*, in which frontal lobe connections to the surrounding brain were severed initially by an open neurosurgical approach called *craniotomy*, using suction to sever the fibers. The demographics of the over 600 patients reported on by Freeman and Watts are not easily summarized. Many were institutionalized but many others were cared for at home and referred by their psychiatrists. The majority were women. All of these patients were considered disabled by their illness. However, Freeman felt the procedure was too costly, being primarily governmentally funded through the state-run mental institutions, and required too much skill to use on a broad scale to empty the wards of the large mental institutions. Freeman was very much a community psychiatrist and saw it as his mission to empty the back wards of state mental hospitals.

Around 1945, Freeman introduced a procedure described by the Italian neurosurgeon Amarro Fiamberti, in which the surgeon introduced a sharp probe (originally an icepick) through the roof of the eye socket (orbit) into the frontal lobe white matter and oscillated it back and forth, thus severing the nerve fibers; this was called a *transorbital lobotomy* (Freeman and Watts, 1950). Watts, who performed the traditional procedure, felt the new procedure violated any sense of neurosurgical dignity. The so-called "icepick lobotomy" could easily be performed, and it is estimated that by 1955 over 40,000 had been done in the United States. Freeman, a nonsurgeon, alone performed or supervised over 3,500 operations in 19 states and 10 foreign countries ("Use of Psychosurgery," 1977). The indications were broad, including almost any patient confined to an institution, predominantly schizophrenics. While as effective as open craniotomy, the procedure was undertaken at a much greater risk of immediate complications resulting in neurologic sequelae, such as paralysis or epilepsy. Long-term psychological results were often associated with intellectual and emotional changes, such as a withdrawn and flattened affect. However, more patients were able to be discharged from the institutions because of the procedure than previously had been possible (Mettler, 1952; Tow, 1955; Petrie, 1952).

With the introduction of the drug chlorpromazine in 1952, use of psychopharmacologic agents (drugs designed to treat the symptoms of psychiatric illness) ended the era of lobotomies. Chlorpromazine resulted in the sedation of agitated patients and alleviation of psychotic behaviors, such that patients could be managed better both in and out of institutions. In the 1960s, with the advent of antidepressant medication, the number of psychosurgical procedures declined even further. Although they were performed far less frequently, they continued to be used from time to time because of their demonstrated beneficial effects in many intractable patients who were not helped by traditional therapy.

In 1947, Ernest Spiegel and Henry Wycis introduced a technique for precisely locating points or targets within the human brain, thereby allowing destruction of specific tissue with minimal disruption of the surrounding brain (Spiegel and Wycis, 1952). This technique, still the technique of choice, is called stereotaxic surgery. Stereotaxis employs precise calculation of locations within the brain using internal, radiographically determined reference points, thus allowing placement of a probe or beam of radiation with great accuracy. At about the same time, John Fulton reasoned that an optimum site of a lesion to treat psychiatric illness should be located in one quadrant of the frontal lobe and could be quite small. Stereotaxic surgery ushered in the modern era of psychosurgery by making possible treatment of psychiatric disease through very small, precisely located lesions.

As knowledge of the limbic structures became more precise, neurosurgeons began directing their efforts to cutting selected fiber tracts that connected the frontal lobes with specific limbic structures by using stereotaxis. Although surgeons could not specify how destruction of small brain areas worked to alleviate the symptoms of psychiatric disease, it did work. Complications from surgery declined significantly. The safety and efficacy of psychosurgery improved greatly. Stereotaxic psychosurgical technique gained in popularity by the late 1960s, when mental-health professionals recognized that the medications used to treat psychic disease did not help everyone and often had significant side effects.

Psychosurgery suffered a dramatic decline in the United States, similar to that coinciding with the advent of psychotropic medication, beginning in the 1970s. Much criticism was directed at those who were performing psychosurgery by those who viewed it as mutilation of the brain. The most vocal opponent was Peter Breggin (Breggin, 1972). Trained in a tradition that denied the authenticity of mental illness as a disease, he argued vehemently that all surgical treatments mutilated the brain and destroyed function. No scientific data were presented to substantiate his claims, but they did serve to raise public awareness about psychosurgery. The case against psychosurgery was aided by the speculation of Vernon Mark and Frank Ervin that the techniques might be helpful in controlling criminal or violent behavior, thereby raising the specter of political control (Mark and Ervin, 1970).

The debate generated a politically stressful environment, with the most vocal groups being against the treatment. There developed a desire on the part of American psychiatrists and neurosurgeons to avoid controversy over this form of treatment. The result was a dramatic decline in the use of these techniques. Between 1949 and 1952 approximately 5,000 lobotomies were performed each year in the United States, largely by itinerant physicians lacking neurosurgical training. The commission established by Congress to investigate psychosurgery estimated that in 1971 and 1972, 140 neurosurgeons had performed a total of approximately 400 to 500 operations a year ("Use of Psychosurgery," 1977). In 1987, Harvard University neurosurgeon Thomas Ballantine reported on a group of 474 psychosurgical patients treated over the previous 25 years (about 18 per year); most procedures had occurred in the late 1960s and early 1970s (Ballantine and Giriunas, 1988). More specific reports from which the current incidence of psychosurgical procedures in the United States might be calculated are lacking.

Current safety and effectiveness

Psychosurgery, in spite of declining frequency due to nonmedical reasons, benefited from the more precise definition and understanding of the types of patients who were likely to be helped by this surgery. This process occurred simultaneously with the development of psychosurgery, as psychiatry made advances in the understanding of mental illness. One important consideration is consent to treatment. Informed consent for mentally ill patients may be possible if the impairment does not extend to rendering the patient "incompetent" in the legal sense. But whether a mentally ill or incarcerated person can ever give a voluntary informed consent is doubtful as mental competence and autonomy are such arbitrary notions. The integrity of the physician is the most effective guarantee of a patient's rights.

Currently, in selecting who should be treated, an appropriate psychiatric diagnosis is required, revealed in symptoms amenable to relief by psychosurgery. These include chronically and severely depressed individuals with a preexisting history of obsessive-compulsive personality traits; chronically anxious patients whose psychic pain is incapacitating; and increasingly incapacitating obsessive-compulsive neuroses associated with depression. All other treatments deemed appropriate for the diagnosis, including the use of appropriate doses of psychopharmacologic medication, should be tried before psychosurgery is contemplated. Incapacity produced by the illness should be disabling and persistent. There should be no contraindications, either physical or mental, to the performance of the procedure.

Technique

Modern stereotaxic psychosurgery consists of producing lesions by heating electrodes in the target areas to coagulate the tissue or, more recently, by the destruction of a target area by focused radiation utilizing either a linear accelerator radiation source or a focusable cobalt radiation source known as the gamma knife. Either technique requires placing the patient into a head frame fixed to the skull with pins inserted under local anesthesia. Some type of imaging—magnetic resonance scanning, computed tomographic scanning, or the introduction of air into the fluid space of the brain for contrast and using radiographs (ventriculography)—defines the target within the brain. When heat is used, a burr hole is placed through the skull over the target area and a probe is introduced into the target. A radio frequency current is applied to the probe and the lesion is produced. The production of the lesion is painless. The radiation lesion technique requires no opening of the skull. The patient is transported to the instrument used and is exposed to a focused beam of radiation. This also is painless. Following the production of the lesion, the patient is returned to the hospital room and usually discharged the following day. The onset of the effects of the heat lesion is virtually immediate, while the radiation may take as long as six months to produce the final result. Both lesions are irreversible.

Targets

Primarily four areas of the limbic system are currently utilized as targets. The procedures, named for the target areas, are cingulotomy, subcaudate tractotomy, limbic leucotomy, and amygdalotomy. Cingulotomy places the lesion in the cingulate gyrus of the brain, located on the inside of the frontal lobes. One or both of these structures may be lesioned, primarily for relief of depression and/or obsession; the procedure has a reported 75 percent recovered or markedly improved result in depression and 56 percent in obsession. Subcaudate tractotomy is performed just below the nucleus of the brain, called the caudate nucleus, in the white-matter fiber tracts connecting with frontal lobe structures. The primary indications are depression, anxiety, and obsession; it has a recovered or improved rate of 68 percent for depression, 63 percent for anxiety, and 53 percent for obsession. Limbic leucotomy is a lesion placed in the white-matter tracts of the frontal lobe connecting to the nucleus called the thalamus. This lesion has been used for depression, anxiety, and obsession, with recovery or improvement in 61 percent for depression, 63 percent for anxiety, and 84 percent for obsession. Amygdalotomy places a lesion in the amygdaloid nucleus of cell bodies located in the temporal lobe and integrally connected to the limbic system structures. Unlike the other targets, amygdalotomy is used primarily for aggression, with a 76 percent markedly improved or recovered outcome (see Maxwell, 1993).

Complications

The incidence of complications for each procedure is extremely low when compared with the morbidity and mortality of the old frontal leucotomy of Freeman and Watts (Mettler, 1952; Tow, 1955; Petrie, 1952). Significant neurologic complications, such as paralysis or epilepsy, and psychological complications, such as persistent behavioral or personality changes, occur in much less than 1 percent of cases (Ballantine and Giriunas, 1982).

The one aspect of the old frontal lobotomy that has remained in the minds of those caring for these patients is the generally placid affect, loss of initiative, and decline in intellectual function that was frequently seen. Reports of neuropsychological studies of patients undergoing modern psychosurgical procedures have indicated no significant damage to higher brain functions such as recognizable personality. Relief of disabling and intractable behavioral symptoms is followed by impressively improved overall function with preservation of personality (Mindus and Jenike, 1992; Bridges, 1990).

However, neuropsychological instruments designed to measure cognition may not be sensitive enough to detect subtle emotional impairments. Currently available methods of testing support the conclusion that limited procedures such as cingulotomy, subcaudate tractotomy, limbic leucotomy, and amygdalotomy result in minimal intellectual and cognitive changes for the patient while reducing disabling symptoms such as depression.

Issues of patient selection

In the 1970s, when violence in the ghettos was a concern, accusations were made by some political activists, black and white, that psychosurgery was being used as a tool of the establishment to exercise political and social control, specifically of minorities and women (Mason, 1973; Carver, 1973). These accusations arose from publicity regarding proposed but never undertaken research projects, to be supported by federal funds, that focused on the psychosurgical treatment of irrational and spontaneously violent behavior arising from epilepsy in the limbic system. In addition, the issue of social control and racism in the application of psychosurgery became public when, with the establishment in Los Angeles of a Center for the Prevention of Violence, one of the researchers who had proposed a study of psychosurgery and violence joined the staff. At about this time, reports of psychosurgery performed on black patients in Mississippi were published (Andy and Jurko, 1972). These were institutionalized, severely disturbed, mentally retarded children; the neurosurgeon defended the practice on the basis that the psychosurgery was indicated medically as a treatment of last resort, and that the preponderance of black patients reflected the composition of the total patient group and not prejudice. There were those in the psychiatric community who felt that the levels of psychiatric care, the availability of qualified staff, and the availability of alternative treatment in this facility were below even minimal standards, thus calling into question the use of psychosurgery. The possibility of de facto racism existed.

No reliable evidence to support charges of intentional racism in the use of psychosurgery has been presented. There is no case of a responsible individual or group claiming that psychosurgery has actually been used for purposes of political action, social control, or acting out of personal prejudices against minority groups or women. However, there are no reliable data with respect to the incidence of psychosurgery performed on whites or blacks, males or females; and such reports as are available give no support to the charge that minority groups of any category have been subjected to operations specifically on the basis of membership in such a group.

With respect to legally committed or otherwise involuntarily institutionalized patients, the issue of valid or proxy consent is a difficult one. However, it is generally acknowledged that there are some patients in this category who may benefit from psychosurgical procedures. As issues of autonomy versus community are studied and elaborated, new ethical grounds for consent in this population should arise (Beauchamp et al., 1994).

Conclusion

There is substantial evidence that current stereotaxic techniques, involving smaller, more discrete lesions in the brain, avoid the unwanted outcomes seen in many patients treated by earlier psychosurgical procedures. In addition, there is sufficient evidence that certain procedures do offer potential benefit to the patient who has failed to respond to other known therapies. These procedures do not appear to produce adverse psychological changes.

JOHN C. OAKLEY

Directly related to this article is the companion article in this entry: ETHICAL ASPECTS. *Also directly related are the entries* ELECTROCONVULSIVE THERAPY; INFORMED CONSENT, *article on* ISSUES OF CONSENT IN MENTAL-HEALTH CARE; MENTAL HEALTH, *article on* MEANING OF MENTAL HEALTH; MENTAL-HEALTH THERAPIES; MENTAL ILLNESS, *article on* CONCEPTIONS OF MENTAL ILLNESS; MENTALLY DISABLED AND MENTALLY ILL PERSONS, *articles on* HEALTH-CARE ISSUES, *and* RESEARCH ISSUES; *and* PATIENTS' RIGHTS, *article on* MENTAL PATIENTS' RIGHTS. *For a further discussion of topics mentioned in this article, see the entries* HARM; HEALTH AND DISEASE, *article on* PHILOSOPHICAL PERSPECTIVES; RESEARCH, UNETHICAL; RESEARCH POLICY, *article on* RISK AND VULNERABLE GROUPS. *Other relevant material may be found under the entries* ALTERNATIVE THERAPIES; COMMITMENT TO MENTAL INSTITUTIONS; DIVIDED LOYALTIES IN MENTAL-HEALTH CARE; MENTAL-HEALTH SERVICES; *and* PSYCHIATRY, ABUSES OF.

Bibliography

ANDY, ORLANDO J., and JURKO, MARION F. 1972. "Thalamotomy for Hyperresponsive Syndrome: Lesions in the Centermedian and Intralaminar Nuclei." In *Psychosurgery: Proceedings of the Second International Conference on Psychosurgery*, pp. 127–135. Edited by Edward Robert Hitchcock, Lauri Laitinen, and Kjeld Vaernet. Springfield, Ill.: Charles C. Thomas.

BALLANTINE, H. THOMAS, and GIRIUNAS, IDA E. 1988. "Treatment of Intractable Psychiatric Illness and Chronic Pain by Stereotactic Cingulotomy." In vol. 2 of *Operative Neurosurgical Techniques: Indications, Methods, and Results*, 2d ed., pp. 1069–1075. Edited by Henry H. Schmidek and William Herbert Sweet. Philadelphia: Saunders.

BEAUCHAMP, TOM L.; BOK, SISSELA; VEATCH, ROBERT M.; and DRESSER, REBECCA. 1994. "Public and Private: Redrawing Boundaries." *Hastings Center Report* (May/June): 18–22.

BREGGIN, PETER K. 1972a. "Psychosurgery for the Control of Violence." *Congressional Record*, 92d Cong., 2d sess., 118, pt. 9:11396–11402.

———. 1972b. "The Return of Lobotomy and Psychosurgery." *Congressional Record*, 118, pt. 5:5567–5577.

BRIDGES, PAUL. 1990. "Psychosurgery Revisited." *Journal of Neuropsychiatry and Clinical Neuroscience* 2, no. 3:326–331.

CARVER, JAMES. 1973. "Psychosurgery: A Matter of Class and Racial Oppression." *Daily World* (New York), October 10.

FREEMAN, WALTER, and WATTS, JAMES W. 1950. *Psychosurgery in the Treatment of Mental Disorders and Intractable Pain*. 2d ed. Springfield, Ill.: Charles C. Thomas.

FULTON, JOHN. 1942. *Physiology of the Nervous System*. New York: Oxford University Press.

———. 1951. *Frontal Lobotomy and Affective Behavior: A Neurophysical Analysis*. New York: W. W. Norton.

FULTON, JOHN, and JACOBSEN, CARLYLE. 1935. "The Functions of the Frontal Lobes; A Comparative Study in Monkeys, Chimpanzees and Man." *Advances in Modern Biology* 4:113–123.

MARK, VERNON H., and ERVIN, FRANK R. 1970. *Violence and the Brain*. New York: Harper & Row.

MASON, B. J. 1973. "Brain Surgery to Control Behavior." *Ebony*, February, pp. 62–64, 76.

MAXWELL, ROBERT E. 1993. "Behavioral Modification." In vol. 2 of *Brain Surgery: Complication Avoidance and Management*, pp. 1557–1565. Edited by Michael L. J. Apuzzo. New York: Churchill Livingstone.

METTLER, FRED A., ed. 1952. *Psychosurgical Problem*. Philadelphia: Blakiston. Early attempt to assess the effects of several procedures, including transorbital lobotomy, performed in the United States.

MINDUS, PER, and JENIKE, MICHAEL A. 1992. "Neurosurgical Treatment of Malignant Obsessive Compulsive Disorder." *Psychiatric Clinics of North America* 15, no. 4:921–938.

MONIZ, EGAS. 1936. *Tentatives opératoires dans le traitement de certaines psychoses*. Paris: Masson.

NATIONAL COMMISSION FOR THE PROTECTION OF HUMAN SUBJECTS OF BIOMEDICAL AND BEHAVIORAL RESEARCH. 1977. "Use of Psychosurgery in Practice and Research." *Federal Register* 42, no. 99:26318–26332.

PAVLOV, IVAN. 1928. *Lectures on Conditional Reflexes*. New York: International Publishing.

PETRIE, ASENATH. 1952. *Personality and the Frontal Lobes: An Investigation of the Psychological Effects of Different Types of Leucotomy*. London: Routledge & Kegan Paul. Early assessment of the effects of the classic leucotomy on intellect, humor, and temperament.

SPIEGEL, ERNEST A., and WYCIS, HENRY T. 1952. *Stereoencephalotomy: Thalamotomy and Related Procedures*. New York: Grune and Stratton.

TOW, PETER MACDONALD. 1955. *Personality Changes Following Frontal Leucotomy: A Clinical and Experimental Study of the Functions of the Frontal Lobe in Man*. London: Oxford University Press. History of the early research on frontal lobe function and the results of a study of its effects on personality.

"Use of Psychosurgery in Practice and Research: Report and Recommendations of the National Commission for the Protection of Human Subjects of Biomedical and Behavioral Research." 1977. *Federal Register* 42, no. 99 (May 23):26318–26332.

VALENSTEIN, ELLIOT S. 1986. *Great and Desperate Cure: The Rise and Decline of Psychosurgery and Other Radical Treatments for Mental Illness*. New York: Basic Books.

II. ETHICAL ASPECTS

As long as patients with problems of feeling, thinking, and behavior are assumed to be capable of making a free and informed decision on the question of a brain operation intended to improve some aspect of their mental state, there is no logical reason to object to such treatment. Ethical and legal problems regarding psychosurgery should arise primarily because of issues relating to consent to treatment, about which there certainly can be argument.

The peculiar problem of psychosurgery arises in part because the organ, the brain, which is the instrument of consent, is also understood to be the source of the disability that requires cure. In itself, this is scarcely an objection. Perhaps no one gives a second thought to the specific justification for obtaining consent to the removal of a brain tumor, even if the patient is confused and a proxy consent is necessary. In contrast, it is plausible that much of the hesitation and obstruction that attend discussions of consent to psychosurgery are based upon unwillingness to view mental illness in the same way as physical illness. Frequently, equality of treatment is denied for all sorts of psychological illness compared with physical illness, as can be seen in numerous insurance policies. With respect to psychosurgery, there is concern that informed consent must depend upon the adequate function of a large part or wide area of the brain, and there is a valid fear that such function is liable to be absent in those to whom the operation is offered.

Even more aptly, it may be supposed that the effect to be abolished is a prime source of virtue, so that if leukotomy (cutting the white matter) abates guilt it may also impair admirable features of the personality. While there can be sympathy with some of these concerns, they are judgmental questions for which practical answers can be demanded. They ought not to operate as a priori justifications for refusing practical treatment to anyone. Sometimes there are practical problems in ensuring that the consent of a particular patient to a particular procedure is genuinely free. Nevertheless, psychosurgery has attracted enough hostile comment from various quarters to lead to the creation of a National

Commission in the United States to look into the topic and related issues after "Widespread expression of public and congressional concern . . . including allegations that these procedures were . . . being used for 'Social Control' of dissidents and violence-prone individuals and . . . were performed disproportionately on members of minority populations" (U.S. Department of Health, Education and Welfare, 1978, p. 53242). Thus, we have to look at the ethical issues against a historical background of success.

The commission demonstrated that there was no substance in the claims being made. For example, only 100 procedures meeting the definition of psychosurgery were being performed annually in the United States in the years leading up to 1977. It also determined that no significant psychological deficits were attributable to the psychosurgery undertaken; that the treatment was efficacious in more than half of the case studies; that there was no evidence that the procedure had been used for psychosocial control; and that only a few operations were conducted on minority or disadvantaged populations. Correspondence with the most active psychosurgeons in the United States revealed that out of 600 patients, only one was black, two were Asian, and six were Hispanic Americans. Between 1970 and 1980 only seven operations were reported to have been performed on children, and only three prisoners underwent psychosurgery. In fact, psychosurgery was largely limited to middle-class individuals. English investigators showed in a cohort of patients from a defined population that psychosurgery provided valuable benefits for a selected small group, particularly those with depression, agoraphobia, obsessional neurosis, and certain aspects of schizophrenia (Hussain et al., 1988).

The ethical aspects of psychosurgery have to do with the conditions under which it is offered.

Axioms and rules

In psychiatric practice, there are some common axioms and some derivative rules. The following may apply to psychosurgery (Merskey, 1991):

1. Ordinarily, medical advice is just advice and the patent is not obliged to follow it. Even the imposition of treatment to save life (e.g., surgical operations for kidney disease or cancer) is only ethically and legally permissible if the patient consents.
2. Children and others in a condition that precludes them from deciding rationally may have decisions made for them by people, usually their next of kin, who have appropriate concern for their interests and welfare.
3. Special care is needed when decisions are made for children and other incompetent persons. Careful scrutiny of the status and motives of the person who makes the decision for the patient is necessary. Given that care, treatment can be ethically undertaken.
4. Ethical actions may or may not be sanctioned by law. The legality of a physician's conduct is a separate issue from its ethical basis.
5. Coercive treatments for the benefit of a third party are unethical and health-care professionals should not use behavior modification, drugs, or lobotomy against an individual's wishes to prevent him or her from hurting someone else.
6. Likewise, coercive treatment for the benefit of society rather than the patient is repugnant to ethical physicians.
7. Patients may consent to treatment that benefits either themselves or others, but there are peculiar difficulties in confirming the presence of free consent in some circumstances, particularly with prisoners.

Overall, the critical issue for the physician is to recognize whether the problem receiving attention is one that is seen by the patient as needing treatment or whether it is seen by others as requiring treatment in the patient's interest. The relationship of physicians to patients is principally based on an implicit contract that the physician will care for the patient provided that the physician is not expected to violate the legal and ethical interests of other people in order to provide that care (Merskey, 1986). Given these presuppositions, the issues surrounding brain surgery can be considered with and without consent in mind.

Brain surgery with consent

The easiest case in which to accept the validity of leukotomy is the relief of severe depression. While leukotomy and related operations such as cingulotomy (destruction of a part of the medial portion of the cerebral hemispheres) are now rarely required for this purpose, a patient with this protracted and life-threatening condition may wish to undergo a surgical operation with relatively small risk in order to relieve the condition. Prior to the introduction of physical methods of treatment, there was a high death rate in patients with severe depression (Huston and Locher, 1948).

When leukotomy was more common in the 1950s and 1960s, a written agreement might not have been obtained—schizophrenic patients are notoriously unwilling to sign documents—but the patient was not actively opposed. Relatives would support the procedure and, at least in Britain, the relatives' consent was accepted as legally sufficient. A large number of chronic schizophrenic patients in some countries were submitted to bilateral standard leukotomy operations under the above conditions. If operations failed to relieve fully the schizophrenic illness, at least they reduced agitation or aggressive outbursts and produced a more manageable state in some extremely disturbed patients. Was this process used for "social control?" The available options included locked or padded rooms and physical restraint. Though most psychiatrists did not regard these options favorably, leukotomy operations were not necessarily undertaken to provide otherwise unattainable control but rather to provide the patient with a quieter and easier life. If the patient did not object, and if he or she was substantially disturbed and likely to benefit from the operation, there could be no reasonable objection to such treatment, given the consent of those most likely to have the patient's best interests at heart. It remains the case that such treatment is still appropriate in the same circumstances.

In addition to the treatment of depression and schizophrenia, stereotactic neurosurgical operations—especially amygdaloidotomy (the amygdala being the grey matter of the brain's frontal lobe)—have been used for the control of aggression, which may be against the patient's own self or directed at others (Kiloh et al., 1974). These are anatomically precise operations performed with the help of X-ray measurements of the skull. For a number of chronic self-mutilators, such an operation was sometimes considered. The recent availability and relatively specific effect of serotonin reuptake inhibitor drugs have eased many patients who were prone to self-damage. The interesting fact that medication might produce such a radical change in self-harm means that the idea of a surgical operation when medication fails can be seen as a logical and reasonable effort to modify an aberrant portion of the brain. Many patients with such tendencies are not intellectually retarded and have no organic brain damage. Yet the fact that most of them can respond to an antidepressant, while others need more radical treatment, suggests that psychosurgery still has a role to play for a few patients.

Psychosurgery for individuals who are dangerous only to others but who might be willing to consent is the most difficult issue in this field. If the patient can consent, one might ask why he or she should not be allowed the treatment? This problem is exemplified by the 1973 case of Kaimowitz v. Department of Mental Health. A patient who had behaved aggressively, but was a prisoner, consented to treatment but was refused it on the grounds that his consent in prison could not be truly free. The patient, who had spent 18 years in prison for murder, had satisfied an "informed consent" review committee comprising a law professor, a priest, and an accountant that he wanted the operation. A suit was brought by an attorney, Kaimowitz, and others belonging to a medical committee for human rights who had never consulted the prisoner. The lawyer appointed by the courts to represent the prisoner thought that the prisoner desperately wanted the operation. Coinciden-

tally, the prisoner's appointed lawyer satisfied the court that his client was held unconstitutionally as a prisoner. He went free, but the discussion continued on the question of whether as a prisoner, he had given free informed consent to psychiatric surgery. The court held that he could not have. Once the prisoner was released, he changed his mind about wanting the operation. According to Robert A. Burt (1975), imprisonment and medical surveillance at least contributed to the prisoner's consent without any attempt having been made by physicians to press the prisoner to agree. Some commentators have argued that no prisoner's consent should be accepted for psychosurgery if its purpose is to alter the type of behavior that caused imprisonment. To guard against the possibility that a prisoner might be deprived of the right to medical care, some framework ought to be contemplated that would provide for exceptions. Exceptions would include independent professional examination of the individual's motives as well as separation of the question of release from the outcome of the operation.

Incompetent patients

Certain incompetent patients might undergo surgery provided that it can be demonstrated that the action is not against their wishes. This would apply particularly to schizophrenic patients, who might accept a surgical operation but would never be able to comprehend or fill out a form requiring them to indicate informed consent. Patients should not undergo surgery if they give the merest hint of refusal.

Children with significant brain damage may benefit from psychosurgery, not so much to treat epilepsy caused by the brain damage as for the reduction of aggressive behavior against either themselves or others (Balasubramaniam and Kanaka, 1975). If the interests of the child are paramount, then the child should not be deprived of the possibility of beneficial surgery, even though he or she is either unable to consent or appears hostile to almost any physical intervention by nursing staff or attendants. This would apply both to patients who gravely damage themselves—and sometimes have been kept for weeks or months in canvas clothing to protect themselves from such inquiry—and to patients who, while retarded and clearly incompetent, attack others if allowed the minimum opportunity for human contact. Such a patient also may benefit if a paternalistic approach to treatment is recognized, acknowledged, and followed.

Notwithstanding, there is no justification for the forcible use of psychosurgery with individuals who are thought to be political prisoners by the family, the patient's proxies, the treating doctor, or indeed any rational contemporary.

In summary, psychosurgery should never be forced, but it might be performed on noncompetent individuals or prisoners without their formal consent, subject to stringent safeguards that require extensive consideration.

HAROLD MERSKEY

Directly related to this article is the companion article in this entry: MEDICAL AND HISTORICAL ASPECTS. *Also directly related are the entries* AUTONOMY; BENEFICENCE; COMPETENCE; PATERNALISM; INFORMED CONSENT, *article on* ISSUES OF CONSENT IN MENTAL-HEALTH CARE; PATIENTS' RIGHTS, *article on* MENTAL PATIENTS' RIGHTS; MENTAL ILLNESS, *article on* CONCEPTIONS OF MENTAL ILLNESS; *and* MENTAL-HEALTH THERAPIES. *For a further discussion of topics mentioned in this article, see the entries* HARM; MENTAL HEALTH, *article on* MEANING OF MENTAL HEALTH; MENTALLY DISABLED AND MENTALLY ILL PERSONS; *and* RESEARCH POLICY, *article on* RISK AND VULNERABLE GROUPS. *Other relevant material may be found under the entries* ALTERNATIVE THERAPIES; COMMITMENT TO MENTAL INSTITUTIONS; DIVIDED LOYALTIES IN MENTAL-HEALTH CARE; ELECTROCONVULSIVE THERAPY; HEALTH AND DISEASE, *article on* PHILOSOPHICAL PERSPECTIVES; MENTAL-HEALTH SERVICES; *and* PSYCHIATRY, ABUSES OF.

Bibliography

BALASUBRAMANIAM, V., and KANAKA, T. S. 1975. "Amygdalotomy and Hypothalamotomy—A Comparative Study." *Confinia Neurologica* 37, nos. 1–3:195–201.

BURT, ROBERT A. 1975. "Why We Should Keep Prisoners from the Doctors." *Hastings Center Report* 5, no. 1:25–34.

FABREGA, HORACIO, JR. 1974. *Disease and Social Behavior: An Interdisciplinary Perspective.* Cambridge, Mass.: MIT Press.

GREENBLATT, STEVEN JAY. 1977. "The Ethics and Legality of Psychosurgery." *New York Law School Law Review* 22, no. 4:961–980.

HUSSAIN, E. S.; FREEMAN, H.; and JONES, R. A. C. 1988. "A Cohort Study of Psychosurgery Cases from a Defined Population." *Journal of Neurology, Neurosurgery, and Psychiatry* 51:345–352.

HUSTON, P. E., and LOCHER, L. M. 1948. "Involutional Psychosis: Course When Untreated and When Treated With ECT." *Archives of Neurology and Psychiatry* 59, no. 3: 385–394.

Kaimowitz v. Department of Mental Health. 1973. Cir. Ct., Wayne City, Mich., Civil Action no. 73-19434-AW (10 July). Reprinted in *Operating on the Mind,* by Willard Gaylin, pp. 185–209.

KILOH, LESLIE G.; GYE, R. S.; RUSHWORTH, R. G.; BELL, D. S.; and WHITE, R. T. 1974. "Stereotactic Amygdaloidotomy for Aggressive Behaviour." *Journal of Neurology, Neurosurgery, and Psychiatry* 37:437–444.

MERSKEY, HAROLD. 1986. "Variable Meanings for the Definition of Disease." *Journal of Medicine and Philosophy* 11, no. 3:215–232.

———. 1991. "Ethical Aspects of the Physical Manipulation of the Brain." In *Psychiatric Ethics,* 2d ed, pp. 185–214. Edited by S. Bloch and P. Chodoff. New York: Oxford University Press.

U.S. DEPARTMENT OF HEALTH, EDUCATION AND WELFARE. PUBLIC HEALTH SERVICE. 1978. "Determination of the Secretary Regarding the Recommendation on Psychosurgery of the National Commission for the Protection of Human Subjects of Biomedical and Behavioral Research." *Federal Register* 43, no. 21:53242–53244.

U.S. NATIONAL COMMISSION FOR THE PROTECTION OF HUMAN SUBJECTS OF BIOMEDICAL AND BEHAVIORAL RESEARCH. 1977. *Report and Recommendations: Psychosurgery [and] Appendix.* Washington, D.C.: U.S. Government Printing Office.

PSYCHOTHERAPY

See MENTAL-HEALTH THERAPIES; *and* PSYCHOANALYSIS AND DYNAMIC THERAPIES.

PUBLICATION POLICIES

See COMMUNICATION, BIOMEDICAL, *article on* SCIENTIFIC PUBLISHING; *and* RESEARCH, UNETHICAL. *See also* FRAUD, THEFT, AND PLAGIARISM.

PUBLIC HEALTH

I. Determinants of Public Health
     Lester Breslow
II. History of Public Health
     John Duffy
III. Philosophy of Public Health
     Dan E. Beauchamp
IV. Public-Health Methods: Epidemiology and Biostatistics
     Colin L. Soskolne

I. DETERMINANTS OF PUBLIC HEALTH

The current preoccupation with medical science and its application as the primary determinant of health derives largely from the enormously successful experience with applying microbiology in the battle against ill health. Identification of specific microorganisms as agents of epidemic communicable diseases, and means of controlling them, aroused expectations of finding "magic bullets" for most of humanity's ills. Further discoveries, such as insulin for diabetes and chemicals effective against certain forms of cancer, have encouraged the notion. Using the term "health provider" to mean a physician epitomizes this view.

However, dependence on medicine as the source of health tends to obscure far more fundamental influences on health. For millennia it has been evident that living conditions and the response to them largely determine people's health. Therefore, people have sought to extend life and improve health not only as individuals but also through communal efforts in the societies of which they are a part. These social efforts to enhance the health of whole populations have come to be called public health, "what we, as a society, do collectively to assure the conditions in which people can be healthy" (Institute of Medicine, 1988, p. 1). In modern times government plays the leading role in this endeavor, supplemented by other endeavors organized to advance the health of the public. Making medical services available to people is only one way in which modern industrialized societies address health challenges; other measures include assuring a healthful environment and encouraging healthful behavior by individuals. To carry out its mission, public health must establish effective linkage with other efforts for social advancement, particularly in welfare and education.

Public health measures its progress by the health status of the population it serves. Thus, knowing the determinants of the public's health (which is also known as public health) is essential to the field.

Advances in health, 1800–2000

The period since 1800 has brought the most spectacular health improvement in human history. From the time of the hunter-gatherers thousands of years ago until the industrial revolution around 1800, Mark Cohen estimates that life expectancy at birth ranged consistently between twenty and fifty years, most commonly about twenty-five to thirty years (Cohen, 1989). At the end of the twentieth century, life expectancy exceeds sixty-five years in most parts of the world and seventy-five years in western Europe, North America, and Japan.

In the United States, for example, life expectancy was only forty-seven years when the twentieth century began. By the late 1980s it had reached seventy-five years, according to the National Center for Health Statistics (1990). To a considerable extent that advance was due to declining infant mortality, from more than 100 per 1,000 in 1900 to less than 10 per 1,000 in the late 1980s, and to the control of communicable diseases, which take their major toll during the early years of life. Since 1960, however, relatively greater extension of life has occurred in the later years. From 1900 to 1960 life expectancy at birth increased twenty-two years, but only one-tenth of that expansion came after age sixty-five. Since 1960, on the other hand, more than half of the five years gained in life expectancy at birth have come beyond age sixty-five.

Table 1 lists specific diseases, and their trends, that have affected residents of the United States since 1900. Medical students in the early 1900s learned about pneumonia as "the old man's friend" and tuberculosis as "the Captain of the Men of Death." Heart disease at the start of the century largely came from rheumatic fever, whereas now atherosclerosis accounts overwhelmingly for heart disease. Population aging considerably influences death rates from cancer and heart disease. Even when adjusted for age, however, cancer mortality has been increasing, mainly because of the twentieth-century epidemic of lung cancer. A rare form of the disease in 1900, respiratory cancer increased to constitute about one-tenth of all cancer deaths in 1950 and almost one-third as the century was closing. Other measures of health status, such as survival to age sixty-five, reveal

TABLE 1. Crude Death Rates per 100,000, Selected Causes, U.S. Registration Area, 1900–1988

Cause of Death	1900	1920	1940	1970	1980	1988
Pneumonia	153	82	25	31	24	32
Tuberculosis	94	113	46	3	1	1
Diphtheria	40	15	1			
Organic heart disease	123	151	296	362	336	312
Cancer	64	83	125	163	184	199
Diabetes	11	16	27	19	15	16

Sources: Forrest E. Linder and Robert D. Grove, *Vital Statistics Rates in the United States, 1900–1940* (Washington, D.C.: U.S. Government Printing Office, 1943), quoted; Edward J. Stieglitz, *A Future for Preventive Medicine* (New York: Commonwealth Fund, 1945); U.S. Bureau of the Census, *Statistical Abstract of the United States, 1990*, 110th ed. (Washington, D.C.: U.S. Dept. of Commerce, Bureau of the Census, 1990).

the role of violence and injury in certain human populations, such as young males in the United States.

Historical determinants of health

Health may be viewed as the human side of a dynamic equilibrium between the organism and its environment; that interface is the place where health is mainly determined.

The genetic structure with which humans enter the world will generally allow survival for about eighty-five years, according to James Fries (1980). In some people, of course, hereditary abnormalities interfere with and/or shorten life, while others live more than eighty-five years in reasonably good health. Beyond these biological influences, since food and oxygen are the most critical elements for human life and since oxygen is only rarely inadequate, nutrition constitutes a paramount factor in health. From earliest times to the present, inadequate food has been a major threat to health. In fact, society has evolved largely to supply enough food for people—for example, through migration and the development of agriculture.

Not infrequently, however, huge numbers of people have been trapped in starvation through ecological and social catastrophes—both in ancient times and more recently, as in the Irish potato blight of the late 1840s and in slavery in the United States, and now in certain African nations and among the homeless in America. Moreover, beyond gross lack of calories, deficiencies of vitamins and other micronutrients cause incalculable damage to health—incalculable because scurvy, rickets, and pellagra may be only the most striking clinical manifestations of severe damage to health.

Industrialization, even though it has improved the standard of living in many respects, has also precipitated some devastating health events. In the early 1800s, when people flocked from the countryside to factory towns and cities in search of a better life, they found crowded housing, gross lack of sanitation, and exhausting work (even for children), as well as food deficiencies. These living conditions produced the "crowd" diseases, epidemics spread by intestinal and respiratory discharges that debilitated many people and caused high mortality. Though all segments of society were affected, the poor suffered then, as throughout history, most severely from the adverse conditions.

While medical science has helped in overcoming the communicable disease epidemics since 1800, other factors have been even more important. John and Sonja McKinley have estimated that at most 3.5 percent of the total decline in mortality (from influenza, pneumonia, diphtheria, whooping cough, and poliomyelitis) since 1900 could be ascribed to medical measures (McKinley and McKinley, 1977). Thomas McKeown has demon-strated that medical science barely affected the decline of tuberculosis (McKeown, 1988).

During the twentieth century a constellation of noncommunicable diseases, led by cardiovascular disease and cancer, has supplanted the epidemic communicable diseases as the foremost health problem in industrialized countries (despite the current public attention to AIDS); and increasingly such noncommunicable diseases are affecting the rest of the world. Again, the circumstances of life and the way people behave in them are the major determinants. For example, the first to indulge in excessive calories, fats, cigarettes, and physical inactivity were affluent men, and accordingly they suffered consequent ischemic heart disease first. Poor men—for example, blacks in the United States—only later had considerable access to those relevant factors; their epidemic of ischemic heart disease came later and is persisting longer.

Major current influences on health

Epidemiological studies have delineated key factors in the rise and the start of the decline of twentieth-century noncommunicable diseases. Most noteworthy, in 1964 an advisory committee to the U.S. surgeon general summarized the growing evidence that "Cigarette smoking is causally related to lung cancer in men . . . the most important of the causes of chronic bronchitis in the United States . . . [and is associated with] . . . a higher death rate from coronary artery disease . . ." (U.S. Surgeon General's Advisory Committee, 1964, pp. 31–32).

Studying a sample of the Alameda County, California, population, Nedra Belloc and Lester Breslow demonstrated the strong relationship of seven health practices to health status and subsequent total mortality: eating moderately, sleeping seven to eight hours, using alcohol moderately if at all, not smoking, eating breakfast, not snacking, and having at least moderate physical activity (Belloc and Breslow, 1972). Men who followed all seven health practices enjoyed physical health equal to that of men thirty years younger who reported two or fewer. Forty-five-year-old men who followed none to three of the health practices had a longevity of sixty-seven years; four to five, seventy-three years; and six to seven, seventy-eight years, thus yielding an advantage of eleven years, depending upon health behavior. Lisa Berkman and Lester Breslow reported further that the extent of one's social network likewise substantially predicted physical health status and mortality (Berkman and Breslow, 1983). A 1974 official Canadian document, the LaLonde Report, proposed a health field concept (LaLonde, 1974). According to the latter, four broad elements comprise the health field: human biology, environment, and lifestyle, and health-care organization. Further, the LaLonde Report asserted that

"Improvements in the [social as well as physical] environment and an abatement in the level of risks imposed upon themselves by individuals, taken together, constitute the most promising ways by which further advances can be made."

The growing emphasis on the way people live as an important health factor in the industrial (and postindustrial) world must be considered carefully in relation to social responsibility for lifestyle. Otherwise, that emphasis can properly be termed "victim blaming." A 1952 report to the president of the United States, *Building America's Health,* noted that "Recognition of the significance of individual responsibility for health does not discharge the obligation of a society which is interested in the health of its citizenry. Such recognition, in fact, increases social responsibility for health" (President's Commission on Health Needs of the Nation, 1952, vol. 1, p. 2). As the Ottawa Charter for Health Promotion stated, "Health promotion is the process of enabling people to increase control over and to improve their health. . . . [It] . . . demands coordinated action by all concerned: by governments, by health and other social and economic sectors, by non-governmental and voluntary organizations, by local authorities, by industry, and by the media" (International World Health Organization Conference, 1986, p. 1).

As it becomes clear that we are able to raise life expectancy to some sort of biological limit, it may well be that public health rather than gross national product (GNP) will constitute the criterion for national success. Using public health as a standard for this success would help illuminate how GNP masks the staggering toll of ill health found among low-income or very poor Americans, many of whom, like American Indians or African Americans, have been disproportionately disadvantaged for generations. Achieving that reorientation of values will require a new approach to the food, alcohol, tobacco, medical, and other industries whose products and services are pertinent to health. Health ethics now entails concern for issues beyond matters in which the physician–patient relationship predominates. How to deal effectively with the "right" to addict young people throughout the world to tobacco and to expose others to one's intoxicated behavior, and similar public-health issues, are coming to the fore. Social action reflecting experience and thought concerning such questions will determine health in the future, just as assuring safe water and milk determined health in the past.

LESTER BRESLOW

Directly related to this article are the other articles in this entry: HISTORY OF PUBLIC HEALTH, PHILOSOPHY OF PUBLIC HEALTH, *and* PUBLIC-HEALTH METHODS: EPIDEMIOLOGY AND BIOSTATISTICS. *Also directly related are* the entries LIFESTYLES AND PUBLIC HEALTH; PUBLIC HEALTH AND THE LAW; HEALTH PROMOTION AND HEALTH EDUCATION; HEALTH SCREENING AND TESTING IN THE PUBLIC-HEALTH CONTEXT; INJURY AND INJURY CONTROL; INTERNATIONAL HEALTH; *and* WARFARE, *article on* PUBLIC HEALTH AND WAR. *For a further discussion of topics mentioned in this article, see the entries* AGING AND THE AGED, *article on* LIFE EXPECTANCY AND LIFE SPAN; EPIDEMICS; FOOD POLICY; *and* RESPONSIBILITY. *This article will find application in the entries* ABUSE, INTERPERSONAL; AGRICULTURE; AIDS; HAZARDOUS WASTES AND TOXIC SUBSTANCES; HOMICIDE; MENTAL-HEALTH SERVICES; OCCUPATIONAL SAFETY AND HEALTH; PROSTITUTION; SEXUALITY IN SOCIETY, *article on* SOCIAL CONTROL OF SEXUAL BEHAVIOR; *and* SUBSTANCE ABUSE, *article on* ALCOHOL AND OTHER DRUGS IN A PUBLIC-HEALTH CONTEXT. *Other relevant material may be found under the entries* HEALTH AND DISEASE, *article on* HISTORY OF THE CONCEPTS; HEALTH POLICY, *article on* POLITICS AND HEALTH CARE; JUSTICE; *and* SOCIAL MEDICINE.

Bibliography

BELLOC, NEDRA B., and BRESLOW, LESTER. 1972. "Relationship of Physical Health Status and Health Practices." *Preventive Medicine* 1, no. 3:409–421.

BERKMAN, LISA L., and BRESLOW, LESTER. 1983. *Health and Ways of Living: The Alameda County Study.* New York: Oxford University Press.

COHEN, MARK N. 1989. *Health and the Rise of Civilization.* New Haven, Conn.: Yale University Press.

FRIES, JAMES. 1980. "Aging, Natural Death, and the Compression of Morbidity." *New England Journal of Medicine* 303, no. 3: 130–135.

INSTITUTE OF MEDICINE (U.S.). COMMITTEE FOR THE STUDY OF THE FUTURE OF PUBLIC HEALTH. 1988. *The Future of Public Health.* Washington, D.C.: National Academy of Sciences.

INTERNATIONAL WORLD HEALTH ORGANIZATION CONFERENCE ON HEALTH PROMOTION. 1986. *Ottawa Charter for Health Promotion.* Ottawa: Author. Sponsored by WHO, Health and Welfare Canada, and Canadian Public Health Association.

LALONDE, MARC. 1974. *A New Perspective on the Health of Canadians: A Working Document.* Ottawa: Government of Canada.

McKEOWN, THOMAS. 1988. *The Origins of Human Disease.* Oxford: Basil Blackwell.

McKINLEY, JOHN B., and McKINLEY, SONJA M. 1977. "The Questionable Contribution of Medical Measures to the Decline of Mortality in the United States in the Twentieth Century." *Milbank Memorial Fund Quarterly* 55, no. 3:405–428.

U.S. DEPARTMENT OF HEALTH AND HUMAN SERVICES. PUBLIC HEALTH SERVICE. CENTERS FOR DISEASE CONTROL and NATIONAL CENTER FOR HEALTH STATISTICS. 1991.

Health, United States, 1990. Hyattsville, Md.: Author.

U.S. PRESIDENT'S COMMISSION ON HEALTH NEEDS OF THE NATION. 1952. *Building America's Health.* 5 vols. Washington, D.C.: U.S. Government Printing Office.

U.S. SURGEON GENERAL'S ADVISORY COMMITTEE ON SMOKING AND HEALTH. 1964. *Smoking and Health: Report.* Public Health Service Pub. no. 1103. Washington, D.C.: U.S. Government Printing Office.

II. HISTORY OF PUBLIC HEALTH

Public health may be defined as the collective action by a community or society to protect and promote the health and welfare of its members. In a world where sickness and accidents were attributed to spirits, the welfare of the tribe and its individual members depended upon paying proper homage to the spiritual realm. Since public-health measures are based upon the level of existing medical knowledge or prevailing assumptions, the observance of taboos and rituals by early tribal societies represents a form of public health. The origins of modern public health lie in efforts to prevent pestilential diseases, but in the past centuries public health has broadened its aims and now applies the findings of social and scientific fields to promoting physical and mental well-being.

Public health in its modern sense arose as a phenomenon of urbanization. As towns and cities emerged, communal living created special problems relating to food, water, sanitation, and disease. In an urban environment, the responsibility for providing safe food and water and disposing of garbage and human wastes could no longer be left to individual initiative, and what were essentially public-health regulations appeared. Both health and aesthetics supplied the motive for these early sanitary regulations, since foul odors were associated with the miasmic theory of disease, a belief that some obnoxious gaseous substance was the cause of epidemic disease.

The classical civilizations evolved relatively sophisticated public health measures. In the second millennium B.C.E. the Minoans developed elaborate plumbing systems that included flush toilets. The great Roman aqueducts that were built between 312 B.C.E. and about 100 C.E., sections of which still survive, are familiar to all; but what is not so well known is that the Roman water systems, at least the one for Rome, differentiated between water for common use and that for drinking. The decline of the Western Roman Empire meant a return to a rural society, and it was not until the rise of towns and cities in the medieval period that public-health measures were reinstituted. The need to live within the town walls for safety intensified crowding and its concomitant sanitary and health problems. In the medieval period fear of two horrible diseases, leprosy and bubonic plague (the Black Death), was responsible for the practice of isolating the sick and instituting quarantines to keep the sickness at bay. Victims of leprosy were literally read out of society, and the first quarantine laws appeared in 1348 in response to the spread of the Black Death.

The late Renaissance and early modern period witnessed two developments that helped pave the way for the institutionalization of public health. The first of these was the concept of mercantilism, which, among other factors, counted population as a source of a nation's wealth. The second was the development of what was termed political arithmetic. Morbidity and mortality statistics are basic to understanding the health of a population and to determining health policy. Two Englishmen, William Petty (1623–1687) and John Graunt (1620–1674), were among the first to recognize this need. They urged the collection of statistics pertaining to health and social matters in order to promote a more healthy and productive population. The astronomer Edmund Halley in 1693 published a life expectancy table that made possible the first life insurance company. Later, life and industrial insurance companies in the United States were to play a role in promoting public health.

John Locke (1632–1704) in 1690 published his classic treatise, *Essay on Human Understanding,* in which he asserted that human beings were the product of their environment. By applying intelligence to social problems and creating a better society, it would be possible to improve humankind. The French philosophers Denis Diderot, Jean Le Rond d'Alembert, Voltaire, and Jean-Jacques Rousseau carried the idea even further by assuming the perfectibility of humanity. Joining this assumption to the mercantilist principle that a growing and healthy population strengthened the power of the state, the "benevolent despots" of the eighteenth century sought to impose public-health measures by fiat. This form of public health, in which administrators issued decrees relating to health and sanitation, was called "medical police" or medical policy; and its leading exponent was Johann Peter Frank, whose six-volume *Complete System of Medical Policy* (1779–1817) dealt with virtually all aspects of public health, from sanitation to the health of workers.

In Britain, the Civil War and the Glorious Revolution of 1688 had made the British people suspicious of the central government; consequently, much administration was kept at the local level. As in the United States, the major impulse for public-health reform came in the nineteenth century and was led by middle-class reformers motivated by a mixture of Christian benevolence, humanitarianism, and rationalism. The dislocations resulting from economic changes in the eighteenth and early nineteenth centuries created a large impoverished class and led to efforts by humanitarians to reduce the enormous mortality among infants, to alleviate the suffering of prisoners and the insane, and to fight against widespread alcoholism among the working class.

By the early nineteenth century, the industrial revolution was drawing thousands of workers from rural areas into crowded city slums, compounding the growing urban sanitary problems. In Britain, the harsh conditions of the poorly paid men, women, and children working long hours in the newly spawned factories and mills came to the attention of several humane individuals, and, under the leadership of Lord Ashley, a series of factory acts was enacted. The first of these, passed in 1833, restricted the working hours of children below the age of eighteen to twelve per day and sixty-nine per week. In the legislative battle for this law, parliamentary hearings drew attention to the atrocious living conditions of the workers and their high rates of sickness and death. The hearings also showed that the excessive use of alcohol and opium was a means of escape for workers condemned to lifelong toil in a brutalizing environment.

Meanwhile, the physicians C. Turner Thackrah, James Philips Kay, Thomas Southwood Smith, and Neil Arnott were drawing attention to the need for health reform. They were fortunate in enlisting Edwin Chadwick (1801–1890) in their cause. Chadwick was a single-minded reformer who dedicated himself to promoting the welfare of the working class. His investigations and reports on behalf of government commissions, culminating in his report for the Health of Towns Commission, were largely responsible for the passage of the Public Health Act of 1848. This measure marks the first step in the institutionalization of public health in the West.

In France the work of Louis René Villerme (1782–1863) roughly paralleled that of Chadwick. Like the latter, his morbidity and mortality statistics demonstrated the close correlation between health and living standards, and led the French government to establish a national public-health advisory committee in 1848. The committee, which included professionals such as physicians, chemists, pharmacists, and veterinarians, was purely an advisory body. Although it dealt with a wide range of public-health issues, from epidemics to industrial health, it was devoid of all powers, and the successive French governments did little to strengthen it during the rest of the century.

The industrial revolution and its concomitant problems arrived late in the United States, but by 1800 cities were beginning to establish temporary boards of health. The chief impetus for these early health agencies came from a series of yellow fever epidemics that struck port cities from South Carolina to New England in the years from 1793 to 1806. These boards were appointed whenever yellow fever threatened or was present. With medical opinion divided as to whether the disease was an imported contagion or the result of a miasma arising from foul, putrefying substances or some other source, the health officials played safe by promptly quarantining incoming vessels and instituting large-scale sanitary programs. Privies were cleaned, dead animals removed from the streets, stagnant pools drained, and slaughterers, tanners, and other members of the "noxious" trades required to cleanse their premises. After 1806 the danger from yellow fever in the region north of Norfolk, Virginia, receded, and health boards virtually disappeared. The appearance in 1832 of the first of three great epidemic waves of Asiatic cholera that swept through the United States revived these temporary boards, but generally they functioned only in times of emergencies.

By the 1830s and 1840s, American cities were beginning to experience the worst aspects of the industrial revolution. Rural Americans and immigrants flooded into urban areas that were ill prepared to handle the influx. Housing and sanitary conditions deteriorated, and morbidity and mortality rose. The movement to remedy these conditions was initiated largely by physicians, most notably by Benjamin W. McCready, whose 1837 essay drew attention to the deplorable health conditions in the workplace and the slums housing the workers, and by John H. Griscom, whose 1845 report, *The Sanitary Condition of the Laboring Population of New York,* laid the basis for establishing the first effective municipal health department in the United States. In other cities, too, physicians led the reform movement: Wilson Jewell in Philadelphia, Edwin Miller Snow in Providence, Edward Jarvis in Boston, and Edward H. Barton and J. C. Simmonds in New Orleans.

The outstanding layman in the early health movement was Lemuel Shattuck of Boston, who pioneered in the collection of vital statistics and promoted sanitary reform. The success of the early reformers in drawing public attention to the need for action led in the 1850s and 1860s to the appearance of civic sanitary organizations and agencies such as the New York Association for Improving the Condition of the Poor. As in England, the public health movement was both a humanitarian and a moral crusade. A few reformers emphasized improving the morals of the poor, but most recognized that immorality and intemperance were closely associated with the crowded and brutally degraded living conditions of the poor.

In 1857, an abortive attempt was made to unite the health reformers at the national level when Wilson Jewell of Philadelphia summoned a national quarantine convention. The original purpose was to respond to the danger from yellow fever, a disease still ravaging southern ports and threatening the Mississippi Valley. In the first meeting the delegates generally agreed on the necessity to standardize state quarantine laws, but many of them felt that the real need was complete sanitary reform. In the following three annual meetings, sentiment among the delegates swung in favor of a program affecting all areas of community health. At the 1860 meeting a resolution was passed suggesting that the delegates form a national health association. The outbreak of the Civil War ended these hopes, and a national organization awaited the postwar years.

Although the Civil War temporarily set back a nationwide organization of public health leaders, it stimulated the health movement. Wartime experiences in army camps and hospitals demonstrated the value of cleanliness and proper food and housing. In addition, the U.S. Sanitary Commission, a civilian body given official status at the outset of the war, introduced thousands of Union soldiers to the principles of personal and public hygiene. Leading members of this commission also played a key role in establishing the New York Metropolitan Board of Health in 1866, an agency that set the pattern for municipal health departments throughout the United States. Four years later, the Massachusetts State Board of Health, the first effective state health agency, came into existence. The founding of the American Public Health Association in 1872 indicated that the institutionalization of public health in the United States was under way.

Until the 1870s, the only action by the federal government relating to health had been the creation of the U.S. Marine Hospital Service in 1798. Although designed to provide medical care for sick sailors, for much of the nineteenth century it served primarily as a form of political patronage. Two yellow fever epidemics, one in 1873 and a major one in 1878 that spread far up the Mississippi River Valley, resulted in the federal government's briefly moving into the area of public health. Responding to widespread alarm, in 1879 Congress established the National Board of Health. The board was given little authority and limited funds, and was expected to act primarily in an advisory capacity. It immediately encountered strong opposition from the U.S. Marine Hospital Service, which was seeking to expand into the health area, and from state and municipal health officials reluctant to surrender any of their authority. The board performed quite well, promoting scientific health studies, assisting local health boards, and encouraging standardization of local quarantine laws. Nonetheless, political pressure led to its demise in 1883. During the nineteenth century Congress voted substantial funds to promote the health of domestic animals and fowls but virtually nothing for human health.

The Progressive movement at the turn of the century promoted political reform, economic efficiency, and social justice and, in the process, gave an impetus to U.S. public health. By the early twentieth century, public health in all developed countries was both professionalized and institutionalized. The bacteriological revolution had provided a new basis for action by health authorities, shifting the emphasis away from sanitation and environmental considerations and toward utilizing the newly developed antitoxins and vaccines to cure and prevent the great epidemic disorders of earlier years. Advances in technology and improvements in civic administration enabled health departments to spin off to separate agencies many former responsibilities, such as street cleaning and garbage removal, inspecting housing, and supervising water supplies and sewage removal. Their place was taken by new concerns: maternal and child care, the health of schoolchildren, the development of laboratory techniques for diagnostic purposes, and the health of people in rural areas. The major gains during the first forty years of the twentieth century were the elimination or drastic reduction of smallpox, measles, diphtheria, scarlet fever, tuberculosis, and other killer diseases.

Until the bacteriological revolution and the advances in basic sciences in the last decades of the nineteenth century, the medical profession, particularly in the United States, was viewed with considerable skepticism. In an effort to improve their status, physicians took an active role in the early public-health movement, and in England and on the Continent they gained control of it. The institutionalization of public health in the United States, however, assumed a different form, in part because the American Public Health Association from its founding in 1872 included sanitary engineers, bacteriologists, and other nonphysician members. In the early twentieth century, as public health moved into the area of school, maternal, and child health, health officials recognized the inadequacy of the medical care available to the lower-income groups and began establishing clinics. The medical profession by this time had gained control of hospitals and medical education, and dominated medical care. Recognizing that clinics represented a threat to the lucrative fee system, the American Medical Association used its political power to force public-health agencies out of direct health care. Health departments in general were restricted to supplying free vaccines to physicians, referring patients screened by public-health doctors or nurses, gathering statistics, and dealing with community health problems.

As the great killer diseases of former times were brought under control in the first forty years of the twentieth century, health authorities began turning their attention to chronic and constitutional disorders and to the long-neglected area of occupational hazards. Although the danger from miasmas had been dismissed, the post–World War II period saw a rising concern over the environment. The thousands of new chemicals polluting the air and water presented subtle but potentially serious dangers to health, and radiation introduced still another possible threat. In addition, stimulated in part by the psychiatric problems uncovered during the war years, public health was broadened to include community mental health.

The development of sulfa drugs and antibiotics in the World War II period seemed to have ended contagious diseases as major public-health problems. Even venereal disorders appeared to be in full retreat by the 1950s. Within another decade the situation began to change. The success of the new "miracle drugs"—such as penicillin—in curing venereal disorders led physicians to prescribe antibiotics for almost every form of infection, whether the cause was bacterial or viral. The result was the rapid creation of resistant strains of pathogenic organisms. The emergence of resistant forms of syphilis and gonorrhea coincided with the sexual revolution of the 1960s and contributed notably to a sharp rise in the incidence of venereal diseases. Since the 1970s new or newly diagnosed disorders such as genital herpes, Legionnaire's disease, Lyme disease, and acquired immunodeficiency syndrome (AIDS) have appeared, further confirming that infectious diseases remain a serious public-health threat.

Of the above disorders, AIDS best epitomizes the interrelationship between the social and biological factors in defining and dealing with disease. In the U.S., public fears aroused by the rising incidence of AIDS have led to the ostracizing of its victims, demands that physicians and health workers be tested, and pressure upon Congress to divert funds from other medical research to investigate AIDS. The public reaction to this new and fatal disorder has antecedents going far back in history. Bubonic plague, smallpox, yellow fever, and Asiatic cholera all evoked a similar response. In the nineteenth century, Asiatic cholera victims were not infrequently dumped from river boats and left to die on the banks. AIDS bears an additional burden because it is equated with sexual immorality, a venereal disorder compounded by its association with homosexuality. Since the eighteenth century any disease associated with sexual activity has been equated with immorality. As late as 1897 Howard Kelly of Johns Hopkins objected in the American Medical Association's annual meeting to a discussion of "the hygiene of the sexual act," on the grounds that the subject "was attended with filth."

AIDS also illustrates the perennial question of the rights of the individual versus those of society. When, as was true for most of history, epidemic diseases were strange, inexplicable occurrences, isolating or casting out the sick or effectively quarantining an infected area was taken for granted. Pesthouses in the colonial period were designed more to protect the town than to provide care for the sick. When inoculation for smallpox was introduced into the United States in 1721, the early

laws forbade its use on the justifiable grounds that it would spread the disease. In the nineteenth century, laws requiring vaccination were bitterly opposed by many citizens, with antivaccination societies flourishing in a number of areas.

Public-health regulations by their nature are designed to restrict certain activities on the part of individuals. The 1867 annual report of the New York City Health Board declared: "The Health Department of a great commercial district which encounters no obstacles and meets no opposition, may safely be declared unworthy of public confidence." The vast majority of health regulations affect private property or place an extra cost on individuals or businesses; hence they have invariably led to protests. In New York and New Orleans, when health officials designated certain buildings as hospitals during yellow fever epidemics, mobs rioted and burned them to the ground. During an 1894 smallpox epidemic in Milwaukee, the Health Department sought to isolate cases and vaccinate all individuals in the infected areas. The result was rioting and the dismissal of the health officer. Health officers are government officials subject to political pressures; they must always seek a balance between what needs to be done and what can be done.

Limiting the right of individuals to practice medicine, requiring vaccinations, setting standards for food processing, and requiring physical examinations for food handlers, or establishing sanitary regulations with respect to housing or other property is an assertion that the community's health transcends individual or property rights. Laws requiring physicians to report contagious diseases have always raised strong objections from the medical profession, whether they involved reporting yellow fever in the eighteenth and nineteenth centuries or venereal disease in the twentieth century. When the New York City Health Department issued an order requiring the reporting of tuberculosis cases, the city's medical societies were outraged and appealed to the state legislature to restrict the powers of the Board of Health. In contrast, when on several occasions the New York City Board of Health ordered the evacuation of many blocks during the early yellow fever outbreaks, no one objected, nor were any protests made in 1907 when the New York City Health Department decided that in the interest of public welfare Mary Mallon (Typhoid Mary) should be kept on North Brother Island in the East River, where she remained until her death in 1938. Since medical experiments on the poor had long been taken for granted, neither physicians nor laymen, black or white, objected to the 1932 Tuskegee syphilis experiment, funded by the U.S. Public Health Service and designed to study the course of untreated syphilis in blacks.

The latter decades of the twentieth century have seen an increasing sensitivity to individual rights. The most obvious example is the deinstitutionalization of the mentally sick, who now constitute a large portion of the homeless. The question arises of whether individuals, the homeless in particular, have the right to refuse treatment for mental illness or contagious disorders. The presence in the community of cases of tuberculosis and other communicable diseases represents a threat both to the individual concerned and to the citizens at large. The main issue—as alcoholism, drug addiction, and smoking illustrate—is not whether the government should regulate individual conduct but the degree to which it does so.

As the United States moves toward revising its health-care system, decisions must be made as to the role of public-health agencies. Maternal and child care for the lowest income groups and preventive medicine have traditionally been in the domain of public health. At present the vaccination of children is left to private medicine or state and local authorities, with the result that thousands of children remain unprotected. These responsibilities should, and probably will, be of major concern in a comprehensive health-care system. In devising a new health system, will public-health departments expand their work in these areas or surrender them? Or should public health be incorporated into a comprehensive health-care system? Whatever the case, serious thought must be given to formulating any major changes in the nation's health-care system.

JOHN DUFFY

Directly related to this article are the other articles in this entry: DETERMINANTS OF PUBLIC HEALTH, PHILOSOPHY OF PUBLIC HEALTH, *and* PUBLIC-HEALTH METHODS: EPIDEMIOLOGY AND BIOSTATISTICS. *Also directly related are the entries* LIFESTYLES AND PUBLIC HEALTH; HEALTH PROMOTION AND HEALTH EDUCATION; *and* HEALTH SCREENING AND TESTING IN THE PUBLIC-HEALTH CONTEXT. *For a further discussion of topics mentioned in this article, see the entries* AIDS, *article on* PUBLIC-HEALTH ISSUES; ENVIRONMENTAL HEALTH; EPIDEMICS; HEALTH-CARE RESOURCES, ALLOCATION OF, *article on* MACROALLOCATION; HOMICIDE; INJURY AND INJURY CONTROL; INSTITUTIONALIZATION AND DEINSTITUTIONALIZATION; MENTAL-HEALTH SERVICES; OCCUPATIONAL SAFETY AND HEALTH; PRISONERS, *article on* HEALTH-CARE ISSUES; PUBLIC HEALTH AND THE LAW; *and* SEXUALITY IN SOCIETY, *article on* SOCIAL CONTROL OF SEXUAL BEHAVIOR. *Other relevant material may be found under the entries* HEALTH-CARE DELIVERY, *article on* HEALTH-CARE SYSTEMS; HEALTH AND DISEASE; HEALTH OFFICIALS AND THEIR RESPONSIBILITIES; HEALTH POLICY, *article on* POLITICS AND HEALTH CARE; INTERNATIONAL HEALTH; *and* SUBSTANCE ABUSE, *article on* ALCOHOL AND OTHER DRUGS IN A PUBLIC-HEALTH CONTEXT.

Bibliography

DUFFY, JOHN. 1953. *Epidemics in Colonial America.* Baton Rouge: Louisiana State University Press.
———. 1968–1974. *A History of Public Health in New York City.* 2 vols. New York: Russell Sage Foundation.
———. 1971. "Social Impact of Disease in the Late Nineteenth Century." *Bulletin of the New York Academy of Medicine,* 2d ser., 47, no. 7:797–810.
———. 1979. "The American Medical Profession and Public Health: From Support to Ambivalence." *Bulletin of the History of Medicine* 53, no. 1:1–22.
———. 1982. "The Physician as a Moral Force in American History." In *New Knowledge in the Biomedical Sciences: Some Moral Implications of Its Acquisition, Possession, and Use,* pp. 3–21. Edited by William B. Bondeson, H. Tristram Engelhardt, Jr., Stuart F. Spicker, and Joseph M. White, Jr. Dordrecht, Netherlands: D. Reidel.
———. 1990. *The Sanitarians: A History of American Public Health.* Urbana: University of Illinois Press.
GRISCOM, JOHN H. 1845. *The Sanitary Condition of the Laboring Population of New York: With Suggestions for Its Improvement. . . .* New York: Harper & Brothers.
LUBOVE, ROY, ed. 1966. *Social Welfare in Transition: Selected English Documents, 1834–1909.* Pittsburgh: University of Pittsburgh Press.
McCULLOCH, SAMUEL C., ed. 1950. *British Humanitarianism: Essays Honoring Frank J. Klingberg.* Philadelphia: Church Historical Society.
MECKEL, RICHARD A. 1990. *"Save the Babies": American Public Health Reform and the Prevention of Infant Mortality, 1850–1929.* Baltimore: Johns Hopkins University Press.
MELOSI, MARTIN V., ed. 1980. *Pollution and Reform in American Cities, 1870–1930.* Austin: University of Texas Press.
ROSEN, GEORGE. 1974. *From Medical Police to Social Medicine: Essays on the History of Health Care,* pp. 120–158. New York: Science History Publications.
———. 1975. *Preventive Medicine in the United States, 1900–1975: Trends and Interpretations.* New York: Science History Publications.
ROSENBERG, CHARLES E. 1962. *The Cholera Years: The United States in 1832, 1849, and 1866.* Chicago: University of Chicago Press.
SHATTUCK, LEMUEL; BANKS, NATHANIEL P., JR.; and ABBOTT, JEHIEL. 1948. *Report of the Sanitary Commission of Massachusetts, 1850.* Foreword by Charles-Edward Amory Winslow. Cambridge, Mass.: Harvard University Press.
STARR, PAUL. 1982. *The Social Transformation of American Medicine: The Rise of a Sovereign Profession and the Making of a Vast Industry.* New York: Basic Books.
WILLIAMS, RALPH CHESTER. 1951. *The United States Public Health Service, 1798–1950.* Washington, D.C.: Commissioned Officers Association, U.S. Public Health Service.
WING, KENNETH R. 1985. *The Law and the Public's Health.* 2d ed. Ann Arbor, Mich.: Health Administration Press.

III. PHILOSOPHY OF PUBLIC HEALTH

Public health is the prevention of disease and premature death through organized community effort. While this community effort is often led by government, many nongovernment and quasi-public institutions play key roles in promoting the public's health. Public health as an idea is one of the most influential of our time, and has been an important force in changing the shape of the modern world and enlarging government's scope, if not its size, since the middle of the nineteenth century. The general idea that government and communities can systematically discover, anticipate, and relieve disease and social distress through collective choice and organization is relatively new in human history. It involves the complex and related developments of collections and analysis of statistics, the understanding of variations in disease patterns in human societies (usually called epidemiology), and government of sufficient scale and capacity to exploit these findings.

Public health's focus on populations and communities is its most distinctive feature and the primary source of its philosophical interest. The community perspective produces a way of thinking about disease and early death and their prevention, that often runs counter to the categories and assumptions of much of modern bioethics and other disciplines as well. Public health as an organized practice views disease and premature death from the standpoint of the community and its capacity for self-examination, reorganization, and modification. The community perspective, far from neglecting the welfare of individuals, strengthens society's ability to discover the causes of disease in individuals, and society's capacity to devise flexible and rapid means for controlling disease and preventable death. Bioethics has been interested mainly in the intersection of the worlds of public health and the individual and his or her autonomy, and far less in public health as a method, seeing this as falling outside its sphere into the world of practice, and into the realm of contingency, experience, and practical action (Dewey, 1929).

Considerations for a philosophy of public health

Public health as a method bears a strong resemblance to pragmatism, with its emphasis on probabilistic and fallibilistic ways of knowing, on exploiting experience and action, and on the centrality of knowing and acting in the context of communities, institutions, and practices (Bernstein, 1992; Rorty, 1982). While it is true that public health has many roots in utilitarianism (the English reformer E. H. Chadwick was once a literary secretary to Jeremy Bentham), public health came of age in the United States and Europe during the late nineteenth century and the early decades of the twentieth century, when the causes and methods for preventing many deadly diseases were discovered.

At the same time, philosophy and the social sciences began to revolt against the formalism of previous centuries (Dewey, 1929), and in both the United States and Europe, in philosophy and the social sciences, the search for fundamental truths gave way to empiricism and pragmatism, to a greater stress on the parallels between social science and philosophy, and to courses of action guided by both results and experience (Feffer, 1993; Anderson, 1990). After World War II there was in the United States a marked retreat to the earlier formalism with the rise of analytic philosophy and the return to social contract ideas, factors in the tendency of bioethics and philosophy to ignore the more pragmatic way of public health. This is not to say that public health as an organized practice needs no further philosophical elaboration or justification, or that it can ignore questions about the limits of health policy in restricting liberty or the coherence of public health's use of the idea of the common good. It is simply to say that public health does not need first to be translated into utilitarianism or contract theory to become a social philosophy.

A philosophy of public health must accomplish four things. First, it must give a central place to the unique approach and method of public health, with its distinctive emphasis on community, and on the central role of the scientific method in formulating courses of action for social improvement. Second, a philosophy of public health must give priority to prevention, and must challenge and revise explanations for health problems with the community perspective, which is essential to effective prevention. Third, a philosophy of public health must set out and defend an adequate definition of the common good, taking into account public health's pursuit of the common well-being—measured in terms of rates of disease and early death—as the object of group or common action. Fourth, while the philosophy of public health must acknowledge the claims of individual autonomy and justify actions that limit liberty and autonomy, it must do so in a way that leaves the community perspective and the common good intact.

Health by design: The idea of prevention

Prevention is the major focus in public health, and it involves as a minimum the imaginative redesign of social environments and communities to better promote health and safety, as well as the replacement of older models of the problems that need to be solved. A major part of the battle in public health, especially in applying public-health methods to modern problems of chronic disease, injury, and alcohol and other drug problems, is to redescribe these problems in terms of the community perspective, countering the individualism, so widely prevalent in much of philosophy and social science, that serves as a powerful obstacle to effective prevention.

Two recent examples make this point. In the case of alcohol, since the 1970s there has been a shift away from purely individual or agent-focused explanations for alcohol problems, based on the capacities, dispositions, and motivations of individuals who drink, and subsequently experience problems, factors like "loss-of-control" over drinking. With the public-health perspective, the focus is on the exposure of whole societies to alcohol, on the varying levels of total consumption among groups, and on such factors as price, hours of sale, and age limits in causing rates of problems. This approach does not seek so much to explain alcoholism (why some people drink addictively) but why rates of alcoholism rise or fall among communities, or over time (Moore and Gerstein, 1981).

In a similar way, highway safety since the early 1960s has witnessed a shift from individual capacities ("driver error," "driver negligence," "failure to yield the right-of-way," and factors beyond the control of agents, such as "acts of God") toward such factors as the exposure of drivers to highway hazards, miles driven annually, types of roads driven on, and the safe or unsafe character of the automobile. Exposure is a key variable in this redescription and often results in counterintuitive insights. For example, researchers have noted that "driver education programs" in the United States probably raise the level of death and injury because they expose more young people to the hazards of driving at an early age.

Public health has many similarities to modern applied systems theory and the policy sciences, with their stress on nonreductionism, on policy or systems knowledge rather than disciplinary knowledge, on systems-level (community-level) analysis, and on promoting change through novel interventions with high leverage potential, often deployed at places located far from the primary cause of the problems.

It is common to find public-health specialists, in their attempt to fashion new means of reducing disease, speaking of "agents," "hosts," and "environments," translating individual descriptions of problems into community descriptions. According to the interpretation of William Haddon, Jr., this framework's "agents" are "exchanges" of hazardous chemicals, ionizing sources, drugs, or kinetic energy, suffered by individual "hosts." The environment is the larger social and physical terrain of hazardous agents and hosts. The purpose of this strange language is to provoke new ways of thinking about old problems, and to give public-health designers free play in their imaginative search for new and innovative ways of reducing dangers, ways that are both effective and ultimately politically feasible. All three elements—hosts, agents, and environment—are potential targets for change and modification, with no priority given any one (Haddon, 1973).

This search for new societal arrangements is often expressed as the search for "conditions" that promote health or prevent disease, a point found in the Institute of Medicine's report *The Future of Public Health,* and its definition of the mission of public health: "the fulfillment of society's interest in assuring the conditions in which people can be healthy" (Institute of Medicine, 1988).

In one way or another, public health concerns collective choice. Public health is about how much alcohol is permitted in society (per capita consumption levels), about the frequency of highway crashes, about the number of drownings in a state or nation, and about the changes in environment, legislation, and public attitudes that will directly affect those statistics. This emphasis on social organization and social arrangements in public health does not reduce public health to a species of social causation. For example, to use the link between general consumption levels and occurrence rates of cirrhosis is not to say that society causes specific individuals to drink heavily or alcoholically. It is to say that because we have learned through scientific studies that society, through alcohol policy, can influence the levels and kinds of problems in society, it is accurate to say that society influences these problems, and can and should seek, within the context of democratic discussion and debate, to sharply reduce them.

Public health and the common good

In the public-health view, the common good in public health means the good of individuals taken together as a group, as communities, or in terms of aggregate health and safety; this aggregate health, expressed as so many thousands of lives saved, is the object of organized government or community effort. The common good does not mean that each individual has the same or identical good in health and safety, or even the same interests. An individual with a genetic predisposition for colon cancer does not have the same interest in health and safety as another who lacks such genetic makeup. Yet both can be said to have a common interest in measures to promote health and safety and to reduce general risks to health and safety that all face, including risks from cancer. This is another way of saying that individuals can face threats to health and safety alone and in groups, using group efforts to reduce those threats.

The common good expressed in aggregate terms does not refer to a good that is separate from, and set over against, the good of the individuals who constitute a group at risk. It is rather that the good of the group is jointly consumed, producing a common benefit of thousands of lives saved and many thousands more who will avoid injury or disease. This common benefit of lives saved (and avoidance of disease) is taken as the expression of the common good and is the object or purpose of collective or common action.

For most public-health problems, the aggregate savings in lives is far smaller than the number of individuals at risk and whose liberty is to be limited. Put another way, and for most public-health problems, the group that benefits from protections is a much smaller subset of the group that is at risk. Thus, all who are at risk and whose liberty is limited by public-health legislation do not benefit; the benefit accrues for an unknown and unaccountable minority of the larger at-risk group. Because this good is expressed in the form of statistical lives, it is viewed as a savings for the community. Thus, it is not wrong to think of public-health measures as undertaken by a community for the sake of a common good, that is, the thousands whose lives will actually be saved. The slogan for public health should not be "The life you save may be your own," but rather, "The lives we save together may include your own."

Geoffrey Rose refers to the fact that communities benefit more from public health than individuals as the "prevention paradox" (Rose, 1985). The prevention paradox states that most modern public-health risks are sufficiently low and widely distributed—indeed, they often stem from mass behavior like driving automobiles, drinking, smoking—and that despite the fact that millions engage in the activity, savings in lives will measure only in the tens of thousands in any period.

Public health and autonomy

Some have used John Stuart Mill's famous point in *On Liberty* that only individuals can know their own good (Mill, 1975) to criticize many public-health measures— such as laws that require people to wear seat belts in automobiles and helmets when riding motorcycles, and requiring fluoride in the water supply—as paternalistic. These laws threaten the autonomy of individuals, and also threaten to usher in an era of vast, paternal, preventive government. Ronald Dworkin argues that "laws that promote the common interest insult no man . . . while laws that constrain one man, on the grounds that he is incompetent to judge are profoundly insulting" (Dworkin, 1977, p. 263). Dworkin is here arguing that seat-belt laws or higher taxes on alcohol are not in the common interest, and are therefore insulting. Unlike Mill, he believes that the class of these kinds of laws and restrictions is actually quite small.

Those who support public-health restrictions on individual liberty, but who wish to avoid a strong paternalist position, can do so in basically two ways. They can argue that public-health measures are only mildly paternalistic. This is the "weak paternalism" thesis (Dworkin, 1972; Feinberg, 1973). In this view, public-health measures are not strongly intrusive, and they save thousands of lives. Most philosophers today seem to embrace this view. The second and more controversial view is that public-health interventions are not at all paternalistic (Beauchamp, 1988) because the good produced

is not a private or individual good, but rather a common good produced by common action. In this view, the citizen sees himself or herself as living in a world in which common action, after public and democratic discussion, often promotes public-health, and while individuals may potentially benefit from these actions, the community or the common good will assuredly benefit.

The differences between these two basically supportive perspectives on most public-health legislation cannot easily be reconciled, but their differences should not be exaggerated. Both sides agree that any restriction on liberty and autonomy needs justification. The only disagreement is over who is benefiting from this restriction and whether the good is private or common.

In the public-health perspective, the conception of autonomy is one of a basic autonomy, not an absolute autonomy. A basic autonomy can be overridden on evidence that restrictions are minimal, acceptable, and will produce a substantial savings in lives. The guardians of basic autonomy are the democratic process and elected officials, such as legislators or chief executives. This makes many nervous, yet the long history of the struggle for public-health legislation is, on balance, reassuring. Because most public-health legislation necessitates the burdens placed on large numbers of individuals, including powerful interests, to benefit small numbers of individuals, the political path to successful public-health legislation is strewn with political roadblocks that are likely powerful deterrents to overzealous public-health activists. This emphasis on relying on the processes of democratic communities reflects the pragmatism of public health as philosophy, and its interest in political theory. Also, Richard Flathman, a political theorist, notes that governments rarely promote the good of a single individual (Flathman, 1966).

Public health and social justice

An enduring theme in public health is the attempt to persuade democratic bodies to legislate rules for economic production and distribution that are safer and more benign. Community public-health interests frequently oppose powerful, well-organized entities such as corporations and interest groups. Public health as an interest of the community often causes deep conflict among elected officials, who are also strongly enjoined to promote economic prosperity.

The struggle for the common health and safety is further complicated by the fact that the redistribution of the burdens of health and safety protection is on behalf of "statistical lives." Thus the struggle of public health has many resemblances to the struggle for social justice in society (Beauchamp, 1976) in that they both work on behalf of the less numerous and less powerful against the power of the market and its masters. The idea of social justice influences public health, for instance, as it battles the human immunodeficiency virus (HIV) epidemic, to modify its traditional methods of fighting epidemics (Bayer, 1988), using new weapons like confidentiality and privacy to fight societal discrimination and prejudice toward the victims of the widespread epidemic.

Democracy, public discussion, and public health

Much of public health is concerned with providing and/or regulating information and education. These activities typically encounter far fewer ethical conflicts than does legislation that limits individual liberty or property in order to promote health and safety. Yet even here the distinctive footprint of public health as a social practice can be detected. Progress against cigarette smoking has been made in the United States during the decades after World War II not so much through regulating or banning smoking as through communicating the discovery by public-health researchers of the links between smoking and disease. The subsequent public discussion and controversies surrounding a series of reports by U.S. surgeons general (and also by health officials in other nations) widely publicized the links between smoking and lung cancer and heart disease. The further publicity surrounding the role of tobacco in public policy and other related controversies produced a growing awareness of smoking as a social problem. This publicity, coupled with the ban on television advertising of cigarettes, produced sharp declines in smoking rates (Warner, 1986), in advance of more recent and controversial moves to ban smoking in public areas.

Here again, the unique emphasis in public health is to use the discovery of threats to the common health as part of the "hubbub" of democracy. Such controversy can be used to affect public opinion and discussion (including a growing social disapproval of smoking) as principal forces for promoting change in individual and mass behavior (Beauchamp, 1988). Public dialogue, in turn, moves public health into the new territories of promoting more information and speech and of countering advertising's role in limiting information.

Conclusion

The idea of public health as philosophy involves the elaboration of its core ideas of promoting fallibilistic and probabilistic ways of knowing, of learning from experience and action, of imaginatively proposing new designs to social environments to promote health and safety, and, above all, of focusing on prevention and community approaches everywhere possible. While public health proponents have been successful in ensuring that their methods are central to the study of health problems, working closely with scientists studying disease from an epidemiological perspective (and in the future from a more molecular and genetic perspective), they have been less successful in having public health's group approach accepted as philosophy. While it is true that public health is one of those "second languages" of community (Bellah et al., 1985), it has yet to be widely appreciated among philosophers and social scientists as a distinctive method with a distinctive philosophical perspective on common health problems, one that bears a strong resemblance to pragmatist perspectives on action and experience.

Finally, as health reform has increasingly dominated the public agenda in the United States, it is likely that public-health lessons will be more widely appreciated for two reasons: to prevent disease and reduce the burden and costs of illness, and, equally important, to remind the larger society that medicine and public health alike promote a common good, a lesson that is central to public health's distinguished history.

DAN E. BEAUCHAMP

Directly related to this article are the other articles in this entry: DETERMINANTS OF PUBLIC HEALTH, HISTORY OF PUBLIC HEALTH, *and* PUBLIC-HEALTH METHODS: EPIDEMIOLOGY AND BIOSTATISTICS. *Also directly related is the entry* PUBLIC HEALTH AND THE LAW, *article on* LEGAL MORALISM AND PUBLIC HEALTH. *For a further discussion of topics mentioned in this article, see the entries* AIDS, *article on* PUBLIC-HEALTH ISSUES; AUTONOMY; ECONOMIC CONCEPTS IN HEALTH CARE; FREEDOM AND COERCION; HEALTH-CARE RESOURCES, ALLOCATION OF, *article on* MACROALLOCATION; HEALTH POLICY, *article on* POLITICS AND HEALTH CARE; HEALTH PROMOTION AND HEALTH EDUCATION; HEALTH SCREENING AND TESTING IN THE PUBLIC-HEALTH CONTEXT; INJURY AND INJURY CONTROL; JUSTICE; LAW AND MORALITY; PATERNALISM; *and* UTILITY. *Other relevant material may be found under the entries* ADVERTISING; ETHICS, *articles on* TASK OF ETHICS, NORMATIVE ETHICAL THEORIES, *and* SOCIAL AND POLITICAL THEORIES; HEALTH AND DISEASE, *articles on* SOCIOLOGICAL PERSPECTIVES, ANTHROPOLOGICAL PERSPECTIVES, *and* PHILOSOPHICAL PERSPECTIVES; HEALTH OFFICIALS AND THEIR RESPONSIBILITIES; PUBLIC HEALTH AND THE LAW, *article on* PHILOSOPHY OF THE LAW OF PUBLIC HEALTH; *and* RIGHTS.

Bibliography

ANDERSON, CHARLES W. 1990. *Pragmatic Liberalism.* Chicago: University of Chicago Press.

BAYER, RONALD. 1988. *Private Acts, Social Consequences: AIDS and the Politics of Public Health.* New Brunswick, N.J.: Rutgers University Press.

BEAUCHAMP, DAN E. 1976. "Public Health as Social Justice." *Inquiry* 13, no. 1:3–14.

———. 1988. *The Health of the Republic: Epidemics, Medicine, and Moralism as Challenges to Democracy.* Philadelphia: Temple University Press.

BELLAH, ROBERT N.; MADSEN, RICHARD; SULLIVAN, WILLIAM M.; SWIDLER, ANN; and TIPTON, STEVEN. 1985. *Habits of the Heart: Individualism and Commitment in American Life.* Berkeley: University of California Press.

BERNSTEIN, RICHARD J. 1992. *The New Constellation: The Ethical-Political Horizons of Modernity/Postmodernity.* Cambridge, Mass.: MIT Press.

DEWEY, JOHN. 1929. *The Quest for Certainty: A Study of the Relation of Knowledge and Action.* New York: Minton, Balch.

DWORKIN, GERALD. 1972. "Paternalism." *Monist* 56, no. 1: 64–84.

DWORKIN, RONALD M. 1977. *Taking Rights Seriously.* Cambridge, Mass.: Harvard University Press.

FEFFER, ANDREW. 1993. *The Chicago Pragmatists and American Progressivism.* Ithaca, N.Y.: Cornell University Press.

FEINBERG, JOEL. 1973. *Social Philosophy.* Englewood Cliffs, N.J.: Prentice-Hall.

FLATHMAN, RICHARD E. 1966. *The Public Interest: An Essay Concerning the Normative Discourse of Politics.* New York: Wiley.

GUSFIELD, JOSEPH R. 1981. *The Culture of Public Problems: Drinking-Driving and the Symbolic Order.* Chicago: University of Chicago Press.

HADDON, WILLIAM, JR. 1973. "Energy Damage and the Ten Countermeasure Strategies." *Journal of Trauma* 13, no. 4:321–331.

INSTITUTE OF MEDICINE. 1988. *The Future of Public Health.* Washington, D.C.: National Academy Press.

MILL, JOHN STUART. 1975. [1850].*On Liberty.* Edited by David Spitz. New York: W. W. Norton.

MOORE, MARK H., and GERSTEIN, DEAN R. 1981. *Alcohol and Public Policy: Beyond the Shadow of Prohibition.* Washington, D.C.: National Academy Press.

RORTY, RICHARD. 1982. *Consequences of Pragmatism: Essays, 1972–1980.* Minneapolis: University of Minnesota Press.

ROSE, GEOFFREY. 1985. "Sick Individuals and Sick Populations." *International Journal of Epidemiology* 14, no. 1: 32–38.

SELZNICK, PHILIP. 1992. *The Moral Commonwealth: Social Theory and the Promise of Community.* Berkeley: University of California Press.

WARNER, KENNETH E. 1986. *Selling Smoke: Cigarette Advertising and Public Health.* Washington, D.C.: American Public Health Association.

IV. PUBLIC-HEALTH METHODS: EPIDEMIOLOGY AND BIOSTATISTICS

Epidemiology is basic to modern public health. It provides, for example, the rational basis for health planning, the justification for allocating funding, and the basis for deciding whether or not to introduce or change preventive health policies. Finally, it plays a fundamental role in making decisions concerning optimal treatment regimens through its involvement in the clinical evaluation process.

Epidemiology is distinct from medical science in that epidemiology's focus is on population health, opposed to medicine's focus on the individual patient. While medicine seeks to heal the individual who, by virtue of being susceptible, becomes ill, epidemiology seeks to identify the underlying cause that results in illness among those who are susceptible. With an underlying cause identified, it becomes possible to intervene at the source of the chain of events that leads to illness among people who are susceptible. Removal of the cause can directly result in preventing those who are susceptible from being exposed to it in the first place and thereby from becoming ill.

Epidemiology focuses on large numbers of people comprising populations or communities. It is a quantitative (as opposed to a qualitative) science whose methods are heavily dependent on the application of biostatistical principles and on advances in biostatistical methods. As with other quantitative sciences, epidemiology requires the counting, classification, and analysis of sizable amounts of data. In order to derive meaning from large amounts of data, statistical techniques are used to produce various kinds of summaries. These techniques are known as biostatistics in the health and/or biological sciences.

Through the early 1940s, prior to the advent of antibiotics at the time of World War II, epidemiologists were occupied almost exclusively with controlling infectious diseases. Success resulted in better control of infectious diseases; improved living standards, especially in developed countries; and increased life expectancy of the population. Consequently, epidemiology expanded from its preoccupation with infectious diseases to include noninfectious diseases.

The notion that noninfectious and, by extension, chronic diseases can be prevented by eliminating their causes, analogous to the prevention of infectious diseases, is a relatively new concept. Hence, the modern role of epidemiology, from the public health perspective, is to identify appropriate interventions for consideration by policymakers for controlling disease at the source and thereby promoting health in the community.

The linking of epidemiology and biostatistics has become a hallmark of modern epidemiology in both its research and its practice areas of activity. Research in epidemiology tends to embrace activities of an experimental nature, while the practice domain tends to focus on disease surveillance and monitoring activities. Regardless of the domain, biostatistics provides the analytic tools used in epidemiology.

Scientific discovery in the laboratory should ultimately have practical application at the bedside. Results of epidemiologic investigations made on a population or on clearly defined subgroups of the population ought to benefit individuals. Because the results of population-based research are couched in terms of probabilities, the application of epidemiologic studies to the individual is not direct. Nevertheless, the identification of risk factor information in the absence of a biologically identified cause of a disease has been instrumental for prevention programs. Furthermore, physicians can apply probabilities in deciding therapeutic options.

The scope of epidemiologic activity

Epidemiologic studies are necessary to provide both valid and reliable data not only concerning the distribution of diseases in populations, but also on the impact of social, economic, environmental, and other factors on the health of populations. In addition, epidemiologic data are often fundamental in making future projections of disease burden, crucial for planning purposes.

Concerning professional ethics, in the physician–patient "medical" relationship, the physician assumes a patient advocacy role; epidemiologists, on the other hand, assume a population/community advocacy role. Ethical guidelines that have been developed for medicine therefore have little relevance to epidemiology. Obligations assumed under these two different models must be explicit for trust to exist between professionals and the public.

Since the 1960s, epidemiology has undergone dramatic growth, paralleling to some extent the growth and development of computers. In North America, for example, the sex distribution and training of epidemiologists has changed over this period. Previously, epidemiologists were predominantly male, but today about half, especially those engaged in research, are women. Also, about half of today's epidemiologists were never trained as physicians.

The absolute numbers of epidemiologists have grown exponentially and the development of advanced computer technology has enabled epidemiologists to work with and share increasingly larger databases and to apply sophisticated multivariate statistical adjustment techniques via the use of computer software. But while technology has led to important advances in epidemiology, the complex issues of ensuring both integrity in science and ethical conduct among scientists have yet to be adequately addressed. There is increasing recognition of the need for guidelines to ensure professional accountability to the public in whose service epidemiologists work.

Classical epidemiology—as distinct from clinical evaluation—is primarily an observational science; it studies the events of daily life among the members of the various subgroups that comprise a community. Unlike controlled experiments, epidemiologic research measures events associated with populations whose lifestyles, work habits, and other characteristics have evolved outside the epidemiologist's control. Because uncontrollable and unknown risk factors can impact study outcomes radically, they must be accounted for if demonstrated contrasts, comparisons, and differences are attributed to these. Epidemiologic methods include various approaches for ensuring appropriate analysis of observational events. Professional epidemiologists are cognizant of the strengths, weaknesses, and limitations of the various methodologic options in light of the complexities associated with the conduct of uncontrolled experiments.

The closest epidemiology comes to the conduct of a controlled experiment is in the randomized controlled trial (RCT). However, RCTs can be justified only on the basis of substantial preexisting information concerning the intervention of interest (e.g., a particular therapy). Preexisting information usually is derived from the conduct of studies utilizing designs that are nonexperimental in nature (i.e., from the realm of natural experiments). Only where justification exists can human beings be subjected to random allocation in a clinical trial. Natural experiments in observational research include descriptive, ecological, retrospective case-control, and prospective cohort designs.

Diseases associated with aging, including cancer, diabetes, and cardiovascular diseases, have required greater attention. Because epidemiology provides the methodology for rational approaches to interventions, epidemiology is fundamental to disease prevention. Interventions based on epidemiological studies have taken the form of health promotion programs, such as campaigns for smoking cessation, no drinking and driving, and condom use in sexual intercourse. The onset in 1981 of the acquired immunodeficiency syndrome (AIDS) pandemic, however, reminded epidemiologists that infectious diseases are not necessarily a thing of the past.

With escalating health-care costs in Canada, the United States, and elsewhere, epidemiology is playing a major role through providing the evaluative methodology for assessing cost-effective interventions for rational health-care planning. Epidemiologists establish health goals by assessing health status indicators for a population; they identify target levels for reduced morbidity, disability, and mortality. These activities have implications for resource allocation which bear directly on the ethical principle of distributive justice. Indeed, numerous jurisdictions are attempting to identify those illnesses for which free health coverage should be provided by the "state" based on prevailing population values. Epidemiology assists in these determinations through expertise in survey methodology, health-status indicators, and disease classification.

From the foregoing, it is clear that epidemiology plays a major role in health-policy decisions, which involve, among others, substantial financial resources. "Health" is big business. Concerns arose during the 1980s about the possible influence of individuals and/or groups whose vested interests could bias outcome(s), motivated by financial profit and/or professional prestige. Conflicting-interest issues have been of concern not only in the interpretation of epidemiologic studies in favor of any one interest group's position but even in limiting or blocking the potential to conduct the best possible epidemiologic study for addressing a health concern.

The legal aspects—in terms of civil, administrative, and criminal law—are profound. With utilitarian goals in mind (i.e., doing the greatest good for the largest number of people), the courts usually have invoked the collective good over individual freedoms (e.g., in legislation concerning vaccination, quarantine, seat belts, and smoke-free public indoor environments in both Canada and the United States).

In general, governments prefer that professions regulate themselves. Professional organizations are expected to do what is necessary to minimize scientific misconduct and ensure professional etiquette among employers, sponsors, colleagues, and clients.

A historic and ongoing concern: Privacy

Any epidemiologic investigation conducted under the auspices of an institution (e.g., a university, hospital, or government office) is likely to be subjected to ethical review by a committee. The committee usually comprises members of various disciplines as well as a lay representative.

Not only can ethics review committees examine the nature of the question to be addressed by the investigation, but they also may determine the appropriateness of the methods being proposed. Generally, however, the main focus tends to be on the possible harms versus benefits to those who will participate in the study; that is, with issues of privacy, informed consent, and confidentiality, and most important, that none of the procedures expected of the subjects/participants will cause them harm.

Scientific peer review concentrates on the aptness of the proposed scientific research methods, including the scientific relevance of the proposed research question, assessment of potential bias and confounding, adequacy of the proposed size of the study and associated statistical power, and recognized limitations impacting on the interpretation of the study. These two distinct but related areas of concern are seldom brought to the attention of a single expert other than the principal investigator, and perhaps also his or her research team. Without the support of both groups, the proposal usually cannot proceed into action.

Because the data epidemiologists rely on can be personally sensitive, governments have enacted privacy legislation to protect its citizens. Only with special permission from the custodians of these data bases can epidemiologists gain access—usually controlled—to the data banks essential to the conduct of health research. Some agencies also impose an oath of secrecy on the researcher.

One protection that researchers are expected to exercise (in their publication of results from access to health records in the public domain) is the anonymity of all persons studied. In addition, the identification of small areas or groups of people must be avoided also to ensure anonymity and thereby the protection of individual privacy. Individual or group stigmatization is to be avoided. Any infringement of the public trust could have repercussions, including legal penalties to the researcher involved. Furthermore, the epidemiologic research enterprise could be placed in jeopardy by engendering a loss of trust in research by the very communities whose support (both financial and possibly also participatory) is needed for investigation purposes.

Professional training, in conjunction with well-publicized guidelines, is likely to minimize any risk of infringement. In addition, the epidemiologist has an obligation not only to respect the right to privacy of personal data, but to ensure that coworkers are equally vigilant. "Whistleblowing" also must be encouraged and those doing so must be protected from any form of reprisal. Most professional ethics guidelines/codes require that attention be drawn to the person who elects to perform contrary to normative standards of professional practice.

In 1991, European Community government officials developed a set of proposals concerning rights to privacy. Unfortunately, if enacted, these proposals could serve to make it virtually impossible to conduct epidemiologic research that depends on access to these data banks. The proposals ensure that personal information provided for one purpose cannot be used for another purpose without prior consent. Similar legislative proposals were mounted in the United States in the mid-1970s, but were defeated. Hence, epidemiologists and biostatisticians worldwide have a duty to remain vigilant of legislative proposals that might, directly or indirectly, adversely impact research for the public's health. They must be organized enough to provide input to such legislative proposals. Ultimately, it is the public-health interest that must prevail.

Current issues

Ethics guidelines.   The first stated need for guidelines on the ethical conduct of epidemiologists was printed in 1985. Despite considerable debate within the profession in North America, through 1987, little movement was made. It was at the International Epidemiological Association's (IEA) 1987 XIth Scientific Meeting in Helsinki, Finland, that the proposal to develop guidelines was adopted. By 1990, further discussion had advanced the thinking on this subject and a first draft of IEA guidelines was published.

A milestone conference on the subject of ethics in epidemiology had stimulated the discussion in 1989. The conference had been organized by the United States' Industrial Epidemiology Forum. The organizers had compiled a set of ethics guidelines and a commentary; these subsequently were published in the conference proceedings in 1991. Since then, the Council for International Organizations of Medical Sciences (CIOMS) has published *International Guidelines for Ethical Review of Epidemiological Studies* together with a compendium conference proceedings which contributed to the development of these guidelines. In addition, CIOMS published *International Ethical Guidelines for Biomedical Research Involving Human Subjects.* (CIOMS, 1991, 1993).

In November 1991, the American College of Epidemiology was accorded the leadership role among the North American epidemiology bodies to further ethics initiatives in this region of the world. Other groups of epidemiologists with specialty interests are contributing to this process (e.g., environmental epidemiologists).

The Industrial Epidemiology Forum's Guidelines, modeled on those developed some years earlier by the International Statistical Institute, are organized as follows:

I. *Obligations to the subjects of research*
   to protect their welfare, ensuring no physical or mental harm through their participation
   to obtain their informed consent, ensuring the fullest possible understanding of any risks and benefits associated with participation
   to protect their privacy, ensuring no stigmatization resulting from information provided through their participation
   to maintain confidential information, ensuring the privacy of the participant

II. *Obligations to society*
   to avoid conflicting interests, recognizing that vested interests could bias research in ways that fail to serve the goal of seeking truth
   to avoid partiality by openly recognizing one's biases
   to widen the scope of epidemiology by teaching its methods to interested candidates
   to pursue responsibilities with due diligence
   to maintain public confidence in the profession by ensuring that both the strengths as well as the limitations of the profession are disclosed

III. *Obligations to funders and employers*
   to specify obligations, ensuring that the values and principles to which epidemiologists are expected to abide are clearly understood
   to protect privileged information, respecting the need of employers and providers of information to have reasonable time to assess the implications of research utilizing their data to their interests prior to disseminating the results from such a study

IV. *Obligations to colleagues*
   to report methods and results for wider peer review
   to confront unacceptable behavior and conditions, ensuring ethical conduct in support of the public interest
   to communicate ethical requirements, thereby ensuring accountability of the profession to the public

Loreen Herwaldt (1993) has extended the guidelines set forth by the Industrial Epidemiology Forum by identifying principles having special relevance to hospital infection control officers and clinical practice.

While guidelines, commentaries, and case studies are recognized as essential to ethical conduct, they are insufficient. They must be taught, learned, discussed, challenged, and revised in light of case studies, if they are to affect behavior. Finally, mechanisms for dealing with allegations of breaches of conduct need to be established with remedies that serve to mitigate any wrongs.

Conflicting interests. Objectivity is required both on the part of the epidemiologist who is proposing a research project or submitting a manuscript for publication and on the part of the scientific peer review committee members. A conflict of interest arises when a reviewer has a vested interest in the subject under review that can either positively or negatively impact on the review decision. When a reviewer has a conflict of interest—whether at the scientific approval stage, the ethics review stage, or the publication stage—this must be declared and such reviewer's comments should be considered in this light in any final decision.

Reviewers have an obligation never to use, or to discuss with others, the ideas conveyed in a proposal/manuscript without full attribution to the person who proposed them. To do otherwise would misappropriate the intellectual property of another. In addition, if the reviewer is in a position to execute another's proposal, whether funded or not, such work should not proceed without the prior written permission of the person whose idea it was.

Screening for disease and HIV antibody. As a means of secondary prevention, early detection of disease through screening programs is well recognized. The AIDS pandemic, however, has presented new challenges well documented by Ronald Bayer and his colleagues, whose concern has been more with the stigmatization of individuals or groups (Bayer et al., 1993). Access to test results by, for example, employers, landlords, or insurance companies has been of concern to infected people who fear job or housing loss and non-insurability. In research involving sexual practices, for example, the investigator requires special legal protection not only to render data inaccessible under subpoena but also to disclose such issues as the sexual abuse of children to child welfare authorities. Since valid responses must be obtained from persons volunteering for research if epidemiologic studies are to be useful, the right to privacy by the person being studied has to be secured in order for the person to participate honestly in the study.

In its initial years, testing for the human immunodeficiency virus (HIV) antibody was intended (together with self-exclusion) to secure the safety of the donated blood supply. Shortly thereafter, however, there were mandates for the testing of population subgroups believed to be at high risk of infection. It was postulated that the HIV antibody test could separate those truly positive from those truly negative, after which one could identify or physically separate the positives from the negatives. (The Cuban model, applied since early in the epidemic, has required that all persons found to be HIV-antibody positive be confined to a common residence and thus be barred from associating with persons who are not HIV-antibody positive.) Unfortunately, no test provides 100 percent sensitivity and specificity for HIV antibody or any other test. Furthermore, a "window period" exists between time of exposure and infection with HIV and the actual development of antibody. This window period can range from about three weeks to several months during which time the individual would test negative when in fact he or she could transmit the virus. This example demonstrates how epidemiology can assist in the rational presentation of facts, thus preventing misinterpretation by the media and/or lobby groups not fully informed of the scientific facts and how to interpret them.

Notification. When special subgroups are identified for a study, the results of that study should be provided to the participants. Specifically, in occupational cohort studies, it is recommended in the United States that study participants be informed of any exposure to health risks uncovered through the study. The question that remains relates to the welfare of other workers who may be exposed to similar risk factors and who therefore could be at the same level of risk as those workers who were actually studied. If the cohort study that initially identified the risk was well-designed, it might be possible to extrapolate the research findings to other subgroups at risk in similar occupations, as well as to former employees. These latter two potentially at-risk groups are not currently included in the United States' National Institute for Occupational Safety and Health (NIOSH) guidelines.

Technologies continue to grow for determining individual susceptibility to illness that arises from workplace exposure to hazardous substances. If employers were privy to such information, they could exclude a job applicant on the grounds of wishing to protect the individual and at the same time to protect themselves from potential litigation. The tension arises between the obligation for full disclosure by the job applicant/worker on the one hand, and the obligation of the employer to provide a safe workplace. Some employers have argued that to render a workplace safe could be economically impractical. The controversy continues. Women, for example, face restrictions on employment in certain industries for fear by employers of liability—based on the existing body of knowledge about exposure to certain substances during pregnancy—if pregnancy should result in any abnormality at birth.

One mechanism for disseminating information involves community participation at all stages of a study, from hypothesis formulation through proposal development, review, conduct, analysis, write-up, and interpretation. In this way, community values are integrated into the research. Some occupational health studies have succeeded simply by establishing steering committees. These include not only scientists but also labor and management. Government involvement on a steering committee may also be appropriate.

Women and minorities. The U.S. National Institutes of Health has stated that research has focused disproportionately on white male subjects (Dresser, 1992). Results from studies on males are generalized to other population subgroups (i.e., to women and racial minorities) when the results, in fact, may not be generalizable. Such inferences may not only be misleading for the health of women and minorities but also could create harm through the potentially inappropriate application of findings from studies on white males to other groups in the United States. Therefore, it has now been mandated in the United States that women and minorities be included in all research programs whenever possible (NIH/ADAMHA, 1991).

It is difficult to quarrel with the concerns and remedies noted above. However, epidemiology is undertaken in populations not only where the problem to be investigated arises but also in populations that are large enough to satisfy statistical considerations. That is, access to exposed populations is what motivates and justifies epidemiologists to design and conduct a study. Statistical power is a function of the prevalence of exposure in a population. If a large enough number of women or minorities is not exposed to a given agent (e.g., chemical or pathogen) of interest, then their inclusion in studies could be unproductive, consequently wasting resources. Clearly, the researcher must be cognizant of the limits to which inferences can be drawn from any study; it is up to those formulating policy, however, to provide the incentives needed to encourage and enable the address of researchable questions of relevance to groups other than white males.

Assessment to date and future directions

Only recently have ethics guidelines been drafted for epidemiologists, whereas statisticians had broached the subject and developed guidelines in the 1980s. Physicians have been concerned with professional standards of practice in North America since the late nineteenth century. Although epidemiologists indeed may be entering the ethics discussion later than their counterparts, the relative recency of the profession must, of course, be considered. In their favor, epidemiologists are making efforts not only to develop ethics guidelines but also to integrate ethics into their teaching programs and into continuing professional education more generally. Ultimately, the expectation is that grass-roots involvement will maximize the likelihood of adherence to guidelines; the greater accountability of the profession to the public in whose interest epidemiology functions will be more assured.

Of growing concern are issues of self-interest and conflicting interests that sometimes take precedence over the public interest. Greater attention is being given to the consequences of research for destructive purposes through possible harm to the ecosystem and the advancement of militarism. Unless the professions are conversant with the principles of ethics, technological advances will continue to outstrip the ability of professions to respond; the professions' role will continue to be one manifesting a *reactive* as opposed to a *proactive* position.

COLIN L. SOSKOLNE

Directly related to this article are the other articles in this entry: DETERMINANTS OF PUBLIC HEALTH, HISTORY OF PUBLIC HEALTH, *and* PHILOSOPHY OF PUBLIC HEALTH. *Also directly related are the entries* PUBLIC HEALTH AND THE LAW; *and* HEALTH SCREENING AND TESTING IN THE PUBLIC-HEALTH CONTEXT. *For a further discussion of topics mentioned in this article, see the entries* COMMUNICATION, BIOMEDICAL, *article on* MEDIA AND BIOETHICS; CONFLICT OF INTEREST; ECONOMIC CONCEPTS IN HEALTH CARE; EPIDEMICS; FRAUD, THEFT, AND PLAGIARISM; INFORMATION DISCLOSURE; INFORMED CONSENT; LICENSING, DISCIPLINE, AND REGULATION IN THE HEALTH PROFESSIONS; MINORITIES AS RESEARCH SUBJECTS; OCCUPATIONAL SAFETY AND HEALTH; PRIVACY AND CONFIDENTIALITY IN RESEARCH; PROFESSION AND PROFESSIONAL ETHICS; PUBLIC POLICY AND BIOETHICS; RESEARCH, UNETHICAL; TECHNOLOGY, *especially the article on* TECHNOLOGY ASSESSMENT; TRUST; UTILITY; WHISTLEBLOWING; *and* WOMEN, *article on* RESEARCH ISSUES. *This article will find application in the entries* AGING AND THE AGED, *article on* HEALTH-CARE AND RESEARCH ISSUES; AIDS, *article on* HEALTH-CARE AND RESEARCH ISSUES; *and* CHILDREN, *article on* HEALTH-CARE AND RESEARCH ISSUES. *For a discussion of related ideas, see the entries* BIOETHICS EDUCATION, *article on* OTHER HEALTH PROFESSIONALS; COMMERCIALISM IN SCIENTIFIC RESEARCH; RESEARCH METHODOLOGY; *and* RESEARCH POLICY. *Other relevant material may be found under the entries* HEALTH CARE, QUALITY OF; *and* HEALTH OFFICIALS AND THEIR RESPONSIBILITIES.

Bibliography

BANKOWSKI, Z.; BRYANT, JOHN H.; and LAST, JOHN M. 1991. *Ethics and Epidemiology: International Guidelines. Proceedings of the XXVth CIOMS Conference, Geneva, Switzerland, 7–9 November, 1990.* Geneva: Council for International Organizations of Medical Sciences.

BAYER, RONALD. 1993. "The Ethics of Blinded HIV Surveillance Testing." *American Journal of Public Health* 83, no. 4:496–497.

BAYER, RONALD; DUBLER, NANCY N.; and LANDESMAN, SHELDON. 1993. "The Dual Epidemics of Tuberculosis and AIDS: Ethical and Policy Issues in Screening and Treatment." *American Journal of Public Health* 83, no. 5:649–654.

BAYER, RONALD, and FAIRCHILD-CARRINO, AMY. 1993. "AIDS and the Limits of Control: Public Health Orders, Quarantine, and Recalcitrant Behavior." *American Journal of Public Health* 83, no. 10:1471–1476.

BAYER, RONALD, and TOOMEY, KATHLEEN E. 1992. "HIV Prevention and the Two Faces of Partner Notification." *American Journal of Public Health* 82, no. 8:1158–1164.

BEAUCHAMP, TOM L.; COOK, RALPH R.; FAYERWEATHER, WILLIAM E.; RAABE, GERHARD K.; THAR, WILLIAM E.; COWLES, SALLY R.; and SPIVEY, GARY H. 1991. "Ethical Guidelines for Epidemiologists." *Journal of Clinical Epidemiology* 44 (suppl. 1):151S–169S.

COUNCIL FOR INTERNATIONAL ORGANIZATIONS OF MEDICAL SCIENCES (CIOMS). 1991. *International Guidelines for Ethical Review of Epidemiological Studies.* Geneva: Author.

———. 1993. *International Ethical Guidelines for Biomedical Research Involving Human Subjects.* Geneva: Author.

DRESSER, REBECCA. 1992. "Wanted: Single, White Male for Medical Research." *Hastings Center Report* 22, no. 1: 24–29.

FAWCETT, ERIC. 1993. "Working Group on Ethical Considerations in Science and Scholarship." *Accountability in Research* 3:69–72.

FAYERWEATHER, WILLIAM E.; HIGGINSON, JOHN; and BEAUCHAMP, TOM L., eds. 1991. "Industrial Epidemiology Forum's Conference on Ethics in Epidemiology." *Journal of Clinical Epidemiology* 44 (suppl.). Special issue.

GORDIS, LEON, and GOLD, ELLEN. 1980. "Privacy, Confidentiality, and the Use of Medical Records in Research." *Science* 207, no. 4427:153–156.

GORDIS, LEON; GOLD, ELLEN; and SELTSER, RAYMOND. 1977. "Privacy Protection in Epidemiologic and Medical Research: A Challenge and a Responsibility." *American Journal of Epidemiology* 105, no. 3:163–168.

HERWALDT, LOREEN A. 1993. "National Issues and Future Concerns." In *Prevention and Control of Nosocomial Infections*, 2d ed. Edited by Richard P. Wenzel. Baltimore: Williams & Wilkins.

HOFFMAN, RICHARD E. 1984. "The Use of Epidemiologic Data in the Courts." *American Journal of Epidemiology* 120, no. 2:190–202.

JOWELL, ROGER. 1986. "The Codification of Statistical Ethics." *Journal of Official Statistics* 2, no. 3:217–253.

LAPPE, MARC. 1986. "Ethics and Public Health." In *Maxcy-Rosenau Public Health and Preventive Medicine*, 12th ed., pp. 1867–1877. Edited by John M. Last. Norwalk, Conn.: Appleton-Century-Crofts.

LAST, JOHN M. 1987. "Ethical Issues in Public Health." In his *Public Health and Human Ecology*, pp. 351–370. East Norwalk, Conn.: Appleton & Lange.

———. 1991. "Guidelines on Ethics for Epidemiologists." *International Journal of Epidemiology* 19, no. 1:226–229.

LILIENFELD, ABRAHAM, and LILIENFELD, DAVID E. 1982. "Epidemiology and the Public Health Movement: A Historical Perspective." *Journal of Public Health Policy* 3, no. 2:140–149.

NATIONAL INSTITUTES OF HEALTH. 1991. "NIH/ADAMHA Policy Concerning Inclusion of Women in Study Populations." *NIH Guide* 20, no. 32:1–3.

ROSE, GEOFFREY. 1985. "Sick Individuals and Sick Populations." *International Journal of Epidemiology* 14, no. 1:32–38.

———. 1989. "High-Risk and Population Strategies of Prevention: Ethical Considerations." *Annals of Medicine* 21, no. 6:409–413.

ROSEN, GEORGE. 1958. *A History of Public Health*. New York: MD Publications.

ROTHMAN, KENNETH J. 1981. "The Rise and Fall of Epidemiology, 1950–2000 A.D." *New England Journal of Medicine* 304, no. 10:600–602.

RUSSEL, ELIZABETH, and WESTRIN, CLAES-GORAN. 1992. "Ethical Issues in Epidemiological Research." In "Medicine and Health: Workshop on Issues on the Harmonization of Protocols for Epidemiological Research in Europe, Florence, June 30 to July 2, 1991." Edited by Manuel Hallen and K. Vuylsteek. Commission of the European Communities, COMAC Epidemiology EUR 14596 EN.

SCHULTE, PAUL A. 1991. "Ethical Issues in the Communication of Results." *Journal of Clinical Epidemiology* 44 (suppl. 1):57S–61S.

SEVERSON, RICHARD K.; HEUSER, LINDA; and DAVIS, SCOTT. 1988. "Recontacting Study Participants in Epidemiologic Research." *American Journal of Epidemiology* 127, no. 6:1318–1320.

SOSKOLNE, COLIN L. 1985. "Epidemiological Research, Interest Groups, and the Review Process." *Journal of Public Health Policy* 6, no. 2:173–184.

———. 1986. "Scientific and Ethical Conflicts in Cancer Studies Involving Human Subjects." *Women and Health* 11, nos. 3–4:197–215.

———. 1989. "Epidemiology: Questions of Science, Ethics, Morality, and Law." *American Journal of Epidemiology* 129, no. 1:1–18.

———. 1991. "Ethical Decision-Making in Epidemiology: The Case Study Approach." *Journal of Clinical Epidemiology* 44 (suppl. 1):125S–130S.

———. 1991–1992. "Rationalizing Professional Conduct: Ethics in Disease Control." *Public Health Reviews* 19, nos. 1–4:311–321.

———. 1992. "Reader Questions Extensive Funding for Women's Health." *New Epidemiology Monitor* 13, no. 10:7.

———. 1993a. "Ethics and Policy Lost in Headline." *New Epidemiology Monitor* 14, no. 1:7.

———. 1993b. "Introduction to Misconduct in Science and Scientific Duties." *Journal of Exposure Analysis and Environmental Epidemiology* 3 (suppl. 1):245–252.

———, ed. 1993c. *Journal of Exposure Analysis and Environmental Epidemiology* 3 (suppl. 1):297–320. Special issue, "Questions from the Delegates and Answers by the Panelists Concerning 'Ethics and Law in Environmental Epidemiology.'"

SOSKOLNE, COLIN L., and LAST, JOHN M. 1993. "CMA Epidemiology Guidelines." *Journal of Occupational Medicine* 35, no. 2:97–98.

STOLLEY, PAUL D. 1985. "Faith, Evidence, and the Epidemiologist." *Journal of Public Health Policy* 6, no. 1:37–42.

SUSSER, MERVYN. 1977. "Judgment and Causal Inference: Criteria in Epidemiologic Studies." *American Journal of Epidemiology* 105, no. 1:1–15.

———. 1985. "Epidemiology in the United States After World War II: The Evolution of Technique." *Epidemiologic Reviews* 7:147–177.

SUSSER, MERVYN; STEIN, ZENA; and KLINE, JENNIE. 1978. "Ethics in Epidemiology." *Annals of the American Academy of Political and Social Science* 437:128–141.

TEICH, ALBERT H., and FRANKEL, MARK S. 1992. *Good Science and Responsible Scientists: Meeting the Challenge of Fraud and Misconduct in Science*. Washington, D.C.: American Association for the Advancement of Science.

TERRIS, MILTON. 1979. "The Epidemiologic Tradition: The Wade Hampton Frost Lecture." *Public Health Reports* 94, no. 3:203–209.

———. 1987. "Epidemiology and the Public Health Movement." *Journal of Public Health Policy* 8, no. 3:315–329.

VINEIS, PAOLO, and SOSKOLNE, COLIN L. 1993. "Cancer Risk Assessment and Management: An Ethical Perspective." *Journal of Occupational Medicine* 35, no. 9:902–908.

WEED, DOUGLAS L., and TROCK, BRUCE. 1988. "Interactions and Public Health Decisions." *Journal of Clinical Epidemiology* 41, no. 2:207–209.

WESTRIN, CLAES-GORAN. 1993. "Ethical, Legal, and Political Problems Affecting Epidemiology in European Countries." *IRB* 15, no. 3:6–8.

WESTRIN, CLAES-GORAN; NILSTUN, TORE; SMEDBY, BJORN; and HAGLUND, BENGT. 1992. "Epidemiology and Moral Philosophy." *Journal of Medical Ethics* 18, no. 4:193–196.

PUBLIC HEALTH AND THE LAW

I. Philosophy of the Law of Public Health
Frank P. Grad
II. Legal Moralism and Public Health
Dan E. Beauchamp

I. PHILOSOPHY OF THE LAW OF PUBLIC HEALTH

Public-health law covers a broad area that regulates activities and facilities to protect human health and that establishes institutions and programs to advance health and well-being. The development of public-health law has long been informed by the shared beliefs, political and philosophical, that provide a reason for government generally—to advance the common good and to protect the health, safety, and welfare of the people. Public-health law has changed over the years to reflect technological, scientific, and medical advances and to respond to newly emerging threats and hazards. Societal and legal developments have in turn created new ethical problems and challenges.

Historical background

In the eighteenth and nineteenth centuries, public health was concerned primarily with protecting the public against communicable disease and preventing epidemics. Concerns for environmental food and waste sanitation, health and safety in the workplace, and other protections we now take for granted arose only late in the nineteenth century and mostly in the early twentieth century. Driven largely by recurring epidemics of cholera, yellow fever, smallpox, typhus, typhoid, dysentery, diphtheria, and scarlet fever, states and municipalities created boards of health to take steps to protect against disease (Rosen, 1958). Because little was known about what caused disease, quarantine, the separation of persons who could infect others, became, in the absence of immunization or other preventive measures, the primary mode of control. As the understanding of bacterial spread of disease grew, other preventive measures followed, including the control of food handlers to prevent typhoid carriers from working in food establishments, the prevention of persons with tuberculosis from working as teachers or nursemaids, and the prohibition of industrial work in the home to prevent the dissemination of tuberculosis through homemade clothing. Other regulations forbade spitting in public places and carrying soiled laundry on public conveyances such as the early subway system in New York (Rosen, 1958).

The basis for early state and local legislation was the state's police power to protect the safety, health, and welfare of the people. The police power is the very reason for the establishment of state governments: to advance the public good and to protect all of us from each other. The police power is a broad and inherent power of government because it is part of the social contract (Bentham, 1969a, 1969b).

The police power had long been relied on even before public health became a concern. For example, the courts relied on police power in 1837 to support a state law authorizing the construction of a second bridge across the Charles River, which interfered with an alleged earlier franchise held by the owners of an old bridge (*Proprietors of Charles River Bridge* v. *Proprietors of Warren Bridge*, 1837). In 1851 the courts relied on police power to uphold state legislation limiting an owner's use of his property in Boston Harbor, when such use would interfere with navigation (*Commonwealth* v. *Alger*, 1851). The police power also provided the basis in 1876 for a state law to regulate grain elevator charges (*Munn* v. *Illinois*, 1876). In all of these instances, the courts relied on the police power to advance the interests of the community.

The broad thrust of the police power to advance and protect community interests was further developed in early public-health cases, upholding the state regulation of retail liquor sales over the objection that such regulation interfered with the use of private property (*Crowley* v. *Christiansen*, 1890). In these early cases, the claims of public interest under the police power overcame the assertion of private property interests protected under constitutional due process. Later cases involving the discriminatory regulation of laundries in wood-frame buildings (*Yick Wo* v. *Hopkins*, 1886) and the establishment of a quarantine district in such a way as to include and burden a larger number of Chinese immigrants (*Jew Ho* v. *Williamson*, 1900) firmly applied the police power to protect public health, safety, and morals while upholding individual interests protected by the Fourteenth Amendment of the U.S. Constitution.

In the twentieth century, public-health law in the United States increasingly dealt with the resolution of the tensions between the exercise of the state police power and protection of personal liberties through the due-process clause of the Fourteenth Amendment and other protections found in the Bill of Rights. In the landmark case *Jacobson v. Massachusetts* (1905), the U.S. Supreme Court upheld the city of Cambridge and the state of Massachusetts in exercising the police power to compel Jacobson to undergo a smallpox vaccination, not for his own protection but to prevent him from infecting others should he himself become infected in the smallpox epidemic in Cambridge. Jacobson argued that the law denied him liberty without due process and denied him the equal protection of the law. The Court upheld the state's exercise of the police power by applying a standard of reasonableness that followed utilitarian principles—the greatest protection for society at the least cost to the individual. Thus, the state's chosen method of control (vaccination) was reasonably adopted to achieve the end sought (an end to the epidemic) and was seen by the Court as a not excessive price to be paid by the individual under the circumstances (cf. Bentham, 1969b).

In cases where the exercise of police power allegedly violated property rights, other analytical approaches have been applied. In some of these, reliance on constitutional principles was not even articulated, because equitable approaches under the common law had long dealt with inappropriate uses of private property. For example, it is a well-established legal principle that citizens have a right to enjoin or abate a nuisance, a condition that is unwholesome or filthy and adversely affects neighboring property owners. The ancient principle of *sic utere tuo ut alienum non laedas* ("use your property so as not to hurt another") was often applied in private disputes and cited in constitutional decisions. States and municipalities began to designate such conditions as abatable nuisances, and public authorities could then prohibit or abate them. Some conditions first considered nuisances were referred to in *Commonwealth v. Alger* (1851), including warehouses for the storage of gunpowder near habitations or highways; wooden buildings of excessive height in populous neighborhoods and similar structures not covered with incombustible materials; buildings used for hospitals for contagious disease; the use of buildings to carry on noxious or offensive trades; and the raising of a dam that causes stagnant waters emitting dangerous fumes to spread over meadows near inhabited villages. A contemporary listing would include garbage dumps, sites for the disposal of hazardous wastes, paint spray plants, and fat-rendering plants. In *Mugler v. Kansas* (1887), the defendant had used his property to operate a brewery—a proscribed use—and was enjoined from using his property in this manner. The equitable rule of *sic utere tuo ut alienum non laedas* also calls for a balancing of equities, that is, a balancing of the benefits denied to the defendant against the benefit derived by the community in stopping undesirable uses of the property.

Expansion of public-health law

With the entry of the federal government into the field of public health in the twentieth century, public-health law expanded greatly, and there were significant changes in the character of the exercise of governmental powers and in the tasks undertaken by public-health law. The federal government has no plenary police powers (e.g., it lacks the power to provide for health, safety, and welfare), and yet the federal government plays a major role in the creation of public-health policies and in their execution through the exercise of particular powers delegated to it by the states under Article I of the U.S. Constitution. These powers include the power to regulate interstate and foreign commerce and the power to tax and spend for the general welfare. The Food, Drug, and Cosmetic Act (FDCA; 21 U.S.C. 301 et seq.), enacted in 1938, demonstrates the use of the federal commerce power in public-health regulation. Congress not only regulates trade and interstate transport of food, drugs, and cosmetics but also authorizes the Food and Drug Administration (FDA) both to set standards and to monitor the standard of quality of the merchandise itself, including the percentage of peanuts by weight in peanut butter and the water content of pastrami shipped across interstate lines. Through the FDA, the federal government also regulates the safety and efficacy of drugs and pharmaceuticals, adopting a detailed mechanism of administrative controls, including the power to adopt standards to inspect pharmacies and to exercise detailed supervision of the entire area of food and drug regulation. Interstate commerce regulation also includes the control of harmful emissions from automobile engines, showing that interstate-commerce controls affecting public health may be designated "environmental controls," though their primary purpose is the advancement of public health. In order to exercise the commerce power, the federal government usually acts directly through a federal agency, such as the FDA or the Environmental Protection Agency (EPA).

Taxing and spending power reflects a less direct exercise of federal powers. An early example of the use of this power in the public-health field was the 1944 Hill Burton Hospital Construction Program (now found in Subchapter IV, 42 U.S.C. 291(a) et seq., on Construction and Modernization of Hospitals and Other Medical Facilities) under which the federal government grants funds to a state or municipality for hospital construction programs and nonprofit community hospitals (Grad, 1990). As a condition of the grant, the state or local government must comply with federal regulations, including facility and personnel requirements, as well as provide free services for indigent persons. Another ongoing grant-in-aid program is the program under Subchapter II of the Federal Water Pollution Control Act Amendments of 1972 for the construction of public waste-treatment works by states and municipalities (33 U.S.C. 1281–1299). This program has helped clean up U.S. waterways and develop improved sewers in U.S. cities. Grant-in-aid programs have been used widely to support infrastructure developments to advance public health. Under grant-in-aid programs, the federal government does not act directly but requires states to pass regulations and carry out construction, enforcement, and compliance activities in order to meet the conditions of the grant.

Federal public-health activities under the commerce power are somewhat analogous to the state exercise of the police power in that they command and control certain activities. Like exercises of the state police power, they must meet the constitutional requirements of due process and equal protection. Their philosophical basis is largely utilitarian, seeking to find a reasonable balance between the public interest and the protection of private entrepreneurial interests in development and property. Federal public-health activities under the taxing and spending power may advance similar concerns, but to the extent that they involve significant distribution of federal funds, other concerns, such as those relating to fairness in distribution, also play a part. John Rawls argues that if the principle of equal liberty is met, as well as the principle of equality of opportunity, the difference principle permits inequalities in the distribution of social and economic goods if those inequalities will benefit everyone, especially the least advantaged (Rawls, 1971). Distribution formulas for the sharing of federal funds by geographic areas and by responding to areas with greater needs meet the Rawls formulation.

Major public-health approaches

There are two major approaches in the protection of public health. The first and older one uses regulatory enforcement programs, ranging from epidemiologic controls and protection against unwholesome living conditions to identification and removal of poisons in the environment. Included are protection of the food and water supplies and protection against hazards and poisons in the workplace. Programs to protect the public against the variety of nuclear hazards from the generation of nuclear energy and efforts to prevent the destruction of the protective stratospheric ozone layer by the dissemination of hydrofluorocarbons and other ozone-destructive gases are also included in this area. Public health now also includes major aspects of environmental protection and occupational health and safety.

Although the field of public-health regulation and enforcement has grown enormously, its expansion is ex-ceeded by the second area of public-health protection, an increasing number and volume of public-health services. The government provides services to advance the health of the public, including the provision of well-baby clinics, family-planning clinics, community mental-health programs, and a variety of government-sponsored research institutions that provide special services. Both regulatory enforcement programs and service programs must meet constitutional requirements. In general, equal protection under the Fourteenth Amendment specifies that the same degree of fairness apply in the provisions of benefits and services as in the imposition of obligations and duties. As a result, government agencies give careful consideration to allocation factors in the distribution of services to determine how priorities ought to be set between public health and other needs and to determine the priority of certain health-related needs over others. Finally, institutions must often determine specific allocations among individuals with different health and other needs (Rawls, 1971). Of course, political considerations, such as pressure from physicians and other service providers or from consumers, including such politically powerful groups as the elderly, also have an effect—sometimes a profound one—on the process.

In addition to direct service programs, Medicare and Medicaid (both established in 1965) pay or reimburse medical costs. Medicare is an offshoot of Social Security, based on a major social insurance initiative. Focused on reimbursement of fees for service, it subsidizes health-care costs of social-security recipients—primarily the disabled and persons sixty-five and older. Initially paid for by employer and employee contributions, Medicare became an entitlement program because employees had secured contractual rights to social insurance through their own contributions. Medicaid is a federal grant-in-aid program, financed by both federal and state contributions, to provide medical care for the "medically indigent," persons whose family income level is so low that it is impossible for them to pay their own medical expenses. Both Medicare and Medicaid are managed federally by the Health Care Financing Administration (HCFA).

Government involvement is dominant in these programs; since government reimburses medical providers for services rendered, it is directly involved in regulating the quality of the services. Medicaid may be viewed as a welfare program that takes the place of earlier, inadequate provision of care for the poor through charitable or public institutions. Medicare, based on contractual entitlements, was created with the initial expectation that employees would die soon after reaching the retirement age of sixty-five. However, the increasing longevity of the covered population and the substantial increase in the cost of health services have led to persistent and loud political criticism. But such programs are hardly novel. State financing of health-care costs began in Germany under Otto von Bismarck in the late nineteenth century, and many European nations, including Great Britain, the Netherlands, the Scandinavian countries, and Austria, have continued to provide health care, though their gross national product and their industrial base are considerably smaller than that of the United States.

In the United States there is no right to health care or to treatment under federal or state law, except insofar as specific reimbursement provisions have been provided by law. There certainly is no constitutional entitlement to health care. However, a number of writers have suggested an egalitarian right to health care, claiming that everyone who has an equal need for health-care services or resources must have equal access to them. This has sometimes been asserted as a corollary of a general egalitarian welfare right, requiring the distribution of resources first to assure that everyone's net welfare over a lifetime is equal (Buchanan, 1989; Veatch, 1981). This expansion of welfare rights, including the right to health care, had not as of 1994 become part of American law. Any such proposal would be promptly rejected by the so-called libertarian point of view, which regards as inappropriate all social ordering that does not rely on the allocation of goods and services by market processes (Buchanan, 1989; Nozick, 1974).

It is difficult to formulate a single philosophical basis for federal involvement in the multiplicity of public-health programs. Twentieth-century federal public-health programs are invariably based on detailed programmatic legislation that not only establishes new rules of law but also creates major new governmental structures to manage the newly emerging areas of governmental control (Grad, 1985). Such new structures are exemplified by the FDA, the EPA, and agencies that manage social insurance programs such as Medicare and Medicaid. In every instance, the agency is given broad rule-making powers to be exercised in accordance with the general purposes indicated in the statute. In statutes to protect society against toxic substances and hazardous waste, the general purpose may be "to protect health and the environment." When it comes to such legislative instructions, one might be tempted to refer to the earlier principle *sic utere tuo ut alienum non laedas* or to the broader principle of preventing harm to others, but this would not be historically or analytically correct, since these earlier principles were intended to govern persons in their private relationships or in their relationships within a relatively small community. Modern public-health programs address broader national or even global problems. Moreover, the emphasis of earlier approaches was generally to prevent harm, while modern program-

matic legislation often seeks to advance public benefits. The utilitarian rationale of protecting the health interests of the public at the least possible cost to the individual seems the most appropriate. The purposes of public-health programs are legislatively defined. Legislation is political and therefore majoritarian in its nature, unlike the judicially established bases for protection under common law, articulated by judges and intended primarily to resolve individual disputes.

Public health and AIDS

The emergence of AIDS (acquired immunodeficiency syndrome) in the 1980s demonstrated the basic tension between the protection of individual rights and the enforcement of broadly applicable police-power measures to protect public health. Another significant challenge was the threat of a multidrug-resistant form of tuberculosis in the late 1980s and 1990s. Communicable diseases are generally reportable under health codes, and such reports to a health department are normally protective of the patient's privacy. Special confidentiality protections are particularly applicable to reports of sexually transmitted diseases and, in earlier times, of tuberculosis. The reason for special privacy protections originated in the protection of the patient against stigma, because a report of certain diseases was regarded as a social disgrace. The knowledge that the report of a communicable disease may result in stigmatization and discrimination was undesirable from the public-health point of view, because patients were less likely to seek treatment if their confidentiality was breached.

When AIDS emerged in 1981, most other communicable diseases had ceased to represent major public-health problems, and the early history of reports to health departments and the possibility of contact investigations to trace potentially exposed persons, particularly in the area of sexually transmitted diseases, had become a forgotten record. Constitutional protection of privacy as a part of due process had been developed earlier in the context of the right of a pregnant woman to choose to terminate pregnancy. Privacy protections, and related protections of personal autonomy, are asserted to protect against the disclosure of HIV (human immunodeficiency virus) status, even though AIDS is by now a reportable disease in each state of the United States.

Since transmission of HIV was at first associated with homosexual intercourse and later with intravenous drug use, there were compelling reasons to protect the identity of persons who were HIV-positive. Privacy protections also interfered with giving notice of exposure and risk to persons who had been exposed, because such information, unless disclosed voluntarily, would inevitably breach the patient's confidentiality. As of 1994, the tension between the desirable protection of the patient's privacy and the public-health commitment to inform exposed persons had not been fully resolved, and halfway measures had sometimes been adopted. In New York State, for instance, the physician of a patient diagnosed as HIV-positive could, but was under no legal compulsion to, inform the patient's spouse or other sexual partners. The problem will not be resolved until public-health education succeeds in lifting the stigma of AIDS or until a cure for the disease is found.

Because persons who are HIV-positive and have a defective immune system are more likely to contract tuberculosis than others, the recurrence of tuberculosis in multidrug-resistant form creates a situation in which the disclosure of a patient's affliction with tuberculosis may be regarded, often erroneously, as an indication of positive HIV status, aggravating the problem of maintaining confidentiality. Privacy is now an aspect of personhood, and protection against the invasion of privacy—in this instance, the invasion of informational privacy—is constitutionally given under the Fifth Amendment (Tribe, 1978). Ethical protection of privacy is based on privacy as an aspect of personhood, protectable to the same extent as a person's physical integrity. Violations of privacy then become ethically justifiable only if disclosure serves a greater good. Thus, whether a patient's HIV status should be disclosed to others depends on the need of such others to know and on the potential uses and benefits that may result from the disclosure (Bayer, 1989).

Genetic privacy

Privacy issues also arise in new areas of public health. Public screening programs for PKU (phenylketonuria), an inborn metabolic defect that causes mental retardation unless promptly controlled by a special diet low in phenylalanine, and sickle-cell anemia have long been part of the law of many state public-health programs. However, the Human Genome Initiative (HGI), a multibillion-dollar federal project to trace and sequence the human genome, as of the mid-1990s was moving issues of privacy protection into the foreground. Information relating to a person's genetic makeup is especially sensitive, because it may provide predictive information as to future health and the risk of having children afflicted with a genetic disease. A person might not want information of this kind disclosed because genetic diseases are still regarded as stigmatizing by much of society. This information also is of substantial economic value to insurance companies and to employers who would rather not have to buy health insurance for employees whose families are at risk of substantial medical expenses. The right to privacy in this connection has been referred to not only as a personal right but as a protectable public good, thus subject to disclosure only for reasons

significant enough to outweigh the value of privacy (Henkin, 1974).

Conclusion

Public-health law is a dynamic developing field, based on established principles and legal tradition, yet contemporary and responsive to current needs. Soundly based on the police power of the state and certain delegated federal powers under the U.S. Constitution, public-health law has experienced a significant expansion in its current inclusion of such fields as the law of mental health, the law of occupational health and safety, major aspects of environmental law, and the growing area of legal developments relating to genetic disease. Although the domain of public-health law has expanded, it has retained its essential purpose of advancing the public good at the least cost to individual freedom.

FRANK P. GRAD

Directly related to this article is the companion article in this entry: LEGAL MORALISM AND PUBLIC HEALTH. *Also directly related are the entries* PUBLIC HEALTH; LAW AND BIOETHICS; *and* LAW AND MORALITY. *For a further discussion of topics mentioned in this article, see the entries* AIDS; CONFIDENTIALITY; ENVIRONMENTAL HEALTH; EPIDEMICS; FREEDOM AND COERCION; GENETIC TESTING AND SCREENING; HARM; HEALTH-CARE FINANCING, *articles on* MEDICARE, *and* MEDICAID; MEDICAL ETHICS, HISTORY OF, *section on* EUROPE, *subsection on* CONTEMPORARY PERIOD; OCCUPATIONAL SAFETY AND HEALTH; PHARMACEUTICS, *article on* PHARMACEUTICAL INDUSTRY; PHARMACY; PRIVACY IN HEALTH CARE; RIGHTS; *and* UTILITY. *For a discussion of related ideas, see the entries* AUTONOMY; CONFLICT OF INTEREST; GENETIC COUNSELING; GENETICS AND THE LAW; HEALTH POLICY; HOMICIDE; JUSTICE; LIFESTYLES AND PUBLIC HEALTH; PATIENTS' RIGHTS; PRIVACY AND CONFIDENTIALITY IN RESEARCH; *and* PUBLIC POLICY AND BIOETHICS.

Bibliography

ARRAS, JOHN, and HUNT, ROBERT. 1983. *Ethical Issues in Modern Medicine.* 2d ed. Palo Alto, Calif.: Mayfield.

BAYER, RONALD. 1989. *Private Acts, Social Consequences: AIDS and the Politics of Public Health.* New York: Free Press.

BEAUCHAMP, TOM L., and CHILDRESS, JAMES F. 1983. *Principles of Biomedical Ethics.* 2d ed. New York: Oxford University Press.

BENTHAM, JEREMY. 1969a. "A Fragment on Government." In *A Bentham Reader,* pp. 55–72. Edited by Mary Peter Mack. New York: Pegasus.

———. 1969b. "An Introduction to the Principles of Morals

and Legislation." In *A Bentham Reader*, pp. 78–144. Edited by Mary Peter Mack. New York: Pegasus.

BUCHANAN, ALLEN. 1989. "Health-Care Delivery and Resource Allocation." In *Medical Ethics*, pp. 291–326. Edited by Robert M. Veatch. Boston: Jones and Bartlett.

Commonwealth v. Alger. 1851. 61 Mass. 53.

Crowley v. Christiansen. 1890. 137 U.S. 86.

GRAD, FRANK P. 1985. "The Ascendancy of Legislation: Legal Problem Solving in Our Time." *Dalhousie Law Journal* 9, no. 2:228–260.

———. 1986. "Public Health Law." In *Public Health and Preventive Medicine*, 12th ed., pp. 1849–1865. Edited by John M. Last. Norwalk, Conn.: Appleton-Century-Crofts.

———. 1990. *The Public Health Law Manual.* 2d ed. Washington, D.C.: American Public Health Association.

HENKIN, LOUIS. 1974. "Privacy and Autonomy." *Columbia Law Review* 74, no. 7:1410–1433.

Jacobson v. Massachusetts. 1905. 197 U.S. 11.

Jew Ho v. Williamson. 1900. 103 F.10 (Circuit Court, N.D. Cal.).

Mugler v. Kansas. 1887. 123 U.S. 623.

Munn v. Illinois. 1876. 94 U.S. 113.

NOZICK, ROBERT. 1974. *Anarchy, State, and Utopia.* New York: Basic Books.

Proprietors of the Charles River Bridge v. Proprietors of the Warren Bridge. 1837. 36 U.S. 420.

RAWLS, JOHN. 1971. *A Theory of Justice.* Cambridge, Mass.: Harvard University Press.

ROSEN, GEORGE. 1958. *The History of Public Health.* New York: MD Publications.

TRIBE, LAURENCE H. 1978. "Rights of Privacy and Personhood." In his *American Constitutional Law*, pp. 886–990. Mineola, N.Y.: Foundation.

VANDEVEER, DONALD, and REGAN, TOM, eds. 1987. *Health Care Ethics: An Introduction.* Philadelphia: Temple University Press.

VEATCH, ROBERT M. 1981. *A Theory of Medical Ethics.* New York: Basic Books.

Yick Wo v. Hopkins. 1886. 118 U.S. 356.

II. LEGAL MORALISM AND PUBLIC HEALTH

Modern public health, which uses organized community effort, law, and regulation to save lives and prevent disease, has long been entangled with legal moralism, which uses the same measures to protect society against behavior that is viewed in some quarters as "offensive, degrading, vicious, sinful, corrupt, or otherwise immoral" (Schur and Bedau, 1974, p. 1). "Morals offenses" have "included mainly sex offenses, such as adultery, fornication, sodomy, incest and prostitution, but also a miscellany of nonsexual offenses" (Feinberg, 1973). Legal moralism has cultural and religious origins, but its deepest roots are in purity rituals codified in religious and secular codes (Douglas, 1966). Purity rituals are avoidance rituals designed to make the environment and the community safe from the threat of uncleanness and contamination and to promote social order. These codes governed diet, sexual conduct, bodily cleanliness, and avoidance of contamination.

In its most expansive expression legal moralism is the belief that these behavioral codes, regulations, and legal proscriptions are foundational to a social order. To the moralist, drug taking, vice, crime, and sexual promiscuity not only harm the self and others but also threaten, through contagion and example, to loosen the bonds that hold society together. It is the connection between the proscribed conduct or practice and the theories about how the spread of this conduct threatens social order that so often results in the confusion of public health and moralism. Because moralism is often expressed in terms of public-health theories of contagion, it has proved difficult to separate the two modes of thought.

The belief that immorality is contagious also often includes the belief that immorality causes disease. Barbara Gutmann Rosenkrantz's authoritative history of public health in Massachusetts cites a review of Lemuel Shattuck's 1850 report on the health of the state, noting that the "sanitary movement does not merely relate to the lives and health of the community; it is also a means of moral reform. . . . The ultimate connection between filth and vice has been noted by all writers upon this subject" (Rosenkrantz, 1972, p. 2).

Moralism in public health arises when society or groups in society respond to a health crisis more by voicing objections to a social practice or to a group engaged in that practice than by rationally assessing the dangers of disease and the best ways to prevent its spread. The parallels between theories of disease causation found in public health and legal moralism are often challenged and overturned by scientific theories of disease causation. While public-health campaigns and officials have often addressed problems moralistically in the past, the long-term trend indicates a separation of the two ways of thinking. Moralism has also suffered attacks from religious groups that emphasize social justice or inwardness more than adherence to religious rules. Finally, moralism is challenged by the modern and postmodern tolerance of a wider range of sexual expression and by the spreading support for political liberties and rights of privacy for all citizens, even those accused of immoral practices.

Moralism's most potent threat to public health comes from the ways in which epidemics and moral dissolution are believed to be inextricably tied together. This entanglement makes the victims of new outbreaks of certain diseases seem a threat to society itself. It also leads to powerful drives to stigmatize and shame the epidemic's victims, in the use of legislation and regulation to invoke shame and public denunciation for a category of persons or in what have been called "status degradation ceremonies" (Garfinkel, 1956). The current struggle in the fight against acquired immunodeficiency syndrome (AIDS) is the best-known contemporary example of the confusion between moralism and public health.

Thus, the purpose of the policies of the United States in incarcerating prostitutes during World War I was not just to prevent the spread of syphilis and venereal disease but also to shame and punish a class of individuals and to close and solidify the ranks of a nation going to war (Brandt, 1987). This moral campaign of imprisonment took priority over the use of new medical treatments for syphilis and gonorrhea, which, while still primitive, were surely more effective.

Modern public-health problems, especially those of a contagious or epidemic nature, provide a constant temptation for legislators, health officials, and the public to confuse the ends of preventing harm to individuals and communities and of proscribing immorality. Yet it would be wrong to conclude that all proscriptions of a practice or behavior are tantamount to moralism. Moralism and social disapproval are not the same thing, even though the latter may be an echo of the former. Social disapproval or even indignation about a practice remains a potent ally of many public-health campaigns.

Public health and alcohol policy

Legal moralism has played a prominent role in alcohol policy, particularly in movements to prohibit all drinking in the United States, in England, and in the Nordic countries. The history of alcohol policy, more than that of most public-health problems, reveals the difficulty in separating health issues from moralizing claims. It also reveals how some of the ways we seek to avoid moralism can be counter to science and to the health and safety of the public.

In the United States, Prohibition, or the outlaw of the manufacture and sale of alcoholic beverages, was enforced from 1917 until 1933. The Prohibition movement is a fascinating intermingling of progressive and scientific thinking, moralism, and religious fundamentalism. For example, the Progressive period in U.S. history (roughly 1890 to 1920) was not just a period when the states began to expand their powers over child labor, over the working conditions of adults, or of assuring safe food and water by strengthening the regulatory power of the states over private property; it was also a period that witnessed the rise of movements to protect the decency and purity of the public through antipornography legislation, crackdowns on prostitution (especially during World War I), and American Prohibition (Brandt, 1987).

There is little doubt that the various reform movements that culminated in the passage of the Prohibition amendment brought to the nation's attention a social problem (drunkenness, the saloon, and an overly powerful liquor interest) that demanded state and federal legislation. Also, the record shows clearly that the results of Prohibition, measured solely in public-health terms, were sharply reduced overall consumption of alcohol and related steep declines in serious public-health problems like cirrhosis, admittance to public hospitals for alcohol-related disorders, and the like (Moore and Gerstein, 1981; Beauchamp, 1980).

The strong secular and progressive side to the movement for Prohibition saw the saloon as a great social problem, one that undermined the public health and safety and promoted domestic violence and crimes against women. Both the movements for women's suffrage and the movement against slavery frequently were headed by leaders who also advocated Prohibition. Yet this began to change in the last decade of the nineteenth century. The women's movement had focused its energies on winning suffrage, and the movement against slavery had long since been replaced by Reconstruction. During the concluding decades of the agitation for Prohibition, the first two decades of the twentieth century, support for Prohibition came primarily from Protestant churches; national Prohibition's justification shifted more and more toward the moralistic claim that drink was the root of most of society's evil. (Moralism is often characterized by inflated claims of the evils or dangers from a substance or a practice, even in very small quantities or isolated and scattered acts.) The intertwining of moralism and public policy, especially for alcohol and drug taking, seems more common in nations where fundamentalist forms of Protestantism that stress adherence to religiously sanctioned behaviors are widespread, or in Muslim nations, where similar fundamentalism obtains; Catholic societies have never had successful Prohibition movements (although temperance movements are found in Ireland).

The backlash to Prohibition produced theories of alcoholism that sought both to deny its moralistic forebears and to establish a new and scientific theory of causation, called the disease concept of alcoholism. This was the belief that alcoholism was caused by an inability to control drinking. In parallel fashion, and also to separate itself from a discredited past, the new alcoholism movement denied the public-health benefits of Prohibition, and as late as the 1960s leading national experts claimed that Prohibition caused people to drink more. The links between what a society drinks generally and the level of alcohol problems were viewed as part of a neoprohibitionist agenda.

The attempt to purge society of moralistic remnants of Prohibition has often been met with surprises. For example, there were strong drives to prohibit alcohol in Norway, Sweden, and Finland during the 1920s and

1930s. Only Sweden avoided Prohibition, in a narrow national referendum vote. In Finland, during the late 1960s and 1970s, the drive to eliminate the rural remnants of their national prohibition legislation of the 1930s led to a sharp relaxation of drinking laws throughout society and the elimination of prohibition in rural areas. The experts believed that restrictions actually encouraged drinking of distilled beverages in unsocialized ways and that by eliminating prohibition, drinking would actually decrease. Yet the measures to liberalize drinking were followed by steep increases in drinking rates and associated problems such as public drunkenness (Beauchamp, 1980). Subsequently, state authorities and their advisers retreated from a too-uncritical relaxation of drinking legislation, shifting the justification for alcohol policy more toward a public-health model that accepted limits on all drinking as a necessary part of a sound policy and as not necessarily moralistic.

Western democracies during the 1970s and 1980s witnessed declines in drinking rates, attributed by experts to a growing cultural conservatism and a widening awareness of the public-health consequences of heavy drinking and high levels of per capita consumption. This new period was likely also solidified by the fact that heavy drinking became socially and even morally undesirable, just as smoking became morally undesirable. While drunkenness and addiction were still viewed less punitively, the public began to register its strong disapproval of heavy drinking, especially when it posed risks to others, such as in drinking and driving, or any drinking at all by teenagers. More broadly, the era when drinking itself was not seen as the problem was replaced with a period in which all drinking remains somewhat under a public-health cloud. The evidence that some forms of drinking might promote a healthier heart has caused that cloud to lift only a little.

Smoking and public health

At the turn of the twentieth century, smoking was treated as morally offensive. Churches proscribed cigarette smoking and urged public action. But the long-term popularity of smoking spread too quickly, and the campaign was eventually abandoned. Soon smoking was regarded as cosmopolitan and modern. Cigarette smoking rates grew and became widely and culturally approved (Warner, 1986). In the 1950s epidemiological studies appeared in the United States and England noting the link between smoking and lung cancer and the possible links with heart disease. The U.S. Surgeon General issued a widely discussed report compiling very strong and extensive research suggesting that smoking was one of the most lethal hazards of our times.

The social climate against smoking began to turn in the late 1960s and 1970s. Antismoking sentiment rose,

and cigarette advertising on television was banned. The risks of smoking for third parties was noted. Communities and entire states began to legislate against smoking in public places. Higher taxes on cigarette smoking were advocated. Smoking rates in most industrial societies fell, but most impressively in the United States. This sharp decline is not only due to the extensive public discussion devoted to the hazards of smoking but also to the growing sense of social and even moral disapproval of smoking by the larger society. This social disapproval was sometimes seen as a resurgence of moralism. But there is scant evidence that the strong current of disapproval against smoking adds up to moralism.

Moralism and the AIDS epidemic

As Allan Brandt notes, the battle against venereal diseases in the first decades of the twentieth century and the rise of AIDS more recently give evidence that moralism remains a powerful element in the social construction of society's definition of these diseases (Brandt, 1987). Early in the twentieth century, syphilis was a symbol of a "society characterized by a corrupt sexuality. Venereal disease has typically been used as a symbol of pollution and contamination, [and of] . . . a decaying social order. Venereal disease makes clear the persistent association of disease with dirt and uncleanness as well" (Brandt, 1987, p. 5).

The most serious challenge to modern public health by legal moralism entered with the AIDS epidemic and HIV-related diseases. Because anal sex and frequent sex with multiple partners heightens the risk of transmission of the HIV virus and because intravenous drug use also seriously elevates the risk of infection from contaminated needles, legislation that seeks to regulate these behaviors—which are widely proscribed in many states—is always open to the charge of moralism.

Early in the epidemic in the United States, bathhouses frequented by homosexual patrons became targets of public-health regulations. Many in the gay community charged that the measures were aimed less at fighting the epidemic than at proscribing homosexuality. These advocates argued, quite plausibly, that the regulations would have little impact on the course of the epidemic in San Francisco or New York, the two cities where conflicts primarily arose. This was because the bathhouses were the site of only a fraction of the proscribed behaviors. Advocates also argued that city officials and state public-health authorities had caved in to political pressures (Bayer, 1991b).

The same charge of moralism and discrimination was also brought when public-health officials attempted to introduce methods of identifying the sexual partners of those who were AIDS victims, or when state medical societies sought legislation to make AIDS and HIV diseases reportable to state health authorities (Bayer, 1991b). (All states require private physicians to report certain communicable diseases to state health officials.) Ronald Bayer, in his book *Private Acts, Social Consequences* (1991b), has provided the best chronicle of the clash between public-health legislation and the civil libertarians defending AIDS victims. As Bayer says, "These two abstractions, liberty and communal welfare, are always in a state of tension in public health policy" (1991b, p. 16).

It is likely, however, that the AIDS epidemic has permanently altered the landscape of public-health policy, and not just in the United States. No longer will it be possible to easily equate public health only with the use of powers to restrict power and liberty to promote the public health or to see the realms of public health and individual liberty as radically distinct. The growing awareness is that a sound public-health policy requires more than restrictions on liberty and property to promote the communal welfare. It also may require the expansion of private liberties and rights for groups suffering social discrimination based on moralism.

Dan E. Beauchamp

Directly related to this article is the companion article in this entry: philosophy of the law of public health. *For a further discussion of topics mentioned in this article, see the entries* Behavior Control; Epidemics; Ethics, *article on* religion and morality; Freedom and Coercion; Health Officials and Their Responsibilities; Homosexuality; Law and Morality; Lifestyles and Public Health; Prostitution; *and* Substance Abuse. *This article will find application in the entry* AIDS, *article on* public-health issues. *For a discussion of related ideas, see the entries* Abuse, Interpersonal; Health Promotion and Health Education; *and* Health Screening and Testing in the Public-Health Context.

Bibliography

Bayer, Ronald. 1991a. "AIDS: The Politics of Prevention and Neglect." *Health Affairs* 10, no. 1:87–97.
———. 1991b. *Private Acts, Social Consequences: AIDS and the Politics of Public Health.* New Brunswick, N.J.: Rutgers University Press. The best discussion and history of these political conflicts.
Beauchamp, Dan E. 1980. *Beyond Alcoholism: Alcohol and Public Health Policy.* Philadelphia: Temple University Press.
———. 1988. *The Health of the Republic: Epidemics, Medicine, and Moralism as Challenges to Democracy.* Philadelphia: Temple University Press.
Brandt, Allan M. 1987. *No Magic Bullet: A Social History of Venereal Disease in the United States Since 1880.* New York: Oxford University Press.
Devlin, Patrick. 1959. *The Enforcement of Morals.* London: Oxford University Press.
Douglas, Mary. 1966. *Purity and Danger: An Analysis of the Concepts of Pollution and Taboo.* London: Routledge.
Feinberg, Joel. 1973. *Social Philosophy.* Englewood Cliffs, N.J.: Prentice-Hall.
Garfinkel, Harold. 1956. "Conditions of Successful Status Degradation Ceremonies." *American Journal of Sociology* 61, no. 5:420–424.
Gusfield, Joseph R. 1963. *Symbolic Crusade: Status Politics and the American Temperance Crusade.* Urbana: University of Illinois Press.
Hart, H. L. A. 1963. *Law, Liberty, and Morality.* New York: Vintage.
Moore, Mark H., and Gerstein, Dean, eds. 1981. *Alcohol and Public Policy: Beyond the Shadow of Prohibition.* Washington, D.C.: National Academy Press.
Rosenkrantz, Barbara Gutmann. 1972. *Public Health and the State: Changing Views in Massachusetts, 1842–1936.* Cambridge, Mass.: Harvard University Press.
Schur, Edwin M., and Bedau, Hugo Adam. 1974. *Victimless Crimes: Two Sides of a Controversy.* Englewood Cliffs, N.J.: Prentice-Hall. Bedau's section of this work is a good discussion of legal moralism.
Shattuck, Lemuel. 1948. *Report of the Sanitary Commission of Massachusetts, 1850.* Cambridge, Mass.: Harvard University Press.
Warner, Kenneth E. 1986. *Selling Smoke: Cigarette Advertising and Public Health.* Washington, D.C.: American Public Health Association.

PUBLIC HEALTH AND LIFESTYLES

See Lifestyles and Public Health.

PUBLIC HEALTH AND WAR

See Warfare, *article on* public health and war.

PUBLIC POLICY AND BIOETHICS

There are at least two ways of understanding the relation of public policy to bioethics. The first focuses on public policy *in* bioethics, which includes the public laws (both statutory and case law), policies, regulations, and guidelines that bear on ethical aspects of medical practice and health care. These are public in the sense that they emanate from some publicly accountable governmental process, as opposed to private or professional policy; in addition, nonpublic institutions like hospitals can adopt their own policies to conform to public policy. In this sense, legal requirements to obtain informed consent for treatment, federal regulations requiring approval of a research protocol by an institution's human subjects committee, and the lack in the United States of any governmental means of ensuring universal access to health care for all citizens represent public policy bearing on ethical aspects of medical and research practice. These would be part of the answer to questions of what public policy *is* with regard to whether patients must consent to their treatment, how human subjects in research are to be protected, and whether all citizens should be guaranteed access to a basic level of health care.

When the relation of public policy to bioethics is understood in this way, the question arises as to the extent to which bioethics issues have been and should be matters of explicit public policy. Physician–patient relations, for example, may be taken to be a largely private matter to be worked out by physicians and patients outside of the public sphere, as they in fact were to a great extent in the early part of the twentieth century, or to be a matter of professional concern by physicians in professional settings, but not the subject of and regulated by public policy. Alternatively, such issues might be seen, as they increasingly were in the United States in the 1970s and 1980s, as an appropriate concern of public policy. Thus, public policy in bioethics includes what governments choose not to do, as well as what they do, in bioethics.

The second understanding of the relation of public policy to bioethics focuses on public-policy bodies that have been influential in shaping bioethics, public policy on bioethics issues, and health-care practice. Understood in this way, the subject is the manner and extent to which bodies like the U.S. President's Commission for the Study of Ethical Problems in Medicine and Biomedical and Behavioral Research (hereafter President's Commission) have shaped bioethics and medicine. Why have the United States and many other countries frequently turned to such bodies in the development of public policy in bioethics? How have such bodies functioned? What has been their impact?

In this article we shall address both of these understandings of the relation between public policy and bioethics. A general thesis of this article is that bioethics and public policy, broadly construed to include both these understandings of the relationship between them, have influenced one another. The field of bioethics has helped shape and has been shaped by both public policy in bioethics and a variety of policymaking institutions in bioethics.

The relation between substantive public policy and bioethics

As bioethics in the United States during the 1970s and 1980s became an area of great public and professional concern, many standard bioethical issues began to be addressed, not just in classrooms or between doctors and patients, but also in explicit public debates and policies. One of the most prominent examples, cardiopulmonary resuscitation (CPR) of patients who have suffered cardiac or respiratory arrest, illustrates a relatively common pattern of this development of public policy on important bioethics issues. First, a new technology was developed; in this case and not atypically, it was a form of life-sustaining treatment. Originally the technology was developed for and applied in a relatively narrow range of cases in which there was clear expected benefit; otherwise healthy people who suffered unexpected cardiac or respiratory arrest were saved. Later it came to be used in a wider range of cases, including many patients for whom its expected success and benefit were questionable. This particular technology came to be used even more widely because the conditions to which it responded—cardiac and respiratory arrest—precluded taking time to make thoughtful decisions about whether to employ it.

Reports of widely varied practices, including some that were ethically problematic at best and certainly did not represent sound general practice, led many hospitals to develop formal policies about resuscitation. This general interest in Do Not Resuscitate (DNR) orders led to both normative and empirical scholarly studies of the use of CPR and DNR orders. Public bodies like the President's Commission addressed the issue and developed recommendations about institutional policies, and the Joint Commission for the Accreditation of Hospitals required institutions to have a policy regarding DNR orders. In this case, a public-policy response to an identified and significant ethical problem in medical practice led to both a public and a professional policy response. DNR policies have also been the focus of a broader debate in bioethics about whether resuscitation should be offered to patients or their surrogates when its use would be futile and, if so, how futility should be defined.

In other cases, public-policy initiatives have sought to increase the use of a practice generally deemed desirable. For example, the Patient Self-Determination Act of 1991 was intended to increase the use of advance directives by requiring institutions receiving federal funds both to inform patients at admission of their rights under state law to use advance directives, and to have policies in place for implementing them.

Public policy regarding life-sustaining treatment and the care of the dying reflects as well as any issue the mutual interaction and development of bioethics scholarship and public policy. The Karen Quinlan case first focused public attention on issues of life-sustaining treatment. In the landmark *Quinlan* ruling in 1976, the New Jersey Supreme Court held that an incompetent patient retained a right to refuse life-sustaining medical care, a right that could be exercised by a surrogate, in this case a parent, acting for the patient. The next fifteen years were filled with intense activity on these issues in both the public-policy and scholarly arenas of bioethics. In addition to books, many articles appeared in bioethics journals like the *Hastings Center Report* and in medical journals like the *New England Journal of Medicine*; at the same time, state courts around the country were addressing many legal cases concerned with life-sustaining treatment and care of the dying. Other public-policy bodies issued extensive studies, as in the President's Commission's report *Deciding to Forgo Life-Sustaining Treatment* (1983a), and briefer policy statements on the subject came from professional bodies like the American Medical Association. The President's Commission's report drew explicitly on a wide range of bioethics scholarly work on life-sustaining treatment decisions, as well as on closely related legal scholarship and health-care research. Court decisions frequently appealed not only to legal scholarship but also to the growing bioethics literature.

The bioethics literature on life-sustaining treatment issues was influenced by these court cases in two important ways. First, the attention many of these legal cases received served as a relatively direct stimulus for much bioethics commentary and analysis of the arguments made in the opinions. Because there was generally little specific statutory law constraining the judicial rulings, they often appealed in part to explicitly ethical arguments. Second, and at a deeper level, the President's Commission's report and many legal decisions greatly influenced debates on life-sustaining treatment and played a major role in the degree and nature of the consensus that emerged during the 1980s. This was true especially on specific issues like the moral importance of differences between stopping and not starting life-sustaining treatment and between ordinary and extraordinary treatment, as well as on broader issues like the nature and importance of the moral values of individual self-determination and well-being in guiding life-sustaining treatment decisions. The issue of forgoing life-sustaining nutrition and hydration is a particularly good illustration. Here, the debate in the bioethics literature began not coincidentally, at about the same time nutrition and hydration cases were being brought to a number of courts. Because the bioethics literature and the court decisions are best understood as profoundly interdependent parts of a single debate on which significant consensus

was emerging, the bioethics literature and court decisions were unlikely to veer in sharply conflicting directions on the permissibility of forgoing nutrition and hydration.

From its inception, bioethics has had a micro focus, especially on individual doctor–patient issues, and a macro focus on ethical issues in health policy, especially justice in health care. The micro issues were predominant in bioethics during the 1970s and much of the 1980s, and will, no doubt, continue to be important. But as health-policy debates in the United States focus on access to health care, containment of health-care costs, and rationing of health care, the macro focus of bioethics is likely to become increasingly prominent. On these macro ethical issues in health policy, the profound interaction of bioethics and public policy is even more evident. Unlike many doctor–patient issues, which could to a significant extent be worked out between individual doctors and patients, questions of justice in health care can be adequately addressed only at an institutional and policy level. Bioethics scholarship on these questions of justice that expects to influence public policy and practice must address questions about the design of social, political, and professional institutions and practices. These are public-policy issues at their very core, which means that we can expect more profound mutual influences between bioethics and public policy in the future.

The role of public policymaking bodies in bioethics

U.S. commissions and efforts.   In 1974 the U.S. Congress established the U.S. National Commission for the Protection of Human Subjects of Biomedical and Behavioral Research (hereafter National Commission). Two important factors led to the creation of this first public, national body to shape bioethics thinking and practice in the United States. First, the character of biomedical research had changed significantly in the preceding three decades. Before World War II, such research was carried out largely in small-scale therapeutic settings in which researchers tended to be well known to and trusted by their patients/subjects and the surrounding community. During and following the war, however, the scale of this research expanded greatly as public expectations about the potential benefits from medical research grew. Biomedical researchers increasingly were distinct from clinicians caring for patients, and the well-known and trusted clinician was replaced by the unknown investigator. Second, public concern with research abuses heightened. The shocking abuses of human subjects by Nazi doctors during World War II had earlier drawn public attention to these issues. In

1966 a member of the faculty of Harvard Medical School, Henry Beecher, published an article in the *New England Journal of Medicine*, detailing twenty-three instances of published research in which the treatment of human subjects was at best ethically problematic. Around the same time some especially egregious cases of research abuse received wide public attention, such as the Tuskegee syphilis study, in which black men infected with syphilis were left untreated in order to study the natural course of the disease.

Since its creation, the National Commission's work has shaped law, federal regulatory oversight, and institutional oversight of research practice. The National Commission consisted of eleven commissioners and a professional staff. It held public hearings, commissioned a wide range of studies and scholarly papers, and eventually issued reports on the use of different groups of human subjects—children, prisoners, the mentally infirm, and fetuses—in research. The legislation establishing the National Commission required the secretary of the U.S. Department of Health, Education, and Welfare to implement the National Commission's recommendations or offer a public justification for not doing so. In some cases, the commission's reports led to virtual elimination of research with particular classes of subjects, such as prisoners, while in other cases, they led to the development of special rules for the involvement of particular classes of subjects, such as children. The final report of the National Commission—the Belmont Report—had great impact on bioethics because it addressed the moral principles that underlay the various reports on particular aspects of research (1978a). Here, the principles of respect for persons, beneficence, and justice were enunciated; these same principles later figured prominently in Tom Beauchamp and James Childress's *Principles of Biomedical Ethics* (1989), probably the most widely read and influential scholarly work in bioethics.

The National Commission stressed the moral principle of respect for persons and its implications: that subjects should be enrolled in research only with their free and informed consent and with their confidentiality properly protected. The work of the National Commission continues to form the ethical basis for the federal government's regulatory oversight of research involving use of human subjects, carried out by the Office for the Protection of Research Risks within the U.S. Department of Health and Human Services (HHS).

When the National Commission concluded its work in 1979, the Congress established the President's Commission, with a substantially broader mandate. During the four years of its existence, it issued ten book-length reports on a wide variety of topics in bioethics, including the definition of death, compensating injured research subjects, genetic screening and counseling, genetic engineering, informed consent in medical treatment, decisions about life-sustaining treatment, access to health care, whistle-blowing in research, and protection of research subjects. Like the National Commission, the President's Commission had public commissioners and a full-time professional staff representing a wide variety of academic disciplines.

Because of the diverse nature of the topics addressed by the President's Commission, its reports had different kinds of impact on bioethics. For example, *Defining Death* (1981) contributed to the great majority of states' adopting a uniform brain-death standard for death; here, the impact was a relatively discrete piece of legislation. On the other hand, the report on informed consent, *Making Health Care Decisions* (1982), had a more diffuse, though no less important, impact in advancing the ideal that physicians and patients share decisions about treatment; here, medical education and the professional ethos for physician–patient relations were affected. *Securing Access to Health Care* (1983b) focused on the ethical problems represented by the fact that more than 20 million Americans were without health insurance. This report had relatively less immediate impact than many others because massive government expenditures were necessary to solve the problem at a time when the political ideology of the new administration in Washington, D.C., was to reduce, not expand, government social programs. Ten years after it was issued, however, it was clear that this report contributed to the public and political recognition in the United States of the ethical problem of access to health care and to understanding the ethical case for government action.

The commission's report *Deciding to Forgo Life-Sustaining Treatment* (1983a) was almost certainly its most influential for several reasons. Following the *Quinlan* decision in 1976, both public and professional attention to this area steadily increased. In addition, new and more widely disseminated life-sustaining medical technology meant that both professionals and the public had had more personal experience with these difficult decisions; individual professionals, health-care institutions, and the public were uncertain about what was ethically acceptable and desirable practice regarding life-sustaining treatment. Finally, implementation of the commission's recommendations did not require major new government expenditures. The commission's recommendations centered on patients' or their surrogates' rights to weigh the benefits and burdens of any available treatment alternative, including the alternative of no treatment, according to the patient's values, and to accept or refuse treatment. The report criticized and offered alternative language for some distinctions that until then had had an important influence on the bioethics literature and on practice, such as the differences between not starting and stopping a life-sustaining treatment and between ordinary and extraordinary treatment.

The report filled a vacuum: Hospitals, courts, and elsewhere sorely needed guidance about ethically acceptable practice. The fact that this report, like the others, was issued by the Presidential Commission, gave its recommendations an unmatched authoritativeness. While the reports of such public bodies as the President's Commission are generally considered of high quality, the very authority they are accorded raises the question of the ethical grounds of that authority, an issue that will be addressed later in this entry.

The National Commission and the President's Commission have been the two most prominent and influential public-policy bodies in the United States focused squarely on bioethics issues. A number of other public or quasi-public bodies, however, also have entered these frays. Subsequent to these national commissions, several states, including New Jersey and New York, established bioethics commissions. In addition, many government bodies and commissions with a broader medical or health policy agenda have had one or more bioethicists among their members and have included bioethics issues as a part of their broader concerns. The Task Force on Organ Transplantation of the HHS addressed ethical issues in the procurement and distribution of scarce organs for transplantation, although the ethical issues were not the main focus of its work. The Office of Technology Assessment of the U.S. Congress has conducted a number of studies that include analyses of the ethical issues, although its mandate precludes it from making policy recommendations. The Institute of Medicine within the National Academy of Sciences has done studies and issued reports on such issues as the growth of for-profit hospitals. Furthermore, many other government organizations and studies whose main focus is not on ethical issues typically now include some discussion of the ethical aspects of their work.

A striking example of the extent to which bioethics in the United States has become an accepted part of the public realm is the Human Genome Project. This $15 billion, fifteen-year project to map and sequence the complete human genome or genetic code has given the ethical implications of government-sponsored research an unprecedented role. At the time the project was being debated in Congress, there was considerable concern about its ethical, social, and legal ramifications. James Watson, the first director of the Center for Human Genome Research at the National Institutes of Health, committed the center to spending at least 3 percent of its total budget on research and public and professional education concerning these legal and bioethical issues.

A last important manifestation of public-policy bodies in bioethics in the United States has been the formation of grass-roots citizen groups in a number of states to address bioethics issues. Such groups have often treated issues of health policy, especially how to set priorities among health-care services with a view to allocating limited funds in government health insurance programs, such as Medicaid. The widely publicized prioritization of health-care services in the state of Oregon made use of such citizen groups.

The United States is not alone in turning to government bodies to address issues of bioethics. Indeed, while the United States has had no national government bioethics commissions since the end of the President's Commission in 1983, countries throughout the world have established them in recent years. Nearly every country in northern and western Europe, as well as a number of eastern European countries, now has a national bioethics commission. Such commissions also exist in a number of countries in the Americas and in Asia and Oceania.

These national bioethics commissions have varied greatly—in their form and membership, in the scope of issues addressed, and in their general effectiveness. For example, the Danish Council of Ethics, established by Parliament in 1988, has followed a populist model, with largely lay members, and has pursued broad educational efforts. In France, the National Consultative Ethics Committee on Life and Medical Sciences has followed a more elite model with scholarly and professional members, high public and professional prestige, and more direct attempts to determine government policy. In Great Britain, government-sponsored groups have addressed ethical policy issues in reports comparable in scope and detail with those of the National Commission and the President's Commission in the United States; the most prominent example in bioethics is the Warnock Report (1985), concerning new reproductive technologies.

Although there is no international bioethics commission as such, both the United Nations, through two of its agencies, and the Council of Europe have created agencies that have been active in bioethics. In 1982 the International Association of Bioethics was formed. Most non-U.S. efforts, however, have been at a national level so that they can reflect a particular society's historical, political, legal, and cultural traditions.

Membership and authority issues. The use of governmental bodies to address public policy in bioethics raises political and ethical questions of membership, function, decision-making methods, and the authority of their recommendations. With regard to membership, there has often been an attempt to balance two concerns: first, that members have relevant expertise on the issues the body will address and that it be representative of the relevant professions and disciplines; second, that members represent their communities in such areas as gender, minority status, and political affiliation. Statutes establishing these bodies often mandate the areas from which members must be drawn.

The membership question is related to the proper function of these bodies and the authority of their recommendations. If these bodies were to provide only the highest-level expertise on the issues of concern, the case for representativeness would be weak, though even then the question of who had expertise in bioethics, and the nature of their expertise, would be more contentious in bioethics than in an area of scientific medicine, like pulmonary function. That has not generally been their sole function, however. They have been viewed as combining such expertise with the role of addressing what public policy should be. This latter role is by its very nature a more political role, which requires representation of groups that have a substantial stake or interest in the policy question at issue, both on ethical grounds and because the group's recommendations must be able to be "sold" in the political process.

The difficulty of using governmental bodies to address deeply divisive ethical and political issues is illustrated by the task force established to address the use of fetal tissue in research. Its recommendations to permit limited use of fetal tissue essentially were ignored by the Bush administration in the late 1980s because the use of fetal tissue was so closely related to the politically contentious issue of abortion. "Right to Life" groups feared any use of fetal tissue could increase or appear to condone abortions. The attempt by the U.S. Congress in the late 1980s to establish a biomedical ethics advisory committee to its Biomedical Ethics Board also failed in large part because of political struggles over abortion.

Representativeness in membership is desirable to ensure that concerns and points of view of significant groups are taken account of for pragmatic reasons, so those groups will support instead of block implementation of the recommendations, and for ethical reasons, so those most affected by the recommended policies have some say about what the policies will be. At the same time, powerful professional groups, such as physicians, have a substantial stake in the policy outcomes about which bioethics commissions typically deliberate and make recommendations. When such professional groups have important or dominant roles with bioethics commissions, they can shape and control the debates, the policy alternatives considered, and the recommendations that emerge from these debates. Thus, in the membership of public-policy bioethics bodies, as well as in the policy process more broadly, representation for affected groups must be balanced with preventing powerful professional groups from controlling and distorting the policy process.

The authority of the recommendations of these public-policy bioethics bodies is more problematic than those of analogous scientific bodies for several reasons. First, as already noted, the nature and even the existence of expertise in ethics generally, and bioethics in particular, is contested to an extent it is not in scientific medicine. Many people believe that ethical claims express attitudes and cannot be shown in principle, much less in practice, to be true or false in the manner that claims about empirical matters of fact can be. By contrast, a consensus conference on the appropriate treatment of pulmonary hypertension or breast cancer may be controversial and involve ethical or value issues, but it is usually thought that expertise in the medical aspects of these treatment issues is not problematic to the extent that bioethics expertise is.

Second, appeals to authority are widely acknowledged to be out of place in ethical reasoning—it is the strength of the arguments, not who makes them, that should persuade us. Because public bodies like the President's Commission typically lack any enforcement powers for their recommendations, their impact ultimately should, and does, lie in their ability to persuade others who do have authority to pass legislation, render court decisions, and make institutional policies, of the wisdom of their recommendations. This has led many such bodies to see their task as articulating and advancing an emerging consensus on the issues it addresses. The President's Commission put great efforts into reaching consensus, and had only one dissent, from a single commissioner, in all of its reports. Moreover, all such bodies will give some weight to arriving at consensus, and as in the more overtly political process, reaching consensus sometimes requires that ethically problematic but politically necessary compromises be made, especially regarding policy recommendations.

Some would argue that the main purpose of such bodies is to sharply delineate the ethical issues, conflicts, and choices. Pragmatic or political compromise, according to this view, should be left to the overtly political process. This is essentially the model pursued by the Office of Technology Assessment in its reports. In this way the ethics body can speak more unequivocally to the ethical issues and not compromise or cut and trim the ethical arguments where it is politically expedient to do so; on the other hand, it probably makes it less effective than it might otherwise be in influencing policy.

Another issue that has received some attention concerning these public bodies is the methodology they do or should employ in their deliberations and in arriving at policy positions on bioethics issues. Albert Jonsen and Stephen Toulmin (1988) have argued that when members of the National Commission addressed concrete cases, they were generally able to arrive at consensus, even when they disagreed strongly on the more general moral principles or theories that underlay their consensus. They contrast their experience with what is sometimes called principlism, in which bioethics, and applied or practical ethics more generally, are seen as beginning with moral principles or theories that are applied in a relatively mechanical, deductive fashion to particular cases or policy choices.

Since providing reasons for concrete moral judgments involves appeal to moral principles or reasons of often substantial generality, public-policy bodies like bioethics commissions should, and in fact often do, work back and forth between concrete cases and more general moral principles. The aim should be to develop a position on the particular ethical and policy issues that is backed by the most plausible, coherent reasons. This can often be a great challenge when political pressures to reach a publicly acceptable compromise conflict with the policy backed by the best ethical reasons.

Conclusion

Bioethics issues have come to receive prominent attention in public policy, and bioethics scholarship has strongly influenced public policy in health care. At the same time, public policy in the form of legal decisions and public-policy bodies have deeply influenced the development of both the field and scholarship of bioethics during the last decades of the twentieth century. As bioethics comes to focus more on broader issues of health policy in coming years, this mutual interaction and influence between public policy and bioethics can only be expected to increase.

DAN W. BROCK

Directly related to this entry are the entries LAW AND BIOETHICS; HEALTH POLICY, *article on* POLITICS AND HEALTH CARE; PUBLIC HEALTH AND THE LAW, *article on* PHILOSOPHY OF THE LAW OF PUBLIC HEALTH; *and* MEDICAL ETHICS, HISTORY OF, *section on* THE AMERICAS, *article on* UNITED STATES IN THE TWENTIETH CENTURY. *For a further discussion of topics mentioned in this entry, see the entries* DEATH, DEFINITION AND DETERMINATION OF, *article on* LEGAL ISSUES IN PRONOUNCING DEATH; DEATH AND DYING: EUTHANASIA AND SUSTAINING LIFE, *article on* PROFESSIONAL AND PUBLIC POLICIES; GENOME MAPPING AND SEQUENCING; HEALTH-CARE RESOURCES, ALLOCATION OF; LICENSING, DISCIPLINE, AND REGULATION IN THE HEALTH PROFESSIONS; *and* PATIENTS' RIGHTS, *article on* ORIGIN AND NATURE OF PATIENTS' RIGHTS. *This article will find application in the entries* DISABILITY, *article on* LEGAL ISSUES; ENVIRONMENTAL POLICY AND LAW; ORGAN AND TISSUE PROCUREMENT; RESEARCH POLICY; STRIKES BY HEALTH PROFESSIONALS; *and* SUBSTANCE ABUSE, *article on* LEGAL CONTROL OF HARMFUL SUBSTANCES.

Bibliography

ADVISORY COMMITTEE TO THE DIRECTOR, NATIONAL INSTITUTES OF HEALTH (U.S.). 1988. *Human Fetal Tissue Transplantation Research Panel: Report of the Advisory Committee.* Vol. 1. Bethesda, Md.: National Institutes of Health.

BEAUCHAMP, TOM L., and CHILDRESS, JAMES F. 1989. *Principles of Biomedical Ethics.* 3d ed. New York: Oxford University Press.

BEECHER, HENRY K. 1966. "Ethics and Clinical Research." *New England Journal of Medicine* 74, no. 24:1354–1360.

BRODY, BARUCH A., ed. 1990. *Journal of Philosophy and Medicine* 15, no. 4:345–448. Special issue, "The Role of Philosophy in Public Policy and Bioethics."

"Commissioning Morality: A Critique of the President's Commission for the Study of Ethical Problems in Medicine and Biomedical and Behavioral Research." 1984. *Cardozo Law Review* 6, no. 2:223–355.

GLOVER, JONATHAN. 1989. *Ethics of New Reproductive Technologies: The Glover Report to the European Commission.* De Kalb: Northern Illinois University Press.

GRAY, BRADFORD H., ed. 1986. *For-Profit Enterprise in Health Care.* Washington, D.C.: National Academy Press.

JENNINGS, BRUCE. 1988. "A Grassroots Movement in Bioethics." *Hastings Center Report* 18, no. 3 (spec. supp., June-July):1–16.

JONSEN, ALBERT R., and TOULMIN, STEPHEN. 1988. *The Abuse of Casuistry: A History of Moral Reasoning.* Berkeley: University of California Press.

Quinlan, In re. 1966. 70 N.J. 10, 355 A.2d 647.

ROTHMAN, DAVID J. 1991. *Strangers at the Bedside: A History of How Law and Bioethics Transformed Medical Decision Making.* New York: Basic Books.

TASK FORCE ON ORGAN TRANSPLANTATION. 1986. *Organ Transplantation: Issues and Recommendations.* Rockville, Md.: U.S. Department of Health and Human Services.

U.S. NATIONAL COMMISSION FOR THE PROTECTION OF HUMAN SUBJECTS OF BIOMEDICAL AND BEHAVIORAL RESEARCH. 1978a. *The Belmont Report: Ethical Principles and Guidelines for the Protection of Human Subjects of Research.* Washington, D.C.: U.S. Government Printing Office.

———. 1978b. *Research Involving Those Institutionalized as Mentally Infirm: Report and Recommendations.* Washington, D.C.: U.S. Department of Health, Education, and Welfare.

U.S. PRESIDENT'S COMMISSION FOR THE STUDY OF ETHICAL PROBLEMS IN MEDICINE AND BIOMEDICAL AND BEHAVIORAL RESEARCH. 1981. *Defining Death: A Report on the Medical, Legal, and Ethical Issues in the Determination of Death.* Washington, D.C.: U.S. Government Printing Office.

———. 1982. *Making Health Care Decisions: A Report on the Ethical and Legal Implications of Informed Consent in the Patient-Practitioner Relationship.* Washington, D.C.: U.S. Government Printing Office.

———. 1983a. *Deciding to Forgo Life-Sustaining Treatment: A Report on the Ethical, Medical, and Legal Issues in Treatment Decisions.* Washington, D.C.: U.S. Government Printing Office.

———. 1983b. *Securing Access to Health Care: A Report on the Ethical Implications of Differences in the Availability of Health Services.* Washington, D.C.: U.S. Government Printing Office.

WARNOCK, MARY. 1985. *A Question of Life: The Warnock Report on Human Fertilisation and Embryology.* Oxford: Basil Blackwell.

QUALITY OF HEALTH CARE

See HEALTH CARE, QUALITY OF.

QUALITY OF LIFE

See LIFE, QUALITY OF. *See also* LIFE.

QUARANTINE AND ISOLATION

See EPIDEMICS.

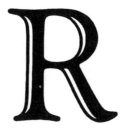

RACE AND RACISM

In the biomedical sciences of the United States and in their wider cultural context, ideas about race and gender play a prominent but unacknowledged role. Despite their apparent universality, concepts of race and gender vary over time and place. Different beliefs about race and gender, and their social results, are found in other cultures past and present. Both are, in fact, cultural constructions, one culture's folk theories of human biological variation. The great variability to be found in racial and gender notions is indicative of their local cultural construction.

Biological and behavioral assertions concerning race are without empirical validity. After decades of research, largely in anthropology, the social and cultural bases of racial conceptions have become clear. Because "race" is a folk-culture concept, it is here used in its ethnographic connotation. While many, perhaps most, cultures of the world do not hold racial theories, such theories are important to consider in discussions of biomedical ethics, especially in the United States. Given the demonstrably negative social, psychological, and health results of the perpetuation of the invidious distinctions represented by racial (and gender) identities and the antipathy generated by their stereotypes, the continued use of racial identities in biomedical work may be said to represent a serious ethical, as well as a biomedical research, problem.

Historical constructions of race

Race is one of a number of popular cultural conceptions about human variability. The Western concept was developed in its present scientific and related lay versions largely in the nineteenth century (Barkan, 1992; Gossett, 1965; Naroll and Naroll, 1973; Stocking, 1968). At its most abstract level, race is an explanation for observed human variation; people differ in appearance because they belong to different races. Behavior is also implicated; people behave differently because they belong to different races. Racism is a set of negative beliefs held by individuals or groups with respect to a population thought to be biologically distinct. Such beliefs about fundamental biological differences came late to the Western world, but not as a result of scientific progress.

The ancients—whether the civilizations of Nubia and Egypt or the later Minoan, Mesopotamian, Greek, and Roman civilizations—held no beliefs about essential human biological or racial differences. There was recognition that people differed in appearance, language, custom, and even ethics (MacIntyre, 1966), but such differences were not considered reflections of immutable, biological differences among humans. Nor could there have existed assertions that biology determined behavior, for most of these civilizations were composed of a variety of physical and cultural types in various stages of assimilation to a titular ethnic identity (e.g., Sherwin-White, 1967). Were this not the case, the ancient empires could not have expanded their numbers through the recruitment of physically and culturally different peoples, for they would have thought them fundamentally different and nonassimilable.

An important step in the development of the notion of race is to be found in the work of the Swedish botanist and taxonomist Carolus Linnaeus (1707–1778). Linnaeus built upon earlier notions of "species," distinct groups of living things that cannot interbreed. Linnaeus proposed a classification comprising six human "groups"; he did not use the term "race." These human groups were understood as neither pure nor (biologically) stable; they were not represented as distinct species. Such an assertion would have been contradicted at the time by considerable evidence of interbreeding of Europeans and other groups. Such empirical evidence was later ignored in the West.

The French naturalist and founder of invertebrate paleontology George Louis Buffon (1707–1788) introduced the term "race" into the biological literature in 1749. The term then did not refer to distinct human groups with separate origins or biologies (Montagu, 1964). Buffon's and Linnaeus's early reflections on human difference regarded such differences, correctly, as representing variations of a single species.

In the eighteenth and nineteenth centuries, English and German philosophy and science began the construction of ideas of fundamental, incommensurate biological differences dividing human groups (Barkan, 1992; Boas, 1940; Gould, 1981). While evolutionist views of monogenesis (a theory of a single origin of all humans) replaced polygenesis (a theory of multiple, separate origins) and creationist views (those based on religious beliefs and not on investigations of the natural world) in Europe, nineteenth-century theories were largely alike in expressing "racist" sentiments, though the sentiments were not recognized as such. Triumphant nineteenth-century evolutionism fitted well in racist science.

Monogenecists assigned to non-Europeans fates of early separation from a "main" line of Europeans. Jean-Baptiste Lamarck (1744–1829) suggested that differences among human groups around the world were to be attributed to the inheritance of acquired characteristics. He implicated the role of the environment in evolutionary change, although he misconstrued the mechanism of biological change.

Non-Europeans, and many eastern and southern Europeans, were believed to have a common origin by many western European scholars, but were seen as less evolved. Some were said to be little different than non-human primates (Barkan, 1992; Stocking, 1968). And some ethnic groups of western Europe created "racial" alliances. English historians of the nineteenth century repeatedly referred to the "rational and freedom-loving" character of the English as racial traits of the Anglo-

Saxon, believed to be a branch of the "German race" (Gossett, 1965). As with the Nazi "race science" of the next century, the notion of the German race excluded most people commonly regarded in the United States as belonging to a "white race" (e.g., the French and other circum-Mediterranean people, Celtic ethnics, the Slavic people) as well as people from what are commonly regarded as other "races" in U.S. ideology—Asians, Africans, and Native Americans.

In England, Sir Francis Galton (1822–1911), the father of statistical manipulation, lent both ideas and methods to racial theories. He coined the term "eugenics," and conceived of this new "science" as a program of "racial" improvement. The idea of group biological improvement was carried to horrendous extremes by Nazi "hygienists." Galton's work on head size and intelligence lent credence to later racist work in the United States as well, such as that of physician Robert Bean of Virginia. His work, in 1906, purportedly showed that parts of the brain were of different sizes in "Whites and Negroes" (in Gould, 1981). He also claimed to have found measurable differences in males and females and between higher and lower classes. His interpretations and biased readings, soon disproved (Gould, 1981), showed the affinity of the ideas of racism, sexism, and elitism in the United States that are also apparent in English science.

Sir Cyril Burt, dean of twentieth-century educational psychology in England, studied twins during the first half of the twentieth century. He purported to show that twins raised apart had the same IQ. It appears he sought scientific proof for the English folk notion that nature determined human abilities such as intelligence. As a consequence, his views were widely received for decades and influenced the establishment of national examinations. The examinations were used to limit the educational opportunities of millions of young people in Britain. In the 1970s, it was discovered that the late scientist had, in fact, fabricated most of his data. He had also fabricated his long-time research assistants, who supposedly collected most of the data, as well as his coauthors (Gould, 1981). The advocates of nature over nurture suffered a heavy blow when this key body of literature was discredited.

In the United States, a multicultural society usually referred to as "multiracial," Burt's elitist arguments were converted to racist (and sexist) theories by his students, psychologists such as Hans Jurgen Eysenck and Jensen (Gould, 1981), as well as others (Fausto-Sterling, 1992). Research aimed at showing that African-Americans and other "minorities" were intrinsically less intelligent than the generic "White race." Within each group, moreover, women were said to be less capable than men. Many flaws appear in this sort of research. One of the major problems is the fact that social labels, such as White and Black, were used to make genetic arguments; the arguments were flimsy because they regularly excluded from consideration profound differences in the social and educational experience of the members of the various social categories. This was done in order to arrive at (prejudged) conclusions of inborn racial differences.

A similar idea concerning mental illness was developed in German psychiatry in the mid-1800s. The leader of nineteenth-century German psychiatry, Wilhelm Griesinger, adopted a biological definition of mental disorders. His dictum was that "mind diseases are brain diseases" (Gilman, 1985). The idea that mental illness was based in biology and not social environment was actually borrowed from German philosophy, which in turn had taken the idea from popular German culture. Griesinger passed on this popular prejudice in his psychiatric science to a follower, Emile Kraepelin. Kraepelin became the twentieth century's father of biological psychiatry and the creator of a racially based "comparative psychiatry" (Gaines, 1992a; Gilman, 1985). This influential figure made the case for the biological basis of major mental diseases such as schizophrenia. His ideas were greatly influential on Nazi and contemporary U.S. biological psychiatry (Barkan, 1992; Gaines, 1992c; Gilman, 1985).

The Nazi "race science" of the 1930s reverted to nineteenth-century polygenesis to explain differences among racial groups and to assert its group's alleged superiority (Montagu, 1964). Some Germans were likewise seen as unfit; they were the disabled, the mentally ill, and the homosexual. In contemporary German society, popular and medical beliefs still express the model of mental illness that considers the mentally ill to be biologically different from "normal" people (Townsend, 1978).

As is evident, both English and German cultures exhibit biological theories of human difference. A brief historical look suggests that the ideas of these two cultures are related. In both systems, differences are held to be intrinsic and groups are hierarchically ranked, allegedly in terms of abilities. In the relatively isolated society of England, the Germanic notion of inherent differences and similarities based upon shared "blood" was doubtless introduced by invading Germanic tribes in the fifth century. The idea remained but was applied to internal social differences within England. This focus transformed the theory of difference based upon blood into the English notion of "breeding" that was and is applied to members of the British (which includes the Celtic peoples) social system. It produced Britain's rigid class systems wherein abilities are said to be differentially inherited by those differing in breeding. This conception of inborn qualities then serves to justify the respective social positions of society's members.

The critique of scientific racism

Evolutionists explained the increasing knowledge of human diversity in biological terms (Barkan, 1992; Gossett, 1965). The allegedly different developmental levels of various societies were said to indicate inferior inborn abilities in the societies' people compared with the usual apex of evolution found in (western) Europe. Eastern Europe, not a direct heir to the Renaissance, has been considered marginal in much of western European thought and totally alien and inferior in Germanic thought. History tells us, however, that Europe was the last of the world's areas to develop the hallmarks of civilization, hallmarks largely borrowed from others who were later alleged to be less evolved than (western) Europeans.

Anthropological arguments. Racist evolutionist ideas, and many not evolutionist, permeated much of medicine, psychology, biology, and other sciences in Europe and the United States at the beginning of the twentieth century. Among the first to lead a concentrated and protracted attack on scientific racism was Franz Boas (1858–1942). A German immigrant, Boas was the foremost anthropologist of his time and the founder of U.S. anthropology. Among many other things, Boas's research demonstrated the plasticity of the human form and the overlap in measurements (anthropometry) of anatomical features previously asserted to be unique to specific racial groups. These findings flatly contradicted the conceptions of races as stable, unchanging, and distinct physical types. Time has continued to enhance our understanding of the enormous plasticity of human biology, a biology so changeable that it has produced all the variations in the human form found in the world in less than 180,000 years.

Boas himself demonstrated how rapidly biology can change, as well as the nonempirical basis of racial differences, by showing that very different anthropometric readings could be obtained from the children of immigrants to the United States when compared with their parents. The cause was the change in environmental factors, especially nutrition. These measurements indicated, according to the current, specific racial measurement norms, that people in the same family appeared to belong to completely different racial groups (Boas, 1940).

Boas also advanced fatal arguments against notions of the relatedness of race to behavior. He showed that so-called races did not exhibit distinct religious, linguistic, or general cultural patterns. People of a variety of races spoke the same language and practiced the same religion. And members of the same race spoke different languages, held different religious beliefs, and otherwise exhibited distinct cultures. Race could not be shown to determine even major forms of human behavior (Boas,

1940; Stocking, 1968). Many of the positions advanced by Boas remain the most powerful antiracist arguments. It is remarkable that he began his assault on scientific racism before 1910, a time when blatantly racist statements were common in science and in the White House (see Brandt, 1985).

Evolutionary schemes were soon generally recognized as based on biased conjecture. There were no empirical bases for the evolutionary stages of Karl Marx, Herbert Spencer, Edward Tylor, or any of the other evolutionary theorists. Boas replaced evolutionist theorizing with the study of the historical diffusion of cultural traits. Historical diffusionism based its arguments on empirical evidence from all the branches of anthropology, physical anthropology, linguistics, archaeology, and sociocultural anthropology as well as from history. Such evidence was used to demonstrate that the current cultural (or physical) features or organization of any group were a result of contact and borrowing from other groups it had encountered. Of less influence in cultural change were innovation and creativity. Cultural arrangements, then, had more to do with a particular history of contact than with innate abilities related to alleged evolutionary stages. This understanding replaced a notion of the evolution of a single human general culture with an understanding of particular cultures' histories.

Evolutionists rank people and cultures from low to high, worst to best. Implicit in evolutionist thinking is the idea of progress, the idea that things are changing for the better. Evolution and progress are unrelated in fact and must be kept separate. Evolutionary change is simply descent with modification; there is no implication of improvement or superiority of later social or biological forms over earlier ones.

But evolutionists depicted some groups, such as Africans, as being near the apes because the groups were perceived as different. They were said to resemble nonhuman primates, such as chimpanzees and apes, who were described as having thick lips, curly hair, and dark skin. This representation has persisted despite the fact that nonhuman primates actually have straight hair covering their rather white skin and are totally lacking lips. That is, nonhuman primates exhibit precisely the characteristics claimed by Europeans as indicative of their own racial superiority.

While racism is still common, though less so than earlier in the twentieth century in the United States, evolutionist notions containing the idea of progress persist. A counter to these ideas is one of Boas's most enduring contributions: his articulation of the notion of "cultural relativism," which is not a theory but a descriptive reaction to wide experience with other cultures. While evolutionists ranked people and cultures, anthropologists after Boas came to see them in relative terms;

cultures were not better or worse than one another, they were simply different. One could not judge a culture using values from another; cultures must be evaluated using internal, not external, criteria. Relativism has become a central tenet of anthropology, the science of culture.

Biomedical sciences often evidence not the relativism of Boas but the hierarchical evaluative thinking indicative of evolutionism. An implicit ranking system appeared in medicine and persists in notions of defects afflicting groups of people. Historians of medicine show that this idea was disseminated by medicine's association of specific illness states with specific ethnic groups (called races) and/or genders (Chesler, 1972; Gilman, 1985; Pernick, 1985). This was but one of many techniques for the pathologization of often fictitious differences.

Difference from an implicit standard, that is, Anglo, male, adult (Gaines, 1992a; Gilman, 1985), in medical and psychiatric thought has been represented as problematic, dangerous, exceptional, pathological, defective, weak, vulnerable, and/or requiring "special" treatment (Gaines, 1992a; Osborne and Feit, 1992). Ultimately, the idea communicated is that culturally defined "others"—in the United States, non-European ethnics, women, and children—are simply, and inherently, "not normal" (Ehrenreich and English, 1973; Gilman, 1985).

One significant problem with the theories about natural racial groups is the fact that the precise number of them has never been agreed upon. Throughout the last century and a half, enumerations of groups said to constitute races fluctuated from author to author. Indeed, the number of racial groups is still changing. A recent example is the creation, starting in the early 1980s, of a Hispanic race.

The dynamics of the numbers of races should not be surprising given that the boundaries created to distinguish among the various groups have no empirical bases. Such discriminations are everywhere the arbitrary choice of an author (Gould, 1981; UNESCO, 1969; Stocking, 1968). The lack of fixed criteria for differentiation is reflected in the changes over time in racial labels of individuals in modern health statistical records (Hahn, 1992), in local and personal history (Domínguez, 1986), and in the ever-changing number of races, a number that varies somewhere between one race and three hundred. The correct number is one.

The heterogeneity of race.   Analyses of biogenetic differences of human groups lead to the recognition of a great variety of characteristics, most of which are shared in various proportions. Local configurations of traits (height, color, etc.) produce a huge number of distinguishable groups. On the African continent, there are about one thousand biologically distinguishable groups, as opposed to races (Hiernaux, 1970). Human groups are not divisible into groups that exhibit unique, nonoverlapping physiological characteristics. Differences in biology are always local differences that are characteristic of a local inbreeding population. What is seen as normal human biology also changes from culture to culture (see Kuriyama, in Leslie and Young, 1993). Just as the cultural elements exhibited by individuals of ethnic groups vary, so does the biology of members of so-called races.

The central problem for racial classifications is that there exist no intrinsically significant human features. Cultures have selected specific features as worthy of concern and hence as criteria of inclusion or exclusion. The selection of any one trait—such as skin, hair, or eye color, body hair, height, weight, religion, or place of birth—as a criterion of group exclusion or inclusion is, by definition, arbitrary. The selected characteristics represent historical attributions of meaning in local cultural contexts, not the expression of universal human nature or physical characteristics.

Racial theories in the United States

Most observers in the United States, whether lay or scientific, believe that observation of racial differences and racial antipathy has existed since time immemorial, being an understandable outcome of the encounter of dissimilar social groups. However, this is understandable only in a specific cultural context and is not an accurate rendering of the history of cultural contact.

The deleterious effect of "racism" on perception and cognition is obvious if the ancestry of U.S. racial groups is examined. Misrepresentations appear in scientific research as well as the popular media. The two—research and media—engage in a kind of cultural conversation that confirms the reality of race. An objective look at the ancestry of members of the major groups in the United States reveals race as a fatal conceptual problem in public health and medical research.

In the United States, most people labeled by self and others as Native Americans are biologically part European; in many cases, they are largely so. Many such individuals also have West African ancestry. Virtually all American "blacks," or African-Americans, are biologically part European. In many if not most cases, more of their ancestors came from Europe than from West Africa. Quite commonly, African-Americans also have Native American ancestry (Blu, 1980; Domínguez, 1986; Gaines, "Medical/Psychiatric Knowledge," in Gaines, 1992a; Hallowell 1976; Naroll and Naroll, 1973; Watts, 1981).

All classificatory whites claiming multigenerational descent in the South can be shown to have West African

ancestry and, very likely, Native American ancestry (Domínguez, 1986; Hallowell, 1976; Naroll and Naroll, 1973). This is not surprising since most of the colonists who settled in the U.S. South were single males. The relatively few unmarried females were generally of lower status and in long-term bond service. Without Native American and African women, European males in the South could not have had offspring. In the move westward into what was northern Mexico, where the Spanish had settled with Native Americans a century before the English came to the East Coast, one finds again that those "Americans" who went were primarily males from the South and the East. For this reason, the descendants of these early settlers in the West (settlers who were themselves illegal immigrants because this was northern Mexico) are today of mixed ancestry, although this is not publicly known.

Another distortion relates directly to Latinos, Mexicans, and other groups of "Hispanics." Latinos are descendants of western European, Native American, and West African peoples. This mixture is what the term "la raza" means: a "race" born of a mixture of elements. Because many Mexicans are actually Indians or partly so, the difference between Native Americans (many of whom are Spanish-speaking) and Hispanics is often only nationality, a matter of sociolegal definition and not biology. In other instances, Hispanics have no Native American ancestry but do have West African along with their western European ancestry. In many Latino groups (such as those of Venezuela and Puerto Rico), West African ancestry is virtually universal.

Despite the very definition of Latino as people of mixed cultural and biological ancestry, this language group has been homogenized in the scientific literature and, in the 1980s, became a discrete biological group, a "race" (Gaines, "Medical/Psychiatric Knowledge," in Gaines, 1992a; Hahn, 1992). In reality, the groups seen as discrete in the United States—white, African-American, Native American, and Latino—are not at all biologically distinct. Indeed, individuals in any of the categories may embody the same mixture of ancestors as do individuals in the others. The difference in the group to which one is assigned depends not on biology but on local context and social history. These groups represent social categories that are unstable and without common biogenetic content.

Variable racial criteria. In considering the referents of the term "race," no fixed criterion exists even within the United States. Many nonbiological criteria are used to identify races. The term is applied, for example, to people from a region or geographical direction, one usually designated from the perspective of Europe (e.g., Asians/Orientals). Another referent of this cultural term "race" is a specific continental location (e.g., African, [Native] American). A new basis for a racial group has also emerged quite recently—language. Hispanic, a new racial identity in the United States, may be attributed on the basis only of a surname; here language is biologized.

Putative skin color is commonly used as a marker of race, for example, white, red, black, brown, yellow. This use of color-as-race continues despite the fact that Asians run the gamut in complexion from white to black, as in southern India. The same range of skin color is found among people labeled black or white in the United States. The lack of real color "lines" produces cases of people who are black but look white or the reverse, as well as many other oddities. In such instances, it is social history (i.e., knowledge of ancestry) that produces assignment to an allegedly biological category.

A final criterion of race in the United States is religion. Judaism is employed to demarcate an allegedly biologically distinct group. But it is clear that Jews conform to the local physiological characteristics of the communities in which they reside (e.g., Germany, Poland, Russia, England, Scandinavia, Spain, France). The Jews in the United States represent a (fictional) biological group created by religious intolerance.

If a cultural approach has some predictive value, one can anticipate that the antipathy of U.S. people toward Arabs in the 1980s and 1990s will likely result in the social construction of yet another historically unknown race—Muslims. (The British have used the term "Wogs.") Some indication of this process may be seen in the descriptions of the 1990s conflict in the former Yugoslavia. The U.S. media described the conflict as between "Muslims, Serbs, and Croats," although the Muslims were themselves either Serbs or Croats whose ancestors converted to Islam.

Because racism clearly influences cognition, perception, and affect (emotion), it could well appear in psychiatric classifications as a specific disorder. Rather than a condition of professional psychiatric concern, racism and its twin, sexism, instead appear as significant implicit elements in psychiatric (mis)diagnosis and (mis)treatment (Adebimpe, 1981; Chesler, 1972; Good, 1993).

The erroneous views of race found in the United States encode several distinct ideas: (1) a fixed number of distinct biological populations, or races, exist in nature; (2) races have distinctive physical, mental, and/or behavioral characteristics; (3) racial characteristics (physical and behavioral) are naturally reproduced over time; and (4) specific group characteristics—physical, mental, and often moral—are hierarchically ranked, that is, some groups are superior to others (Boas, 1940; Gould, 1981; Stocking, 1968; Montagu, 1964). These assumptions, however, are not the only extant racial views of human difference.

Cultural systems of racial classification beyond the United States

Some writers have argued that capitalism, with a need for cheap labor and for justifying expropriation of land and resources, provided the political context and motivation that drove science to create a defensible basis in biology for immoral acts such as slavery and genocide (Rex and Mason, 1988). Certainly, Europeans' encounters with Native Americans and imported West Africans affected their constructions of human difference (Gossett, 1965). However, it appears more likely that racial views are a form of "ethnobiology," a cultural classificatory theory about the nature of human variability (Gaines, 1992a), because some racial ideologies predate capitalism. As well, various capitalist countries exhibit distinctive notions of race. Their differing views have resulted in very different treatment of those designated as belonging to different races.

Race in Europe.   Both English and German science and society produced biological constructions of affinity and difference (Gaines, 1992a). Those who are alike share a common "blood" in Germany and "breeding" in England. Those of the same blood constitute a "race." This German belief is a kind of biological essentialism. It is a much more exclusive notion of race than that found in the United States. It is in reality a kind of ancient kinship theory, a theory of a coherent, related descent group (Gaines, 1992a) that later merged with evolutionist ideas. As such, it is much narrower than U.S. notions. In contemporary Germany, the cultural system of group membership based upon descent from a common ancestor continues. It determines social identity as well as citizenship and suitability to hold political office, for non-Germans cannot hold office or become citizens.

The same system of social classification is found in Alsace, the culturally Germanic northeastern province of France. The biological German system exists alongside a very different, French cultural system that determines ethnic identity by other means. It accords in-group identity to those sharing French civilization and culture. Membership is primarily based on language, not appearance or place of birth (Gaines, 1992a). The term "race" in France thus refers to people who share a particular language and civilization. Both can be acquired, but the latter only by means of the former. Anyone can become French; being French is a linguistic/existential state, not a biological one as in the case of the German system.

The so-called racist groups of France may be seen as "culturalists"; their targets are not races but culturally distinct groups, such as unassimilated Muslims. French-speaking sub-Saharan Africans are not targets of the

French racism. North Africans have been historically white even though their complexions run the gamut from black to pale. The conflicts in France thus cannot be based upon race, though they are reported as such in the U.S. media where cultural differences are always interpreted as "racial differences."

Race in Japan and South Africa.   In Japan, a modern, industrial, and scientific society, a conception of human races exists that differs from that of the United States. Japanese sciences hold, and offer evidence to support, that the Japanese are a race distinct from Koreans, Chinese, the indigenous Ainu people, and the outcast Eta group (DeVos and Wagatsuma, 1966). In contrast, U.S. science and society hold that all these people from the East constitute a single biological race, along with South Asians, Indonesians, Filipinos, and others. These people do not evidence a common language, culture, or physical appearance, so the U.S. cultural system converts a geographical designation of people, borrowed from Europe, into an "Asian race."

In South Africa, there exists yet another system that classifies "racial groups." There, before the official collapse of apartheid, a sociolegal system was in place that distinguished four groups: Black, White, Asian, and Coloured. All people with ancestry in more than one of the first three groups were categorized as Coloured. Chinese were Asian, but Japanese were White. Each group historically has had different rights and privileges (see Schwartz, in Gaines, 1992a). All have equal status, at least legally, in the new South Africa.

In the United States, unlike South Africa, science and society ignore mixed ancestry and label individuals as wholly belonging to the least prestigious group of his or her parents, that is, to one exclusive category or another. In medical research, epidemiological studies, and clinical practice, people of mixed ancestry—that is, most Americans—are treated as if they had no ancestry except (West) African, Native American, Asian, or European. Designations are assumed to refer to homogeneous, distinct biological groups. If "admixture" is noted, researchers tend to ignore European ancestry and focus on genetic "vulnerabilities" deriving only from the subject's putative "minority" ancestry (Duster, 1990; Gaines, 1985; Wailoo, 1991).

In the United States, virtually all people called black or African-American, a term coined by anthropologist Melville Herskovits, would be classified in South Africa as Coloured because of their mixed ancestry (West African, western European, Native American). Indeed, all U.S. residents who claim long lines of U.S. antecedents would be likewise classified because they too have mixed ancestry. The same would hold true for most Native Americans and Latinos. Ironically then, the major U.S. "racial" groups, those with major anti-pathies and conflicts enduring over centuries based on their "racial differences," all would be classified in South Africa as belonging to the same racial group—Coloured.

Race as a key variable in biomedical research and practice

The ideas of race enumerated above underlie almost all medical and psychiatric research in the United States that pertains to group differences other than age or sex (Gaines, 1992a; Hahn, 1992; Robbins and Regier, 1991; Osborne and Feit, 1992). Remarkably, these beliefs concerning the existence or homogeneity of human populations called "races" have not the slightest scientific (or logical) basis; no empirical evidence has ever existed for the differentiation of humanity into broad racial groups (Gould, 1981; Montagu, 1964; UNESCO, 1969). In reality, thousands of biologically distinct human groups exist (Hiernaux, 1970; Montagu, 1964; Naroll and Naroll, 1973; Watts, 1981).

Assertions of the biological bases of differences among races are used to justify caste systems; that is, the results of oppression, discrimination, and poverty are commonly used to justify further discrimination and prejudice (Boas, 1940; DeVos and Wagatsuma, 1966; Naroll and Naroll, 1973; Thomas and Sillen, 1972). As is shown below, medical research, theory, and practice often play this same role in U.S. society and thereby serve as "scientific" justification for the persistence of popular conceptions of racial difference and of racism (Brandt, 1985; Gilman, 1985; Duster 1990).

Racial groups are mental constructs. As mental constructs they cannot evidence medical conditions. Yet "one of the most common methodological blunders in scientific studies of the significance of racial differences in the United States is the tacit acceptance of this phantasmic notion of race as the basis for establishing research samples" (Harris, 1968, p. 264). Given this, it can be noted that a folk medicine, or "ethnomedicine," is largely a creation of cultural beliefs. Its practices serve to reinforce and even justify those beliefs. Such is precisely the nature of medical research on group differences in the United States. This supportive role may be seen in research on afflictions said to appear only in certain populations.

The myth of race-specific diseases.   In biology or psychology, research science is used to reach conclusions that are in fact a priori assumptions; "prejudice not . . . documentation dictates conclusions" (Gould, 1981 p. 80). In today's medical and scientific community, expressed ideas concerning ethnic and gender inferiority are largely implicit. They are replaced in the medical literature by vague assertions such as vulnerability, susceptibility, tendency, increased risk, and difference.

One aspect of this discourse that constructs and maintains racial difference concerns "race-specific diseases." Since it is believed that races are distinct groups with their own biologies, it stands to reason that they would exhibit particular diseases. Sickle-cell anemia is a case in point.

At the beginning of the twentieth century, sickle-cell anemia was found originally through laboratory analysis of the blood of five patients—two European-Americans, two "mulattos" (in the parlance of the time, persons of mixed European and West African ancestry, but very largely the former), and one "Negro" (who doubtless was also part European). The findings were reported in the medical literature, however, as a condition found only in Negroes (Wailoo, 1991). In fact, this condition has existed in most world populations including the Mediterranean, Middle Eastern, Indian, Filipino, and South American. Instructively, the condition is not found among people in eastern, southern, or central Africa. Rather, it is found largely in West Africa, the ancestral area of most people in the Americas with African ancestry. Clearly, the condition is not a "racial disease" but rather a characteristic of some local populations.

Tay-Sachs disease is said to be a Jewish disease. In fact, it is a disorder found in a specific local population of the eastern Mediterranean from which some Jews, as well as Arabs, came. Jews not from this area, and not descended from people who were, have no risk of developing the disorder. The same is true of the so-called Portuguese disease, a degenerative, fatal neurological disease said to afflict Portuguese people. The afflicted are in reality descended from a single person (one Joseph) who carried the gene causing the disease. It is purely by chance that the antecedent person was Portuguese. Unrelated Portuguese are not at risk for developing the disease. In Tay-Sachs and the Portuguese diseases, specific sites of affliction are generalized to all in the racial category of the afflicted. "Local biologies" (Gaines, 1992a) are ignored in favor of "racial" ones.

The medical assertion that certain diseases are peculiar to specific races is without merit. The fiction is maintained through a number of techniques. Findings in a single person of a racial group are regularly generalized to all members of that putative group (Brandt, 1978; Wailoo, 1991); a part is made to stand for a whole. For example, a clinical finding that Indians in Britain required lower therapeutic levels of certain psychotropic medications became the basis for research comparing "Asians" and "Caucasians" (Lin et al., 1990; Lin et al., 1986; Mendoza et al., 1992).

Tendencies discerned in research are commonly reinterpreted to suggest significant differences in research on hypertensive medications; "diuretics are best for 'blacks' and beta-blockers for 'whites.'" Since members in neither group have common ancestry in the United States, such stereotypes can limit diagnosis of problems to groups "known" to be afflicted; others are then overlooked, misdiagnosed, or considered to be exceptions. As such, they do not challenge the stereotype, though logically such exceptions should call into question the very notion of racial distinctiveness.

Despite the absence of any scientific basis, the idea of race represents the basic population variable, aside from age and sex, on which inquiries focus and in terms of which results are interpreted and recommendations made. The huge body of literature on race-specific problems and racial comparisons are actually of unknown scientific value, though they represent a rich corpus for cultural study.

As long as medical science continues in its archaic racial folk beliefs, its claims to objective, acultural, and disinterested status in the health field are seriously compromised. Because these and gender beliefs are purely popular, modern medical sciences appear as cultural medicines, ethnomedicines, albeit professional ones (Gaines, 1992c; Hahn and Gaines, 1985). The validity of racial conceptions has been challenged and its use compromised. The continued use of racial conceptions in biomedical research and practice looms as a central conceptual and methodological problem in the biomedical sciences.

Consequences of racial beliefs. Common to intentional and unintentional discriminatory motivations is the unstated theory that ancestry in nonwhite groups "taints" the individual, not only determining identity but also causing disease. This is the implicit pathologization of perceived "difference" typical in research on high blood pressure and diabetes as well as a variety of other conditions (Cowie et al., 1989; Harris, 1991; Jones and Rice, 1987). Affliction is attributed to the fact that the individuals are "minority," by which is meant biologically different and therefore "defective."

Considering the study of diabetes in African-Americans more closely, it is found that while no risk factors and very few cases of diabetes exist in West Africa, individuals classified as African-Americans are still commonly said to be at "high risk" for developing the disease because of their "racial or ethnic ancestry." The presence of diabetes in these populations has other probable causes that are normally overlooked in research. They are (1) the European genetic background of the African-Americans; (2) poverty and related poor nutrition caused by discrimination; and (3) the high animal-fat content of the dominant northern European diet.

Racial thinking leads researchers to ignore oppression, racism, and discrimination—all of which can implicate the researchers themselves—as well as other cultural and biological factors. Research is confined to allegedly biological problems existing as defects within the afflicted. The real biogenetic makeup of individuals goes unanalyzed while their social identity is blamed for their illness.

Research on the treatments of choice and treatment recommendations in U.S. biomedicine demonstrates that medical and psychiatric diagnoses and therapeutic choices are often made on the basis of patients' social identity, be it race, class, or gender rather than objective need (Brandt, 1985; Ehrenreich and English, 1973; Gilman, 1985; Good, 1993; Lindenbaum and Lock, 1993; Osborne and Feit, 1992). Historically, this includes the differential use of anesthesia; the poor didn't need it but the wealthy did, as they were more delicate! (Pernick, 1985).

The form of intervention in psychiatry, pharmacotherapy, and psychotherapy is today heavily dependent on racial and/or sexual stereotypes rather than on empirical psychiatric signs or symptoms (Katz, 1985; Gaines, 1982, 1992a, 1992c; Littlewood, 1982). Blacks and Hispanics are often seen as belonging to that group of patients termed "psychologically unsophisticated" or "not psychologically minded" (e.g., Leff, 1981; MacKinnon and Michels, 1971; Sudack, 1985). Psychopharmacotherapy is seen as more "appropriate" for such patients than forms of "talk" therapy.

It should be recalled that U.S. psychiatry in the nineteenth century "found" that psychiatric disorders afflicted black slaves who otherwise "unaccountably" ran away from their masters. This is a historical version of a biological psychiatry and posits that all conditions are biological and will ultimately yield to somatic interventions. Environment, in this view, can be discounted or its consideration delayed until suspected "biological components" can be studied.

In medical research, behavior is also related to race. Medical researchers often choose research topics that implicate behaviors judged as immoral or incautious when dealing with minority populations, for example, number of sex partners, unwed mothers, and drug addiction (Gaines, 1985; Osborne and Feit, 1992). In this way, medical research also becomes moral research and supports blame-the-victim thinking.

In the psychiatric literature, neo-evolutionist racial theories lurk behind some assertions. Certain groups, such as the English, are said to be more evolved and psychologically normal (see Leff, 1981). In this view, somatization is allegedly less evolved and is characteristic of less developed "traditional" or "primitive" societies. The position inserts a cultural view of emotion and thought into a not-too-implicit neo-evolutionist scheme.

In the West, emotions are believed to be natural, universal, and distinct from cognition. But anthropological research has shown that specific emotions are not universal nor are they naturally distinct from cognitive or bodily states and functions (see Good et al., Lutz,

Obeyesekere, Schieffelin, in Kleinman and Good, 1985). While highly valued in a very few cultures, psychologization of distress is not "natural," but rather a learned, shared, and transmitted cultural approach (Kleinman, 1988). Psychologization is not found in many areas of Europe itself, for example, the Mediterranean and eastern Europe (Gaines, 1992c; Gaines and Farmer, 1986; see Good et al. in Kleinman and Good, 1985), or in China, Japan, or India (Kleinman and Good, 1985; Leslie and Young, 1993).

Research on racial differences provides the scientific bases for the maintenance of popular and scientific racial ideology in the United States. This ideology clearly leads to differential evaluation of social actors in medical and nonmedical contexts. As such, biomedical practices can be said to contribute to the social problems caused by racism. These problems include unequal access and poor medical outcomes (Good, 1993). The use of racial categories in biomedical research and practice, then, may be seen to breach the medical profession's own primary ethical injunction "to do no harm."

Genes, race, and violence. Biomedicine conceives of its domain as the discovery and manipulation of nature (see Gordon, in Lock and Gordon, 1988). Its wider culture perceives nature as something to be dominated and controlled (Pike, 1992). Ideas of nature, as well as those of difference and inferiority that are encoded in racial and gender identities, greatly affect practice and research in U.S. biomedical sciences. Classes of people believed to be closer to nature are seen as requiring control and guidance, even domination. Such people—among them women, children, non-Anglo or non-Germanic European ethnics (e.g., French, Italian, Spanish, Celtic, and Slavic people), Africans and their descendants, Native Americans, Hispanics, Pacific Islanders—are, in the United States, rather widely believed to be emotional, and therefore dangerous, unpredictable, and wild. Comments about "natural abilities" (intuitive, musical, irrational, fierce, shrewd) or characteristics of particular groups indicate their closeness to nature; they, like animals, are thought to be dominated by instinct and irrationality, not by "reason," a European cultural and masculine virtue (Chesler, 1972; Fausto-Sterling, 1992; Kleinman and Good, 1985; Pike, 1992).

The imputation of wildness, impulsiveness, and irrationality is doubtless a culturally constituted defensive projection of aggression that actually exists in the dominant group (Gilman, 1985; Pike, 1992). It is used to justify control, domination, and even extermination, as with Africans and Native Americans in the United States and non-German ethnics and the disabled in World War II Germany.

A similar logic appears in contemporary U.S. society. Urban violence, born of repression, discrimination, violence, and poverty, is recast as "genetic predispositions to violence or criminality" in individuals and the groups to which they are ascribed, especially after periods of civil unrest. However, rather obvious examples of genetic predispositions toward criminality and violence in the dominant group are regularly ignored as are centuries of clear provocations of African-Americans.

If researchers were indeed interested in a dispassionate evaluation of genetic components of violence and criminality, it would be appropriate to study people descended from generations of individuals all of whom have committed crimes of a serious nature. In the United States, such a population would be the many immigrants from Russia or Germany, as well as their offspring. Another group of subjects would be the descendants of slave traders and owners. Mass murderers and serial killers in the United States and Europe are virtually always white; their relatives would be suitable subjects of biological research on white criminality. These data might suggest some genetic basis for the inheritance of violent tendencies, if one were to think in "racial" terms. But researchers on violence and its causes regularly ignore such evidence. It appears that violence and criminality are possible genetic predispositions only when they appear in individuals belonging to specific low-status racial groups.

Race and clinical studies.   That racial groups are considered unequally in U.S. biomedical science and society is clearly demonstrated by the infamous and tragic Tuskegee syphilis study. In 1932, the U.S. Public Health Service (PHS) began a prospective study of syphilis infection among four hundred rural Alabamans who were black male sharecroppers. The researchers asserted that the study could be a "natural experiment" because it was assumed (for racist reasons) that "such people" were all infected and would not seek treatment for their condition (Brandt, 1978). For these reasons, the PHS argued that it could observe the natural history of syphilis infection in these black men. As it happened, the subjects, who had been unknowingly selected, began to seek treatment almost immediately.

Rather than provide health care, the PHS initiated a vast conspiracy to prevent the subjects from receiving care from any source. It conspired with local and state health officials, clinics and hospitals, and the U.S. Army, in which some of the men had enlisted, to prevent disclosure to the subjects of their diagnosis and to prevent treatment of their affliction.

Despite the fact that the natural experimental premise was invalidated in short order, this horrendous project continued over four decades until 1972, when public outcries finally stopped it. Until that time, however, the study was often reported in the medical literature without raising ethical concerns about informed consent, the sometimes fatal use of these human subjects, or the conspiracy to prevent them from receiving efficacious treatments (Brandt, 1978, 1985).

Aside from specific research projects that indicate differential concern for specific groups in the United States, "minorities" in day-to-day medical settings are often underdiagnosed for problems that could be treated (e.g., heart disease) and overdiagnosed for others. For example, blacks are regularly misdiagnosed with schizophrenia. These misdiagnoses lead to confinement and inappropriate pharmacological regimens. Loss of freedom and improper use of powerful psychotropic medications may themselves lead to chronicity in the illnesses that are left untreated, illnesses that led the patient to the attention of health professionals in the first place (see Adebimpe, 1981; Mukherjee et al., 1983; Bell and Mehta, 1980; Good, 1993). This is one means by which medicine creates chronicity of particular disorders as well as increases in the reported incidence of these disorders in a specific population. The circular logic is completed by the subsequent tendency to diagnose in an individual a disorder that is reported as "common" in members of his or her racial or ethnic group.

It is important for a full understanding of the role of racial classifications in the biomedical field to see it as part of a cultural system. This allows for the recognition of both the clearly concerned altruistic practitioners and researchers and the profoundly troubling aspects of racial thought in biomedical practices. In this view, the problems of racial thinking may be seen to arise frequently from the use of popular racial notions by force of tradition—tradition in the Weberian sense, wherein it is one source of authority for human action (Weber, 1978). The use of racial categories is thus not necessarily racist.

Conclusions

The U.S. version of human biology is a folk biology that assumes that social categories—"races"—are reflections of nature rather than culture. As a result, biomedical work, as well as public health care, is conducted and interpreted in these terms. In clinical practice in U.S. medicine, every patient record begins with three basic bits of information thought to be of critical importance: age, race, and gender (e.g., "A thirty-seven-year-old black female presented with . . ."). This is a significant part of the discourse of medicine that reconfirms the cultural conceptions that race, age, and sex are natural and empirical realities that make a difference.

Specific forms of communalism, such as racism and sexism, are intrinsic to U.S. society. As a result, they are fundamentally part of its medical institutions, because U.S. medicine is a reflection of the culture that created it. Culturally specific prejudice makes U.S. biomedicine an expression of a particular culture and its history. That culture has held and still expresses empirically problematic and ultimately unethical conceptualizations of human variation. However, neither contemporary medicine nor society remains monocultural; different ethnic and gender voices are being heard advocating what may be seen as more cultural and therefore humane and equal medical-research concerns and treatment. In many scientific fields, the lessons learned from the Nazi atrocities—as well as the inclusion of Jews, African-Americans, and women into collegial relations—has helped to reduce scientific racism and sexism since the 1950s (Barkan, 1992). Trends of pluralism begun then continue and expand.

Modern biomedical thought in the United States appears to lag in its understanding of the bases of human differences. The basis is culture, not biology. Even though racial terms are now often exchanged for ethnic ones, the problems persist in biomedicine and related sciences. Ethnicity has a cultural referent, and race has a putatively biological one. The two terms are incommensurate and cannot be used interchangeably.

Intentionally or unintentionally, biomedicine conserves, employs, and disseminates racial and gender-biased conceptions in its theory and practice. Such actions may be seen to derive both from habit and from nefarious intent. Comparisons are at the heart of science. U.S. science, along with U.S. popular society, has always thought that comparisons of black versus white or other races are the more or less "natural" ones to make in a "multiracial" society. Some others yet seek to show one group's superiority over others.

Biomedical enterprises will surely be subject to increasing ethical and practical criticism in the future "both from without and within its cultural tradition by those it fails to serve and those it serves to fail" (Gaines, 1992c). The growing understanding of the cultural biases of the professional medicines (and sciences) of the world suggests that medicines, like their particular medical ethics, reflect local cultural realities. A pluralistic medicine is needed in a multicultural country such as the United States. In such a country, a single medical voice may easily lead to, if not generate, bioethical conflicts. A medicine without cultural understandings, unreflective of its own cultural foundations, is inadequate, and an inadequate medicine cannot be of great help in a multicultural society.

ATWOOD D. GAINES

Directly related to this entry are the entries BIOLOGY, PHILOSOPHY OF; EUGENICS; HUMAN NATURE; GENETICS AND RACIAL MINORITIES; GENETICS AND HUMAN SELF-UNDERSTANDING; *and* SEXISM. *For a further discussion of topics mentioned in this entry, see the entries* BEHAVIORISM, *article on* HISTORY OF BEHAVIORAL PSYCHOLOGY; EVOLUTION; FEMINISM; GENETICS AND HUMAN BEHAVIOR; HOMOSEXUALITY; JUSTICE; *and* PSYCHIATRY, ABUSES OF. *Other relevant material may be found under the entries* EUGENICS AND RELIGIOUS LAW; GENETIC COUNSELING; GENETICS AND ENVIRONMENT IN HUMAN HEALTH; GENETICS AND THE LAW; GENETIC TESTING AND SCREENING, *article on* ETHICAL ISSUES; MEDICAL GENETICS, *article on* ETHICAL AND SOCIAL ISSUES; RESEARCH, UNETHICAL; *and* RESEARCH BIAS.

Bibliography

ADEBIMPE, VICTOR R. 1981. "Overview: White Norms and Psychiatric Diagnosis of Black Patients." *American Journal of Psychiatry* 138, no. 3:279–285.

BARKAN, ELAZAR. 1992. *The Retreat of Scientific Racism: Changing Concepts of Race in Britain and the United States Between the World Wars.* Cambridge: At the University Press.

BELL, CARL C., and MEHTA, HARSHAD. 1980. "The Misdiagnosis of Black Patients with Manic Depressive Illness." *Journal of the National Medical Association* 72, no. 2: 141–145.

BLU, KAREN I. 1980. *The Lumbee Problem: The Making of an American Indian People.* Cambridge: At the University Press.

BOAS, FRANZ. 1940. *Race, Language and Culture.* New York: Free Press.

BRANDT, ALLAN M. 1978. "Racism and Research: The Case of the Tuskegee Syphilis Study." *Hastings Center Report* 8, no. 6:21–29.

———. 1985. *No Magic Bullet: A Social History of Venereal Disease in the United States Since 1880.* Oxford: Oxford University Press.

CHESLER, PHYLLIS. 1972. *Women and Madness.* San Diego: Harcourt Brace Jovanovich.

COWIE, CATHERINE C.; PORT, FRIEDRICH K.; WOLFE, ROBERT A.; SAVAGE, PETER J.; MOLL, PATRICIA P.; and HAWTHORNE, VICTOR M. 1989. "Disparities in Incidence of Diabetic End Stage Renal Disease According to Race and Type of Diabetes." *New England Journal of Medicine* 321, no. 16:1074–1079.

DEVOS, GEORGE A., and WAGATSUMA, HIROSHI. 1966. *Japan's Invisible Race: Caste in Culture and Personality.* Berkeley: University of California Press.

DOMÍNGUEZ, VIRGINIA R. 1986. *White by Definition: Social Classification in Creole Louisiana.* New Brunswick, N.J.: Rutgers University Press.

DUSTER, TROY. 1990. *Backdoor to Eugenics.* New York: Routledge.

EHRENREICH, BARBARA, and ENGLISH, DEIRDRE. 1973. *Complaints and Disorders: The Sexual Politics of Sickness.* Old Westbury, N.Y.: Feminist Press.

FAUSTO-STERLING, ANNE. 1992. *Myths of Gender: Biological Theories About Women and Men.* 2d ed. New York: Basic Books.

GAINES, ATWOOD D. 1985. "Alcohol: Cultural Conceptions and Social Behavior Among Urban 'Blacks.'" In *The American Experience with Alcohol: Contrasting Cultural Per-*

spectives, pp. 171–197. Edited by Linda A. Bennett and Genevieve M. Ames. New York: Plenum.

————. 1992a. "From DSM-I to III-R: Voices of Self, Mastery and the Other: A Cultural Constructivist Reading of U.S. Psychiatric Classification." *Social Science and Medicine* 35, no. 1:3–24.

————. 1992b. "Medical/Psychiatric Knowledge in France and the United States: Culture and Sickness in History and Biology." In *Ethnopsychiatry: The Cultural Construction of Professional and Folk Psychiatries*, pp. 171–201. Edited by Atwood D. Gaines. Albany: State University of New York Press.

————, ed. 1992c. *Ethnopsychiatry: The Cultural Construction of Professional and Folk Psychiatries*. Albany: State University of New York Press.

GAINES, ATWOOD D., and FARMER, PAUL. 1986. "Visible Saints." *Culture, Medicine and Psychiatry* 10, no. 3:295–330.

GILMAN, SANDER L. 1985. *Difference and Pathology: Stereotypes of Sexuality, Race, and Madness*. Ithaca, N.Y.: Cornell University Press.

GOOD, BYRON J. 1993. "Culture, Diagnosis and Comorbidity." *Culture, Medicine and Psychiatry* 16, no.4:427–446.

GOSSETT, THOMAS F. 1965. *Race: The History of an Idea in America*. New York: Schocken.

GOULD, STEPHEN JAY. 1981. *The Mismeasure of Man*. New York: W. W. Norton.

HAHN, ROBERT A. 1992. "The State of Federal Health Statistics on Racial and Ethnic Groups." *Journal of the American Medical Association* 267, no. 2:268–273.

HAHN, ROBERT A., and GAINES, ATWOOD D., eds. 1985. *Physicians of Western Medicine: Anthropological Approaches to Theory and Practice*. Dordrecht, Netherlands: D. Reidel.

HALLOWELL, A. IRVING. 1976. "American Indians, White and Black: The Phenomenon of Transculturalization." In his *Contributions to Anthropology: Selected Papers of A. Irving Hallowell*, pp. 498–529. Chicago: University of Chicago Press.

HARRIS, MARVIN. 1968. "Race." In vol. 9 of *International Encyclopedia of the Social Sciences*, pp. 263–269. Edited by David L. Sills. New York: Macmillan.

————. 1991. "Epidemiological Correlates of NIDDM in Hispanics, Whites, and Blacks in the U.S. Population." *Diabetes Care* 14, no. 7:639–648.

HIERNAUX, JEAN. 1970. "The Concept of Race and the Taxonomy of Mankind." In *The Concept of Race*, pp. 29–44. Edited by Ashley Montagu. New York: Free Press.

JONES, WOODROW, and RICE, MITCHELL R., eds. 1987. *Health Care Issues in Black America: Policies, Problems, and Prospects*. New York: Greenwood.

KLEINMAN, ARTHUR. 1988. *Rethinking Psychiatry: From Cultural Category to Personal Experience*. New York: Free Press.

KLEINMAN, ARTHUR, and GOOD, BYRON, J., eds. 1985. *Culture and Depression: Studies in the Anthropology and Cross-Cultural Psychiatry of Affect and Disorder*. Berkeley: University of California Press.

LEFF, JULIAN P. 1981. *Psychiatry Around the Globe: A Transcultural View*. New York: Marcel Dekker.

LESLIE, CHARLES M., and YOUNG, ALLAN, eds. 1993. *Paths to Asian Medical Knowledge*. Berkeley: University of California Press.

LIN, KEH-MING; POLAND, RUSSELL E.; and CHEN, C. 1990. "Ethnicity and Psychopharmacology: Recent Findings and Future Research Directions." In *Family, Culture and Psychobiology*. Edited by Eliot Sorel. New York: Legas.

LIN, KEH-MING; POLAND, RUSSELL E.; and LESSER, IRA M. 1986. "Ethnicity and Psychopharmacology." *Culture, Medicine and Psychiatry* 10, no. 2:151–165.

LINDENBAUM, SHIRLEY, and LOCK, MARGARET M., eds. 1993. *Knowledge, Power and Practice: The Anthropology of Medicine and Everyday Life*. Berkeley: University of California Press.

LITTLEWOOD, ROLAND. 1982. *Aliens and Alienists: Ethnic Minorities and Psychiatry*. Harmondsworth, U.K.: Penguin.

LOCK, MARGARET M., and GORDON, DEBORAH R., eds. 1988. *Biomedicine Examined*. Dordrecht, Netherlands: Kluwer.

MacINTYRE, ALASDAIR C. 1966. *A Short History of Ethics*. New York: Macmillan.

MacKINNON, ROGER A., and MICHELS, ROBERT. 1971. *The Psychiatric Interview in Clinical Practice*. Philadelphia: W. B. Saunders.

MENDOZA, RICARDO; SMITH, MICHAEL W.; POLAND, RUSSELL E.; LIN, KEH-MING; and STRICKLAND, TONY L. 1992. "Ethnic Psychopharmacology: The Hispanic and Native American Perspective." *Psychopharmacology Bulletin* 27, no. 4:449–461.

MONTAGU, ASHLEY. 1964. *Man's Most Dangerous Myth: The Fallacy of Race*. 4th ed., rev. Cleveland: World.

MUKHERJEE, SUKDEB; SHUKLA, SASHI; WOODLE, JOANNE; ROSEN, ARNOLD M.; and OLARTE, SILVIA. 1983. "The Misdiagnosis of Schizophrenia in Bipolar Patients: A Multiethnic Comparison." *American Journal of Psychiatry* 140, no. 12:1571–1574.

NAROLL, RAOUL, and NAROLL, FRADA, eds. 1973. *Main Currents in Cultural Anthropology*. New York: Appleton-Century-Crofts.

OSBORNE, NEWTON G., and FEIT, MARVIN D. 1992. "The Use of Race in Medical Research." *Journal of the American Medical Association* 267, no. 2:275–279.

PERNICK, MARTIN S. 1985. *A Calculus of Suffering: Pain, Professionalism, and Anesthesia in Nineteenth-Century America*. New York: Columbia University Press.

PIKE, FREDRICK B. 1992. *The United States and Latin America: Myths and Stereotypes of Civilization and Nature*. Austin: University of Texas Press.

REX, JOHN, and MASON, DAVID J., eds. 1988. *Theories of Race and Ethnic Relations*. Cambridge: At the University Press.

ROBINS, LEE N., and REGIER, DARREL A., eds. 1991. *Psychiatric Disorders in America: The Epidemiologic Catchment Area Study*. New York: Free Press.

SHERWIN-WHITE, ADRIAN NICHOLAS. 1967. *Racial Prejudice in Imperial Rome*. Cambridge: At the University Press.

STOCKING, GEORGE W. 1968. *Race, Culture and Evolution: Essays in the History of Anthropology*. New York: Free Press.

SUDAK, HOWARD S., ed. 1985. *Clinical Psychiatry*. St. Louis, Mo.: W. H. Green.

THOMAS, ALEXANDER, and SILLEN, SAMUEL. 1972. *Racism and*

Psychiatry: A Comparison of Germany and America. Secaucus, N.J.: Citadel.

TOWNSEND, JOHN MARSHALL. 1978. *Cultural Conceptions and Mental Illness.* Chicago: University of Chicago Press.

UNESCO. 1969. *Race and Science.* New York: Columbia University Press.

WAILOO, KEITH. 1991. "'A Disease *sui generis*': The Origins of Sickle-Cell Anemia and the Emergence of Modern Clinical Research, 1904–1924." *Bulletin of the History of Medicine* 65, no. 2:185–208.

WATTS, ELIZABETH S. 1981. "The Biological Race Concept and Diseases of Modern Man." In *Biocultural Aspects of Disease,* pp. 3–23. Edited by Henry Rothschild and Charles F. Chapman. New York: Academic Press.

WEBER, MAX. 1978. *Economy and Society.* Vol. 1. Edited by Guenther Roth and Claus Wittich. Berkeley: University of California Press.

RAPE

See ABUSE, INTERPERSONAL; *and* WOMEN, *article on* HEALTH-CARE ISSUES.

RATIONING OF HEALTH CARE

See HEALTH-CARE RESOURCES, ALLOCATION OF.

RECOMBINANT DNA RESEARCH

See GENE THERAPY.

REFUSAL TO TREAT

See AIDS, *article on* HEALTH-CARE AND RESEARCH ISSUES. *See also* BENEFICENCE; *and* PROFESSIONAL–PATIENT RELATIONSHIP, *article on* ETHICAL ISSUES.

REFUSAL OF TREATMENT

See DEATH AND DYING: EUTHANASIA AND SUSTAINING LIFE; PATIENTS' RIGHTS; *and* RIGHTS, *article on* RIGHTS IN BIOETHICS.

REHABILITATION MEDICINE

Rehabilitation medicine encompasses medical, psychosocial, and vocational interventions provided to persons who have experienced some type of functional impairment. Individuals receiving rehabilitation services may have been born with a disabling condition, such as cerebral palsy, spina bifida, muscular dystrophy, or mental retardation; or they may have acquired disability from stroke, spinal cord injury, polio, amputation, cardiovascular disease, acquired immune deficiency syndrome (AIDS), or traumatic brain injury. They may receive rehabilitation treatments at a traditional acute-care hospital, at a hospital specializing in rehabilitation, or at a post-acute facility, sometimes called a "transitional" or "independent living" facility. Increasingly, individuals receive rehabilitation services in their homes through home health agencies or visiting nurses (DeLisa, 1988).

Consumers of rehabilitation medicine, especially if their disabilities are acquired rather than congenital, invariably experience intense feelings of anger, rage, helplessness, and worthlessness (Gunther, 1971). Ethical problems arise from the way disability disrupts one's capacity to make autonomous choices and decisions and to develop and sustain meaningful social relationships. The transformation of a self that experiences profound alienation resulting from a disability to a self that can productively engage the world is the ultimate challenge of rehabilitation and prompts many of its ethical considerations.

Certain aspects of contemporary rehabilitation medicine derive from treatment strategies, dating back to the 1920s, for managing job-related injuries. A series of developments associated with World War II, however, shaped rehabilitation medicine as it is known today. Widespread use of penicillin resulted in the survival of seriously injured soldiers. The resultant crowding of nursing homes and chronic-care facilities created an imperative to return wartime casualties either to the front or to meaningful civilian life. President Franklin Roosevelt, himself no stranger to rehabilitation, wrote to Secretary of War Henry Stimson in 1944 that "No overseas casualty [shall] be discharged from the armed forces until he [sic] has received the maximum benefit of hospitalization and convalescent facilities, which must include physical and psychological rehabilitation, vocational guidance, prevocational training and resocialization." Toward the war's end, financier Bernard Baruch and physicians who included Howard Rusk and Henry Kessler established Veterans Administration hospitals that would translate the war experience of rehabilitation into civilian life. Their vision evolved into the comprehensive multidisciplinary approach of rehabilitation that is known today (Berkowitz, 1981).

Admission to a rehabilitation facility, typically a few weeks or months after acute hospitalization, anticipates that the individual is medically stable and not at serious risk of a life-threatening episode. Most important, patients admitted to rehabilitation facilities are deemed to have sufficient capacity and "rehabilitation potential" to engage in various therapeutic programs aimed at restoring as much functional ability as possible (Purtilo, 1992). Absence of rehabilitation potential may result in the individual's admission to a long-term-care facility.

Contemporary rehabilitation interventions focus on reducing the disabling effects of physical impairments (e.g., poor motor control, loss of sensorimotor skills, muscle weakness, loss of sensation, paralysis, loss of bowel and bladder control); cognitive impairments (e.g., poor concentration, memory, attention, insight, information processing, problem solving); or behavioral impairments (e.g., emotional disorganization, poor emotional expression, inability to engage in goal-directed behavior, poor interpersonal skills). Because the patient's impairments often appear in combinations or clusters, rehabilitation medicine involves an array of specialized therapies and services to assist patients in overcoming their often multiple functional limitations (Keith, 1991).

In acute rehabilitation hospitals, treatments are typically provided by a specially designated team of professionals that, depending on the nature and extent of the patient's impairments, may include a physiatrist (a physician who specializes in physical medicine and rehabilitation), a rehabilitation nurse, a physical therapist, an occupational therapist, a specialist in communicative disorders, a recreational therapist, a psychologist, a social-service specialist, a spiritual adviser, an orthotist/prosthetist, a vocational rehabilitation counselor, and perhaps a rehabilitation engineer (Lyth, 1992). Length of stay for rehabilitation patients varies according to medical need and the extent of health insurance. Stroke patients commonly spend two to six weeks in acute rehabilitation (Parfenchuck et al., 1990); persons with serious brain injury may spend one to four months (Cope and Hall, 1982); and persons with spinal cord injury may spend three to five months (Apple, 1992).

Bioethical issues

Because the scope of rehabilitation medicine is so broad, and because other entries will focus on bioethical aspects of disability that either follow from or are independent of an individual's formal stay in an in-patient rehabilitation facility, this entry will discuss certain bioethical aspects of rehabilitation medicine as they derive from the provider–patient relationship. Examining how rehabilitation relationships form and evolve illuminates how bioethical ideals such as autonomy, nonmaleficence, beneficence, and justice occur in the context of treating persons with serious disability. The provider–patient models whose bioethical ramifications will be discussed below are the contractual, paternal, educational, and empowering models.

The contractual model.   The contractual model usually refers to the clinician and the patient developing a mutual understanding and accord on the nature of and need for treatment, its probable benefits and risks, and so forth. Informed consent is central in such discussions; the provider of services assumes certain contractual responsibilities to inform and secure consent to treat the patient, while the patient's consent implies an agreement to the conditions of treatment, including reasonable compliance with the treatment program, remunerating the provider, and so on (Caplan et al., 1987).

The rehabilitation patient's engagement in treatment is not passive, as it would be in an acute, surgical scenario. Active and eventually self-directed, it focuses on learning and performing a variety of functional tasks, such as walking, dressing, toileting, and bathing. Nevertheless, the contractual model in acute rehabilitation is immediately qualified by the fact that many rehabilitation patients have sustained organic impairments that substantially interfere with their cognitive ability to make autonomous decisions. Some patients may not be able to concentrate on, understand, evaluate, or process information well enough to make choices and decisions congruent with their welfare. Or the patient may be psychologically devastated by the onset of disability and unwilling to participate in therapy. Certain rehabilitation patients may experience serious cognitive disorganization accompanied by frightened, anxious feelings and regression to childlike levels of behavior, especially with respect to managing their feelings and impulses (Rosenthal, 1987).

Although rehabilitation is defined as elective treatment, many patients do not elect it at all. The onset of a disability like stroke, spinal cord injury, or brain injury can be so abrupt and severe that many rehabilitation patients begin to comprehend the nature and extent of their disability only *after* they have been medically stabilized and referred to the rehabilitation environment. There the patient, confronted with the functional challenges that the disability has imposed, may begin to try to make sense out of what has happened and to deal with the fact that some of his or her life expectations may have to be modified. To the extent that patients are cognitively or psychologically unable to manage these situations, their capacity to make autonomous choices is problematic (Purtilo, 1988). Furthermore, the individual who is discharged directly from an acute hospital to a rehabilitation facility, and only then begins to realize his or her circumstances, has not voluntarily assumed the promissory role that is implicit in the contractual model. To view such a patient's subsequent resistance to or noncompliance with the rehabilitation effort as a violation of a contractual agreement overlooks the fact that the patient may never have reflected on or consented to rehabilitation in the first place.

In sum, the contractual model's presumption of an autonomous self who can voluntarily and insightfully contemplate, assume, and fulfill a variety of promises and obligations is hardly congruent with the reality of the acute rehabilitation environment for many patients. From what has been implied above, a more probable model of care, at least in the early stages of recovery from a neurological event, is the one that will be examined next: the paternalistic model.

The paternalistic model.   Paternalism has been defined as "the interference with a person's liberty of action justified by reasons referring exclusively to the welfare, good, happiness, needs, interests or values of the person being coerced" (Dworkin, 1972, p. 65). Once the prevailing model in provider–patient relationships, paternalism has since 1970 come under increasing fire, both from the patient-rights' movement and in the literature of bioethics. Compelling legal justifications for paternalism now condone overriding a patient's decision only when the decision would pose serious harm to the patient or to identifiable others (Jonsen et al., 1992). In acute rehabilitation, justified paternalism is usually predicated on the patient's impaired cognition or psychological disorganization. As Arthur Caplan observed, "If it is true that time is essential in allowing patients to accommodate to the reality of severe impairment, then this would seem . . . at least for some patients in some settings, to allow for the presence of paternalistic medical care" (1988, p. 315).

Paternalism in acute rehabilitation frequently appears when patients resist complying with their therapeutic program. Patients may object to the time at which they must rise in the morning to begin therapy, the nature and intensity of their therapies, their diet, the kinds of medications they require, the aesthetics of their hospital room, the personalities of other patients in their room, the date of discharge, or the discharge site. Alternatively, some rehabilitation patients will insist on engaging in activities that pose harm to them, such as trying to walk unassisted despite poor balance or muscle weakness.

Paternalistic interventions in certain instances—such as refusing to comply with a clinically depressed, suicidal patient's request for privacy—are easily justified. Paternalism cannot serve as the preferred provider–patient relationship, however, for at least three reasons. First, justifying a paternalistic intervention in rehabilitation on the basis of a patient's cognitive or psychological impairment requires an objective determination of that impairment. If the rehabilitation patient exhibits profoundly impaired memory, extreme confusion, or very poor judgment, he or she has a doubtful claim to self-determination. Yet providers may disagree on which of the patient's decisions are sufficiently problematic to justify a paternalistic decision. Richard Wanlass and his

colleagues (1992) showed that rehabilitation clinicians do not consistently or reliably apply the labels "mild," "moderate," and "severe" to cognitively impaired patients; Vivian Auerbach and John Banja (1993) found that considerable discrepancy exists among physicians, mental-health professionals, and lawyers in distinguishing competent from incompetent decisions made by persons with traumatic brain injury; and Bruce Caplan (1983) noted a marked disparity between patient and provider ratings of the patient's mood. In cases of considerable professional disagreement about a patient's "competence" to make decisions or the severity of a patient's cognitive impairment or mood disorder, it is not possible to justify overriding the patient's decision *on those bases.*

A second reason for rejecting a thoroughgoing paternalism in rehabilitation is that providers with paternalistic attitudes risk misinterpreting resistance to therapy as "noncompliant" or "unmanageable." Whatever their therapeutic value, such attitudes and behaviors may indicate the provider's need to be in control (McKnight, 1989). When patients resist the provider's ministrations, the provider may become angry or exhibit behaviors destructive to the therapeutic relationship (Gunther, 1987). What may appear to be noncompliant patient behaviors may in fact be the patient's attempt to assert himself or herself, an attempt that perhaps ought to be applauded as an expression of the patient's striving for independence rather than discouraged as inappropriate behavior.

A third reason for rejecting paternalism is that it ultimately runs counter to the rehabilitation ideal of independence. If the goal of rehabilitation is to help the person's movement toward functional independence, then patients ought to begin learning how to assume control of their lives in the rehabilitation environment. Consequently, the rehabilitationist who excludes the patient's input or interest in defining goals and making decisions is stifling the very behavior and attitude he or she is supposed to be cultivating. Indeed, because a profound change in one's bodily image and functional capacity can so seriously affect one's self-image and identity, the ultimate goal of rehabilitation may well be to bring patients to accept themselves as persons with disability and empower them with the necessary will and information to engage the world on somewhat new terms (Banja, 1992).

The educational model.   Empowerment depends in part on various kinds of information the patient will need to function as autonomously as possible. Newly disabled persons require information on and training in managing their activities of daily living (e.g., bathing, grooming, feeding, toileting, and so on); they may also need to learn about creative recreational opportunities, financial planning, social skills training, problem solving, accessing community resources, sexual enjoyment, using community transportation, assertiveness, and perhaps vocational planning or training. Patients should also learn about their rights as rehabilitation consumers before and after rehabilitation discharge: that they have the right to request reasonable changes in the personnel of their teams; that disclosures of otherwise confidential information may occur, for example, to family members or third-party payers; how rehabilitation termination is decided and what evidence is used to determine the nature and length of the rehabilitation; and how they are protected by legislation, such as the Americans with Disabilities Act (Caplan et al., 1987).

Providing this information responds to the same ethical principles requiring that information be imparted to an individual about to undergo surgery. In the latter case, information is treatment-specific, while in the former, the information addresses a host of functional issues. But whereas consent to surgical procedures pertains only to the intervention at issue, consent to rehabilitation reflects a disabled person's willingness to manage his or her life. If no effort is made to stimulate the rehabilitation patient's will to use that information or to *be* autonomous, then the rehabilitation effort may ultimately fail. Rehabilitation providers not only must convey important information but also must seek to deepen the patient's appreciation of its value and encourage the patient to use it.

The empowerment model.   Able-bodied persons frequently confess to being uncomfortable around and having negative feelings toward individuals with disability. Persons with disability are therefore often isolated, deprived, discriminated against, and generally assigned to dependent roles. Ironically, even public programs presumed to assist persons with disability toward autonomy and independence sometimes foster dependency (McKnight, 1989). Persons who receive services from such programs frequently complain of feeling dehumanized, subservient, devalued, and ostracized. Studies of the psychodynamic aspects of relationships among program personnel and clients suggest that program staff may develop a narcissistic feeling of authority from these relationships that is threatened by their clients' acting independently (Mullins, 1989). Consequently, it is not surprising that such programs may be perceived by clients as unhealthy.

According to the empowerment model, which is moored in principles of social justice, the goal of rehabilitation is to facilitate the rehabilitation consumer's access to social goods. Necessary elements of this access involve social attitudes and measures that aim at equalizing opportunity. Because persons with disability face limitations on normal functioning, justice theorists like Norman Daniels (1985) argue that a society ought to assume certain duties to make up for the fact that an unequal distribution of disabilities among citizens unfairly handicaps the disabled person's attempts to satisfy his or her life needs. Legislation such as the Americans with Disabilities Act, which calls for reforms in hiring practices, barrier-free architecture, handicapped-accessible public transportation, and the implementation of communication devices in business operations for employees who are speech- or hearing-impaired, is highly responsive to the goal of empowerment.

The robust sense of autonomy explicit in the empowerment model transcends clinical objectives that stop at restoring functional ability. In seeking to enhance the individual's power to control his or her life, the empowerment model aims at liberating the individual's self by respecting and advocating the individual's right to his or her choices, preferences, and decisions. From a therapeutic standpoint, therefore, the provider may have to honor the patient's preferences even if they contradict the therapist's, allow the patient to take reasonable decision-making risks, and be prepared to assist when the patient fails. Most important, the therapist must provide the patient with the tools necessary to seize, maintain, and enjoy control of his or her life.

Because many rehabilitation patients are depressed and despondent over the onset of their disability, various empowering models or strategies have been formulated by mental-health professionals (O'Hara and Harrell, 1991). A key ethical challenge for the therapist is determining when patients are reasonably ready or "competent" to gainsay therapeutic recommendations, or when patients can "reasonably" assume the risks inherent in the enjoyment of their moral and constitutional liberties and freedoms (Purtilo, 1988). Meeting this kind of challenge requires an acute sensitivity on the therapist's part in judging when certain types of paternalistic interventions are warranted versus when patients may assume control and responsibility. While the empowerment model may not object to vesting decision-making authority in the provider at the beginning of rehabilitation, in ideal cases that power is increasingly channeled to the consumer as rehabilitation discharge nears. The goal is for patients to realize their right to engage the world on their terms and to enjoy the self-esteem and dignity of risk that derives from doing so (O'Hara and Harrell, 1991).

Familial and social obligations

Families play a critical role during the rehabilitation process, not only supporting their loved ones but also learning how to accommodate their needs after rehabilitation discharge. The nature and extent of familial duty that occurs by virtue of a member's becoming disabled is nevertheless problematic. Overwhelmed by the financial and personal toll that caring for someone with serious disability poses, families may feel that the burdens imposed on them by the individual's care needs are unreasonable. If the family defaults, does an individual's misfortune in sustaining a disability impose special obligations on society? The extent to which the disabled person's family assumes the responsibilities of care depends on the family's love, sense of values, and willingness to sacrifice, rather than on legal or constitutional mandates (Callahan, 1988). If both family and society repudiate a duty to care for the person with disability, then the rehabilitation itself is jeopardized

The future of allocating rehabilitation services requires a moral consensus about what disability within human life means and whether and to what extent society has a duty to accommodate the needs of persons with disability. Because such a consensus about disability does not yet exist in contemporary American society, rehabilitation medicine is available largely on the basis of the ability to pay (Brody, 1988). Shrinking financial resources may preclude the provision of rehabilitation resources to those who desperately need but cannot afford them. Although condoning such a situation in an egalitarian society seems ethically repugnant (Purtilo, 1992), a marked reluctance, if not downright hostility, exists toward imposing social obligations—such as increased tax revenues—to improve care for persons with disabilities. In the face of moral arguments that the burdens resulting from disability should be lightened by spreading them as widely and equitably as possible, libertarians counter that because "I am not my brother's keeper," others' disability and its rehabilitation are not their concern (Will, 1986).

To the extent, however, that able-bodied persons accept the idea of valid social roles for persons with disabilities, social stigmas that have interfered with the latter's participation in mainstream American life may diminish. The implementation of the Americans with Disabilities Act may facilitate this change in attitude because it insists that greater opportunities be made available for persons with disability to enter the economic mainstream of American life. Furthermore, demographic projections indicate an astonishing rate of growth among elderly persons in the United States, many of whom will require rehabilitation services at some point in their lives. To the extent that they can influence the political will, access to rehabilitation resources may expand rather than shrink through legislative enactments.

If moral arguments are not sufficient to justify the allocation of rehabilitation services, certain purely material considerations might compel an examination of the merits of rehabilitation medicine. Extensive research indicates that the social costs of disability without rehabilitation are staggering (Brooks, 1991; Davidoff et al., 1991). Reimbursement for rehabilitation services might be straightforward and noncontroversial, then, simply because of its cost-effectiveness.

Appeals to self-interest may also sustain an interest in rehabilitation's merit. As medical technology and improved lifestyle choices result in increased longevity, the need for rehabilitation services will doubtless increase. To the extent that living longer increases the probability of a disabling neurological or musculoskeletal impairment, Americans might seek to protect their own access to rehabilitation services by advocating an entitlement to such access for everyone else.

In any case, rehabilitation's objective of securing independence for its consumers fits admirably into an egalitarian culture's sociopolitical aspirations. Independence for persons with disability is the same thing as independence for the able-bodied: the ability to enjoy life as a chooser of ends and to participate in a just and democratic society. Much to its credit, and perhaps more than any other medical specialty, the ethos of rehabilitation medicine embodies these cherished ideals of individual freedom and liberty.

JOHN D. BANJA

Directly related to this entry is the entry DISABILITY, *article on* HEALTH CARE AND PHYSICAL DISABILITY. *For a further discussion of topics mentioned in this entry, see the entries* ALLIED HEALTH PROFESSIONS; CHRONIC CARE; COMPETENCE; FAMILY; HEALTH-CARE FINANCING; HEALTH-CARE RESOURCES, ALLOCATION OF, *article on* MICROALLOCATION; INFORMED CONSENT; LIFE, QUALITY OF; LONG-TERM CARE; PROFESSIONAL–PATIENT RELATIONSHIP; RIGHTS, *article on* RIGHTS IN BIOETHICS; *and* TEAMS, HEALTH-CARE. *For a discussion of related ideas, see the entries* AUTHORITY; AUTONOMY; BENEFICENCE; CONFIDENTIALITY; JUSTICE; *and* PATERNALISM. *Other revelant material may be found under the entries* HEALTH-CARE DELIVERY, *article on* HEALTH-CARE INSTITUTIONS; LAW AND BIOETHICS; *and* MENTALLY DISABLED AND MENTALLY ILL PERSONS. *See also the* APPENDIX (CODES, OATHS, AND DIRECTIVES RELATED TO BIOETHICS), SECTION III: ETHICAL DIRECTIVES FOR OTHER HEALTH-CARE PROFESSIONS, OCCUPATIONAL THERAPY CODE OF ETHICS *of the* AMERICAN OCCUPATIONAL THERAPY ASSOCIATION, *and* CODE OF ETHICS AND GUIDE FOR PROFESSIONAL CONDUCT *of the* AMERICAN PHYSICAL THERAPY ASSOCIATION.

Bibliography

APPLE, DAVID F., JR. 1992. "Spinal Cord Injury." In *Rehabilitation Medicine: Contemporary Clinical Perspectives*, pp. 149–171. Edited by Gerald F. Fletcher, John Banja, Brigitta Jann, and Steven Wolf. Philadelphia: Lea & Febiger.

AUERBACH, VIVIAN S., and BANJA, JOHN D. 1993. "Competency Determinations." In vol. 2 of *Medical-Psychiatric Practice*, pp. 515–535. Edited by Alan Stoudemire and Barry S. Fogel. Washington, D.C.: American Psychiatric Press.

BANJA, JOHN. 1992. "Ethics in Rehabilitation." In *Rehabilitation Medicine: Contemporary Clinical Perspectives*, pp. 269–298. Edited by Gerald F. Fletcher, John Banja, Brigitta Jann, and Steven Wolf. Philadelphia: Lea & Febiger.

BERKOWITZ, EDWARD D. 1981. "The Federal Government and the Emergence of Rehabilitation Medicine." *Historian* 43, no. 4:530–545.

BRODY, BARUCH A. 1988. "Justice in the Allocation of Public Resources to Disabled Citizens." *Archives of Physical Medicine and Rehabilitation* 69, no. 5:333–336.

BROOKS, NEIL. 1991. "The Effectiveness of Post-Acute Rehabilitation." *Brain Injury* 5, no. 2:103–109.

CALLAHAN, DANIEL. 1988. "Families as Caregivers: The Limits of Morality." *Archives of Physical Medicine and Rehabilitation* 69, no. 5:323–328.

CAPLAN, ARTHUR L. 1988. "Informed Consent and Provider–Patient Relationships in Rehabilitation Medicine." *Archives of Physical Medicine and Rehabilitation* 69, no. 5: 312–317.

CAPLAN, ARTHUR L.; CALLAHAN, DANIEL; and HAAS, JANET. 1987. "Ethical and Policy Issues in Rehabilitation Medicine." *Hastings Center Report* 17, no. 4 (spec. suppl.): 1–20.

CAPLAN, BRUCE. 1983. "Staff and Patient Perception of Patient Mood." *Rehabilitation Psychology* 28, no. 2:67–77.

COPE, D. NATHAN, and HALL, KARYL. 1982. "Head Injury Rehabilitation: Benefit of Early Intervention." *Archives of Physical Medicine and Rehabilitation* 63, no. 9:433–437.

DANIELS, NORMAN. 1985. *Just Health Care*. New York: Cambridge University Press.

DAVIDOFF, GARY N.; KEREN, OFER; RING, HAIM; and SOLZI, PABLO. 1991. "Acute Stroke Patients: Long-Term Effects of Rehabilitation and Maintenance of Gains." *Archives of Physical Medicine and Rehabilitation* 72, no. 11:869–873.

DELISA, JOEL A., ed. 1988. *Rehabilitation Medicine: Principles and Practice*. Philadelphia: Lippincott.

DWORKIN, GERALD. 1972. "Paternalism." *Monist* 56, no. 1: 64–84.

GUNTHER, MEYER S. 1971. "Psychiatric Consultation in a Rehabilitation Hospital: A Regression Hypothesis." *Comprehensive Psychiatry* 12, no. 6:572–585.

———. 1987. "Catastrophic Illness and the Caregivers: Real Burdens and Solutions with Respect to the Role of the Behavioral Sciences." In *Rehabilitation Psychology Desk Reference*, pp. 219–243. Edited by Bruce Caplan. Rockville, Md.: Aspen.

JONSEN, ALBERT R.; SIEGLER, MARK; and WINSLADE, WILLIAM J. 1992. *Clinical Ethics: A Practical Approach to Ethical Decisions in Clinical Medicine*, 3d ed., pp. 40–65. New York: McGraw-Hill.

KEITH, ROBERT A. 1991. "The Comprehensive Treatment Team in Rehabilitation." *Archives of Physical Medicine and Rehabilitation* 72, no. 5:269–274.

LYTH, JANALEE REINEKE. 1992. "Models of the Team Approach." In *Rehabilitation Medicine: Contemporary Clinical Perspectives*, pp. 225–242. Edited by Gerald F. Fletcher,

John Banja, Brigitte Jann, and Steven Wolf. Philadelphia: Lea & Febiger.

McKNIGHT, JOHN L. 1989. "Do No Harm: Policy Options That Meet Human Needs." *Social Policy* 20, no. 1:5–14.

MULLINS, LARRY L. 1989. "Hate Revisited: Power, Envy, and Greed in the Rehabilitation Setting." *Archives of Physical Medicine and Rehabilitation* 70, no. 10:740–744.

O'HARA, CHRISTIANE C., and HARRELL, MINNIE. 1991. *Rehabilitation with Brain Injury Survivors: An Empowerment Approach*. Gaithersburg, Md.: Aspen.

PARFENCHUCK, THOMAS A.; PARZIALE, JOHN R.; LIBERMAN, JOAN R.; BUTCHER, ROBERT P.; and AHERN, DAVID K. 1990. "The Evolution of an Acute Care Hospital Unit to a DRG-Exempt Rehabilitation Unit: A Preliminary Communication." *American Journal of Physical Medicine and Rehabilitation* 69, no. 11:11–15.

PURTILO, RUTH B. 1988. "Ethical Issues in Teamwork: The Context of Rehabilitation." *Archives of Physical Medicine and Rehabilitation* 69, no. 5:318–322.

———. 1992. "Whom to Treat First, and How Much Is Enough?" Ethical Dilemmas That Physical Therapists Confront As They Compare Individual Patients' Needs for Treatment." *International Journal of Technology Assessment in Health Care* 8, no. 1:26–34.

ROSENTHAL, MITCHELL. 1987. "Traumatic Head Injury: Neurobehavioral Consequences." In *Rehabilitation Psychology Desk Reference*, pp. 37–63. Edited by Bruce Caplan. Rockville, Md.: Aspen.

WANLASS, RICHARD L.; REUTTER, SUSAN L.; and KLINE, AMY E. 1992. "Communication Among Rehabilitation Staff: 'Mild,' 'Moderate,' or 'Severe' Deficits?" *Archives of Physical Medicine and Rehabilitation* 73, no. 5:477–481.

WILL, GEORGE F. 1986. "For the Handicapped, Rights but No Welcome." *Hastings Center Report* 16, no 3:5–8.

RELIGIOUS ETHICS

For an overview of the topic, see ETHICS, *article on* RELIGION AND MORALITY. *Various religious traditions are discussed in* AFRICAN RELIGION; BUDDHISM; CONFUCIANISM; EASTERN ORTHODOX CHRISTIANITY; HINDUISM; ISLAM; JAINISM; JUDAISM; NATIVE AMERICAN RELIGIONS; PROTESTANTISM; ROMAN CATHOLICISM; SIKHISM; *and* TAOISM. *Special practical topics in religious ethics include* ABORTION, *section on* RELIGIOUS TRADITIONS; BODY, *article on* CULTURAL AND RELIGIOUS PERSPECTIVES; DEATH, *articles on* EASTERN THOUGHT, *and* WESTERN RELIGIOUS THOUGHT; ENVIRONMENT AND RELIGION; EUGENICS AND RELIGIOUS LAW; HEALING; MENTAL HEALTH, *article on* MENTAL HEALTH AND RELIGION; *and* POPULATION ETHICS, *section on* RELIGIOUS TRADITIONS. *Professional issues are discussed in* PASTORAL CARE.

RENAL DIALYSIS

See KIDNEY DIALYSIS. *See also* ARTIFICAL ORGANS AND LIFE-SUPPORT SYSTEMS.

RENAL TRANSPLANTATION

See Organ and Tissue Transplants. *See also* Organ and Tissue Procurement.

REPRODUCTIVE TECHNOLOGIES

I. INTRODUCTION

The development of effective and imaginative approaches to the management of human infertility has focused public attention on the techniques themselves and on their ethical and legal implications. Although differing widely in their complexity, these methods have one characteristic in common: the separation of human reproduction from the act of coitus. An understanding of these reproductive technologies is essential to an overall consideration of ethical issues surrounding them.

Artificial insemination

Artificial insemination involves the mechanical placement of spermatozoa into the female reproductive tract. Inseminations are separated into two broad categories: those utilizing the semen of the husband or designated partner (AIH) and those employing semen of a third party, or donor insemination (DI). Since the ethical and moral issues surrounding AIH and DI take on different dimensions, each will be considered separately.

AIH constitutes effective treatment when, for whatever reason, the male partner is unable to ejaculate within the vagina. Some males are unable to ejaculate during coitus but can ejaculate through masturbation or the use of vibratory stimuli. Certain anatomical abnormalities result in faulty semen placement. Hypospadias,

a penile abnormality in which the opening of the urethra is located a distance from the tip of the glans penis, causes the ejaculate to be deposited at the periphery of the vagina even when the penis is well within. Retrograde ejaculation is a condition usually caused by a complication of prostatic surgery resulting in the formation of a channel that causes the ejaculate to be directed away from the penis and retrograded into the bladder. After ejaculation, semen for artificial insemination can be recovered from the bladder by catheterization.

Normal vaginal intercourse may be precluded by congenital or acquired vaginal abnormalities. In rare cases, the vagina is constricted as the result of in utero exposure to the hormone diethylstilbestrol (DES) or possibly by past trauma. Psychological problems in the male or female or both may interfere with normal coital exchange.

In recent years, AIH has been recommended when the semen displays deficiencies in numbers of sperm or their ability to move. Laboratory techniques have been developed to separate and concentrate the most active spermatozoa. These are then introduced into the uterine cavity, closer to the site of fertilization. Intrauterine insemination has been used with variable results in cases of male infertility and in couples with unexplained infertility (Blasco and Mastroianni, 1991).

Techniques of obtaining semen. Semen for use in artificial insemination is usually obtained by masturbation. An alternate possibility is intercourse using a plastic condom. Coitus interruptus is not recommended, as the first portion of the ejaculate, which contains the majority of active, motile spermatozoa, is sometimes lost. In cases of obstruction of the vas deferens, which serves as the conduit for spermatozoa, spermatozoa have been obtained surgically from the epididymis, the storage depot for spermatozoa. Specimens so obtained have been used successfully for both the gamete intrafallopian tube transfer (GIFT) procedure and in vitro fertilization (IVF).

Timing of the insemination. Placement of spermatozoa should be timed to coincide with the twelve hours immediately preceding ovulation. Approximately twenty-four hours before ovulation, increased levels of luteinizing hormone (LH) can be detected in the urine, using a color indicator to predict ovulation. The day-to-day development of the egg-containing ovarian follicle can be monitored with pelvic ultrasound. To enhance the accuracy of ovulation timing still further while causing the release of additional eggs for fertilization, the use of human gonadotropins to induce ovulation has become increasingly popular.

Insemination and sex selection. Insemination has also been used in an effort at sex selection. Various treatments have been recommended to separate the X-chromosome-bearing (female-producing) from the

Y-chromosome-bearing (male-producing) spermatozoa. Success rates in the production of male offspring in the 80 percent range are claimed (van Kooij and van Oost, 1992). Such techniques are useful in animal husbandry but do not yield a consistently satisfactory success rate in humans. Sex selection would be useful to avoid a sex-linked genetic disease. Sex preselection based solely on preference for a boy or a girl has much wider social implications.

Donor insemination.   Donor insemination was mentioned as a method of treating infertility in the nineteenth century. As DI has become more widely used, the legal climate has become more favorable and the status of the offspring much less uncertain. With this has come awareness of the importance of careful counseling and the use of appropriate permission forms. There has not yet been a case in U.S. law in which the anonymous sperm donor has been assigned parental responsibility.

The clinical indications for donor insemination are related mainly to deficiencies in the semen. The most clear-cut cases are those in which the male partner suffers from azoospermia (no spermatozoa). Indications have been extended to include those in whom some spermatozoa are present but the quality of the specimen is poor. Known hereditary disorders in the male partner, such as Huntington's disease, Tay-Sachs, or hemophilia, are also indications for DI.

In vitro fertilization (IVF) has widened the possibility of conception with severely deficient semen. Donor insemination is sometimes used in IVF when there is failure of fertilization using the male partner's specimen.

Evaluation of the couple for donor insemination.   A couple considering donor insemination should be thoroughly counseled. If either partner has reservations, it is wise to accept these at face value and encourage consideration of other options, including adoption. The man's fertility should be thoroughly evaluated, and efforts made to correct any abnormalities. The woman also should be thoroughly evaluated for factors that might contribute to infertility. Both partners are usually required to review and sign a detailed informed-consent form.

Selection and screening of donors.   In most circumstances, the donor is anonymous. Occasionally there is a request that a close relative (usually a brother or even a father) be used. In such cases, the couple should be encouraged to consider carefully the potential for future familial conflicts. Analysis of donor semen should meet the normal standards for fertility (American Fertility Society, 1986). The donor should be in excellent health and be screened for any family history of genetic disorders. Serologic tests for syphilis and serum hepatitis B antigen are obtained initially and after six

months. The genitalia are cultured for gonorrhea and chlamydia. An initial screening for the AIDS virus antibodies is performed and repeated after six months because the antibody test for AIDS may not turn positive until several months after infection. Most centers now use frozen semen exclusively. If a donor is providing repeated specimens, periodic reevaluation of his health status is essential. Clinics should maintain records of pregnancies and set a limit on the number of pregnancies any one donor may produce. To decrease the possibility of consanguinity in a given population, an arbitrary limit of ten or fewer pregnancies is recommended.

It is important to maintain confidential donor records, including all of the information on the screening procedures, so that it is available on an anonymous basis if it is needed for medical reasons in the future.

Technique of insemination.   The standard insemination involves placing the specimen, thawed if it has been frozen, into the cervical canal by means of a small, flexible cannula. As the vaginal speculum is removed, the remainder of the specimen is placed in the vagina, at the outer cervical canal. The patient remains supine for twenty minutes or so. The specimen may be held in place with a cervical cap, which is removed four to six hours after insemination. For intrauterine insemination, a plastic cannula is passed through the opening of the cervix into the uterine cavity, where the concentrated, pretreated (i.e., washed) spermatozoa are deposited.

Cryopreservation of semen.   Since the first successful insemination with freeze-stored semen in 1953, this technique has had a significant impact on clinical practice. In the 1970s, formal semen banks were established, largely to address the needs for long-term preservation of the specimens of men who had undergone vasectomy. Semen also is preserved prior to chemotherapy or radiation, which might result in sterility. Although there is no formal reporting system, information accumulated over the years has failed to uncover an increased incidence of genetic defects among the offspring resulting from insemination with cryopreserved semen.

The response of spermatozoa to cryopreservation is unpredictable and varies on an individual basis. Some specimens freeze well and others do not. The pregnancy rate is lower overall with frozen semen. The only reliable way to determine whether a specimen is suitable for cryopreservation is to cryopreserve it, thaw it, and evaluate the impact of the procedure on the quality of sperm motility. Specimens are usually stored in individual straws or small vials so that fractions may be thawed while the remainder is preserved for future use. The Ethics Committee of the American Fertility Society has determined that cryopreservation of human semen is ethically and medically acceptable, but does speak of the lack of uniformity in standards among sperm banks and of the importance of establishing certification standards (American Fertility Society, 1986). Most large university centers use only cryopreserved semen for donor insemination.

In vitro fertilization

In vitro fertilization and embryo transfer (IVF-ET) is increasingly common in infertility practice (Society for Assisted Reproductive Technology, 1993). Initially used exclusively in women with damaged fallopian tubes, the indications for IVF-ET have been extended to include male factor infertility and cases in which no cause for the infertility can be uncovered. Much as artificial insemination separates procreation from the coital act, in vitro fertilization separates fertilization from the normal maternal environment, allowing the initial phases of development to occur outside the reproductive tract, followed by transfer of the embryo into the uterus. The first successful in vitro fertilization was carried out in a normally ovulating woman whose tubes had been surgically removed. A single egg (ovum, oocyte) was obtained by aspiration at the time of laparoscopy. The oocyte was fertilized in vitro and transferred to the uterus after two days.

In later developments, the ovaries were stimulated with human urinary gonadotropins to induce development of several follicles, each containing an ovum, in a given cycle. This approach is now standard. Follicular development is followed by means of blood estrogen levels, and the size of the growing follicles is measured by ultrasound. When the follicles are judged ready for ovulation, a second hormone, human chorionic gonadotropin (hCG), is administered to induce ovulation. This causes further development of the follicles and the maturing of oocytes within them. The oocytes complete their first division in a process referred to as meiosis, releasing half their complement of chromosomes in a small, round structure, the first polar body. The maternal chromosomes are now ready for the second meiotic division, which occurs after the ovum has been penetrated by the spermatozoa. Within two to three hours of the expected time of ovulation, the oocytes are aspirated from their follicles.

In the early phases of IVF development, this was carried out with the aid of the laparoscope. The procedure required general anesthesia and involved placing a telescope through the umbilicus for visualization of the pelvic structures. The oocytes were obtained by needle aspiration. Today, ova are obtained by ultrasound-guided transvaginal aspiration. This procedure can be done without general anesthesia, and the overall approach to in vitro fertilization is greatly simplified.

Another major clinical problem in the early phases of IVF development was that occasionally a patient would ovulate before the oocytes could be obtained, and the cycle would have to be canceled. Analogues of the gonadotropin-releasing hormone (GnRH) are now used to prevent this. These analogues are capable of blocking the release of the patient's pituitary gonadotropins, and the ovaries can be brought under the complete control of exogenously administered hormones. The number of follicles that develop varies from patient to patient, and even in the same patient from one cycle to the next. By and large, the aim is to obtain as many oocytes as possible in a given treatment cycle, especially if the couple has selected cryopreservation as a possible option.

IVF treatment is both physically and emotionally demanding. Several visits for hormone determinations and ultrasound are required. Ovum recovery, although relatively safe, is not without complications. Rarely ovarian infection occurs, which can further compromise the fertility status of the patient. This point is particularly pertinent when oocytes are being obtained for donation.

A freshly ejaculated semen specimen is obtained for insemination. The ova are placed in individual containers and mixed with spermatozoa that have been prepared by separating them from the semen and incubating them in a solution designed to enhance their fertilizability. It is useful to have a cryopreserved semen specimen on hand in the event that a fresh specimen cannot be obtained when needed. The inseminated ova are cultured for approximately twenty-four hours and then inspected for evidence of fertilization.

Much has been learned about human fertilization through in vitro fertilization. When it is removed from the woman's body, the ovum is surrounded by layers of small, loosely packed cells, the cumulus oophorus. An inner layer of more densely arranged cells, the corona radiata, immediately surrounds the oocyte. These cells interface with the zona pellucida, a translucent protein shell that immediately surrounds the egg. Penetration past these barriers is accomplished through a sequence of interactions between spermatozoa and the ovum and its layers (Kopf and Gerton, 1990). When the spermatozoon reaches the zona pellucida, a series of chemical communications occurs. These condition the spermatozoon so that it can penetrate through the zona pellucida. Once past the zona, the spermatozoon attaches to the egg membrane and is then incorporated into the egg cytoplasm, the tail along with the head. The head is then transformed into a pronucleus. The second polar body is released and the nucleus of the egg is transformed into a pronucleus. The pronuclei then join and the chromosomes are intermingled in preparation for the first cell division. Twenty-four hours after insemination, there are two pronuclei and two polar bodies. This constitutes evidence that the penetration has been successful and fertilization is in process. After two days, the embryo has developed to the four-to-eight-cell stage and is ready for transfer into the uterus.

Embryo transfer. The dividing embryos are incorporated into the end of a catheter that is then passed through the cervical opening into the uterine cavity, where they are discharged. The pregnancy rate is progressively improved if more than one embryo is transferred. If more than four are transferred, there is a greatly increased possibility of multiple pregnancy. Twins are not a problem, but triplets or more greatly increase the possibility of fetal loss. Therefore, in many IVF programs no more than four fertilized oocytes are transferred. The availability of cryopreservation has made such decisions easier.

The issue of when meaningful human life begins is pivotal in any discussion of IVF. The fertilization process is a complex series of events. The spermatozoon must be exposed to the environment of the female reproductive tract for a period of time before it acquires the ability to penetrate the layers surrounding the recently ovulated oocyte. This process, referred to as "capacitation," takes between one and two hours in the human. It is reproduced in vitro in the fluids utilized for sperm preparation. The series of events involving penetration through the zona pellucida requires complex chemical communication between sperm and egg. After the spermatozoon has penetrated into the cytoplasm, completion of fertilization, although increasingly probable, is not assured.

The events that follow, including the formation and subsequent fusion of the pronuclei, occupy more than twenty-four hours. In the natural sequence of events, the conceptus remains in the fallopian tube for approximately three days. At the eight-to-sixteen-cell stage, it is transported into the uterus. There it develops into a fluid-filled structure, the blastocyst, that attaches to the uterine lining, or endometrium, on the sixth to seventh day after fertilization. The blastocyst is incorporated into the endometrium and invades blood vessels. Development occurs rapidly thereafter, but it is not until the fourteenth day that it develops unique characteristics. This coincides with the formation of the primitive streak, a linear region that can be identified on the early embryonic disk; it signals the beginning of the development of a distinct category of cells. Until this point, there is the potential for division into identical twins. Each of the individual cells in the early conceptus has the potential to develop into a complete adult. On or about day five or six, specialized cells, the trophoblasts, are formed. They provide the point of attachment for the placenta and are essential to the nourishment of the growing embryo. The Ethics Committee of the American Fertility Society applies the term "pre-embryo" to the conceptus through the first two weeks of gestation (Ethics Committee, American Fertility Society, 1986). It takes the position that the moral status of the pre-embryo is different from that of either the unfertilized eggs and spermatozoa or the later stages in embryonic development.

Cryopreservation of pre-embryos. Techniques for freeze-preserving pre-embryos have contributed to the success of human in vitro fertilization and embryo transfer. The incidence of multiple pregnancy, which increases dramatically if more than four pre-embryos are transferred, can be reduced with the availability of cryopreservation. Pre-embryos not transferred during the treatment cycle can be utilized in subsequent spontaneous ovulation cycles. When pregnancy occurs in the initial treatment cycle and pre-embryos have been cryopreserved, a number of future options must be considered. These issues should be reviewed and decisions made before the pre-embryos are frozen. Patients whose response to stimulation clearly indicates that more than four oocytes will be recovered should consider their options well in advance of ovum recovery. Those who for whatever reason, including deeply felt moral reservations, choose not to cryopreserve may wish to have sperm added to no more than four oocytes and have all of the fertilized specimens transferred. Remaining ova can be disposed of in their unfertilized state. Another alternative short of cryopreservation is to fertilize all available ova and select only the best of the resulting pre-embryos, as determined by their appearance and rate of cell division, for replacement, discarding the remainder.

The standard consent form should contain a detailed description of the possibilities to consider if a decision is made to cryopreserve human pre-embryos. As far as is known, cryopreservation of human pre-embryos is not associated with adverse fetal effects. Generally it is agreed that the pre-embryos will be frozen and stored for use in subsequent cycles. Unforeseen situations can occur, such as failure of equipment, although backup freezer systems and liquid-nitrogen holding facilities are usually available in the event of such an occurrence.

In most major centers, the disposition of unused frozen pre-embryos is reviewed in advance of cryopreservation. Handling of these pre-embryos is subject to the couple's joint disposition. They agree that if one partner is unwilling or unable to assume responsibility for the fertilized eggs, the responsibility reverts to the other partner. If that person is not willing or able to assume ownership, the hospital or clinic usually reserves the right to dispose of the pre-embryos in accordance with policies in existence at the time.

Micromanipulation of oocytes and embryos in vitro

Instruments have been developed to allow manipulation of gametes and pre-embryos under magnification. These techniques of micromanipulation have been used extensively in laboratory mammals. More recently they have been applied to human eggs, spermatozoa, and pre-embryos. When the oocyte is not penetrated by spermatozoa that are otherwise apparently normal, micromanipulation can be used to insert a spermatozoon mechanically through the zona pellucida into the space between the zona and the oocyte (subzonal insertion or SUZI) or directly into the oocyte itself (intracytoplasmic sperm insertion or ICSI). Pregnancies that would otherwise be impossible can occur as a result of this procedure.

Micromanipulation has been extended to pre-embryos. It has been suggested that the second polar body, the cell that is released from the ovum at the time it is penetrated by the spermatozoon, be removed for chromosome analysis in an effort to determine whether the embryo is genetically normal. This approach could be used in couples at risk of genetic abnormalities and would avoid the onus of a decision to terminate the pregnancy later on. Individual cells have been removed from the embryo for analysis without apparent harm (Tarin and Handyside, 1993). Other possibilities may eventually emerge, including the removal and storage of individual cells as clones of the embryo that is transferred. Many of these approaches have not yet attained clinical practicality, but they raise moral, ethical, and legal issues that it would be wise to address now.

Gamete intrafallopian tube transfer

The procedure referred to as gamete intrafallopian tube transfer (GIFT) involves the transfer of freshly recovered ova and conditioned spermatozoa into the fallopian tubes. Thus, fertilization actually occurs in vivo. GIFT is not applicable to all infertility patients. Those with damaged or absent fallopian tubes are obviously not candidates. GIFT has been recommended for couples with unexplained infertility and women with extratubal disease, such as pelvic adhesions or endometriosis. The success rate following GIFT, 30–35 percent, is roughly twice that of in vitro fertilization (Society for Assisted Reproductive Technology, 1993). Although fertilization occurs within the fallopian tube, GIFT is certainly assisted reproductive technology and is clearly separated from the coital act. When more than four ova are recovered at the time of a GIFT procedure, one or more are usually fertilized in vitro and cryopreserved for transfer in subsequent cycles. Transfer of the ova and spermatozoa into the fallopian tubes is usually carried out by means of laparoscopy. Techniques employing ultrasound-guided transuterine transfer are being developed to obviate laparoscopy.

Surrogate gestational mothers

Human in vitro fertilization has opened the possibility that the resulting pre-embryos can be transferred to a woman other than the woman providing the oocytes. The second woman, referred to variously as a surrogate carrier, a womb mother, a placental mother, or a surrogate gestational mother, provides the gestational but not the genetic component of that pregnancy. Usually arrangements are made for the couple whose egg and sperm produced the embryo to adopt the newborn.

In another type of surrogacy, a husband's spermatozoa are used to inseminate a woman other than his wife. This surrogate mother carries the gestation to term. Agreement is reached before the procedure is carried out that the contracting couple will have custody of the resulting child.

In everyday infertility practice, there are circumstances that seem to justify these procedures. Consider a woman who was born without a uterus but with normal, functioning ovaries. Her husband is normally fertile. The patient's sister had a tubal sterilization after three pregnancies and is healthy in every way. The patient's sister's husband is entirely in agreement with the patient's sister's desire to act as a gestational surrogate mother. Oocytes are obtained from the patient, they are fertilized with her husband's spermatozoa, and the pre-embryos are transferred to her sister's uterus. In this situation we are virtually 100 percent confident that the pregnancy resulted from the procedure and is not an accidental result of coitus between the surrogate and her husband. The offspring is the genetic product of the husband and wife and has no direct genetic relationship to the patient's sister.

Other cases involve the use of a surrogate mother who contributes 50 percent of the chromosomal makeup of the offspring; this represents a more complex situation. The birth mother who clearly is genetically related to the offspring will be giving up her newborn child (hers in terms of both birth process and genetics). Indications for the use of a surrogate gestational mother include any condition in which there are functioning ovaries but an absent or nonfunctioning uterus. The uterus may be congenitally absent or may have been removed because of disease; it may be nonfunctional as a result of in utero DES exposure. A surrogate carrier may also be considered if pregnancy is ill-advised for reasons of maternal health. Another issue concerns responsibility for the child in the event that it is abnormal or damaged as a result of premature birth or birth trauma. There are also issues of the health status and behavior of the surrogate gestational mother during pregnancy. One must consider the impact of drugs or alcohol and the possibility of transmission of diseases. Finally, there is the issue of payment to the surrogate gestational mother. The possibility for exploitation certainly exists.

Oocyte donation

The clinical indications for the use of donor ova usually are rather straightforward. They include premature menopause and the inability of the wife to produce genetically normal oocytes. On the surface, the ethical issues surrounding the use of donor oocytes should be no different from those involved in the use of donor semen. They are compounded, however, by the risks involved in obtaining oocytes compared with obtaining a semen specimen. For example, ovarian infection could occur following ovum retrieval, which could result in permanent sterility (Tureck et al., 1993). In addition to the cost of the procedures, which is usually borne by the couple requiring the oocytes, there is also the question of payment to the donor for her time, pain, and suffering.

In contrast to spermatozoa, oocytes are difficult to cryopreserve; hence, menstrual cycle coordination between the recipient and the donor is required. Alternatively, donor oocytes may be fertilized with the husband's sperm, and the pre-embryos cryopreserved for future transfer. Sources of donor oocytes include the excess eggs from patients undergoing in vitro fertilization, oocytes obtained incidental to an operative procedure such as a sterilization, or a specific donation by a relative or close friend. Increasingly, the source of the eggs is a paid "volunteer." The availability of this technology allows pregnancy in women who are well past the ordinary childbearing age (Sauer et al., 1990, 1993).

Conclusion

The techniques employed in what is known as the "new assisted reproductive technologies" are varied and challenging. They range in complexity from seemingly straightforward artificial insemination to micromanipulation of ova, spermatozoa, and pre-embryos—and perhaps, in the future, to treatment of genetic disease by gene insertion in vitro. Just as the techniques vary, so do the ethical issues surrounding them. In no other field is there a greater opportunity for interaction among the physician–scientist, ethicist, moral theologian, social scientist, and legal scholar.

LUIGI MASTROIANNI, JR.

Directly related to this article are the other articles in this entry: SEX SELECTION; ARTIFICIAL INSEMINATION; IN VITRO FERTILIZATION AND EMBRYO TRANSFER; SURROGACY; CRYOPRESERVATION OF SPERM, OVA, AND EMBRYOS; ETHICAL ISSUES; *and* LEGAL AND REGULATORY ISSUES. *For a further discussion of topics mentioned in this article, see the entries* CRYONICS; FETUS; *and* LIFE. *This article will find application in the entries* EUGENICS, *article on* ETHICAL ISSUES; FERTILITY CONTROL; MATERNAL–FETAL RELATIONSHIP; *and* WOMEN, *article on* HEALTH-CARE ISSUES. *Other relevant material may be found under*

the entries ADOPTION; *and* MARRIAGE AND OTHER DOMESTIC PARTNERSHIPS.

Bibliography

AMERICAN FERTILITY SOCIETY. 1986. "New Guidelines for the Use of Semen Donor Insemination." *Fertility and Sterility* 46 (suppl. 2):95S–110S.

BLASCO, LUIS, and MASTROIANNI, LUIGI, JR. 1991. "Intrauterine Insemination in the Treatment of Infertility: Evaluation and Preparation of Semen." *Assisted Reproduction Reviews* 1, no. 2:72–75.

ETHICS COMMITTEE. AMERICAN FERTILITY SOCIETY. 1986. "Ethical Considerations of New Reproductive Technology." Report of *Fertility and Sterility* 46 (Suppl. 1).

KOPF, GREGORY S., and GERTON, GEORGE L. 1990. "The Mammalian Sperm Acrosome and the Acrosome Reaction." In *The Biology and Chemistry of Mammalian Fertilization*, pp. 153–203. Edited by Paul M. Wasserman. Boca Raton, Fla.: CRC Press.

SAUER, MARK V.; PAULSON, RICHARD J.; and LOBO, ROGERIO A. 1990. "A Preliminary Report on Oocyte Donation Extending Reproductive Potential to Women over 40." *New England Journal of Medicine* 323, no. 17:1157–1160.

———. 1993. "Pregnancy After Age 50: Application of Oocyte Donation to Women After Natural Menopause." *Lancet* 341, no. 8841:321–323.

SOCIETY FOR ASSISTED REPRODUCTIVE TECHNOLOGY. AMERICAN FERTILITY SOCIETY. 1993. "Assisted Reproductive Technology in the United States and Canada: 1991 Results from the Society for Assisted Reproductive Technology Generated from the American Fertility Society Registry." *Fertility and Sterility* 59, no. 5:956–962.

TARIN, JUAN J., and HANDYSIDE, ALAN H. 1993. "Embryo Biopsy Strategies for Preimplantation Diagnosis." *Fertility and Sterility* 59, no. 5:943–952.

TURECK, RICHARD W.; GARCIA, CELSO-RAMON; BLASCO, LUIS; and MASTROIANNI, LUIGI, JR. 1993. "Perioperative Complication Arising After Transvaginal Oocyte Retrieval." *Obstetrics and Gynecology* 81, no. 4:590–593.

VAN KOOIJ, ROELOF J., and VAN OOST, BERNARD A. 1992. "Determination of Sex Ratio for Spermatozoa with a Deoxyribonucleic Acid-Probe and Quinacrine Staining: A Comparison." *Fertility and Sterility* 58, no. 2:384–386.

VAN STEIRTEGHEM, A.; JORIS, H.; LIU, J.; NAHY, Z.; TOURNAYE, H.; LEIBAERS, I.; and DEVROEY, P. 1993. "Assisted Fertilization by Subzonal Insemination and Intracytoplasmic Sperm Injection." In *Gamete and Embryo Quality: The Proceeding of the Fourth Organon Round Table Conference, Thessaloniki, Greece, 24–25 June*, pp. 117–124. Edited by Luigi Mastroianni, Jr., H. J. T. Coelingh Bennick, S. Suzuki, and H. H. M. Vemer. Carnforth, U.K.: Parthenon.

II. SEX SELECTION

Sex selection may be performed at three stages before birth: (1) before conception, by separation of X- (female) and Y- (male) bearing sperm; (2) before implantation of an embryo in the womb, by use of in vitro fertilization and embryo selection; and (3) after a pregnancy is established, by prenatal diagnosis and selective abortion of fetuses of the sex not desired. Preconception methods of sex selection have not proved reliable. Most of these depend on separation of X- and Y-bearing sperm, which may somewhat increase the odds of conceiving a child of the desired sex but does not guarantee a particular result. Preimplantation embryo selection could offer an alternative to parents who would find abortion for sex selection morally objectionable. Embryos not implanted could be frozen and stored rather than being destroyed. Although technically possible, this method will likely appeal to few, because of its high cost and the low success rate of in vitro fertilization (Robertson, 1992). Thus, around the world, most sex selection before birth occurs through prenatal diagnosis, including amniocentesis, chorionic villus sampling, or ultrasound, followed by selective abortion. Ultrasound, although not definitive, may show the male genitals; its major use is for parents who desire a son and who are willing to abort a fetus that is not clearly male.

Sex selection may be morally justifiable in some cases to give parents the option of avoiding the births of males with serious genetic disorders, usually called X-linked disorders, that a healthy mother can transmit to her sons but not to her daughters. These include hemophilia and some forms of muscular dystrophy. A male fetus whose mother carries a gene for an X-linked disorder has a 50 percent chance of having the disorder. Some X-linked disorders cannot be diagnosed before birth. Identification of fetal sex gives parents the option of selective abortion of male fetuses who are at 50 percent risk of having severe medical problems. This use of prenatal diagnosis falls within medically accepted uses of prenatal diagnosis to provide parents with information on which to make decisions about fetuses with serious genetic disorders.

Most sex selection has no relationship to genetic disorders. It is solely for the sex desired by the parents. Two ethical issues are involved. The first is whether families should be able to choose the sex of their children, and if so, under what conditions. The second is whether abortion is justified as a means to this end. Although about one-third of the U.S. public favors use of preconception methods of sex selection (Dixon and Levy, 1985), relatively few (5 percent) approve of prenatal testing and abortion for this purpose (Singer, 1991). A substantial minority (38 percent), however, would approve the use of abortion for sex selection if a couple already had three children of the same sex, regardless of whether these were boys or girls (Singer, 1991).

Direct requests for prenatal diagnosis for sex selection have been few in Western nations, in view of (1) the absence of a strong cultural preference for children of a particular sex, and (2) personal and cultural objections to the use of abortion for this purpose. Although the majority of Americans believe that abortion should be available to others in a wide variety of situations, including sex selection, few would use it themselves (Wertz et al., 1991). In any case, the numbers of requests for prenatal diagnosis for sex selection cannot be documented in Western nations, because few parents make open requests.

Medical professionals in the United States appear increasingly willing to perform prenatal diagnosis for those making requests for sex selection, however. According to a 1975 survey of 149 clinically oriented geneticists and counselors, 15 percent would recommend amniocentesis for sex selection in general and 28 percent would do so for a couple with one girl who wanted to have only two children and who wanted to be sure that their final child would be a son who could carry on the family name (Fraser and Pressor, 1977). In 1985, 62 percent of 295 doctoral-level geneticists in the United States would either perform prenatal diagnosis (34 percent) or offer a referral (28 percent) for a couple with four daughters who desired a son and who would abort a female fetus (Wertz and Fletcher, 1989b, 1989c, 1990). Substantial percentages in some other nations would also perform prenatal diagnosis for this couple, including 60 percent in Hungary, 52 percent in India, 47 percent in Canada, 38 percent in Sweden, 33 percent in Israel, 30 percent in Brazil, 29 percent in Greece, and 24 percent in the United Kingdom. A 1990 survey, using the same question, found that 85 percent of master's-level genetic counselors in the United States would either arrange for prenatal diagnosis or a referral (Pencarinha et al., 1991).

In giving reasons for acceding to parents' requests, many geneticists in the 1985 survey said that sex selection was a logical extension of parents' acknowledged rights to choose the number, timing, spacing, and genetic health of their children. These geneticists regarded withholding any service, including sex selection, as medical paternalism and an infringement on patient autonomy. Those who would refuse prenatal diagnosis said that it was a misuse of scarce medical resources designed to look for serious genetic abnormalities, that sex was not a disease, or that they disapproved of the abortion of a normal fetus. Most regarded sex selection as a private procedure involving only the interests of doctor and patient, rather than as a procedure that could affect the wider society or the status of women. Few, except for geneticists in India, mentioned the societal implications of sex selection. Women, who comprised 35 percent of doctoral-level geneticists in the United States, were twice as likely as men to say that they would actually perform prenatal diagnosis for the couple with four daughters in the case above (Wertz and Fletcher, 1989b, 1989c, 1990).

Most requests for sex selection in developed nations are probably covert, with women requesting prenatal diagnosis on the basis of anxiety about the health of the fetus. Most geneticists in the United States (89 percent) and around the world (73 percent) would perform prenatal diagnosis for an anxious woman aged twenty-five with no medical or genetic indications for its use (Wertz and Fletcher, 1989b, 1990). Parents are usually asked if they wish to know the fetal sex, though some clinics do not provide the information unless specifically requested (Wertz and Fletcher, 1989c). In effect, sex selection as facilitated by prenatal diagnosis is therefore available to most families.

For some women having prenatal diagnosis for medically indicated reasons, such as maternal age over thirty-five, knowledge of fetal sex may present a troubling or even unwelcome possibility for choice. For example, a woman aged forty with three sons, whose pregnancy is unexpected and who has always wanted a daughter, could decide to have prenatal diagnosis, which is medically indicated by her age and genetic risk, and to find out the fetus's sex before deciding whether to continue the pregnancy. Knowledge about fetal sex affects abortion decisions among some women (about 16 percent) having prenatal diagnosis on the basis of advanced maternal age, especially if the pregnancy was not intended (Sjögren, 1988).

The major use of prenatal diagnosis for sex selection occurs in those developing nations where there is a strong preference for sons. In some nations, such as India, the majority of prenatal diagnostic procedures are performed for sex selection rather than detection of fetal abnormalities. Ultrasound, although not always accurate, is affordable even to villagers and poses no risk to the mother. In many nations of Asia, sex selection contributes to an already unbalanced sex ratio occasioned by neglect of female children. An estimated sixty to one hundred million women are "missing" from the world's population (Sen, 1990), including twenty-nine million in China and twenty-three million in India. Whereas in the United States, the United Kingdom, and France, there are 105 women to every 100 men, and in Africa and Latin America the proportions of women and men are roughly equal, in much of Asia, including Pakistan, Afghanistan, Turkey, Bangladesh, India, and China, there are fewer than 95 women for every 100 men (United Nations, 1991). Families desire sons for economic reasons. In these nations, where most people have no social security or retirement pensions, sons are responsible for caring for parents in their old age. Daughters usually leave the parental family to live with their husbands and help care for their parents-in-law. Even if a daughter stays in the parental home, she sel-

dom has the earning power to support her parents. In some nations, a daughter represents a considerable economic burden because her family must pay a dowry to her husband's family in order to arrange a marriage. A son's religious duties at his parents' funerals, though often cited as a reason for son preference in India, are of lesser importance than economic factors. These religious duties can be performed by other male relatives. As elsewhere in the world, cultural sex stereotypes and sexism also play a role in the desire for sons.

Ethical arguments in favor of sex selection in general, including preconception selection, are that (1) sex choice would enhance the quality of life for a child of the "wanted" sex; (2) sex choice would provide a better quality of life for the family that has the sex balance it desires; (3) sex choice would provide a better quality of life for the mother, because she would undergo fewer births and her status in the family would be enhanced; and (4) sex choice would help to limit the population (Warren, 1985). According to these arguments, families that have the sex "balance" that they desire would be happier. Children of the "unwanted" sex, usually female, would be spared the abuse, neglect, and early death that is their documented fate in some developing nations (Verma and Singh, 1989) and that may occur to a less obvious extent elsewhere. Women would not be abused by their husbands for not bearing children of the desired sex. Women would not suffer repeated pregnancies and births in order to produce at least one child of the desired sex, usually a son. Families would not have more children than they could afford in order to have a child of the desired sex. Many families in developing nations would prefer to have at most two children. These couples could limit their family size and still have a son to support them in their old age, instead of continuing to have children until they have a son. The threat of world overpopulation might recede.

Each of the arguments above can be effectively countered. Arguments that sex selection will lead to a better quality of life for families, children, or women are comprehensible only in the context of a sexist society that gives preferential treatment to one sex, usually the male. Instead of selecting sex, it should be possible to improve quality of life by making society less sexist. Although sex selection could prevent some abuse of unwanted female children and their mothers in the short run, it does not correct the underlying abuses, namely the social devaluation of women in many parts of Asia and the gender stereotyping of children of both sexes in the rest of the world.

There is no good evidence that sex selection will reduce population growth in developing nations. Most families try to have the number of children that is most economically advantageous. If they could select sex, and if one sex presented an economic advantage over the other, some families might have more children—all of the advantaged sex—than they would have had in the absence of sex selection. Education of women in developing nations and increased opportunities for their employment outside the home are probably more effective means of reducing population growth than sex selection. In developed nations, sex selection will likely have no effect on population size, because most families do not have more children than they wish in order to have a child of a particular sex (Dixon and Levy, 1985).

Arguments against all types of sex selection are based on the premise that all sex selection, including selection for the "balanced family" desired in most Western nations, helps to perpetuate gender stereotyping and sexism (Overall, 1987; Warren, 1985). Sex selection violates the principle of equality between the sexes (U.S. President's Commission, 1983). In a nonsexist society, there should be no reason to select one sex over the other. Michael Bayles has examined concerns that might be put forward for sex preference, including replacing oneself biologically, carrying on the family name, rights of inheritance, or jobs requiring either men or women. He points out that none of these reasons are valid (Bayles, 1984). A child's sex does not make that child biologically any more "my" child than a child of the other sex. In modern societies, women as well as men can carry on the family name, inherit estates, and carry out most jobs. Conversely, men can care for children, elderly parents, or relatives with disabilities, tasks that usually fall on women in developed nations and that could in the future lead to a preference for daughters. Mary Anne Warren points out that even in a nonsexist society, however, there would remain a natural desire for the companionship of a child of one's own sex (Warren, 1985). This is not a strong argument in favor of sex selection. Any activity that a parent can enjoy with a child of one sex, such as sports, vacations, or hobbies, can be enjoyed with a child of the other sex.

Another argument against sex selection is that it could increase gender inequalities, even in developed nations where parents usually prefer sons and daughters equally. Although these preferences are slight, there is evidence that in the United States families would prefer that the firstborn be a boy or that they have two sons and a daughter if they are to have three children (Pebley and Westhoff, 1982). Firstborns tend to receive more economic advantages than laterborns. A society in which firstborns tended to be sons would tend to give more power to males.

There are additional arguments against sex selection if it takes place after conception. Prenatal diagnosis for this purpose is a misuse of a costly, and in some nations scarce, medical resource. If use of prenatal diagnosis for sex selection becomes widespread, this could discredit all uses of prenatal diagnosis, including use to detect serious disorders in the fetus. Sex selection undermines the major moral reason that justifies prenatal diagnosis—giving parents information on which to make decisions about fetuses with serious and untreatable genetic disorders. Using prenatal diagnosis to select sex could lead toward selection on cosmetic grounds, such as height, weight, or eye, hair or skin color, if analysis for such characteristics in the fetus ever becomes technically possible. Some parents would select for such purposes, especially for weight (Wertz et al., 1991).

Laws prohibiting sex selection could do more harm than good in most nations, because such laws could lead to further interference with reproductive freedom. Some would argue that instead of focusing on sex selection, societies should work toward equality of the sexes and against gender stereotyping, including the stereotyping of fetuses (Rothman, 1986), and should establish a moral climate against sex selection of any kind. Sex selection is not a medical service; doctors are not forced to accede to patient requests or offer referrals. Doctors could also consider withholding information about fetal sex, although this puts control into the hands of doctors and could lead to a resurgence of medical paternalism.

In nations where sex selection has become a social problem, however, laws may be useful as interim measures to prevent widespread abuses of prenatal diagnosis, at least until women achieve equality. Even if laws cannot be adequately enforced, they may be symbolically important in establishing the equality of women (Verma and Singh, 1989; Wertz and Fletcher, 1989c). Long-range solutions are education for women and equality in the work force. Societies generally place higher value on women if their work is recognized as productive (which usually means work outside the home), if they have some economic rights, and if there is an awareness of the social changes necessary to overcome inqualities. In developing nations, women's longevity and the ratio of women to men are in direct parallel with women's participation in the work force (Sen, 1990). Thus in sub-Saharan Africa, where many women work outside the home, women outnumber men, while in Pakistan, India, and Bangladesh, where relatively few women work outside the home, there are fewer women than men. The solution to sex selection in these nations seems to lie in women's entry into the paid work force.

It is important to seek solutions to the problem of sex selection now, because it has the potential power to change entire societies. If preconception methods become available, societies and individuals may act on their preferences with little possibility of legal or moral restraint. Sex selection could further unbalance the already unbalanced sex ratio in many parts of the world and could lead to greater numbers of "missing women." Professionals need to reconsider a trend toward honoring all patient requests, including sex selection. Prospective parents need to reconsider the consequences of unlimited choice.

DOROTHY C. WERTZ

Directly related to this article are the INTRODUCTION *and other articles in this entry:* ARTIFICIAL INSEMINATION; IN VITRO FERTILIZATION AND EMBRYO TRANSFER; SURROGACY; CRYOPRESERVATION OF SPERM, OVA, AND EMBRYOS; ETHICAL ISSUES; *and* LEGAL AND REGULATORY ISSUES. *For a further discussion of topics mentioned in this article, see the entries* ABORTION; GENETIC COUNSELING; GENETIC TESTING AND SCREENING; LIFE, QUALITY OF; POPULATION ETHICS, *section on* ELEMENTS OF POPULATION ETHICS; POPULATION POLICIES, *section on* STRATEGIES OF FERTILITY CONTROL; *and* WOMEN. *For a discussion of related ideas, see the entries* EUGENICS; INFORMATION DISCLOSURE; PATERNALISM; PERSON; RIGHTS; *and* SEXISM. *Other relevant material may be found under the entries* FAMILY; FERTILITY CONTROL; FETUS; *and* MATERNAL–FETAL RELATIONSHIP.

Bibliography

BAYLES, MICHAEL D. 1984. *Reproductive Ethics.* Englewood Cliffs, N.J.: Prentice-Hall.

DIXON, RICHARD D., and LEVY, DIANE E. 1985. "Sex of Children: A Community Analysis of Preferences and Pre-Determination Attitudes." *Sociological Quarterly* 26, no. 2:251–271.

FRASER, F. CLARKE, and PRESSOR, C. 1977. "Attitudes of Counselors in Relation to Prenatal Sex-Determination Simply for Choice of Sex." In *Genetic Counseling.* Edited by H. Lubs and F. de la Cruz. New York: Raven Press.

OVERALL, CHRISTINE. 1987. *Ethics and Human Reproduction: A Feminist Analysis.* Boston: Allen and Unwin.

PEBLEY, ANNE R., and WESTHOFF, CHARLES F. 1982. "Women's Sex Preferences in the United States: 1970 to 1975." *Demography* 19, no. 2:177–189.

PENCARINHA, DEBORAH; BELL, N.; EDWARDS J.; and BEST, R. G. 1991. "Study of the Attitudes and Reasoning of M.S. Genetic Counselors Regarding Ethical Issues in Medical Genetics." *American Journal of Human Genetics* 49 (suppl.):326.

ROBERTSON, JOHN A. 1992. "Ethical and Legal Issues in Preimplantation Genetic Screening." *Fertility and Sterility* 57, no. 1:1–11.

ROTHMAN, BARBARA KATZ. 1986. *The Tentative Pregnancy: Prenatal Diagnosis and the Future of Motherhood.* New York: Viking.

SEN, AMARTYA. 1990. "More Than 100 Million Women Are Missing." *New York Review of Books,* December 20, pp. 61–66.

SINGER, ELEANOR. 1991. "Public Attitudes Toward Genetic Testing." *Population Research and Policy Review* 10, no. 3:235–255.

SJÖGREN, BERIT. 1988. "Parental Attitudes to Prenatal Information About the Sex of the Fetus." *Acta Obstetrica et Gynecologia Scandinavia* 67, no. 1:43–46.

UNITED NATIONS. 1991. *The World's Women, 1970–1990: Trends and Statistics.* New York: Author.

U.S. PRESIDENT'S COMMISSION FOR THE STUDY OF ETHICAL PROBLEMS IN MEDICINE AND BIOMEDICAL AND BEHAVIORAL RESEARCH. 1983. *Screening and Counseling for Genetic Conditions. A Report on the Ethical, Social, and Legal Implications of Genetic Screening, Counseling, and Education Programs.* Washington, D.C.: U.S. Government Printing Office.

VERMA, ISHWAR C., and SINGH, BALBIR. 1989. "Ethics and Medical Genetics in India." In *Ethics and Human Genetics: A Cross-Cultural Perspective,* pp. 250–270. Edited by Dorothy C. Wertz and John C. Fletcher. Berlin: Springer-Verlag.

WARREN, MARY ANNE. 1985. *Gendercide: The Implications of Sex Selection.* Totowa, N.J.: Rowman & Allanheld.

WERTZ, DOROTHY C., and FLETCHER, JOHN C. 1989a. "Ethical Decision-Making in Medical Genetics: Women as Patients and Practitioners in Eighteen Nations." In *Healing Technology: Feminist Perspectives,* pp. 221–244. Edited by Kathryn Strother Ratcliff. Ann Arbor: University of Michigan Press.

———. 1989b. *Ethics and Human Genetics: A Cross-Cultural Perspective.* Heidelberg: Springer-Verlag.

———. 1989c. "Fatal Knowledge? Prenatal Diagnosis and Sex Selection." *Hastings Center Report* 19, no. 3:21–27.

———. 1990. "Medical Geneticists Confront Ethical Dilemmas: Cross-Cultural Comparisons Among 18 Nations." *American Journal of Human Genetics* 46, no. 6:1200–1213.

WERTZ, DOROTHY C.; ROSENFIELD, JANET M.; JANES, SALLY R.; and ERBE, RICHARD W. 1991. "Attitudes Toward Abortion Among Parents of Children with Cystic Fibrosis." *American Journal of Public Health* 81, no. 8:992–996.

III. ARTIFICIAL INSEMINATION

There are two distinct approaches to artificial insemination (AI). Homologous artificial insemination, known by the acronym AIH (artificial insemination, husband), uses a husband's sperm to inseminate his wife. Heterologous artificial insemination (AID, for artificial insemination, donor) uses sperm from a man other than the woman's husband. Traditionally, AID has been used by married couples so that the wife can bear a child in cases of the husband's infertility or genetic incompatibility between the couple. AID is now also used by single women who desire to have a child but do not have a marital or other stable heterosexual partner, or by a woman in a life partnership with another woman. AID also is used in implementing a surrogacy agreement under which a woman will bear a child to be relinquished to the semen donor or a third party after birth.

Background

A relatively simple process, until some two decades ago AID in the United States was practiced largely in an aura of secrecy and with little regulation despite complex legal questions that could stem from it. This situation reflected prevailing attitudes that discouraged public discussion of private sexual practices. Legislators shied from regulation because of aversion to controversy, the perception that the practice was limited, and a sense of futility because the legal problems seemed insoluble without broad reform of legitimacy and paternity laws at a time when family-law reform was not a pressing issue.

Social, legal, and scientific developments since the 1970s have led to more critical focus on AI and the legal and ethical issues it raises. Effective birth-control methods and legal abortion, along with social and economic changes enabling more single mothers to keep their children rather than relinquish them for adoption, sharply reduced the number of healthy neonates available for adoptive placement. At the same time, vastly expanded scientific knowledge about genetics and wider popular awareness of the impact of hereditary disease increased demand for artificial insemination from couples seeking to avoid genetic conditions or diseases. AI usage and acceptance increased significantly as a result, though past secrecy practices and their vestiges make it difficult to quantify the extent of the increase. A 1978 study based on practitioner responses to a questionnaire estimated between 6,000 and 10,000 births annually through AID in the United States. A broader study by the Office of Technology Assessment (OTA) of the U.S. Congress in 1986–1987 indicated that there were 30,000 births through AID and 35,000 through AIH during a comparable period one decade later (U.S. Congress, OTA, 1988).

AI was once the only alternative for effecting conception other than through coitus. Practices such as in vitro fertilization and surrogate embryo transfer now represent other choices, though they are far more technology-dependent. Among new terms introduced to reflect the expanded options (and avoid confusion with AIDS), "assisted conception" is currently the most widely accepted; it was chosen by the National Conference of Commissioners on Uniform State Laws for its 1988 Uniform Act on Status of Children of Assisted Conception, a model statute that has generated little legislative response. AID remains the most popular procedure and the one for which physician involvement or significant technical assistance is least needed.

Selecting and testing donors

Many problems and concerns associated with AI have stemmed from broad physician discretion to select patients and donors and to determine whether and how to screen them. Until recently there were no clearly accepted guidelines, and individual attitudes and values of practitioners still can control whether a person will be accepted for AI. Similarly, a practitioner may choose potential donors on the basis of individual views about ap-

propriate "matching." Because of the secrecy long characterizing AID practice, established medical standards based on custom that might be used in tort actions are lacking.

The 1978 study mentioned earlier revealed that screening for genetic anomalies and even communicable disease was surprisingly lax among many practitioners. There was also disparity in the numbers of women inseminated by the sperm of one donor, with some responses raising concern about the potential for accidental incest. The later OTA study (U.S. Congress, OTA, 1988) revealed improvement in these practices, with a major testing change in response to concern about transmission of AIDS to impregnated women through semen from seropositive donors. This has since led to increased testing of donors as well as recordkeeping on the parties; with the aura of secrecy lifting, expanded donor screening to deal with more than concern about AIDS seems inevitable.

Attempts to "medicalize" AID

Despite the lack of clear standards for physicians, some states have attempted to "medicalize" AID through statutes providing that it can be performed only by licensed physicians. This type of regulation is considered futile by many because of the ease with which the process can be effected without medical assistance as well as understandable reluctance to prosecute a woman for performing the insemination herself. More problematic are some state statutes that provide for terminating a sperm donor's parental rights only if AID is performed by a physician, making it possible for a donor to assert paternity in other circumstances. The ethical objection to this form of law is that the penalty is borne as much or more by the child as by a parent.

Designating the physician as gatekeeper without established guidelines or standards has led to legal and practical problems. A Virginia physician who performed AID using his own semen without his patients' knowledge or agreement was convicted of criminal fraud. But such a scenario leaves many unanswered questions, including whether it is ethical for a physician who satisfies basic health and genetic requirements to use his semen if nothing is done to mislead the patient and there is disclosure and consent.

Further difficulties have been raised by physician failure to adhere to statutory requirements that can enable parental status to be fixed clearly. For example, most state laws on artificial insemination address only the circumstance of AID for a married woman with her husband's consent; some of these require that consent be in writing, and some instruct the physician to file a copy of it with a specified legal agency. Courts have confronted cases in which a physician failed to obtain written consent and situations in which a husband questioned the continued nature of his consent when conception occurred only after a lengthy period.

Reflecting long-standing legal concern for upholding the legitimacy of children, some courts have found that oral consent can provide adequate compliance even in the face of a statutory provision for written consent, and others have determined that a physician's failure to file the consent agreement with a designated state agency according to the statutory mandate does not affect a child's legitimate status if consent has in fact been obtained.

Establishing paternity

Until several decades ago, results of blood tests could serve only to rule out paternity except in highly unusual cases, and even then they were usable only in a limited number of situations. There was a strong legal presumption that a child born to a married woman cohabiting with her husband was his legitimate offspring, and in many jurisdictions neither spouse could give testimony that would render a child illegitimate. Fathers of illegitimate children were considered to have little constitutional protection regarding assertion of parental rights, particularly if the mother was married to someone else. Not surprisingly, it was then widely believed that under almost any predictable scenario a successful challenge of the husband's being the father would be extremely unlikely if an AID practitioner kept no records and carefully matched the blood types of all the parties. Some physicians sought further to lessen the odds of successful legal challenge by mixing a sterile husband's sperm with that of an anonymous donor. Dubbed "confused" or "combined" artificial insemination (CAI), the practice was a form of medical/legal gamesmanship undertaken on the questionable premise that it would overcome the presumption of paternity of a husband in courts of a state with no statute legitimizing offspring of consensual AID by married couples. CAI is largely discredited today. However, a woman may be inseminated with the sperm of different donors during a particular AID cycle.

Earlier assumptions that paternity would not be challenged or could not be established affirmatively have proved to be unrealistic. Tissue typing now permits affirmative proof of paternity to a high degree of probability. The presumption of legitimacy is far easier to challenge, and legal limitations on the testimony of husbands and wives have eroded substantially. Concurrent with these developments, fathers of illegitimate children have been accorded greater constitutional protection of their parental rights. With the recent shift to record-keeping because of concern about HIV transmission, information about donors should be more accessible to courts unless statutes are enacted to preclude this.

Risk awareness

Given the uncertainty still prevalent in many situations and the differing state laws, questions are now being raised about whether physicians should tell their patients about potential legal problems. Laws determining what information a physician must disclose to a patient generally come from tort law governing informed consent. Criteria may vary between states, but a patient ordinarily should be informed about the risks of serious harm that a procedure poses, as well as feasible alternative strategies.

However, it must be recognized that informed-consent law developed in the context of disclosure of health risks and medical alternatives. The risks most likely to deter a patient from choosing AID, in contrast, are largely legal, including questions about kinship status, whether a sperm donor might assert parentage, and confidentiality in the event of legal actions such as divorce. Another legal hazard is that siblings related by half blood through a common sperm donor might marry without awareness of their kinship. If the relationship were discovered, such a marriage would automatically be void under most state laws without the need for an annulment.

Adoption, one of the most feasible alternatives to AID, is a legal rather than a medical procedure. Judicial expansion of the doctrine of informed consent or specific legislation thus might be necessary to legally require communication of such nonmedical information. However, the medical need for disclosure might be based on potential psychological harm to the child, the mother, or the husband. Even so, although a physician seemingly has an ethical obligation to advise that there may be serious legal risks as well as a legal alternative, it is unclear and probably doubtful that there is a legally enforceable duty to make such disclosure.

The special case of AIH

Paternity concerns associated with AID are obviated by AIH. At one time questions of legitimacy were raised in the courts in the context of marriages annulled for impotence (inability to copulate) after birth of an AIH child. Today most jurisdictions have laws providing that a biological child of the parties to a void or voidable marriage is deemed their legitimate offspring.

The Ethics Committee of the American Fertility Society has concluded that AID is acceptable for demonstrated medical indications such as male infertility, husband's genetic disorder, or ejaculatory dysfunction. However, in its 1986 and 1990 reports, it noted that questions remain about the efficacy of AIH in a number of instances, including manipulation for the purpose of sex selection, and that use of AIH for such uncertain purposes should be regarded as a clinical trial.

Sperm banking

Until recently sperm banking received little regulatory attention. The American Fertility Society now provides specific guidelines dealing with donor screening, and though they have no statutory authority, they should become increasingly important in establishing standards of practice that may be used in legal actions.

A widely recommended current practice to avoid HIV transmission is to test a donor at the time semen is taken and to retest six months later. This provides an illustration of the newly expanded recordkeeping.

Cryopreservation, used in sperm banks, offers prospect of posthumous use of a donor's sperm. With AIH, this could continue family lineage; it also could create genealogical nightmares and raise complex testamentary issues in both AIH and AID because of the pervasive emphasis on biological parentage in estate law. Model language in the Uniform Act on Status of Children of Assisted Conception would assure that a sperm donor is not the father of a child conceived after his death.

Today some men have sperm cryopreserved before undergoing chemotherapy or entering an occupation with radiation hazards, making questions about posthumous use of donor sperm likely to increase. Surprisingly little attention has been paid to this potential issue by donors and sperm banks at the time deposits are made.

Further ethical and religious objections and concerns

An early and long-standing objection to artificial insemination is its "unnaturalness," whether accomplished through AIH or AID. A further concern is that it separates procreation from sexual expression, and thus a child born as a result of the procedure does not stem from a true conjugal relationship. An opposing view is that rational human control over nature is a major human achievement and that the new technology and understanding can benefit mankind. Variations between these arguments present differing views about determining the circumstances under which assisted conception can be deemed morally justifiable.

Some opponents regard AID as ethically tantamount to adultery. Others who would not categorize it as adultery nevertheless object because of concern that it could lead to adultery by a married woman wishing to have a child and using third-party sperm without medical intervention. Trial courts in Canada (1921) and the United States (1954) suggested that AID might even constitute legal adultery, though subsequent cases have followed the opposing tack of a Scottish judge who opined that insemination could be performed by the woman herself, and there is no legal concept of self-adultery.

Another objection has been based on the reliance on masturbation for collecting donor semen. For the Roman Catholic Church, this is particularly objectionable; because the procedure replaces rather than facilitates the conjugal act, it is a sign of the dissociation of the sexual union and procreation. The Roman Catholic Church has further condemned AID as contrary to the unity of marriage and conjugal fidelity, which demand that a child be conceived in marriage (Catholic Church, 1987).

There has been disagreement within Judaism over the ethical implications of AI. Many commentators express the view that AIH is permissible in limited circumstances if certain halakic guidelines are respected, but some rabbis have objected on the theory that it is a sin to emit sperm other than in its permitted place. AID is more widely opposed, particularly among Orthodox rabbinical authorities, both because it might be regarded as adultery and because the practice could lead to intermarriage between half siblings (see, e.g., Lasker, 1988).

Objections to use of AID by unmarried heterosexual couples, same-sex couples, or single women center on the question of whether it is morally justifiable to utilize assisted conception for others than a family who otherwise would be unable to procreate safely if at all. This objection is complicated by ethical and legal debate about what constitutes a family. The most widespread legislative approach has been to facilitate AID for married couples by providing a method for them to proceed with some guarantee that they will have exclusive parental rights. By omitting reference to nonmarried couples, other parties are relegated to the use of basic rules on paternity and legitimacy that were not designed to deal with AID.

In addition to uncertainty about parent–child status, fear of identifying AID with selective breeding caused the practice to be wrapped in a shroud of secrecy. Selective breeding became an especially objectionable popular concern after revelations about the goal of a "master race" under the National Socialist regime in Germany. Even so, at least one sperm bank in the United States has been established to accept donations from persons of superior intellect, such as Nobel laureates. According to newspaper accounts, the mother of one of the first offspring born through AID with such sperm previously had lost custody of children for abusing them by trying to drive them to intellectual success.

Impact on children.   The fact that AID produces an offspring that is genetically linked to one person in a couple makes this alternative more attractive than adoption to many couples, even though the same ethical problems do not exist for those who adopt because they are dealing with a child already in being. While it is accepted practice to tell adopted children about their special status at an early time and in a manner designed to make them feel wanted rather than rejected, parents may choose not to tell their children about conception through AID. Today's more extensive recordkeeping and major strides in establishing paternity significantly increase the chances that a child will learn about AID parentage. This might result from medical testing, but there also is evidence that many couples utilizing AID discuss this with third parties, increasing the likelihood that a child may learn of it even if the parents remain silent.

Given the pattern of increasing willingness to depart from a long accepted pattern of confidentiality for adoptions (at least for those effected through state or private agencies), it seems inevitable that demands for similar treatment will be raised for children of AID now that paternity is more readily determinable through records and testing.

Payment for semen.   The term "sperm donor" is a misnomer because compensation of persons supplying semen has been a long-standing practice, whether the intermediary is an AID practitioner or a commercial sperm bank. Views about the morality of selling body parts and recent statutes banning some such sales raise the question of whether payments for semen should be continued. Statutes prohibiting organ sales usually exempt regenerative tissue or semen. But the 1986 report by the Ethics Committee of the American Fertility Society recommends that semen should not be purchased. Similarly, the 1979 draft recommendations of the Council of Europe with regard to artificial insemination would forbid payment to semen donors except for reimbursement of expenses.

Aside from the ethical objection to making a commodity of human tissue (and particularly semen), there is the health concern of avoiding encouragement of persons with infectious or hereditary diseases to sell their semen, a situation analogous to that of blood donors. The state of Oregon provides that a man who is aware that he has a transmissible disease or defect should not donate semen. However, the only means for enforcing the prohibition seemingly would be through a damage action against a donor by one acquiring the disease or defect through the donor's knowing violation.

Access to AI: How much personal autonomy in a legal context?   Though existence of a broad right to procreate—an especially strong recognition of personal autonomy—has been asserted by persons seeking to enforce surrogacy contracts in which a third party's womb is utilized, it also might be raised by someone denied access to AID for use outside surrogacy. The paucity of judicial attention to the latter may reflect both the wide access to medical assistance for AID and the fact that it can be accomplished without such access. A federal appeals court in 1990 denied a male prisoner's request to facilitate procreation with his wife through AIH. However, because prisoners sustain some recognized diminution of their legal rights during imprisonment, this particular limitation on use of AIH does not serve to define the parameters of any right to procreate through AIH or AID in other contexts.

A few states have sought to assure greater access to AI by requiring that issuers of health insurance with obstetrical coverage provide coverage at least for basic procedures in reproductive assistance that could include AI.

Ethical and political divisions

Popular attention has been captured by surrogacy and more exotic assisted-conception techniques, but AI remains the most widely used. And it still presents serious issues in need of resolution. The key problem in AI from a legal standpoint is that under many current state laws, parentage and legitimacy remain unclear because even statutes that seek to clarify such issues are often narrow in scope. To no small extent this situation results from objections to use of AI by unmarried persons, including same-sex couples. Ultimately these issues may be resolved only in the context of a broader review of rights based on nonbiological relationship in matters such as child custody and adoption. However, failure to deal with serious status problems because of religious or ethical disagreement seems inconsistent with family-law approaches in areas such as divorce, where it is recognized that the civil law provides basic guidelines that should not obstruct the tenets of individual religious groups who are free to follow their own beliefs.

WALTER WADLINGTON

Directly related to this article are the INTRODUCTION *and other articles in this entry:* SEX SELECTION; IN VITRO FERTILIZATION AND EMBRYO TRANSFER; SURROGACY; CRYOPRESERVATION OF SPERM, OVA, AND EMBRYOS; ETHICAL ISSUES; *and* LEGAL AND REGULATORY ISSUES. *For a further discussion of topics mentioned in this article, see the entries* ADOPTION; AIDS, *article on* PUBLIC-HEALTH ISSUES; AUTONOMY; CHILDREN, *articles on* RIGHTS OF CHILDREN, *and* CHILD CUSTODY; CONFIDENTIALITY; CRYONICS; FAMILY; HOMOSEXUALITY, *article on* ETHICAL ISSUES; INFORMED CONSENT, *article on* MEANING AND ELEMENTS OF INFORMED CONSENT; LABORATORY TESTING; MARRIAGE AND OTHER DOMESTIC PARTNERSHIPS; ORGAN AND TISSUE PROCUREMENT, *article on* ETHICAL AND LEGAL ISSUES REGARDING LIVING DONORS; RIGHTS; *and* SEXUALITY IN SOCIETY. *Other relevant material may be found under the entries* EUGENICS; EUGENICS AND RELIGIOUS LAW; GENETIC ENGINEERING, *article on* HUMAN GENETIC ENGINEERING; LAW AND MORALITY; *and* NATURE.

Bibliography

ANDREWS, LORI B., and DOUGLASS, LISA. 1991. "Alternative Reproduction." *Southern California Law Review* 65, no. 1:623–682.

CATHOLIC CHURCH. CONGREGATION FOR THE DOCTRINE OF THE FAITH. 1987. *Instruction on Respect for Human Life in Its Origin and on the Dignity of Procreation.* Vatican City: Author.

CURIE-COHEN, MARTIN; LUTTRELL, LESLEIGH; and SHAPIRO, SANDER. 1979. "Current Practice of Artificial Insemination by Donor in the United States." *New England Journal of Medicine* 300, no. 11:585–590.

ETHICS COMMITTEE. AMERICAN FERTILITY SOCIETY. 1986. "Ethical Considerations of the New Reproductive Technologies." *Fertility and Sterility* 46, no. 3 (suppl. 1):1S–94S.

———. 1990. "Ethical Considerations of the New Reproductive Technologies." *Fertility and Sterility* 53, no. 6 (suppl. 2):1S–109S.

FINEGOLD, WILFRED J. 1976. *Artificial Insemination.* 2d ed. Springfield, Ill.: Thomas.

———. 1980. *Artificial Insemination with Husband Sperm.* Springfield, Ill.: Thomas.

GIBSON, ELIZABETH L. 1991. "Artificial Insemination by Donor: Information, Communication and Regulation." *Journal of Family Law* 30, no. 1:1–44.

GLOVER, JONATHAN. 1989. *Ethics of New Reproductive Technologies: The Glover Report to the European Commission.* De Kalb: Northern Illinois University Press.

KNOPPERS, BARTHA M., and LeBRIS, SONIA. 1991. "Recent Advances in Medically Assisted Conception: Legal, Ethical, and Social Issues." *American Journal of Law and Medicine* 17, no.4:329–361.

LASKER, DANIEL J. 1988. "Kabbalah, Halakah, and Modern Medicine: The Case of Artificial Insemination." *Modern Judaism* 8, no. 1:1–14.

LEACH, W. BARTON. 1962. "Perpetuities in the Atomic Age: The Sperm Bank and the Fertile Decedent." *American Bar Association Journal* 48, no. 10:942–944.

MACKLIN, RUTH. 1991. "Artificial Means of Reproduction and Our Understanding of the Family." *Hastings Center Report* 21, no. 1:5–11.

NATIONAL CONFERENCE OF COMMISSIONERS ON UNIFORM STATE LAWS. Annual. *Matrimonial, Family and Health Laws.* Vol. 9 of *Uniform Laws Annotated.* St. Paul, Minn.: West.

NEW SOUTH WALES LAW REFORM COMMISSION. 1986. *Artificial Conception: Human Artificial Insemination.* Sydney: Author.

ONTARIO LAW REFORM COMMISSION. 1985. *Report on Human Artificial Reproduction and Related Matters.* Toronto: Ministry of the Attorney General.

SHANNON, THOMAS A., and CAHILL, LISA SOWLE. 1988. *Religion and Artificial Reproduction: An Inquiry into the Vatican "Instruction on Respect for Human Life in Its Origin and on the Dignity of Procreation."* New York: Crossroad.

U.S. CONGRESS. OFFICE OF TECHNOLOGY ASSESSMENT (OTA). 1988. *Artificial Insemination: Practice in the United States: Summary of a 1987 Study.* Washington, D.C.: Author.

WADLINGTON, WALTER. 1970. "Artificial Insemination: The Dangers of a Poorly Kept Secret." *Northwestern University Law Review* 64, no. 6:777–807.

———. 1983. "Artificial Conception: The Challenge for Family Law." *Virginia Law Review* 69, no. 2:465–514.

WIKLER, DANIEL, and WIKLER, NORMA J. 1991. "Turkey-Baster Babies: The Demedicalization of Artificial Insemination." *Milbank Memorial Fund Quarterly* 69, no. 1: 5–40.

IV. IN VITRO FERTILIZATION AND EMBRYO TRANSFER

In in vitro fertilization (IVF), a woman's ovaries are stimulated with fertility drugs to produce multiple eggs. The physician monitors the woman's response by examining urine samples, blood samples, and ultrasound imaging. After giving her an injection to control the timing of the egg release, the physician retrieves the eggs in one of two ways. In a laparoscopy, done under general anesthesia, the surgeon aspirates the woman's eggs through a hollow needle inserted into the abdomen, guided by a narrow optical instrument called a laparoscope. In the more recently developed transvaginal aspiration, done with local anesthesia, the physician inserts the needle through the woman's vagina, guided by ultrasound.

After they are retrieved, the eggs are placed in separate glass dishes and combined with prepared spermatozoa from the woman's partner or a donor. The dishes are placed for twelve to eighteen hours in an incubator designed to mimic the temperature and conditions of the body. If a single spermatozoon penetrates an egg, IVF has occurred.

A fertilized egg subdivides into cells over a period of forty-eight to seventy-two hours. Microscopic in size, it is generally called a pre-embryo or an embryo after it has divided into two or more cells. When the embryos have divided into four to sixteen cells, they are placed in a hollow needle (catheter) that is inserted into the woman's vagina. The embryo or embryos are released into the woman's uterus in the procedure known as embryo transfer. Implantation in the uterine wall, if it takes place, will occur within days after transfer; a pregnancy is detectable about two weeks after the transfer.

In established IVF clinics, the odds that a continuing pregnancy and birth will occur after embryo transfer are 20–30 percent. Because problems can arise at all stages of IVF, such as the inability to retrieve eggs or secure fertilization, the odds are less if they are calculated from the time fertility drugs are first given. Data from several national registries indicate a delivery rate of 9–13 percent if calculated from the starting point of hormonal stimulation (Cohen, 1991). The birthrates tend to cluster among clinics, so that some clinics account for a large percentage of the total births while others have few or no deliveries (Medical Research International, 1992). Tens of thousands of embryo transfers are carried out each year internationally, and thousands of babies have been born. Clinicians reported over 12,000 deliveries following IVF in one five-year period (1985–1990), and in one country (the United States) alone (Medical Research International, 1992).

Present and future variations

The first birth following IVF occurred in England in 1978 (Steptoe and Edwards, 1978). The technique was originally designed to circumvent blocked or damaged fallopian tubes in women trying to become pregnant. During the late 1970s and early 1980s, physicians combined the male partner's sperm and the female partner's eggs and transferred the embryos shortly after fertilization. If the couple had a large number of embryos, physicians either transferred all at once, which created the risk of a multiple pregnancy, or disposed of extra embryos, which wasted the embryos and was morally problematic.

The start of embryo freezing in the early 1980s has given physicians greater control over the number of embryos transferred at once. Two to four embryos are transferred in the first IVF cycle and the remaining embryos, if any, are frozen for later thawing and transfer. Embryo freezing saves the woman from the hormonal stimulation of repeated start-up IVF cycles, and it allows embryo transfer when the woman's body has returned to a more natural state. By enabling the transfer of a small number of embryos at once, it reduces the odds of a multiple pregnancy and the subsequent risk this poses to the woman and the fetuses. Controlled transfer of embryos is arguably less morally problematic than the selective abortion of fetuses in a large multiple pregnancy. The birth of the first infant to have been frozen as an embryo took place in Australia in 1984. Embryo freezing is now a routine option in IVF.

Another variation that has increased the flexibility of IVF is the use of donated sperm, eggs, and embryos to circumvent fertility problems such as low sperm count in the male partner, lack of ovulation in the female partner, or lack of fertilization with the couple's own eggs and sperm, or to help couples at high risk avoid passing on a serious genetic disorder to their children. Sperm and embryo donation are more straightforward than egg donation, which is complicated by the need to synchronize the menstrual cycles of the donor and recipient. Women are either paid for their services in donating eggs or they donate in the course of their own medical treatment. In addition, some women donate eggs for their sisters or other close relatives. Donation of eggs or sperm raises questions about, among other things, confidentiality of medical records, the child's sense of identity, and the psychological well-being of the donor.

The embryos in IVF can be transferred to a surrogate if the genetic mother does not have a uterus or cannot carry a child to term for other reasons. Although the surrogate is usually unrelated, there have been instances of embryo transfer to the sister or even the mother of a woman who cannot carry a fetus to term. In the latter case, the surrogate is the child's gestational mother and genetic grandmother.

Sperm microinjection is another technique used in connection with IVF. If the male partner has low sperm count or poor sperm quality, a healthy spermatozoon can be manually inserted into the egg with special microinstruments. This alternative to sperm donation allows the transfer of embryos genetically related to the couple. This and other microsurgical procedures remain experimental and infrequent.

Another procedure for IVF is the examination of sperm, eggs, and embryos for chromosomal and genetic abnormalities. Preimplantation diagnosis has been conducted on an experimental basis in the United States, Britain, and other European countries. It is being developed for couples at high risk for passing to their children a genetic disorder such as cystic fibrosis or Tay-Sachs disease but who will not terminate a pregnancy and are therefore not candidates for prenatal screening.

Preimplantation diagnosis includes polar-body analysis (analyzing the DNA of the first polar body of the human egg), trophectoderm biopsy (examining extraembryonic cells surrounding the inner cell mass), and embryo biopsy (removing a single cell from a four- or eight-cell embryo). It also includes chromosomal analysis to select only female embryos for transfer to couples who are at high risk for passing on a sex-linked disease, such as hemophilia, to male children. Pregnancies and births have been reported following embryo biopsy and sex preselection. Many variables remain to be worked out in preimplantation diagnosis, and physicians urge caution before expanding it in the IVF setting (Trounson, 1992). Correcting genetic flaws after they have been diagnosed is a distant, though foreseeable, possibility (Verlinksy et al., 1990).

Ethical issues in IVF

A recurring and unresolved issue in IVF involves the status of the embryo (McCormick, 1991). The Ethics Advisory Board, set up by the U.S. Department of Health, Education and Welfare, and later disbanded without its recommendations' being acted on, issued a report in 1979 stating that "The human embryo is entitled to profound respect, but this respect does not necessarily encompass the full legal and moral rights attributed to persons" (U.S. Department of Health, Education and Welfare, 1979, p. 107). The Warnock Commission issued a report in Britain in 1984 that also accorded the embryo a "special status," though not the same status "as a living child or adult" (Warnock, 1985).

The notion that the embryo is an entity with a special status deserving special respect is contested by those who regard the embryo as fully a human being from the moment of conception. An instruction issued by the Vatican concluded that the "human being must be respected—as a person—from the very first instant of his existence" (Catholic Church, 1987; Shannon and Cahill, 1988). The unique genetic makeup of the embryo, among other things, is given as evidence of its individuality.

Beliefs about the embryo's status are central to conclusions about what in IVF is permissible and what is not. Some observers who regard the embryo as a human being believe IVF is ethically acceptable provided all embryos are transferred and given a chance to survive. Others believe external fertilization is always immoral. If the embryo is regarded as a human being, it has "full human rights," including the right not to be experimented upon without its consent (Ramsey, 1972a, 1972b). Even if one regards IVF as no longer experimental, the conclusion of immorality still extends to IVF's variations, which begin as experimental procedures posing the risk of higher-than-normal embryo loss.

If, on the other hand, the embryo is regarded as only potentially a human, fewer ethical strictures on IVF techniques apply. The Ethics Advisory Board concluded that IVF was ethically acceptable for married couples and that research on human embryos was acceptable provided the research was designed to establish IVF safety, would yield "important scientific information," complied with federal laws protecting research subjects, and proceeded only with the consent of tissue donors. No research was to take place beyond the fourteenth day after fertilization. After fourteen days, the embryo begins to develop an embryonic disk or "primitive streak" and is no longer capable of spontaneous twinning, which means it is on the way to becoming a single individual.

IVF has been criticized as a fundamentally dehumanizing technique that takes place in a laboratory, involves the scientist as a third party, is geared to the production of human beings, and is aimed at conquering nature and producing a "quality" child (Kass, 1985). The language of IVF and its business and marketing overtones contribute to a situation in which tissues and children are treated as commodities to be produced and in which intimacy is devalued (Lauritzen, 1990). The Vatican instruction concluded that IVF is unnatural because the sperm are secured by masturbation and the union takes place outside the body. Tissue donation is

especially illicit, as it is "contrary to the unity of marriage, [and] to the dignity of the spouses" (Catholic Church, 1987).

Some feminists have expanded on this theme by criticizing laboratory conception as an intervention that divides reproduction—once a continuous process taking place naturally within the woman's body—into discrete and impersonal parts subject to a male-dominated medical profession (Arditti et al., 1984). They argue that in IVF, women are perennial research subjects in an unending set of techniques that have significant emotional costs (Williams, 1989); that IVF benefits men and compromises women; and that it curtails women's autonomy and magnifies gender-based power differences in society (Wikler, 1986). Other feminists support IVF if it is bounded by feminist ethics and if it builds women's control over reproduction rather than taking it away (Sherwin, 1989).

IVF's variations challenge notions of the family, the interests of the potential child, the distribution of societal resources, and the rights of prospective parents. Tissue donation from relatives creates new biological if not legal relationships—for example, when a sister donates an egg to a sister for IVF or a brother donates sperm for his brother's IVF attempt. Embryo freezing creates the prospect of some embryos being stored indefinitely or transferred in a later generation, possibly endangering the resulting child's sense of identity. It also sets the stage for custody disputes and conflicts over the disposition of unwanted embryos (*Davis v. Davis*, 1992).

Embryo diagnosis for genetic defects raises safety questions for the embryo and potential child. Conceivably, it will lead to screening for many genetic problems and not just the life-threatening disorders envisioned now. On the one hand, discarding embryos after tests reveal a genetic abnormality might be less morally contentious than aborting pregnancies, at least for those who believe the embryo has a lesser status than a fetus. On the other hand, discarding "defective" embryos may blunt societal sensibilities and invite fertile couples into the costly and uncertain IVF procedure. The ability to preselect embryos according to sex raises concerns that the technique will be used for nonmedical reasons to give couples a child of their preferred gender, which may be male (Wertz and Fletcher, 1989).

IVF is highly selective in the people it can help. An expensive procedure covered by few insurance companies, it is available primarily to affluent couples. Critics question the wisdom of directing scarce resources to an elective and costly procedure with low odds of success (Callahan, 1990). Others advise paying more attention to preventing infertility in the first place (Blank, 1988). Aggressive marketing of IVF, including marketing that distorts success rates to make them seem greater than they actually are, arguably creates needs by making couples feel they ought to try IVF because it is there to try and by interfering with alternatives such as adoption or stopping efforts to conceive.

Concerns about the support of IVF and embryo research have been integrated into formal policy in a number of countries (Knoppers and LeBris, 1991). For example, the British Human Embryology and Fertilisation Act of 1990 created a licensing authority to conduct on-site visits to clinics in which human embryos are manipulated, review research proposals, and ensure that quality control is maintained in the laboratories (Morgan and Lee, 1991). A restrictive law in Germany, by contrast, makes criminal a range of techniques not therapeutic for the embryo, including sex preselection for nonmedical reasons ("German Embryo Protection Act," 1991). Among the international documents relating to embryo manipulations are a recommendation from the Parliamentary Assembly of the Council of Europe that the Council of Ministers provide a "framework of principles" governing embryo and fetal research ("Parliamentary Assembly," 1989) and a set of principles relating to IVF and its variations ("Council of Europe," 1989).

Fifteen states in the United States mention embryos in their statutes, but legislators passed most laws with abortion and fetuses in mind rather than IVF and embryos. Some of these laws would presumably make embryo research illegal, but their constitutionality has not been tested (Robertson, 1992). In 1989 the U.S. Supreme Court reviewed Missouri's abortion statute but declined to address the constitutionality of the statute's preamble that "the life of each human being begins at conception" (*Webster* v. *Reproductive Health Services,* 1989). This definition of personhood appears to contradict the Court's abortion rulings, but by leaving it untouched, the Court left the embryo's legal status unclear.

Several states have passed laws mandating insurance coverage for IVF under certain conditions (U.S. Congress, Office of Technology Assessment, 1988). The federal government does not fund proposals involving human embryos; by law, research must be reviewed by an ethics board ("Protection of Human Subjects," 1975), but no board has replaced the Ethics Advisory Board, which was disbanded in 1979. This has led to a de facto funding moratorium.

Conclusion

Prior to and in the years following the first successful use of IVF, critics argued that it challenged the sanctity of marriage and family, posed the threat of psychological and physical harm to unborn children, involved the immoral destruction of human embryos, made women experimental pawns in research in which men asserted control over reproduction, and introduced the senseless creation of people in an era of overpopulation. It was also said to admit no clear stopping point, use scarce medical resources, and amount to an elective technique that did not cure infertility.

Supporters argued that IVF would spare couples the psychological trauma of infertility, meet the needs of tens of thousands of women with blocked fallopian tubes, lead to knowledge that would help ensure healthy children, and preserve the family by bringing children to couples who truly want them. They responded to criticism by saying IVF was no more unnatural than cesarean births, should not be diminished merely because it did not cure infertility, posed no apparent risks to children, and was not immoral, in that embryos were only potential human beings.

Today, basic IVF has shifted from experimental to standard medical practice. It is widely available, is regarded as safe, and is the only viable way women with blocked fallopian tubes can conceive a baby genetically related to them. New technical additions ensure, however, that external fertilization will remain at center stage in the ongoing bioethics debate over reproductive technologies.

The lasting unanswered questions relate to the high value placed on genetic parenthood, equitable access to techniques across race and class, the impact of laboratory conception on women's control over reproduction, and whether priority ought to be placed on conception in a time when discussions are directed to ways of reducing the gap in medical services available to richer and poorer citizens.

Perhaps most significant, however, is the matter of the limits to be placed on reproductive technologies. It appears that the scope of refinements is nearly endless. Should substantive and procedural limits be placed by government on any of IVF's variations? If so, which, and why? Understanding the reasons for placing limits is as important as understanding the reasons laboratory conception is pursued with such intensity in the first place.

ANDREA L. BONNICKSEN

Directly related to this article are the INTRODUCTION *and other articles in this entry:* SEX SELECTION; ARTIFICIAL INSEMINATION; SURROGACY; CRYOPRESERVATION OF SPERM, OVA, AND EMBRYOS; ETHICAL ISSUES; *and* LEGAL AND REGULATORY ISSUES. *Also directly related are the entries* FETUS; *and* GENETIC TESTING AND SCREENING, *articles on* PREIMPLANTATION EMBRYO DIAGNOSIS, CARRIER SCREENING, *and* ETHICAL ISSUES. *For a further discussion of topics mentioned in this article, see the entries* CHILDREN, *article on* CHILD CUSTODY; CONFIDENTIALITY; CRYONICS; FAMILY; FEMINISM; GENETIC ENGINEERING, *article on* HUMAN GENETIC ENGINEERING; HEALTH-CARE

RESOURCES, ALLOCATION OF; MATERNAL–FETAL RELATIONSHIP, *article on* ETHICAL ISSUES; PERSON; RIGHTS; *and* TECHNOLOGY, *article on* PHILOSOPHY OF TECHNOLOGY. *For a discussion of related ideas, see the entry* ABORTION. *Other relevant material may be found under the entries* EUGENICS; EUGENICS AND RELIGIOUS LAW; LIFE; NATURE; PUBLIC POLICY AND BIOETHICS; RESEARCH, UNETHICAL; RESEARCH POLICY; *and* WOMEN, *article on* HEALTH-CARE ISSUES.

Bibliography

ARDITTI, RITA; KLEIN, RENATE DUELLI; and MINDEN, SHELLY, eds. 1984. *Test-Tube Women: What Future for Motherhood?* London: Pandora Press.

BLANK, ROBERT H. 1988. *Rationing Medicine.* New York: Columbia University Press.

CALLAHAN, DANIEL. 1990. *What Kind of Life: The Limits of Medical Progress.* New York: Simon & Schuster.

CATHOLIC CHURCH. CONGREGATION FOR THE DOCTRINE OF THE FAITH. 1987. *Instruction on Respect for Human Life in Its Origin and on the Dignity of Procreation: Replies to Certain Questions of the Day.* Doctrinal statement of the Vatican (March 10). Vatican City: Author.

COHEN, JEAN. 1991. "The Efficiency and Efficacy of IVF and GIFT." *Human Reproduction* 6, no. 5:613–618.

"Council of Europe Publishes Principles in the Field of Human Artificial Procreation." 1989. *International Digest of Health Legislation* 40, no. 4:907–912.

Davis v. Davis. 1992. 18 Fam.L.Rptr. 2029 (Tenn.).

"German Embryo Protection Act (October 24, 1990)" (Gesetz zum Schutz von Embryonen [Embryonenschutzgesetz— ESchG]). 1991. *Human Reproduction* 6, no. 4:605–606.

KASS, LEON. 1985. *Toward a More Natural Science: Biology and Human Affairs.* New York: Free Press.

KNOPPERS, BARTHA M., and LEBRIS, SONIA. 1991. "Recent Advances in Medically Assisted Conception: Legal, Ethical and Social Issues." *American Journal of Law and Medicine* 27, no. 4:329–361.

LAURITZEN, PAUL. 1990. "What Price Parenthood?" *Hastings Center Report* 29, no. 2:38–46.

MCCORMICK, RICHARD A. 1991. "Who or What Is the Preembryo?" *Kennedy Institute of Ethics Journal* 1, no. 1:1–15.

MEDICAL RESEARCH INTERNATIONAL, SOCIETY FOR ASSISTED REPRODUCTIVE TECHNOLOGY (SART), and AMERICAN FERTILITY SOCIETY. 1992. "In Vitro Fertilization–Embryo Transfer (IVF-ET) in the United States: 1990 Results from the IVF-ET Registry." *Fertility and Sterility* 57, no. 1:15–24.

MORGAN, DEREK, and LEE, ROBERT G. 1991. *Blackstone's Guide to the Human Fertilisation and Embryology Act, 1990.* London: Blackstone Press.

"Parliamentary Assembly of Council of Europe Adopts Recommendation on Use of Human Embryos and Foetuses for Research Purposes." 1989. *International Digest of Health Legislation* 40, no. 2:485–491.

"Protection of Human Subjects: Fetuses, Pregnant Women, and In Vitro Fertilization." 1975. *Federal Register* 40:150 (8 Aug.) pp. 33525–33552. Codified in 45 C.F.R. 46, especially section 204(d).

RAMSEY, PAUL. 1972. "Shall We 'Reproduce'? I. The Medical Ethics of In Vitro Fertilization." *Journal of the American Medical Association* 220, no. 10:1346–1350.

———. 1972b. "Shall We 'Reproduce'? II. Rejoinders and Future Forecast." *Journal of the American Medical Association* 220, no. 11:1480–1485.

ROBERTSON, JOHN A. 1992. "Ethical and Legal Issues in Preimplantation Genetic Screening." *Fertility and Sterility* 57, no. 1:1–11.

SHANNON, THOMAS, A., and CAHILL, LISA SOWLE. 1988. *Religion and Artificial Reproduction: An Inquiry into the Vatican "Instruction on Respect for Human Life in Its Origin and on the Dignity of Human Reproduction."* New York: Crossroad.

SHERWIN, SUSAN. 1989. "Feminist Ethics and New Reproductive Technologies." In *The Future of Human Reproduction,* pp. 259–271. Edited by Christine Overall. Toronto: Women's Press.

STEPTOE, PATRICK C., and EDWARDS, ROBERT G. 1978. "Birth After the Reimplantation of a Human Embryo." *Lancet* 2, no. 8085:366.

TROUNSON, ALAN L. 1992. "Preimplantation Genetic Diagnosis—Counting Chickens Before They Hatch?" *Human Reproduction* 7, no. 5:583–584.

U.S. CONGRESS. OFFICE OF TECHNOLOGY ASSESSMENT. 1988. *Infertility: Medical and Social Choices.* OTA-BA-358. Washington, D.C.: U.S. Government Printing Office.

U.S. DEPARTMENT OF HEALTH, EDUCATION AND WELFARE. ETHICS ADVISORY BOARD. 1979. *Report and Conclusions: HEW Support of Research Involving Human In Vitro Fertilization and Embryo Transfer.* Washington, D.C.: U.S. Government Printing Office.

VERLINSKY, YURY; PERGAMENT, EUGENE; and STROM, CHARLES. 1990. "The Preimplantation Genetic Diagnosis of Genetic Diseases." *Journal of in Vitro Fertilization and Embryo Transfer* 7, no. 1:1–5.

WARNOCK, MARY. 1985. *A Question of Life: The Warnock Report on Human Fertilisation and Embryology.* Oxford: Basil Blackwell.

Webster v. Reproductive Health Services. 1989. 492 U.S. 490.

WERTZ, DOROTHY C., and FLETCHER, JOHN C. 1989. "Fatal Knowledge? Prenatal Diagnosis and Sex Selection." *Hastings Center Report* 19, no. 3:21–27.

WIKLER, NORMA JULIET. 1986. "Society's Response to the New Reproductive Technologies: The Feminist Perspectives." *Southern California Law Review* 59, no. 5:1043–1057.

WILLIAMS, LINDA S. 1989. "No Relief Until the End: The Physical and Emotional Costs of In Vitro Fertilization." In *The Future of Human Reproduction,* pp. 120–138. Edited by Christine Overall. Toronto: Women's Press.

V. SURROGACY

Surrogacy, a reproductive arrangement involving three or more persons, typically comes into play for several reasons: when the female member of a married couple is unable to conceive a child, or unable to gestate a child for physical and/or psychological reasons; or, though able to conceive and gestate a child, unwilling to do so for some medical reason—for example, a genetic disease that she does not wish the child to inherit—or even for some strictly personal reason—for example, a schedule interruption that would interfere with her career. If she and her husband desire to rear a child to whom they are at least 50 percent genetically related, they may decide to seek a woman who is willing to carry a pregnancy to term for them. Less typically, unmarried couples may seek the services of a surrogate mother for reasons similar to those of married couples. So, too, may single women and single men, with the specific aim of single-parenting a child genetically related to them.

There are two types of surrogate mothers: those who gestate an embryo genetically related to them (partial surrogacy) and those who gestate an embryo genetically unrelated to them (full surrogacy) (Singer and Wells, 1985, p. 96). In cases of partial surrogacy, a woman agrees (1) to be artificially inseminated with the sperm of a man who is not her husband; (2) to carry the subsequent pregnancy to term for a fee (commercial surrogacy) or out of generosity (noncommercial surrogacy); and (3) to relinquish the child at birth to the couple or single person. Although the contractual arrangements are the same in cases of full surrogacy, the medical ones are not since the woman gestates an embryo that is not genetically hers.

Although it is tempting to substitute the term "gestational mother" for the term "surrogate mother," so as not to prejudge which of two or more women is indeed the moral and/or legal mother of a child, such relabeling is conceptually confusing. Not all gestational mothers are surrogate mothers. For example, although a woman to whom an embryo is donated is her child's gestational mother, she is not her child's surrogate mother. What makes a gestational mother a surrogate mother is that she both begins and ends her pregnancy with the intention of relinquishing the baby to someone else.

Moral arguments for and against surrogacy

In addition to traditional arguments for and against surrogacy, there are several feminist ones. Relying largely on Kantian perspectives and/or natural-law perspectives, often related to official Roman Catholic teachings (Shannon and Cahill, 1988), traditional opponents of surrogacy object to it for five reasons. First, they claim that surrogacy is unnatural since it involves techniques like artificial insemination by donor (AID) and/or in vitro fertilization (IVF), both of which are "artificial" means to the "natural" end of procreation. Second, they note that the surrogate mother offers not simply her gestational services but herself as a human person. Thus,

only someone who is morally prepared to endorse slavery should morally endorse surrogacy. Third, they argue that just as a prostitute degrades herself when she offers herself as a sex object, a surrogate mother degrades herself when she offers herself as a reproductive container. Fourth, they maintain that introducing a third party into the process of procreation weakens the marital relationship. A woman might fantasize about the "potency" of the man who artificially inseminated her, and a man might marvel at the "fecundity" of the surrogate mother, regarding her as somehow better than his infertile wife. Fifth, they insist that surrogacy erodes the mother–child relationship, since the surrogate mother deliberately becomes pregnant with the intention of giving up the child (Krimmel, 1983). When she does this for a fee, her act becomes indistinguishable from "baby-selling," a practice that most moralists condemn as a form of slavery.

Traditional proponents of surrogacy maintain that their opponents base their case on faulty reasoning. First, they note that if the line between the "natural" and the "artificial" separates moral from immoral practices, then society ought to forbid intravenous feeding—an "unnatural" way of eating—as well as in vitro fertilization—an "unnatural" way of procreating. Second, they observe that since someone cannot buy something that already belongs to him, a genetic father cannot buy his genetic child from the woman who gestated it. Third, they claim that it is no more degrading to offer one's sexual or reproductive services to others than it is to offer one's "brain power" or "muscle power" to them. Fourth, they object that a surrogate mother does not necessarily jeopardize the marital relationship of the couple who hire her. She intrudes on them only as much as they permit her to do so. Fifth, they argue that there is nothing inherently wrong with intentionally and voluntarily procreating a child that one does not plan to parent, provided that those who do plan to parent the child have the child's best interests at heart.

Invoking both utilitarian reasoning, according to which an action is right if it maximizes the utility (pleasure or happiness) of those affected by the action, and contractarian reasoning, according to which contracts freely entered into ought to be honored, traditional proponents of surrogacy make one final observation on its behalf. They note that surrogacy is simply a new form of "collaborative reproduction"—that is, a mode of reproduction that requires more or other than the energies, efforts, and endowments of a couple (Robertson, 1983). Since society has not morally condemned genetic parents for soliciting and/or accepting other people's help in rearing their children (for example, through such social arrangements as adoption, step-parenting, foster-parenting, wet-nursing, and babysitting), they argue that society ought not to morally condemn genetic parents who require other people's assistance in bearing their children.

Feminist arguments for and against surrogacy seek to correct the male biases that often limit traditional pro and con arguments. These biases may be manifest in any number of ways, but they often appear "in rationalizations of women's subordination, or in disregard for, or disparagement of, women's moral experiences" (Jaggar, 1992, p. 361). Although there are various diverging feminist positions on surrogacy, three lines of thought are particularly prominent.

Liberal feminists, who believe that women's liberation depends on women having the same educational, political, and economic opportunities and rights as men, argue that women, provided they do not harm anyone in the process, should be permitted to use whatever reproduction-controlling and/or reproductive-aiding technologies they need to live as men's equals. Preventing a woman from working as a surrogate mother, or from hiring a surrogate mother, violates her reproductive freedom just as much as preventing a woman from using birth control or having an abortion.

In contrast to liberal feminists, *Marxist feminists,* who believe that women's liberation depends on the destruction of a capitalist system that makes some people the economic pawns of other people, argue that when a woman offers her reproductive services not as a gift but as a commodity, her action is most likely coerced. For the most part, surrogate mothers who sell their reproductive services are considerably poorer than the men and/or women who buy them. Unable to support herself and/or her family, a woman will sometimes sell the only thing she has of value: her body. To say that a woman "chooses" to do this, says the Marxist feminist, is simply to say that when a woman is forced to choose between poverty and exploitation, she sometimes chooses exploitation as the lesser of two evils. Although most surrogate mothers should not be blamed for their choice, it is an unfree one that results in their degradation, and no decent society can sit idly by as some women are reduced to "baby-making" machines.

Radical feminists, who believe that women's liberation ultimately depends not only on a political and economic revolution but also on a sexual revolution capable of radically transforming male and female gender roles, deepen the Marxist feminist analysis of exploitation to include noneconomic exploitation. Whereas Marxist feminists emphasize that under capitalism there is always a price high enough to entice even the most resistant person to sell what is most precious, radical feminists emphasize that, frequently, women agree to serve as surrogate mothers simply because they wish to be recognized as "good"—that is, generous, loving, altruistic—

women. Traditionally, the more sacrificial a woman is, the more society praises her. It matters not how much she hurts herself in the process.

Radical feminists also urge that far from being "collaborative," surrogacy is a reproductive arrangement that creates divisions among persons, but especially among women. Relatively rich persons hire relatively poor women to meet their reproductive needs, adding childbearing services to the child-rearing services that economically disadvantaged women have traditionally provided to economically privileged persons. Worse, reproductive technologists sort women into three classes: genetic mothers, gestational mothers, and social mothers. In the future, no one woman will beget, bear, and rear a child. Rather, genetically superior women will beget embryos in vitro; strong-bodied surrogate mothers will carry these "test-tube babies" to term; and sweet-tempered women will rear these newborns from infancy to adulthood (Corea, 1985).

Public-policy approaches to surrogacy

Several public-policy approaches to surrogacy have been articulated, ranging from its criminalization to its strict enforcement as a matter of contract. In 1985 the United Kingdom passed the Surrogacy Arrangements Act, which make serving as a surrogacy broker a criminal offense. Lawyers, physicians, and social workers—as well as certain newspaper and media personnel—are subject to fines and/or imprisonment if they initiate or participate in commercial surrogacy arrangements (Surrogacy Arrangements Act, 1985). Those who favor the criminalization of commercial surrogacy concede that even noncommercial surrogacy involves the possibility that some people will use other people as means to their own ends. However, they insist that such exploitation becomes significantly probable and not simply possible whenever financial interests are involved. The main problem with criminalizing surrogacy arrangements, be they commercial or noncommercial, is that such a stratagem may constitute an unjustified restriction on procreative freedom. If an individual or couple cannot have a genetically related child without the assistance of a surrogate mother, then, arguably, the state must show that there is no less restrictive way to prevent the harms that surrogacy allegedly causes.

Less restrictive ways to regulate surrogacy include its assimilation into adoption law and its enforcement as a matter of contract. Those who recommend that surrogacy be assimilated into adoption law argue that there is little difference between making arrangements to adopt a woman's baby as soon as she knows she is pregnant and making arrangements to adopt a woman's baby shortly before she becomes pregnant. Therefore, the same rules that govern adoption should govern surrogacy arrangements. Adoption rules permit payment, but only for the woman's reasonable medical expenses. Moreover, the adopting couple may pull out of the negotiations at any time before the adoption papers are signed; and the woman who plans to relinquish her child is given an opportunity after its birth to change her mind. Perhaps the strongest argument in favor of the adoption approach is that it harmonizes with the long-standing legal view that the woman who gives birth to a child is that child's mother. Thus, lawyer George Annas insists that whether or not the surrogate mother is genetically related to the child, the state should recognize her as the child's legal mother because "she will definitely be present at the birth, easily and certainly identifiable, and available" to care for the child (Annas, 1988, p. 24).

Nevertheless, despite all of surrogacy's similarities to adoption, it remains fundamentally different. As feminist Phyllis Chesler sees it, adoption is a child-centered practice whereby adults, willing to give children the kind of love they need to thrive, take into their homes and hearts children who are already conceived or born. In contrast, surrogacy is an adult-centered practice whereby children are deliberately conceived and brought into existence so that adults can have someone to love (Chesler, 1988). Worse, by insisting on a 50 percent genetic link, the child becomes genetically prearranged rather than unconditionally accepted (as adopted children are).

In contrast with those who seek to regulate surrogacy through adoption law, those who seek to regulate it through contract law regard surrogacy as a business transaction between consenting adults for reproductive services. Supporters of the contract approach claim that all disputes between surrogate mothers and contracting persons should be regarded as breaches of contract to be remedied either by a specific performance or a damages approach. Under the specific performance approach, for example, the state would take the child away from a balking surrogate mother, remanding the child's custody to its legal parent or parents (that is, the contracting person or persons). In contrast, under the damages approach, the state would require a balking surrogate mother to pay monetary damages to the contracting person or persons in lieu of relinquishing the child.

Whatever its theoretical merits, the damages approach suffers from practical disadvantages. For example, since most surrogate mothers are poor compared with those who contract for their services, they may not be able to pay the damages assessed against them; and, even if they are able to pay the assessed damages, the money will not adequately compensate the relatively rich but childless contracting person or persons. However, the greatest objection to any contract approach to surrogacy, whether it favors specific performance or

damages, is that if the law enforces surrogacy arrangements as it enforces any contract, it may contribute to the view that children are just another consumer good to be bought and sold at will.

Social perspectives on surrogacy

When one looks at surrogacy arrangements worldwide, one is led to conclude that such arrangements are ordinarily negotiated by relatively privileged infertile persons who have the $25,000 or more to pay both the surrogate broker's and the surrogate mother's fees. Although one hears about relatively poor people reproducing a child "collaboratively" and "altruistically," for the most part the people who participate in such arrangements are family members and/or friends. In any event, some commentators have observed that the issue is not whether surrogacy is commercial or noncommercial. Rather, the issue is why, given a burgeoning world population, infertile people are frantically seeking ways to add to its numbers. After all, there is something ironic about infertile people seeking to augment their reproductive powers through artificial insemination, in vitro fertilization, and surrogacy arrangements even as fertile people seek to control their reproductive powers through contraception, abortion, and sterilization.

But even if people have a right to procreate or not procreate children who are genetically related to them, society needs to ask itself why, with very rare exceptions, genetic connection is viewed as the ultimate determinant of parenthood. Because (full) surrogacy permits a split between begetting and bearing a child, it forces society to reconsider the role that genes should play in assigning parental rights and responsibilities. It can, in fact, be claimed that what makes one a parent is not so much a genetic contribution to a child as it is a gestational connection or parental relationship to him or her.

In addition to inviting society to focus on the necessary and sufficient conditions for parenthood, surrogacy invites society to ask itself some profoundly disturbing questions about procreative freedom. Is it "liberating" for infertile persons to believe that unless they can produce a child genetically related to them, their lives will be without real joy? Similarly, is it "liberating" for a woman to sell her reproductive services to anyone who wishes to pay for them, even if she must regard herself as an incubator? Finally, is it "liberating" for children to be "sold" by surrogate mothers who do not want a relationship with them and/or to be "bought" by persons who do want a relationship with them, provided, as many surrogacy contracts stipulate, they are born without disease or defect?

As attractive as is the ideal of collaborative parenting—a state of affairs in which two or more people, able fully to share all parental blessings and burdens, together beget, bear, *and* rear a child—it is an ideal that is particularly difficult to achieve in a racist, sexist, and classist society. Until society comes to terms with the full implications of procreative freedom, it must use its powers of moral persuasion and legal coercion to eliminate any exploitative aspects of surrogacy. Certainly, society must pay particular attention to the interests of women and children as it seeks to formulate good public policies for the regulation of an arrangement that transforms a number of our most fundamental relationships, including parenthood.

ROSEMARIE TONG

Directly related to this article are the INTRODUCTION *and other articles in this entry:* SEX SELECTION; ARTIFICIAL INSEMINATION; IN VITRO FERTILIZATION AND EMBRYO TRANSFER; CRYOPRESERVATION OF SPERM, OVA, AND EMBRYOS; ETHICAL ISSUES; *and* LEGAL AND REGULATORY ISSUES. *For a further discussion of topics mentioned in this article, see the entries* ADOPTION; CHILDREN, *articles on* RIGHTS OF CHILDREN, *and* CHILD CUSTODY; FAMILY; FEMINISM; JUSTICE; MARRIAGE AND OTHER DOMESTIC PARTNERSHIPS; MATERNAL–FETAL RELATIONSHIP; PROSTITUTION; ROMAN CATHOLICISM; *and* UTILITY. *Also directly related is the entry* FETUS, *article on* PHILOSOPHICAL AND ETHICAL ISSUES. *Other relevant material may be found under the entries* FERTILITY CONTROL; LAW AND MORALITY; NATURE; PUBLIC POLICY AND BIOETHICS; RIGHTS; *and* SEXUALITY IN SOCIETY.

Bibliography

ANDREWS, LORI B. 1988. "Position Paper: Alternative Modes of Reproduction." In *Reproductive Laws for the 1990s*, pp. 361–403. Edited by Sherrill Cohen and Nadine Taub. Clifton, N.J.: Humana Press.

———. 1990. "The Aftermath of Baby M: Proposed State Laws on Surrogate Motherhood." In *Ethical Issues in the New Reproductive Technologies*, pp. 186–201. Edited by Richard T. Hull. Belmont, Calif.: Wadsworth.

ANNAS, GEORGE J. 1988. "Death Without Dignity for Commercial Surrogacy: The Case of Baby M." *Hastings Center Report* 18, no. 2:23–24.

BAYLES, MICHAEL D. 1990. "Genetic Choice." In *Ethical Issues in the New Reproductive Technologies*, pp. 241–253. Edited by Richard T. Hull. Belmont, Calif.: Wadsworth.

CAPRON, ALEXANDER M., and RADIN, M. S. 1988. "Choosing Family Law over Contract Law as a Paradigm for Surrogate Motherhood." *Law, Medicine, and Health Care* 16, nos. 1–2:34–43.

CHESLER, PHYLLIS. 1988. *The Sacred Bond: The Legacy of Baby M.* New York: Times Books.

COREA, GENA. 1985. *The Mother Machine.* New York: Harper & Row.

DAVIS, PEGGY C. 1988. "Commentary: Reproductive Technologies from Artificial Insemination to Artificial Wombs. Alternative Modes of Reproduction: The Locus and Determinants of Choice." In *Reproductive Laws for the 1990s*, pp. 421–431. Edited by Sherrill Cohen and Nadine Taub. Clifton, N.J.: Humana Press.

HULL, RICHARD, T., ed. 1990. *Ethical Issues in the New Reproductive Technologies.* Belmont, Calif.: Wadsworth.

JAGGAR, ALISON M. 1992. "Feminist Ethics." In *Encyclopedia of Ethics*, pp. 361–370. Edited by Lawrence Becker and Charlotte Becker. New York: Garland.

KASS, LEON. 1983. "'Making Babies' Revisited." In *Ethical Issues in Modern Medicine*, pp. 407–413. Edited by John Arras and Robert Hunt. Palo Alto, Calif.: Mayfield.

KETCHUM, SARA ANN. 1987. "New Reproductive Technologies and the Definition of Parenthood: A Feminist Perspective." In *Feminism and Legal Theory: Women and Intimacy.* Madison: Institute for Legal Studies, University of Wisconsin Madison.

KRIMMEL, HERBERT T. 1983. "The Case Against Surrogate Parenting." *Hastings Center Report* 13, no. 5:35–39.

O'BRIEN, MARY. 1981. *The Politics of Reproduction.* Boston: Routledge and Kegan Paul.

OVERALL, CHRISTINE. 1987. *Ethics and Human Reproduction: A Feminist Analysis.* Boston: Allen and Unwin.

RICH, ADRIENNE. 1976. *Of Woman Born: Motherhood as Experience and Institution.* New York: Norton.

ROBERTSON, JOHN A. 1983. "Surrogate Mothers: Not So Novel After All." *Hastings Center Report* 13, no. 5:28–34.

ROTHMAN, BARBARA KATZ. 1989. *Recreating Motherhood: Ideology and Technology in a Patriarchal Society.* New York: Norton.

SHANNON, THOMAS A., and CAHILL, LISA SOWLE. 1988. *Religion and Artificial Reproduction: An Inquiry into the Vatican "Instruction on Respect for Human Life in Its Origin and on the Dignity of Human Reproduction,"* pp. 140–177. New York: Crossroad.

SINGER, PETER, and WELLS, DEANE. 1985. *Making Babies: The New Science and Ethics of Conception.* New York: Scribner.

SPALLONE, PATRICIA, and STEINBERG, DEBORAH LYNN, eds. 1987. *Made to Order: The Myth of Reproductive and Genetic Progress.* Oxford: Pergamon.

Surrogacy Arrangements Act (United Kingdom). 1985. Ch. 49, p.2(1)(a)(b)(c).

VI. CRYOPRESERVATION OF SPERM, OVA, AND EMBRYOS

The technical ability to freeze sperm, embryos, and eventually ova for long periods and then thaw them without destroying their biologic potential offers several new reproductive options for both fertile and infertile individuals. It makes the donation of eggs, sperm, or embryos to treat infertility a more efficient and safe procedure. It also allows individuals and couples to preserve sperm, eggs, and embryos to protect against future reductions in gametic viability due to age, disease, or occupational exposure, and permits posthumous reproduction to occur.

As with any technological deviation from the natural mode of conception, these techniques raise both medical questions of safety and efficacy and ethical, legal, and social questions about prohibition, restriction, or regulation of these practices. Once cryopreservation is medically established as safe and effective, its ethical, legal, and social acceptability depends on a general acceptance of noncoital and assisted means of reproduction, with specific issues relating to the particular technique in question.

Sperm

Cryopreservation of sperm is now well established medically and socially as a commercial enterprise. Sperm banking occurs as an aspect of infertility practice, or as an option for men who foresee damage to their gametes as a result of disease or occupational exposure. In the former case, a commercial sperm bank recruits sperm providers, screens them medically and socially, and usually pays them a fee for their sperm (technically they are vendors rather than donors of sperm though the latter word is commonly used to describe their role). The sperm is then distributed to doctors or others who practice artificial insemination with donor sperm, who in turn resell or distribute it to recipients.

A main legal and ethical issue with regard to this practice is the duty of the sperm bank to screen sperm donors and their sperm for infectious diseases, including the human immunodeficiency virus (HIV). Guidelines of the American Fertility Society, the main professional organization of physicians treating infertility, now recommend that donated sperm be screened for HIV diseases. Because there may be a six-month gap before HIV transmission shows up on antibody screening tests, screening requires that the donated sperm be quarantined for six months so that a second test can be performed on a sample to ensure that it is not HIV-infected. Failure to screen in this way is unethical and could make the sperm bank legally liable for transmission of HIV to recipients and offspring.

There are no laws that restrict to whom sperm banks may sell their sperm, and in the United States, the buying and selling of sperm is not generally covered by federal or state laws against selling organs, though several European countries prohibit the practice. Thus a bank could sell sperm to a single woman or representative organizations for use in inseminating single women. Despite fears that a bank or physician who provides sperm to an unmarried woman could be held liable for financial support of a child born as a result, no such legal liability has yet been imposed. While some persons find artificial insemination of single women to be unethical, and the practice is prohibited in some countries, it can allow

women who otherwise could not bear children to reproduce, and unmarried women who are committed to reproduction in this way have been shown to be able childrearers.

Commercial sperm banks also provide service to individuals or couples who wish to store sperm for later use because of treatment of disease, occupational exposure, or fear of later impotence. Because no legislation specifically applies to this practice, its legal status would depend upon basic contract law. The depositor would be entitled to keep the sperm in the bank and retrieve it under conditions specified in the contract of deposit. Thus sperm could be released to the depositor or to his designee posthumously, if that is envisaged, and the bank would perhaps have no obligation to maintain the sperm past a specified time if failure to pay storage charges should occur. Clear specification of rights and duties in the original contract is essential. While posthumous release of stored sperm to the appropriate designee could lead to the birth of a child without a rearing father, this situation is similar to the insemination of an unmarried woman and should be treated similarly. Whether a child born posthumously will be able to share in a deceased's estate is a matter of state inheritance law that does not affect the ethical, legal, or social acceptability of the practice.

The bank would, of course, have a legal duty to return the correct sperm to the depositor. At least one case has arisen in which the bank returned the wrong sperm, which led to the birth of a child who was not of the same race as the depositor. In such instances, suits for damages are likely to be successful. An important issue will concern damages, because there is no way to establish that in fact the lost gametes would have implanted and produced a child. In addition, some states regulate the operation of sperm banks as medical or clinical laboratories to protect the health and safety of consumers of their services.

Many of the issues that arise with commercial sperm banks would also apply to physicians who recruit sperm donors directly. They too would have ethical and legal duties of reasonable care to assure that donors have been tested for genetic and infectious disease. They would also be free to inseminate single women and use sperm posthumously, if that is the clear intention of the parties.

Ova

The ability to freeze and then successfully thaw ova has not yet been developed, due to the larger size of the ovum and the great amount of fluid in it. Once this ability is developed, egg banking will occur.

Frozen ova have less ethical significance than frozen embryos. Once the technical ability to freeze and thaw ova safely is developed, they will play an important role in enabling women to initiate pregnancies through in vitro fertilization (IVF), which involves hormonal stimulation of the ovaries to produce ova, often many more than are needed for fertilization at that time; freezing the extra ova will minimize the need for additional cycles of egg retrieval. Rather than inseminate all eggs retrieved in a cycle of IVF treatment, many couples will prefer to freeze extra eggs, which can then be thawed and inseminated for later attempts at pregnancy. Cryopreservation of ova, rather than embryos, may thus become the preferred method of storage.

Once ova freezing and banking begins, the same issues that currently arise with cryopreservation of sperm will occur. Commercial ova banks, which may be associated with sperm and embryo banks or exist independently, will be established. No doubt such banks will both buy or procure eggs from women and then resell them to doctors and couples in need of an egg donation. The main issues will then concern what the precise arrangement is between the donor and the bank concerning subsequent use, whether the bank will be responsible for genetic and infectious disease screening, and whether the bank will be responsible for any rearing costs of offspring.

With eggs that have been frozen for subsequent use in initiating pregnancy in an infertile couple, the agreement between the woman or couple and the storage facility will be of paramount importance. The depositor of the eggs will be the owner and will control release or discard of cryopreserved ova within the limits of the storage facility's policies. Thus the contract between the depositor and the facility would largely control deposits of eggs prior to disease treatment or occupational exposure or to use then or at a later time. As long as the depositor has paid storage charges, she would be entitled to have the eggs stored, to expect reasonable care to be taken in their maintenance, and to have the eggs released, transferred, or discarded as directed. Posthumous release and use of stored eggs should be as acceptable as posthumous release and use of stored sperm. As with sperm banking, failure of payment could lead to the bank taking the eggs out of storage, but it would not be entitled to transfer them to other persons in lieu of payment unless there were a specific agreement to that effect. Professional or even legislative regulation of ova banking to ensure standards of health and safety can also be expected.

Embryos

Cryopreservation of embryos (sometimes referred to as preimplantation embryos or "pre-embryos") is now a well-established adjunct to IVF programs. Standard IVF treatment often produces more eggs than can be safely fertilized and placed in the uterus at one time. Rather than fertilize only the number of eggs that could be

safely transferred or fertilize all retrieved eggs and discard the surplus, cryopreservation allows all eggs to be fertilized, a safe number such as two or three placed in the uterus, and the rest frozen for later use. At a later time, the frozen embryos can be thawed and placed in the uterus, donated to others, or discarded. Although the success rate is not as great as with fresh embryos, the pregnancy rate of both fresh and frozen embryos from a single egg-retrieval cycle is 15 to 20 percent greater than the rate from use of fresh embryos alone. Until the ability to freeze and thaw ova is developed, the excess eggs retrieved in a cycle of IVF treatment are likely to be inseminated and then cryopreserved for use during a later cycle.

The main issues that arise with cryopreservation of embryos concern the ethical and legal status of embryos and the locus of dispositional authority over frozen embryos. While some persons have argued that embryos are persons or moral subjects with all the rights of persons, and others claim that embryos are merely tissue with no special status or rights, a wide ethical and legal consensus in the United States, Europe, and Australia views embryos as "deserving of special respect, though not the respect due persons." As a result, embryos may be created, frozen, donated, and even discarded or used in research when there is a valid need to treat infertility or pursue a legitimate scientific goal and rules concerning consent of the gamete providers and institutional review board approval have been followed.

With regard to dispositional authority over frozen embryos, it is now well established that the couple providing the gametes has dispositional authority within the limits of state law and the conditions of storage set by the IVF program or storage facility. If they agree to have embryos created from their gametes cryopreserved, they are "owners" of the embryos and may decide on any disposition of frozen embryos that their agreement with the storage facility and applicable statutes permit.

Since the frozen gametes are the joint property of the persons providing the gametes, their joint consent is needed for disposition until they relinquish or transfer their dispositional authority to others. To maximize their control over embryos and to introduce administrative efficiency into the operation of embryo banking, they should also give written directions at the time of storage for disposition of frozen embryos in the future if the providers have died, divorced, are unavailable for decision, or are unable to agree between themselves on disposition.

In such cases, the IVF program or embryo bank should be able to rely on this prior agreement in decisions concerning stored embryos. This will give advance control to the parties and clear directions to the bank and minimize costly disputes about what to do with stored embryos. Although no court has yet been faced with a case directly involving a disputed contract, there have been cases recognizing the right of the depositing couple to remove their frozen embryo from a bank against the bank's wishes. There is also legal authority recognizing the validity of such advance contracts for disposition in case disputes arise.

The *Davis* v. *Davis* case (1992) illustrates the wisdom of giving effect to the prior agreement. A couple had frozen seven embryos pursuant to their efforts to have children via IVF. They subsequently decided to divorce but could not agree on disposition of the frozen embryos. The husband opposed thawing them and using them to start pregnancy, while the wife insisted that she or another person have them placed in her. The Tennessee Supreme Court finally resolved this issue by ruling that an agreement between the parties for disposition in the case of divorce would have been binding, and that in the absence of such an agreement, the relative burdens and benefits of a particular solution must be examined. In that case if the party wishing to retain the embryos had other means of obtaining embryos, such as by going through IVF again with a new partner, that party's wish to have children could still be satisfied without foisting unwanted parenthood on the party who wished that the embryos not be used. On the other hand, if there was no other way for that party to be reasonably able to produce embryos, so that the existing embryos were the last resort or chance to have offspring, then they should be entitled to use them. In that case, fairness would require that the objecting party not have to provide child support. In the facts presented to it, the court ruled in favor of the husband, who did not want frozen embryos implanted after divorce, because the wife had alternative ways to reproduce.

Ethical and legal codes for assisted reproduction in other countries have not yet addressed the problem that arose in the *Davis* case. A country could take the position that all embryos must be preserved, or that provision of gametes for IVF is a commitment to have all resulting embryos placed in the uterus. However, the American preference to have the parties control disposition in the case of divorce or disposition by prior agreement might also be recognized, for it maximizes the procreative liberty of the parties directly involved.

The authority of the gamete providers over the disposition of frozen embryos can be limited by law or the policies of the banks or facilities where frozen embryos are stored. For example, some European countries (Spain and Germany) prohibit embryo discard and research, while others (Great Britain, for example) limit the period of storage to a maximum of ten years or the reproductive life of the woman, whichever is longer. While U.S. legislation on these issues is largely absent, the Ethics Committee of the American Fertility Society (1986) has recommended a similar maximum period of storage, and individual embryo banks and programs for

religious or administrative reasons have imposed limitations on dispositions that involve discard, donation, or release of frozen embryos to other programs. As long as the storage facility makes clear its restrictions on disposition of frozen embryos, it may impose these restrictions on couples who request storage of embryos at that facility.

Conclusion

Cryopreservation of sperm, ova, and embryos offers individuals options to extend or enhance their reproductive ability and should presumptively be recognized as adjuncts of their procreative liberty. If this view is accepted, principles of informed consent and contract will inform and regulate most of the transactions and activities that occur with cryopreserved gametes and embryos. In some cases legislation to protect the parties' wishes and ensure the health and viability of stored gametes and embryos may also be desirable.

JOHN A. ROBERTSON

Directly related to this article are the INTRODUCTION *and other articles in this entry:* SEX SELECTION; ARTIFICIAL INSEMINATION; IN VITRO FERTILIZATION AND EMBRYO TRANSFER; SURROGACY; ETHICAL ISSUES; *and* LEGAL AND REGULATORY ISSUES. *Also directly related is the entry* CRYONICS. *For a further discussion of topics mentioned in this article, see the entries* FETUS; PERSON; RIGHTS; *and* WOMEN, *article on* HEALTH-CARE ISSUES. *Other relevant material may be found under the entries* FAMILY; FUTURE GENERATIONS, OBLIGATIONS TO; HEALTH SCREENING AND TESTING IN THE PUBLIC-HEALTH CONTEXT; LAW AND BIOETHICS; MARRIAGE AND OTHER DOMESTIC PARTNERSHIPS; *and* ORGAN AND TISSUE PROCUREMENT, *article on* ETHICAL AND LEGAL ISSUES REGARDING LIVING DONORS.

Bibliography

Davis v. Davis. 1992. 842 S.W.2d 588 (Tenn.).

ETHICS COMMITTEE. AMERICAN FERTILITY SOCIETY. 1986. "Ethical Considerations of the New Reproductive Technologies." *Fertility and Sterility* 46, no. 3 (suppl. 1): 1S–94S.

ROBERTSON, JOHN A. 1986. "Embryos, Families, and Procreative Liberty: The Legal Structure of the New Reproduction." *Southern California Law Review* 59, no. 4:939–1041.

———. 1990. "In the Beginning: The Legal Status of Early Embryos." *Virginia Law Review* 76, no. 3:437–517.

U.S. CONGRESS. OFFICE OF TECHNOLOGY ASSESSMENT. 1988. *Infertility: Medical and Social Choices.* Washington, D.C.: Author.

U.S. DEPARTMENT OF HEALTH, EDUCATION AND WELFARE. ETHICS ADVISORY BOARD. 1979. *HEW Support of Research*

Involving Human In Vitro Fertilization and Embryo Transfer.
Fed. Register 35, 033.

VII. ETHICAL ISSUES

The introduction of in vitro fertilization (IVF) in 1978 sparked anew an intense ethical debate about the use of innovative reproductive technologies that had raged a decade earlier (McCormick, 1978). Questions were raised about whether these technologies would harm children and parents and alter people's understanding of the meaning of procreation, family, and parenthood. Gradually the controversy subsided as healthy children were born from these procedures; committees in at least eight countries issued statements indicating that they considered the use of IVF ethically acceptable in principle (Walters, 1987). Arguably, one reason for this readiness to embrace IVF and other new reproductive techniques was that they enabled couples to create offspring in a way that seemed an extension of the natural way of procreating. Although IVF involved joining sperm and ovum in a glass dish, the resulting embryo, once implanted, went through a natural period of gestation that culminated in the birth of a child. A second reason was that these technologies, with the exception of artificial insemination by donor, allowed people to have children who were genetically their own. Louise Brown, the first child created through IVF, resulted from the union of the gametes of her biological parents. Third, the children born of these new means of reproduction were born into traditionally structured families. These techniques were assumed to have been developed for use by married couples who, with the new baby, would form what was ordinarily defined as a nuclear family.

In the 1990s, these rationales for accepting novel reproductive technologies are being challenged by medical advances and a changing social environment. Human intervention in the procreative process has become more frequent, more complex, and more highly technological. Oocytes can be removed surgically from one woman and, after fertilization, transferred to another in the procedure of oocyte donation. Women can lend their wombs to others for the incubation of children who have no genetic connection to such "surrogates." Embryos created in vitro can be cryopreserved and stored for use in future years by their genetic parents or by others. Consequently, it is difficult to argue that such innovative measures are mere extensions of the natural way of reproducing. Parthenogenesis (stimulating an unfertilized egg to develop and produce offspring by mechanical or chemical means), cloning (deriving genetically identical organisms from a single cell or very early embryo), and ectogenesis (maintaining the fetus completely outside the body) are on the horizon. Furthermore, third, fourth, and fifth parties, such as oocyte donors, surrogate mothers, and (some suggest) even fetuses and cadavers, are joining sperm donors to assist those who are childless to have offspring. New forms of assisted reproduction are increasingly being used to create children who are not tied to those who will raise them by biological or hereditary links. Finally, these technologies are no longer used almost exclusively to create traditional nuclear families. Unmarried heterosexual and homosexual couples and single women and men now have greater access to them. Such scientific and social changes give new emphasis to the older unresolved ethical questions about the uses of these technologies and raise new questions.

Ethical questions raised by the use of the new reproductive technologies

The initial ethical question created by these technologies is whether they ought to be used at all. Different religious traditions vary tremendously in their judgments about the licitness of the use of these novel techniques. The Roman Catholic church declared the use of new reproductive technologies morally unacceptable (Catholic Church, 1987) because they separate the procreative, life-giving aspects of human intercourse from the unitive, lovemaking aspects, and these, according to Catholic teachings, are morally inseparable in every sexual act. The creation of a child should involve the convergence of the spiritual and physical love of the parents; fertilization outside the body is "deprived of the meanings and the values which are expressed in the language of the body and in the union of human persons" (Catholic Church, 1987, p. 28).

Certain other religious groups, such as the Lutheran, Anglican, Jewish, Eastern Orthodox, and Islamic, view some of these methods as ethically acceptable because God has encouraged human procreation (Lutheran Church, 1981; Episcopal Church, 1982; Feldman, 1986; Harakas, 1990; Rahman, 1987). According to these bodies, it is sufficient that love and procreation are held together within the whole marital relationship; each act of sexual intercourse need not be open to the possibility of conception. Still other religious groups hold that there is no necessary moral connection between conjugal sexual intercourse and openness to procreation, and consequently they accept the use of the new reproductive technologies with few qualifications (Smith, 1970; Simmons, 1983; General Conference, 1985). In Hindu thought, for instance, although there is no authoritative teaching on this subject, the mythologies of ancestors appear to allow IVF, oocyte donation, embryo implantation, and surrogacy (Desai, 1989).

Feminists, too, are split about the use of the new reproductive technologies. Some argue that these novel methods define and limit women in ways that demean them, for example, as "fetal containers." They maintain that the desire of many women, both fertile and infertile, for children is, in large part, socially constructed (Bartholet, 1992; Williams, 1992). The cultural imperative to have children drives infertile women to undergo physically, emotionally, and financially costly treatment. They are thrust into the hands of a predominantly male medical establishment that uses women as "living laboratories" whose body parts they manipulate without regard to the consequences (Rowland, 1992). Male experts sever what was once a continuous process of gestation and childbirth for women into discrete parts, thereby fragmenting motherhood (Corea, 1985).

In contrast, other feminists argue that the new reproductive technologies enhance the status of women by providing them with an increased range of options. By circumventing infertility and providing women with alternative means of reproducing, these technologies extend reproductive choices and freedoms (Jaggar, 1983; Andrews, 1984; Macklin, 1994). In their view, the charge that surrogacy exploits women is paternalistic because it questions women's ability to know their own interests and to make informed, voluntary, and competent decisions (Macklin, 1990); women have the ability and right to control their bodies and to make autonomous choices about their participation in such practices, these feminists argue.

Some people recommend adoption over the use of the new reproductive technologies because they view the latter as physically and emotionally debilitating and unlikely to succeed, whereas adoption, while not easy, provides a home and family for children in need (Bartholet, 1993). Yet adoption is a second choice for many infertile couples because of its perceived drawbacks. These include the declining number of healthy children available for adoption, the long and emotionally draining wait, the expense, and the difficult and often frustrating system with which adoptive parents must deal (Lauritzen, 1993). Although the use of assisted reproduction presents some of the same problems as adoption, it offers what some infertile couples consider distinct advantages: It allows them to have children who are genetically related to at least one of them and (except in the case of surrogacy) makes the experience of pregnancy and birth available to the woman. The desire to reproduce through lines of kinship and to connect to future generations exerts a powerful influence, as does the hope of experiencing the range of fulfilling events associated with pregnancy and childbirth (Overall, 1987).

Individual choice, substantial harm, and community values

A central issue in the debate about the use of reproductive technologies concerns the scope that should be given to individual discretion over their use. Some phil-

osophical commentators, emphasizing personal autonomy, enunciate a broad moral right to reproduce by means of these technologies (Bayles, 1984; Brock, 1994). They borrow from legal discussions of the right to reproduce, which some legal theorists take to include the liberty to use methods of assisted reproduction (Robertson, 1986; Elias and Annas, 1987). To limit individual choice about noncoital means of reproduction, the state must show that the use of specific reproductive technologies threatens substantial harm to participants and the children born to them (Robertson, 1988). The philosophers influenced by such legal positions maintain that individuals have great leeway in their choice of whether to procreate, with whom, and by what means. They have a right to enter into contractual arrangements giving them access to these technologies and to utilize third parties in their reproductive efforts. Those who take this approach concede that substantial adverse effects on others, particularly the children, would justify restricting individual use of assisted reproduction.

Since the primary reason for accepting these innovative methods is to bring children into the world, a major consideration in assessing them is whether or not they harm these children. Critics contend that these techniques may cause social and psychological problems to the resulting children because of confusion they engender over divided biological parentage and the social stigmatization to which they may be subjected (Callahan, 1988). John Robertson responds that this criticism is logically incoherent. When the alternative is nonexistence, he argues, it is better for the children to have been born—even though they may experience some harm from the means used to bring them into the world—than never to have existed at all (Robertson, 1986). In most cases, the difficulties they face are not so great as to render life a complete loss.

There are several problems with this influential response. One is that it justifies allowing almost any harm to occur to children born as a result of the use of these techniques in that it can almost always be said they are better off alive. Moreover, this argument presupposes that these children are waiting in a world of nonexistence to be summoned into existence and that they would be harmed by not being born. Since children do not exist at all prior to their arrival in this world, there are no children who could be harmed by not being born. When we say that it is better for a child to have been born, we do not compare that child's current existence with a previous one. Instead, we make an after-the-fact judgment that life is a good for an already existing child, even though that child may have suffered some harm from the technology used to bring him or her into the world. Critics of the use of the new reproductive technologies, however, make a before-the-fact judgment about children who do not exist, but who might. They maintain that it would be wrong to bring children into the world if they would suffer certain substantial harms as a result of the methods by which they are created. This is a logically coherent claim that justifies considering whether the new reproductive technologies severely damage children born as a result of their use.

The criterion of avoiding substantial harm, while valid, may provide inadequate ethical constraints on various ways of employing the new reproductive arrangements. The criterion is derived from a position that especially prizes individuality, liberty, and autonomy—quite possibly at the cost of values that are served by the building of families and communities, and by accounting for the common good (Cahill, 1990). Taking respect for individual freedom as the primary value, according to Allen Verhey, runs the danger of reducing the value of persons to their capacities for rational choice and denying the significance of the communities that shape them. People are not just autonomous individuals, they are also members of communities, some of which are not of their own choosing. Freedom is insufficient for an account of the good life in the family. Thus, it may be morally legitimate to recommend limits to individual choice about assisted reproductive techniques, not only to protect the children born of these methods but also to uphold basic community values. What is at issue, he suggests, is what kind of society we are and want to become (Verhey, 1989).

Ethical issues related to the introduction of third parties

The introduction of third parties into procreative acts, according to some critics, imperils the very character of society by threatening the nuclear family, the basic building block of U.S. society (Ethics Committee, 1986; Callahan, 1988). Religious commentators and groups, in particular, have expressed concern about the effect of the use of gamete donors and surrogates on the relation between married couples within the nuclear family. Richard McCormick, a Roman Catholic theologian, argues that when procreation takes place in a context other than marriage (as when single women use artificial insemination by donor, for example) and another's body is used to achieve conception (as in the case of surrogacy, for example), total dedication to one's spouse is made more difficult; in Roman Catholic terminology, it also violates "the marriage covenant wherein exclusive, nontransferable, inalienable rights to each other's person and generative acts are exchanged" (Ethics Committee, 1986, p. 82).

In Islamic law, artificial insemination by donor is rejected on grounds that the use of the sperm of a man other than the marriage partner confuses lineage and might also constitute a form of adultery because a third party enters into the procreative aspect of the marital relation. The practice is highly controversial in the Jewish religion because (1) some consider it a form of adultery; (2) some take the resulting child to be illegitimate; and (3) if the donor is unknown, the practice might eventually result in incestuous marriage between siblings. Most other religious groups that have commented on surrogacy also reject it because it depersonalizes motherhood and risks subjecting surrogates and procreation itself to commercial exploitation. Such practices will lead people to regard children as products who, in Oliver O'Donovan's terms, are "made" rather than "begotten" (O'Donovan, 1984).

Those who wish to counter concerns about adultery distinguish between adultery and the use of a gamete or womb contributed by a third party to assist a married couple to have a child. A necessary element of adultery, they contend, is sexual intercourse; neither gamete donation nor surrogacy involves sexual contact between the recipient and the donor. Moreover, unlike adultery, no element of unfaithfulness need inhere in participation in gamete donation. Indeed, a couple may participate in gamete donation just because they have a strong commitment to their marriage, rather than out of disdain for it (Lauritzen, 1993). When only one parent can contribute genetically to the procreation of a child, but both can nourish and nurture a child, this argument runs, it is ethically acceptable for them to have a child by means of third-party collaboration.

The use of third parties in the provision of the new reproductive technologies leads to confused notions of parentage, critics note, since it severs the connection between the conceptive, gestational, and rearing components of parenthood. It can be difficult to predict who will be declared the rearing parent in different reproductive scenarios, despite the fact that they embrace the same set of facts. For instance, in IVF followed by embryo transfer, the woman who gestates an embryo provided by someone else is considered the mother of the resulting child, but in artificial insemination by donor she is not. Those who respond to this criticism, in attempting to develop a consistent ethical basis for awarding the accolade of parenthood, give priority either to the interests of the children born of these technologies or to those of their adult progenitors.

Those who view the interests of the children as of prime importance argue that genetic connections should constrain the freedom to choose parental status in that biological kinship relations are important to children's development and self-identity (Callahan, 1988). Purposefully to break the link between procreation and rearing, these commentators maintain, harms children born of these procedures because it obscures their identity within a family lineage. Indeed, it has been argued that the biological relationship between gamete donors and the children who result from their contributions carries an obligation for donors to support and nurture those children (Callahan, 1992). Respondents observe that it is not considered wrong to separate the genetic and rearing components of parenthood in such well-established arrangements as adoption, stepparenting, blended families, and extended kin relationships. This precedent suggests that, although the genetic relation may be important, it is not essential to parenthood. Caring for and raising a child are of greater significance for parenthood than providing the genetic material or gestational environment, according to this view. Consequently, the rearing parent should have moral priority over the genetic parent in the interests of the child (Lauritzen, 1993). Others focus on the interests of the parents when the choice is between the genetic and the gestational mother, and they contend that the gestational mother should prevail because of her greater physical and emotional contribution and the risks of childbearing (Elias and Annas, 1986).

Parents who are not the biological progenitors of the children they raise and those who provide them with gametes often fear social stigmatization. This raises the question of whether anonymity and secrecy should be used to envelop all who participate in the use of the new reproductive technologies for their own protection. Anonymity has to do with concealing the identity of the donor; secrecy has to do with concealing the fact that recipients have participated in gamete donation. The practice of artificial insemination by donor has historically been carried out in secrecy with anonymous donors to protect family and donor privacy; oocyte donation, which began with openness about the identity of donors, is moving in that direction as well. The major argument against this development takes the interests of the children as primary and contends that since the personal and social identity of children is dependent on their biological origins, they ought to know about their genetic parents (National Bioethics Consultative Committee, 1989). Several countries that accept this argument have adopted regulations allowing children, when they reach maturity, to gain access to whatever information is available about donors who contributed to their birth.

Technologies of assisted reproduction, especially those involving third parties, facilitate the creation of models of family that depart significantly from the traditional nuclear family. As single persons, homosexual couples, and unmarried heterosexual couples increasingly gain access to these technologies, both religious and secular bodies express concern about weakening mutual commitment within the family and about the welfare of the resulting children. Sherman Elias and George Annas observe that "it seems disingenuous to argue on the one hand that the primary justification for noncoital reproduction is the anguish an infertile married couple suffers because of the inability to have a 'traditional family,' and then use the breakup of the traditional family

unit itself as the primary justification for unmarried individuals to have access to these techniques" (Elias and Annas, 1986, p. 67). The Warnock Report, developed by a commission of inquiry into the use of artificial means of reproduction in Great Britain in 1984, concluded that "the interests of the child dictate that it should be born into a home where there is a loving, stable, heterosexual relationship and that, therefore, the deliberate creation of a child for a woman who is not a partner in such a relationship is morally wrong" (Warnock, 1985, p. 11).

Some psychologists claim that children who grow up in these nontraditional families will suffer psychological and social damage because they will lack role models of both genders and may consequently develop an impaired view of sexuality and procreation (McGuire and Alexander, 1985). Moreover, they argue, two parents are better able than one to cope with the demands of childrearing. Other studies have been used to vindicate the opposite conclusions (McGuire and Alexander, 1985). Since few studies have been carried out on the consequences for children of atypical family arrangements that emerge when the new reproductive technologies are employed, it is difficult to provide any clear evidence to support or undermine these opposing contentions. A further concern voiced is that using new reproductive technologies to assist single people and homosexual couples to have children involves a misuse of medical capabilities because these methods are not being employed to overcome a medical problem but to circumvent biological limits to parenthood.

To others, however, the use of new methods of assisted reproduction by single people and homosexual couples mirrors the reality that U.S. society has begun to move away from the nuclear family (Glover, 1989). They see the inclusion of homosexual parents within the meaning of family as a move toward greater equality in a society in which those who are homosexual suffer from prejudice and discrimination. If single people and homosexual couples can offer to a child an environment that is compatible with a good start in life, the *Glover Report to the European Commission* maintains, they ought to have access to these techniques, but it is appropriate for those providing them to make some inquiries before proceeding (Glover, 1989). The Royal Commission on New Reproductive Technologies of Canada approved of allowing infertility clinics to provide single heterosexual and lesbian women access to donor insemination on grounds that no reliable evidence could be found that the environment in families formed by these gamete recipients is any better or any worse for the children than in families formed by heterosexual couples (Canada, Royal Commission on New Reproductive Technologies, 1993).

Ethical issues related to commodification

A concern of special ethical significance is that the introduction of third parties into some of the new reproductive techniques carries with it the danger of commodification of human beings, their bodies, and their bodily products. Giving payment of any sort to surrogates and gamete donors, some argue, risks making them and the children produced with their assistance fungible objects of market exchange, alienating them from their personhood in a way that diminishes the value of human beings (Radin, 1992). Third parties who assist others to reproduce should be viewed as donors of a priceless gift for which they ought to be repaid in gratitude, but not in money.

Others argue that persons have a right to do what they choose with their bodies and that when they choose to be paid, their reimbursement should be commensurate with their services (Robertson, 1988). The value of respect for persons is not diminished by using surrogates and gamete donors for the reproductive purposes of others if those third parties are fully informed about the procedure in which they participate and are not coerced into participating—even when they are paid (Harris, 1992). There is a presumption on all sides that third parties should not be specifically compensated for their gametes, wombs, or babies. Several groups that have considered the matter, though, such as the Warnock Committee in Great Britain (Warnock, 1985) and the Waller Committee in Australia (Victoria, 1984), allow third-party payment for out-of-pocket and medical expenses. The American Fertility Society goes further when it maintains that gamete donors should be paid for their direct and indirect expenses, inconvenience, time, risk, and discomfort (Ethics Committee, 1990). It would be unfair and exploitive not to pay donors for their time and effort, John Robertson argues (Robertson, 1988).

Offering large amounts of money to third parties incommensurate with the degree of effort and service that these persons provide may diminish the voluntariness of their choice to participate in assisted reproduction, particularly when they have limited financial means. There is concern that a new economic underclass might develop that would earn its living by providing body parts and products for the reproductive purposes of those who are better off economically. This would violate the principle of distributive justice, which requires that society's benefits and burdens be parceled out equitably among different groups (Macklin, 1994). However, if poor women and men have voluntarily and knowingly accepted their role in these reproductive projects, it could be seen as unjustifiably paternalistic to deny them the opportunity to earn money. The possibility of exploitation of the poor must be weighed "against a possible step toward their liberation through economic gain" from a new source of income connected to innovative methods of reproduction (Radin, 1987).

Ethical issues related to the uses of embryos, fetuses, and cadavers

When the process of fertilization is external, the embryo becomes accessible to many forms of intervention. During the brief extracorporeal, in vitro period, embryos can be frozen, treated, implanted, experimented on, discarded, or donated. Theoretically, embryos that result from IVF could be cryopreserved for generations, so that a woman could give birth to her genetic uncle, siblings could be born to different sets of parents, or one sibling could be born to another. A 1993 experiment in which human embryos were split reawakened concerns about these sorts of possibilities, which had remained dormant since a mid-1970s controversy about cloning human beings (National Advisory Board, 1994). (Cloning, either by transplanting the nucleus from a differentiated cell into an unfertilized egg from which the nucleus has been removed or by splitting an embryo at an early stage when its cells are still undifferentiated, results in individuals who are genetically identical to the original from which they are cloned.)

Advocates of embryo splitting view it as a way of obtaining greater numbers of embryos for implantation in order to enhance the chances of pregnancy for those who are infertile (Robertson, 1994). Critics claim that cloning in any form negates what we view as valuable about human beings, their individuality and uniqueness. It risks treating children as fungible products to be manipulated at will, rather than as unique, self-determining individuals. These critics maintain that twinning that occurs in nature is an unavoidable accident that does not involve manipulation of one child-to-be to produce a duplicate (McCormick, 1994). Defenders of cloning respond that the similarity of identical twins does not diminish their uniqueness or their sense of selfhood. In any case, cloned individuals would not be identical in that the genome does not fully determine a person's identity. Environmental factors, such as family upbringing and the historical context, weigh heavily in influencing the expression of genes (National Advisory Board, 1994).

It is the potential for abuse of cloning that disturbs most critics. The possibility of cryopreserving cloned embryos suggests the option of implanting cloned embryos and bringing them to term should their already-born twin need a tissue or organ transplant. In another scenario, embryos derived from parents who are likely to produce "ideal specimens" would be cloned and sold on a "black market." Critics condemn such potential applications of cloning because they diminish the value of embryos and of human beings by treating them as objects available for any use by others (National Advisory Board, 1994). They are concerned that the deep desire of the infertile for children, in combination with scientific zeal and market forces, will create strong pressure to clone embryos without a view to the ethical considerations involved.

In 1993 scientists in the United Kingdom announced the possibility of using for infertility treatment eggs and ovaries taken from aborted fetuses (Carroll and Gosden, 1993). The eggs could be fertilized in vitro and then transferred into infertile women who lack viable eggs; the ovaries could be transplanted directly into women to mature and produce eggs. This would help meet the shortage of oocytes for those who lack their own. Such uses of aborted fetuses, however, are highly contentious and strike some as grotesque. Many who object to abortion on ethical grounds maintain that this procedure, like other forms of fetal tissue use, would encourage the practice. Moreover, it seems self-contradictory for a woman to consent to abortion and at the same time consent to become a grandmother. Children created by this procedure, it could be argued, would know little about their genetic heritage or about their mother, other than that she was a dead fetus, and would therefore be at risk of both psychological and social harm.

Female cadavers provide another potential source of oocytes for those who are infertile. It has been proposed that women consider donating their ovaries for use by others after their death, much as individuals donate organs such as kidneys and livers (Seibel, 1994). It may soon be possible to collect immature eggs from cadavers, mature and fertilize them in vitro, and then transfer them into infertile women. This procedure would have an advantage over the use of eggs from aborted fetuses in that the recipient would be able to learn the medical and genetic history of the adult donor. An argument for this practice is that it would allow the continuation of the family's biological heritage and serve to console the grieving family because some aspect of their deceased relative will have been preserved. Postmortem recovery of eggs would be done with the consent of the donor and would therefore respect individual rights and allow freedom of choice for individuals and their close relatives.

This proposal is grounded in an analogy between organ and gamete donation. Yet gamete donation is different in that it involves the provision of an essential factor for bringing a child into existence; it is not life-saving but life-giving. The interests of the resulting children, consequently, provide a major consideration to be taken into account in determining whether such procedures ought to be pursued. The difficulty noted earlier in connection with the introduction of third parties arises in this instance as well. Children develop their identity and self-understanding, in part, through their relation-

ships with their biological parents. Consequently, they might face serious psychological and social harm if one of their biological parents were a cadaver. Indeed, this concern amounts to a central social concern as well, in that the prospect of using gametes derived from the newly dead in order to create children endangers our perception of the respect due to the dead human body and our view of procreation as ideally grounded in an interpersonal relationship between living persons.

Ethical issues related to access and justice

Although those able to procreate naturally can decide whether and when to do so, the choice to reproduce among those who need medical assistance to do so is more limited. In part, this is because they enter a health-care system in which providers have responsibilities both to candidates for infertility treatment and to the resulting child, because they are assisting in the creation of a new human being. Although physicians have a special obligation to respect the autonomy and freedom of those who are candidates for treatment, they are not obligated to provide them with all treatments that they request (Chervenak and McCullough, 1991). As one of several groups of gatekeepers of the new reproductive technologies, some physicians use a medical-indications criterion to bar access to these technologies to some patients, as when, for example, the physical risk of pregnancy is too great. Yet many physicians find that they cannot easily separate medical indications from indications that are psychological, social, and ethical. Questions requiring judgments that go beyond those that are strictly medical arise in many situations. These questions include possible treatment for candidates who wish to create "designer babies" of a certain sex, intelligence, and/or race; couples who want to use a surrogate mother for frivolous reasons related to personal convenience; infertile single women who request access to both oocyte and sperm donation in lieu of adoption; women of advanced reproductive age who want to have children despite the risk to their own health; and couples who appear severely dysfunctional and prone to violence and child abuse. Physicians are not usually trained to address ethical questions that arise in such situations. Because physicians have personal and professional biases and are part of a largely unregulated and profitable infertility industry, it might be appropriate to assign the gatekeeper role to a specially trained group of professionals who are not physicians. Another possibility is to utilize guidelines for the use of the new reproductive technologies prepared by physician professional associations, institutional ethics committees, private-sector ethics boards, public ethics commissions, and state and national regulatory agencies; such guidelines should address not only medical but social, psychological, and ethical issues (Cohen, 1994; Fletcher, 1994).

Public-policymakers and private health-care insurance regulators also affect who gains access to the new reproductive technologies. If they define infertility treatment as a response to a disease rather than to a social need, a case for financial support of the new reproductive technologies can be made. Because infertility is a physical condition that impairs normal function, many commentators regard it as something like a disease, the victims of which are in need of help from medical science (Overall, 1987). However, it can also be argued that since reproductive technologies do not correct the condition causing infertility, they do not constitute medical treatment for a disease. Yet many well-accepted treatments do not correct the underlying condition but only its symptoms or disabilities. Given the importance to many people of having a biological child and the fact that normal functioning allows this, the claim has been made that infertility should be treated as a disease on a par with other physical impairments. Historically, the "barren" woman or man has not been accorded sympathy; the availability of infertility treatment might disarm similar current discriminatory attitudes toward those who are infertile.

Even if infertility were defined as a disease, however, this would not indicate that its treatment would be ethically mandatory. The U.S. health-care system does not have infinite resources and cannot provide everyone with every desired or desirable health service. Should the new reproductive technologies be subject to more severe criteria for funding than are set for other medical techniques? Because infertility is a physical dysfunction with significant effects on the life plans of those it affects, it can be contended that a just society should include reproductive technologies among the range of treatments covered. The opposing argument is that the costs of such treatment and its relatively low likelihood of success do not justify its inclusion.

A related issue arises from the fact that only a limited range of people—those with greater financial resources—benefit from the new reproductive technologies. Access depends on economic factors, culture, race, and social class. Those in the United States who are poor have little access to specialty services such as infertility clinics because public and private insurers provide limited coverage. If poor people participate at all in the use of these technologies, they do so as surrogates or occasionally as oocyte donors. Thus, the use of new reproductive technologies has potential for creating further unjust schisms in our society between rich and poor and between one subculture and another.

As long as IVF services and gametes are in short supply, questions will arise about how to select candidates from among those who seek access to the new methods of assisted reproduction. Those persons who are infertile or who carry a serious genetic disease may have a greater first claim than those who are not infertile but who wish to use these methods to select the features of their children or as a matter of personal convenience. This is because the need of the former is a more basic need, directly related to the goal of remedying a difficulty in normal species functioning. A more refined set of rationing priorities would take account of such factors as the number of children an individual or a couple already has; whether they have a support system in place to assist them to care for a child adequately; and the greater medical risk to certain recipients of treatment, such as women of advanced reproductive age. These considerations would be grounded in the interests of the potential children and of their would-be parents, as well as in the need to distribute the number of children among couples in an equitable way.

Conclusion

Behind many of the ethical issues raised by the new reproductive technologies lie difficult questions about the importance of genetic parenthood, the nuclear family, and the welfare of children, as well as the role that society should play in overseeing the creation of its citizens. Perplexity about how to resolve these questions is due, in part, to the speed with which these technologies are being developed. There is a growing concern that they are being created too rapidly, before the old technologies, such as artificial insemination, have been integrated into the ethical and social fabric. As the rate of reproductive change accelerates, the ability to provide ethical safeguards for the creation and use of the new reproductive technologies diminishes. This may be the most persuasive reason to provide some form of direction and regulation of the new reproductive technologies that incorporates defensible ethical limits to their use.

CYNTHIA B. COHEN

Directly related to this article are the INTRODUCTION *and other articles in this entry:* SEX SELECTION; ARTIFICIAL INSEMINATION; IN VITRO FERTILIZATION AND EMBRYO TRANSFER; SURROGACY; CRYOPRESERVATION OF SPERM, OVA, AND EMBRYOS; *and* LEGAL AND REGULATORY ISSUES. *Also directly related are the entries* GENETIC TESTING AND SCREENING, *articles on* PREIMPLANTATION EMBRYO DIAGNOSIS, *and* PRENATAL DIAGNOSIS; FEMINISM; JUSTICE; *and* WOMEN, *article on* HEALTH-CARE ISSUES. *For a further discussion of topics mentioned in this article, see the entries* ABORTION, *section on* CONTEMPORARY ETHICAL AND LEGAL ASPECTS, *article on* CONTEMPORARY ETHICAL PERSPECTIVES; FAMILY; FERTILITY CONTROL; FUTURE GENERATIONS, OBLIGATIONS TO; *and* MARRIAGE AND OTHER DOMESTIC PARTNERSHIPS.

Other relevant material may be found under the entries CRYONICS; EUGENICS; GENETIC COUNSELING; ORGAN AND TISSUE PROCUREMENT; SEXUALITY IN SOCIETY; *and* TECHNOLOGY.

Bibliography

ANDREWS, LORI. 1984. *New Conceptions: A Consumers' Guide to the Newest Infertility Treatments.* New York: St. Martin's Press.

BARTHOLET, ELIZABETH. 1992. "In Vitro Fertilization: The Construction of Infertility and of Parenting." In *Issues in Reproductive Technology I: An Anthology,* pp. 253–260. Edited by Helen Bequaert Holmes. New York: Garland.

———. 1993. *Family Bonds, Adoption and the Politics of Parenting.* Boston: Houghton Mifflin.

BAYLES, MICHAEL D. 1984. *Reproductive Ethics.* Englewood Cliffs, N.J.: Prentice-Hall.

BROCK, DAN W. 1994. "Reproductive Freedom: Its Nature, Bases, and Limits." In *Health Care Ethics: Critical Issues,* pp. 43–61. Edited by John F. Monagle and David C. Thomasma. Gaithersburg, Md.: Aspen.

CAHILL, LISA SOWLE. 1990. "The Ethics of Surrogate Motherhood: Biology, Freedom, and Moral Obligation." In *Surrogate Motherhood: Politics and Privacy,* pp. 151–164. Edited by Larry O. Gostin. Bloomington: Indiana University Press.

CALLAHAN, DANIEL. 1992. "Bioethics and Fatherhood." *Utah Law Review* 1992:735–746.

CALLAHAN, SIDNEY. 1988. "The Ethical Challenge of the New Reproductive Technology." In *Medical Ethics: A Guide for Health Care Professionals,* pp. 26–37. Edited by John F. Monagle and David C. Thomasma. Rockville, Md.: Aspen.

CANADA. ROYAL COMMISSION ON NEW REPRODUCTIVE TECHNOLOGIES. 1993. *Proceed with Care: Final Report of the Royal Commission on New Reproductive Technologies.* 2 vols. Ottawa, Canada: Author. See especially Vol. 2.

CARROLL, JOHN, and GOSDEN, ROGER G. 1993. "Transplantation of Frozen-Thawed Mouse Primordial Follicles." *Human Reproduction* 8, no. 8:1163–1167.

CATHOLIC CHURCH. CONGREGATION FOR THE DOCTRINE OF THE FAITH. 1987. *Instruction on Respect for Human Life in Its Origin and on the Dignity of Procreation: Replies to Certain Questions of the Day.* Washington, D.C.: United States Catholic Conference.

COHEN, CYNTHIA B. 1994. "In Search of a Variety of Bioethics Forums." *Politics and the Life Sciences* 13, no. 1:82–84.

COREA, GENA. 1985. *The Mother Machine: Reproductive Technologies from Artificial Insemination to Artificial Wombs.* New York: Harper & Row.

DESAI, PRAKASH N. 1989. *Health and Medicine in the Hindu Tradition: Continuity and Cohesion.* New York: Crossroad.

ELIAS, SHERMAN, and ANNAS, GEORGE J. 1986. "Social Policy Considerations in Noncoital Reproduction." *Journal of the American Medical Association* 225, no. 1:62–68.

———. 1987. "Reproductive Liberty." In their *Reproductive Genetics and the Law,* pp. 143–167. Chicago: Year Book Medical.

EPISCOPAL CHURCH. GENERAL CONVENTION. 1982. *Journal of the General Convention of the Protestant Episcopal Church in the United States of America.* New York: Author. See Res. A067, Sec. C158.

ETHICS COMMITTEE. AMERICAN FERTILITY SOCIETY. 1978. "Reproductive Technologies: Ethical Issues." In *Encyclopedia of Bioethics,* Vol. 4, pp. 1454–1464. Edited by Warren T. Reich. New York: Macmillan and Free Press.

———. 1990. "Ethical Considerations of the New Reproductive Technologies." *Fertility and Sterility* 53, no. 6, supplement 2:1S–104S.

FELDMAN, DAVID M. 1986. *Health and Medicine in the Jewish Tradition: L'hayyim—to Life.* New York: Crossroad.

FLETCHER, JOHN. 1994. "On Restoring Public Bioethics." *Politics and the Life Sciences* 13, no. 1:84–86.

GENERAL CONFERENCE. MENNONITE CHURCH. 1985. *Human Sexuality in the Christian Life: A Working Document for Study and Dialogue.* Scottdale, Pa.: Faith and Life Press and Mennonite Publishing House.

GLOVER, JONATHAN. 1989. *Ethics of New Reproductive Technologies: The Glover Report to the European Commission.* De Kalb: Northern Illinois University Press.

HARAKAS, STANLEY SAMUEL. 1990. *Health and Medicine in the Eastern Orthodox Tradition: Faith, Liturgy, and Wholeness.* New York: Crossroad.

HARRIS, JOHN. 1992. *Wonderwoman and Superman: The Ethics of Human Technology.* Oxford: Oxford University Press.

JAGGAR, ALISON M. 1983. *Feminist Politics and Human Nature.* Totowa, N.J.: Rowman & Allanheld.

LAURITZEN, PAUL. 1993. *Pursuing Parenthood: Ethical Issues in Assisted Reproduction.* Bloomington: Indiana University Press.

LUTHERAN CHURCH. MISSOURI SYNOD. COMMISSION ON THEOLOGY AND CHURCH RELATIONS. SOCIAL CONCERNS COMMITTEE. 1981. *Human Sexuality: A Theological Perspective.* St. Louis, Mo.: Concordia.

MACKLIN, RUTH. 1990. "Is There Anything Wrong with Surrogate Motherhood? An Ethical Analysis." In *Surrogate Motherhood: Politics and Privacy,* pp. 136–150. Edited by Larry O. Gostin. Bloomington: Indiana University Press.

———. 1994. *Surrogates and Other Mothers: The Debates over Assisted Reproduction.* Philadelphia: Temple University Press.

McCORMICK, RICHARD A. 1986. "Ethical Considerations of the New Reproductive Technologies." *Fertility and Sterility* 46, no. 3, supplement 1:82.

———. 1994. "Blastomere Separation: Some Concerns." *Hastings Center Report* 24, no. 2:664–667.

McGUIRE, MAUREEN, and ALEXANDER, NANCY J. 1985. "Artificial Insemination of Single Women." *Fertility and Sterility* 43, no. 2:182–184.

NATIONAL ADVISORY BOARD ON ETHICS IN REPRODUCTION. 1994. "Report on Human Cloning Through Embryo Splitting: An Amber Light." *Kennedy Institute of Ethics Journal* 4, no. 3:251–282.

NATIONAL BIOETHICS CONSULTATIVE COMMITTEE (AUSTRALIA). 1989. *Reproductive Technology: Record Keeping and Access to Information: Birth Certificates and Birth Records of Offspring Born as a Result of Gamete Donation. Final Report to Australian Health Ministers.* Canberra, Australia: Author.

O'DONOVAN, OLIVER. 1984. *Begotten or Made?* Oxford: At the Clarendon Press.

OVERALL, CHRISTINE. 1987. *Ethics and Human Reproduction: A Feminist Analysis.* Boston: Allen & Unwin.

RADIN, MARGARET JANE. 1987. "Market-Inalienability." *Harvard Law Review* 100, no. 8:1849–1937.

RAHMAN, FAZLUR. 1987. *Health and Medicine in the Islamic Tradition: Change and Identity.* New York: Crossroad.

ROBERTSON, JOHN A. 1986. "Embryos, Families, and Procreative Liberty: The Legal Structure of the New Reproduction." *Southern California Law Review* 59, no. 4: 939–1041.

———. 1988. "Technology and Motherhood: Legal and Ethical Issues in Human Egg Donation." *Case Western Reserve Law Review* 39, no. 1:1–38.

———. 1994. "The Question of Human Cloning." *Hastings Center Report* 24, no. 2:6–14.

ROWLAND, ROBYN. 1992. *Living Laboratories. Women and Reproductive Technologies.* Bloomington: Indiana University Press.

SIMMONS, PAUL D. 1983. *Birth and Death: Bioethical Decision-Making.* Philadelphia: Westminster.

SMITH, HARMON L. 1970. *Ethics and the New Medicine.* Nashville, Tenn.: Abingdon Press.

U.S. DEPARTMENT OF HEALTH, EDUCATION AND WELFARE. ETHICS ADVISORY BOARD. 1979. *HEW Support of Research Involving Human in Vitro Fertilization and Embryo Transfer: Report and Conclusions.* Washington, D.C.: Author.

VERHEY, ALLEN. 1989. "On Having Children and Caring for Them: Becoming and Being Parents." In *Christian Faith, Health, and Medical Practice,* pp. 178–183. Edited by Hessel Bouma III, Douglas Diekema, Edward Langerak, Theodore Rottman, and Allen Verhey. Grand Rapids, Mich.: W. B. Eerdmans.

VICTORIA. COMMITTEE TO CONSIDER THE SOCIAL, ETHICAL, AND LEGAL ISSUES ARISING FROM IN VITRO FERTILIZATION. 1984. *Report on the Disposition of Embryos Produced by in Vitro Fertilization.* Melbourne, Australia: Author. Chaired by Louis Waller.

WALTERS, LEROY. 1987. "Ethics and the New Reproductive Technologies: An International Review of Committee Statements." *Hastings Center Report* 17, no. 3 (spec. suppl.):3–9.

WARNOCK, MARY. 1985. *A Question of Life: The Warnock Report on Human Fertilisation and Embryology.* Oxford: Basil Blackwell.

WILLIAMS, LINDA S. 1992. "Biology or Society? Parenthood Motivation in a Sample of Canadian Women Seeking in Vitro Fertilization." In *Issues in Reproductive Technology I: An Anthropology,* pp. 261–274. Edited by Helen Bequaert Holmes. New York: Garland.

VIII. LEGAL AND REGULATORY ISSUES

Reproductive freedom is not a simple concept. Encompassing far more than abortion, it also includes the choice of whether and with whom to procreate, how many times to procreate, and by what means. It includes the choice of the social context (e.g., marital, communal, or solitary) in which the reproduction takes place and, to some extent, the characteristics of the children people will have (gender, presence or absence of certain disease). It is grounded, for some moral philosophers, in self-determination, individual welfare, and equality of expectation and opportunity (Brock, 1992).

Noncoital reproduction, that is, reproduction achieved despite the absence of sexual intercourse, allows single, homosexual, and infertile people to start and rear families. Often, it entails such controversial techniques as extracorporeal maintenance of an embryo, screening and storage of gametes, or the reproductive assistance of men and women who do not plan to maintain a relationship with the child they help to conceive or gestate.

Thus, new reproductive technologies enable individuals to exercise more reproductive choices. This, in turn, invites exploration of the depths of cultural relativism and the meaning of genetic linkage; the preference for the heterosexual couple as the paradigm for family life; the role of the state as the regulator versus facilitator of individual aspirations; and the role of the state and the professional as the gatekeeper to the technologies that permit people to circumvent infertility or conventional forms of procreation.

Under U.S. law, states can outlaw or regulate certain aspects of reproductive technologies. Areas for possible state intervention include protection of the extracorporeal embryo; protection of patients (and their resulting children) who seek to use reproductive technologies; regulation of contract (i.e., "surrogate") motherhood; definition of family forms and familial relationships in light of gamete transfers and use of contract birth mothers; and limitation on commercialization of the techniques. But the extent to which states can ban or regulate noncoital reproduction depends on the extent to which procreation is protected by state and federal constitutions, and the extent to which ancillary practices, such as payment for gametes or services of a contract mother, are viewed as part of the act of procreation or as independent acts of commercial negotiation.

In the United States, the more zealously procreation is guarded by constitutional guarantees and the more broadly the definition of procreation is drawn, the more compelling and narrowly drawn must be state efforts to restrict use of noncoital procreation. Those restrictions, when they exist, will be manifested in both common law and statutory law, usually with regard to the fields of contracts, property, or family law. Because the details of such law vary tremendously from state to state, this article focuses primarily on the overarching constitutional issues that limit state policymaking and lawmaking in this field, and compares national responses.

Is there an affirmative right to procreate?

The right to procreate, that is, the right to bear or beget a child, appears to be one of the rights implied by the U.S. Constitution. It is grounded in both individual liberty (*Skinner v. Oklahoma*, 1942) and the integrity of the family unit (*Meyer v. Nebraska*, 1923), and is viewed as a "fundamental right" (*Griswold v. Connecticut*, 1965), one that is essential to notions of liberty and justice (*Eisenstadt v. Baird*, 1972).

The U.S. Supreme court has not explicitly considered whether there is a positive right to procreate—that is, whether every individual has a right to actually bear or beget a child and thereby has a claim on the community for necessary assistance in this endeavor. It has, however, considered a wide range of related issues, including the right of a state to interfere with procreative ability by forcible sterilization (*Skinner v. Oklahoma*, 1942), the right of individuals to prevent conception or to terminate a pregnancy (*Roe v. Wade*, 1973; *Webster v. Reproductive Services*, 1989; *Planned Parenthood v. Casey*, 1992), and the right of individuals to rear children in nontraditional family groups (*Moore v. City of East Cleveland, Ohio* 1977).

Since the 1942 *Skinner* decision, lower courts have accepted the notion that states may not forcibly sterilize selected individuals unless such a policy can withstand strict constitutional scrutiny. The basis for requiring this level of scrutiny is the assertion that the "right to have offspring," like the right to marry, is a "fundamental," "basic liberty." Further, the *Skinner* and *Eisenstadt* decisions arguably hold that the right to use contraception or to be free of unwarranted sterilization is an aspect of individual, rather than marital, privacy. As stated in *Eisenstadt*: "If the right to privacy means anything, it is the right of the individual, married or single, to be free of unwarranted government intrusion into matters so fundamentally affecting a person as the decision to bear or beget a child" (*Eisenstadt v. Baird*, 1972).

But the right to privacy is no longer the primary justification for abortion rights, or, by extension, reproductive rights. The 1992 *Planned Parenthood v. Casey* decision specifically based its opinion on "liberty" (rather than privacy) rights, and concluded that abortion remains protected from state efforts to prohibit abortion. The emphasis on "liberty" language changes the focus of abortion rights from one of limitations on governmental power (as discussed in "privacy"-based decisions) to one of individual control of one's person. The opinion attempts to explain why abortion is an essential "liberty" for women because it permits control of one's body and one's personal destiny.

Justice Antonin Scalia's dissent mocks this attempt. After reciting the list of phrases used elsewhere by his colleagues, such as "a person's most basic decision," "a most personal and intimate choice," "originat[ing] within the zone of conscience and belief," "too intimate and personal for state interference," Scalia complains that "the same adjectives can be applied to many forms of conduct that this Court . . . has held are not entitled to constitutional protection—because, like abortion, they are forms of conduct that have long been criminalized in American society. Those adjectives might be applied, for example, to homosexual sodomy, polygamy, adult incest, and suicide" (p. 785).

Scalia's dissent highlights the potentially far-reaching implications of what the plurality has written regarding the fundamental importance of controlling one's fertility. The *Casey* plurality opinion lays out an argument for reexamining the 1879 *Reynolds v. U.S.* decision (upholding the power of the state to outlaw polygamous marriage) and the 1986 *Bowers v. Hardwick* decision (upholding the power of the state to criminalize homosexual behavior), a task critical to determining if states can restrict noncoital reproduction to married couples. It also lays the groundwork for cases sure to arise concerning prenatal diagnosis, sex selection, cloning, and (ultimately) parthenogenesis.

What can states do to regulate reproductive technologies?

Even assuming that constitutional protection for procreation remains grounded in a fundamental rights analysis, possibilities remain for areas of state regulation of who may use noncoital reproduction and how they may proceed. First, many aspects of noncoital reproduction arguably do not amount to "procreation," and therefore are more amenable to state control. Donor gametes and surrogacy do not permit an infertile person to procreate; rather, they allow fertile persons to reproduce without partners or to bypass the infertility of their partners.

Artificial insemination by donor (AID), for example, can be used by single or lesbian women who want to become pregnant but who find the thought of sexual intercourse with a man distasteful. Almost half the states in the United States have statutory language governing AID that appears to ignore the possibility of such a use, leaving the legal status of the donor-father unclear (U.S. Congress, Office of Technology Assessment [OTA], 1988b). Canada and France have also had national commissions recommend that single and lesbian women be barred from using donor insemination in order to conceive (Liu, 1991; McLean, 1992). Because such women could physically procreate without donor insemination, albeit with great discomfort, it can be argued that such restrictions do not impinge upon a fundamental right to procreate and are therefore potentially tolerable.

Of course, the restrictions would still be subject to challenges based on the unequal treatment of single or lesbian women as compared with the married, heterosexual population. AID for a married couple in which the husband is infertile is also nothing more than a medical alternative to the social solution of adultery; the AID itself does not enable the infertile man to procreate. Nevertheless, in Canada, France, and much of the United States, this form of AID is viewed as therapeutic, seemingly because the "unit" of infertility (i.e., the "patient") is seen as a monogamous, married, heterosexual couple, not as an unmarried individual.

In typical surrogacy arrangements, in which the husband is fertile and the wife infertile, the surrogacy arrangement, like AID, does not permit the infertile wife to procreate, nor is the fertile husband unable to procreate without resorting to surrogacy. Rather, surrogacy allows the husband to procreate without committing adultery and with some assurance, as in the AID scenario, that the couple will be able to retain exclusive custody of the resulting child. As with AID, such a use of contract motherhood is viewed as therapeutic by many. While even this use of surrogacy has engendered opposition ranging from criminalization to mere unenforceability in countries such as Australia, Canada, England, and France, and in some portions of the United States, it has never encountered the same degree of approbation as the so-called surrogacy of convenience, in which a rearing mother finds it useful to hire someone else to carry the child (Liu, 1991; McLean, 1992).

Indeed, much of the debate surrounding the most famous surrogacy case in the United States, *Baby M* (1988), focused on whether the rearing mother had declined to become pregnant due to career concerns and undue worry about her health, or rather due to legitimate concern that pregnancy would seriously worsen her multiple sclerosis. This debate exemplifies the increased willingness of the American public to regulate or ban surrogacy when it is not perceived as a cure for a medical problem such as infertility, a sentiment reflected in the constitutional analysis that permits greater state regulation where the right to procreate is not directly implicated.

Egg donation to a woman who cannot ovulate but who can carry to term does not technically allow the recipient to procreate, as she will not "reproduce" in the genetic sense. But it does allow her to experience pregnancy and childbirth, which for women are intimately associated with genetic procreation. In terms of both biological significance (gestation is, of course, a biological activity) and emotional impact, this would seem to be close to procreation, even in its more narrow definition. Thus, it is difficult to categorize this activity in terms of whether it allows an infertile person to "procreate."

Despite this fact, there is considerable hesitation about permitting egg donation. Whereas sperm donation is widely accepted, egg donation entails significantly more medical discomfort and even risk on the part of the donor. This in turn raises the specter, at least in the United States, of increased payments for the donation. For some, such payments represent an undue incentive to undergo medical risks, as well as an unacceptable commercialization of human gametes. Nevertheless, at least in California, there is a thriving egg donation practice.

Even those aspects of noncoital reproduction that clearly involve procreation can be regulated or banned, if there is a sufficiently compelling state interest. It is true that artificial insemination by husband (AIH), and in vitro fertilization (IVF) using a couple's own gametes (whether or not a contract mother is hired to carry the child to term), permit an otherwise infertile man or woman to procreate genetically. By bypassing the fallopian tube defect or permitting intrauterine insemination of the husband's concentrated semen, these techniques actually help infertile individuals to participate in the act of reproduction. But a compelling state interest in the protection of embryos and fetuses, for example, could justify significant restraints on even AIH and IVF.

Is there a compelling state "interest" in embryos and fetuses?

The most likely claim for a compelling state purpose to outlaw or regulate IVF is that of protection for the extracorporeal embryo, whether or not accompanied by a contract with a gestational surrogate.

The *Webster* v. *Reproductive Services* (1989) and *Planned Parenthood* v. *Casey* (1992) decisions indicate that the U.S. Supreme Court is now quite tolerant of symbolic legislative statements concerning the sanctity of embryonic life and of significant restrictions on the exercise of constitutionally protected rights, such as abortion, in the name of protecting these early life forms. It seems likely that the court would uphold state statutes, such as the one in Louisiana, that regulates management of extracorporeal embryos. Such restrictions may include prohibiting nontherapeutic experimentation on the embryo, embryo discard, and unnecessary creation of "surplus" embryos for the purpose of experimentation. It might also attempt to regulate transfer of embryos. By declaring that life begins at conception, as was done in the Missouri statute upheld in *Webster*, and by equating the rights of embryos to the rights of children, states could demand that embryo transfers be viewed as adoptions.

This was the approach taken by the trial court in the case of *Davis* v. *Davis* (1992), a Tennessee divorce case that struggled with determining the legal status of several frozen embryos that were left over from unsuccessful IVF treatments and became the subject of a divorce dispute. Characterizing the question as one of child custody, and viewing the embryos as children, the trial court then awarded custody to the parent whose actions would be in the best interests of the embryos. By assuming that embryos have "interests," and then defining one of those interests as an interest in being born, the trial court awarded the embryos to the wife, who intended to have them implanted in her womb in the hope of bringing them to term.

By contrast, the appellate court backed away from the characterization of the embryos as "children" and the resulting "best interests" analysis. Without ever explicitly calling the embryos property, the court proceeded to treat them as property held jointly by the couple, and thereby concluded that disposition of the embryos must be by agreement because each party had an equal property interest in them.

The Tennessee Supreme Court reviewed available models for disposition of the embryos when unanticipated contingencies arise. Those models range from a rule requiring, at one extreme, that all embryos be used by the gamete-providers or be donated for uterine transfer (such as is required under an as yet unchallenged Louisiana statute), and, at the other extreme, that any unused embryos be automatically discarded. The Tennessee Supreme Court, when it considered the *Davis* case, was aware of the *Planned Parenthood* v. *Casey* (1992) decision, which reiterated the *Roe* (1973) holding that a state may express an "interest" in a fetus. Unfortunately, like *Roe*, *Planned Parenthood* v. *Casey* fails to identify *what* this interest might be or *why* it arises, leaving the *Davis* court with little guidance on how to extend the state interest argument to nonabortion settings.

Numerous commentators have struggled to identify this state interest (Joyce, 1988; Tooley, 1984). Many begin with the premise that a sufficiently detailed biological understanding of embryo potential will yield an answer:

> [E]very living individual being with the natural potential, as a whole, for knowing, willing, desiring, and relating to others in a self-reflective way is a person. But the human zygote is a living individual (or more than one such individual) with the natural potential, as a whole, to act in these ways. Therefore the human zygote is an actual person with great potential. . . . (Joyce, 1988, p. 169)

But others argue that the genetic blueprint of a person cannot be entitled to the same moral standing as that of the person himself or herself, because any inherent "right" to live is premised on the idea that it is in the "interest" of the entity to continue existing (Tooley, 1984). Where, as with a zygote, there is no self-concept, there can be no "interest" in continuing to exist, no "desire" to continue to exist, and therefore no "right" to continue to exist.

Such an argument refutes the *Davis* trial court's treatment of the frozen embryos as children with an interest in being brought to term. But the appellate court's assumption that they must therefore be treated as property is equally unjustified. Society may choose nonetheless to grant rights to the zygote or fetus, for any number of reasons, if such steps do not unduly impinge on another liberty recognized by society, such as the liberty of men and women to control their reproductive futures.

In fact, Justice John Paul Stevens takes on this issue in his concurring opinion in *Planned Parenthood* v. *Casey:*

> Identifying the State's interests—which the States rarely articulate with any precision—makes clear that the interest in protecting potential life is not grounded in the Constitution. It is, instead, an indirect interest supported by both humanitarian and pragmatic concerns. Many of our citizens believe that any abortion reflects an unacceptable disrespect for potential human life and that the performance of more than a million abortions each year is intolerable; many find third-trimester abortions performed when the fetus is approaching personhood particularly offensive. The State has a legitimate interest in minimizing such offense. . . . These are the kinds of concerns that comprise the State's interest in potential human life. (*Planned Parenthood* v. *Casey,* 1992, 120 L. Ed. 2d 674 at p. 739)

Struggling with the task of expressing a state interest in embryonic life without unduly impinging upon the reproductive rights of adult men and women, the Tennessee Supreme Court in the *Davis* case concluded that embryos are neither children nor property, but occupy an intermediate status based on their potential for development. This, in turn, would not convey a right to be born under either state or federal constitutional law but would demand some protections. These include implantation where possible, freedom from unnecessary creation or destruction, and dignified management.

The Tennessee court's characterization of an intermediate status for embryos is the most intriguing part of the opinion, as it did not present a coherent theory of that status and its implications. There are, of course, models of intermediate property status. Animals, for example, are treated as property with no "right to life," but at the same time are protected from cruel and painful treatment by their owners. Works of art may be owned, but "moral rights" possessed by the artist in some jurisdictions prohibit defacing or destroying the art. Land may be owned subject to numerous restrictions on use that would permanently destroy some publicly valued attribute. Which, if any, of these models describes the intermediate status held by the embryos? And on what basis? This is indeed the key question left totally unanswered by the Tennessee court. As it stands, though the opinion gives some narrow, nearly regulatory guidance to IVF clinics, it offers little to those wondering in general whether other restraints on embryo creation and management are in order.

Other countries have struggled with the same dilemma. Most often, as in England and Australia, the compromise solution is chosen, in which limited experimentation is permitted on unavoidably abandoned embryos. Deliberate creation of embryos for the purpose of experimentation is frowned upon. Occasionally a stricter view is adopted, as in Germany, where embryo experimentation is simply banned. Generally, however, where embryos are to be created in order to permit implantation and gestation, even extracorporeal maintenance or embryo freezing is tolerated (U.S. Congress, OTA, 1988b; Liu, 1991; McLean, 1992).

What is the state interest in the children conceived noncoitally?

Related to state interest in the protection of extracorporeal embryos is its interest in protecting the children born following noncoital conception. This takes its most frequent form in suggestions for limiting use of these technologies to married couples, on the theory that being born into a single-parent home is harmful to a child. On this basis, almost two-thirds of physicians surveyed in 1987 and a number of states either explicitly or implicitly deny artificial insemination services to unmarried women (U.S. Congress, OTA, 1988a, 1988b).

While some may deplore this practice, the fact that unmarried persons are not considered a "suspect" class in constitutional jurisprudence (i.e., they are not considered a class in need of special protection from discriminatory legislation because they are fully able to use the political system to protect their interests), means that such discriminatory practices are largely immune to constitutional challenge as an abridgment of their right to equal protection of the laws. Unless procreation, and specifically the use of artificial insemination, is viewed as a fundamental right, such persons will be limited to challenges under state and federal civil rights statutes in their pursuit of equal access to these technologies.

To the extent that the right to procreate implies a right to create a family, constitutional law from the nineteenth century remains unchallenged in its support for criminalization of family forms, such as polygamy, that fly in the face of Western European tradition. While there have been twentieth-century cases in support of broadening the definition of "family," there has not yet been any case in which the right to marry is extended beyond a heterosexual couple. Thus, whatever the right to privacy entails, it does not appear to guar-

antee the right to form familial relationships that achieve the same legal recognition as that bestowed by marriage.

Generally, current interpretations of constitutional law appear to support the assertion that for married couples there is a right to privacy embedded in the wording and history of the constitution and that such privacy extends to reproductive decision making free from unwarranted governmental intrusion. While case law suggests that individuals are entitled to this privacy in equal measure, judicial hostility to claims of a right by homosexuals to marry or engage in sexual activity (*Bowers v. Hardwick*, 1986), by minors to have unrestricted access to abortion (*Hodgeson v. Minnesota*, 1990), and by physicians to give full information concerning abortion (*Rust v. Sullivan*, 1991) suggest limitations on Supreme Court extension of this right.

Indeed, much of the state activity concerning contract motherhood has been directed at protecting the children conceived through these arrangements. In the event a surrogate changes her mind, a custody dispute can break out between the birth mother and the genetic father. Reluctant to extend parental status to the adopting mother without terminating the parental status of the birth mother, but also determined to see the child placed in the safest home, courts have been in a quandary. Most often the solution has been to refuse to use the contract as the basis for a custody decision, and instead to rely on traditional family notions of child welfare. Next, courts have generally refused to terminate the birth mother's status as a presumptive legal parent. But despite these findings, most courts also award custody to the genetic father and his wife, as it is this couple who is usually better able financially and socially to convince the court that they can provide a secure home for the baby (U.S. Congress, OTA, 1988b; McLean, 1992).

Other concerns regarding contract motherhood

Another state interest in surrogacy stems from the fact that the contracts typically entail promises by the contract mother to refrain from certain behaviors such as drinking, smoking, or the use of illicit drugs, as well as affirmative promises to follow prescribed prenatal care regimes and to undergo prenatal testing for fetal health. Enforcing such contract promises raises constitutional issues, requiring a relinquishment of significant autonomy on the part of the contract mother. This is particularly true with regard to promises to follow prescribed medical care, which may entail submission to invasive tests and even surgery, in the case of cesarean sections.

Surrogacy also raises the specter that the hiring couple might gain what amounts to a property interest in the body of the contract mother. This is particularly true where gestational surrogacy is employed, and the child the contract mother is carrying is genetically related to the hiring parents but not to her. At least one court has been known to issue a "prenatal adoption" order, in which the hiring husband and wife were declared the legal parents of the fetus still within the gestational mother's body (*Smith* v. *Jones*, 1988). In such a case, the hiring parents would have a legally recognized interest in the development of the fetus. Indeed, as parents they might have a legal duty to protect the fetus from harm, as has been confirmed by cases that hold pregnant women criminally liable for behaviors that threaten fetal health. How to protect fetuses while not compromising the physical integrity and legal autonomy of the gestational mother poses a significant constitutional challenge.

Gestational surrogacy also raises fundamental questions about the definition of parenthood, particularly of motherhood. While the law has consistently given preference to biological parents over nonbiological parents, with specific exceptions carved out for adoption and AID, it has never before been forced to consider the definition of "biological." As of the mid-1990s, only one state has considered the problem. In California, a dispute developed between a couple (the Calverts) whose gametes had been used to conceive a child who was subsequently brought to term by a hired gestational contract mother named Anna Johnson. The trial and appellate courts both concluded that the genetic relationship, which defines "natural" parent for men, would define the "natural" parent for women. The two lower courts specifically rejected the notion that gestation is a biological relationship formed by the indisputable fusing of maternal and fetal well-being during the nine months of pregnancy that could equally well form the basis for defining the "natural" mother.

California's lower court decisions in *Johnson* v. *Calvert* (1991), stating that a gestational mother is no more than a foster parent to her own child, are almost without precedent worldwide. Only Israel, bound by unique aspects of religious identity law, has adopted a genetic definition of motherhood. Every other country that has examined the problem—including the United Kingdom, Germany, Switzerland, Bulgaria, and even South Africa with its race-conscious legal structure—has concluded that the woman who gives birth is the child's mother.

The California Supreme Court's 1993 opinion on *Johnson* v. *Calvert* declined to find either the genetic or the gestational mother to be the definitive "natural" parent. Instead, it chose to view either relationship as a presumptive form of natural parenthood. Then it specifically declined the invitation to have the law reflect what had actually happened, that is, the birth of a child

with two biological mothers, one gestational and the other genetic. Agreeing that acknowledging more than one natural mother would be, as the trial court stated, a "recipe for crazymaking," the California Supreme Court said that whichever of the two biologically related women had been the intended mother would then be declared the "natural" mother. It continued by stating that in the event that the gestational and genetic mothers are not the same person, and that the intended mother is neither the genetic nor gestational parent, she would nonetheless be considered the "natural" mother. Thus the court avoided what is at base the most interesting question raised by the use of reproductive technologies: the possibility of declaring more than one woman to be a "natural" parent of a child. To do so, of course, would require escaping the confines of the heterosexual couple as the paradigm for a family and acknowledging that some people become parents by virtue of genetic connection, others by gestational connection, and still others by contract—whether a marital contract with a genetic or gestational parent, or a reproductive technology contract that creates relationships with children conceived with donor gametes or carried to term by contract mothers.

What is the state interest in access to quality services?

A final and overarching area of state interest lies in consumer access and protection. Only a handful of states have legislation mandating insurance coverage for the most expensive of these technologies, IVF. Those states, including Arkansas, Hawaii, Maryland, Massachusetts, Texas, and Wisconsin, have responded to political pressure from organized medicine as well as from infertility support groups. But no state has yet asserted that insurance coverage is required by virtue of the fact that procreation is a fundamental right that may, for some people, be exercised only when using an expensive technology. Indeed, in the context of abortion services, the Supreme Court has made clear that states may forbid Medicaid or other public funding of such services, although they are clearly linked to the exercise of a fundamental right. In fact, the *Webster* decision upheld a state prohibition on the use of public facilities for abortion services, even when no public funds are used.

Where IVF and other reproductive technology services are being provided, however, the state may well choose to regulate them for the sake of protecting patients from unscrupulous practices. These may include misleading advertising, inadequate facilities, insufficiently trained personnel, and negligent screening of gamete donors for genetic and infectious diseases that might be transmitted to recipients. Even in the exercise of a fundamental right, the state may enforce regulations designed to protect the patient.

Another consumer issue involves the regulation of commercialization of reproductive technologies. Although sperm donation has continued apace in countries where no payment is permitted, most commentators agree that the availability of donor gametes and contract mothers in the United States would be severely reduced if commercialization were prohibited. Nonetheless, even when viewing access to reproductive technologies as an exercise of freedom to procreate, several state courts have concluded that there is ample state authority to prohibit commercialization (*Doe* v. *Kelley*, 1981; *Baby M*, 1988). The basis for this conclusion can vary. One line of argument, focusing on surrogacy, characterizes it either as baby-selling or the sale of parental rights, both of which traditionally have been forbidden despite significant libertarian arguments in favor of free markets for both. These prohibitions on selling children or parental rights would easily extend to prohibitions on the sale of embryos, if embryos are characterized as children. Prohibitions on the sale of semen and ova probably could be justified on the same basis as the current prohibitions on organ sales, despite the same line of libertarian arguments.

Other arguments in favor of prohibiting commercialization focus on the effect such activities have on public morals, on the creation of property interests in the bodies of others, and on the fear that the creation of an industry surrounding the sale of gametes, embryos, and reproductive services will create a class of professional breeders. A 1987 survey of surrogacy brokers by the OTA revealed significant discrepancies in economic and educational backgrounds of those who hire contract mothers and those who work as contract mothers (U.S. Congress, OTA, 1988a), leading to the conclusion that the two groups would be unlikely to wield equal bargaining power during the preconception contract negotiations or during postbirth custody disputes.

All of these arguments would probably fail if subjected to the strict scrutiny brought to bear on state interference with a fundamental right. But the reluctance of U.S. courts to view commercialization of reproductive services as an expression of procreative freedom reduces the degree of scrutiny to which state restrictions are subjected. Any rational state purpose will suffice if the restriction interferes with a privilege rather than a fundamental right.

Conclusion

The legal and regulatory issues surrounding reproductive technologies concern the ability of a government to ban or restrict noncoital reproduction because it may harm embryos, children, consumers, or public morals. Where governments choose not to ban the practice, they may wish to regulate it, for example, by limiting what types of prospective parents may use it, which adults will be related to the resulting children, and what kinds of ancillary practices—such as research or commercialization—will be permitted. In the United States, the details of such regulation are a function of state legislation and the resolution of novel cases by the courts. But the federal Constitution places significant limits on how far such legislation or judicial lawmaking may interfere with the opportunity of individuals to exercise procreative choice.

R. ALTA CHARO

Directly related to this article are the INTRODUCTION *and other articles in this entry:* SEX SELECTION; ARTIFICIAL INSEMINATION; IN VITRO FERTILIZATION AND EMBRYO TRANSFER; SURROGACY; CRYOPRESERVATION OF SPERM, OVA, AND EMBRYOS; *and* ETHICAL ISSUES. *For a further discussion of topics mentioned in this article, see the entries* ABORTION; ADOPTION; CHILDREN, *article on* CHILD CUSTODY; CONFIDENTIALITY; FETUS; LAW AND BIOETHICS; LIFE; LIFESTYLES AND PUBLIC HEALTH; MARRIAGE AND OTHER DOMESTIC PARTNERSHIPS; MATERNAL–FETAL RELATIONSHIP; PRIVACY IN HEALTH CARE; RIGHTS; *and* WOMEN, *article on* HEALTH-CARE ISSUES. *For a discussion of related ideas, see the entries* FREEDOM AND COERCION; *and* PATERNALISM. *Other relevant material may be found under the entries* FAMILY; FERTILITY CONTROL; EUGENICS; *and* HEALTH-CARE RESOURCES, ALLOCATION OF, *article on* MICROALLOCATION.

Bibliography

Baby M, In re. 1988. 109 N.J. 396, 537 A.2d 1227.

Bowers v. *Hardwick.* 1986. 106 S. Ct. 2841.

BROCK, DAN W. 1992. "Fertility, Contraception, and Reproductive Freedom." Presented at the Meeting on Women, Equality, and Reproductive Technology, United Nations University, World Institute for Development and Economic Research, Helsinki, Finland, August 2–6.

CAPRON, ALEXANDER MORGAN. 1987. "So Quick Bright Things Come to Confusion." *American Journal of Law and Medicine* 13, nos. 2–3:169–187.

CHARO, R. ALTA. 1990. "Legislative Alternatives for Surrogate Mothering." *Journal of Law, Medicine, and Health Care* 17, no. 1:93–114.

Davis v. *Davis.* 1992. 842 S.W.2d 588 (Tenn.).

Doe v. *Kelley,* 1981. 106 Mich. App. 169.

Eisenstadt v. *Baird.* 1972. 92 S. Ct. 1029.

Griswold v. *Connecticut.* 1965. 381 U.S. 479, 483.

HANNA, KATHI E., ed. 1991. *Biomedical Politics.* Washington, D.C.: National Academy Press.

HILL, JOHN L. 1991. "What Does It Mean to be a 'Parent'? The Claims of Biology as the Basis for Parental Rights." *New York University Law Review* 66, no. 2:353–420.

Hodgeson v. Minnesota. 1990. 110 S. Ct. 2926.

Johnson v. Calvert. 1991. 851 P.2d 776 (Cal. Sup. Ct.); 12 Cal.App.4th 977 (1993).

JOYCE, ROBERT E. 1988. "Personhood and the Conception Event." In *What Is a Person?* pp. 199–211. Edited by Michael F. Goodman. Clifton, N.J.: Humana.

KNOPPERS, BARTHA M., and LEBRIS, SONIA. 1991. "Recent Advances in Medically Assisted Conception: Legal, Ethical and Social Issues." *American Journal of Law and Medicine* 17, no. 4:329–361.

LIPPMAN, ABBY. 1991. "Prenatal Genetic Testing and Screening: Constructing Needs and Reinforcing Inequities." *American Journal of Law and Medicine* 17, nos. 1–2: 15–50.

LIU, ATHENA. 1991. *Artificial Reproduction and Reproductive Rights.* Brookfield, Vt.: Dartmouth.

MCLEAN, SHEILA, ed. 1992. *Law Reform and Human Reproduction.* Brookfield, Vt.: Dartmouth.

Meyer v. Nebraska. 1923. 262 U.S. 390, 401, 402.

Moore v. City of East Cleveland, Ohio. 1977. 431 U.S. 494.

OVERALL, CHRISTINE. 1987. *Ethics and Human Reproduction: A Feminist Analysis.* Boston: Allen & Unwin.

Planned Parenthood v. Casey. 1992. 112 S. Ct. 2791.

Reynolds v. United States. 1879. 98 U.S. 113.

ROBERTSON, JOHN A. 1989. "Technology and Motherhood: Legal and Ethical Issues in Human Egg Donation." *Case Western Reserve Law Review* 39, no. 1:1–38.

———. 1990. "In the Beginning: The Legal Status of Early Embryos." *Virginia Law Review* 76, no. 3:437–517.

Roe v. Wade. 1973. 410 U.S. 113.

Rust v. Sullivan. 1991. 111 S. Ct. 1759.

SCHULTZ, MARJORIE MAGUIRE. 1990. "Reproductive Technology and Intent-Based Parenthood: An Opportunity for Gender Neutrality." *Wisconsin Law Review* 1990, no. 2:297–398.

Skinner v. Oklahoma ex rel. Williamson. 1942. 62 S. Ct. 1110.

Smith & Smith v. Jones & Jones. 1986. 85-532014 DZ, Detroit, Mich. (3rd Cir.).

TOOLEY, MICHAEL. 1984. "In Defense of Abortion and Infanticide." In *The Problem of Abortion,* 2d ed., pp. 120–134. Edited by Joel Feinberg. Belmont, Calif.: Wadsworth.

U.S. CONGRESS. OFFICE OF TECHNOLOGY ASSESSMENT (OTA). 1988a. *Artificial Insemination: Practice in the U.S.: Summary of a 1987 Survey.* Washington, D.C.: Author.

———. 1988b. *Infertility: Medical and Social Choices.* Washington, D.C.: Author.

WAGNER, WILLIAM J. 1990. "The Contractual Reallocation of Procreative Resources and Parental Rights: The Natural Endowment Critique." *Case Western Reserve Law Review* 41, no 1:1–202.

Webster v. Reproductive Services. 1989. 109 S. Ct. 3040.

YOON, MIMI. 1990. "The Uniform Status of Children of Assisted Conception Act: Does It Protect the Best Interests of the Child in a Surrogate Arrangement?" *American Journal of Law and Medicine* 16, no. 4:525–553.

RESEARCH, BEHAVIORAL AND BIOMEDICAL

See INFORMED CONSENT, *article on* CONSENT ISSUES IN HUMAN RESEARCH; RESEARCH, HUMAN: HISTORICAL ASPECTS; RESEARCH METHODOLOGY; *and* RESEARCH POLICY.

RESEARCH, HUMAN: HISTORICAL ASPECTS

In Western civilization, the idea of human experimentation, of evaluating the efficacy of a new drug or procedure by outcomes, is an ancient one. It is discussed in the writings of Greek and Roman physicians and in Arab medical treatises. Scholars like Avicenna (980–1037) insisted that "the experimentation must be done with the human body, for testing a drug on a lion or a horse might not prove anything about its effect on man" (Bull, 1959, p. 221). But records of how often ancient physicians conducted experiments, with what agents, and on which subjects, are very thin. The most frequently cited cases involve testing the efficacy of poisons on condemned prisoners, but the extent to which other human research was carried on remains obscure.

Experimentation was frequent enough to inspire a discussion of the ethical maxims that should guide would-be investigators. Moses Maimonides (1135–1204), the noted Jewish physician and philosopher, instructed colleagues always to treat patients as ends in themselves, not as means for learning new truths. Roger Bacon (1214–1294) excused the inconsistencies in therapeutic practices on the following grounds:

> It is exceedingly difficult and dangerous to perform operations on the human body. The operative and practical sciences which do their work on insensate bodies can multiply their experiments till they get rid of deficiency and errors, but a physician cannot do this because of the nobility of the material in which he works; for that body demands that no error be made in operating upon it, and so experience [the experimental method] is so difficult in medicine. (quoted in Bull, 1959, p. 222)

Human experimentation in early modern Western history

Human experimentation made its first significant impact on medical practice through the work of the English country physician Edward Jenner (1749–1823). Observing that dairy farmers who had contracted the pox from swine or cows seemed to be immune to the more virulent smallpox, Jenner set out to retrieve material from their pustules, inject the material into another person, and see whether the recipient could then resist challenges from smallpox materials. The procedure promised to be less dangerous than the more standard one of inoculating people with small amounts of smallpox that had been introduced into Europe and America from the Ottoman Empire in the first half of the eighteenth century.

In November 1789, Jenner inoculated his son, then about a year old, with swinepox. When this intervention proved ineffective against a challenge of smallpox, Jenner tried cowpox several months later with another subject. As he recalled: "The more accurately to observe the progress of the infection, I selected a healthy boy, about eight years old, for the purpose of inoculation for the cow-pox. The matter . . . was inserted . . . into the arm of the boy by means of two incisions" (Jenner, 1798, pp. 164–165). A week later Jenner injected him with smallpox, and noted that he evinced no reaction. The cowpox had rendered him immune to smallpox. One cannot know whether the boy was a willing or unwilling subject or how much he understood of the experiment. But this was not an interaction between strangers. The boy was from the neighborhood, Mr. Jenner was a gentleman of standing, and the experiment did have potential therapeutic benefit for the subject.

For most of the nineteenth century, human experimentation throughout western Europe and the United States was a cottage industry, with individual physicians trying out one or another remedy on neighbors or relatives or on themselves. One German physician, Johann Jorg (1779–1856), swallowed varying doses of seventeen different drugs in order to analyze their effects. Another, Sir James Young Simpson (1811–1870), an Edinburgh obstetrician who was searching for an anesthesia superior to ether, in November 1847 inhaled chloroform and awoke to find himself lying flat on the floor (Howard-Jones, 1982). Perhaps the most extraordinary self-experiment was conducted by Werner Forssman. In 1929 he passed a catheter, guided by radiography, into the right ventricle of his heart, thereby demonstrating the feasibility and the safety of the procedure.

The most unusual nineteenth-century human experiment was conducted by the American physician William Beaumont (1785–1853) on Alexis St. Martin. A stomach wound suffered by St. Martin healed in such a way as to leave Beaumont access to the stomach and the opportunity to study the action of gastric juices. To carry on this research, which was very important to the new field of physiology, Beaumont had St. Martin sign an agreement, not so much a consent form as an apprenticeship contract. Under its terms, St. Martin bound himself to "serve, abide, and continue with the said William Beaumont . . . [as] his covenant servant," and in return for board, lodging, and $150 a year, he agreed "to assist and promote by all means in his power such phil-

osophical or medical experiments as the said William shall direct or cause to be made on or in the stomach of him" (Beaumont, 1980, pp. xii–xiii).

The most brilliant human experiments of the nineteenth century were conducted by Louis Pasteur (1822–1895), who demonstrated an acute sensitivity to the ethics of his investigations. Even as he conducted his animal research to identify an antidote to rabies, he worried about the time when it would be necessary to test the product on a human being. "I have already several cases of dogs immunized after rabic bites," he wrote in 1884. "I take two dogs: I have them bitten by a mad dog. I vaccinate the one and I leave the other without treatment. The latter dies of rabies: the former withstands it." Nevertheless, Pasteur continued, "I have not yet dared to attempt anything on man, in spite of my confidence in the result. . . . I must wait first till I have got a whole crowd of successful results on animals. . . . But, however I should multiply my cases of protection of dogs, I think that my hand will shake when I have to go on to man" (Vallery-Radot, 1926, pp. 404–405).

The fateful moment came some nine months later when his help was sought by a mother whose nine-year-old son, Joseph Meister, had just been severely bitten by what was probably a mad dog. Pasteur agonized as to whether to carry out what would be the first human trial of his rabies inoculation. He consulted with two medical colleagues, had them examine the boy, and at their urging and on the grounds that "the death of the child appeared inevitable, I resolved, though not without great anxiety, to try the method which had proved consistently successful on the dogs." With great anxiety he administered twelve inoculations to the boy, and only weeks later did he become confident of the efficacy of his approach and the "future health of Joseph Meister" (Vallery-Radot, 1926, pp. 414–417).

Claude Bernard (1813–1878), professor of medicine at the College of France, not only conducted groundbreaking research in physiology, but also composed an astute treatise on the methods and ethics of experimentation. "Morals do not forbid making experiments on one's neighbor or one's self," Bernard argued in 1865. Rather, "the principle of medical and surgical morality consists in never performing on man an experiment which might be harmful to him to any extent, even though the result might be highly advantageous to science, i.e., to the health of others." To be sure, Bernard did allow some exceptions; he sanctioned experimentation on dying patients and on criminals about to be executed, on the grounds that "they involve no suffering of harm to the subject of the experiment." But he made clear that scientific progress did not justify violating the well-being of any individual (Bernard, 1927, p. 101).

Anglo-American common law recognized both the vital role of human experimentation and the need for physicians to obtain the patient's consent. As one English commentator explained in 1830: "By experiments we are not to be understood as speaking of the wild and dangerous practices of rash and ignorant practitioners . . . but of deliberate acts of men from considerable knowledge and undoubted talent, differing from those prescribed by the ordinary rules of practice, for which they have good reason . . . to believe will be attended with benefit to the patient, although the novelty of the undertaking does not leave the result altogether free of doubt." The researcher who had the subject's consent was "answerable neither in damages to the individual, nor on a criminal proceeding. But if the practitioner performs his experiment without giving such information to, and obtaining the consent of this patient, he is liable to compensate in damages any injury which may arise from his adopting a new method of treatment" (Howard-Jones, 1982, p. 1430). In short, the law distinguished carefully between quackery and innovation, and—provided the investigator had the subject's agreement—research was a legitimate and protected activity.

With the new understanding of germ theory in the 1890s and the growing professionalization of medical training in the next several decades, the amount of human experimentation increased and the intimate link between investigator and subject weakened. Typically, physicians administered a new drug to a group of hospitalized patients and compared their rates of recovery with past rates or with those of other patients who did not have the drug. (Truly random and blinded clinical trials, wherein a variety of patient characteristics were carefully matched and where researchers were kept purposely ignorant of which patient received the new drug, did not come into practice until the 1950s.) Thus, German physicians tested antidiphtheria serum on thirty hospitalized patients and reported that only six died, compared to the previous year at the same hospital when twenty-one of thirty-two patients died (Bull, 1959). In Canada, Frederick G. Banting and Charles Best experimented with insulin therapy on diabetic patients who faced imminent death, and interpreted their recovery as clear proof of the treatment's efficacy (Bliss, 1982). So too, George R. Minot and William P. Murphy tested the value of liver preparations against pernicious anemia by administering them to forty-five patients in remission and found that they all remained healthy so long as they took the treatment; the normal relapse rate was one-third, and three patients who on their own accord stopped treatment relapsed (Bull, 1959). It is doubtful if many of these subjects were fully informed about the nature of the trial or formally consented to participate. They were, however, likely to be willing subjects since they were in acute distress or danger and the research had therapeutic potential.

As medicine became more scientific, some researchers did skirt the boundaries of ethical behavior in experimentation, making medical progress—rather than the subject's welfare—the goal of the research. Probably the most famous experiment in this zone of ambiguity was the yellow-fever work of Walter Reed (1851–1902). When he began his experiments, mosquitoes had been identified as crucial to transmission but their precise role was unclear. To understand more about the process, Reed began a series of human experiments in which, in time-honored tradition, the members of the research team were the first subjects (Bean, 1982). It soon became apparent that larger numbers of volunteers were needed and no sooner was the decision reached than a soldier happened by. "You still fooling with mosquitoes?" he asked one of the doctors. "Yes," the doctor replied. "Will you take a bite?" "Sure, I ain't scared of 'em," responded the man. And in this way, "the first indubitable case of yellow fever . . . to be produced experimentally" occurred (Bean, 1982, pp. 131, 147).

After one fellow investigator, Jesse William Lazear, died of yellow fever from purposeful bites, the other members, including Reed himself, decided "not to tempt fate by trying any more [infections] upon ourselves." Instead, Reed asked American servicemen to volunteer, and some did. He also recruited Spanish workers, drawing up a contract with them: "The undersigned understands perfectly well that in the case of the development of yellow fever in him, that he endangers his life to a certain extent but it being entirely impossible for him to avoid the infection during his stay on this island he prefers to take the chance of contracting it intentionally in the belief that he will receive . . . the greatest care and most skillful medical service." Volunteers received $100 in gold, and those who actually contracted yellow fever received a bonus of an additional $100, which, in the event of their death, went to their heirs (Bean, 1982, pp. 134, 147). Although twenty-five volunteers became ill, none died.

Reed's contract was a step along the way to more formal arrangements with human subjects, complete with enticements to undertake a hazardous assignment. But the contract was also misleading, distorting in subtle ways the risks and benefits of the research. Yellow fever was said to endanger life only "to a certain extent"; the likelihood that the disease might prove fatal was unmentioned. And on the other hand, the prospect of otherwise contracting yellow fever was presented as an absolute certainty, an exaggeration that aimed to promote recruitment.

Some human experiments in the pre–World War II period in the United States and elsewhere used incompetent and institutionalized populations for their studies. The Russian physician V. V. Smidovich (publishing in 1901 under the pseudonym Vikentii Veresaev) cited more than a dozen experiments, most of them conducted in Germany, in which unknowing patients were inoculated with microorganisms of syphilis and gonorrhea (Veresaev, 1916). George Sternberg, the Surgeon General of the United States in 1895 (and a collaborator of Walter Reed), conducted experiments "upon unvaccinated children in some of the orphan asylums in . . . Brooklyn" (Sternberg and Reed, 1895, pp. 57–69). Alfred Hess and colleagues deliberately withheld orange juice from infants at the Hebrew Infant Asylum of New York City until they developed symptoms of scurvy (Lederer, 1992). In 1937, when Joseph Stokes of the Department of Pediatrics at the University of Pennsylvania School of Medicine sought to analyze the effects of "intramuscular vaccination of human beings . . . with active virus of human influenza," he used as his study population the residents of two large state institutions for the retarded (Stokes et al., 1937, pp. 237–243). There are also many examples of investigators using prisoners as research subjects. In 1914, for example, Joseph Goldwater and G. H. Wheeler of the U.S. Public Health Service (PHS) conducted experiments to understand the causes of pellagra on convicts in Mississippi prisons.

One of the few instances of an individual investigator being taken to task for the ethics of his research involved Hideyo Noguchi (1876–1928) of the Rockefeller Institute for Medical Research. He was investigating whether a substance he called luetin, an extract from the causative agent of syphilis, could be used to diagnose syphilis; through the cooperation of fifteen New York physicians, he used 400 subjects, most of them inmates in mental hospitals and orphan asylums and patients in public hospitals. Before administering luetin to them, Noguchi and some of the physicians did first test the material on themselves, with no ill effects. But no one, including Noguchi, informed the subjects about the experiment or obtained their permission to do the tests.

Noguchi's work was actively criticized by the most vocal opponents of human experimentation during those years, the antivivisectionists. They were convinced that a disregard for the welfare of animals would inevitably promote a disregard for the welfare of humans. As one of them phrased it: "Are the helpless people in our hospitals and asylums to be treated as so much material for scientific experimentation, irrespective of age or consent?" (Lederer, 1985, p. 336). Despite their opposition, such experiments as Noguchi's did not lead to prosecutions, corrective legislation, or formal professional codes. The profession and the wider public were not especially concerned with the issue, perhaps because the practice was still relatively uncommon and mostly affected disadvantaged populations.

Research at war

The transforming event in the conduct of human experimentation in the United States was World War II. Between 1941 and 1945, practically every aspect of American research with human subjects changed. What were once occasional and ad hoc efforts by individual practitioners now became well-coordinated, extensive, federally funded team ventures. At the same time, medical experiments that once had the aim of benefiting their subjects were now frequently superseded by experiments whose aim was to benefit others, specifically soldiers who were vulnerable to the disease. Further, researchers and subjects were far more likely to be strangers to each other, with no sense of shared purpose or objective. Finally, and perhaps most importantly, the common understanding that experimentation required the agreement of the subjects, however casual the request or general the approval, was superseded by a sense of urgency so strong that it paid scant attention to the issue of consent.

In the summer of 1941, President Franklin Roosevelt created the Office of Scientific Research and Development (OSRD) to oversee the work of two parallel committees, one devoted to weapons research, the other—the Committee on Medical Research (CMR)—to combat the health problems that threatened the combat efficiency of American soldiers. Thus began what one participant called "a novel experiment in American medicine, for planned and coordinated medical research had never been essayed on such a scale" (Keefer, 1969, p. 62). Over the course of World War II, the CMR recommended some 600 research proposals, many of them involving human subjects, to the OSRD for funding. The OSRD, in turn, contracted with investigators at some 135 universities, hospitals, research institutes, and industrial firms. The accomplishments of the CMR effort required two volumes to summarize (the title, *Advances in Military Medicine,* did not do justice to the scope of the investigations); and the list of publications that resulted from its grants took up seventy-five pages (Andrus, 1948). All told, the CMR expended some $25 million. In fact, the work of the CMR was so important that it supplied not only the organizational model but also the intellectual justification for creating, in the postwar period, the National Institutes of Health.

The CMR's major concerns were dysentery, influenza, malaria, wounds, venereal diseases, and physical hardships (including sleep deprivation and exposure to frigid temperatures). To create effective antidotes required skill, luck, and numerous trials with human subjects, and the CMR oversaw the effort with extraordinary diligence. Dysentery, for example, proliferated under the filth and deprivation endemic to battlefield conditions, and no effective inoculations or antidotes existed. With CMR support, investigators undertook laboratory research and then, requiring sites for testing their therapies, turned to custodial institutions where dysentery was often rampant (OSRD, 1944b). Among the most important subjects for the dysentery research were the residents of the Ohio Soldiers and Sailors Orphanage in Xenia, Ohio; the Dixon, Illinois, institution for the retarded; and the New Jersey State Colony for the Feeble-Minded. The residents were injected with experimental vaccines or potentially therapeutic agents, some of which produced a degree of protection against the bacteria but, as evidenced by fever and soreness, were too toxic for common use.

Probably the most pressing medical problem the CMR faced immediately after Pearl Harbor was malaria, "an enemy even more to be feared than the Japanese" (Andrus, 1948, vol. 1, p. xlix). Not only was the disease debilitating and deadly, but the Japanese controlled the supply of quinine, one of the few known effective antidotes. Since malaria was not readily found in the United States, researchers chose to infect residents of state mental hospitals and prisons. A sixty-bed clinical unit was established at the Manteno, Illinois, State Hospital; the subjects were psychotic, backward patients who were purposefully infected with malaria through blood transfusions and then given antimalarial therapies (OSRD, 1944a). With the cooperation of the commissioner of corrections of Illinois and the warden at Stateville Prison (better known as Joliet), one floor of the prison hospital was turned over to the University of Chicago to carry out malaria research and some 500 inmates volunteered to act as subjects. Whether these prisoners were truly capable of consenting to research was not addressed by the researchers, the CMR, or prison officials. Almost all the press commentary was congratulatory, praising the wonderful contributions the inmates were making to the war effort.

In similar fashion, the CMR supported teams that tested anti-influenza preparations on residents of state facilities for the retarded (Pennhurst, Pennsylvania) and the mentally ill (Michigan's Ypsilanti State Hospital). The investigators administered the vaccine to the residents and then, three or six months later, purposefully infected them with influenza (Henle, 1946). When a few of the preparations appeared to provide protection, the Office of the Surgeon General of the U.S. Army arranged for the vaccine to be tested by enrollees in the Army Specialized Training Program at eight universities and a ninth unit made up of students from five New York medical and dental colleges.

Because the first widespread use of human subjects in medical research for nontherapeutic purposes occurred under wartime conditions, attention to the consent of the subject appeared less relevant. At a time when the social value attached to consent gave way before the necessity of a military draft and obedience to commanders' orders, medical researchers did not hesitate to use the incompetent as subjects of human experimentation. One part of the war machine conscripted a soldier, another part conscripted a human subject, and the same principles held for both. In effect, wartime promoted teleological as opposed to deontological ethics;

"the greatest good for the greatest number" was the most compelling precept to justify sending some men to be killed so that others might live. This same ethic seemed to justify using institutionalized retarded or mentally ill persons in human research.

Human research and the war against disease

The two decades following the close of World War II witnessed an extraordinary expansion of human experimentation in medical research. Long after peace returned, many of the investigators continued to follow wartime rules, this time thinking in terms of the Cold War and the war against disease. The utilitarian justifications that had flourished under conditions of combat and conscription persisted, in disregard of principles of consent and voluntary participation.

The driving force in post–World War II research in the United States was the National Institutes of Health (NIH). Created in 1930 as an outgrowth of the research laboratory of the U.S. Public Health Service, the NIH assumed its extraordinary prominence as the successor agency to the Committee on Medical Research (Swain, 1962). In 1945, its appropriations totaled $700,000. By 1955, the figure had climbed to $36 million, and by 1970, $1.5 billion, a sum that allowed it to award some 11,000 grants, about one-third requiring experiments on humans. In expending these funds, the NIH administered an intramural research program at its own Clinical Center, along with an extramural program that funded outside investigators.

The Clinical Center assured its subjects that it put their well-being first. "The welfare of the patient takes precedence over every other consideration" (NIH, 1953a). In 1954, a Clinical Research Committee was established to develop principles and to deal with problems that might arise in research with normal, healthy volunteers. Still, the relationship between investigator and subject was casual to a fault, leaving it up to the investigator to decide what information, if any, was to be shared with the subject. Generally, the researchers did not divulge very much information, fearful that they would discourage patients from participating. No formal policies or procedures applied to researchers working in other institutions on studies supported by NIH funds.

The laxity of procedural protections pointed to the enormous intellectual and emotional investment in research and to the conviction that the laboratory would yield answers to the mysteries of disease. Indeed, this faith was so great that the NIH would not establish guidelines to govern the extramural research it supported. By 1965, the extramural program was the single most important source of research grants for universities and medical schools, by the NIH's own estimate, supporting between 1,500 and 2,000 research projects involving human research. Nevertheless, grant provisions included no stipulations about the ethical conduct of human experimentation and the universities did not fill the gap. In the early 1960s, only nine of fifty-two American departments of medicine had a formal procedure for approving research involving human subjects and only five more indicated that they favored this approach or planned to institute such procedures (Frankel, 1972).

One might have expected much greater attention to the ethics of human experimentation in the immediate postwar period in light of the shadow cast by the trial of the German doctors at Nuremberg. The atrocities that the Nazis committed—putting subjects to death by long immersion in subfreezing water, deprivation of oxygen to learn the limits of bodily endurance, or deliberate infection by lethal organisms in order to study the effects of drugs and vaccines—might have sparked a commitment in the United States to a more rigorous regulation of research. (Japanese physicians also conducted experiments on prisoners of war and captive populations, but their research was never subjected to the same judicial scrutiny.) So too, the American research efforts during the war might have raised questions of their own and stimulated closer oversight.

The Nuremberg Code of 1946 itself might have served as a model for American guidelines on research with human subjects. Its provisions certainly were relevant to the medical research conducted in the United States. "The voluntary consent of the human subject is absolutely essential," the code declared. "This means that the person involved should have legal capacity to give consent." By this principle, the mentally disabled and children were not suitable subjects for research—a principle that American researchers did not respect. Moreover, according to the Nuremberg Code, the research subject "should be so situated as to be able to exercise free power of choice" (Germany [Territory Under . . .], 1947, p. 181), which rendered at least questionable the American practice of using prisoners as research subjects. The Nuremberg Code also stated that human subjects "should have sufficient knowledge and comprehension of the elements of the subject matter involved as to make an understanding and enlightened decision" (Germany [Territory Under . . .], 1947, p. 181), thus ruling out the American practice of using the mentally disabled as subjects.

Nevertheless, with a few exceptions, neither the Code nor these specific practices received sustained analysis before the early 1970s. Only a handful of articles in medical or popular journals addressed the relevance of Nuremberg for the ethics of human experimentation in the United States. Perhaps this silence reflected an eagerness to repress the memory of the atrocities. More likely, the events described at Nuremberg were not perceived by most Americans as relevant to their own practices. From their perspective, the Code had nothing to do with science and everything to do

with Nazis. The guilty parties were seen less as doctors than as Hitler's henchmen (Proctor, 1988).

In the period 1945–1965, several American as well as world medical organizations did produce guidelines for human experimentation that expanded upon the Nuremberg Code. Most of these efforts, however, commanded little attention and had minimal impact on institutional practices whether in Europe or in the United States (Ladimer and Newman, 1962). The American Medical Association, for example, framed a research code that called for the voluntary consent of the human subject, but it said nothing about what information the researchers were obliged to share, whether it was ethical to conduct research on incompetent patients, or how the research process should be monitored (Requirements for Experiments on Human Beings, 1946). In general, investigators could do as they wished in the laboratory, limited only by what their consciences defined as proper conduct and by broad, generally unsanctioned statements of ethical principle.

The World Medical Association in 1964 issued the Helsinki Declaration, stating general principles for human experimentation, and has revised that document four times. The declaration is modeled on the Nuremberg Code, requiring qualified investigators and the consent of subjects. The 1975 revision recommended review of research by an independent committee (Annas and Grodin, 1992).

How researchers exercised discretion was the subject of a groundbreaking article by Henry Beecher, professor of anesthesia at Harvard Medical School, published in June 1966 in the *New England Journal of Medicine*. His analysis, "Ethics and Clinical Research," contained brief descriptions of twenty-two examples of investigators who risked "the health or the life of their subjects," without informing them of the dangers or obtaining their permission. In one case, investigators purposefully withheld penicillin from servicemen with streptococcal infections in order to study alternative means for preventing complications. The men were totally unaware that they were part of an experiment, let alone at risk of contracting rheumatic fever, which twenty-five of them did. Beecher's conclusion was that "unethical or questionably ethical procedures are not uncommon" among researchers. Although he did not provide footnotes for the examples or name the investigators, he did note that "the troubling practices" came from "leading medical schools, university hospitals, private hospitals, governmental military departments . . . government institutes (the National Institutes of Health), Veterans Administration Hospitals, and industry" (Beecher, 1966).

Two of the cases that Beecher cited were especially important in provoking public indignation over the conduct of human research. One case involved investigators who fed live hepatitis virus to the residents of Willowbrook, a New York State institution for the retarded, in order to study the etiology of the disease and attempt to create a protective vaccine against it. The other case involved physicians injecting live cancer cells into twenty-two elderly and senile hospitalized patients at the Brooklyn Jewish Chronic Disease hospital without telling them that the cells were cancerous, in order to study the body's immunological responses.

Another case that sparked fierce public and political reactions in the early 1970s was the Tuskegee research of the U.S. Public Health Service. Its investigators had been visiting Macon County, Alabama, since the mid-1930s to examine, but not to treat, a group of blacks who were suffering from secondary syphilis. Whatever rationalizations the PHS could muster for not treating blacks in the 1930s, when treatment was of questionable efficacy and very complicated to administer, it could hardly defend instructing draft boards not to conscript the subjects for fear that they might receive treatment in the army. Worse yet, it could not justify its unwillingness to give the subjects a trial of penicillin after 1945 (Jones, 1981).

During the 1950s and 1960s, not only individual investigators but government agencies conducted research that often ignored the consent of the subjects and placed some of them at risk. Many of these projects involved the testing of radiation on humans. Part of the motivation was to better understand human physiology; even more important, however, was the aim of bolstering the national defense by learning about the possible impact of radiation on fighting forces. Accordingly, inmates at the Oregon State Prison were subjects in experiments to examine the effects on sperm production of exposing their testicles to X rays. Although the prisoners were told some of the risks, they were not informed that the radiation might cause cancer. So too, terminally ill patients at the Cincinnati General Hospital underwent whole-body radiation, in research supported by the U.S. Department of Defense, not so much to measure its effects against cancer but to learn about the dangers radiation posed to military personnel. During this period, the Central Intelligence Agency also conducted research on unknowing subjects with drugs and with psychiatric techniques in an effort to improve interrogation and brainwashing methods. It was not until the 1980s that parts of this record became public, and not until 1994 that the full dimensions of these research projects were known.

Regulating human experimentation

The cases cited by Beecher and publicized in the press over the period 1966 to 1973 produced critical changes in policy by the leadership of the NIH and the U.S. Food and Drug Administration (FDA). Both agencies were especially sensitive to congressional pressures and feared that criticisms of researchers' conduct could lead to severe budget cuts. They also recognized that the traditional bedrock of research ethics, the belief that investigators were like physicians and should therefore be trusted to protect the well-being of their subjects, did not hold. To the contrary, there was a conflict of interest between investigator and subject: One wanted knowledge, the other wanted cure or well-being.

Under the press of politics and this new recognition, the NIH and the FDA altered their procedures. The fact that authority was centralized in these two agencies, which were at once subordinate to Congress and superordinate to the research community, guaranteed their ability to impose new regulations. Indeed, this fact helps explain why the regulation of human experimentation came first and more extensively to the United States than to other developed countries (Rothman, 1991).

Accordingly, in February 1966, and then in revised form in July 1966, the NIH promulgated through its parent body, the PHS, guidelines covering all federally funded research involving human experimentation. The order of July 1, 1966, decentralized the regulatory apparatus, assigning "responsibility to the institution receiving the grant for obtaining and keeping documentary evidence of informed patient consent." It then mandated "review of the judgment of the investigator by a committee of institutional associates not directly associated with the project." Finally it defined, albeit very broadly, the standards that were to guide the committee: "This review must address itself to the rights and welfare of the individual, the methods used to obtain informed consent, and the risks and potential benefits of the investigation" (Commission on Health Science and Society, 1968, pp. 211–212). In this way and for the first time, decisions traditionally left to the conscience of individual physicians came under collective surveillance.

The new set of rules was not as intrusive as some investigators feared, or as protective as some advocates preferred. At its core was the superintendence of the peer review committee, known as the Institutional Review Board (IRB), through which fellow researchers approved the investigator's procedures. With the creation of the IRB, the clinical investigator could no longer decide unilaterally whether the planned intervention was ethical, but had to answer formally to colleagues operating under federal guidelines. The events in and around 1966 accomplished what the Nuremberg trials had not: They moved medical experimentation into the public domain and revealed the consequences of leaving decisions about clinical research exclusively to the individual investigator.

The NIH response focused attention more on the review process than on the process of securing informed consent. Although it recognized the importance of the principle of consent, it remained skeptical about the ultimate feasibility of the procedure. Truly informed consent by the subject seemed impossible to achieve ostensibly because laypeople would not be able to understand the risks and benefits inherent in a complex research protocol. In effect, the NIH leadership was unwilling to abandon altogether the notion that doctors should protect patients and to substitute instead a thoroughgoing commitment to the idea that patients could and should protect themselves. Its goal was to ensure that harm was not done to the subjects, not that subjects were given every opportunity and incentive to express their own wishes (Frankel, 1972).

The FDA was also forced to grapple with the problems raised by human experimentation in clinical research. With a self-definition that included a commitment not only to sound scientific research (like the NIH) but to consumer protection as well, the FDA did attempt to expand the prerogatives of the consumer—in this context, the human subject. Rather than emulate the NIH precedent and invigorate peer review, it looked to give new meaning and import to the process of consent.

In the wake of the reactions set off by Beecher's article, the FDA, on August 30, 1966, issued a "Statement on Policy Concerning Consent for the Use of Investigational New Drugs on Humans." Distinguishing between therapeutic and nontherapeutic research, in accord with various international codes like the Helsinki Declaration, it now prohibited all nontherapeutic research unless the subjects gave consent. When the research involved "patients under treatment," and had therapeutic potential, consent was to be obtained except in what the FDA labeled the "exceptional cases," where consent was not feasible or not in the patient's best interest. "Not feasible" meant that the doctor could not communicate with the patient (its example was when the patient was in a coma); and "not in the best interest" meant that consent would "seriously affect the patient's disease status" (its example here was the physician who did not want to divulge a diagnosis of cancer) (Curran, 1969, pp. 558–569).

In addition, the FDA, unlike the NIH, spelled out the meaning of consent. To give consent, the person had to have the ability to exercise choice and to have a "fair explanation" of the procedure, including an understanding of the experiment's purpose and duration, "all inconveniences and hazards reasonably to be expected," what a controlled trial was (and the possibility of the use of placebos), and any existing alternative forms of therapy available (Curran, 1969, pp. 558–569).

The FDA regulations represented a new stage in the balance of authority between researcher and subject. The blanket insistence on consent for all nontherapeu-

tic research would have prohibited many of the World War II experiments and eliminated most of the cases on Beecher's roll. The FDA's definitions of consent went well beyond the vague NIH stipulations, imparting real significance to the process. To be sure, ambiguities remained. The FDA still confused research and treatment, and its clauses governing therapeutic investigations afforded substantial discretion to the doctor-researcher. But authority tilted away from the individual investigator and leaned, instead, toward colleagues and the human subjects themselves.

The publicity given to the abuses in human experimentation, and the idea that a fundamental conflict of interest characterized the relationship between the researcher and the subject, had an extraordinary impact on those outside of medicine, drawing philosophers, lawyers, and social scientists into a deeper concern about ethical issues in medicine. Human experimentation, for example, sparked the interest in medicine of Princeton University's professor of Christian ethics, Paul Ramsey. Ethical problems in medicine "are by no means technical problems on which only the expert (in this case, the physician) can have an opinion," Ramsey declared, and his first case in point was human experimentation. He worried that the thirst for more information was so great that it could lead investigators to violate the sanctity of the person. To counter the threat, Ramsey had two general strategies. The first was to make medical ethics the subject of public discussion. We can no longer "go on assuming that what can be done has to be done or should be. . . . These questions are now completely in the public forum, no longer the province of scientific experts alone" (Ramsey, 1970, p. 1). Second, and more specifically, Ramsey embraced the idea of consent; consent, in his formulation, was to human experimentation what a system of checks and balances was to executive authority, that is, the necessary limitation on the exercise of power. "Man's capacity to become joint adventurers in a common cause makes the consensual relationship possible; man's propensity to overreach his joint adventurer even in a good cause makes consent necessary. . . . No man is good enough to experiment upon another without his consent" (Ramsey, 1970, pp. 5–7).

Commissioning ethics

The U.S. Congress soon joined the growing ranks of those concerned with human experimentation and medical ethics. In 1973, it created the National Commission for the Protection of Human Subjects of Biomedical and Behavioral Research, whose charge was to recommend to federal agencies regulations to protect the rights and welfare of subjects of research. The idea for such a commission was first fueled by an awareness of the awesome power of new medical technologies, but it gained congressional passage in the wake of newly uncovered abuses in human experimentation, most notably the Tuskegee syphilis studies.

The U.S. National Commission for the Protection of Human Subjects was composed of eleven members drawn from "the general public and from individuals in the fields of medicine, law, ethics, theology, biological science, physical science, social science, philosophy, humanities, health administration, government, and public affairs." The length of the roster and the stipulation that no more than five of the members could be researchers indicated how determined Congress was to have human experimentation brought under the scrutiny of outsiders. Senator Edward Kennedy, who chaired the hearings that led to the creation of the commission, repeatedly emphasized this point: Policy had to emanate "not just from the medical profession, but from ethicists, the theologians, philosophers, and many other disciplines." A prominent social scientist, Bernard Barber, predicted, altogether accurately, that the commission "would transform a fundamental moral problem from a condition of relative professional neglect and occasional journalistic scandal to a condition of continuing public and professional visibility and legitimacy. . . . For the proper regulation of the powerful professions of modern society, we need a combination of insiders and outsiders, of professionals and citizens" (Commission on Health Science and Society, 1968, part IV, pp. 1264–1265).

Although the National Commission was temporary rather than permanent, and advisory (to the Secretary of Health, Education, and Welfare), without any enforcement powers of its own, most of its recommendations became regulatory law, tightening still further the governance of human experimentation. It endorsed the supervisory role of the IRBs and successfully recommended special protection for research on such vulnerable populations as prisoners, mentally disabled persons, and children. It recommended that an Ethical Advisory Board be established within the Department of Health and Human Services to deal with difficult cases as they arose. This board was inaugurated in 1977 but expired in 1980, leaving a gap in the commission's plan for oversight of research ethics. However, the Office for Protection from Research Risks at NIH exercised vigilance over institutional compliance with research regulations. Finally, the commission issued the Belmont Report, a statement of the ethical principles that should govern research, namely, respect for autonomy, beneficence, and justice. This document not only had an influence on research ethics but on the emerging discipline of bioethics (U.S. National Commission for the Protection of Human Subjects of Biomedical and Behavioral Research, 1979).

Conclusion

In the United States, and to a growing degree in other developed countries, many of the earlier practices that had raised such troubling ethical considerations have been resolved. Oversight of research has been accomplished without stifling it, and without violating the prerogatives of research subjects. Almost everyone who has served on IRBs, or who has analyzed the transformation that their presence has secured on medical experimentation, will testify to their salutary impact. To be sure, the formal composition and decentralized character of these bodies seem to invite a kind of back-scratching, mechanistic review of colleagues' protocols, without the kind of adversarial procedures that would reveal every risk in every procedure. Similarly, IRB review of consent forms and procedures rarely takes the concern from the committee room onto the hospital floor to inquire about the full extent of the understanding of subjects who consent to participate. Nevertheless, IRBs do require investigators to be accountable for the character and severity of risks they are prepared to let others run, knowing that their institutional reputation may be harmed if they minimize or distort it. This responsibility unquestionably has changed investigators' behavior, and social expectations of them. To be sure, abuses may still occur. IRBs must be ready to minimize the amount of risk involved in certain protocols so as to enable researcher-colleagues to pursue their investigations. But they happen considerably less often now that IRB regulation is a fact of life. Scientific progress and ethical behavior turn out to be compatible goals.

DAVID J. ROTHMAN

For a further discussion of topics mentioned in this entry, see the entries AUTOEXPERIMENTATION; COMPETENCE; INFORMATION DISCLOSURE; INFORMED CONSENT; MENTALLY DISABLED AND MENTALLY ILL PERSONS, *article on* RESEARCH ETHICS; MILITARY PERSONNEL AS RESEARCH SUBJECTS; RESEARCH, UNETHICAL; *and* RESEARCH ETHICS COMMITTEES. *For a discussion of related ideas, see the entries* AUTHORITY; AUTONOMY; BIOETHICS; CONFLICT OF INTEREST; FREEDOM AND COERCION; HARM; LAW AND BIOETHICS; *and* LAW AND MORALITY. *Other relevant material may be found under the entries* MINORITIES AS RESEARCH SUBJECTS; MULTINATIONAL RESEARCH; PRISONERS, *article on* RESEARCH ISSUES; PRIVACY AND CONFIDENTIALITY IN RESEARCH; RESEARCH BIAS; RESEARCH METHODOLOGY; RESEARCH POLICY; *and* WARFARE, *articles on* NUCLEAR WARFARE *and* CHEMICAL AND BIOLOGICAL WARFARE. *See also the* APPENDIX (CODES, OATHS, AND DIRECTIVES RELATED TO BIOETHICS), SECTION IV: ETHICAL DIRECTIVES FOR HUMAN RESEARCH.

Bibliography

ANDRUS, EDWIN C.; BRONK, D. W.; CARDEN, G. A., JR.; KEEFER, C. S.; LOCKWOOD, J. S.; WEARN, J. T.; and WINTERNITZ, M. C., eds. 1948. *Advances in Military Medicine Made by American Investigators Under CMR sponsorship.* Boston: Little, Brown. For a summary of the work of the Committee on Medical Research, see the foreword to vol. 1.

ANNAS, GEORGE J., and GRODIN, MICHAEL A. 1992. *The Nazi Doctors and the Nuremberg Code: Human Rights in Human Experimentation.* New York: Oxford University Press.

BAXBY, DERRICK. 1981. *Jenner's Smallpox Vaccine: The Riddle of Vaccinia Virus and Its Origin.* London: Heinemann Educational Books.

BEAN, WILLIAM B. 1982. *Walter Reed: A Biography.* Charlottesville: University of Virginia Press.

BEAUMONT, WILLIAM. 1980. [1833]. *Experiments and Observations on the Gastric Juice and Physiology of Digestion.* Birmingham, Ala.: Classics of Medicine Library.

BEECHER, HENRY K. 1966. "Ethical and Clinical Research." *New England Journal of Medicine* 274, no. 24:1354–1360.

BERG, KARE, and TRANOY, KNUT E., eds. 1983. *Proceedings of Symposium on Research Ethics.* New York: Alan Liss.

BERNARD, CLAUDE. 1927. *An Introduction to the Study of Experimental Medicine.* Translated by Henry Copley Greene. New York: Macmillan.

BLISS, MICHAEL. 1982. *The Discovery of Insulin.* Chicago: University of Chicago Press.

BULL, J. P. 1959. "The Historical Development of Clinical Therapeutic Trials." *Journal of Chronic Diseases* 10, no. 3:218–248.

COMMISSION ON HEALTH SCIENCE AND SOCIETY. 1968. Hearings of 90th Congress, 2d session.

CURRAN, WILLIAM J. 1969. "Governmental Regulation of the Use of Human Subjects in Medical Research: The Approach of Two Federal Agencies." *Daedalus* 98, no. 2:542–594.

CUSHING, HARVEY. 1925. *The Life of Sir William Osler.* Oxford: At the Clarendon Press.

FOX, RENÉE. 1959. *Experiment Perilous: Physicians and Patients Facing the Unknown.* Glencoe, Ill.: Free Press.

FRANKEL, MARK S. 1972. *The Public Health Service Guidelines Governing Research Involving Human Subjects.* Monograph no. 10. Washington, D.C.: Program of Policy Studies in Science and Technology, George Washington University.

GERMANY (TERRITORY UNDER ALLIED OCCUPATION, 1945–1955: U.S. ZONE) MILITARY TRIBUNALS. 1947. "Permissible Medical Experiments." In vol. 2 of *Trials of War Criminals Before the Nuremberg Tribunals Under Control Law No. 10,* pp. 181–184. Washington, D.C.: U.S. Government Printing Office.

HENLE, WERNER; HENLE, GERTRUDE; HAMPIL, BETTYLEE; MARIS, ELIZABETH P.; and STOKES, JOSEPH, JR. 1946. "Experiments on Vaccination of Human Beings Against Epidemic Influenza." *Journal of Immunology* 53, no. 1:75–93.

HOWARD-JONES, NORMAN. 1982. "Human Experimentation in Historical and Ethical Perspectives." *Social Science Medicine* 16, no. 15:1429–1448.

JENNER, EDWARD. 1910. [1798]. "Vaccination Against Smallpox." In *Scientific Papers,* pp. 145–220. Edited by Charles W. Eliot. New York: P. F. Collier.

JONES, JAMES. 1981. *Bad Blood.* New York: Free Press.

KATZ, JAY; CAPRON, ALEXANDER M.; and GLASS, ELEANOR SWIFT. 1972. *Experimentation with Human Beings.* New York: Russell Sage Foundation.

KEEFER, CHESTER S. 1969. "Dr. Richards as Chairman of the Committee on Medical Research." *Annals of Internal Medicine* 71, supplement 8:61–70.

LADIMER, IRVING, AND NEWMAN, ROGER. 1963. *Clinical Investigation in Medicine: Legal, Ethical, and Moral Aspects.* Boston: Law-Medicine Institute of Boston University.

LEDERER, SUSAN. 1985. "Hideyo Noguchi's Luetin Experiment and the Antivivisectionists." *Isis* 76, no. 1:31–48.

———. 1992. "Orphans as Guinea Pigs." In *In the Name of the Child: Health and Welfare, 1880–1940.* Edited by Roger Cooter. London: Routledge.

MCNEIL, PAUL M. 1993. *The Ethics and Politics of Human Experimentation.* Cambridge: At the University Press.

NATIONAL INSTITUTES OF HEALTH. 1953a. *Handbook for Patients at the Clinical Center.* Publication no. 315. Bethesda, Md.: Author. See especially p. 2.

———. 1953b. *The National Institutes of Health Clinical Center.* Publication no. 316. Washington, D.C.: U.S. Government Printing Office. See especially p. 13.

NUMBERS, RONALD L. 1979. "William Beaumont and the Ethics of Experimentation." *Journal of the History of Biology* 12, no. 1:113–136.

OFFICE OF SCIENTIFIC RESEARCH AND DEVELOPMENT (OSRD). COMMITTEE ON MEDICAL RESEARCH (CMR). 1943. National Archives of the United States, Record Group 227: Contractor Records, S. Mudd, University of Pennsylvania (Contract 120, Final Report), March 3.

———. 1944a. Contractor Records, University of Chicago, Contract 450, Report L2, Responsible Investigator Dr. Alf S. Alving, Bimonthly Progress Report, August 1.

———. 1944b. Contractor Records, University of Pennsylvania, Contract 120, Responsible Investigator Dr. Stuart Mudd, Monthly Progress Report 18, October 3.

PROCTOR, ROBERT N. 1988. *Racial Hygiene: Medicine Under the Nazis.* Cambridge, Mass.: Harvard University Press.

RAMSEY, PAUL. 1970. *The Patient as Person: Explorations in Military Ethics.* New Haven, Conn.: Yale University Press.

"Requirements for Experiments on Human Beings." 1946. *Journal of the American Medical Association* 132:1090.

ROTHMAN, DAVID J. 1991. *Strangers at the Bedside.* New York: Basic Books.

STERNBERG, GEORGE M., and REED, WALTER. 1895. "Report on Immunity Against Vaccination Conferred upon the Monkey by the Use of the Serum of the Vaccinated Calf and Monkey." *Transactions of the Association of American Physicians* 10:57–69.

STOKES, JOSEPH, JR.; CHENOWETH, ALICE D.; WALTZ, ARTHUR D.; GLADEN, RALPH G.; and SHAW, DOROTHY. 1937. "Results of Immunization by Means of Active Virus of Human Influenza." *Journal of Clinical Investigation* 16, no. 2:237–243. This was one in a series of investigations that used institutionalized populations.

SWAIN, DONALD C. 1962. "The Rise of a Research Empire: NIH, 1930 to 1950." *Science* 138, no. 3546:1233–1237.

U.S. NATIONAL COMMISSION FOR THE PROTECTION OF HUMAN SUBJECTS OF BIOMEDICAL AND BEHAVIORAL RESEARCH. 1979. *The Belmont Report: Ethical Principles and Guidelines for Protection of Human Subjects of Research.* Washington, D. C.: Author.

VALLERY-RADOT, RENÉ. 1926. *The Life of Pasteur.* Translated by Henriette C. Devonshire. New York: Doubleday.

VERESAEV, VIKENTII V. 1916. [1901]. *The Memoirs of a Physician.* Translated by Simeon Linden. New York: Knopf.

RESEARCH, UNETHICAL

Unethical research is a concept inevitably relative to accepted views concerning research's ethical requirements. For Claude Bernard, an early French exponent of the scientific method in medicine who felt that the principle underlying medical morality requires that persons not be harmed, paradigm cases of unethical research are studies that offer their subjects risks that exceed their potential benefits (Bernard, 1957). The Nuremberg Tribunal, by stating in its first principle of ethical research that the subject's free consent is absolutely essential, added as paradigmatic cases of unethical research those studies performed upon unconsenting persons (Germany [Territory Under Allied Occupation, . . .], 1947). U.S. regulations that require an equitable selection of research subjects imply that a study that is otherwise ethical (e.g., a study with an acceptable risk–benefit ratio and whose subjects have freely consented) becomes unethical when it unfairly draws its research population from persons disadvantaged by reason of race, religion, or dependency, among others ("Federal Policy," 1991).

Examples of unethical research

Whichever ethical requirement may be chosen, the history of human research offers grim examples of its violation. During World War II, German researchers performed a large number of experiments in concentration camps and elsewhere. Subject-victims of Nazi research were predominantly Jews, but also included Romanies (Gypsies), prisoners of war, political prisoners, and others (Germany [Territory Under Allied Occupation . . .], 1947; Caplan, 1992). Nazi experimental atrocities included investigation of quicker and more efficient means of inducing sexual sterilization (including clandestine radiation dosing and unanesthetized male and female castration) and death (an area of study Leo Alexander [1949] termed "thanatology," which includes studies of techniques for undetectable individual assassination—i.e., murder that mimics natural death—as well as mass murder). Among the best-known cases were the hypothermia experiments, which investigated mechanisms of death by freezing and means of preventing it. These studies, motivated by the loss of German pilots over the North Sea, included immersing prisoners in freezing water and observing freezing's lethal physiological pathways.

Beginning in 1932, the U. S. Public Health Service funded a study of the natural progression of untreated syphilis in black men. Four hundred subject-victims were studied, along with 200 uninfected control subjects. The study, whose first published scientific paper appeared in 1936, continued until a newspaper account of it appeared in 1972. Its subject-victims were uninformed or misinformed about the purpose of the study, as well as its associated interventions. For example, participants were told that painful lumbar punctures were given as treatment, when in fact treatment for syphilis was withheld even after the discovery of penicillin (Brandt, 1978; Jones, 1981).

Numerous other examples of unethical research may be cited, though they have received far less attention. A New Zealand study on women that began in 1966 and was active for at least ten years had macabre similarities to the Tuskegee study. It concerned the natural history of untreated cervical carcinoma in situ (i.e., cancer that had not spread), and as in Tuskegee, its subject-victims were both uninformed and had treatment withheld for the study's duration (Paul, 1988). Parallel to the Nazi studies during World War II were those conducted by Japan. They included experimental attacks with biological weapons on at least eleven Chinese cities, and studies conducted on subject-victims that included efforts to induce gas gangrene by exploding fragmentation bombs near the exposed limbs and buttocks of 3,000 prisoners of war who were housed at a detention center known as Unit 731 (McNeill, 1993; Williams and Wallace, 1989).

Much unethical research comes to light only many years after its conduct, as is true of unethical military research conducted by the United States during and immediately following World War II. At that time, over 60,000 U.S. servicemen were involuntarily enrolled in studies involving exposure to chemical warfare agents (mustard gas and lewisite); at least 4,000 of them were exposed to high concentrations in field experiments and test chambers (Institute of Medicine, 1993).

Information about experiments on human radiation response supported by the U.S. government beginning in 1945 came to public attention in 1993. In one study, conducted from 1945 to 1947, eighteen patients considered to be terminally ill were injected with high doses of plutonium to determine how long it is retained in the human body. Military secrecy surrounding atomic energy precluded informed consent. Rather than telling subject-victims they would receive an injection of radioactive plutonium, the investigators told subjects they would receive a "product." Experiments on intellectually handicapped teenagers in a Massachusetts institution involved feeding the subjects very small amounts of radioactive iron and calcium to study the body's absorption of these materials. While the radiation exposure in these studies was low and unlikely to result in harm, the subject-victims were all incompetent, and their parents, who consented on their behalf, were simply asked by the institution to agree to "nutritional experiments." In reaction to news accounts of these and other studies, orders were issued in 1993 to declassify documents relating to unethical exposure of U.S. service personnel and citizens to radiation from atomic-weapons testing after World War II; in 1994 President Bill Clinton appointed a panel to guide a federal investigation into the radiation studies (Mann, 1994).

Several themes emerge from the known examples of unethical research. Such studies are likely to be done using disenfranchised or disadvantaged populations as subjects. In the absence of public outcry, unethical research may continue for many years, despite the fact that readers of the scientific literature in many cases have had access to all the facts they need to expose unethical practice (see Beecher, 1966). The larger and more egregious studies are especially likely to have been motivated by national security concerns and funded by the military.

Use of data from unethical research

Very early sources reflect differing views on the permissibility of making medical or other use of information derived from unethical practices. The Babylonian Talmud (Shabbat 67b) states that the prohibition on Amorite practices (pagan sorcery) does not forbid actions done for the sake of healing, and it cites several cases of permitted incantations and sympathetic magic. Robert Burton quotes Paracelsus's *De occulta philosophia* to similar effect: "It matters not whether it be God or the Devil, Angels or unclean Spirits cure him, so that he be eased" (Burton, 1628, p. 7). By contrast, Thomas Aquinas prohibits "inquiring of demons concerning the future." Even if demons should know scientific truths, he writes, it is improper to "enter into fellowship" with them in this way (Aquinas, 1947).

A large variety of empirical and ethical arguments have been marshaled to oppose the use of data from unethical research. Empirical arguments, which depend upon the facts of particular cases, question the scientific

reliability of such data. For example, Robert Berger, through a close analysis of the Nazi hypothermia data, claims that even by then-current scientific standards, the information is unreliable (Berger, 1990). He describes incomplete and contradictory data reporting, the absence of a controlling scientific protocol, and the control of the research program by scientifically untrained personnel (including Heinrich Himmler, Commander of the SS). In fact, the principal investigator, Sigmund Rascher, had a previous record of deception and was arrested in 1944 and charged with crimes that included scientific fraud. Some commentators argue that such data may be used, but only when the information is exceptionally reliable and useful. Most or all instances known of data gathered unethically, however, fail to meet this test (see Schafer, 1986).

Ethical arguments opposing use of the data are especially numerous. From a consequentialist point of view, unethical studies should be "punished" by "non-use," to discourage future investigators tempted to resort to unethical research practices. Other theories of punishment may be appealed to as well: As a matter of justice, it is argued that unethical investigators should not be rewarded by having the data from their studies used. By expunging the records of unethical research, the society of scientists expresses its solemn condemnation of the methods employed to acquire it; failing to do so would make science complicit with the research studies. Appropriate symbolism may call for the "burial" of this data, as it calls for the burial of the subject-victims from whom the data was derived (see Caplan, 1992; Martin, 1986; Post, 1988).

Rebuttals of these ethical arguments are equally numerous, relying upon the premise that data from unethical research studies may be valuable in principle: Any coincidence between "good science" and "good ethics," these writers argue, is only contingently true. As a practical matter, it is argued, the most serious instances of unethical research could not have been deterred by the punishment of non-use; some of the most heinous research studies were commissioned by governments, especially national security apparatuses. Punishment should be visited upon the investigators who engaged in unethical research; by withholding the use of data, current patients whose care might have been improved by use of that data are made to bear the brunt. Arguments from complicity are rejected because there is no causal connection between the prior acquisition of the data and its current use (the Nazis did not gather information about hypothermia in anticipation of its use by Canadian researchers a generation later); and because the current use of the data, far from being a continuation of the Nazi project, is for humanitarian purposes antithetical to the original Nazi intentions. In that way, the symbolism associated with the use of these data is seen to have a positive, redemptive value, while retaining the data's possible value to science and society (Freedman, 1992; Greene, 1992).

The debate about the use of data from unethical studies should distinguish the different ways scientific results can be used. Three different meanings for data use have been suggested: reference to data, for example, by scientific publication or citation, to serve as grounding for a scientific argument; reliance upon data in establishing or validating a practice, scientific or technological (including clinical); and using data as suggestive of further areas for inquiry (Freedman, 1992). This last meaning, while the most common in practice, has been the least debated; it is unlikely that data, once disclosed, could fail to be used in this way.

Much debate has centered on the first meaning, use of data through publication or citation. Kristine Moe found that the Nazi hypothermia studies had been referenced at least forty-five times in the medical literature (Moe, 1984). The New England Journal of Medicine, among other publications, has taken the position that it will not publish studies considered unethical by its editor; moreover, it will allow references to unethical research only in articles that focus on ethical condemnation of the research in question (Ingelfinger, 1973). Robert J. Levine has argued that a preferable stance would permit the publication of scientifically sound but ethically questionable research, while requiring the simultaneous publication of editorial discussion of the ethical issues raised (Levine, 1986).

Use of data in the second sense, as grounding scientific or ethical practices, was central to a 1988 controversy. While considering air pollution regulations on phosgene, a chemical used in plastics manufacture and a component of pesticides, the U. S. Environmental Protection Agency (EPA) withdrew an analysis that made reference to data derived from Nazi experiments after some EPA scientists circulated a protest letter (Sun, 1988). Phosgene was a component of some chemical weapons, and the Nazis had studied the response of French prisoners to various levels of phosgene exposure. EPA officials, while recognizing scientific and technical flaws in the data's collection and reporting, held the data to be useful additions to the existing animal toxicology information. Nazi data is often said not to be generalizable to a normal population because it was derived from prisoners under horrible conditions of privation. However, even this aspect of the data was applicable because the EPA's recommendations were designed to minimize risk to those most physiologically vulnerable. Those opposed to use of the data presented arguments based on both fact and value. The data were said to be valueless because of their omission of consideration of

vital variables like sex and weight of subject-victims. In addition, some agency scientists felt that data derived from this source, however valuable, should never be used.

In the majority of cases, the scientific value and impact of unethical research has been modest. Ethically, however, the Nazi, Tuskegee, and other studies have loomed large in raising both public awareness and ethical standards for the conduct of research. Unethical research has found its main use in ethics.

BENJAMIN FREEDMAN

For a further discussion of topics mentioned in this entry, see the entries FRAUD, THEFT, AND PLAGIARISM; INFORMATION DISCLOSURE; INFORMED CONSENT, *especially the article on* CONSENT ISSUES IN HUMAN RESEARCH; MILITARY PERSONNEL AS RESEARCH SUBJECTS; *and* MINORITIES AS RESEARCH SUBJECTS. *This entry will find application in the entries* AGING AND THE AGED, *article on* HEALTH-CARE AND RESEARCH ISSUES; CHILDREN, *article on* HEALTH-CARE AND RESEARCH ISSUES; COMMERCIALISM IN SCIENTIFIC RESEARCH; FETUS, *article on* FETAL RESEARCH; GENETICS AND HUMAN BEHAVIOR, *article on* SCIENTIFIC AND RESEARCH ISSUES; MENTALLY ILL AND MENTALLY DISABLED PERSONS, *article on* RESEARCH ISSUES; MULTINATIONAL RESEARCH; PRISONERS, *article on* RESEARCH ISSUES; PRIVACY AND CONFIDENTIALITY IN RESEARCH; RESEARCH ETHICS COMMITTEES; SEX THERAPY AND SEX RESEARCH; STUDENTS AS RESEARCH SUBJECTS; *and* WARFARE, *articles on* NUCLEAR WARFARE, *and* CHEMICAL AND BIOLOGICAL WARFARE. *For a discussion of related ideas, see the entries* AUTHORITY; COMPETENCY; ETHICS; FREEDOM AND COERCION; HARM; TRUST; *and* UTILITY. *See also the* APPENDIX (CODES, OATHS, AND DIRECTIVES RELATED TO BIOETHICS), SECTION IV: ETHICAL DIRECTIVES FOR HUMAN RESEARCH.

Bibliography

ALEXANDER, LEO. 1949. "Medical Science Under Dictatorship." New England Journal of Medicine 241, no. 2:39–47.

AQUINAS, THOMAS. 1947. "Whether It Is Unlawful to Practice the Observance of the Magic Art." In vol. 2 of Summa Theologica, pp. 1608–1609 (II-II, q. 96). Translated by the Fathers of the English Dominican Province. New York: Benziger Brothers. See especially the reply to "Objection 3."

BEECHER, HENRY K. 1966. "Ethics and Clinical Research." New England Journal of Medicine 274, no. 24:1354–1360.

BERGER, ROBERT L. 1990. "Nazi Science—The Dachau Hypothermia Experiments." New England Journal of Medicine 322, no. 20:1435–1440.

BERNARD, CLAUDE. 1957. An Introduction to the Study of Experimental Medicine. Translated by Henry Copley Green. New York: Dover. 1957.

BRANDT, ALLAN M. 1978. "Racism and Research: The Case of the Tuskegee Syphilis Study." Hastings Center Report 8, no. 6:21–29.

BURTON, ROBERT. 1961. [1628]. The Anatomy of Melancholy. London: J. M. Dent.

CAPLAN, ARTHUR L., ed. 1992. When Medicine Went Mad: Bioethics and the Holocaust. Totowa, N.J.: Humana Press.

"Federal Policy for the Protection of Human Subjects; Notices and Rules." 1991. Federal Register 56, no. 117 (June 18):18081–28032.

FREEDMAN, BENJAMIN. 1992. "Moral Analysis and the Use of Nazi Experimental Results." In When Medicine Went Mad: Bioethics and the Holocaust, pp. 141–154. Edited by Arthur L. Caplan. Totowa, N.J.: Humana Press.

GERMANY (TERRITORY UNDER ALLIED OCCUPATION, 1945–1955: U.S. ZONE) MILITARY TRIBUNALS. 1947. "Permissible Medical Experiments." In vol. 2 of Trials of War Criminals Before the Nuremberg Tribunals Under Control Law no. 10, pp. 181–183. Washington, D.C.: U.S. Government Printing Office.

GREENE, VELVL. 1992. "Can Scientists Use Information Derived from the Concentration Camps?" In When Medicine Went Mad: Bioethics and the Holocaust, pp. 155–170. Edited by Arthur L. Caplan. Totowa, N.J.: Humana Press.

INGELFINGER, FRANZ J. 1973. "Ethics of Experiments on Children." New England Journal of Medicine 288, no. 15:791–792.

INSTITUTE OF MEDICINE (U.S.) COMMITTEE TO SURVEY THE HEALTH EFFECTS OF MUSTARD GAS AND LEWISITE. 1993. Veterans at Risk: The Health Effects of Mustard Gas and Lewisite. Edited by Constance M. Pechura and David P. Rall. Washington, D.C.: National Academy Press.

JONES, JAMES H. 1981. Bad Blood: The Tuskegee Syphilis Experiment. New York: Free Press.

LEVINE, ROBERT J. 1986. Ethics and Regulation of Clinical Research. 2d ed. Baltimore, Md.: Urban & Schwarzenberg.

MANN, CHARLES C. 1994. "Radiation: Balancing the Record." Science 263:470–473.

MARTIN, ROBERT M. 1986. "Using Nazi Scientific Data." Dialogue 25:403–411.

McNEILL, PAUL M. 1993. The Ethics and Politics of Human Experimentation. New York: Cambridge University Press.

MOE, KRISTINE. 1984. "Should the Nazi Research Data Be Cited?" Hastings Center Report 14, no. 6:5–7.

PAUL, CHARLOTTE. 1988. "The New Zealand Cervical Cancer Study: Could It Happen Again?" British Medical Journal 297, no. 6647:533–539.

POST, STEPHEN G. 1988. "Nazi Data and the Rights of Jews." Journal of Law and Religion 6, no. 2:429–433.

SCHAFER, ARTHUR. 1986. "On Using Nazi Data: The Case Against." Dialogue 25, no. 3:413–419.

SUN, MARJORIE. 1988. "EPA Bars Use of Nazi Data." Science 240, no. 4848:21.

WILLIAMS, PETER, and WALLACE, DAVID. 1989. Unit 731: Japan's Secret Biological Warfare in World War II. New York: Free Press.

RESEARCH BIAS

In scientific research, whether in the behavioral, biomedical, or physical sciences, investigators rarely admit that data have been gathered and interpreted from a particular perspective. Research in biology, chemistry, and physics, centered on the physical, natural world, is presumed "objective"; therefore, the term "perspective" is not applied to it. The reliability and repeatability of data gathered and hypotheses tested using the scientific method convince researchers that they are obtaining unbiased information. The passive voice in which scientific articles are written, coupled with the emphasis upon trying to eliminate values held by the individual scientist, leads scientists to believe that they investigate natural phenomena as neutral observers without a perspective.

Identifying bias

In the behavioral sciences, the difficulties of studying complex, changing interactions among living beings led to investigations of possible sources of bias. For example, the gender, race, class, and even presence of a researcher during an interview have been shown to influence the responses of the interviewee (Oakley, 1981). Researchers sought to apply the scientific method to problems in the behavioral sciences, in an attempt to eliminate bias.

Like all scholars, scientists hold, either explicitly or implicitly, certain beliefs concerning their enterprise. Most scientists believe, for example, that the laws and facts gathered by scientists are constant, providing that experiments have been done correctly. But historians of science posit that the individuals who make observations and create theories are people who live in a particular country at a certain time in a definable socioeconomic condition, and that their situations and mentalities impinge on their discoveries. Aristotle "counted" fewer teeth in the mouths of women than in those of men—adding this dentitional inferiority to all the others he asserted characterized women (Arditti, 1980). Galen, having read the book of Genesis, "discovered" that men had one less rib on one side than women did (Webster and Webster, 1974). Neither is true, and both would be refuted easily by observation of what would appear by today's standards to be easily verifiable facts. Thus, what we take to be facts can vary depending upon the theory or paradigm—the specific problematics, concepts, theories, language, and methods—guiding the scientist.

Most scientists, feminists, and philosophers of science recognize that no individual can be entirely neutral or value-free. To some, "objectivity is defined to mean independence from the value judgements of any particular individual" (Jaggar, 1983, p. 357). The paradigms themselves, however, also are far from value-free. The values of a culture, in the historical past and the present society, heavily influence the ordering of observable phenomena into a theory. The worldview of a particular society, time, and person limits the questions that can be asked, and thereby the answers that can be given. Therefore, the very acceptance of a particular paradigm that appears to cause a "scientific revolution" within a society may depend upon the congruence of that theory with the institutions and beliefs of the society (Kuhn, 1970). Scholars suggest that Darwin's theory of natural selection was ultimately accepted by his contemporaries (whereas they did not accept similar theories as described by Alfred Russel Wallace and others) because Darwin emphasized the congruence between the values of his theory and those held by the upper classes of Victorian Britain (Rose and Rose, 1980).

Not only what is accepted, but what and how we study, have normative features. Helen Longino (1990) has explored the extent to which methods employed by scientists can be objective (not related to individual values) and lead to repeatable, verifiable results while contributing to hypotheses or theories that are congruent with nonobjective institutions and ideologies of the society: "Background assumptions are the means by which contextual values and ideology are incorporated into scientific inquiry" (1990, p. 216). For example, scientists may calculate rocket trajectories and produce bombs that efficiently destroy living beings without raising the ethical questions of whether the money and effort for this research to support the military could be better spent on other research questions that might be solved by using similar objective methods.

Unintended research bias

Given the high costs of sophisticated equipment, maintenance of laboratory animals and facilities, and salaries for qualified technicians and researchers, virtually no behavioral or biomedical research is undertaken today without governmental or foundation support. The choice of problems for study in medical research is substantially determined by a national agenda that defines what is worthy of study, that is, worth funding. As Marxist (Zimmerman, et al., 1980), African-American (McLeod, 1987), and feminist (Hubbard, 1983; 1990) critics of scientific research have pointed out, the scientific research undertaken in the United States reflects the societal bias toward the powerful, who are overwhelmingly white, middle/upper class, and male. Members of Congress who appropriate the funds for the National Institutes of Health (NIH) and other federal agencies that support research are overwhelmingly white, middle/upper class, and male; thus they may be more likely to vote funds for research that they view as beneficial to health needs (as defined from their perspective). The same descriptors—white, middle/upper class, and male—characterize the individuals in the theoretical and decision-making positions within the medical and scientific establishments that set priorities and allocate funds for research. This lack of diversity among Congressional and scientific leaders may allow unintentional, undetected flaws to bias the research in terms of what we study and how we study it.

Examples from research studies demonstrate that unintentional bias may be reflected in at least three stages of application of the scientific method: (1) choice and definition of problems to be studied; (2) methods and approaches used in data gathering, including whom we choose as subjects; and (3) theories and conclusions drawn from the data.

Choice and definition of problems to be studied. Four widely publicized examples demonstrate that sex differences are *not* routinely considered as part of the question asked. In a longitudinal study of the effects of cholesterol-lowering drugs, for example, gender differences were not determined because the drug was tested on 3,806 men and no women (Hamilton, 1985). The Multiple-Risk Factor Intervention Trial (1990) examined mortality from coronary heart disease in 12,866 men only. The Health Professionals Follow-up Study (Grobbee et al., 1990) looked at the association between coffee consumption and heart disease in 45,589 men. The Physicians' Health Study (Steering Committee of the Physicians' Health Study Group, 1989) found that low-dose aspirin therapy reduced the risk of myocardial infarction in 22,071 male physicians.

Many of these studies, including the Physicians' Health Study, were flawed not only by the factor of gender but also by factors of race and class. Susceptibility to cardiovascular disease is known to be affected by lifestyle factors such as diet, exercise level, and stress, which are correlated with race and class. Since physicians in the United States are not representative of the overall male population with regard to lifestyle, the results may not be applicable to most men.

Designation of certain diseases as particular to one gender, race, or sexual orientation not only cultivates ignorance in the general public about transmission or frequency of the disease; it also results in research that does not adequately explore the parameters of the disease. Some diseases that affect both sexes are identified as "male" diseases. Heart disease is the best example of a disease so designated because heart disease occurs more frequently in men at younger ages than in women. Most of the funding for heart disease has been appropriated for research on predisposing factors for the disease (such as cholesterol level, lack of exercise, stress, smoking, and weight) using white, middle-aged middle-class males.

This "male disease" designation has meant that very little research has been directed toward high-risk groups of women. Heart disease is a leading cause of death in older women (Kirschstein and Merritt, 1985), who currently live on average of eight years longer than men (Boston Women's Health Book Collective, 1984). It is also frequent in poor black women who have had several children (Manley et al., 1985). Virtually no research has explored predisposing factors for these groups, who fall outside the disease definition established from a male perspective.

Recent data indicate that the initial designation of AIDS as a disease of male homosexuals, drug users, and Haitian immigrants not only has resulted in homophobic and racist stereotypes but also has induced the failure of many Americans to understand that AIDS can be transmitted heterosexually. This designation has also led researchers and health-care practitioners to study inadequately the etiology of AIDS and underdiagnose AIDS in women (Norwood, 1988). Women, particularly black and Hispanic women, constitute the group in which AIDS is currently increasing most rapidly, the women appear to manifest AIDS with different symptoms than men. As late as 1992 the Centers for Disease Control Case Definition failed to include gynecologic conditions and other symptoms related to AIDS in women (Rosser, 1991).

Research on conditions specific to females and people of color tends to receive low priority, funding, and prestige. Some examples include dysmenorrhea, incontinence in older women, and nutrition in postmenopausal women. Effects of exercise level and duration upon alleviation of menstrual discomfort, and length and amount of exposure to video display terminals that may result in the "cluster pregnancies" of women giving birth to deformed babies in certain industries, also have received low priority. Although women make up half the population and receive more than half the health care, in 1988 the NIH allocated only 13.5 percent of its total budget to research on illnesses of major consequence for women (Narrigan, 1991). The $500 million Women's Health Initiative of NIH in 1992 began to address this issue. An initial survey on the health of women of color revealed that little research has been done on the effects of reproductive health issues in women of different races. The survey found that women of color felt "undervalued, underserved, underinsured" (Huckshorn, 1991).

These types of bias raise ethical issues. Health-care practitioners treat the majority of the population, which consists of females and minorities, based on information gathered from clinical research in which women and minorities have not been included. Bias in research thus leads to further injustice in health-care diagnosis and treatment.

Approaches and methods used in data gathering. Using the male as the "basic experimental subject not only ignores the fact that females may respond differently to the variable tested; it also may lead to less accurate models even for the male. Models that simulate functioning complex biological systems more accurately may be derived using female rats as subjects in experiments. Scientists like Joan Hoffman (1982) have questioned the tradition of using male rats or primates as subjects. With the exception of insulin and the hormones of the female reproductive cycle, traditional endocrinological theory assumed that most of the twenty-odd human hormones are kept at a constant level in both males and females. Thus, the male of the species, whether rodent or primate, was chosen as the experimental subject because of this noncyclicity. However, new techniques of measuring blood hormone levels have demonstrated episodic, rather than steady, patterns of secretion in virtually all hormones in both males and females. As Hoffman points out, the rhythmic cycle of hormone secretion as portrayed in the cycling female rat appears to be a more accurate model for the secretion of most hormones (Hoffman, 1982).

When women are used as experimental subjects, often they are treated as less than fully human. In his attempts to investigate the side effects of nervousness and depression attributable to oral contraceptives, Joseph Goldzieher gave dummy pills to seventy-six women who sought treatment at a San Antonio clinic to prevent further pregnancies (Goldzieher et al., 1971a; 1971b). None of the women was told that she was participating in research or receiving placebos (Veatch, 1971). The women in Goldzieher's study were primarily poor, multiparous Mexican-Americans. Research that raises similar issues about the ethics of informed consent was carried out on poor Puerto Rican women during the initial phases of testing the effectiveness of "the pill" as a contraceptive (Zimmerman et al., 1980). Data from 1990 have revealed routine testing of pregnant women for HIV positivity without their informed consent at certain clinics (Marte and Anastos, 1990), and subsequent pressure on women who are HIV-positive to abort their fetuses despite the fact that seroconversion from mother to fetus is only 25–30 percent (Selwyn et al., 1989).

Frequently it is difficult to determine whether these women are treated disrespectfully and unethically due to their gender or whether race and class are more significant variables. From the Tuskegee syphilis experiment (1932–1972), in which the effects of untreated syphilis were studied in 399 men over a period of 40 years (Jones,

1981), it is clear that men who are black and poor may not receive appropriate treatment or information about the experiment in which they are participating. Scholars (Dill, 1983; Ruzek, 1988) have begun to explore the extent to which gender, race, and class become complex, interlocking variables that may affect access to and quality of health care.

Using only a particular discipline's established methods may result in approaches that fail to reveal sufficient information about the problem being explored. This may be a difficulty for research surrounding medical problems particularly important to women, people of color, and homosexual males. Pregnancy, childbirth, menstruation, menopause, lupus, sickle-cell disease, AIDS, and gerontology represent health-care issues for which the methods of one discipline are clearly inadequate.

Methods that cross disciplinary boundaries or include combinations of methods traditionally used in separate fields may provide more appropriate approaches. For example, heart disease is caused not only by genetic and physiological factors but also by social/psychological factors such as smoking and stress. Jean Hamilton (1985) has called for interactive models that draw on both the social and the natural sciences to explain complex problems.

Theories and conclusions drawn from the data. Emphasis upon traditional disciplinary approaches that are quantitative and maintain the distance between observer and experimental subject supposedly removes the bias of the researcher. Ironically, to the extent that these "objective" approaches are synonymous with a particular approach to scientific phenomena, they may introduce bias.

First, theories may be presented in androcentric, ethonocentric, or class-biased language. An awareness of language should aid experimenters in avoiding the use of terms such as "tomboyism" (Money and Erhardt, 1972), "aggression," and "hysteria," which reflect assumptions about sex-appropriate behavior (Hamilton, 1985). Researchers should use evaluative terms such as "prostitute" with caution. Often the important fact for AIDS research is that a woman has multiple sex partners or is an IV drug user, rather than that she has received money for sex. The use of such terms as "prostitute" may induce bias by promoting the idea that women are vectors for transmission to men when, in fact, the men may have an equal or greater number of sex partners to whom they are transmitting the disease. Even more important, by emphasizing AIDS in "prostitutes," health-care practitioners are able to distance themselves and their patients from the risk of AIDS. This may also lead to practitioners treating prostitutes as less than human and underdiagnosing AIDS in women who are not prostitutes. Focus on group characteristics such as "prostitute"

or "poor, black, unmarried woman" repeats the initial mistake of identifying the disease by group rather than by behavioral risk.

Once a bias in terminology is exposed, the next step is to ask whether that terminology leads to a constraint or bias in the theory itself. Theories and conclusions drawn from medical research may be formulated to support the status quo of inequality for oppressed groups. Not surprisingly, the androcentric bias in research that has led to exclusion of women from the definitions and approaches to research problems may result in differences in management of disease and access to health-care procedures based on gender. In a 1991 study in Massachusetts and Maryland, John Z. Ayanian and Arnold M. Epstein (1991) demonstrated that women were significantly less likely than men to undergo coronary angioplasty, angiography, or surgery when admitted to the hospital with a diagnosis of myocardial infarction, unstable or stable angina, chronic ischemic heart disease, or chest pain. This significant difference remained even when the variables of race, age, economic status, and other chronic diseases (such as diabetes and heart failure) were controlled. A similar study (Steingart et al., 1991) revealed that women have angina before myocardial infarction as frequently and with more debilitating effects than men, yet they are referred for cardiac catheterization only half as often. Gender bias in cardiac research has therefore been translated into bias in management of disease, leading to inequitable treatment for life-threatening conditions in women.

Recognizing the possibility of bias is the first step toward understanding the difference it makes. Perhaps white male researchers have been less likely to see flaws in and question biologically deterministic theories that provide scientific justification for their superior status in society because they gain social power and status from such theories. Researchers from outside the mainstream (women and people of color, for example) are much more likely to be critical of such theories because they lose power from those theories.

In order to eliminate bias, the community of scientists undertaking research needs to include individuals from backgrounds of as much variety and diversity as possible with regard to race, class, gender, and sexual orientation (Rosser, 1988). Only then is it less likely that the perspective of one group will bias research design, approaches, subjects, and interpretations.

SUE V. ROSSER

For a further discussion of topics mentioned in this entry, see the entries AIDS; FEMINISM; RACE AND RACISM; *and* WOMEN, *article on* RESEARCH ISSUES. *This entry will find application in the entries* AGING AND THE AGED, *article on* HEALTH-CARE AND RESEARCH ISSUES; ANIMAL REsearch; Children, *article on* health-care and research issues; Commercialism in Scientific Research; Fetus, *article on* fetal research; Genetics and Human Behavior, *article on* scientific and research issues; Informed Consent, *especially the article on* consent issues in human research; Mentally Ill and Mentally Disabled Persons, *article on* research issues; Military Personnel as Research Subjects; Minorities as Research Subjects; Multinational Research; Prisoners, *article on* research issues; Privacy and Confidentiality in Research; Research, Unethical; Research Ethics Committees; Science, Philosophy of; Sex Therapy and Sex Research; *and* Students as Research Subjects. *Other relevant material may be found under the entries* Research, Human: Historical Aspects; Research Methodology; Research Policy; *and* Value and Valuation. *See also the* Appendix (Codes, Oaths, and Directives Related to Bioethics), section iv: ethical directives for human research.

Bibliography

Arditti, Rita. 1980. "Feminism and Science." In *Science and Liberation*, pp. 350–368. Edited by Rita Arditti, Pat Brennan, and Steven Cavrak. Boston: South End Press.

Ayanian, John Z., and Epstein, Arnold. 1991. "Differences in the Use of Procedures Between Women and Men Hospitalized for Coronary Heart Disease." *New England Journal of Medicine* 325:221–225.

Boston Women's Health Book Collective. 1984. *The New Our Bodies, Ourselves: A Book by and for Women.* New York: Simon and Schuster.

Dill, Bonnie T. 1983. "Race, Class and Gender: Prospects for an All-Inclusive Sisterhood." *Feminist Studies* 9, no. 1:131–150.

Goldzieher, Joseph W.; Moses, Louis E.; Averkin, Eugene; Scheel, Cora; and Taber, Ben Z. 1971a. "Nervousness and Depression Attributed to Oral Contraceptives: A Double-Blind, Placebo-Controlled Study." *American Journal of Obstetrics and Gynecology* 111, no. 8: 1013–1020.

———. 1971b. "A Placebo-Controlled Double-Blind Crossover Investigation of the Side Effects Attributed to Oral Contraceptives." *Fertility and Sterility* 22, no. 9:602–623.

Grobbee, Diederick E.; Rimm, Eric B.; Giovannucci, Edward; Colditz, Graham; Stampfer, Meir; and Willett, Walter. 1990. "Coffee, Caffeine, and Cardiovascular Disease in Men." *New England Journal of Medicine* 323, no. 15:1026–1032.

Hamilton, Jean. 1985. "Avoiding Methodological Biases and Policy-Making Biases in Gender-Related Health Research." In vol. 2 of *Women's Health: Report of the Public Health Service Task Force on Women's Health Issues*, pp. 54–64. Edited by Ruth L. Kirschstein and Doris H. Merritt. Washington, D.C.: U.S. Dept. of Health and Human Services, Public Health Service.

Hoffman, Joan C. 1982. "Biorhythms in Human Reproduction: The Not-So-Steady States." *Signs: Journal of Women in Culture and Society* 7, no. 4:829–844.

Hubbard, Ruth. 1983. "Social Effects of Some Contemporary Myths About Women." In *Women's Nature: Rationalizations of Inequality*, pp. 1–8. Edited by Marian Lowe and Ruth Hubbard. New York: Pergamon Press.

———. 1990. *The Politics of Women's Biology*. New Brunswick, N.J.: Rutgers University Press.

Huckshorn, Kristin. 1991. "Minority Women Lack Facts on Health Care." *The State*, September 25, p. A-3.

Jaggar, Alison M. 1983. *Feminist Politics and Human Nature.* Totowa, N.J.: Rowman & Allanheld.

Jones, James H. 1981. *Bad Blood: The Tuskegee Syphilis Experiment.* New York: Free Press.

Kirschstein, Ruth L., and Merritt, Doris H., eds. 1985. *Women's Health: Report of the Public Health Service Task Force on Women's Health Issues.* Vol. 2. Washington, D.C.: U.S. Dept. of Health and Human Services, Public Health Service.

Kuhn, Thomas S. 1970. *The Structure of Scientific Revolutions.* 2d ed. Chicago: University of Chicago Press.

Longino, Helen. 1990. *Science as Social Knowledge: Values and Objectivity in Scientific Inquiry.* Princeton, N.J.: Princeton University Press.

Manley, Audrey; Lin-Fu, Jane S.; Miranda, Magdalena; Noonan, Alan; and Parker, Tanya. 1985. "Special Health Concerns of Ethnic Minority Women." In vol. 2 of *Women's Health: Report of the Public Health Service Task Force on Women's Health Issues*, pp. 37–47. Edited by Ruth L. Kirschstein and Doris H. Merritt. Washington, D.C.: U.S. Dept. of Health and Human Services.

Marte, Carola, and Anastos, Kathryn. 1990. "Women—the Missing Persons in the AIDS Epidemic: Part II." *Health/PAC Bulletin* 20, no. 1:11–23.

Money, John, and Erhardt, Anke. 1972. *Man and Woman, Boy and Girl: The Differentiation and Dimorphism of Gender and Identity from Conception to Maturity.* Baltimore: Johns Hopkins University Press.

Multiple Risk Factor Intervention Trial Research Group. 1990. "Mortality Rates After 10.5 Years for Participants in the Multiple Risk Factor Intervention Trial: Findings Related to A Priori Hypotheses of the Trial." *Journal of the American Medical Association* 263, no. 13: 1795–1801.

Narrigan, Deborah. 1991. "Research to Improve Women's Health: An Agenda for Equity." *Network News: The Newsletter of the National Women's Health Network*, March/April/May, pp. 3, 9.

Norwood, Chris. 1988. "Women and the 'Hidden' AIDS Epidemic." *Network News: Newsletter of the National Women's Health Network*, November–December, pp. 1, 6.

Oakley, Ann. 1981. "Interviewing Women: A Contradiction in Terms." In *Doing Feminist Research*, pp. 30–61. Edited by Helen Roberts. London: Routledge & Kegan Paul.

Reingold, Nathan, and Rothenberg, Marc, eds. 1987. *Scientific Colonialism: A Cross-Cultural Comparison.* Washington, D.C.: Smithsonian Institution Press.

Rose, Hilary, and Rose, Stephen. 1980. "The Myth of the Neutrality of Science." In *Science and Liberation*, pp. 17–

32. Edited by Rita Arditti, Pat Brennan, and Steve Cavrak. Boston: South End Press.

ROSSER, SUE V. 1988. "Good Science: Can It Ever Be Gender-Free?" *Women's Studies International Forum* 11, no. 1: 13–19.

———. 1991. "AIDS and Women." *AIDS Education and Prevention* 3, no. 3:230–240.

RUZEK, SHERYL. 1988. "Women's Health: Sisterhood Is Powerful, but So Are Race and Class." Keynote address delivered at Southeast Women's Studies Association Annual Conference. University of North Carolina-Chapel Hill, February 27.

SELWYN, PETER A.; SCHOENBAUM, ELLIE E.; DAVENNY, KATHERINE; ROBERTSON, VERNA J.; FEINGOLD, ANAT R; SHULMAN, JOANNA F.; MAYERS, MARGUERITE M.; KLEIN, ROBERT S.; FRIEDLAND, GERALD H.; and ROGERS, MARTHA F. 1989. "Prospective Study of Human Immunodeficiency Virus Infection and Pregnancy Outcomes in Intravenous Drug Users." *Journal of the American Medical Association* 261, no. 9:1289–1294.

STEERING COMMITTEE OF THE PHYSICIANS' HEALTH STUDY GROUP. 1989. "Final Report on the Aspirin Component of the Ongoing Physicians' Health Study." *New England Journal of Medicine* 321:129–135.

STEINGART, RICHARD M.; PACKER, MILTON; HAMM, PEGGY; COGLIANESE, MARY ELLEN; GERSH, BERNARD; GETTMAN, EDWARD M.; SOLLANO, JOSEPHINE; KATZ, STANLEY; MOYE, LEM; BASTA, LOFTY L.; LEWIS, SANDRA J.; GOTTLEIB, STEPHEN S.; BERNSTEIN, VICTORIA; McEWAN, PATRICIA; JACOBSON, KIRK; BROWN, EDWARD J.; KUKIN, MARRICK L.; KANTROWITZ, NIKI E.; and PFEFFER, MARC A. 1991. "Sex Differences in the Management of Coronary Artery Disease." *New England Journal of Medicine* 325, no. 4:226–230.

VEATCH, ROBERT M. 1971. "Experimental Pregnancy." *Hastings Center Report* 1:2–3.

WEBSTER, DOUGLAS, and WEBSTER, MOLLY. 1974. *Comparative Vertebrate Morphology.* New York: Academic Press.

ZIMMERMAN, B., et al. 1990. "People's Science." In *Science and Liberation*, pp. 299–319. Edited by Rita Arditti, Pat Brennan, and Steve Cavrak. Boston: South End Press.

RESEARCH ETHICS COMMITTEES

The Declaration of Helsinki (1989) establishes as the international standard for biomedical research involving human subjects this requirement: "Each experimental procedure involving human subjects should be clearly formulated in an experimental protocol which should be transmitted for consideration, comment and guidance to a specially appointed committee independent of the investigator and sponsor . . ." (Article I.2). In most of the world this committee is called the research ethics committee (REC). In the United States, federal law assigns to the committee the name institutional review board, and the authority and responsibility for approving or disapproving proposals to conduct research involving human subjects (Robertson, 1979a). In Canada, the research ethics board has similar authority to approve or disapprove research proposals, not merely to offer "consideration, comment and guidance" (Medical Research Council of Canada, 1987, p. 48).

History

The Nuremberg Code (1949) and the original Declaration of Helsinki (1964) make no mention of committee review; these documents placed on the investigator all responsibility for safeguarding the rights and welfare of research subjects. The first mention of committee review in an international document was in the Tokyo revision of the Declaration of Helsinki (1975).

In the United States, the first federal document requiring committee review was issued on November 17, 1953. Entitled "Group Consideration for Clinical Research Procedures Deviating from Accepted Medical Practice or Involving Unusual Hazard," its guidelines applied only to research conducted at the newly opened Clinical Center at the National Institutes of Health (Lipsett et al., 1979). We know very little about peer review in other institutions in the 1950s other than that it existed at least in some medical schools. In 1961 and again in 1962, questionnaires were sent to American university departments of medicine. Approximately one-third of those responding reported that they had committees, and one-quarter either had or were developing procedural documents (Curran, 1970).

On February 8, 1966, the surgeon general of the U.S. Public Health Service (USPHS) issued the first federal policy statement requiring research institutions to establish the committees that subsequently came to be known as RECs (Curran, 1970). This policy required recipients of USPHS grants in support of research involving human subjects to specify that

> the grantee institution will provide prior review of the judgment of the principal investigator or program director by a committee of his institutional associates. This review shall assure an independent determination: (1) Of the rights and welfare of the . . . individuals involved, (2) Of the appropriateness of the methods used to secure informed consent, and (3) Of the risks and potential medical benefits of the investigation. . . .

The evolution of the federal government's charges to the committee and of its recognition of the need for diversity of committee membership was reflected in several revisions of its policy between 1966 and 1969 (Veatch, 1975; R. Levine, 1986); these will be discussed further.

Purpose

The purpose of the REC is to ensure that research involving human subjects is designed to conform to relevant ethical standards. Historically, the REC's primary focus was on safeguarding the rights and welfare of individual research subjects, concentrating on the plans for informed consent and the assessment of risks and anticipated benefits. In 1978, the National Commission for the Protection of Human Subjects of Biomedical and Behavioral Research (National Commission) added a requirement that the REC ensure equitableness in the selection of research subjects (R. Levine, 1986). The National Commission was concerned primarily with protecting vulnerable subjects from bearing a disproportionately large share of the burdens of research. Subsequently, as participation in some types of research became perceived as a benefit, RECs also assumed responsibility for ensuring disadvantaged person equitable access to such benefits (C. Levine, 1988).

A source of continuing controversy is whether the REC has an obligation to approve or disapprove the scientific design of research protocols (R. Levine, 1986). Those who argue that they do or should have such an obligation point out that the leading ethical codes establish a requirement for good scientific design. Moreover, they argue, the REC's obligation to determine that risks to subjects are reasonable in relation to anticipated benefits necessarily relies on a prior determination that the scientific design is adequate, for if it is not, there will be no benefits and any risk must be considered unreasonable.

Opponents to assigning such an obligation to the REC, while conceding these two points, argue that the REC is not designed to make expert judgments about the adequacy of scientific design. RECs are generally competent to appraise the value of the science—what the Nuremberg Code calls "the humanitarian importance of the problem to be solved"—but not the validity of the methods or the results (Freedman, 1987; Veatch, 1975). In general, responsibility for assessment of scientific validity is, and ought to be, delegated to committees designed to have such competence—such as scientific review committees either within the institution or at funding agencies such as the National Institutes of Health (R. Levine, 1986).

Membership

The surgeon general's 1966 memo called for prior review by "a committee of [the investigator's] associates," what was commonly called "peer review." As of 1968, 73 percent of committees were limited in membership to immediate peer groups: scientists and physicians (Curran, 1970).

On May 1, 1969, USPHS guidelines were revised to indicate that a committee constituted exclusively of biomedical scientists would be inadequate to perform the functions now expected of it: "The membership should possess . . . competencies necessary in the judgment as to the acceptability of the research in terms of institutional regulations, relevant law, standards of professional practice and community acceptance."

Regulations of the U.S. Department of Health and Human Services (DHHS), first promulgated in 1974 and since revised several times, maintain the spirit of the 1969 policy and in addition require gender diversity; at least one nonscientist (e.g., lawyer, ethicist, member of the clergy); and at least one member who is not affiliated with the institution (commonly and incorrectly called a "community representative"). Persons having conflicting interests are to be excluded; this concern is also reflected in the Declaration of Helsinki's requirement of a "committee independent of the investigator and sponsor."

According to Robert Veatch (1975), the REC is an intermediate case between two models of the review committee: The "interdisciplinary professional review model," made up of diverse professionals such as doctors, lawyers, scientists, and clergy, brings professional expertise to the review process, while the "jury model . . . reflects the common sense of the reasonable person" (p. 31). In the jury model "expertise relevant to the case at hand is not only not necessary, it often disqualifies one from serving on the jury" (p. 31). Veatch concedes that in order to perform all of its functions, the REC requires both professional and jury skills. However, he argues that the presence of professionals makes it more difficult for the REC to be responsive to the informational needs of the reasonable person or to be adept at anticipating community acceptance.

John Robertson (1979b) would correct the "structural bias" of professional domination by introducing a "subject surrogate," an expert advocate for the subjects' interests. DHHS regulations require that if an REC "regularly reviews research that involves a vulnerable category of subjects . . . consideration shall be given to the inclusion of . . . [persons who know] about and [are] experienced in working with these subjects." For research involving prisoners, the regulations require that at least one member of the REC be either a prisoner or a prisoner representative. There is unresolved controversy over whether persons with AIDS should be appointed to serve on all RECs that review research in the field of HIV infection (C. Levine et al., 1991).

Locale

In the United States the first RECs were established in the institutions where research was conducted. The 1966 surgeon general's policy statement required a committee of "institutional associates." In 1971 the Food and Drug Administration (FDA) promulgated regulations that required committee review only when regulated research was conducted in institutions; hence their name, institutional review committee. Regulations proposed in 1973 by the Department of Health, Education and Welfare, forerunner of DHHS, also reflected a local setting in their term "organizational review board." In 1974 the National Research Act established a statutory requirement for review by a committee to which it assigned the name "institutional review board," a compromise between the two names then extant.

RECs are required to comply with federal regulations when reviewing activities involving FDA-regulated "test articles" such as investigational drugs and devices, and when reviewing research supported by federal funds (Robertson, 1979a). Moreover, all institutions that receive federal research grants and contracts are required to file "statements of assurance" of compliance with federal regulations. In these assurances virtually all institutions voluntarily promise to apply the principles of federal regulations to all research they conduct, regardless of the source of funding.

These points notwithstanding, each REC has a decidedly local character. Most have local names, such as "human investigation committee" or "committee for the protection of human subjects." Each is appointed by its own institution, and each makes its own interpretation of the requirements of federal regulations. For example, at one university medical students are forbidden to serve as research subjects, while at another, involvement of medical students as research subjects is sometimes required as a condition of approval (R. Levine, 1986).

The National Commission recommended that RECs should be "located in institutions where research . . . is conducted. Compared to the possible alternatives of a regional or national review . . . local committees have the advantage of greater familiarity with the actual conditions . . ." (1978, pp. 1–2). The National Commission envisioned the local REC as an ally of the investigator in safeguarding the rights and welfare of research subjects, as well as a contributor to the education of both the research community and the public.

The FDA's change in regulations in 1981 to require REC review of all regulated research, regardless of where it was done, created a problem for the many physicians who were conducting investigations in their private offices; many of these physicians had no ready access to RECs. In response, private corporations developed "noninstitutional review boards" (NRBs) (Herman, 1989). Although there are theoretical reasons to question the validity of reviews by NRBs, they appear to be performing satisfactorily.

In 1986, the FDA began to waive the requirement for local REC review of some protocols designed to evaluate, or to make available for therapeutic purposes, investigational new drugs, particularly those intended for the treatment of HIV infection. In such cases RECs were offered the option of accepting review by a national committee as fulfilling the regulatory requirement for REC review. Such practices have caused some commentators to question the strength of the government's commitment to the principle of local review.

Internationally, there is much less commitment to the importance of local review. The International Ethical Guidelines for Biomedical Research Involving Human Subjects (1993), promulgated by the Council for International Organizations of Medical Sciences, require REC approval for all research involving human subjects and recognize the validity of review at a regional or, "in a highly centralized administration," a national level. In many European countries, RECs are regional (McNeill, 1989).

Several commentators have expressed concern that in the United States the local institution has too much power in protection of human research subjects. John Robertson (1979b), for example, alerts us to "the danger . . . that research institutions will use [RECs] to protect themselves and researchers rather than subjects"; others point to the close associations between RECs and risk-management offices in many institutions as evidence that RECs are being used in this manner.

Criticisms

Before 1962, "a general skepticism toward the development of ethical guidelines, codes, or sets of procedures concerning the conduct of research" prevailed in the medical research community (Curran, 1970, p. 408). In the 1970s several biomedical scientists were harshly critical of the REC system, claiming that it tended to stifle creativity and impede progress (R. Levine, 1986); survey research, however, showed that only 25 percent of biomedical researchers agreed with the statement that "The review . . . is an unwarranted intrusion on the investigator's autonomy—at least to some extent" (National Commission, 1978, p. 75). Behavioral and social scientists were considerably less accepting of review, claiming that their research activities were much less likely than those of the biomedical scientist to harm subjects. Some argued that since all they did was talk with subjects, review was an unconstitutional constraint on their freedom of speech (R. Levine, 1986).

According to Peter Williams (1984), RECs do an inadequate job of ensuring that risks will be reasonable in relation to anticipated benefits. This is inevitable for three reasons:

1. Federal regulations on this standard are written in vague language, in contrast to the clearer direction provided for protecting subjects' rights. Moreover, since the regulations permit consideration of the long-range effects of applying knowledge as benefits

but not as risks, they create a bias in favor of approval.

2. The membership of the committee, dominated as it is by professionals, is likely to place a higher value than laypersons would on the benefit of developing new knowledge.

3. Groups confronted with choices involving risks may be either more or less cautious or "risk aversive" than the average of individuals within the group; this is known as the "risky shift" or "group polarization phenomenon." Peter Williams (1984) and Robert Veatch (1975) believe that in the context of RECs, the groups are likely to be more tolerant of higher levels of risk than they would be as individuals.

Several commentators have proposed that RECs could enhance their effectiveness by sending members to the sites of the actual conduct of research to verify compliance with protocol requirements (Robertson, 1979b) or to supervise consent negotiations (Robertson, 1982). Others respond that while such activities should be done when there are reasons to suspect problems in specific protocols, routine monitoring activities might be detrimental to the successful functioning of the committee by eroding its support within the institution (R. Levine, 1986).

Evaluation

Critics of the REC system claim that there is little or no objective evidence that REC review prevents the conduct of inadequate research. For example, a national survey of RECs revealed that the rate of rejection of protocols is less than one in one thousand (National Commission, 1978). Supporters of the system respond that the actual rejection rate is much higher if one includes protocols withdrawn because investigators refuse to modify them as required by RECs. Moreover, rejection rates may be a poor indicator of the REC's quality; protocols may be improved in anticipation of the REC's requirements, and investigators, fearing rejection, may decide not to submit proposals they think might be rejected.

It is very difficult to evaluate the REC's performance objectively; satisfactory subjective evaluations can be made only by experienced REC members and administrators (R. Levine, 1986). Jerry Mashaw concludes in his excellent theoretical analysis of RECs:

> If [the REC] is to do its core job well, we must live with its inevitable incompetence at other tasks. Moreover, we must also live with the rather vague regulatory standards and with the continuing inability of the federal funding agencies to know for sure whether [RECs] are functioning effectively. If we would have wise judges and paternalistic [skilled in protecting subjects' rights

and welfare interests] professionals, we can neither specifically direct nor objectively evaluate their behavior. (1981, p. 22)

ROBERT J. LEVINE

For a further discussion of topics mentioned in this entry, see the entries INFORMED CONSENT, *article on* CONSENT ISSUES IN HUMAN RESEARCH; *and* PUBLIC POLICY AND BIOETHICS. *This entry will find application in the entries* AGING AND THE AGED, *article on* HEALTH-CARE AND RESEARCH ISSUES; CHILDREN, *article on* HEALTH-CARE AND RESEARCH ISSUES; COMMERCIALISM IN SCIENTIFIC RESEARCH; FETUS, *article on* FETAL RESEARCH; GENETICS AND HUMAN BEHAVIOR, *article on* SCIENTIFIC AND RESEARCH ISSUES; MENTALLY ILL AND MENTALLY DISABLED PERSONS, *article on* RESEARCH ISSUES; MILITARY PERSONNEL AS RESEARCH SUBJECTS; MULTINATIONAL RESEARCH; PRISONERS, *article on* RESEARCH ISSUES; PRIVACY AND CONFIDENTIALITY IN RESEARCH; RESEARCH, UNETHICAL; RESEARCH BIAS; SEX THERAPY AND SEX RESEARCH; *and* STUDENTS AS RESEARCH SUBJECTS. *For a discussion of ethics committees in animal research, see the entries* ANIMAL RESEARCH, *article on* LAW AND POLICY; *and* VETERINARY ETHICS. *Other relevant material may be found under the entries* LAW AND BIOETHICS; RESEARCH, HUMAN: HISTORICAL ASPECTS; RESEARCH METHODOLOGY; RESEARCH POLICY; *and* RIGHTS, *article on* RIGHTS IN BIOETHICS. *See also the* APPENDIX (CODES, OATHS, AND DIRECTIVES RELATED TO BIOETHICS), SECTION IV: ETHICAL DIRECTIVES FOR HUMAN RESEARCH.

Bibliography

ANNAS, GEORGE. 1991. "Ethics Committees: From Ethical Comfort to Ethical Cover." *Hastings Center Report* 21, no. 3:18–21.

COUNCIL FOR INTERNATIONAL ORGANIZATIONS OF MEDICAL SCIENCES. 1993. *International Ethical Guidelines for Biomedical Research Involving Human Subjects.* Geneva: Author.

CURRAN, WILLIAM J. 1970. "Governmental Regulation of the Use of Human Subjects in Medical Research: The Approach of Two Federal Agencies." In *Experimentation with Human Subjects,* pp. 402–454. Edited by Paul A. Freund. New York: George Braziller.

FREEDMAN, BENJAMIN. 1987. "Scientific Value and Validity as Ethical Requirements for Research: A Proposed Explication." *IRB* 9, no. 6:7–10.

HERMAN, SAMUEL S. 1989. "A Noninstitutional Review Board Comes of Age." *IRB* 11, no. 2:1–6.

LEVINE, CAROL. 1988. "Has AIDS Changed the Ethics of Human Subjects Research?" *Law, Medicine and Health Care* 16, nos. 3–4:167–173.

LEVINE, CAROL; DUBLER, NANCY N.; and LEVINE, ROBERT J. 1991. "Building a New Consensus: Ethical Principles and

Policies for Clinical Research on HIV/AIDS." *IRB* 13, nos. 1–2:1–17.

LEVINE, ROBERT J. 1986. *Ethics and Regulation of Clinical Research.* 2d ed. Baltimore: Urban and Schwarzenberg.

LIPSETT, MORTIMER B.; FLETCHER, JOHN C.; and SECUNDY, MARIAN. 1979. "Research Review at NIH." *Hastings Center Report* 9, no. 1:18–21.

MASHAW, JERRY L. 1981. "Thinking About Institutional Review Boards." In *Whistleblowing in Biomedical Research: Policies and Procedures for Responding to Reports of Misconduct.* The President's Commission for the Study of Ethical Problems in Medicine and Biomedical and Behavioral Research. pp. 3–22. Washington, D.C.: U.S. Government Printing Office.

McNEILL, PAUL M. 1989. "Research Ethics Committees in Australia, Europe, and North America." *IRB* 11, no. 3: 4–7.

MEDICAL RESEARCH COUNCIL OF CANADA. 1987. *Guidelines on Research Involving Human Subjects.* Ottawa: Author.

NATIONAL COMMISSION FOR THE PROTECTION OF HUMAN SUBJECTS OF BIOMEDICAL AND BEHAVIORAL RESEARCH. 1978. *Report and Recommendations: Institutional Review Boards.* Publication no. (OS) 78-0008. Washington, D.C.: Department of Health, Education and Welfare.

ROBERTSON, JOHN A. 1979a. "The Law of Institutional Review Boards." *UCLA Law Review* 26:484–549.

———. 1979b. "Ten Ways to Improve IRBs." *Hastings Center Report* 9, no. 1:29–33.

———. 1982. "Taking Consent Seriously: IRB Intervention in the Consent Process." *IRB* 4, no. 5:1–5.

VEATCH, ROBERT M. 1975. "Human Experimentation Committees: Professional or Representative?" *Hastings Center Report* 5, no. 5:31–40.

WILLIAMS, PETER C. 1984. "Success in Spite of Failure: Why IRBs Falter in Reviewing Risks and Benefits." *IRB* 6, no. 3:1–4.

RESEARCH METHODOLOGY

I. Conceptual Issues
    Kenneth F. Schaffner
II. Controlled Clinical Trials
    Loretta M. Kopelman

I. CONCEPTUAL ISSUES

Research in medicine, in the biomedical sciences, and in science in general is defined as "studious inquiry or examination; *esp*: investigation or experimentation aimed at the discovery and interpretation of facts, revision of accepted theories or laws in the light of new facts, or practical application of such new or revised theories or laws" (Merriam-Webster, 1983, p. 1002). The U.S. federal government's Common Rule for human-subject investigation (hereafter CR) echoes Webster's definition; according to the CR, "*Research* means a systematic investigation, including research development, testing, and evaluation, designed to contribute to generalizable knowledge" ("Protection of Human Subjects," 1993, pt. 46, sec. 102). Research can refer to investigations that involve intentional manipulation of the objects studied, frequently termed "experimental" studies, as well as those inquiries that collect data generated by naturally occurring events, or "observational" studies. This article focuses on the burdens and benefits scientific research has on human subjects (or perhaps better, on trial participants) and on society, as well as on laboratory animals. Research methodology comprises those general principles and designs used to describe valid and effective inquiries into nature, which includes humans. Research methodology has philosophical, scientific, and social dimensions.

General aspects of research methodology

Beginning with Plato and Aristotle, philosophers have proposed a number of different though quite general approaches to scientific method. René Descartes and Francis Bacon wrote on the subject in the seventeenth century, but the study of scientific method received its most systematic treatments in the work of the nineteenth-century philosophers and scientists William Whewell, Stanley Jevons, and John Stuart Mill (1959), who forcefully re-presented the methods of agreement, difference, concomitant variation, and others that continue to influence contemporary philosophers; frequently these are referred to as Mill's Methods. Philosophers of science have continued to stimulate the imagination of practicing scientists. Since the early 1960s, Sir Karl Popper's "falsificationist" approach, T. S. Kuhn's account of revolutionary scientific changes as "paradigm shifts," and the latter's criticisms of traditional rational and gradualist methodology have been cited in a number of scientific research articles.

Research methodology also involves more specific scientific components, including the analysis of different laboratory methodologies (e.g., molecular approaches and pure culture techniques); the utility of various "animal models" of diseases; and the characterization and assessment of the strengths of distinct study designs, ranging from the report of an individual case to the randomized controlled clinical trial. These scientific components may involve a considerable amount of sophisticated mathematical and statistical analysis. In this article, both the philosophical and the scientific dimensions of research methodology will be pursued in the context of questions that they raise for bioethics.

A final major aspect of research methodology is the important "social" dimension of systematic empirical investigations. By this term we intend to signify the ethical, legal, political, and religious aspects of research methodology. More specifically, this rubric treats various moral implications of scientific investigation, including vulnerable or hitherto ignored subject populations (e.g., the disabled and women), from both descriptive and normative perspectives, as well as significant interactions among the philosophical, scientific, and social themes.

The scope of research

Biomedical and behavioral investigations.   Biomedical research (generally understood as also including behavioral research in the psychological and social sciences) covers a broad array of disciplines. The term "biomedical" is itself intended to bridge the gap between the more fundamental, "pure," or "basic" sciences, such as physiology and biochemistry, and the more "applied" sciences, such as pathology and pharmacology. This interpretation, however, leaves the more "clinical" sciences, such as anesthesiology and medicine, less connected with the meaning of science than is appropriate. Better, perhaps, to follow a more expansive definition as found in *Webster's Ninth New Collegiate Dictionary,* which gives as one definition of "biomedical": "Of, relating to, or involving biological, medical, and physical science" (Merriam-Webster, 1983, p. 153). *Dorland's Medical Dictionary* (26th ed.) offers as its preferred meaning "biological and medical" (Dorland, 1985, p. 169). In accordance with this expanded characterization of the term, virtually all of the natural, behavioral, and social sciences, as well as engineering, can be conceived of as biomedical sciences if the intent is to place them in the service of advancing generalizable knowledge in the domains of medicine and health care (Levine, 1978).

Basic science and clinical science.   A common division is found in the departmental organization in medical schools distinguishing between basic sciences, such as microbiology (but also including more applied sciences such as pharmacology), and the clinical sciences such as medicine and oncology, whose practitioners spend much of their time and effort working with patients. It must not be forgotten that studies employing systems ranging from in vitro ("test tube") inquiries through research on bacterial viruses to animal-model investigations comprise the bulk of research in the biomedical sciences. Preliminary research on new drug therapies, as well as investigations into human immunodeficiency virus (HIV) pathophysiology, fall into this category. In addition, in recent years there has been heightened awareness of the ethical problems generated by the use of animals in biomedical research, and thus it is appropriate to comment briefly on this basic science dimension of research methodology.

In 1976 an important study investigated the type of research that led to the ten most important advances in the treatment of cardiovascular and pulmonary diseases (Comroe and Dripps, 1976). The investigators used a broad definition of "clinically oriented" research; studies involving animals, tissues, or cells (including cell fragments) were included in the definition if the author mentioned a possible clinical application even briefly. In spite of this expansive definition, some 41 percent of key articles involved in the development of these ten clinically relevant advances were not clinically oriented; that is, they reported on basic science research. This finding suggests that supporting only "targeted" or "mission-oriented" research is likely to have adverse effects on clinical research advances.

Another intensive investigation, conducted in 1985 by the National Research Council's Committee on Models for Biomedical Research, examined the nature of research methodology in the biomedical sciences and underscored the intimate and reciprocal relationship between research generally characterized as "clinical" and research generally characterized as "basic" (National Research Council, 1985). This report introduced the general notion of a "biomatrix," which was defined as a "complex body, or matrix, of interrelated biological knowledge built from studies of many kinds of organisms, biological preparations, and biological processes at various levels" (National Research Council, 1985, p. 2). Within such a multidimensional matrix, biomedical research involves "many-many modeling" in which analogous features at various levels of aggregation (e.g., molecules, cells, and organs) are related to each other across various species. The committee suggested that an "investigator considers some problem of interest—a disease process, some normal physiological function, or any other aspect of biology or medicine. The problem is analyzed into its component parts, and for each part and at each level, the matrix of biological knowledge is searched for analogous phenomena. . . . Although it is possible to view the processes involved in interpreting data in the language of [simple] one-to-one modeling, the investigator is actually modelling back and forth onto the matrix of biological knowledge" (National Research Council, 1985, p. 67). The Comroe and Dripps study, as well as the council's report, thus indicate that clinically relevant advances emerge from research sources beyond those involving human subjects.

Before innovations can be tested on humans, ethical codes and governmental regulation require research involving chemical, cell-fragment, cell, tissue, and intact-animal-model systems. The Nuremberg Code (1947–1948), for example, recommends that human experimentation should be based on the results of animal experimentation (Beauchamp and Childress, 1979). The Declaration of Helsinki (1964, revised in 1975) requires that "biomedical research involving human subjects must conform to generally accepted scientific principles and should be based on adequately performed laboratory and animal experimentation . . ." (Beauchamp and Childress, 1979, p. 290). These requirements are based on the belief that such inquiries will assist in identifying interventions that are both safer and more effective by the time they are finally applied to human subjects. In the biomedical sciences, including studies involving human subjects, biological diversity and the number of systems that strongly interact in living organisms create considerable complexity. Researchers must often pay special attention to ensuring the (near) identity of the organisms under investigation, except for those differences that are the focus of the scientist's inquiry.

Biomedical investigations involving virtually identical laboratory organisms can yield precise and often nonstatistical results that can then be utilized in more variable human populations. As is discussed in the section below on various study designs, human variability of both genetic and environmental sources will typically require the extensive use of statistical methodologies to uncover generalizable knowledge that is clinically applicable. In more rigidly controllable laboratory experiments—for example, in the rapidly advancing area of molecular genetics—biomedical scientists can often employ the classical methods of experimental inquiry, referred to earlier as "Mill's Methods." These methods can be thought of as attempting to discover the causal structure of the world, and in their application scientists endeavor to identify and compensate for possible confounding factors that, if ignored, can lead to mistaken inferences about causes and effects. Thus all natural scientists attempt to compensate for interfering and extraneous factors, frequently by setting up a control comparison or a control group. Such controls are a direct implementation of what Mill termed the "method of difference" and Claude Bernard, the notable nineteenth-century French scientist and methodologist, the "method of comparative experimentation." The method of difference may be stated in a form similar to that in which Mill presented it:

> Suppose that in Case 1 some phenomenon occurs, and in Case 2, that is identical with Case 1 *except for one factor*, the phenomenon does *not* occur. Then the single difference between the two cases is the effect of that phenomenon, or the cause of that phenomenon, or an indispensable part of the cause of that phenomenon. (See Mill, 1959, p. 256, for his original language)

Claude Bernard felt this focus on only one difference was far too stringent and reformulated the experimental idea as his method of "comparative experimentation":

> Physiological phenomena are so complex that we could never experiment at all rigorously on living animals if we necessarily had to define all the other changes we might cause in the organism on which we were operating. But fortunately it is enough for us completely to isolate the one phenomenon on which our studies are brought to bear, separating it by means of comparative experimentation from all surrounding complications. Comparative experimentation reaches this goal by adding to a similar organism, used for comparison, all our experimental changes save one, the very one which we intend to disengage. (Bernard, 1957, pp. 127–128)

Bernard referred to comparative experimentation as "the true foundation of experimental medicine."

General ethical issues associated with research on human subjects

The principal ethical controversies in biomedical (including behavioral and social) research have emerged from studies involving human subjects. Before discussing the general ethical requirements of studies involving human subjects, however, it is important to describe briefly the often contentious debate about the terms used to distinguish between different kinds of standard medical practice and research, among them "therapeutic research," "nontherapeutic research," "innovative treatments," and "experimentation."

Terminological considerations. It is a fundamental tenet of medical ethics that the well-being of human subjects should be protected. This tenet, together with another general ethical principle frequently associated with the name of philosopher Immanuel Kant, to treat oneself or another human being always as an end and never merely or only as a means, requires that a human research subject be expected to obtain some direct benefit from the investigation, or, if not, to waive such benefit on the basis of a free and informed consent. (This Kantian injunction is sometimes characterized as a principle of "respect for persons.") The need to clarify the therapeutic/nontherapeutic distinction in the light of such principles should be evident.

Thoughtful scholars have generally agreed about the difficulty of drawing a clear distinction between research and accepted practice, but have differed about the usefulness of various terms proposed to assist with this task. Some (Fried, 1978) find the distinction between therapeutic and nontherapeutic experimentation "crucial," whereas others (Capron, 1978) find it is better phrased as one between beneficial and nonbeneficial experimentation. Robert Levine, an authority on research involving human subjects, contends that the expressions "therapeutic research," "nontherapeutic research," and "experimentation" (in human subject contexts) are "unacceptable" and "illogical" (Levine, 1986, p. 8). The problem arises in part because it is fairly common that a diagnostic and therapeutic plan involve some variation from the textbook norm, and because it is in only rare cases that biomedical research conveys absolutely no benefit on its subjects.

Levine suggests that we employ the term "nonvalidated practices" as a more encompassing term for "innovative therapies," acknowledging that it is the uncertainty associated with variation in the outcomes of diagnostic and therapeutic maneuvers that is the principal issue (Levine, 1986, p. 4). This suggestion seems to have been accepted in much of the recent literature, though frequently the narrower term "nonvalidated therapy" is also employed. Though no definitive algorithm can be provided that will unambiguously differentiate the various inquiries and activities discussed in the preceding paragraph, the general proposal that appears to emerge from the discussion involves three elements. First, the intent of the investigator is critical in determining whether the intervention (or the withholding of an intervention) is to be characterized as primarily beneficial to the subjects or as contributing to generalizable knowledge. A surgeon employing a novel suturing technique in an attempt to save a patient from bleeding to death does not evidence any intent of beginning a research project to evaluate a new operative technique. Second, the degree of variation from standard practice figures in this determination, and this may depend as well on the degree of possible harm that the intervention entails. Even small variations associated with significant harm are more likely to be seen as nonvalidated in contrast to small variations with minor adverse consequences. For example, a physician may believe that he or she must try a powerful immunosuppressive drug, usually used only in the case of potential organ-transplant rejection, to help a patient suffering with severe rheumatoid arthritis. The dangers associated with such drugs and the departure from their normal use argues that this would be a "nonvalidated practice." Finally, there is the element of uncertainty, the degree of likelihood of a particular outcome or set of outcomes. These include both anticipated and unintended effects (side effects). Again, the example just cited of the immunosuppressive drug would be relevant here because of the difficulty of anticipating the effects of powerful drugs on systems as complex as the immune system.

For interventions from which the researcher intends to produce new general knowledge, that represent significant departures from accepted practice, and about which there is reasonable uncertainty regarding consequences, including intended outcomes, it would seem mandatory that the researchers develop a formal research protocol to be assessed by an appropriate institutional review board (IRB). Such a multidimensional "sliding scale," possibly with thresholds that could be specified in particular areas of clinical investigation, may be the best possible mechanism for determining whether to require IRB review in this complex area.

Ethical requirements for research on human subjects. As noted in the preceding section, general principles requiring free and informed consent and a net balance of benefits over harms for the individual subject (unless this is waived by the subject in the interests of greater social benefits) will be assumed in all research contexts, and the present section will examine additional details regarding these requirements. Furthermore, however, in order both to safeguard research subjects and ensure that the resources used will generate valuable knowledge, a research study must conform to scientifically validated principles of design. To begin with, a prospective research project must be evaluated in terms of the risks of harm—physical, psychological, and social—to the subject(s), as well as in terms of the benefits that are likely to accrue to participants. Only studies in which the expected benefits outweigh the expected harms are morally permissible. Further, there must be no alternative and less risky means for the subject to obtain the anticipated benefits. Subjects must be selected equitably, with special sensitivity to the problems faced by vulnerable populations, such as children, prisoners, pregnant women, mentally disabled persons, or educationally disadvantaged persons. In recent years the practice of "community consultation" has developed, which involves meetings with representatives of the at-large subject community (e.g., HIV-infected individuals) to "assure a suitable balancing of the relevant values [such as respect for persons, individual beneficence and justice] in the design and conduct of a clinical trial" (Levine et al., 1991, p. 10).

An investigator must also obtain the legally effective informed consent of the subject or of the subject's legally authorized representative. Such consent must be voluntary and not obtained by coercive measures. The consent must be informed; this means that the investigator must specify the purposes of the research and how long the subject is expected to participate and provide a nontechnical description (in terms readily understandable to the subject) of any procedures to be followed, as well as a designation of procedures considered untested or experimental. The subject must also be provided with a description of any reasonable foreseeable risks or discomforts as well as reasonably anticipated benefits. Alternative procedures or courses of treatment that may be advantageous to the participant must be disclosed. Subjects are also to be provided with a statement about the extent of confidentiality of their records and, for research involving more than minimal risk, an explanation of what, if any, compensation or treatments will be available in the event of injury. According to the CR, subjects must be informed about whom to contact for answers about any questions or injuries that may arise in the course of or as a consequence of the research. They are to be told that their participation is voluntary and that they may refuse to participate or may withdraw from participation without any penalty or loss of benefits to which they would normally be entitled ("Protection of Human Subjects," 1993). Should the investigator come to believe in the course of the research that harm to the patient has become likely, the patient should be so informed and withdrawn from the project. The above requirements underscore the point that informed consent should not be conceived of only as a one-time event, but is best construed as an ongoing process involving clinical investigators and trial participants.

In certain types of behavioral and social-science research, investigators have maintained that scientifically valid conclusions can be obtained only if the subjects are kept uninformed or even deliberately deceived about the nature of the research. In a well-known example of this type of research, Stanley Milgram's studies on obedience to authority, subjects were falsely told they were causing pain to another human as part of a learning experiment. A majority of subjects proceeded to escalate the level of fictiously inflicted pain to "agonizing" levels on the instructions of the investigator. Subsequently, when the subjects were informed about this feature of themselves as part of the debriefing, they experienced severe, and in some cases, prolonged anxiety reactions (Milgram, 1963). Milgram defended his study against criticism and reported that most of the subjects had a positive view of their participation (Milgram, 1964).

The ethics of such studies continue to be controversial. Levine notes that he himself chairs an IRB that occasionally approves deceptive studies but generally disapproves of deception (Levine, 1986). Various guidelines regarding deceptive research methods have been published (American Psychological Association, 1982). An alternative view of such research is urged by Tom Beauchamp and James Childress (1989), who recommend that such studies be disapproved if significant risk is involved and if subjects are not informed that they are being placed at risk.

In response to many unethical research practices, ranging from Nazi atrocities before and during World War II to well-documented cases in the United States, the U.S. government has mandated a set of formal procedures to ensure compliance with ethical requisites. Institutions involved in research on human subjects are required to have their investigations reviewed and approved by institutional review boards (IRBs) whose composition, procedures, and record-keeping requirements are well-defined in law and governmental regulations. However, the determination by a duly con-

stituted IRB that these ethical requirements have been satisfied does not always resolve the ethical and practical stresses generated by research on human subjects. It should be noted, however, that the determination by a duly constituted IRB of the satisfaction of these ethical requirements does not in all cases resolve all ethical and practical stresses generated by research on human subjects. A number of authors have discerned a deeply rooted dilemma that the physician as healer and the physician as researcher confronts in a search for generalizable knowledge employing human subjects. This dilemma has its source partly in the respect-for-persons principle cited above and partly in the ethical principle that the physician should do what is best for his or her patient. The dilemma is also most clearly evident in the context of the randomized controlled clinical trial but can also arise in less stringent research designs, which it will be necessary to discuss before turning to an account of this troublesome research predicament.

Study designs

The spectrum of study designs in biomedical and behavioral research. Diverse research designs guide research in the biomedical, behavioral, and clinical sciences. Since this topic can easily become quite technical and mathematically abstruse, this article presents only a general introduction to this subject. (For specialized information including indications when, and why, one design is preferable to another, see works on clinical epidemiology and monographs devoted to specific research designs, e.g., Feinstein, 1986; Fletcher et al., 1982; Hulley and Cummings, 1988; Lilienfeld and Lilienfeld, 1980; and Sackett et al., 1985.)

The chart depicted in Figure 1 can be used as a guide to the various research designs found in clinical research. (This figure is based in part on Lilienfeld and Lilienfeld, 1980, p. 192, and in part on Fletcher et al., 1982, p. 193.) To these designs should also be added the "case report" and the "case series," in which a biomedically interesting individual's (or small group of similar individuals') situation is described. Some writers characterize the case report or case series as another design; others view such a small series as conductible using any of the designs described in the chart below. (The use of small numbers of subjects in any trial design, however, raises concerns that errors of interpretation are likely because of chance events. Problems generated by chance events in biomedical research are analyzed using the tools of mathematical statistics.)

The "interval of data collection" refers to the period of time during which data are collected. If one or more populations are studied over a period of time, the study is described as a "longitudinal" one. Alternatively, we may wish to collect information within one time slice,

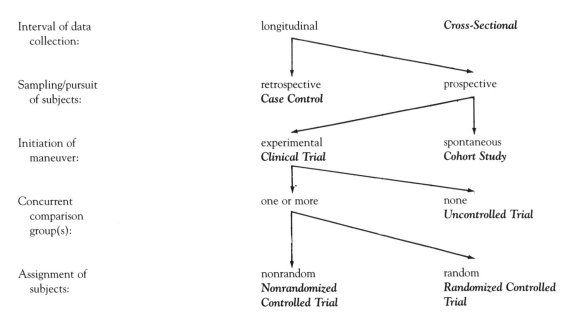

FIGURE 1. The epidemiological study: various research designs used to establish causation in medicine.

yielding a "cross-sectional" study. Moving to the next line, the investigator may collect data by looking back in time—for example, inquiring (or reviewing chart records) to learn whether the population was exposed to a specific agent. At least one control group is assembled to provide a comparison, again retrospectively. This "case control" design is the type of approach that Arthur Herbst and his colleagues employed in his pioneering inquiry into the causes of vaginal cancer in daughters of mothers who had been given diethylstilbestrol (DES), a synthetic estrogen believed to help prevent miscarriages, during their pregnancies (Herbst et al., 1971). The case-control type of study is generally thought to be open to a number of potential errors, termed "biases." Potentially confounding elements therefore need to be monitored carefully.

If the putative active difference between the comparison groups, such as the administration of a new drug, is intentionally introduced by the investigators, a study is characterized as "experimental." If the suspected active difference occurs by accident or is chosen by the subjects—for example, a subject's decision to begin cigarette smoking or to reduce blood cholesterol by diet—the investigation is termed a "cohort" study. A longitudinal prospective experimental study is a clinical trial, but such trials may or may not involve a comparison control group. Good examples of uncontrolled types of clinical trials are Phase I and Phase II investigations of new drugs, though occasionally a Phase II investigation may involve randomized controls (see Byar et al., 1990). Phase I studies look at the metabolism and toxicity of new drugs, often in normal subjects, and Phase II

inquiries test for preliminary efficacy of a drug or a procedure. The terms "Phase I" and "Phase II" were introduced in 1977 by the U.S. Food and Drug Administration (FDA). (For details of the procedures by which toxicity and efficacy of interventions are evaluated, see Gilman et al., 1980, chapter 68.)

A Phase III investigation is almost always a "randomized controlled trial." Randomization refers to the process of assigning a patient to one rather than another treatment (or to the control group) by the flip of a coin or a more mathematically sophisticated but analogous procedure of using a table of random numbers. The randomized controlled clinical trial (hereafter RCT) refers to that form of investigation that involves (1) one or more treatment groups and a control group that will typically receive a placebo (an inert substance) or the standard therapy (i.e., the traditionally accepted therapy); (2) randomized assignment of patients to the two or more groups (possibly after stratification or subgrouping based on known factors that will make a difference) sometimes referred to as "arms" of the trial; and (3) often a single- or double-blind design in which the assignments of the agents or procedures being tested are not known to the patients (single-blind) or possibly also to the treating health professionals (double-blind). In one unusual exception to that rule, the trial of the anti-HIV drug didanosine, or ddI, the whole experimental cohort were given ddI; these subjects were compared with "historical," or retrospectively identified, control subjects (Waldholz, 1992; FDA, 1991).

Considerable debate has occurred about the methodological value and the ethical significance of randomization in controlled clinical trials. Various types of studies described above differ in their "strength," that is, their ability to detect what is actually causing the changes that are being observed. The case series is traditionally the weakest of the research designs; other designs, in order of increasing strength, are the case-controlled study, the cohort study, and the randomized clinical trial. The principal reason for the increase in design strength is the decrease in the likelihood of "bias," or lack of comparability of the matched populations, as one moves from case series through to the randomized controlled clinical trial.

There are many types of bias, and some of them are quite subtle (Sackett, 1979). A major source of bias is selection or susceptibility bias, in which the groups compared have distinctly different outcome probabilities (more specifically, different prognostic likelihoods for the study's endpoint). This type of bias can occur within the study, or it can arise as part of the selection process and affect the generalizability of a study's results. In this type of situation, unrepresentative individuals are selected, and subgroups drawn from the unrepresentative class are then assigned to the arms of the study. An example of this type of bias would occur if only the sickest patients in a study were given the new drug and the better-off patients were assigned standard therapy (or a placebo). Another source of noncomparability is performance bias, in which the interventions in the trial are not reasonably equal. An example would be if the patients receiving the new drug were monitored much more closely and treated for concurrent health problems with no such monitoring and treatment being provided to the control group. A third type of bias is "confounding" bias, in which another, unsuspected causal variable "travels along" with the putative causal variable and actually accounts for the outcome. This could occur in a study to determine the effects of alcohol consumption on lung function, if alcohol drinkers were also much more likely to be smokers and the effect of smoking was not considered by the investigators. Other significant types of bias are detection or measurement bias, where the outcome event is detected differently in the comparison groups—for example, if the test group received MRIs and the control group standard X rays—and transfer bias, in which subject dropouts or reassignments may yield differences in outcome. The arguments for randomization in clinical investigations typically cite the ability of randomized assignment to decrease the likelihood of bias because, many maintain, randomizing will average together, and thus cancel out, factors that are not suspected by the investigators to affect the outcome.

Historical controls in trials involving life-threatening illness. A vigorous debate has arisen in connection with the need for controls of new therapies for life-threatening illnesses, such as acquired immuno-deficiency syndrome (AIDS) and some forms of cancer. The argument against using any concurrent control subjects who would, in the absence of any standard therapy, receive a placebo is that individuals in the control group would face certain death. One proposal is to treat as many affected subjects as possible with the new regimen and use knowledge about earlier untreated individuals as a comparison to assess the safety and efficacy of the new treatment. This would be a case-controlled study using historical controls. Regarding historical controls there are two generally opposing views developed in the literature. One side (e.g., Chalmers et al., 1972) contends that there are good arguments for always beginning the use of a new therapy with an RCT. On the other side there are theorists (e.g., Freireich and Gehan, 1979) who contend that RCTs are highly overrated and that more extensive use of historical controls is desirable. Most commentators' sentiments appear to take a middle position, and it should be recalled that for drug trials, a three-phase investigation is required by the FDA, beginning with tests for toxicity and proceeding to RCTs only in Phase III.

A prominent international group of statisticians recently proposed that the only situations in which an uncontrolled trial (i.e., a trial in which *all* the participants receive the new therapy) is justified had to meet five rather stringent conditions:

> (1) there must be no other treatment appropriate to use as a control; (2) there must be sufficient experience to ensure that the patients not receiving therapy will have a uniformly poor prognosis; (3) the therapy must not be expected to have substantial side effects that would compromise the potential benefit to the patient; (4) there must be a justifiable expectation that the potential benefit to the patient will be sufficiently large to make the interpretation of the results of a nonrandomized trial unambiguous; and (5) the scientific rationale for the treatment must be sufficiently strong that a positive result would be widely accepted. (Byar et al., 1990, p. 1344)

Satisfaction of all these conditions should ensure the conclusion that a new therapy should be provided via an uncontrolled trial. The same considerations also support the need for wider availability of therapies in like situations. Concerns about HIV and AIDS have forced significant changes in the traditional perception of clinical trials. Where life-threatening diseases are involved, such trials become points of access to a possibly efficacious treatment rather than a means of ascertaining the safety and efficacy of treatments.

Meta-analysis. Human variability, based on both genetics and environment, requires the extensive use of statistical methodologies to uncover generalizable, clinically applicable knowledge. This is in contrast to laboratory investigations in which virtually identical organisms yield cleaner and often "deterministic" results. Besides the variability of the subjects studied, many sources of bias such as the ones described can also lead to incorrect research conclusions.

Under these circumstances, researchers have turned increasingly to a method of clinical trial pooling and interpretation that seems to provide a better means of inferring correct conclusions from repeated clinical investigations. This methodology, known as meta-analysis, uses a set of formal statistical techniques to aggregate a group of separate but similar studies. In contrast to the widely employed scientific practice of summing up such studies qualitatively in a review article, meta-analysis purports to fulfill this summarizing function quantitatively and thus more precisely and objectively. Meta-analysis has been practiced for many years in a variety of scientific disciplines, from physics to the biomedical and the behavioral sciences, but only since the early 1980s has it had a major impact in the clinical arena, particularly in the areas of cardiovascular disease and obstetrics and gynecology (Chalmers et al., 1989; Mann, 1990).

Simple introductions as well as accessible authoritative accounts of the methodology are available. (See Mann, 1990, for an introduction, and Rosenthal, 1991, for a more comprehensive overview.) The technique remains controversial even as its use in biomedicine escalates exponentially.

Conclusion. This article has reviewed a number of conceptual issues associated with current research methodology in the biomedical sciences. We have looked at research in the basic sciences, such as biochemistry and microbiology, but have concentrated on the clinical sciences, such as medicine, oncology, and virology, since it is in the latter that ethical issues affecting human subjects arise. Scientific research on humans takes place in the context of a complex web of ethical and legal requirements, and the interplay between methodological and ethical/legal components of research has been examined. Ethical and regulatory principles (primarily as affecting U.S. research) have been presented, and several conceptual issues regarding scientific inquiry have been outlined, including different types of research designs. This article is limited to an introduction to these issues, which become very technical in their details; references to further reading have been provided.

Although scientific methodology has a venerable history, many current issues are of much more recent vintage. In point of fact, the randomized controlled clinical trial (RCT) is essentially a post–World War II invention, and the discipline of meta-analysis is a creature of the late 1980s and 1990s. New issues will continue to arise as better methodologies and improved safeguards for human subjects are sought, and the reader is urged to consult on-line bibliographic services, such as the BIOETHICS database at the U.S. National Library of Medicine, in addition to references provided in this article, to keep up to date with a continuously evolving subject.

KENNETH F. SCHAFFNER

Directly related to this article is the other article in this entry: CONTROLLED CLINICAL TRIALS. *Also directly related are the entries* INFORMED CONSENT, *article on* CONSENT ISSUES IN HUMAN RESEARCH; PRIVACY AND CONFIDENTIALITY IN RESEARCH; RESEARCH BIAS; RESEARCH ETHICS COMMITTEES; RESEARCH POLICY; RESEARCH, HUMAN: HISTORICAL ASPECTS; *and* RESEARCH, UNETHICAL. *This article will find application in the entries* ANIMAL RESEARCH; AUTOEXPERIMENTATION; MINORITIES AS RESEARCH SUBJECTS; *and* MULTINATIONAL RESEARCH. *Other relevant material may be found under the entries* ACADEMIC HEALTH CENTERS; COMMUNICATION, BIOMEDICAL, *article on* SCIENTIFIC PUBLISHING; FRAUD, THEFT, AND PLAGIARISM; RIGHTS; *and* SEX THERAPY AND SEX RESEARCH. *See also the* APPENDIX (CODES, OATHS, AND DIRECTIVES RELATED TO BIOETHICS), SECTION IV: ETHICAL DIRECTIVES FOR HUMAN RESEARCH.

Bibliography

AMERICAN PSYCHOLOGICAL ASSOCIATION. 1982. *Ethical Principles in the Conduct of Research with Human Participants.* Washington, D.C.: Author.

BEAUCHAMP, TOM L., and CHILDRESS, JAMES F. 1979. *Principles of Biomedical Ethics.* 1st ed. New York: Oxford University Press.

———. 1989. *Principles of Biomedical Ethics.* 3d ed. New York: Oxford University Press.

BERNARD, CLAUDE. 1957. [1865]. *An Introduction to the Study of Experimental Medicine.* Translated by Henry C. Green. New York: Dover.

BYAR, DAVID P., SCHOENFELD, DAVID A.; GREEN, SYLVAN B., et al. 1990. "Design Consideration for AIDS Trials." *New England Journal of Medicine* 323, no. 19:1343–1348.

CAPRON, ALEXANDER M. 1978. "Human Experimentation: Basic Issues." In vol. 2 of *Encyclopedia of Bioethics,* pp. 692–699. Edited by Warren T. Reich. New York: Macmillan.

CHALMERS, JAIN; ENKIN, MURRAY; KEIRSE, MARK; and ENKIN, ELEANOR, eds. 1989. *Effective Care in Pregnancy and Childbirth.* New York: Oxford University Press.

CHALMERS, THOMAS C.; BLOCK, JEROME; and LEE, STEPHANIE. 1972. "Controlled Studies in Clinical Cancer Research." *New England Journal of Medicine* 287, no. 2:75–78.

COMROE, JULIUS H., JR., and DRIPPS, ROBERT D. 1976. "Scientific Basis for the Support of Biomedical Science." *Science* 192, no. 4235:105–111.

DORLAND, W. A. NEWMAN. 1985. *Dorland's Illustrated Medical Dictionary,* 26th ed. Philadelphia: W. B. Saunders.

FEINSTEIN, ALVIN R. 1986. *Clinical Epidemiology: The Architecture of Clinical Research.* Philadelphia: W. B. Saunders.

FLETCHER, ROBERT H.; FLETCHER, SUZANNE W.; and WAGNER, EDWARD H. 1982. *Clinical Epidemiology: The Essentials.* Philadelphia: Williams & Wilkins.

FOOD AND DRUG ADMINISTRATION (U.S.). 1977. *General Considerations for the Clinical Evaluation of Drugs.* DHEW Publication No. (FDA) 77-3040. Washington, D.C.: U.S. Government Printing Office.

———. 1991. "Summary Minutes of Antiviral Drugs Advisory Committee" (July 18/19). Meeting #6, Bethesda Holiday Inn, Bethesda, Md. Available from FDA on request.

FREIREICH, EMIL, and GEHAN, EDMUND. 1979. "The Limitations of the Randomized Clinical Trial." In *Cancer Drug Development*—Part B, pp. 277–310. Edited by Vincent T. De Vita and Harris Busch. Methods of Cancer Research, vol. 17. New York: Academic Press.

FRIED, CHARLES. 1978. "Human Experimentation: Philosophical Aspects." In vol. 2 of *Encyclopedia of Bioethics,* pp. 699–702. Edited by Warren T. Reich. New York: Macmillan.

GOODMAN, LOUIS S., and GILMAN, ALFRED G., eds. 1980. *Goodman and Gilman's The Pharmacological Basis of Therapeutics.* 6th ed. New York: Macmillan.

HERBST, ARTHUR L.; UHLFELDER, HOWARD; and POSKANZER, DAVID C. 1971. "Adenocarcinoma of the Vagina: Association of Maternal Stilbestrol Therapy with Tumor Appearance in Young Women." *New England Journal of Medicine* 284, no. 16:878–881.

HULLEY, STEPHEN B.; CUMMINGS, STEVEN R.; and BROWNER, WARREN S., eds. 1988. *Designing Clinical Research: An Epidemiologic Approach.* Baltimore, Md.: Williams & Wilkins.

LEVINE, CAROL; DUBLER, NANCY N.; and LEVINE, ROBERT J. 1991. "Building a New Consensus: Ethical Principles and Policies for Clinical Research on HIV/AIDS." *IRB* 13, nos. 1–2:1–17.

LEVINE, ROBERT J. 1978. "Biomedical Research." In vol. 4 of *Encyclopedia of Bioethics,* pp. 1481–1492. Edited by Warren T. Reich. New York: Macmillan.

———. 1986. *Ethics and Regulation of Clinical Research.* 2d ed. New Haven, Conn.: Yale University Press.

LILIENFELD, ABRAHAM M., and LILIENFELD, DAVID E. 1980. *Foundations of Epidemiology.* New York: Oxford University Press.

MANN, CHARLES 1990. "Meta-Analysis in the Breech." *Science* 249:476–480.

MILGRAM, STANLEY. 1963. "Behavioral Study of Obedience." *Journal of Abnormal Psychology* 67, no. 4:371–378.

———. 1964. "Issues in the Study of Obedience: A Reply to Baumrind." *American Psychologist* 19, no. 11:848–852.

MILL, JOHN STUART. 1959. [1843]. *A System of Logic.* London: Longmans, Green and Co.

NATIONAL RESEARCH COUNCIL. COMMITTEE ON MODELS FOR BIOMEDICAL RESEARCH. 1985. *A New Perspective.* Washington, D.C.: National Academy Press.

"Protection of Human Subjects." 1993. Code of Federal Regulations. Title 45, pt. 46.

ROSENTHAL, ROBERT 1991. "Meta-Analysis: A Review." *Psychosomatic Medicine* 53, no. 3:247–271.

SACKETT, DAVID L. 1979. "Bias in Analytic Research." *Journal of Chronic Diseases* 32, nos. 1–2:51–63.

SACKETT, DAVID L.; HAYNES, R. BRIAN; and TUGWELL, PETER. 1985. *Clinical Epidemiology: A Basic Science for Clinical Medicine.* Boston: Little, Brown.

U.S. FEDERAL GOVERNMENT. 1991. Federal Policy for the Protection of Human Subjects (45 CFR 46). *Federal Register,* vol. 56, 117:28013–28.

U.S. PRESIDENT'S COMMISSION FOR THE STUDY OF ETHICAL PROBLEMS IN MEDICINE AND BIOMEDICAL AND BEHAVIORAL RESEARCH. 1983. *IRB Guidebook.* Washington, D.C.: United States Government Printing Office.

WALDHOLZ, MICHAEL. 1992. "Bristol-Meyers Guides AIDS Drug Through a Marketing Minefield." *Wall Street Journal,* October 10, pp. A1 and A7.

Webster's Ninth New Collegiate Dictionary. 1983. Springfield, Mass.: Merriam-Webster.

II. CONTROLLED CLINICAL TRIALS

In the last half of the twentieth century, clinical trial methodology fundamentally transformed the nature of biomedical research. During this period, investigators developed ways to avoid subtle biases in research design and adapt methods of statistical analysis to empirical research. The story of the progressive sophistication of biomedical research, however, does not begin in clinics or hospitals but in a cornfield. Ronald A. Fisher (1890–1962), the famous British statistician, biologist, and eugenicist, devised methods for testing hypotheses about how to improve crops (Gigerenzer et al., 1989). He divided fields into two or more groups, making them as similar as possible in composition and treatment. His goal was to isolate the effects of the one different feature on the individuals studied. For example, would a fertilizer given to some of the corn improve yield? Differences between groups could then be expressed as probabilities about whether outcomes are due to chance or their different treatment. By studying more individuals for longer periods, confidence increases that variations between group outcomes are due to their different treatment.

In the late 1940s Fisher and others began to adapt and refine these pioneering principles for use with human research. Since that time investigators have used clinical-trial methods to evaluate virtually everything affecting patients: therapies, diagnostic techniques, prevention of illnesses, vaccines, counseling, health delivery systems, and even the benefits of classical music, pets, and humor on health. For example, people were divided into large groups; some got a daily aspirin and others a placebo or an inert substance. This helped ensure that groups were treated alike even down to the number of pills that they were given. The group receiving aspirin suffered fewer heart attacks (Steering Committee, 1989). Like methods developed in agricultural research, the goal is to compose and treat groups as similarly as possible except for one feature under study. Investigators attempt to identify other features that are likely to affect outcomes and stratify or distribute individuals with those features equally between groups. For example, the healthiest individuals (people, pigs, or parsnips) should be stratified equally among the groups since health often affects outcomes.

To help further ensure that groups are similar, investigators generally use another method, randomization (nonhuman choice), such as random numbers, to assign individuals to groups. For example, suppose that investigators want to study the influence of coffee upon alertness. They know other things affect alertness, such as people's interest in the subject or their intelligence, and they try to stratify people with these variables equally between groups. But investigators also know many other features affect alertness, such as people's sleeping, eating, or television-watching habits. Unable to identify all such variables or distribute people with similar features equally between groups, investigators try to minimize the impact of these "nuisance" variables and achieve uniform groups through randomization. Even simple random methods, like flipping a coin to determine group assignments, help ensure that people with distinctive features that could affect results do not cluster in one group. The larger the groups, the more likely that randomization will produce similar groups. The goal of randomization is to combat bias in group assignments by distributing individual characteristics whose effects are unknown equally among the study arms to minimize their influence. In human studies, randomized clinical trials (RCTs) use random assignment to eliminate through equal distribution the effects of such variables as nutritional habits, beliefs, attitudes, behavior, ancestry, or education in correlating the variable under investigation with observed effects. Nonrandomized trials generally seem second best because of the risk of bias in the formation of the groups.

Investigators use other methods in addition to randomization and stratification to make groups similar and eliminate bias. In single-blind studies, subjects do not know their group assignment, thereby minimizing the effects of their beliefs and expectations about the different modes of treatment. They should be treated so similarly that they cannot know which treatment they receive. Investigators' subconscious beliefs, preferences, or attitudes may also affect how they take care of individuals or evaluate outcomes. Believing one medicine works best, for example, may affect their estimates of how individuals respond. To combat such biases, investigators may use double-blind designs where the group assignments are kept from both subjects and investigators until after the trial so that investigators' own views will not contaminate the study's results.

Impartial studies can expose the flaws of common wisdom, the errors of standard practice, and the harms or benefits of treatments. For example, in the 1940s and early 1950s doctors believed that giving copious amounts of oxygen to premature infants prevented death and brain damage. By 1953 this common wisdom was being challenged by clinical trials and by 1954 the link between the lavish use of oxygen and blindness from retrolental fibroplasia (RLP) was clearly established (Silverman, 1980). Other studies uncovered previously unforeseen adverse drug reactions. For example, systematic testing of commonly used antibiotics showed that premature infants receiving sulfisoxazole (gantrisin) had a much higher incidence of death and retardation than other groups. Further investigation revealed that premature infants could not metabolize and detoxify bilirubin thus causing kernicterus, or neurological damage to the brain (Behrman and Vaughan, 1987). In addition to discrediting standard therapies, clinical trials also account for many treatment advances. In three decades of continual evaluation of alternative therapies through clinical trials, childhood leukemia went from a uniformly fatal disease to an often curable illness. RCTs also demonstrated that coronary artery bypass surgery was ineffective for many of the diseases for which it had been widely used.

In a controlled clinical trial, investigators compare the outcomes for patients getting one treatment with those who do not get the treatment. This allows investigators to separate the treatment's effects from other influences. The U.S. Department of Health and Human Services cites five kinds of control groups distinguished, in part, upon whether the comparison is a historical control group (where patients' outcomes are compared with records from past patients) or a concurrent control group (where patients' outcomes are compared with patients currently being treated): (1) placebo concurrent control; (2) dose comparison, concurrent control; (3) no treatment concurrent control; (4) active treatment concurrent control; and (5) historical control. Investigators often regard the double-blind RCT with concurrent control group getting a placebo as the gold standard because it offers the greatest assurances that differences between groups have not been distorted by people's different diagnosis criteria, treatments, observations, measurements, or expectations.

Despite clinical trials' social utility, nagging moral concerns persist about how to reconcile RCTs with traditional physicians' duties and established patients' rights. Unlike corn, patients have legitimate preferences about how they want to be treated and doctors have responsibilities to try to give patients care designed to meet their individual needs, goals, and desires. Controlled trials restrict people's choices and limit the ways therapies can be adapted for them by the methodologies of stratification, randomization, inflexible interventions, eligibility requirements, and single-blinded or double-blinded study designs. Some favor changing what are considered to be patients' rights or therapists' duties thereby making it easier to do studies, while others propose changes in the trials, especially in RCTs. Still others conclude either that all RCTs are unethical or that RCTs must be reviewed individually to assess their acceptability.

Physicians as scientists

When physicians enroll patients in clinical trials, they help patients collectively by gaining knowledge, but may lose flexibility in tailoring treatments for individual patients. This can create a conflict between doctors' roles as scientists dedicated to conducting the best studies to gain knowledge and as healers dedicated to adapting treatments to each patient's needs, goals, and values. To address this potential conflict, most clinicians and ethicists agree that a clinical trial is not morally acceptable unless it meets the uncertainty principle, taken to mean here that as the trial begins, and after a comprehensive review of the literature about what treatments benefit a certain group, impartial, reasonable, and informed people of good will agree that (1) for all treatments currently being given and compared there is sufficient evidence that the therapeutic success rate is acceptably high; (2) it is uncertain whether any one of the treatments being tested is any better than any of the others; and (3) no study arm provides what is known to be inferior care. (This problem does not arise for research with corn since no one worries if, in testing the benefits of one treatment, some corn gets what is believed to be inferior care.) Physicians, then, should not agree to compare therapies if they have reason to believe a patient might thereby obtain inferior care (Byar et al., 1990; Chalmers et al., 1972; Kopelman, 1986; Ellenberg, 1984; Levine et al., 1991; Shaw and Chalmers, 1970; Zelen, 1990). Most physicians apparently agree and will not enroll patients in trials if they believe it will harm their patients or the doctor–patient relationship (Taylor et al., 1984). Despite wide agreement that the uncertainty principle must be fulfilled, substantive disagreements remain about how to use it.

Balancing benefits and burdens. One controversy about how to use the uncertainty principle concerns what values to employ in deciding if treatments are equally good. Investigators tend to measure equality among treatments in terms of easily quantified outcomes such as survival after cancer treatments or reduction of blood pressure. Patients and some clinicians, however, also consider how treatments affect the quality of patients' lives and if they think it makes them feel better (Levine et al., 1991). Views, therefore, about what

treatments are equally good differ when people regard different things as relevant benefits and burdens. Hence nausea, hair loss, sexual impotence, weakness, extra costs, inconvenience, or more hospital visits may be more important outcomes from a patient's perspective than from an investigator's perspective in determining when treatments are equally good.

Clinician preference. Another controversy about how to use the uncertainty principle may be called "the problem of clinician preference," or: Should conscientious clinicians with any preference at all for one treatment arm enroll their patients in a clinical trial? Some argue that clinicians have a duty to provide what they believe to be the best available care for patients; consequently, as long as physicians have *any* preference about which treatment is best for their patients, they should not enroll their patients in clinical trials (Fried, 1974; Gifford, 1986; Waldenstrom, 1983). It is rare that clinicians have no preference whatsoever about what is best for their patients, especially for the treatment of serious illnesses where the outcomes, conveniences, risks, and possible benefits are different. Moreover, if asked, patients will often have preferences even if the clinicians do not, and this could break the tie for doctors. Consequently, these critics find trials, especially RCTs, generally unethical.

Philosopher Benjamin Freedman tries to solve the problem of clinician preference by distinguishing between "theoretical equipoise" and "clinical equipoise" (Freedman, 1987). Theoretical equipoise is an epistemic (cognitive) state where the evidence is exactly balanced that treatments are of equal value. Clinical equipoise, in contrast, is that state in which the community of expert clinicians is undecided as to the preferred treatment for the given population as determined by the study's eligibility criteria; the study should be designed to disturb clinical equipoise and to terminate when it is achieved. Freedman argues that clinical equipoise is a more useful way to understand that treatments are equally useful for a particular group and thus that the uncertainty principle has been reached. To decide this, the treatment that the particular clinician prefers should not be the focus. Instead, the focus should be on what the community of clinicians believe to be equally good treatments for some condition when their respective benefits and burdens are assessed. A clinician may have a preference for one treatment but respect colleagues with different views. Thus, as the trial begins, treatments (including any placebo arm) must be in clinical equipoise, or regarded as having equal merit by the community of expert clinicians in treating some condition for a certain group. Disagreements should be expected in a rapidly advancing field like medicine and help justify why trials are important.

This solution presupposes agreement about who should be in the community of expert clinicians deciding which treatments are equally good. Disputes arise over this, however; some people insist, for example, that there ought to be many perspectives, including those of investigators, clinicians, and lay advocates, to represent patients' sometimes different values, and others disvalue the views of any but the most acclaimed clinical investigators (Kopelman, 1994).

Starting trials.   Disagreements can erupt about the overall benefits of the new treatments or investigational new drugs when compared with standard care. To justify the time, energy, risks, and expense of testing a new therapy for some condition by means of an RCT, investigators must produce preliminary evidence of its safety, efficacy, and proper dose. Some reasonable and informed people are likely to be more impressed with these findings than others, especially for serious diseases with no established treatments (Levine, 1991). Consequently, they disagree about if or when trials should begin.

Ending trials.   The goal of a study is to learn whether different treatments are equally good for certain conditions. But justification for claiming to know something is a matter of degree, and there can be substantial disagreements about the pragmatic matter of where to draw the line for the purpose of saying that we know treatments are or are not equally good. Investigators should adopt rules about when to stop at the outset of a study; generally they do not release preliminary data, but there are some exceptions. A panel is often charged with monitoring the data and deciding if trials should be ended early because people in one arm of the study are doing far worse than others. For example, azidothymidine (AZT) was first tested against a placebo in a double-blind RCT to see if it helped patients with acquired immunodeficiency syndrome (AIDS). Doctors and nurses believed they knew from the abatement of symptoms which patients were getting AZT and which were getting a placebo. After several months, 16 of the 137 patients on the placebo arm died while only 1 of the 145 patients receiving AZT died. The trial was ended and all received AZT (Beauchamp and Childress, 1989).

Deciding when to stop a trial is not an entirely scientific or mathematical decision. It is, in large part, a pragmatic or moral decision. Investigators, panels, and journal editors typically require a probability of at most 0.05 (five chances in a hundred) that the observed results between groups occurred by chance, as a ground for holding that "sufficient evidence" exists to say they "know" that the groups are different. Although the 0.05 standard is a reasonable and well-established convention, it should not be misunderstood. As Daniel Wikler (1981) and Loretta Kopelman (1986, 1994) have argued, it is at best a moral trade-off between continuing the study so long that some people receive obviously suboptimal care and stopping so early that some people

are harmed because insufficiently verified treatments are adopted or discredited. Some will draw that line differently, especially where treatments are tested for serious illnesses with few other means of treatment, as in AIDS research (Kopelman, 1994).

Eligibility criteria and cooperation.   Another problem about how to use the uncertainty principle arises when investigators disagree with clinicians or patients about who should be eligible for studies (Dresser, 1992). Doctors sometimes object to these criteria and the subsequent exclusions in a way that undermines cooperation with investigators (Kopelman, 1994). For example, to gain access for their patients into a study and the kind of superior care (often free) it holds, clinicians may "reinterpret" the eligibility criteria (profiles investigators distribute for inclusion of potential subjects). For example, AZT, the first effective drug to treat AIDS, was initially tested for safety and efficacy against a placebo in a double-blind RCT, as has been mentioned. Some doctors falsified eligibility criteria to try to enroll their patients so that they gained a 50 percent chance of receiving the treatment they believed (correctly in this case) would help their patients (Levine, 1988). Rumors also persisted that some doctors knew that patients enrolled in the placebo-control arm of the trial were simultaneously using AZT obtained from sources not connected to the trial. This study illustrates tensions that can exist between the physician's role as patient advocate and as an investigator. Falsifying eligibility criteria or not monitoring cooperation can help individual patients, yet threatens the collective well-being of patients by distorting trial results.

Patients as subjects

To enroll in studies, people or their guardians must give informed consent, or authorization that is competent, adequately informed, and voluntary. Assuming that people are competent to give consent and do so voluntarily, what do they need to know to give informed consent for clinical studies?

Generally they must be told about the study's nature, purpose, duration, procedures, and foreseeable risks and benefits. Moreover, they need to know about any alternative treatments, inconveniences, additional costs, and extra procedures or hospitalizations resulting from enrollment. They must also be told of their right to withdraw from the study at any time should they agree to participate (US CFR, 1983). If the study design includes different groups, randomization, or placebos, for example, prospective subjects need to be informed. Consent for therapy or research requires giving people all information that a reasonable person would want to know in order to make a choice.

These widely recognized consent requirements create tensions in relation to the goals of clinical trials. For example, suppose in testing treatments, one study arm uses surgery with medical management resulting in a faster recovery if there are no complications, and the other study arm uses medical management alone, with fewer risks but a slower recovery. If distinctive groups have special preferences, such as the elderly preferring medical management and the young surgery, then the study of the different treatment results could be biased through self-selection. Thus, there is a difficulty that may be called "the problem of subject preference," or: How can people's preferences be accommodated while preserving the scientific integrity of the RCT? Consider three possible solutions (Kopelman, 1994).

(1) Defenders of strict methods. Some criticize traditional informed-consent doctrine as unrealistic, too individualistic, and shortsighted because it gives too much weight to individual choice and makes it hard to conduct good studies (Tobias, 1988; Zelen, 1979, 1990). Physicians and health-care professionals, they argue, have a duty to take proper care of patients, but are not typically required to educate them about these technical and complex matters; patients should get good treatment given by conscientious professionals, but do not need to know how, when, or why investigators evaluate their treatments. Most patients cannot understand the investigation's complexities, they argue, and would be harmed by learning of the uncertainties about what care is best or that they are being studied. Investigators should be free to design the best possible trials consistent with good care, they argue, and the current understanding of patients' rights disrupts clinical trials thereby slowing medical progress. If people have only the right to good care and not the right to refuse to be enrolled in a study, it would be easier for investigators to conduct research and minimize problems of bias introduced by people's preferences. For example, Marvin Zelen devised schemas where patients give their consent for a treatment without knowing that it was selected by a random method and/or that they are in a study; other designs prerandomize people to group assignments before consent is sought (Zelen, 1979, 1990).

In this view therapists and investigators should have more authority to decide what information shall be given to patients or their representatives and when people will be enrolled in clinical trials. Such paternalism, however, garners legal and moral criticism (Ellenberg, 1984, 1992; Kopelman, 1986, 1994). It not only denies people self-determination, but, without pertinent information, people do not have means to protect their own well-being. The doctrine of informed consent developed because many patients and activists want impartial information and want to participate in choices about their care, especially about when they will serve as research

subjects. For example, statistician Susan Ellenberg criticizes Zelen's prerandomization schemas where patients are assigned to groups before consent is sought. She argues that this threatens impartiality in gaining consent, risking that the informational sessions will be shaped to enhance the benefits and minimize the risks of each individual assignment (Ellenberg, 1984, 1992).

(2) Critics of strict methods. These critics object to clinical trials for putting collective benefits over individual rights and welfare. Charles Fried (1974) and Daniel Wikler (1981) agree that it is hard to conduct studies, especially RCTs, and fulfill informed-consent doctrine, but conclude that consent must be defended as the more important social practice. A society can thrive without medical advances, but not without liberties. Although trials have increased medical knowledge enormously, consent is a central way to protect our civil liberties. They are skeptical that people give genuine informed consent. These critics maintain that investigators do not tell, and most patients do not understand, that at some point in the trial it may become apparent that some groups are getting suboptimal care (Wikler, 1981). Investigators, they argue, put medical advances ahead of subject-patient rights and welfare because those rights typically violate physicians' duties to their patients (Fried, 1974; Gifford, 1986; Marquis, 1986; Wikler, 1981). These critics understand the physicians' duty, or what some call the "therapeutic obligation," as the duty to provide patients with what their doctors believe is the best available care. This statement of physicians' duty or the therapeutic obligation, however, presumes that physicians know which treatment is best; often, there is no treatment known to be best. Moreover, it is paternalistic to assume that it is up to physicians to choose what is best for people. The doctrine of informed consent developed because people want to be able to learn about their options and make choices themselves.

(3) Research as a cooperative venture. In contrast to these two positions holding that we must choose between good trials and good informed consent, other commentators argue that clinical trials, including RCTs, can be cooperative ventures between patients and investigators (Freedman, 1987; Kopelman, 1986, 1994; Levine et al., 1991; Levine, 1986, 1988). They believe that investigators and patients should work together with candor, respect, and trust about the goals and means of the research. They maintain that with proper consent some studies (but not all) are morally justifiable. Kopelman argues that no general approval should be given for RCTs because some designs are incompatible with established patients' rights. Other designs may be acceptable for some studies, but not for others, when judged in terms of people's rights and the structural integrity of the RCT (Kopelman, 1986).

Critics of this view doubt that studies can be cooperative ventures between investigators and patients, given their unequal knowledge or power (Tobias, 1988; Wikler, 1981; Zelen, 1979). Most patients, they claim, cannot be partners because they do not understand the benefits or burdens of their treatment options, let alone the scientifically rigorous methodology used in testing.

Subjects may have to be regarded as partners in a cooperative venture, however, if investigators expect people to enroll and cooperate. People can defeat trials if they do not identify with the investigators' goals. In one case investigators were testing whether patients infected with human immunodeficiency virus (HIV) who were not yet showing symptoms of AIDS would benefit from AZT. At the end of the trial, researchers estimated that 9 percent of the patients in the placebo arm had been taking AZT. If more patients in the placebo group had secretly taken AZT, investigators might have judged a beneficial drug ineffective and refused to release it for this use (Merigan, 1990). These patients, facing a life-threatening disease, found a way to get the drug they believed useful and inadvertently jeopardized a clinical trial and the welfare of future patients. Poor cooperation results when the subjects fail to identify with the goals of the study, do not understand its importance, or are asked to risk too much in terms of health and convenience. Generally, subject cooperation is at its highest when the study involves simple, clear directions, mild diseases, and few inconveniences (Spilker, 1992).

Patient advocacy

As studies have become more refined and successful, patients or their advocates increasingly want a say in how trials are done and who is eligible to participate. Most biomedical research study populations exclude people of color, women, and children. Despite recent directives to redress this, women and others remain remarkably underrepresented (Dresser, 1992). Advocates argue that this is unfair because enrollment in trials often provides people the only available access to adequate care or promising investigational new drugs. For example, children with AIDS initially could not get AZT because only adults could be enrolled in studies. Even after some studies showed that AZT was beneficial for treatment of adults, regulations initially forbade its prescription for children because it had not been tested with them (Pizzo, 1990). Moreover, a study excluding people of color, females, and children focuses upon a narrow range of the patient population (adult white males), making it uncertain whether the results of a study apply to other groups. There may be differences among groups; if there are, variations might be due to nature, nurture, or a combination of both. A study on depression, for example, conducted exclusively with white men, leaves uncertainty as to whether the results would be the same for other groups who have different social standing, burdens, genes, or physiologies. More flexible eligibility requirements, advocates argue, would give all groups access to new treatments and would also yield results that more accurately reflect the entire patient population. Opponents respond that this would make it harder to ensure that groups are comparable with regard to baseline factors such as prognosis.

Patient-advocacy groups also demand more access to preliminary information about the safety and efficacy of different modes of care. They want less secrecy regarding early trends, especially where patients have few treatment options for serious diseases. Many patients with severe or chronic diseases, or their families, have learned to follow closely relevant research, and they want greater access to promising new treatments.

These proposals have generated a variety of responses (Byar et al., 1990; Levine et al., 1991; Merigan, 1990; Schaffner, 1986; "Expanded Availability," 1990). For example, programs make some investigational new treatments more available by means of expanded access or parallel track ("Expanded Availability," 1990). In the past, there was a single way, or "track," for patients to get certain investigational new treatments, namely, participate in the study as a subject. Some people could not be subjects because they lived too far from the study site(s). Others failed to meet investigators' requirements, and such exclusions were sometimes particularly infuriating to clinicians and patients when these criteria were tied to age, gender, or prognosis (Kopelman, 1994). New programs expanded access or offered a "parallel track" to make it possible for some patients who are not subjects to have investigational new treatments. Patients with HIV-related diseases, for example, can sometimes obtain investigational new treatments even though they are not enrolled as trial subjects. Some investigators recommend this approach when there are no therapeutic alternatives, when the drugs are being tested, when there is some evidence of their efficacy, when there are no unreasonable risks for the patient, and when the patient cannot participate in the RCT (Byar et al., 1990). This solution presupposes that there is agreement about who should make these verdicts. Community representation on panels that make these decisions may be reassuring to groups advocating more openness.

These and other proposals allow greater flexibility, but also may make it harder to conduct and interpret the results (Ellenberg, 1984; Merigan, 1990). For example, if patients can get the investigational new treatment without enrolling in the RCT, they may refuse to participate. Thus, even if these proposed changes are adopted, the problem of the tension between an individual and collective interest in conducting trials may not be solved. The balance may merely be shifted.

Uncertainty

The moral problems surrounding trials are often framed in terms of knowledge and power. Investigators want control of studies to conduct careful trials and learn how to help patients collectively. Patients and their doctors want optimal information and choice about treatment modalities to help individual patients. Yet discomfort with uncertainty may also underlie the uneasiness with clinical trials. To conduct them investigators must admit that they do not know what treatment is best and must accept a mode of care selected by chance. They have to lower their defenses enough to admit that hunches are not knowledge. When the stakes seem high, this realization represents an extraordinarily difficult psychological adjustment, even for such well-educated people as oncologists and oncology nurses faced with making choices for themselves or their families about whether to enroll in an RCT (Belanger et al., 1991).

When researchers consider the adoption of procedures such as copious amounts of oxygen for premature infants (later found to cause blindness), a high premium is placed on protection of the public from someone's idea of "promising" new treatments; however, when they think of drugs that have proved to help sustain or improve people's lives, a high premium is placed on early access. Who should decide the optimal degree of testing or protection needed in order to establish the safety and efficacy of drugs before they are available? This question of access versus protection is a social and moral decision, not just a scientific matter. It is not unlike the decision about how much inspection of foods or buildings is necessary in order to protect the public. When the stakes are high, as in fatal or chronically degenerative diseases with no promising treatments, the disputes about when to begin or end trials are sometimes a tangle of scientific, moral, social, political, statistical, and medical problems.

LORETTA M. KOPELMAN

Directly related to this article is the other article in this entry: CONCEPTUAL ISSUES. *For a further discussion of topics mentioned in this article, see the entries* AIDS, *article on* HEALTH-CARE AND RESEARCH ISSUES; CHILDREN, *article on* HEALTH-CARE AND RESEARCH ISSUES; INFORMED CONSENT, *especially the article on* CONSENT ISSUES IN HUMAN RESEARCH; MINORITIES AS RESEARCH SUBJECTS; PATIENTS' RIGHTS; PLACEBO; RESEARCH BIAS; RESEARCH POLICY; RIGHTS; VALUE AND VALUATION; *and* WOMEN, *article on* RESEARCH ISSUES. *This article will find application in the entries* ANIMAL RESEARCH; FETUS, *article on* FETAL RESEARCH; *and* MULTINATIONAL RE-

SEARCH. *For a discussion of related ideas, see the entries* CONFLICT OF INTEREST; HARM; INFORMATION DISCLOSURE; INTERPRETATION; JUSTICE; PRIVACY AND CONFIDENTIALITY IN RESEARCH; PROFESSIONAL–PATIENT RELATIONSHIP; RISK; *and* UTILITY. *Other relevant material may be found under the entries* AGING AND THE AGED, *article on* HEALTH-CARE AND RESEARCH ISSUES; ANIMAL WELFARE AND RIGHTS; GENETICS AND HUMAN BEHAVIOR, *article on* SCIENTIFIC AND RESEARCH ISSUES; MENTALLY DISABLED AND MENTALLY ILL PERSONS, *article on* RESEARCH ISSUES; MILITARY PERSONNEL AS RESEARCH SUBJECTS; PRISONERS, *article on* RESEARCH ISSUES; RESEARCH, HUMAN: HISTORICAL ASPECTS; RESEARCH, UNETHICAL; RESEARCH ETHICS COMMITTEES; SEX THERAPY AND SEX RESEARCH; *and* STUDENTS AS RESEARCH SUBJECTS. *See also the* APPENDIX (CODES, OATHS, AND DIRECTIVES RELATED TO BIOETHICS), SECTION IV: ETHICAL DIRECTIVES FOR HUMAN RESEARCH.

Bibliography

BEAUCHAMP, TOM L., and CHILDRESS, JAMES L. 1989. *Principles of Biomedical Ethics.* 3d ed. Oxford: Oxford University Press.

BEHRMAN, RICHARD E., and VAUGHAN, VICTOR C., III. 1987. *Nelson Textbook of Pediatrics.* 13th ed. Philadelphia: W. B. Saunders.

BELANGER, DANIEL; MOORE, MALCOLM; and TANNOCK, IAN. 1991. "How American Oncologists Treat Breast Cancer: An Assessment of the Influence of Clinical Trials." *Journal of Clinical Oncology* 9, no. 1:7–16.

BYAR, DAVID P.; SCHOENFELD, DAVID A.; GREEN, SYLVAN B.; AMATO, DAVID A.; DAVIS, ROGER; DE GRUTTOLA, VICTOR; FINKELSTEIN, DIANNE M.; GATSONIS, CONSTANTINE; GELBER, RICHARD D.; LAGAKOS, STEPHEN; LEFKOPOULOU, MYRTO; TSIATIS, ANASTASIOS A.; ZELEN, MARVIN; PETO, JULIAN; FREEDMAN, LAURENCE S.; GAIL, MITCHELL; SIMON, RICHARD; ELLENBERG, SUSAN S.; ANDERSON, JAMES R.; COLLINS, RORY; PETO, RICHARD; and PETO, TIM. 1990. "Design Considerations for AIDS Trials." *New England Journal of Medicine* 323, no. 19: 1343–1348.

CHALMERS, THOMAS C.; BLOCK, JEROME B.; and LEE, STEPHANIE. 1972. "Controlled Studies in Clinical Cancer Research." *New England Journal of Medicine* 287, no. 2: 75–78.

DRESSER, REBECCA. 1992. "Wanted: Single, White Male for Medical Research." *Hastings Center Report* 22, no. 1: 24–29.

ELLENBERG, SUSAN S. 1984. "Randomization Designs in Comparative Clinical Trials." *New England Journal of Medicine* 310, no. 21:1404–1408.

———. 1992. "Randomized Consent Designs for Clinical Trials: An Update." *Statistics in Medicine* 11, no. 1: 131–132.

"Expanded Availability of Investigational New Drugs Through a Parallel Track Mechanism for People with AIDS and

HIV-Related Disease." 1990. *Federal Register* 55, no. 98 (May 21):20856–20860.

FREEDMAN, BENJAMIN. 1987. "Equipoise and the Ethics of Clinical Research." *New England Journal of Medicine* 317, no. 3:141–145.

FRIED, CHARLES. 1974. *Medical Experimentation: Personal Integrity and Social Policy.* New York: American Elsevier.

GIFFORD, FRED. 1986. "The Conflict Between Randomized Clinical Trials and the Therapeutic Obligation." *Journal of Medicine and Philosophy* 11, no. 4:347–366.

GIGERENZER, GERD; SWIJTINK, ZENO; PORTER, THEODORE; DASTON, LORRAINE; BEATTY, JOHN; and KRÜGER, LORENZ, eds. 1989. *The Empire of Chance: How Probability Changed Science and Everyday Life.* Cambridge: At the University Press.

KOPELMAN, LORETTA M. 1986. "Consent and Randomized Clinical Trials: Are There Moral or Design Problems?" *Journal of Medicine and Philosophy* 11, no. 4:317–345.

———. 1994. "How AIDS Activists Are Changing Research." In *Health Care Ethics: Critical Issues,* pp. 199–209. Edited by David C. Thomasma and John F. Monagle. Gaithersburg, Md.: Aspen.

LEVINE, CAROL; DUBLER, NANCY N.; and LEVINE, ROBERT J. 1991. "Building a New Consensus: Ethical Principles and Policies for Clinical Research on HIV/AIDS." *IRB* 13, nos. 1–2:1–17.

LEVINE, ROBERT J. 1986. *Ethics and Regulation of Clinical Research.* 2d ed. Baltimore: Urban and Schwarzenberg.

———. 1988. "Uncertainty in Clinical Research." *Law, Medicine and Health Care* 16, nos. 3–4:174–182.

MARQUIS, DON. 1986. "An Argument That All Prerandomized Clinical Trials Are Unethical." *Journal of Medicine and Philosophy* 11, no. 4:367–383.

MERIGAN, THOMAS C. 1990. "You Can Teach an Old Dog New Tricks: How AIDS Trials Are Pioneering New Strategies." *New England Journal of Medicine* 323, no. 19: 1341–1343.

PIZZO, PHILIP A. 1990. "Pediatric AIDS: Problems Within Problems." *Journal of Infectious Diseases* 161, no. 2:316–325.

"Protection of Human Subjects." 1993. *Code of Federal Regulations.* Title 45, Pt. 46.

SCHAFFNER, KENNETH F. 1986. "Ethical Problems in Clinical Trials." *Journal of Medicine and Philosophy* 11, no. 4: 297–315.

SHAW, LAWRENCE W., and CHALMERS, THOMAS C. 1970. "Ethics in Cooperative Trials." *Annals of the New York Academy of Sciences* 169, art. 2:487–495.

SILVERMAN, WILLIAM A. 1980. *Retrolental Fibroplasia: A Modern Parable.* New York: Grune and Stratton.

SPILKER, BERT. 1992. "Methods of Assessing and Improving Patient Compliance and Clinical Trials." *IRB* 14, no. 3:1–6.

STEERING COMMITTEE OF THE PHYSICIANS' HEALTH STUDY RESEARCH GROUP. 1989. "Final Report on the Aspirin Component of the Ongoing Physicians' Health Study." *New England Journal of Medicine* 321:129–135.

TAYLOR, KATHRYN M.; MARGOLESE, RICHARD G.; and SOSKOLNE, COLIN L. 1984. "Physicians' Reasons for Not Entering Eligible Patients in a Randomized Clinical Trial of Surgery for Breast Cancer." *New England Journal of Medicine* 310, no. 21:1363–1367.

TOBIAS, JEFFREY STUART. 1988. "Informed Consent and Controlled Trials." *Lancet* 2, no. 8621:1194.

WALDENSTROM, JAN. 1983. "The Ethics of Randomization." In *Research Ethics,* pp. 143–149. Edited by Kare Berg and Knut Erik Tranoy. New York: Alan R. Liss.

WIKLER, DANIEL. 1981. "Ethical Considerations in Randomized Clinical Trials." *Seminars in Oncology* 8, no. 4:437–441.

ZELEN, MARVIN. 1979. "A New Design for Randomized Clinical Trials." *New England Journal of Medicine* 300, no. 22:1242–1245.

———. 1990. "Randomized Consent Designs for Clinical Trials: An Update." *Statistics in Medicine* 9, no. 6:645–656.

RESEARCH POLICY

I. GENERAL GUIDELINES

The phrase "research policy" has two basic meanings when applied to biomedical research. The first meaning refers to policy that establishes a program for a general course or plan of action intended to reach a desired target or goal. In biomedical research, the goal or target is usually specified in terms of a program relevant to the diagnosis, prevention, treatment, or cure of a specific disease or condition. The second meaning of research policy refers to policy that imposes conditions or restraints on biomedical research investigators or their institutions. Although policies that establish programs can be readily distinguished from policies that constrain actions, both types of policy often originate in the same legislative action. For example, the law (P.L. 93-348) that established a program for research training grants also required regulations for the protection of human subjects. However, even when both policies originate from the same law, they are implemented by processes that are decidedly different from one another.

Policy development is sometimes called "applied ethics." And, at its best, policy development represents a successful attempt to discern and apply common or widely held public moral standards to programs or activities of a government. The development of public policy frequently embodies values that can be defended by sound ethics and is often crafted with the assistance of ethicists. Despite these observations, policy development is seldom orderly, rarely internally consistent, and usually represents a compromise between competing views.

U.S. biomedical research policy is, for the most part, either created by the Congress in the form of programs administered by federal agencies or established by the agencies themselves to administer their programs. Most agencies that support biomedical research pattern their policies on the models of the National Institutes of Health (NIH) and the Department of Health and Human Services (HHS) within which the NIH is located. The reason for policy dominance by the NIH is that it is the primary health-research agency of the U.S. government. In fiscal year 1993, for example, 83 percent of all federal biomedical research funds were dispensed through NIH programs. The remaining 17 percent of federal biomedical research funds were distributed through fifteen other departments and agencies that conducted or supported biomedical research. Because the budget of the NIH is so large in comparison with that of other agencies and because the NIH is the largest supporter of biomedical research in the world, its policies tend to be followed in the United States, where they are legally enforced, as well as abroad, where they are not binding. A brief history of the NIH from a policy perspective will throw light on U.S. biomedical research policies.

The development of the NIH and the growth of targeted policy

The U.S. government has supported biomedical research since 1887 when it provided funds to the Staten Island Hygienic Laboratory of Joseph Kenyoun, M.D., for the study of cholera and other infectious diseases. In 1918 Congress enacted the Chamberlain-Kahn Act, its first targeted legislative initiative, for the study of venereal diseases at the Hygienic Laboratory. In 1930, Congress directed that the Hygienic Laboratory be expanded, moved to the Washington, D.C., area, and renamed the National Institutes of Health. The addition and separation of categorical institutes began when the Bone-Magnuson Act of 1937 created the National Cancer Institute, within the NIH. Bone-Magnuson served as a prototype for future health research legislation. It identified a target, created a program, authorized funding, and required an advisory council to provide peer review for research awards. The legislation also provided for the training of research investigators, called for the coordination of federal and state agencies, and allowed funding of research outside the United States.

The NIH expanded rapidly following World War II. Budgets rose dramatically between 1946 and 1969 and gradually after that time. Between 1946 and 1949, the NIH budget grew from $180,000 to more than $800 million. By 1993 the NIH had a budget of $9.8 billion and a projected budget of more than $11 billion for 1994. By 1993 the agency had become a federation of seventeen research institutes, four research centers, two support divisions, and the National Library of Medicine. Fifteen of the seventeen institutes were categorical, that is, their research mission was targeted or directed by Congress. Some research was targeted at diseases (e.g., the National Institute of Diabetes and Digestive and Kidney Diseases), some was targeted at organ systems (e.g., the National Eye Institute), some was targeted at conditions (e.g. the National Institute on Aging), and some was targeted at processes (e.g., the National Institute of Child Health and Human Development). By selecting targets and appropriating only for research designed to meet those targets, Congress directly controlled the directions taken by the life sciences in the United States.

The growth of targeted policies

U.S. policy decisions concerning the level of support and the targets of biomedical research are arrived at, primarily, through the federal budget process. Its four phases are (1) authorization—the legislative process by which the U.S. Congress establishes a program and sets dollar limits for its support; (2) appropriation—the process by which the Congress designates actual amounts of money to be spent on authorized programs; (3) allocation—the procedure used by the executive branch to distribute the money to federal programs; (4) obligation—the actual expenditure of the money.

For example, in a given year the U.S. Congress might authorize the establishment of a dental caries research program to be supported at a level of no more than $100 million per year for each of the subsequent three fiscal years. The actual appropriation might be set at $25 million in the first year, $50 million in the second, and $75 million in the third. In the first year, the allocation process would assign the $25 million of appropriated money to the National Institute for Dental Research (NIDR), an institute within the NIH. The NIDR would obligate the $25 million to the dental caries program. The dental caries program director might obligate 50 percent of the money to grants-in-aid (grants), 33 percent to contracts, and 10 percent to cooperative agreements. The remainder, about 7 percent, might be obligated to support program management expenses. Although the mechanisms of research support (grants, contracts, and cooperative agreements) differ, all obligated research monies would be dedicated to the prevention, diagnosis, treatment, or cure of dental caries. The budget process is repeated each year for each program (programs are often referred to as "line items" in the budget). Over time, this process expresses and implements the broad policy goals.

The budget process sets policy by answering the following questions: (1) What fraction of federal revenues will be dedicated to biomedical research? (2) What categories of research will be supported and what categories will not be supported? (3) How much money will be allocated to each research target? (4) If the appropriation for one medical research program is increased, will that increase be derived from general revenues (new money) or diverted (pirated) from other programs?

Targeted public policies arrived at annually through the highly politicized budget process were, for many years, criticized by segments of the scientific community on the grounds that politically popular targets rather than scientific opportunities were dictating the course and the goals of biomedical research. Even proponents of a targeted approach to biomedical research support argued that political targets should be set, not by political whim, but by a Congress that is responsive to mortality and morbidity data relevant to each disease and sensitive to social costs and public fears associated with various diseases.

In the years following World War II, when the NIH was rapidly expanding, a major segment of the annual budget allocation for biomedical research was appropriated under the authorization of section 301 of the Public Health Service Act. Section 301 did not specify targets for research dollars, nor did it put time or dollar limits on the authorized research. As a consequence, appropriations were often lacking in specificity, leaving the NIH free to obligate funds in support of those research projects judged by the peer review system to be scientifically meritorious. General authorizations under Section 301, coupled with allocation guided by peer review, were considered by many in the scientific community as the most rational public policy for funding research. However, as research budgets have increased since World War II, so has the tendency to define specific policy targets for biomedical research. Very little research is currently appropriated under the general authority of section 301; funding usually takes place under categorical program authorizations.

Although research dollars are targeted under increasingly specific authorizing legislation, the research community has won a major concession from the Congress. In 1985, NIH director Dr. Donald S. Frederickson worked out an agreement with the Senate Budget Committee to provide the NIH with funds for six thousand investigator-initiated, or "R01," grants each year. Since then, the peer-review system recommends funding for those R01 grant applications that it considers to have the highest scientific potential for providing a knowledge base necessary for reaching a goal or target set by the Congress. Most R01 awards support basic research.

Although they may be funded under, for example, cancer or diabetes targets, they generate research that often turns out to relate to a target other than the one under which they are funded. R01 grants allow investigators to exercise wide discretion and creativity in conducting research. The investigator-initiated grant arrangement represents an effective policy compromise between non-targeted awards and the targeted program authorizations established by the Congress.

> The success of NIH, contrasted with the dismal failure of the Superfund (which had little research or scientific input), is a case history for all who need to learn the lesson of making policy without scientific input. If government officials want to solve some of these very difficult problems, they can do so with policy that uses scientific, not emotional standards. . . . If the research is to flower, a strong investigator-initiated atmosphere on the NIH model must be generated by other government agencies, and a willingness for flexibility and adventure must be the attitude of the scientists. (Koshland, 1994)

U.S. policies that impose restrictions on research

Policies that impose limits or restrictions on biomedical research may be enjoined by the Congress at any stage in the budget process. For example, the Congress, in authorizing programs and appropriating funds for research in human reproductive biology, dictated a strict prohibition on any use of appropriated funds for abortion research. One result of the policy was that RU-486, a compound widely used in France and England to effect abortions, has been ruled off-limits for U.S.-funded researchers who wish to study its abortifacient effects in humans. Nevertheless, RU-486 has been investigated in government-supported research targeted at the prevention and cure of cancer.

The policy not to fund abortion research applies directly only to government-funded programs, but it has indirectly affected behavior in the private sector. For example, approval to market RU-486 for commercial use in the United States has not yet been sought by the firm that owns the patent.

Congress may also prohibit funding to institutions that do not comply with federal policies. Typically, it does not create regulations specifically for biomedical research. Rather, it imposes general restrictions on institutions that receive funding from any federal programs. When applied to institutions that receive research awards, these regulations function as a condition of an award. In other words, an institution is not eligible for funding unless it has assured the awarding agency that it is in compliance with applicable laws and regulations. Examples of this kind of policy include laws and regulations governing civil rights, the disabled, sex discrimination, sexual harassment, and the maintenance of a drug-free workplace.

Congress is not alone in having authority to set policy. The president, the Office of Management and Budget, and federal department and agency heads may also shape research policy through administrative directives. Just as congressional policy sometimes places conditions on awards, so does policy that has been initiated through the executive branch. For example, in 1988 the secretary of HHS restricted federally funded research involving the transplantation of tissue derived from aborted fetuses. The ban on fetal-tissue research applied only to research projects funded by the HHS. However, it had a chilling effect on similar kinds of research in the private sector. The policy ban on fetal-tissue transplant research remained in force, despite contrary recommendations of an advisory panel, until lifted by executive order in 1993.

Research policies outside the United States

In contrast to the U.S. system, Canada, the United Kingdom, Scandinavia, Germany, Japan, Australia, and most other industrialized countries designate a fixed percentage of their total health budgets to support biomedical research. Research "set-aside" funds are assigned to specific research projects by quasigovernmental agencies called Medical Research Councils (MRCs) that rely on peer review to decide how to distribute the money. The distribution of federal research monies in these countries lies outside of their national parliaments and is therefore arguably less politicized and less targeted than the U.S. procedures. Once a total budget figure is established, decisions concerning what research is to be supported pass to the MRC.

While research investigators operating with government funds in these countries generally exercise wider discretion and are subject to less policy direction and regulation than U.S. scientists, the amount and relative size of expenditures of public money dedicated to research has been consistently lower than in the United States. In addition, public accountability for use of the research funds has also lagged behind that of the United States.

One can only speculate what impact a unified economic community might have on the level of governmental support of biomedical research in Europe. There have been few indications to suggest that research will be funded centrally in Europe. Nevertheless, in order to avoid unnecessary duplication of research, such a policy will almost certainly be considered for some large research projects. Whether or not arrangements are made for central funding of biomedical research, it seems likely that funds will, for the foreseeable future, continue to be allocated through well-established and highly respected national MRCs.

In Europe, a shift to central authority over policies that impose restrictions or limitations on biomedical research is probable. Uniformity of constraints is desired by both politicians and scientists. Agreement on non-binding guidelines has already occurred in areas such as the protection of human subjects, the care and use of laboratory animals, and the appropriate use of recombinant DNA technology. The principal difficulty with central authority over research policies is associated with policy oversight, enforcement, and sanctions. These issues are, by their very nature, problematic. When they are coupled with questions relating to national versus regional jurisdiction, they become doubly difficult. The European community will be sharply challenged to find a credible and workable way to impose restrictions on research within the framework of the newly developing political structures.

Policies for the protection of human subjects

In 1966, the U.S. surgeon general issued the first policy for the protection of human subjects involved in research supported by the Public Health Service (PHS). This policy was revised several times and reissued in 1971 by the Department of Health, Education and Welfare (HEW). The policy required institutions that conduct research involving human subjects to provide assurances that the rights and welfare of subjects would be protected not only in research funded by the department but in all research involving human subjects that is conducted by the institutions. In response to the National Research Act of 1974 (P.L. 93-348), the policy was revised and reissued as a regulation (45 CFR 46) with the force of law.

The National Research Act also required the secretary of HEW to create the National Commission for the Protection of Human Subjects of Biomedical and Behavioral Research. The commission, which served from 1974 to 1978, outlined recommendations for strengthening existing research regulations to provide additional protections for vulnerable populations, including pregnant women, human fetuses, children, prisoners, and people with mental disabilities. In 1978 the commission also issued the Belmont Report: Ethical Principles and Guidelines for the Protection of Human Subjects of Research (U.S. National Commission, 1978). The report stressed the ethical importance of the principles of respect for persons, beneficence, and justice as a context for compliance with federal regulations.

All recommendations of the commission were accepted by HEW and transformed into regulatory form. Virtually every institution in the United States subscribed to the Belmont principles. Basic regulations reflecting the commission's recommendations (45 CFR 46 Subpart A) were reissued in 1981, and the final additional protections for vulnerable research subjects were promulgated in stages through 1983 by HHS (formerly HEW). Key features of the regulations include review by local institutional review boards of research projects that involve human subjects to assure that informed consent will be elicited from each subject; that research risks will be reasonable in the light of expected benefits; and that subjects will be recruited in an equitable fashion.

The National Commission was succeeded by the U.S. President's Commission for the Study of Ethical Problems in Medicine and Biomedical and Behavioral Research. In 1981, that commission recommended that the HHS regulations be extended to provide protections for all human subjects involved in research funded by any department or agency of the federal government. In 1991, the Common Federal Rule was promulgated by sixteen departments and agencies of the federal government; it is the only example of a regulation promulgated simultaneously by all relevant segments of the U.S. government.

Research involving human gene therapy must comply with the Common Rule, but in addition it must be reviewed and approved by a national recombinant DNA advisory committee (RAC). That committee has issued "points to consider" for the guidance of investigators preparing research proposals involving human gene therapy. The first such project was approved in 1991. By the end of 1993, more than thirty such projects had been approved under the RAC's policy.

Humane care and use of laboratory animals

The first Public Health Service (PHS) policy for the protection of laboratory animals was issued in 1963 and was revised many times prior to being reissued in 1986 (P.L. 99-158). Not only does the policy include detailed provisions for the care and use of animals involved in research conducted or supported by PHS agencies, but it serves as the basis for provisions in the relevant sections of the regulations issued by the U.S. Department of Agriculture (USDA) under the Animal Welfare Act amendments of 1985 (P.L. 99-196). Thus, the policy governing laboratory animals involved in research funded by the federal government and the regulations governing the care and use of animals involved in research in the private sector have been harmonized.

Inclusion of women and minorities in research

In response to growing perceptions that biomedical research has, since World War II, addressed more health problems in men than in women and more health problems in the white population than in minority populations, the NIH has developed a policy to ensure the inclusion of women and members of minority groups in biomedical research. The NIH policy requires that women and minorities be included in NIH-supported clinical research unless a clear and compelling justification is provided to the director of the funding component. An increase in the cost of conducting the research or analyzing the data is not considered to be sufficient to justify an exception to the policy. It is clear that the recruitment of women and minorities as research subjects and the analysis of data for gender-specific and minority-specific applications of research findings will continue to be significantly increased.

Scientific misconduct and conflict of interest

The scientific community has been plagued by the conduct of some research investigators who have deviated from the standards of sound, ethical research. Charges of plagiarism, deliberate mismanagement of data, and false credits for publication have been raised with increasing frequency. In some instances, guilt has been established and the NIH has imposed sanctions. The NIH has developed a policy requiring awardee institutions to train researchers in ethics and to demonstrate that they have developed standards that are adequately promulgated and enforced.

Associated with allegations of misconduct have been allegations that some investigators tainted the credibility of their research by conducting it under the cloud of actual or apparent conflicts of interest. For example, conflict-of-interest allegations were made concerning the credibility of at least thirteen researchers who provided data in a multicentered study of treatment for myocardial infarction. The investigators all held stock in a pharmaceutical house that stood to make, or lose, a considerable amount of money depending on the outcome of the trial. The NIH and other federal agencies have prepared policy statements governing conflicts of interest on the part of research investigators and research institutions.

Conclusion

Public policies governing biomedical research will always remain in tension with the inner-directed goals of the research itself. Sometimes the tension produces major controversies. In other situations, sound public policy reduces conflict. Despite ongoing tension, the public policies that both support and constrain biomedical research, particularly in the United States, have produced a flowering of biological knowledge unprecedented in human history. The privilege of receiving public support is conditioned on compliance with public policy and accountability to the public.

CHARLES R. MCCARTHY

Directly related to this article are the other articles in this entry: RISK AND VULNERABLE GROUPS, *and* SUBJECT SELECTION. *For a further discussion of topics mentioned in this article, see the entries* ANIMAL RESEARCH; ANIMAL WELFARE AND RIGHTS; CHILDREN, *article on* HEALTH-CARE AND RESEARCH ISSUES; CONFLICT OF INTEREST; ETHICS; FRAUD, THEFT, AND PLAGIARISM; GENETICS AND HUMAN BEHAVIOR, *article on* SCIENTIFIC AND RESEARCH ISSUES; HEALTH-CARE RESOURCES, ALLOCATION OF, *article on* MACROALLOCATION; INFORMED CONSENT, *especially the article on* CONSENT ISSUES IN HUMAN RESEARCH; MINORITIES AS RESEARCH SUBJECTS; RESEARCH, UNETHICAL; RESEARCH BIAS; RESEARCH METHODOLOGY; VALUE AND VALUATION; *and* WOMEN, *article on* RESEARCH ISSUES. *This article will find application in the entries* COMMERCIALISM IN SCIENTIFIC RESEARCH; RESEARCH, HUMAN: HISTORICAL ASPECTS; *and* RESEARCH ETHICS COMMITTEES. *For a discussion of related ideas, see the entries* JUSTICE; PRIVACY AND CONFIDENTIALITY IN RESEARCH; *and* RISK. *Other relevant material may be found under the entries* AGING AND THE AGED, *article on* HEALTH-CARE AND RESEARCH ISSUES; AIDS, *article on* HEALTH-CARE AND RESEARCH ISSUES; FETUS, *article on* FETAL RESEARCH; MENTALLY DISABLED AND MENTALLY ILL PERSONS, *article on* RESEARCH ISSUES; MILITARY PERSONNEL AS RESEARCH SUBJECTS; MULTINATIONAL RESEARCH; PRISONERS, *article on* RESEARCH ISSUES; SEX THERAPY AND SEX RESEARCH; *and* STUDENTS AS RESEARCH SUBJECTS. *See also the* APPENDIX (CODES, OATHS, AND DIRECTIVES RELATED TO BIOETHICS), SECTION IV: ETHICAL DIRECTIVES FOR HUMAN RESEARCH.

Bibliography

BARON, CHARLES H. 1985. "Fetal Research: The Question in the States." *Hastings Center Report* 15, no. 2:12–16.

BLANK, ROBERT H., and BONNICKSEN, ANDREA L., eds. 1993. *Debates over Medical Authority/New Challenges in Biomedical Experimentation.* Vol. 2 of *Emerging Issues in Biomedical Policy.* New York: Columbia University Press.

CHASE, MARILYN. 1989. "Bad Chemistry: Mixing Science, Stocks, Raises Question of Bias in the Testing of Drugs." *Wall Street Journal,* January 26, pp. A1, A6.

COHN, VICTOR. 1973. "NIH Vows Not to Fund Fetus Work." *Washington Post,* April 13, pp. A1, A8.

COUNCIL ON ETHICAL AND JUDICIAL AFFAIRS. AMERICAN MEDICAL ASSOCIATION. 1991. "Gender Disparities in Clinical Decision Making." *Journal of the American Medical Association* 266, no. 4:559–562.

ETHICS ADVISORY BOARD. U.S. DEPARTMENT OF HEALTH, EDUCATION AND WELFARE. 1979. *HEW Support of Research Involving in Vitro Fertilization and Embryo Transfer: Report and Conclusions.* Washington, D.C.: U.S. Government Printing Office.

ETHICS COMMITTEE. AMERICAN FERTILITY SOCIETY. 1990.

"Ethical Considerations of the New Reproductive Technologies." *Fertility and Sterility* 53, no. 6 (suppl. 2):1S–104S.

FADEN, RUTH R.,; BEAUCHAMP, TOM L.; and KING, NANCY M. P. 1986. *A History and Theory of Informed Consent.* New York: Oxford University Press.

"Federal Policy for the Protection of Human Subjects; Notices and Rules." 1991. *Federal Register* 56, no. 117 (June 18):28001–28032.

HEALY, BERNADINE; CAMPEAU, LUCIEN; GRAY, RICHARD; HERD, J. ALAN; HOOGWERF, BYRON; HUNNINGHAKE, DONALD; KNATTERUD, DONALD; STEWART, WILLIAM; WHITE, CARL; and the INVESTIGATORS OF THE POST CORONARY ARTERY BYPASS GRAFT SURGERY CLINICAL TRIAL. 1989. "Conflict-of-Interest Guidelines for a Multicenter Clinical Trial of Treatment After Coronary-Artery Bypass-Graft Surgery." *New England Journal of Medicine* 320, no. 14:949–951.

HUMAN FETAL TISSUE TRANSPLANTATION RESEARCH PANEL. 1988. *Report of the Human Fetal Tissue Transplantation Research Panel.* 2 vols. Bethesda, Md.: National Institutes of Health.

KING, PATRICIA, and AREEN, JUDITH. 1988. "Legal Regulation of Fetal Tissue Transplantation." *Clinical Research* 36, no. 3:205–208.

KOSHLAND, DANIEL E., JR. 1994. "Strategic Goals on an NIH Model." *Science* 263, no. 5150:1071.

LEVINE, ROBERT J. 1986. *Ethics and Regulation of Clinical Research.* 2d ed. Baltimore: Urban & Schwarzenberg.

MASTROIANNI, ANNA C.; FADEN, RUTH R.; and FEDERMAN, DANIEL D., eds. 1994. *Women and Health Research: Ethical and Legal Issues of Including Women in Clinical Studies.* Washington, D.C.: National Academy Press.

MATHIEU, DEBORAH, ed. 1988. *Organ Substitution Technology: Ethical, Legal, and Public Policy Issues.* Boulder, Colo.: Westview.

NIH Data Book: Basic Data Relating to the National Institutes of Health. 1993. Washington, D.C.: U.S. Government Printing Office.

PERRY, SEYMOUR. 1987. "The NIH Consensus Development Program: A Decade Later." *New England Journal of Medicine* 317, no. 8:485–488.

PRIMACK, JOEL R., and VON HIPPEL, FRANK. 1974. *Advice and Dissent: Scientists in the Public Arena.* New York: Basic Books.

REDMAN, ERIC. 1973. *The Dance of Legislation.* New York: Shannon & Schuster.

RELMAN, ARNOLD S. 1980. "The New Medical-Industrial Complex." *New England Journal of Medicine* 303, no.17: 963–970.

ROTHMAN, DAVID J. 1991. *Strangers at the Bedside: A History of How Law and Bioethics Transformed Medical Decision-making.* New York: Basic Books.

STRICKLAND, STEPHEN P. 1972. *Politics, Science and Dread Disease: A Short History of the United States Medical Research Policy.* Cambridge, Mass.: Harvard University Press.

U.S. DEPARTMENT OF HEALTH AND HUMAN SERVICES AND THE U.S. DEPARTMENT OF ENERGY. 1990. *Understanding Our Genetic Inheritance: The U.S. Human Genome Project: The First Five Years, FY 1991–1995.* Bethesda, Md.: U.S.

Department of Health and Human Services, Public Health Service, National Institutes of Health, National Center for Human Genome Research.

U.S. NATIONAL COMMISSION FOR THE PROTECTION OF HUMAN SUBJECTS OF BIOMEDICAL AND BEHAVIORAL RESEARCH. 1978. *The Belmont Report: Ethical Principles and Guidelines for the Protection of Human Subjects of Research.* Washington, D.C.: Author.

WALTERS, LEROY. 1975. "Ethical and Public Policy Issues in Fetal Research." In *Report and Recommendations: Research on the Fetus: Appendix.* (OS) 76–128. Washington, D.C.: U.S. Government Printing Office.

II. RISK AND VULNERABLE GROUPS

There are two groups of people considered to be vulnerable research subjects. First, people lacking capacity to give informed consent are vulnerable because they depend on others to protect them. Particularly children and those severely impaired by mental illness or retardation are regarded as vulnerable because they lack capacity to give informed consent. Second, people who are likely to be coerced or manipulated are vulnerable because fear, ignorance, or pressure may account for their agreement to participate. Institutionalized persons, prisoners, members of the military, students, hospital staff, laboratory assistants, and pharmaceutical personnel are frequently cited as vulnerable to coercion or manipulation (U.S. Public Health Service, 1991; CIOMS, 1993). In addition, the indigent and desperate may be unduly tempted into study participation by large financial remunerations. Because the informed participation of vulnerable subjects is problematic, enrolling them in research protocols often requires special justification and safeguards (CIOMS, 1993; Protection of Human Subjects, 1991; Levine, 1986).

Vulnerability to coercion and manipulation

There has been some consensus, at least in theory, about how to protect the rights and welfare of competent adults who are vulnerable to coercion or manipulation. First, since the right to consent is grounded in its utility, fairness, and the right of self-determination, studies should be reviewed to ensure that consent is voluntary and that the risks of research are not unfairly distributed to vulnerable groups (CIOMS, 1993; Protection of Human subjects, 1991). This evaluation should be conducted by panels known as institutional review boards (IRBs) or research ethics committees (RECs). The views of RECs and IRBs, however, may differ from those of the vulnerable subjects. One remedy is to assemble a group of prospective subjects and conduct a group consultation. Robert Levine writes, "In recent years it has become increasingly apparent that meetings with assemblies of prospective subjects serves much more than the

purposes of efficacy in recruitment. They also accomplish the goals of reducing individual intimidation and learning about the value judgment of productive subjects" (1986, p. 91).

Second, most agree that the greater the vulnerability and risk to competent adults, the more specific protections should be adopted; where it is difficult to supervise the voluntariness of vulnerable people's consent, they should receive special regulatory protection. For example, because prisoners live in settings that are inherently coercive, the U.S. government stipulates research regulations for prisoners (Protection of Human Subjects, 1991, subpart C). Studies with more than a minimal risk or that do not hold out benefit to prisoners (individually or as a class) require demonstrated utility, special safeguards, experts' approval, and authorization from the secretary of health and human services. These restrictions make biomedical research with prisoners difficult to justify because there are no diseases unique to them as a class. Given their extraordinary living conditions, however, social or behavioral studies might gain approval.

A third area of general agreement about protecting vulnerable competent adults from coercion or manipulation concerns the importance of avoiding interference with people's self-determination or unjustified paternalism. There is less consensus, however, on how to do this. Some guidelines, such as the U.S. federal regulations "Protection of Human Subjects" regard pregnant women as particularly susceptible to pressure and coercion. The guidelines instruct IRBs: "When some or all of the subjects are likely to be vulnerable to coercion or undue influence such as children, prisoners, pregnant women, mentally disabled persons, or economically or educationally disadvantaged persons, additional safeguards have been included in the study to protect the rights and welfare of these subjects" (1991, III(b)). The U.S. Public Health Service Consultation on International Collaborative Human Immunodeficiency Virus (U.S. Public Health Service, 1991), include pregnant and nursing women on their list of possibly vulnerable groups. The goal of these guidelines is to protect the fetuses and newborns, as well as pregnant and nursing women, from research risk. Such policies are controversial when women cannot participate and research is a woman's only or best means to gain access to investigational drugs or therapy. It may be an unfair denial of benefits to rule that women cannot be considered as subjects. First, they are denied the benefits of learning about how drugs affect them as a group. Second, men of reproductive age are not excluded from drug studies; yet many drugs cause changes in male germ cells that are mutagenic. Consequently, the restriction of opportunities for women to participate in research just because they are or might become pregnant has drawn sharp criticism (CIOMS, 1993). Where there is a conflict between the health needs of the mother and that of the fetus, an important consensus is developing that the mother should be at liberty to resolve it herself (CIOMS, 1993). Restrictions to protect the fetus sometimes rest upon poorly founded assumptions about what causes harm to the fetus or that these measures are needed to ensure that pregnant women will protect their fetuses. Informed consent from any woman, however, presupposes that she is informed of the likely harms or benefits, including that to her fetus. Pregnancy and nursing make women neither incapable of consent, like children, nor vulnerable to coercion or manipulation, like students and prisoners.

Other competent people may also resent paternalistic restrictions of their liberties. Impoverished people, including students, may willingly volunteer as subjects in studies that have risks but pay well. They may argue that if fighter pilots receive high pay for taking risks, civilians, too, should have the choice to obtain high pay for taking research risks. But others fear that high payment inherently constitutes undue influence (CIOMS, 1993).

Thus, when vulnerable people are competent, disagreements abound concerning what specific restrictions on their choices are fair, promote their well-being, and respect their self-determination. Too little protection risks their exploitation; too much protection risks unjustified paternalism. Before limiting the liberty of competent people, we should use community consultation with members of the potentially vulnerable group to consider if they want such protection, if the probability and magnitude of harm warrant constraints, and if the restrictions are the least invasive to secure their well-being.

Lacking capacity to give consent

As with the competent people, the ethical basis for research policy with persons lacking capacity to give informed consent concerns promoting their self-determination, fair treatment, and well-being. There are four important policy options offering different approaches to balancing what is fair, most protective of incompetent people's well-being, and most respectful of whatever self-determination they have or may develop. These four policies represent different regulative ideals because they balance these primary values differently, and because they offer different authority principles (stating who decides) and guidance principles (substantive directions about how decisions should be made). The remaining discussion will focus on these options.

The "surrogate," or "libertarian," solution. One policy allows the same sort of research with people who lack capacity to give consent as with other subjects,

if guardians consent. Since guardians have the authority to choose the mode of care, religion, and schooling for their dependents, then, according to this view, guardians should determine whether their charges participate in research.

Critics argue that guardians have no authority to volunteer another for studies that are hazardous or that do not hold out benefit for them (Ramsey, 1970; Levine, 1986; Kopelman, 1989). Guardians have authority insofar as they promote the well-being of those under their care and prevent, remove, or minimize harms to them. Volunteering to put oneself in harm's way to gain knowledge may be morally admirable. But volunteering to put another in harm's way is not admirable, and violates the guardian's protective role. Critics argue that allowing guardians to enroll their charges in potentially harmful experiments wrongs the charges, sets a dangerous precedent, and has a brutalizing effect upon society.

The "no consent–no research," or "Nuremberg," solution. Another policy forbids enrolling people as research subjects without their consent. This view is maintained in the first international research statement, the Nuremberg Code. It states, "The voluntary consent of the human subject is absolutely essential." It goes on to define consent—in a way that has become fairly standard—as requiring legal capacity, free choice, and understanding of "the nature, duration, and purpose of the experiment; the methods and means by which it is conducted; all inconveniences and hazards reasonably to be expected; any effects upon his health or person which may possibly come from participation in the research" (Germany [Territory Under Allied Occupation . . .], 1947).

Composed at the end of World War II, the Nuremberg Code stands as an international response to the horrible, involuntary medical studies done by Nazi physicians in which many unwilling subjects and prisoners were killed or permanently maimed (Proctor, 1988). It is uncertain if it was intended as a comprehensive code for research (McCormick, 1974). If it is taken as a general policy, however, subjects who lack capacity to give informed consent cannot serve as research subjects.

Critics argue that this policy option would cripple medical advances for people who cannot give consent, turning them into "therapeutic orphans" (Shirkey, 1968; McCormick, 1974; Levine, 1986). Children, retarded persons, and those incapacitated by mental illness have unique medical problems; thus, studies with normal adult volunteers may be inapplicable. Normal adults cannot serve as subjects in studies comparing treatments for schizophrenia, manic-depression, or lung disease in premature infants. To test the safety and efficacy of many standard, innovative, or investigational treatments for distinctive groups, some members of the groups have to be subjects in controlled testing.

The "no consent–only therapy," or "Helsinki," solution. A third policy permits persons who lack the capacity to give informed consent to be enrolled as research subjects if the studies are therapeutic and if guardians consent. This view is represented in the next major international code for research to follow the Nuremberg Code, the World Medical Assembly's Declaration of Helsinki, written in 1964 and revised in 1975, 1983, and 1989. It states, "In the case of legal incompetence, informed consent should be obtained from the legal guardian in accordance with national legislation" (I[11]). The incompetent person must agree as well, when able to do so. The code allows research with incompetent people, but "only to the extent that medical research is justified by its potential diagnostic or therapeutic value for the patient" (II[6]). If, however, the medical research is nontherapeutic, then "the subjects should be volunteers" (III[2]). People who cannot volunteer cannot be subjects in nontherapeutic studies.

This policy option distinguishes *clinical or therapeutic research* (studies seeking generalizable knowledge and intending to provide medically acceptable therapy for the individual) from *nontherapeutic biomedical research* (studies seeking generalizable knowledge and not intended as therapy to benefit the individual directly). Therapeutic studies attempt to benefit the person through prevention, diagnosis, or treatment of disease. Thus, drawing the line at therapeutic research for people who lack capacity to give informed consent seems to defenders to be a good solution to the problem of when to permit incompetent people to serve as subjects (Ramsey, 1970).

One difficulty with this third option concerns the difficulty of classifying studies as therapeutic or nontherapeutic in a way that is not arbitrary or misleading. Therapeutic studies often have features that are not a part of routine therapy, such as extra tests, hospitalizations, or visits to the doctor. If these nontherapeutic features increase costs, risks, or inconvenience to the patient, classifying the study as "therapeutic" may be arbitrary and misleading. Moreover, this classification can be misleading if people assume therapeutic studies are always safe or beneficial. Labeling something "therapeutic" may mask risk, inconvenience, costs, or nonbeneficial features, creating an inappropriate bias for participation.

A second problem is that it seems unreasonable to prohibit important research that is not hazardous, especially when it offers nontherapeutic benefits to subjects. Subjects would be neither harmed nor wronged if they gained from the experience, liked participating, and were not at risk of harm. Children may enjoy and learn from participating in nontherapeutic studies in which they are asked to do such things as stack similar blocks or identify animals from sounds they make. These nontherapeutic studies could be important for establishing

criteria of normal vision and hearing. Adults who are not legally competent may also enjoy and learn from serving as research subjects in nontherapeutic studies. For example, they might like an outing to a research facility, meeting the investigators or learning about the study. In addition, they can benefit indirectly from nontherapeutic studies.

For a study to be therapeutic, it must have *direct* benefit to subjects. This rules out even low-risk studies with only *indirect* benefits to incompetent persons. This option, for example, impedes the formation of standards about typical growth and development. Such standards presuppose carefully tested criteria distinguishing people with developmental delays or impairments from those with normal growth and development. Establishing such norms requires collecting and analyzing data on the growth and development of large numbers of children. Such safe but important research, however, is forbidden under this policy because it is not therapeutic. Even though these studies establishing norms for growth and development are safe, they are nontherapeutic because they are designed not to benefit the subjects directly but to gain generalizable knowledge. If children stack blocks at play, it is not research; if people test views about how they stack blocks, it is research but may be no more burdensome to the child. Thus, when nontherapeutic studies are needed to promote the well-being of incompetent people as a *group*, and involve little or no risk of harm or inconvenience to them, it seems hard to understand how they are harmed or wronged by participation.

There are other far-reaching consequences of the Helsinki rule stipulating that when medical research is nontherapeutic, "The subjects should be volunteers—either healthy persons or persons or patients for whom the experimental design is not related to the patient's illness" (III[2]). It prohibits epidemiological studies and the investigation of the natural history of disease when there are no therapies. These are among the most important methods for collecting information, so this policy, if adopted, would have grave consequences.

The initial justification for excluding persons who lack the capacity to give informed consent from nontherapeutic research was to honor their rights and protect their welfare. Safe, nontherapeutic research, however, seems neither unfair nor a violation of the rights or welfare of people who lack the capacity to give consent. Failing to do safe but important studies might be unfair and violate their rights and welfare, since it fails to consider all their needs.

Some question if the Declaration of Helsinki was meant to be interpreted so literally that it disallows all nontherapeutic biomedical research studies with persons who cannot give consent (McCormick, 1974). If it was not meant to be taken literally, why has this policy remained through four versions?

The "risk–benefit," or "U.S. federal regulation," solution.   A fourth approach allows research on procedures or interventions with incompetent persons when the research holds out direct benefit to them or does not place them at unwarranted risk of harm, discomfort, or inconvenience. Defenders of the fourth option should clarify what risk is unwarranted. This policy uses risk assessment to set priorities between the social utility of encouraging studies and the protection of people's rights of self-determination and well-being. To try to set priorities between the social utility of such studies and respect and protection of incompetent people, this option stipulates that the greater the risk, the more rigorous and elaborate the procedural protection and consent requirements. The U.S. Federal Regulations ("Protection of Human Subjects," 1991) reflect this fourth policy option in the codes for research with children adopted in 1983, and those proposed in 1978 (but never adopted) for institutionalized people with mental impairment or retardation. The Council for International Organizations of Medical Science has adopted a similar standard (CIOMS, 1993). On this fourth option, therapy is one of the intended benefits that should be taken into account in a risk analysis. Whenever possible, the incompetent persons should give their assent to participate. Assent means affirmative agreement, not just lack of objection.

There are advantages to focusing directly upon the likely benefits and harms of procedures or intervention being studied. First, there are benefits other than therapy that may play a role in deciding if it is reasonable to serve as a subject. A safe, nontherapeutic study that increases a child's understanding of a sibling's chronic illness, for example, might have important lessons about empathy for the child. Those giving consent need to know, of course, the nature and magnitude of the intended benefits (such as education or therapy) or risks of harms associated with the study. Second, calling something "therapeutic" can create the unwarranted idea that participating in the study is in a person's best interest. Risk assessment can reveal hazards, inconveniences, and costs in therapeutic studies that some reasonable people would prefer to avoid.

Using a likely-harms-to-benefits calculation, the U.S. regulations specify four categories of research for children ("Protection of Human Subjects," 1991). IRBs or RECs can approve research that they judge to be in the first three categories, including studies that have no more than a minor increase over a minimal risk and studies that hold out benefit to the subjects. They cannot approve studies that have more than a minor increase over a minimal risk and that do not hold out benefit for the subjects, and must seek approval from the federal government to conduct them. As in the case of

the guidelines for prisoners cited earlier, procedural safeguards increase with risk.

There are no final guidelines in the United States for research on those institutionalized as mentally infirm, but there is a proposal about how to treat those institutionalized with impairments like mental illness, senility, psychosis, mental retardation, or emotional disturbances (U.S. Department of Health, Education and Welfare, 1978a, 1978b). It is similar to that proposed for children, except that it allows incompetent adults more authority to decline to participate in studies. The consent or assent of those institutionalized with such impairments must be sought. None who refuse may be enrolled in any study that does not hold out direct benefit without authorization from the courts.

Unfortunately, this fourth policy option has difficulties. Key terms have vague definitions, permitting broad interpretations about what risks of harm are warranted and what constitutes a benefit. For example, the pivotal concepts of "minimal risk" and "a minor increase over a minimal risk" are problematic (Kopelman, 1989). The regulations state that "'minimal risks' means that the probability and magnitude of harm or discomfort anticipated in the proposed research are not greater in and of themselves than those ordinarily encountered in daily life or during the performance of routine physical or psychological examinations or tests" (Protection of Human Subjects, 1991, 102 i). The Council for International Organizations of Medical Science has adopted a similar definition (1993).

The first part of the definition is vague because daily risks include dangers from living in cities, riding in cars, flying in airplanes, and being in a world filled with nuclear and conventional weapons. Do we know the nature, probability, and magnitude of these "everyday" hazards well enough to serve as a baseline to estimate research risk? It seems easier to determine whether asking a four-year-old to stack blocks is a minimal-risk study than to determine the nature, probability, and magnitude of whatever risks people normally encounter in their daily lives.

The second part of the definition seems to set a standard for physical interventions that have a minimal risk. The test is whether the activity is like that of a routine examination. Accordingly, IRB or REC members may not approve *as minimal risk* research such procedures as X rays, bronchoscopy, spinal taps, or cardiac catheterization because they are not part of routine examinations. IRBs and RECs, however, can approve studies that have a *minor increase over minimal risk,* and some of these procedures have been approved as having a minor increase over a minimal risk. Thus, no definition has been given for the crucial upper limit of risk that can be approved by IRBs or RECs.

Finally, this definition of "minimal risk" offers no guidance about how to assess *psychosocial risks* such as invasion of privacy, breach of confidentiality, labeling, and stigmatization. In "routine" visits, doctors and nurses "ordinarily encounter" discussions of family abuse, sexual preference, and diagnoses that could affect reputations or the ability to get jobs or insurance.

Without clear standards for risk assessment, how effective are these guidelines? A survey of pediatric department chairs and pediatric research directors (Janofsky and Starfield, 1981) found considerable differences of opinion about whether procedures such as venipuncture, arterial puncture, and gastric and intestinal intubation are hazardous. For example, most regarded arterial puncture to have a "greater than minimal risk"; but between 8 and 24 percent thought it had less than a minimal risk, depending on the child's age. An editorial in the *Journal of Pediatrics* found such variation "cause for concern" and said that better standards of risk assessment are needed (Lascari, 1981).

In short, this policy fails to clarify crucial standards about what constitutes a risk, a benefit, or how to balance them. For example, the National Institutes of Health appointed a nine-member review board to assess whether a study of the safety and efficacy of synthetic growth hormone (hGH) was in compliance with federal research guidelines (1992). Eighty children whose adult height was projected to be at or below the first percentile could participate with their parents' consent. The children receive injections three times a week for four to seven years (six hundred to eleven hundred injections), half getting hGH and, for comparison, the other half receiving salt water, an ineffective placebo. Neither the doctors, nor the parents, nor the children know who gets water and who gets the growth hormone. Each year all the children come to the National Institutes of Health to undergo a variety of tests, including physicals, X rays, nude photographs, and psychological evaluations. Of the nine panelists, a majority held there was a minor increase over minimal risk, but this risk was offset by the health benefits of being in the study. Two others judged there was no benefit to offset the risks, inconvenience, and discomfort to those getting water rather than hGH, but the study was important enough to be justified. One panelist (this author) argued that a study of a terrible disease might justify these risks for the group getting water injections; but shortness is no disease, and so the risk is unwarranted.

If there is any consensus that the fourth approach represented by the U.S. rules and CIOMS is the best way to set priorities between the need to protect the rights and welfare of people who lack the capacity to give informed consent with the need to encourage research, it may mask different understandings of what constitutes an acceptable risk of likely-harms-to-benefits ratio.

Conclusion

IRBs and RECs should continue to play an important role in protecting vulnerable subjects while making it possible to continue important research. Without safeguards, vulnerable subjects risk exploitation. Excessive restrictions, however, have dangers as well. They can thwart the advance of knowledge needed to improve medical care for the groups they seek to protect. Where potential subjects are capable of giving legal consent but are vulnerable to pressure or manipulation, their consent should be monitored to see if it is coerced or manipulated, and regulations should be sought only when they can be justified. There is general agreement that competent adults should serve as research subjects whenever possible, and that when people who lack capacity to give consent are enrolled as subjects in biomedical research, the study should be related to their health-care needs. The guardian's consent should be obtained; and, if possible, the assent or permission of the person lacking capacity to consent should also be sought. Since there are difficulties with each of the four policies regarding subjects lacking capacity to give informed consent, IRBs and RECs will have to consider issues of utility, fairness, and protection without entirely satisfactory guidance.

LORETTA M. KOPELMAN

Directly related to this article are the other articles in this entry: GENERAL GUIDELINES, *and* SUBJECT SELECTION. *For a further discussion of topics mentioned in this article, see the entries* CHILDREN, *article on* HEALTH-CARE AND RESEARCH ISSUES; FREEDOM AND COERCION; INFORMED CONSENT, *especially the article on* CONSENT ISSUES IN HUMAN RESEARCH; MATERNAL–FETAL RELATIONSHIP; MENTALLY DISABLED AND MENTALLY ILL PERSONS, *article on* RESEARCH ISSUES; PRISONERS, *article on* RESEARCH ISSUES; PRIVACY AND CONFIDENTIALITY IN RESEARCH; RESEARCH ETHICS COMMITTEES; RESEARCH METHODOLOGY; RISK; *and* WOMEN, *article on* RESEARCH ISSUES. *This article will find application in the entries* AGING AND THE AGED, *article on* HEALTH-CARE AND RESEARCH ISSUES; ANIMAL RESEARCH; ANIMAL WELFARE AND RIGHTS; FETUS, *article on* FETAL RESEARCH; MILITARY PERSONNEL AS RESEARCH SUBJECTS; MINORITIES AS RESEARCH SUBJECTS; *and* STUDENTS AS RESEARCH SUBJECTS. *For a discussion of related ideas, see the entries* AUTONOMY; COMPETENCE; CONFLICT OF INTEREST; HARM; JUSTICE; PATERNALISM; *and* UTILITY. *Other relevant material may be found under the entries* AIDS, *article on* HEALTH-CARE AND RESEARCH ISSUES; GENETICS AND HUMAN BEHAVIOR, *article on* SCIENTIFIC AND RE-

SEARCH ISSUES; MULTINATIONAL RESEARCH; RE-
SEARCH, HUMAN: HISTORICAL ASPECTS; RESEARCH,
UNETHICAL; *and* RESEARCH BIAS. *See also the* APPENDIX
(CODES, OATHS, AND DIRECTIVES RELATED TO BIOETH-
ICS), SECTION IV: ETHICAL DIRECTIVES FOR HUMAN RE-
SEARCH.

Bibliography

COUNCIL FOR INTERNATIONAL ORGANIZATIONS OF MEDICAL
SCIENCE (CIOMS). 1993. *International Ethical Guidelines
for Biomedical Research Involving Human Subjects.* Geneva,
Switzerland: Author.

GERMANY (TERRITORY UNDER ALLIED OCCUPATION, 1945–
1955: U.S. ZONE) MILITARY TRIBUNALS. 1947. "Permissible Medical Experiments." In vol. 2 of *Trials of War
Criminals Before the Nuernberg Tribunals Under Control
Law No. 10,* pp. 181–183. Washington, D.C.: U.S. Government Printing Office.

JANOFSKY, JEFFREY, and STARFIELD, BARBARA. 1981. "Assessment of Risk in Research on Children." *Journal of Pediatrics* 98, no. 5:842–846.

KOPELMAN, LORETTA M. 1989. "When Is the Risk Minimal
Enough for Children to Be Research Subjects?" In *Chil-
dren and Health Care: Moral and Social Issues,* pp. 89–99.
Edited by Loretta M. Kopelman and John C. Moskop.
Dordrecht, Netherlands: Kluwer.

LASCARI, ANDRÉ D. 1981. "Risks of Research on Children."
Journal of Pediatrics 98, no. 5:759–760.

LEVINE, ROBERT J. 1986. *Ethics and Regulation of Clinical Research.* 2d ed. Baltimore: Urban & Schwarzenberg.

McCORMICK, RICHARD A. 1974. "Proxy Consent in the Experimental Situation." *Perspectives in Biology and Medicine*
18, no. 1:2–20.

NATIONAL INSTITUTES OF HEALTH. HUMAN GROWTH HOR-
MONE PROTOCOL REVIEW COMMITTEE. 1992. *Report of the
NIH Human Growth Hormone Protocol Review Committee.*
Bethesda, Md.: Author.

PROCTOR, ROBERT. 1988. *Racial Hygiene: Medicine Under the
Nazis.* Cambridge, Mass.: Harvard University Press.

RAMSEY, PAUL. 1970. *The Patient as Person: Explorations in
Medical Ethics.* New Haven, Conn.: Yale University Press.

SHIRKEY, HARRY C. 1968. "Therapeutic Orphans." *Journal of
Pediatrics* 72, no. 1:119–120.

U.S. DEPARTMENT OF HEALTH, EDUCATION AND WELFARE.
NATIONAL COMMISSION FOR THE PROTECTION OF HUMAN
SUBJECTS OF BIOMEDICAL AND BEHAVIORAL RESEARCH.
1978a. *Research Involving Those Institutionalized as Mentally Infirm: Report and Recommendations,* DHEW Publication (05) 78–0006. Washington, D.C.: Author.

———. 1978b. *Appendix to Report and Recommendations, Re-
search Involving Those Institutionalized as Mentally Infirm.*
DHEW Publication no. (OS–78–0007). Washington,
D.C.: Author.

U.S. PUBLIC HEALTH SERVICE. 1991. "Consultation on International Collaborative Human Immunodeficiency Virus
(HIV) Research." *Law, Medicine and Health Care* 19, nos.
3–4:259–263.

WORLD MEDICAL ASSEMBLY. 1989. "The Declaration of Helsinki: Recommendations Guiding Medical Doctors and
Biomedical Research Involving Human Subjects." *Law,
Medicine, and Health Care* 19, nos. 3–4:264–265. Adopted
by the 18th World Medical Assembly, Helsinki, Finland,
in 1964; amended in 1975, 1983, and 1989.

III. SUBJECT SELECTION

Selecting individuals to participate in research involves
not only scientific decisions about appropriate entry criteria but also ethical decisions about the distribution of
benefits and burdens. The U.S. National Commission
on the Protection of Human Subjects of Biomedical
and Behavioral Research (U.S. National Commission,
1979) cited three ethical principles as the foundation of
research ethics. The first, respect for persons, and the
second, beneficence, have been analyzed more often
and in greater depth than the third, justice. Investigators, regulators, and institutional review boards (IRBs)
are accustomed to applying the principle of beneficence
by examining the risk–benefit ratio and applying the
principle of respect for persons by examining informed
consent. But the third principle—the selection of subjects as a matter of justice—has often been considered
last and in only one of its aspects, the protection of vulnerable groups from exploitation as subjects. This situation is changing as persons and groups previously
excluded from research on grounds of vulnerability seek
access to what they perceive as research benefits, primarily the opportunity to try new drugs for serious and
life-threatening illnesses.

According to the U.S. National Commission, justice is relevant to the selection of subjects at two levels:
the social and the individual. At the individual level,
"researchers [should] exhibit fairness: thus, they should
not offer potentially beneficial research only to some
patients who are in their favor or select only 'undesirable' persons for risky research" (1979, p. 7). At the social level, "distinctions [should] be drawn between
classes of subjects that ought, and ought not, to participate in any particular kind of research, based on the
ability of members of that class to bear burdens and on
the appropriateness of placing further burdens on already
burdened persons" (U.S. National Commission, 1979,
p. 7). Specifically, on the grounds of social justice,
classes of subjects should be ranked (e.g., adults before
children) and some classes of potential subjects (e.g.,
prisoners and the institutionalized mentally infirm)
should be selected only under certain conditions and
perhaps not at all.

Very few philosophers or other scholars have proposed standards by which to establish priorities in the
selection of subjects. Hans Jonas proposed a "descending order of permissibility" for the "conscription" of sub-

jects (Jonas, 1970). In his view, researchers themselves should be the first to test a new therapy, in that they can best understand the risks and benefits. Believing that very sick or dying patients are particularly vulnerable to researchers' invitations, Jonas opposed using them in research not directly related to their care.

Another approach has been to assert an obligation to participate in biomedical research. Arthur Caplan (1984) argued that research is a form of voluntary social cooperation that generates obligations of fairness and reciprocity. If a competent individual voluntarily seeks care in a hospital or institution that conducts biomedical research, he or she benefits from research and should share in its costs (i.e., participate). This obligation is a general one, not an obligation to volunteer for the first available trial or any particular trial.

Selecting the least vulnerable

Underlying these different views is the assumption that research is risky or at least burdensome. If this is true, subjects should be selected in a way that protects those whose social, demographic, or economic characteristics make them particularly vulnerable to coercion and exploitation. Volunteering for research is seen as either a duty to be discharged or an altruistic act to be applauded. This emphasis on protecting vulnerable persons is understandable, given the signal event in the modern history of clinical research ethics—the cruel and often fatal experiments performed on unconsenting prisoners by Nazi doctors in World War II (Caplan, 1992). Public opinion in the United States also was shaped by the revelations of unethical experiments such as the Tuskegee Syphilis Study of poor black sharecroppers (Jones, 1993), the Willowbrook hepatitis B studies at an institution for mentally retarded children (Rothman, 1982), and the Jewish Chronic Disease Hospital studies in which live cancer cells were injected into uninformed elderly patients (Katz et al., 1972). The most influential single article was one by Henry Knowles Beecher, a respected anesthesiologist, in the *New England Journal of Medicine*; it described a series of studies at major research institutions that placed subjects at risk and failed to obtain informed consent (Beecher, 1966; Rothman, 1991).

The view of research as inherently risky and of research subjects as inherently needing protection began to change in the early 1980s. Why? First, consider research at the level of individuals. The empirical question of the actual risk in most research studies has been answered: quite low. The U.S. President's Commission for the Study of Ethical Problems in Biomedical and Behavioral Research asked three large research institutions to summarize their experience with research-related injuries (U.S. President's Commission, 1982). Each group

found a very low incidence of adverse effects. In one institution, out of more than 8,000 subjects involved in 157 protocols, only 3 adverse effects were reported, including 2 headaches after spinal taps. Some of these reassuring results may be due to the vigilance of IRBs and investigators in reducing the likelihood of risk in designing and implementing studies. While risk is always an element that subjects should consider when deciding whether to enter a study, it is often no longer the paramount issue.

Sharing the benefits of research

Even more important, the benefits side of the equation has assumed greater weight in individual decision making. Patients and advocacy groups are demanding more autonomy and less paternalism in the selection of subjects. Desperately ill patients forcefully argue that they are willing to trade a higher level of risk for the potential benefits of promising new procedures, devices, or drugs. Advocates for women and children point out that the typical exclusion or underrepresentation of these populations in clinical trials means that the drugs, when approved, will be prescribed for them with little direct data about dosage, efficacy, or side effects. These trends have been spurred by the vigorous, sometimes confrontational, efforts of persons with the acquired immunodeficiency syndrome (AIDS). This advocacy also has stressed the inclusion of groups with poor access to trials, mainly women and minorities (C. Levine, 1988, 1993).

Increased emphasis on women's health issues has provided some information on subject recruitment. Examining the inclusion of women in clinical trials, the U.S. General Accounting Office reviewed the practices of the National Institutes of Health (NIH) and the Food and Drug Administration (FDA) (Nadel, 1990; U.S. General Accounting Office, 1992). In both instances women were found to be underrepresented. The FDA review found that women were represented in every clinical trial of the fifty-three drugs approved by the FDA in the previous three and a half years. However, for more than 60 percent of the drugs, the proportion of women in the trial was less than the proportion of women with the relevant disease. Women were particularly underrepresented in trials of cardiovascular drugs, even though cardiovascular disease is the leading cause of death in women.

In arguing for wider inclusion criteria in clinical trials, patient advocates and some clinicians have noted that in the interest of good medical care, drugs should be tested on the populations that will use them. This belief runs counter to the more traditional research view of subject selection, which focuses on testing drugs in a small, homogeneous population in order to detect differences in efficacy and side effects as rapidly as possible.

Even with broadened inclusion criteria, not all patients who want access to promising new agents can be enrolled in clinical trials because they fail to meet the inclusion criteria, they live too far from a research center, or the trials are already closed. Several other mechanisms have been developed, such as the "parallel track," in which qualified patients who cannot enroll in clinical trials may obtain a promising drug through their physician ("Expanded Availability," 1992). Community-based research, especially in cancer and AIDS, also has made clinical trials more accessible to patients.

The NIH has formalized the movement toward broader selection of subjects by mandating that its research grant recipients include appropriate numbers of women and minorities (Kirschstein, 1991). The 1993 NIH Revitalization Act (P.L. 103-43) extended the revised NIH policy by requiring the NIH director to ensure that women and members of minority groups are included in each federally funded project. The director may waive the requirement if the inclusion is inappropriate for health reasons, the purpose of the research, or any other circumstance. Cost, however, is not a permissible reason to fail to include women and members of minority groups.

This trend has limits, however. The inclusion of pregnant women in clinical trials is still controversial unless the trial is specifically designed to benefit the fetus, such as trials to prevent maternal–fetal transmission of the human immunodeficiency virus (HIV), which is associated with AIDS. Some of the objections to including pregnant women rely on ethical concerns about, for example, placing at risk a fetus, who cannot consent. Most of the concerns are based on fears of legal liability should the fetus be born with an injury that might be attributed to the investigational drug. Other subject groups for which protection is still deemed essential include children (Levine, 1991) and prisoners and mentally ill persons. Still other groups sometimes cited as vulnerable include elderly people, military personnel, pharmaceutical company employees, and medical students. Although some conditions and some protocols might be coercive, in general these individuals can make choices voluntarily. Special procedures have been set up in some instances to ensure voluntariness (see, e.g., Winter, 1984, on the U.S. Department of Defense).

From the societal perspective, equitable selection of subjects means that the groups bearing the burdens of research should also share in its benefits. Opponents of research in prisons argue that the fruits of the research—newly approved drugs—are rarely available in that setting. Similarly, although many drug trials have been carried out in Third World countries, these nations are often so poor or so lacking in health-care services that they cannot afford to provide the tested drugs to their citizens.

More recently, representatives of Third World countries and of poorly served communities in the United States have been demanding a greater role in the distribution of benefits (Lurie et al., 1994; National Commission on AIDS, 1992; Thomas and Quinn, 1991). Their agreement to participate in clinical drug trials is sometimes conditioned on a promise from trial sponsors to provide something of benefit to the population—the drug, if it proves efficacious, or the health infrastructure needed to deliver the therapy. Efficacy trials for vaccines, which require thousands of subjects, cannot be conducted without the goodwill and participation of a community's leaders. Community consultation, in which investigators and community spokespersons collaborate on the design and implementation of a trial, is becoming a frequent strategy for ensuring that the concerns of the pool of potential subjects and their representatives are addressed.

Recognizing the importance of social justice in the distribution of burdens and benefits, the World Health Organization (WHO) and the Council for International Organizations of Medical Sciences (CIOMS) guidelines for international research state:

> Before undertaking research involving subjects in underdeveloped communities, whether in developed or developing countries, the investigator must ensure that:
> • persons in underdeveloped communities ordinarily will not be involved in research that might equally well be carried out in developed communities;
> • the research is relevant to the health needs and responsive to the priorities of the community. (WHO-CIOMS, 1993)

The commentary on this guideline states: "If any product is to be developed, such as a new therapeutic agent, clear understandings should be reached about whether and how the product, once developed, will be made available to members of the community in which the research was conducted" (WHO-CIOMS, 1993, pp. 38–39).

The equitable selection of subjects now includes an assessment of both the need for protecting vulnerable individuals and groups and the importance of allowing them maximum choice in making the ultimate decision to participate. In the future, even more emphasis will be placed on the equitable distribution of the benefits of research.

CAROL LEVINE

Directly related to this article are the other articles in this entry: GENERAL GUIDELINES, *and* RISK AND VULNERABLE GROUPS. *For a further discussion of topics mentioned in this article, see the entries* AIDS, *article on* HEALTH-CARE AND

RESEARCH ISSUES; AUTONOMY; BENEFICENCE; CHILDREN, article on HEALTH-CARE AND RESEARCH ISSUES; ECONOMIC CONCEPTS IN HEALTH CARE; FETUS, article on FETAL RESEARCH; INFORMED CONSENT, especially the article on CONSENT ISSUES IN HUMAN RESEARCH; JUSTICE; MATERNAL–FETAL RELATIONSHIP; MINORITIES AS RESEARCH SUBJECTS; MULTINATIONAL RESEARCH; RESEARCH, UNETHICAL; RESEARCH BIAS; RESEARCH ETHICS COMMITTEES; RESEARCH METHODOLOGY; and WOMEN, article on RESEARCH ISSUES. This article will find application in the entries AGING AND THE AGED, article on HEALTH-CARE AND RESEARCH ISSUES; MENTALLY DISABLED AND MENTALLY ILL PERSONS, article on RESEARCH ISSUES; MILITARY PERSONNEL AS RESEARCH SUBJECTS; PRISONERS, article on RESEARCH ISSUES; and STUDENTS AS RESEARCH SUBJECTS. For a discussion of related ideas, see the entries COMPETENCE; FREEDOM AND COERCION; OBLIGATION AND SUPEREROGATION; PATERNALISM; and RACE AND RACISM. Other relevant material may be found in the entries ANIMAL RESEARCH; PRIVACY AND CONFIDENTIALITY IN RESEARCH; and RESEARCH, HUMAN: HISTORICAL ASPECTS. See also the APPENDIX (CODES, OATHS, AND DIRECTIVES RELATED TO BIOETHICS), SECTION IV: ETHICAL DIRECTIVES FOR HUMAN RESEARCH.

Bibliography

BEECHER, HENRY K. 1966. "Ethics and Clinical Research." New England Journal of Medicine 274, no. 24:1354–1360.

CAPLAN, ARTHUR L. 1984. "Is There a Duty to Serve as a Subject in Biomedical Research?" IRB 6, no. 5:1–5.

———, ed. 1992. When Medicine Went Mad: Bioethics and the Holocaust. Totowa, N.J.: Humana.

"Expanded Availability of Investigational New Drugs Through a Parallel Track Mechanism for People with AIDS and Other HIV-Related Disease." 1992. Federal Register 57, no. 73 (April 18):13250–13259.

JONAS, HANS. 1970. "Philosophical Reflections on Experimenting with Human Subjects." In Experimentation with Human Subjects, pp. 1–31. Edited by Paul A. Freund. New York: George Braziller.

JONES, JAMES H. 1993. Bad Blood: The Tuskegee Syphilis Experiment. New and expanded ed. New York: Free Press.

KATZ, JAY; CAPRON, ALEXANDER M.; and GLASS, ELEANOR SWIFT, eds. 1972. Experimentation with Human Beings: The Authority of the Investigator, Subject, Professions, and State in the Human Experimentation Process. New York: Russell Sage Foundation.

KIRSCHSTEIN, RUTH L. 1991. "Research on Women's Health." American Journal of Public Health 81, no. 3:291–293.

LEVINE, CAROL. 1988. "Has AIDS Changed the Ethics of Human Subjects Research?" Law, Medicine and Health Care 16, nos. 3–4:167–173.

———. 1991. "Children in HIV/AIDS Clinical Trials: Still Vulnerable After All These Years." Law, Medicine and Health Care 19, nos. 3–4:231–237.

———. 1993. "Women as Research Subjects: New Priorities, New Questions." In Emerging Issues in Biomedical Policy: An Annual Review, pp. 169–188. Edited by Robert H. Blank and Andrea L. Bonnicksen. New York: Columbia University Press.

LEVINE, ROBERT J. 1984. "What Kinds of Subjects Can Understand This Protocol?" IRB 6, no. 5:6–8.

———. 1988. Ethics and Regulation of Clinical Research. 2d ed. New Haven, Conn.: Yale University Press.

LURIE, PETER; BISHAW, MAKONNEN; CHESNEY, MARGARET A.; COOKE, MOLLY; LEMOS FERNANDES, MARIA EUGENIA; HEARST, NORMAN; KATONGOLE-MBIDDE, EDWARD; KOETSAWANG, SUPORN; LINDAN, CHRISTINA P.; MANDEL, JEFFREY; MHLOYI, MARVELLOUS; and COATES, THOMAS J. 1994. "Ethical, Behavioral, and Social Aspects of HIV Vaccine Trials in Developing Countries." Journal of the American Medical Association 271, no. 4:295–301.

NADEL, MARK V. 1990. National Institutes of Health: Problems Implementing Policy on Women in Study Populations. Statement of Mark V. Nadel, Associate Director, National and Public Health Issues, Human Resources Division, Before the Subcommittee on Health and the Environment, Committee on Energy and Commerce, House of Representatives. GAO/T–HRD–90–38. Washington, D.C.: U.S. General Accounting Office.

NATIONAL COMMISSION ON AIDS. 1992. The Challenge of HIV/AIDS in Communities of Color. Edited by Linda C. Humphrey and Frances Porcher. Washington, D.C.: Author.

ROTHMAN, DAVID J. 1982. "Were Tuskegee and Willowbrook 'Studies in Nature'?" Hastings Center Report 12, no. 2: 5–7.

———. 1991. Strangers at the Bedside: A History of How Law and Bioethics Transformed Medical Decision Making. New York: Basic Books.

THOMAS, STEPHEN B., and QUINN, SANDRA CROUSE. 1991. "The Tuskegee Syphilis Study, 1932 to 1972: Implications for HIV Education and AIDS Risk Education Programs in the Black Community." American Journal of Public Health 81, no. 11:1498–1504.

U.S. CONGRESS. 1993. National Institutes of Health Revitalization Amendment. Public Law 103-43. Washington, D.C.: Author.

U.S. GENERAL ACCOUNTING OFFICE. 1992. Women's Health: FDA Needs to Ensure More Study of Gender Differences in Prescription Drug Testing: Report to Congressional Requesters. GAO/HRD–93–17. Washington, D.C.: Author.

U.S. NATIONAL COMMISSION FOR THE PROTECTION OF HUMAN SUBJECTS OF BIOMEDICAL AND BEHAVIORAL RESEARCH. 1979. The Belmont Report: Ethical Principles and Guidelines for the Protection of Human Subjects of Research. Washington D.C.: U.S. Government Printing Office.

U.S. PRESIDENT'S COMMISSION FOR THE STUDY OF ETHICAL PROBLEMS IN MEDICINE AND BIOMEDICAL AND BEHAVIORAL RESEARCH. 1982. Compensating for Research Injuries: A Report on the Ethical and Legal Implications of Programs to Redress Injuries Caused by Biomedical and Behavioral Research. Washington, D.C.: Author.

WORLD HEALTH ORGANIZATION AND COUNCIL FOR INTERNATIONAL ORGANIZATIONS OF MEDICAL SCIENCES (WHO-

CIOMS). 1993. "International Ethical Guidelines for Biomedical Research Involving Human Subjects." Geneva: Author.

WINTER, PHILIP E. 1984. "Human Subject Research Review in the Department of Defense." *IRB* 6, no. 3:9–10.

RESPONSIBILITY

Responsibility has emerged as a central ethical category, directing attention to human beings as moral actors. It highlights the importance for ethical understanding of self-conscious moral commitments, discretion in moral judgment, personal strengths necessary to effective action, a wise use of the power and authority of societal offices, and accountability to oneself and to fellow human beings, perhaps also to God, for moral judgment and action. Discussions of responsibility do not displace systematic treatments of moral principles, laws, and rules; neither do they set aside critical studies of values worthy of promotion in human affairs. They recast these inquiries in terms of the personal lives and social roles of human beings.

Themes associated with responsibility have long been prominent in philosophical and religious discourse, though in different conceptual forms. Especially important are accounts of the moral and intellectual virtues, of moral character, and of the obedient or resolute wills of the upright (Aristotle, 1934; Aquinas, 1966; Calvin, 1957; Kant, 1949; cf. Cohen, 1972). Also relevant are themes elaborated in conceptions of moral law, including natural law; in notions of the orders of nature or creation; in interpretations of divine commandments and ordinances; and in treatments of God's covenant with Israel, or of the Christian idea of a new covenant in Jesus Christ (Aristotle, 1934; Aquinas, 1966; Brunner, 1937; Häring, 1961). Contemporary accounts of responsibility weave these classic themes together in ways that take account of modern social realities, and that utilize theories of action provided by the human sciences.

In regard to modern realities, the concept of responsibility corresponds to social complexity, which routinely generates problems with more features than any system of moral rules can encompass. It fits well with advanced technologies and high levels of specialization, where expert knowledge and skill are indispensable to moral judgment. Responsibility takes account of open spaces within democratic and free-market settings for individuals and groups to follow independent initiatives in the pursuit of cherished social goals. It accords with modern social theory, which conceives of social institutions—the state, business enterprises, special-interest associations, even families and religious bodies—as the constructions of autonomous individuals contracting for mutual advantage. Finally, responsibility can accommodate reflections on the moral ambiguities of the social and organizational contexts that structure human activity. In respect to each of these characteristics, themes relating to responsibility take on considerable importance.

The concept of responsibility enjoys prominence, then, because it can draw together a wide range of ethical ideas in a fashion pertinent to contemporary social existence. For some thinkers it serves as the unifying principle of a comprehensive ethical theory (cf. Niebuhr, 1963; Jonsen, 1968). Responsibility virtually becomes the first principle of ethics, so that the admonition "Be responsible!" conveys all that needs to be said about the moral life (Jonsen, 1968; cf. Glatzer, 1966). The theoretical task is to unfold the dimensions of responsibility in their bearing on personal and social processes.

The dimensions of responsibility appear both in the personal lives of individuals and in the roles, positions, and offices that order social institutions. All of these dimensions may not be explicit in a particular ethical theory, though most enter into discussion at some point. For religious thinkers, responsibility includes relationship to God, which uncovers a theological basis for ethical understanding.

Duties

At the most elementary level, responsible persons are those who recognize and carry out their duties. Duties define the moral requisites of human social existence: what we normally must do, no matter what else we might hope to accomplish, and what we normally may not do, regardless of our larger objectives. Moral duties can be qualified or set aside only when exceptional steps are necessary to secure the values they are designed to protect. Thus, medical procedures normally may not be performed without a patient's informed consent, even if the patient's life is at risk. However, in a medical emergency, they may be performed without consent, provided the patient is unable to respond and there is no one present with authority to decide on his or her behalf.

Duties are formulated as laws, regulations, and rules, perhaps in conjunction with underlying moral principles. Responsible persons abide by moral principles in their personal lives. They pay special attention to principles and rules linked to their social roles: parent, spouse, physician, research scientist, junior executive at a medical center, senator. They support collective efforts to uphold moral standards that order human activities in institutional contexts (cf. Beauchamp and Childress, 1994). For those who are religious, moral duties may derive their ultimate authority from divine purposes.

Tasks

Within the constraints of moral principles and rules, responsibility consists in the reliable performance of assumed or assigned tasks. We may speak of our tasks as our responsibilities. Responsible persons know what needs to be done, they appreciate its significance, they proceed on their own, they get the job done, and they do it well (Jonsen, 1968).

Some tasks are broad and open-ended: sustaining a good marriage; bearing and nurturing children; promoting the public good as a citizen, public servant, or professional. Others are specialized, such as the practice of pediatric medicine. Some may be narrowly focused, for example, the execution of insurance claims. Even specialized tasks lack clear limits. When do physicians know enough to be confident that they are providing optimal care for their patients? When have they done enough to promote life, health, and healing? Responsible persons maintain standards of excellence in relation to expectations associated with their social roles. Those who are religious may further connect their tasks with a vocation to serve a wider, divine purpose in all areas of their lives.

General well-being

In conjunction with explicit moral commitments and role-determined assignments, responsible persons strive for just, fair, and good conditions where they live and work. They seek to bring about and maintain states of affairs that favor human well-being, perhaps the well-being of all creatures. Similarly, they resist and, where possible, seek to change circumstances that do harm to fellow human beings, even to other living creatures. They strive to improve the execution of tasks, and to see that basic moral imperatives are honored in everyday social interactions. Those who are religious may be sustained in their quest for a greater good by their hope in the promises of God.

Thus, a physician's responsibility does not end with patient care or with professional relationships wherein standards of quality care are maintained. It includes a public interest in the health-care system as a whole, and in its ability to provide appropriate services for all people. More broadly, it embraces the promotion of human health in basic life patterns.

Commitment

Responsibility is about personal commitment. It expresses human care about the moral life (cf. Fingarette, 1967). Those who are responsible claim their duties and tasks as their own, as ways of acting that are internal to

who they have become and are becoming (Gustafson, 1975; cf. Jonsen, 1968).

Classic ethical theories dealt with commitment either in terms of moral virtues (Aristotle, 1934; Aquinas, 1966) or in terms of the resolute will (Calvin, 1957; Kant, 1949; cf. Novak, 1974). Moral virtues are habits, stable ways of acting that accord with the good. They derive their energy from passions that have been "perfected" through disciplined practice, until an actor is disposed to do the good as a kind of "second nature." In terms of normative content, the central moral virtue is justice, the disposition to grant to each person what he or she is due.

In Judaism and in Reformed Protestant thought, the basic commitment to do the good has been defined not as habit or disposition but as volition, a self-conscious determination to do one's duty in all things. Here the aim is not to shape the passions but to control them. Immanuel Kant gave these latter traditions philosophical form by speaking of the unqualified value of the "good will," that is, the will ever ready to do what the moral law commands (Kant, 1949).

Modern psychological theories generally set aside accounts of the self that isolate discrete virtues or particular psychic functions, such as the will. They portray the self as a complex, dynamic process in which a centered unity can be only a relative achievement (cf. Wallwork, 1991). Post-Freudian thinkers place special emphasis on the formative power of human relationships in these complex dynamics (cf. Erikson, 1968; Winnicott, 1965; Kohut, 1977; Chodorow, 1978). Thus, our moral commitments are integral to the relational bonds that form and sustain us as human beings. We come to understand these commitments through our life stories, including both family stories and the stories of communities to which we belong. It is by means of narrative that we apprehend and claim our moral identities (Taylor, 1991; Ricoeur, 1992).

Psychological perspectives substantially inform ethical discussions of responsibility (cf. Fingarette, 1967; Rouner, 1992; Wallwork, 1991; Taylor, 1991). They render more intelligible seemingly irrational features of human behavior: individuals acting in socially inappropriate ways or in ways that work against their self-conscious purposes (cf. Fingarette, 1967). They help us grasp dynamics that leave some persons virtually incapable of consistent care for the good, and hence unable to respond to concrete situations with moral sensitivity. In other instances, persons may profess moral concern, yet find themselves internally torn, deeply ambivalent, or emotionally empty. They lack focused energy to carry out the good they claim to honor.

In classic thought, such cases either revealed bad habits, called vices (Aristotle, 1934; Aquinas, 1966), or they represented the bondage of the will to sinful inclinations (Augustine, 1953; Calvin, 1957; Luther, 1957; cf. Kant, 1949). Modern perspectives introduce notions of pathology to account for this "irresponsible" behavior. They offer neither moral admonition nor judgment but therapy, a supportive relationship wherein a skilled professional helps a patient gain insight into the internal conflicts that impel him or her to destructive behavior. Therapy provides resources for self-discovery that open the way to mature moral concern (cf. Fingarette, 1967; Wallwork, 1991). Through processes of self-discovery we reconnect with values and relationships that give identity and significance to human life.

Moral commitment involves social roles and offices. Responsible persons incorporate into their personal identities moral principles and values that are linked to positions they occupy. Social roles, like social institutions, are invariably marred by moral ambiguities. They gain their moral import from the fact that despite their ambiguity, they serve a greater good, at least by minimizing harm. Responsible actors seek to advance the moral promise of their offices while resisting their morally questionable tendencies.

Strength

Responsibility presumes that we have the personal strengths and the requisite skills to carry out our duties and to perform our tasks. Classic traditions of moral virtue and volition focus on distinctively moral strengths. In volitional approaches, the pivotal strength is willpower, the determination to control any fears, desires, even natural inclinations, that might distract us from our duty. Those who are religious seek divine support for moral rectitude.

In theories of virtue, moral strength derives from an ability to harness the passions in the service of purposive activity (Aristotle, 1934; Aquinas, 1966). On the one hand, responsibility requires personal toughness, perseverance, courage. These strengths stem from a natural, organic combativeness that through practice has been shaped into a virtue. If we lack such strength, the pressures, threats, and risks common to social existence will force us to shrink from the proper performance of basic tasks and duties. For example, a physician might remain silent after witnessing a senior colleague's failure to observe minimal professional standards in practice. Although the physician cares about standards, he or she cannot bear the stresses of a formal complaint. Courage equips us to follow through on our commitments, even those that entail danger.

On the other hand, responsibility requires self-control, the ability to restrain our wants, desires, and feelings when they dispose us to betray our commitments. Here, too, we develop self-control or temperance through practice. We learn to shape our wants and desires to accord with the larger good toward which we aspire. Without self-control we are unreliable. Our desires continually override good judgment, perhaps even impelling us to harmful actions (cf. Aristotle, 1934; Aquinas, 1966).

Because of an attraction to a patient, a psychiatrist violates sexual boundaries that define professional relationships. A research scientist falsifies research data or makes improper use of the findings of others in order to advance his or her career. In the interest of increased income, a specialist in internal medicine proposes medical procedures of dubious merit to a dying patient. Responsibility requires the discipline to restrain our wants for the sake of our moral integrity.

Modern psychological theories deal with similar phenomena, although with greater emphasis on the complex dynamics, including interpersonal relationships, that figure so prominently in our makeup. As a result, moral strengths appear less as matters of personal accomplishment and more as functions of self-formation in relationships. As inherently social beings, we derive both courage and self-control from human bonds that cohere with our moral purposes (cf. Kohut, 1977; Chodorow, 1978; Rouner, 1992; Glatzer, 1966).

Personal strengths are not limited to emotional resources or volitional restraints. They embrace intellectual capacities, general and specialized knowledge, competence in oral and written communication, self-confidence, self-esteem, the mastery of skills crucial to typical tasks, physical strength and agility, energy, stamina, and manual dexterity.

We may not associate all of these elements with the moral life, yet they profoundly affect a person's ability to act. The responsible life includes, therefore, a commitment to cultivate native talents and abilities, and to devise ways of mitigating disabilities. Similarly, social responsibility requires policies that enhance human potential for effectiveness: opportunities for education and advanced training; specialized equipment and physical arrangements for persons hampered by "handicapping conditions"; nondiscriminatory practices regarding race, gender, ethnic origin, age, religious identification, and sexual orientation.

Responsibility for personal strengths includes self-care and discipline in holding personal and professional commitments to manageable levels. Mistakes, indiscretions, intemperate and abusive behavior, even addictive and self-destructive patterns, are more likely when we habitually overextend ourselves. Personal strengths are indispensable to the good we are disposed to do. They also allow us to broaden our moral commitments, perhaps to assume leadership in promoting the common good.

Power

The human capacity to act derives from social offices and positions as well as from personal strengths (cf. Brunner, 1937; Bonhoeffer, 1955). Responsible persons are attentive to power dynamics that operate in their interactions with colleagues, associates, and employees, as well as with patients, clients, customers, and users of services. They resist abuses of power in these interactions and draw upon the resources of their offices to promote justice and the common good. They model fairness and concern for general well-being in their own activities; they commend similar practices by others.

Judgment

Responsibility involves sound judgment about the good to be done in concrete situations. Our ability to judge depends upon stable moral commitments and personal strengths to act on those commitments. It is affected by the perceptions of those to whom we are closely related, and also by interests that structure our business, professional, and political activities. Yet judgment is still a distinct skill, a "practical intellectual virtue" cultivated through practice (Aristotle, 1934; Aquinas, 1966).

Moral judgment operates in a number of ways, all of which involve the creative imagination and accumulated practical wisdom of morally mature individuals. It consists in the interpretation and application to concrete cases of laws, regulations, and rules that define moral duties (cf. Ramsey, 1970). These regulations may be borne by the common culture or the culture of professional practice; they may also be codified in public law or in the operating procedures of complex organizations, such as hospitals. The task is to discern what is at stake in these regulations so that they can appropriately inform particular moral judgments. Interpretation generally leads to a search for principles that disclose what is morally at stake in various regulations, for example, the claim that these regulations protect conditions essential to human existence and well-being.

By their very nature, principles, laws, and rules are abstract. It is not uncommon, therefore, to confront cases that are not adequately covered by existing regulations. Moral judgment may then consist in the construction of new rules that can inform our responses to these problem cases. The new rules may represent reformulations or extensions of familiar standards. They may consist of novel directives derived from elemental moral principles. The goal is to furnish stable guidelines for dealing with an emerging class of cases in the context of changing social circumstances. Bioethics continually confronts such challenges as it responds to enlarged technical capacities within biomedical practice.

Some cases are sufficiently distinct that they are best treated as exceptions to the rules. Moral judgment then entails adapting the rules to take account of variables that define the exception. Through experience, we learn to distinguish genuine exceptions from sets of cases that expose problems with existing rules. For the latter, we must rethink the rules, devising fresh formulations suited to the new cases.

In many life contexts, such as biomedical practice, we regularly deal with so many specific variables that general principles and rules cease to prove helpful as guides to moral judgment. Especially important are cases where conflicting values and disvalues are likely to result from any conceivable course of action, such as the treatment of the terminally ill or experiments with promising medical procedures that invariably have negative side effects. Practical wisdom for handling such cases emerges through experience accumulated in the treatment of similar cases. By evaluating a significant number of cases, we increase our ability to isolate variables pertinent for assessing each new case. This pattern of moral judgment is continuous with classic traditions of casuistry, or case reasoning. Casuistry locates moral judgment in the comparative study of recognizable classes of cases that require human decision and action (cf. Jonsen and Toulmin, 1988). Medical centers now institutionalize casuistic thinking through case conferences and regular consultations with specialists and advisers.

Responsiveness

H. Richard Niebuhr (1963) dramatizes the social matrix of action. We act in response to actions upon us and in anticipation of further responses to our own actions in ongoing social interactions. In this interactive framework, moral judgment involves responsiveness, self-conscious attempts to draw upon the perceptions and experiences of others in our own deliberations (cf. Gilligan, 1982). Responsiveness is best realized in conversation among representative actors in a situation. The conversation is not primarily an occasion for debate, in which the stronger positions defeat the weaker until the most cogent prevails. Its purpose is to facilitate vision. It may confirm widely held judgments, yet it may uncover matters that have been concealed, clarify phenomena that have been obscured, and bring to awareness considerations previously passed over.

Responsiveness begins with the attempt to understand "what is going on." It does not presume that the morally important issues in a situation are obvious. Through conversation we surface the pivotal issues and construct ways of portraying them to ourselves and others. Historical studies and social analyses inform these efforts. The account we provide of the situation sets the stage for a consideration of appropriate responses.

Responsive judgments are guided by the notion of what is "fitting." The fitting action may be largely self-evident once we have grasped what is morally at stake in a situation. Yet it may emerge only gradually, through the thoughtful balancing of multiple variables with their negative and positive features. Moral imagination and discernment are as important to this balancing process as are conceptual precision and logical rigor. The reasoning involved, moreover, is often more akin to weaving a tapestry than to forging a chain. Various strands of thinking supplement, complement, and perhaps clash with one another within a complete configuration. A fitting response is integral to that configuration. It consists of the most promising means of negotiating multiple considerations. For Niebuhr, fitting actions are also responses to God, the center of values that bestows authority on all values.

Responsiveness gains moral urgency from the partial, even distorted, nature of all human viewpoints. Biases rooted in special interests plague our most sincere efforts to promote justice. For example, a white male medical establishment gave lower priority to breast cancer than to prostate cancer. In studying heart disease, it focused on male rather than female subjects. Exalting scientific advances and technical achievements, the U.S. health-care system institutionalizes almost unlimited care for those with comprehensive health coverage while failing to offer basic care for the poor. Other biases—racial, ethnic, religious—have distorted biomedical practices from time to time. We overcome socially mediated biases by responsiveness to the voices of those previously left out of the conversation.

Responsiveness is not merely a personal trait. It can be incorporated into professional, organizational, and institutional practices. We can create contexts for exchanges of views among peers, colleagues, coworkers, support staff, and volunteers. We can regularly seek information from those who receive medical services: patients, clients, consumers, constituents. Within a particular organization, these exchanges promote collaboration on common projects, facilitate coordination among interrelated activities, and enhance both quality and efficiency in performance. As a dimension of responsibility, responsiveness contributes to good management. Similarly, professionals routinely respond to peer judgments through associations, convocations, conferences, and publications, as well as through regular consultations and case conferences. Ideally, they also elicit the active participation of clients to whom they offer their services.

Responsiveness in moral judgment is especially pertinent to the formation of public policy, such as debates about health-care reform. These debates begin with at-

tempts to interpret "what is going on" and move to proposals for the "fitting" response (Niebuhr, 1963). In the United States, controversial policy issues are rarely resolved by a new public consensus on the proper treatment of pressing social problems. Practical accomplishments require compromise. To gain support for new directions in policy, public actors accommodate the special interests of competing groups. In so doing, they consent to measures that fall short of their larger goals. The search for acceptable compromises is crucial to public responsibility.

Accountability

Responsibility embraces accountability for judgments and actions (cf. Jonsen, 1968). Because our actions affect the lives of fellow human beings, we have to answer to others for what we do. We must be able to give an account of our intentions and of their moral bases that is credible within the relevant conversational context, whether it be familial, communal, professional, or public. Responsible persons seek feedback from others because they are conscientious about quality performance. Structures of accountability may be formalized in well-defined review processes, including disciplinary hearings, and civil and criminal actions. Yet they also operate in everyday human interactions.

The morally committed have a strong sense of accountability to self. Conscience names the dynamism whereby we answer to ourselves for our fidelity to our commitments. If we violate our own normative standards, we feel guilt. If others have been disadvantaged or harmed by our actions, we recognize a need to apologize, perhaps to make restitution. In religious contexts, accountability involves answering to God as the source and ground of the moral life. We confess our failures, seek forgiveness, and pray for strength to renew our commitments.

Responsibility includes a readiness to hold others accountable for their actions, in the interest of the common good. It will not suffice to be conscientious only about our own actions. Because substantive moral commitments are requisite to human existence and well-being, we must hold one another accountable to those commitments. Accountability is especially important for professionals, who alone are adequately equipped to assess the performances of peers. Likewise, we are obliged to promote mutual accountability in the organizational and communal contexts in which we normally live and work; this includes support for appropriate disciplinary hearings and criminal proceedings.

The notion of accountability directs us to revisit all of the dimensions of responsibility, though with a focus on our obligation to nurture, model, encourage, cultivate, and teach responsibility to fellow human beings, especially the children, youth, and young adults of a coming generation.

Thomas W. Ogletree

Directly related to this entry are the entries Casuistry; Conscience; Emotions; Ethics, *articles on* normative ethical theories, social and political theories, *and* religion and morality; Interpretation; Narrative; *and* Virtue and Character. *For a discussion of related ideas, see the entries* Authority; Care; Compassion; Competence; Feminism; Fidelity and Loyalty; Literature; Love; Metaphor and Analogy; *and* Value and Valuation. *This entry will find application in the entries* Bioethics Education, *the* introduction *and article on* secondary and postsecondary education; Clinical Ethics; Health Officials and Their Responsibilities; *and* Profession and Professional Ethics.

Bibliography

Aquinas, Thomas. 1966. *Treatise on the Virtues.* Translated by John A. Oesterle. Notre Dame, Ind.: University of Notre Dame Press.

Aristotle. 1934. *Nicomachean Ethics.* Translated by Harold Rackham. New York: G. P. Putnam.

Augustine. 1953. "On Free Will." In *Augustine: Earlier Writings.* Selected and translated by John H. S. Burleigh. Philadelphia: Westminster Press.

Beauchamp, Tom L., and Childress, James F. 1994. *Principles of Biomedical Ethics.* 4th ed. New York: Oxford University Press.

Bonhoeffer, Dietrich. 1955. *Ethics.* Translated by Neville H. Smith. New York: Macmillan.

Brunner, Emil. 1937. *The Divine Imperative: A Study in Christian Ethics.* Translated by Olive Wyon. London: Lutterworth Press.

Calvin, John. 1957. *Institutes of the Christian Religion.* Translated by John Allen. Grand Rapids, Mich.: Eerdmans.

Chodorow, Nancy. 1978. *The Reproduction of Mothering: Psychoanalysis and the Sociology of Gender.* Berkeley: University of California Press.

Cohen, Hermann. 1972. *Religion of Reason: Out of the Sources of Judaism.* Translated by Simon Kaplan. New York: Frederick Ungar.

Erikson, Erik. 1968. *Identity: Youth and Crisis.* New York: Norton.

Fingarette, Herbert. 1967. *On Responsibility.* New York: Basic Books.

Gilligan, Carol. 1982. *In a Different Voice: Psychological Theory and Women's Development.* Cambridge, Mass.: Harvard University Press.

Glatzer, Nahum N., ed. 1966. *The Way of Response: Martin Buber, Selections from His Writings.* New York: Schocken.

Gustafson, James M. 1975. *Can Ethics Be Christian?* Chicago: University of Chicago Press.

Häring, Bernard. 1961. *The Law of Christ: Moral Theory for Priests and Laity.* 3 vols. Translated by Edwin G. Kaiser. Westminster, Md.: Newman Press.

Harron, Frank; Burnside, John W.; and Beauchamp, Tom L. 1983. *Health and Human Values.* New Haven, Conn.: Yale University Press.

Jonsen, Albert R. 1968. *Responsibility in Modern Religious Ethics: A Guide to Making Your Own Decisions.* Washington, D.C.: Corpus Books.

Jonsen, Albert R., and Toulmin, Stephen E. 1988. *The Abuse of Casuistry: A History of Moral Reasoning.* Berkeley: University of California Press.

Kant, Immanuel. 1949. *Fundamental Principles of the Metaphysics of Morals.* Translated by Thomas K. Abbott. Indianapolis, Ind.: Bobbs-Merrill.

Kohut, Heinz. 1977. *The Restoration of the Self.* New York: International Universities Press.

Luther, Martin. 1957. "The Freedom of the Christian, 1520." In *Career of the Reformer: I.* Vol. 31 of *Luther's Works.* Translated by W. A. Lambert and revised by Harold J. Grimm. Philadelphia: Muhlenberg Press.

Niebuhr, H. Richard. 1963. *The Responsible Self: An Essay in Christian Moral Philosophy.* New York: Harper & Row.

Novak, David. 1974. *Law and Theology in Judaism.* 2 vols. New York: Ktav.

Ramsey, Paul. 1970. *The Patient as Person: Explorations in Medical Ethics.* New Haven, Conn.: Yale University Press.

Ricoeur, Paul. 1992. *Oneself as Another.* Translated by Kathleen Blamey. Chicago: University of Chicago Press.

Rouner, Leroy S., ed. 1992. *Selves, People, and Persons: What Does It Mean to Be a Self?* Notre Dame, Ind.: University of Notre Dame Press.

Taylor, Charles. 1991. *The Ethics of Authenticity.* Cambridge, Mass.: Harvard University Press.

Wallwork, Ernest. 1991. *Psychoanalysis and Ethics.* New Haven, Conn.: Yale University Press.

Winnicott, Donald W. 1965. *The Maturational Process and the Facilitating Environment.* New York: International Universities Press.

RIGHTS

I. Systematic Analysis
   Carl Wellman
II. Rights in Bioethics
   Ruth Macklin

I. SYSTEMATIC ANALYSIS

Rights are of practical importance primarily, although not exclusively, because of the duties they imply. Thus, many jurists and moral philosophers have maintained the logical correlativity of rights and duties. The strong form of this doctrine asserts that every right implies a correlative duty and every duty implies a correlative right. For example, the creditor's right to be paid logically implies the debtor's duty to pay, and the debtor's duty to pay logically presupposes the creditor's right to be paid. But the duties of charity seem to invalidate this strong thesis. Although a wealthy person has a moral duty to contribute to those in need, no poor individual or charitable organization has a correlative right to receive a contribution, because the donor has the right to choose how to distribute his or her charitable donations.

This instance suggests a weaker form of the doctrine of the correlativity of rights and duties. Although every right implies some correlative duty, not every duty implies a correlative right. Even this thesis may be too strong. Physicians licensed in Missouri have a right to practice in any community in that state. But this implies neither that the residents of Missouri have a duty to enable them to practice medicine by becoming their patients nor that the state has a duty not to interfere with their practice by drafting them to serve in the Missouri National Guard. Presumably, the physicians' right to practice implies that they should not be arbitrarily prevented from exercising this right, but the content of any implied duty need not be correlative with or as extensive as the physicians' liberty to practice medicine in Missouri. In short, although rights do imply duties, the exact logical relations between rights and duties remain controversial.

The nature of rights

The essential connection between rights and duties suggests that rights might be equivalent to duties. John Austin (1885) defined a legal right as a relative legal duty. Thus, the creditor's right to be paid is the debtor's duty of payment to the creditor and nothing more. The concept of a right is that of a duty thought of from the perspective of the party to whom that duty is owed. John Stuart Mill (1861) similarly conceived of a moral right as a relative moral duty, a moral duty owed to the person who would be harmed by its nonperformance.

Joel Feinberg (1980) has argued that any reduction of rights to duties omits what is most distinctive of and valuable in rights, namely, claiming. To have a right is to be in a position to demand that to which one is entitled, much as one can claim one's coat by presenting a claim check to the attendant at a cloakroom. He defines a right as a valid claim. A legal right is a claim, the recognition of which is justified by some system of legal rules; a moral right is a claim justified by the principles of an enlightened conscience.

H. L. A. Hart (1982) maintains that what is distinctive about rights is that they determine the proper distribution of freedom. My right to paint my house purple is my liberty to paint my house purple or not to do so as I choose, together with a protective perimeter of duties of others not to interfere with my choice, for example, by stealing the purple paint I have purchased or trespassing upon my property and battering me. Thus, Hart defines a right as a protected choice.

Neil MacCormick (1977) objects that many of our most fundamental rights allow no room for free choice. Under U.S. law, one's constitutional right not to be enslaved cannot be waived by one who might choose to escape from abject poverty by becoming the slave of some benevolent master. He defines a right as a protected interest. The content of any right is something that is presumed to be in one's interest, and the function of rights is to secure the possession of these goods to each and every individual right-holder.

A rather different interest theory of rights has been proposed by Joseph Raz (1986). He defines a right as an interest-based reason sufficient for the imposition of some duty or duties upon others. Thus, he conceives of rights in terms of their role in practical reasoning; they function as intermediate conclusions between the individual interests upon which they are grounded and the duties they imply.

Ronald Dworkin (1977) also conceives of rights in terms of their role in practical reasoning, especially in the justification of political decisions. Although every action of the government requires some justification, an appeal to the public welfare is usually sufficient. But when some law or state action infringes upon a right of some individual, this justification is no longer adequate. He therefore defines a right as an individual trump over social utility. Accordingly, the function of rights is to provide special protection to the individual against any government action aimed at maximizing some social goal or set of social goals.

If there is any consensus in these very different conceptions of rights, it is that the concept of a right is essentially distributive, that is, rights are ascribed to and possessed by each individual or entity in a group separately rather than collectively. Whereas the many benefits and harms to various affected parties of any action are summed together in the act's total utility, each individual person has his or her own right that demands respect independently of the rights or welfare of any other individuals.

Possessors of rights

Any theory about the nature of rights implies something about the kinds of beings that could possess a right. If a right really is a protected choice, then any ascription of rights to a being incapable of free choice would be, as Hart (1955) points out, empty. One of the reasons that MacCormick (1977) adopts a protected-interest theory of rights is to explain how newborn infants, who are incapable of choice but do have interests, can possess moral and legal rights. Still, his theory implies that only beings with interests could possibly be right-holders.

The immediate implications of some conception of rights are often unacceptable to a moral philosopher or a morally sensitive person. For example, Feinberg defines a right as a valid claim and explains what it is to have a claim in terms of the activity of claiming. This seems to imply that only a being capable of claiming could possess a right. Although Feinberg (1980) recognizes that infants are incapable of claiming anything as their due, he believes that they clearly do have legal and moral rights. How is this possible? Adults, normally parents or guardians, can claim their rights for them. Thus, he extends the range of possible right-holders by maintaining that a right-holder can be represented by someone else. But what kind of a being can be represented? His answer is that only when a being has interests can another act on his or her behalf. On the basis of this principle he ascribes rights to children and even some nonhuman animals, but denies that plants or mere physical objects could possess rights.

What of human fetuses? Fetuses are surely incapable of free choice or of claiming and probably do not yet possess any interests. Therefore, most theories of the nature of rights seem to imply that they could not be rightholders. One way to extend the possession of rights to fetuses, however, is to appeal to their potentiality for claiming or interests or personhood or whatever is required by one's conception of a right. Because the human fetus already possesses the qualification for being a right-holder in potentiality, it already has at least some capacity to possess rights. At the other end of life, some argue that the dead can have rights because, while alive, they had interests that survive their death, for example, interests in their reputations or in having their wills respected.

Tom Regan (1983) uses two lines of reasoning to extend the ascription of rights from human beings to nonhuman animals. One argument begins with our ascriptions of rights to humans. He points out that the usual hypotheses about what qualifies one to possess rights, such as rationality or personhood, fail to explain our firm judgments that, for example, brain-damaged children or very senile patients have rights. Regan argues that any criterion broad enough to be consistent with our moral convictions about the rights of humans will imply that some animals can also possess rights. Another argument begins with our recognition that some of our duties concerning animals are direct duties, duties owed to animals. For example, we have a duty not to cause animals to suffer unnecessarily, not in order to prevent ourselves from becoming callous to human suffering, as Immanuel Kant (1959) suggested, but for the sake of the animals themselves. Regan then argues that

the best explanation of our direct duties to animals is the hypothesis that they are grounded on the rights of animals. What gives animals as well as humans the inherent value that confers rights is not merely being alive, but having a life that fares well or ill for them. No consensus about the kinds of beings that could possess rights has yet emerged.

The grounds of rights

The grounds of anyone's right are the reasons why he or she has that right, the qualifications of the right-holder together with the norms that confer the right. Everyone agrees that the law grounds legal rights, that it is the rules and regulations of any legal system that confer legal rights upon those subject to that system. There is, however, room for disagreement about the precise nature of those laws.

Hart (1955) maintains that the law consists of a set of social rules practiced in some society and applied in its courts. He maintains that a legal right arises from the application of some legal rule to a particular case. Dworkin (1977) argues that the adjudication of hard cases, cases where no valid legal rule implies any clear decision, requires an appeal to legal principles. Unlike a legal rule that either decides a case or is completely inapplicable, a legal principle can have more or less weight and may conflict with other legal principles that also apply to any hard case. He concludes that our fundamental legal rights are grounded on principles rather than rules.

There is also debate about whether every posited rule or principle is legally valid. Suppose that a legislature enacts a statute purporting to legitimize slavery. Would this statute confer on anyone a genuine legal right to own another human being? Thomas Aquinas would have argued that it does not because an unjust law is no law at all. Law can impose duties and confer rights only by virtue of being a dictate of reason, and no command that conflicts with the natural law, the moral law evident to reason, can be rational. Austin (1885) rejected any such natural-law theory. What the law is, is one thing; what it ought to be, another. Hence, any law posited by legislation that commands a relative duty thereby confers a valid legal right.

There is considerably more disagreement about the grounds of moral rights. The view first enunciated by William of Ockham (1285–1349) and most familiar in the political theory of John Locke (1960) is that natural law, the moral rules commanded by God and self-evident to human reason, grounds moral rights much as the law posited by human legislators and judges confers legal rights. Skepticism about the existence of any divine legislator and doubts about the self-evidence of any moral rules have gradually made this traditional theory less credible than heretofore.

Mill (1861) defined a moral right in terms of a relative moral duty and argued that utility is the ground of our duties. Because our fundamental moral obligations are actions that tend to promote the happiness or mitigate the unhappiness of all those affected by them, those individuals who would be harmed by our failure or refusal to so act have moral rights to the performance of those duties owed to them.

Dworkin (1977) and others object that to ground moral rights upon social utility is to deprive rights of their primary function of protecting the individual against mistreatment inflicted to maximize social goals. MacCormick (1977) and Raz (1986), in somewhat different ways, preserve the essentially distributive nature of rights, without severing their connection with human well-being, by holding that individual interests ground moral rights. Not all of one's interests confer rights, of course, only those interests of sufficient importance to impose upon others some duty or duties to promote, or at least not damage, those interests.

Kant (1959) denied that goals, whether they be social utility or individual interests, can impose the categorical imperative of duty. Our fundamental moral obligation is to treat all persons, all rational agents, as ends in themselves and not merely as means to some ulterior end. Accordingly, most contemporary Kantians ground moral rights upon respect for persons, that is, upon the dignity of each individual moral agent.

Moral rights have traditionally been correlated with the duties of justice, in contrast with the duties of charity that are not owed to any particular individual. John Rawls (1971) has argued that the principles of justice are those principles concerning the basic structure of the political and economic institutions of their society that would be chosen by rational individuals in the "original position," roughly a position in which no person can impose his or her will upon another or predict what place he or she will have in the society to be regulated by those principles. Thus, the basic moral rights of the individual are grounded, not on any actual agreement, but on a hypothetical contract to which the members of any society would agree unanimously, were they fully rational and choosing under ideal conditions. Each of these theories of the grounds of rights needs further development, and none of them has yet achieved general acceptance.

Classes of rights

The basic categories are institutional rights that are conferred by some sort of organization or social convention, and moral rights that are conferred by moral grounds independent of human beliefs or practices. (To be sure,

some philosophers deny that there are any noninstitutional rights, but moral rights figure prominently in many ethical and political theories.) The most important species of institutional rights are legal rights conferred by the rules or principles of some legal system; the most fundamental species of moral rights are human rights (traditionally called natural rights) that one possesses simply by virtue of being human and whether or not they are recognized by the institutions of one's society. (In a secondary sense, human rights are those rights conferred upon all human beings by some legal system, most notably in those nations that have ratified the European Convention on Human Rights [Council of Europe, 1990].) Human rights are contrasted with every species of special moral rights that one possesses by virtue of some special status, for example as a citizen, or as a doctor, or as a subject of biomedical research.

Many jurists and moral philosophers adopt conceptual distinctions introduced by Wesley Newcomb Hohfeld (1919) to distinguish between claim rights, liberty rights, power rights, and immunity rights. The creditor has a claim against the debtor to payment if and only if the debtor has a duty to the creditor to pay the amount owed. A man has a liberty to grow a beard simply because he has no duty not to do so. A patient has a power to render surgery permissible because the patient has the ability, by consenting to be operated on, to confer upon the surgeon the liberty to operate. An owner has an immunity against having his or her property given away by another because no unilateral act of another would constitute a donation of one's property.

Another important distinction, applying primarily to claim rights, is that between positive and negative rights. A positive right is one that implies a positive duty of some second party, a duty to do some sort of action; a negative right imposes a negative duty, a duty not to act in some specific manner. Thus, one who has medical insurance typically has a positive right to be reimbursed for medical expenses, and every patient has a negative right not to be operated upon without consent. Our labels for rights are often misleading in this respect. For example, the patient's right "not to be abandoned" is probably a positive right that imposes upon one's physician the duty either to provide necessary medical care or to arrange for someone else to provide such care.

Rights in political theory

Conceptions of the ideal society and of the authority of government are determined to a considerable degree by the place of rights in one's social and political philosophy. Libertarians regard individual liberty as inviolable and advocate a minimal government and a laissez-faire economic system. They tend to make rights, whether thought of as natural rights along Lockean lines or as utilitarian social institutions, central to their theory. They give primacy to the individual rights to life, liberty, and property, and conceive of these as negative rights, rights that others not deprive one of life, interfere with one's liberty of thought or action, or take away one's property or the free use thereof.

Liberals also regard individual liberty as central to their political theory, although they conceive of liberty and assess its value in various ways. They typically advocate democratic political institutions, including a set of basic civil rights, to set constitutional limits on the powers of government. Many regard these civil rights as legal protections of more fundamental human rights. They tend to affirm a wider range of rights than libertarians and to recognize that individual rights impose positive as well as negative duties upon others. Thus, one's right to due process might impose a duty upon the state to provide an impoverished person with legal counsel as well as a duty not to prejudice a jury. Some, but not all, liberals supplement the traditional civil and political rights with a set of social and economic rights, such as the right to social security or to an adequate standard of medical care.

Communitarians insist that the cultural traditions and social practices of a community are necessary for the full development of our human capacities and the realization of our well-being. Therefore, they reject the "atomism" of traditional natural-rights theory. Because individuals are not born autonomous moral agents and could not become fully human in a state of nature, they cannot possess any absolute human rights independent of and holding against society. Because human motivation is not exclusively egoistic and rationality is not confined to maximizing one's own self-interest, the authority of government is not derived from any social contract between completely independent individuals. Communitarians believe that their criticisms undermine, not only libertarian theories of rights like Robert Nozick's (1974), derived from Locke's (1960) natural law philosophy, but also liberal theories of rights like those of Dworkin (1977), who conceives of rights as trumps against social goals, and Rawls (1971), who grounds basic rights in a hypothetical contract entered into by individuals in an original (presocial) position.

Although their philosophies may vary in fundamental ways, all feminists oppose the oppression of women and believe that the previously neglected experiences and contributions of women will enrich moral, social, and political theory. In their struggle for social and political equality, most early feminists campaigned for equal civil rights and appealed to women's equal human rights. Without renouncing these rights, some recent feminists have become more critical of traditional theories of rights and more dubious of the appeal to rights as an instrument to eradicate the oppression of women.

Elizabeth Wolgast (1987) has argued that the social atomism of natural-rights theory is contrary to the experience of women, who find the substance of their lives, for better or worse, to consist primarily in their interpersonal relations with those close to them. The equality of civil and human rights presupposes an abstract justice of universal moral rules inconsistent with the ethics of very particular responsibilities in concrete contexts that better fits the experience of caregivers such as wives and mothers. Although equal rights are supposed to protect the weak, women often find themselves unable to claim their moral rights against husbands or physicians upon whom they are economically or medically dependent.

Carol Smart (1989) points out that it is often hazardous for a woman to appeal to her rights in a legal system dominated by males. This is partly because rights oversimplify complex power relations; for example, a battered wife is usually physically weaker than her husband and may lack the skills to enable her to leave "his" home and support herself. Again, the appeal to any right can often be met by an appeal to some counterright; although a wife has a right not to be molested, her husband has a right to live in "his" home and to see "his" children. Because each individual right-holder must prove that her right has been violated, even a number of court cases will fail to remedy a widespread social harm affecting large numbers of women.

Mary Ann Glendon (1991) adds that the U.S. dialect of rights talk impoverishes political discourse. Because rights are asserted as absolutes with an unqualified peremptory content, our rights talk heightens social conflict and inhibits dialogue that might resolve our social problems. Its emphasis upon individual demands and silence about our responsibilities to others renders it deficient in dealing with the distress of the poor, the homeless, the unemployed, and the marginalized members of our society. Its presupposition of the lone rights-bearer neglects the dimension of sociability so important for human character, competence, and civic virtue. For example, formulating problems of family rights in terms of the rights of the individual members of the family ignores the social and economic conditions that families require in order to flourish.

Where are we now in our systematic analysis of rights? We have several coherently developed conceptions of the nature of a right and enough discussion to identify the strengths and weaknesses of each. Available theories of the kinds of beings that could possess rights are more scarce and less satisfactory; only Joel Feinberg's (1980) appeal to interests and a few responses to it are very rigorous. Although pronouncements about the grounds of rights, especially moral rights, are common enough, plausible theories that are clearly explained and systematically defended are almost totally lacking. Finally, criticisms of theories of rights by communitarians and feminists have revealed, not so much defects in rights themselves, as important aspects of our legal, political, and moral life neglected by traditional and even much recent jurisprudence and ethical theory.

CARL WELLMAN

Directly related to this article is the companion article in this entry: RIGHTS IN BIOETHICS. *For a further discussion of topics mentioned in this article, see the entries* ANIMAL WELFARE AND RIGHTS, *article on* ETHICAL PERSPECTIVES ON THE TREATMENT AND STATUS OF ANIMALS; ETHICS; FEMINISM; FETUS, *article on* PHILOSOPHICAL AND ETHICAL ISSUES; NATURAL LAW; PERSON; UTILITY; *and* WOMEN. *This article will find application in the entries* FUTURE GENERATIONS, OBLIGATIONS TO; HEALTH-CARE RESOURCES, ALLOCATION OF; PATIENTS' RESPONSIBILITIES; *and* PATIENTS' RIGHTS. *For a discussion of related ideas, see the entries* AUTONOMY; FREEDOM AND COERCION; JUSTICE; LAW AND BIOETHICS; *and* OBLIGATION AND SUPEREROGATION. *See also the* APPENDIX (CODES, OATHS, AND DIRECTIVES RELATED TO BIOETHICS), SECTION I: DIRECTIVES ON HEALTH-RELATED RIGHTS AND PATIENT RESPONSIBILITIES.

Bibliography

AUSTIN, JOHN. 1885. *Lectures on Jurisprudence; or, The Philosophy of Positive Law.* 5th ed. London: John Murray.

BENN, STANLEY I. 1967. "Rights." In vol. 7 of *Encyclopedia of Philosophy,* pp. 195–199. Edited by Paul Edwards. New York: Macmillan.

COUNCIL OF EUROPE. 1990. *European Convention on Human Rights.* Strasbourg, France: Author.

DWORKIN, RONALD M. 1977. *Taking Rights Seriously.* Cambridge, Mass.: Harvard University Press.

FEINBERG, JOEL. 1980. *Rights, Justice, and the Bounds of Liberty; Essays in Social Philosophy.* Princeton, N.J.: Princeton University Press.

GLENDON, MARY ANN. 1991. *Rights Talk: The Impoverishment of Political Discourse.* New York: Free Press.

HART, H. L. A. 1955. "Are There Any Natural Rights?" *Philosophical Review* 64, no. 2:175–191.

———. 1982. *Essays on Bentham: Studies in Jurisprudence and Political Theory.* Oxford: At the Clarendon Press.

HOHFELD, WESLEY NEWCOMB. 1919. *Fundamental Legal Conceptions as Applied in Judicial Reasoning; and Other Legal Essays.* New Haven, Conn.: Yale University Press.

KANT, IMMANUEL. 1959. *Foundations of the Metaphysics of Morals and What Is Enlightenment?* Translated by Lewis White Beck. Indianapolis, Ind.: Bobbs-Merrill.

LOCKE, JOHN. 1960. *Two Treatises of Government.* Rev. ed. Edited by Peter Laslett. Cambridge: At the University Press.

MACCORMICK, D. NEIL. 1977. "Rights in Legislation." In *Law, Morality and Society: Essays in Honour of H. L. A. Hart,* pp. 189–209. Edited by P. M. S. Hacker and J. Raz. Oxford: At the Clarendon Press.

MILL, JOHN STUART. 1969. *Utilitarianism.* In vol. 10 of *Collected Works.* Toronto: University of Toronto Press.

NOZICK, ROBERT. 1974. *Anarchy, State, and Utopia.* New York: Basic Books.

RAWLS, JOHN. 1971. *A Theory of Justice.* Cambridge, Mass.: Harvard University Press.

RAZ, JOSEPH. 1986. *The Morality of Freedom.* Oxford: At the Clarendon Press.

REGAN, TOM. 1983. *The Case for Animal Rights.* Berkeley: University of California Press.

SMART, CAROL. 1989. "The Problem of Rights." In her *Feminism and the Power of Law,* pp. 138–159. London: Routledge.

TAYLOR, CHARLES. 1979. "Atomism." In *Powers, Possessions and Freedom: Essays in Honour of C. B. MacPherson,* pp. 39–61. Edited by Alkis Kontos. Toronto: University of Toronto Press.

THOMSON, JUDITH JARVIS. 1990. *The Realm of Rights.* Cambridge, Mass.: Harvard University Press.

WADE, FRANCIS C. 1975. "Potentiality in the Abortion Discussion." *Review of Metaphysics* 29, no. 2:239–255.

WOLGAST, ELIZABETH HANKINS. 1987. "Wrong Rights." In her *The Grammar of Justice,* pp. 28–49. Ithaca, N.Y.: Cornell University Press.

II. RIGHTS IN BIOETHICS

Rights in bioethics are a subclass of the broader notion of moral and legal rights described in the preceding article. Some rights in bioethics are both moral and legal, such as the right of patients to be informed about and grant permission for recommended medical treatments. This and other rights of patients have been recognized in judicial rulings or statutes enacted by legislatures, and in philosophical ethics applied to medical practice and research. Some rights in bioethics have the status of *moral rights merely,* for example, the claim that there exists a right to health care. That claim asserts a moral right, implying that a corresponding legal right ought to exist. As of early 1993, the U.S. federal government had not enacted legislation that would legally establish the claim to a right to health care. Many other nations legally guarantee a right to health care for all citizens.

Rights as claims

Even when claims asserting moral rights in bioethics are backed up by laws, those laws can be overturned or restricted and new laws enacted, thus altering the legal rights while leaving the claims about moral rights intact. One prominent example is the claim in support of a woman's right to terminate a pregnancy. Moral claims asserting a woman's right to control her own body were made before the 1973 ruling in *Roe v. Wade.* In that case the U.S. Supreme Court declared that the constitutional "right of privacy . . . is broad enough to encompass a woman's decision whether or not to terminate her pregnancy." However, in its 1989 decision in *Webster* v. *Reproductive Health Services,* the Supreme Court restricted that constitutional right by indicating that it would allow states to place additional conditions on the circumstances in which a woman may exercise her right.

Alterations in legal rights also occur in statutes. An example is that of laws pertaining to HIV infection. At the beginning of the AIDS epidemic, claims about the rights of people with HIV infection were asserted but not legally supported. By the late 1980s, however, many states had passed legislation granting people the right not to have their blood tested for HIV infection without their knowledge and consent, laws ensuring a right to confidentiality of people with HIV infection, as well as the right not to be discriminated against because of their HIV-positive status.

The area of *moral rights merely* tends to be more problematic than the sphere of legal rights. It is generally easier to put forward relevant and cogent reasons or evidence in support of the claim that a legal right exists than it is to justify a claim about the existence of a disputed moral right. That is because legal rights are written down in statutes, found in the Constitution and interpreted by the courts, and appear in judicial opinions that declare the common law, while moral rights asserted as mere claims may lack widespread support or other objective evidence of their existence.

In both the legal and moral domains, rights may be surrounded by inescapable vagueness, even when the existence of a right is not in dispute. For example, patients are normally held to have a right to confidentiality in the physician–patient relationship. Yet even legal requirements concerning confidentiality are rarely stated in the form of absolutes. If a patient confides to a psychiatrist an intention to harm another person and the therapist has some grounds for believing that the patient will carry out the stated intention, must the therapist maintain confidentiality or can a breach be justified? A well-known precedent was set in 1974 in the case of *Tarasoff* v. *The Regents of the University of California,* which established a psychotherapist's "duty to warn" or to take other preventive steps if the therapist knows or should know that a patient poses a danger to others.

Another difficulty lies in the correct ordering of rights in situations when more than one right can be claimed. For example, the patient's right to confidentiality normally prevents a physician from disclosing a patient's diagnosis without the consent of the patient. But suppose the patient's blood has been tested for HIV antibodies and the result is positive. The patient requests that the physician not disclose this fact to his wife. One claim asserts that a person at risk of acquiring a lethal infection has a right to that information, so the wife should be told; the competing claim asserts the patient's right to confidentiality, prohibiting the physician

from disclosing to the wife. Laws in some states permit but do not require a physician to disclose HIV information to a spouse or other known sex partner. These examples illustrate the problems that can surround legal as well as moral rights.

The language of rights can also generate confusion. A deeply cherished right in free societies is the right to life, which prohibits innocent people from being killed by the state and promises state protection against other threats to the lives of citizens. However, "the right to life" has taken on a new meaning since being adopted by groups with a political agenda. In the sphere of bioethics, those beliefs include a nearly absolute prohibition of abortion, as well as opposition to practices such as termination of life support and honoring living wills. Most "right to life" groups do not include opposition to the death penalty as part of their political agenda. This can be explained by their concern for "innocent" life, thereby excluding from those deserving protection people who have been convicted of crimes. By casting their moral position in terms of a "right to life," these groups make it appear that anyone who favors a woman's right to an abortion or a patient's right to have life support withdrawn must therefore reject the proposition that people have a right to life. The confusion stems from applying a general moral claim asserting the "right to life" to a highly controversial area like abortion, and to honoring living wills, which is a widely accepted practice.

The growth of the field of bioethics has been accompanied by a multitude of claims about rights. However, as long ago as 1914 Justice Benjamin Cardozo established an important judicial precedent when he articulated the right of patients to consent to treatment: "Every human being of adult years and sound mind has a right to determine what shall be done with his own body; and a surgeon who performs an operation without his patient's consent commits an assault, for which he is liable in damages" (*Schloendorff* v. *New York Hospital*). Yet even that extension into the medical sphere of the fundamental human right to be free from bodily assault established only the patient's right to *consent* to invasive medical procedures. Not until 1957, in the landmark decision in *Salgo* v. *Leland Stanford Jr. University Board of Trustees,* did a court rule that patients have a right to *informed* consent, thereby obligating physicians to disclose certain information about the procedures to be carried out before seeking the patient's consent.

A different historical current following World War II culminated in the right of research subjects (including patients enrolled in clinical studies) to voluntary, informed consent to serve as a subject of human experimentation. The atrocities committed by the Nazis in the name of biological and medical research led to the promulgation in 1948 of the Nuremberg Code, which mandated that subjects of experimentation must grant their fully voluntary and informed consent to any request from a researcher to participate in a medical experiment. Exposés of unethical research carried out by respected phsyician-researchers in the United States heightened the awareness of the medical community, the federal government, and members of the public, eventually leading to the drafting of regulations governing federally funded research involving human subjects (Rothman, 1991). Although the wording of these regulations is not always framed in the language of rights, the clear intent is to ensconce the moral rights of research subjects in law. In addition to informed consent regarding the purpose, procedures, risks, benefits, and alternatives to participation, these rights include the right to refuse to participate in research, the right to withdraw at any time without prejudice to ongoing or future medical care, and the right to confidentiality.

Rights claims in bioethics have been made on behalf of patients generally (Annas, 1989), as well on behalf of special populations or classes of patients: children, people who are mentally ill or mentally retarded, the elderly, prisoners, and certain classes of patients such as people with AIDS. Since it is only women who can become pregnant, the right of women throughout the world to obtain safe, legal abortions has been a major concern. As a moral right, the right to an abortion is claimed under the broader right of a woman to "control her own body," or under the right to self-determination.

Recently in the United States, rights have been claimed on behalf of women and minorities in the realm of biomedical research. Stemming from observations that women and minorities have been underrepresented in a large number of clinical investigations, this claim asserts their right to equitable access to medical treatments still in the experimental stage. More generally, claims have been made for the inclusion of much larger numbers of women in biomedical research, since past studies have yielded information that can reliably be used to benefit only men with health problems. Underlying these claims asserting the rights of special populations is a demand for equitable treatment and for recognition of basic human attributes.

In an earlier era, when physicians maintained greater authority in their relationship with patients and fewer rights of patients had been explicitly recognized, there was little need for doctors to issue claims about their own rights. As the right of patients to have their autonomy respected has become widely acknowledged, rights claimed by physicians have begun to increase. A small number of physicians has claimed the right to refuse to perform invasive procedures on patients known or suspected to be HIV-infected, on the grounds that physicians should not be required to undergo unreason-

able risks to their life or health. A somewhat larger number of doctors has asserted their "right to know" a patient's HIV status, in order that they may take proper precautions to avoid becoming infected. Dr. Neal Rzepkowski, an HIV-infected physician who was forced to resign his position as an emergency room physician when his infection became known, claimed his "right to work" in denying that patients have the right to know about his HIV status. Some physicians now claim the right to decline to provide treatments they deem "futile," arguing that respect for patients' autonomy does not require doctors to comply with whatever patients may demand.

Prominent examples of rights

The previous article describes two basic categories of rights: institutional rights conferred by some sort of organization or social convention, and moral rights, of which human rights are the most fundamental species. The following are among the most prominent examples of rights in bioethics falling under both of these basic categories.

The "right to die." The "right to die" has been presented to courts as part of the right of privacy and as an expression of patients' right to refuse treatment (Rhoden, 1988). Yet the phrase "the right to die" illustrates how confusing the language of rights can become. What may be referred to in the moral language of rights as "the right to die" must, in the legal domain, be placed into a different category, since no legally established right to die exists. Moreover, since most of the circumstances in which this right is claimed involve patients' or their families' request to withhold or withdraw life-sustaining treatment, the most accurate expression of this right is "the right to refuse medical treatment." To go beyond that well-established moral and legal right is to assert the right to assisted suicide or to have active euthanasia performed. Although claims to these latter rights have been asserted and the initiatives appeared on election ballots in the state of Washington in 1991 and in California in 1992, as of early 1993 there were no statutes in the United States that grant individuals the right to assisted suicide or to active euthanasia.

Recent years have witnessed the expansion of a patient's right to refuse medical treatment to cover a future time when they have lost their mental capacity. The first legislative enactment in this area was the Natural Death Act, passed by the California legislature in 1976. The right to decide about future medical treatment falls into the larger category known as "advance directives," which can be executed in the form of a living will or by appointing a health-care agent whose authority goes into effect when the patient loses decisional capacity. All fifty states now have legislation recognizing patients' rights in the form of a living will, appointment of a health-care agent, or both. The legal right of relatives to refuse life-sustaining treatment for a patient who has not executed a living will or health-care proxy remains unclear, although a moral right has been claimed by many who argue that an incapacitated patient's relatives are best situated to decide about the appropriateness of continued medical treatment (Rhoden. 1988).

The right to liberty. The category of liberty rights includes a number of prominent examples in bioethics. Several court decisions in the 1970s established a number of rights for individuals involuntarily confined on grounds of "dangerousness to self or others." The chief moral reason for challenging involuntary commitment to a mental institution is that the practice constitutes an infringement of individual liberty. Such challenges are based on the claim that the right to liberty has priority over other rights in cases where rights conflict (Szasz, 1963). In the case of *Wyatt* v. *Stickney* (1972), the court listed many subsidiary rights of individuals confined in mental institutions. These included a right to the least restrictive conditions necessary for treatment, the right to be free from isolation, the right not to be subjected to experimental research without consent, the right to a comfortable bed and privacy, the right to adequate meals, and the right to an individualized treatment plan with a projected timetable for meeting specific goals.

A second prominent appeal to a liberty right is found in the U.S. Supreme Court's ruling in 1990 in *Cruzan* v. *Director, Missouri Department of Health*, the first "right to die" case to come before the Court. Nancy Cruzan was a young woman who had remained in a persistent vegetative state for several years following an automobile accident. Her parents eventually requested that artificially administered nutrition and hydration be withdrawn, a request that was denied by the Missouri Supreme Court on grounds that "clear and convincing" evidence of the patient's wishes was lacking. Although the U.S. Supreme Court held that the Constitution does not preclude a state from requiring clear and convincing evidence of an incompetent patient's wishes to forgo life-sustaining treatment, the Court's opinion nevertheless assumed that autonomous patients have a constitutionally protected "liberty interest" in refusing unwanted medical treatment.

The U.S. Supreme Court again invoked liberty rights in its ruling in a 1992 abortion case, *Casey* v. *Planned Parenthood Association of Southeastern Pennsylvania*. Although the Court did allow states to impose some restrictions on a woman's right to an abortion, it upheld the constitutional right to an abortion established in *Roe* v. *Wade*. However, in *Casey* the Court did not refer to the right to privacy but, instead, to basic rights of liberty found in the liberty clause of the Four-

teenth Amendment, as well as in past cases that recognized rights to bodily integrity and "a person's most basic decisions about family and parenthood."

Rights in declarations, codes, and bills. There is a middle ground between legally established rights and *moral rights merely*. It consists of rights claims issued by trade or professional associations, such as the American Hospital Association, and national or international organizations like the World Health Organization and the United Nations. Also in this middle ground are statements that assert the rights of special populations, such as children, the handicapped, or the mentally retarded. These declarations and bills lack the force of law, but they can nonetheless establish a strong societal presumption in favor of recognizing the moral rights asserted in them.

The American Hospital Association first proclaimed a set of patients' rights in its 1973 statement "A Patient's Bill of Rights," which listed twelve specific rights (the statements comprising these rights have undergone periodic revisions since the 1973 version). Some patients' rights are cast in a general form, such as the first right affirmed: "The patient has the right to considerate and respectful care." What remains unclear about the "Patients' Bill of Rights" is the recourse that patients have if their stated rights are violated. Unlike legally established rights, there is typically no clear procedure or publicly known method by which a patient can bring grievances against the hospital or its staff, or obtain remedies when rights have been violated.

The principles stated in the Constitution of the World Health Organization include a central claim about rights: "The enjoyment of the highest attainable standard of health is one of the fundamental rights of every human being without distinction of race, religion, political belief, economic or social condition." The WHO Constitution also includes a statement about the responsibility of governments for the health of their people. If there is a correlativity of rights and duties, this governmental responsibility can be viewed as embodying a correlative *duty* implied by the stated fundamental *right* of every human being to the highest attainable standard of health.

An example of a declaration of rights aimed at a special population is the Declaration of General and Special Rights of the Mentally Handicapped, which was adopted by the International League of Societies for the Mentally Handicapped in 1968 and in modified form by the General Assembly of the United Nations in 1971. The main precept of this and related documents is that mentally retarded persons are held to have all the fundamental rights of anyone else of their age and nationality. Among these are the right to education and training appropriate to developmental status, the right to guardianship or other form of protective advocacy, and the right to marry and to procreate. This last clause gives rise to a potential conflict of rights in places where laws permit involuntary sterilization of mentally retarded persons, including the provision that parents may consent to sterilization on behalf of their mentally retarded offspring.

Another international statement claiming the existence of rights was agreed upon by the representatives of 136 governments in the World Population Plan of Action in Bucharest in 1974: "All couples and individuals have the basic right to decide freely and responsibly the number and spacing of their children and to have the information, education and means to do so." As is true of other examples, the rights enumerated in this statement of reproductive rights imply the existence of correlative duties on the part of some agency, most probably a government, to guarantee their fulfillment.

Problems in assessing rights claims in bioethics

Problems in assessing rights claims fall into different categories, of which two leading types are discussed here: (1) the status of entities to which rights are attributed and (2) conflicts of rights.

Bearers of rights.   This class of problems concerning the evaluation of rights claims arises out of the need to determine what properties are essential in order to qualify as a bearer of rights. Disagreements abound concerning the status of entities to which rights are attributed: Is the fetus a creature to whom rights can properly be ascribed? Can rights be ascribed only to humans, or are nonhuman animals appropriate bearers of rights? Are nonexistent entities, such as future generations or an individual's not yet conceived children, ones to which rights can correctly be attributed? In this last example, different actions or policies might rest on the answers to questions about the bearers of rights. Some claims about the rights of future generations address environmental concerns, as in assertions that future generations have a right to clean air and water. If such a right does exist, then present generations have certain obligations to refrain from acts of pollution that might not harm existing populations but would pose a hazard long in the future. Another claim holds that an individual's (or couple's) future progeny has a right not to be afflicted with an inherited genetic disorder. If that right exists, then the individual or couple with a heritable disorder could have an obligation to refrain from procreating.

The debate over the fetus as a bearer of rights has several layers. At the most fundamental level, the question is whether an entity resulting from fertilization of a human egg by human sperm at any point during the nine-month gestational period properly can be said to have rights. Although different kinds of rights might be claimed on behalf of the fetus, the one that has received the most attention is the right to life. The debate on this issue is closed on one side by those who contend that rights begin at the moment of birth but not before. For others, who argue that at some stage of its development a fetus acquires rights, the problem shifts into the next category—conflicts of rights.

Disputes over the proper bearers of rights are not limited to embryos and fetuses, but also include animals. One side argues that only human entities can properly be said to have rights, while opponents contend that nonhuman beings qualify. Animal rightists claim that the lives of animals are as valuable as those of humans, and that animals have inherent rights that give rise to correlative duties on the part of humans. An intermediate view is held by animal welfarists, who deny that animals have rights yet maintain that animals deserve humane treatment when they are raised and slaughtered for food or used in laboratory experiments. In this view, humans have duties to animals grounded on their welfare, or their capacity to suffer.

Conflicts of rights.   Problems arise in both the moral and the legal domains when rights come into conflict. A well-known conflict appears in the context of abortion, pitting the alleged right to life of the fetus against the right of the pregnant woman to self-determination, or the right to control her own body. But there are other conflicts in the maternal–fetal domain as well. If an obstetrician recommends a cesarean section in the hope of obtaining a better outcome for the infant-to-be, the pregnant woman may decide not to undergo the increased risk to herself of a surgical delivery. She may then seek to exercise her right to refuse treatment, a right embodied in the broader right to informed consent to treatment. The woman's right would then conflict with the alleged right of the fetus—its "right to life" or its "right to be born healthy," depending on whether its life or health was in jeopardy. It is sometimes held that it is not the rights of the fetus that pose this conflict but, rather, those of the child-to-be. That is still problematic, since it is open to question whether entities that do not yet exist (such as the "child-to-be") can properly be said to have rights.

Two situations noted earlier illustrate the potential for conflicts of rights. The first is that of people who are involuntarily committed to mental institutions on grounds that they are likely to commit acts of violence. The right of a person who has committed no crime to remain free is pitted against society's right to protection when the individual is judged "dangerous to others." The second situation is an HIV-positive individual's right to confidentiality, which may clash with the right of a sex partner or needle-sharing partner to information that might prevent acquisition of a fatal condition.

Advances in medical technology have created conflicts of rights that are unprecedented or rarely encountered. An example is the range of new reproductive technologies and practices: in vitro fertilization, freezing of embryos, and surrogacy. The practice of surrogacy can result in disputes over who has a right to the infant when a woman who has served as a surrogate is unwilling to give up the child after birth. The biological father can claim a right to the child on grounds of his paternity and also on the basis of the contractual agreement in which the surrogate promised to give up the child at birth. The surrogate can claim a right to the child on the same genetic basis when she has been artificially inseminated. Even when she serves only as a "gestational surrogate," she might claim a right to the infant because of her contribution through nine months of gestation and during labor and childbirth. Reasonable people disagree about which claims about rights in disputed surrogacy arrangements have greater validity, and state statutes and court cases have yielded contradictory answers to this question (Gostin, 1990).

Another advance in medical technology, the capability to freeze and store embryos for future use, can create a conflict of rights between the gamete contributors. In one case, a couple who had created and frozen seven embryos for possible future implantation into the woman decided to divorce. A legal battle ensued (*Davis* v. *Davis*, 1992), with each member of the couple claiming a right with respect to the embryos. The wife sought control of the embryos, contending that it might be her only chance to have her own biological children, while the husband sought veto power over her decision on the grounds that it would impose on him the burdens of unwanted parenthood. Although a lower court awarded the embryos to the woman, who sought to implant them, that decision was later reversed. The Tennessee Supreme Court said that the "issue centers on the two aspects of procreational autonomy—the right to procreate and the right to avoid procreation." The court ruled that "the party wishing to avoid procreation should prevail, assuming that the other party has a reasonable possibility of achieving parenthood by means other than the use of the pre-embryos in question."

Another case involved a dispute between an in vitro fertilization (IVF) program and a couple over custody of a frozen embryo. In the case of *York* v. *Jones* (1989), a couple who had been using the services of the IVF program at the Jones Institute in Norfolk, Virginia, moved to California and wanted to transport their remaining frozen embryo to a Los Angeles program. The Virginia program refused to grant permission. The court denied the clinic's efforts to dismiss the couple's lawsuit, thus resolving the question in favor of the couple's right to remove the embryo for transfer to another IVF program. The case did not address the question of whether control over frozen embryos should be construed as a custody or a property right.

In all these examples of conflicts, debates rage over which rights ought to take precedence. Regardless of the evidence or reasons put forward relevantly and cogently in support of such claims, decisions concerning the priority of one person's rights over those of another are likely to remain controversial when the rights in conflict appear to be legitimate. To resolve any conflict of rights, a judgment must be made about which rights weigh more heavily or under precisely what conditions the rights of one person take precedence over the rights of another. When conflicts are brought to court, a judge may resolve the issue, but judicial decisions at one level are sometimes overturned by a higher court, and courts at the same level have been known to reverse themselves at a later time.

Conclusion

In addition to the bioethics rights discussed in this article, numerous others have been claimed on behalf of all people as well as particular groups. It is evident that some of the rights claimed in bioethics are difficult if not impossible to fulfill, since it is not within the power of any single individual or even a government to take all the necessary steps to satisfy them. But as with any moral ideal, rights claims in bioethics serve an important function in setting forth the human needs and conditions requisite for attaining a just society.

RUTH MACKLIN

Directly related to this article is the companion article in this entry: SYSTEMATIC ANALYSIS. *Also directly related are the entries* PATIENTS' RIGHTS; CHILDREN, *article on* RIGHTS OF CHILDREN; *and* LAW AND BIOETHICS. *For a further discussion of topics mentioned in this article, see the entries* ANIMAL WELFARE AND RIGHTS, *article on* ETHICAL PERSPECTIVES ON THE TREATMENT AND STATUS OF ANIMALS; FETUS, *article on* PHILOSOPHICAL AND ETHICAL ISSUES; FUTURE GENERATIONS, OBLIGATIONS TO; *and* REPRODUCTIVE TECHNOLOGIES, *articles on* IN VITRO FERTILIZATION AND EMBRYO TRANSFER, SURROGACY, *and* CRYOPRESERVATION OF SPERM, OVA, AND EMBRYOS. *This article will find application in the entries* ABORTION, *articles on* CONTEMPORARY ETHICAL ISSUES, *and* LEGAL AND REGULATORY ISSUES; AIDS, *article on* PUBLIC-HEALTH ISSUES; COMMITMENT TO MENTAL INSTITUTIONS; DEATH AND DYING: EUTHANASIA AND SUSTAINING LIFE, *article on* ETHICAL ISSUES; INFORMED CONSENT, *articles on* LEGAL AND ETHICAL ISSUES OF CONSENT IN HEALTH CARE (*with its* POSTSCRIPT), *and* CONSENT ISSUES IN HUMAN RESEARCH; PROFESSIONAL-PATIENT RELATIONSHIP, *article on* ETHICAL ISSUES; *and* WOMEN, *article on* RESEARCH ISSUES. *See also the* APPEN-

DIX (CODES, OATHS, AND DIRECTIVES RELATED TO BIOETHICS), SECTION I: DIRECTIVES ON HEALTH-RELATED RIGHTS AND PATIENT RESPONSIBILITIES; *and* SECTION IV: ETHICAL DIRECTIVES FOR HUMAN RESEARCH, NUREMBERG CODE.

Bibliography

AMERICAN HOSPITAL ASSOCIATION. 1973. *A Patient's Bill of Rights.* Chicago: Author. Approved by the American Hospital Association's House of Delegates, February 6, 1973. Copyrighted in 1975 by the AHA.

ANNAS, GEORGE J. 1989. *The Rights of Patients: The Basic ACLU Guide to Patient Rights.* 2d ed. Carbondale: Southern Illinois University Press.

Casey v. Planned Parenthood Association of Southeastern Pennsylvania. 1992. 60 U.S. 4795.

Cruzan v. Director, Missouri Department of Health. 1990. 110 S. Ct. 2841.

Davis v. Davis v. King. 1989. Fifth Jud. Ct., Tennessee, E-14496, Sept. 21 (Young, J.); *Davis v. Davis.* 1992. 1992 Tenn. LEXIS 400 (June 1); *petition for rehearing denied in part and granted in part on other grounds,* 1992 Tenn. LEXIS 622 (November 23).

GOSTIN, LARRY, ed. 1990. *Surrogate Motherhood: Politics and Privacy.* Bloomington: Indiana University Press.

RHODEN, NANCY K. 1988. "Litigating Life and Death." *Harvard Law Review* 102, no. 12:375–446.

Roe v. Wade. 1973. 410 U.S. 113. 35 L. Ed. 2d 147. 93 S. Ct. 705.

ROTHMAN, DAVID. 1991. *Strangers at the Bedside: A History of How Law and Bioethics Transformed Medical Decision Making.* New York: Basic Books.

Salgo v. Leland Stanford, Jr., University Board Trustees. 1957. 317 P.2d 170. 181.

Schloendorff v. New York Hospital. 1914. 211 N.Y. 125. 105 E. 92.

SZASZ, THOMAS S. 1963. *Law, Liberty and Psychiatry: An Inquiry into the Social Uses of Mental Health Practices.* New York: Macmillan.

Tarasoff v. The Regents of the University of California. 1976. 551 P.2d 334, 17 Cal.3d 425, Supreme Court of California, *en banc,* July 1.

Webster v. Reproductive Health Services. 1989. 492 U.S. 490, 109. S. Ct. 3040.

Wyatt v. Stickney. 1972. 344 F. Supp. 373 (M.D. Ala.).

York v. Jones. 1989. 717 F. Supp. 421 (E.D. Va.).

RISK

"Risk" most commonly refers to an adverse future event that is not certain but only probable. Sometimes the term is used to name any uncertain future event, positive or negative, and frequently it is used to mean the likelihood of future harm being realized. For purposes of this entry, "risk" has the first standard meaning. Any risk has two components: the magnitude of negativity (including kind, degree, duration, and timing) and the probability of occurrence. Risk assessment—determining the possible negative consequences of actions and events—both identifies negativities and calculates their probabilities. The positive counterpart of risk is the probable benefit, and we name a situation "lucky" whenever some impending risk is not realized. The likelihood of any materialization of risk and the chance of its lucky nonrealization stand in an inverse relation; taken together, they add to a probability of one.

The concepts of risk and probability raise difficult and fundamental questions of ontology, or the nature of being, and epistemology, or the nature of knowledge, that cannot be examined here. However, important ethical questions are also involved. What, for instance, is the conceptual relation between morality and luck? A deep gap exists between two opposing views; one sees the moral life as independent of, and immune to, luck, and the other sees, contrarily, morality as deeply and intrinsically subject to luck (see Nussbaum, 1986; Williams, 1981). Less fundamental though no less important problems have to do with how to evaluate risks and, consequently, the moral permissibility of risk-bearing actions. Which risks are acceptable and which are not? Who should decide? How should risks and benefits be fairly distributed? These are essential questions to both general and medical ethics.

Ethics and theories of decision making under risk

Theories of decision making describe how people actually make decisions or, more often, propose criteria for rational decision making. These theories usually focus on decisions persons make concerning their own affairs—a realm of behavior some scholars consider falling under the reign of morality. But even for scholars with different views, plausible criteria of rationality in self-related decision making are nevertheless relevant to morality: Sometimes, people (e.g., physicians) may have a moral duty to help others (e.g., patients) in rational decision making, and to question or sometimes even to disregard decisions that are clearly irrational. Moreover, one should expect that the structural criteria of good decision making do not differ between self-regarding and other-regarding decisions, and it is precisely in terms of structural characteristics that decisional rationality is commonly seen (see Nida-Rümelin, 1993). Since risks—or benefits that are only probable—whether known or unknown, whether involving self, identified others, or statistical others, are faced by everyone in all spheres of human decision making, risk assessment provides a major subject of decision theory.

Risk assessments. Decisions to be made between alternatives with calculable probabilities of harms (or benefits) are called "decisions under risk"; those to be made where probability values cannot be ascribed to all considered outcomes are referred to as "decisions under uncertainty"; finally, whenever someone has to decide upon unpredictable outcomes, he or she is called "ignorant" (in the technical sense). Such ignorance is, of course, an element of our decisions all the time. However, we commonly frame decision alternatives as either positively realizing certain desired and undesired outcomes or as negatively not realizing them; in this way, outcomes (either positive or negative) that are completely unknown in fact get "swallowed" by this complete though underdetermined characterization of outcomes. Without this maneuver, we would be paralyzed in most daily decision making.

Practical problems with risk taking, then, start with identifying harms and benefits and, more specifically, with calculating probabilities, and continue on to decision making, taking into account the risks or uncertainties thus determined. Determining probabilities is a matter of natural or experimental observation, theorizing, and inductive extrapolation. What people in fact act on are not statistical probabilities out in the world but personally perceived probabilities. These personal probabilities may result from calculations involving various factors other than knowledge of the best available statistical probabilities: idiosyncratic beliefs, personal experience, skepticism, or ignorance, for example.

Decision making with known probability values for the various alternatives is considered standard decision theory, or Bayesian theory (named after the eighteenth-century mathematician Thomas Bayes). This theory describes as rational a strategy that calculates net expected utilities and then chooses that course of action which maximizes expected utility. It is hereby presupposed that utilities can be ascribed to any of an action's possible outcomes—remaining, however, noncommittal as to what counts as good or harmful. Calculating an action alternative's expected utility results from summing up all possible harms and benefits, multiplied by the various probability values.

The most plausible examples come from the areas of lottery and gambling, where utilities are given as simple and commensurable monetary gains or losses. Take, for instance, a lottery with the alternatives A (paying $8 for a chance of 1 in 10 to gain $100) and B (paying $100 for a chance of 2 in 10 to win $500). Expected utilities come out as follows:

A: $0.9(-\$8) + 0.1(\$100 - \$8) = \$2$;
B: $0.8(-\$100) + 0.2(\$500 - \$100) = \$0$.

Thus a preference for alternative A turns out to be the rational choice. Even in this simplistic example one

can, however, think of circumstances under which B would be the rational choice instead, for example, someone who desperately needs exactly $400 (the difference between best bet and lottery price in B), but who is basically indifferent to a loss of $100. In this case, the Bayesian theorem can be salvaged by introducing personal utilities that do not parallel the monetary values. However, there are other challenges—apparent paradoxes in actual or conceivable decision making by otherwise rational people—that leave the debate open as to whether these situations can still be readjusted to Bayesianism by appropriate reinterpretations of either effective personal utilities or personal probabilities (see Broome, 1991; Gärdenfors and Sahlin, 1988; Moser, 1990; Nida-Rümelin, 1993).

There are, however, indisputable exceptions to the rationality of maximizing expected utilities (Rescher, 1983). One of them would be realized by any case that includes the prospect of an outcome that is evaluated as an incomparably greater loss for oneself or for others than any other possible alternative. After envisaging such a catastrophe, it would be absolutely reasonable, or even morally obligatory, to opt out of quantitative risk analysis. Nobody would rationally choose, nor should one impose, the risk of a catastrophe for some relatively minor benefit. Another necessary exception to maximizing the expected utility concerns extremely low, "effectively zero" probabilities. Here again, rationality requires us to do without complete quantitative comparison and simply to dismiss those numberless but sufficiently remote disastrous possibilities. The threshold of effective zeroness, however, is likely to be a matter of ongoing dispute. More important, there may well be a conflict between avoiding catastrophes and dismissing remote probabilities. It is precisely this kind of conflict that fuels, for instance, the battle on genetic germ-line therapy, where some people insist on the catastrophic character of possible, uncontrollable side effects to whole generations, whereas others think the probability of such events will eventually be "effectively zero."

The need to ascribe (dis)utilities to alternative outcomes entails, finally, the problem of the incommensurability of certain harms or goods, which may make it impossible to identify the preference for one action alternative as most rational. However, even without catastrophes, effective zeroness, or incommensurability, maximization of expected utility is not necessarily the most rational strategy. Often people prefer either "playing safe"—choosing that option whose worst outcome is still the relative best (i.e., "maxi-min" strategy, or maximizing the minimum)—or "gambling"—choosing the option with the highest possible gain (i.e., "maxi-max, or maximizing the maximum).

Decision making under uncertainty is when a person is unable to ascribe probability values to some of the possible outcomes. In this case, it is often possible to calculate "uncertainty ranges" and, hence, ranges of expectations. Here the alternative strategies are once again "playing safe" (risk aversive), "gambling" (high risk), or a middle-ground strategy that chooses the option with the "best" range midpoint. Rationality can do no more than point out these alternatives. Which alternative someone ought to pick is irreducibly a matter of his or her personal attitude toward risk taking.

Protection against relativity. Given these three person- and context-sensitive variables—(1) evaluation of harm; (2) personal probability; and (3) personal risk attitude—is there any protection against total relativity in what good decision making means? Rationality requires that, at least where only an individual's own well-being is at stake, his or her evaluations of both outcomes and probabilities be in some sense consistent, stable over time, and susceptible to corrections when confronted with new information (Rescher, 1983). People tend irrationally to disregard those probabilities that are low or relate to distant events or that overemphasize recent experience. This kind of behavior may be correctable after appropriate information has been received. This may in turn impose an ethical obligation on others to provide relevant information in order to aid rational decision making.

More often than not, people's actions also have some impact on the actions or the well-being of others. This leads decision theory (here, game theory) into the area of mutual cooperation and into questions about risk rationality (see discussions and interpretations of prisoners' dilemma-type situations in Gärdenfors and Sahlin, 1988; Moser, 1990; Nida-Rümelin, 1993; Rescher, 1983). In addition, the other-regarding side of actions now indisputably raises questions about rational decision making in morally relevant cases.

Transferring the standards of expected utility theory—Bayesian or revised—to questions of morally good decision making is not a technical move but rather the adoption of a specific type of ethical theory. What is adopted is a structurally teleological or consequentialist ethic (one that determines what ought or ought not to be done to others entirely by the pursuit of expected good) where nature and relative weight of harms and goods are still open, subject to an additional theory of value. Hence, debates over the acceptability of some variant of expected utility theory in morally relevant situations have their roots in the very foundations of what counts as an acceptable type of ethical theory (see Broome, 1991; Nida-Rümelin, 1993).

When standard expected utility theory is applied to decisions involving others' well-being, problems that have already been identified in the one-person scenario reappear in aggravated form. Evaluation of negativities and choice among risk strategies are now to be justified

from a third-person point of view. Certain kinds of harm to others, such as those violating basic moral rights, arguably may be exempted from risk calculation much like potentially catastrophic outcomes in self-regarding decision making.

Additionally, emerging problems that are genuinely moral relate to the question of interpersonal incommensurability of goods; to the value of fair distribution rather than mere aggregation of harms, risks, and benefits; and finally, to the possibility that the value of some goods or harms may also vary with the context in which they occur. As an example of the last, it cannot simply be rejected as irrational that we would pay much more money to prevent a (statistical) death through lack of adequate emergency medical care than to prevent a (statistical) death by safety improvements in, say, highway traffic. Obviously, many people consider access to medical care (morally) more important than the provision of traffic safety, notwithstanding their respective life-saving potentials (Rescher, 1983).

When confronted with decisions that include risks to others, there are thus obligations to (a) choose at least a "conservative" risk strategy, (b) not neglect that the weight of a negativity may vary relative to different persons or contexts, and (c) pay attention to whatever counts as a fair distribution of risks. With all these caveats, calculation of risks will resemble only faintly the usual concept of cost–benefit analysis, of which risk–benefit analysis is a subset.

Health-related risks in medical care and public policy

The risks and probable benefits to human life and health have implications for three distinct levels of action and decision making: first, for research activities that identify and measure health effects, for example, of toxic substances, environmental influences, or medical interventions; second, for public policy, for example, with regard to public risk management (regulating substances, determining safety standards, handling tobacco advertising, or funding medical research), or health-care planning; and third, for individual treatment decisions. All these decisions involve issues of protection against possibly occurring disease, dysfunction, disability, pain, or premature death, or else of improvement or at least nondeterioration where such harm already exists.

Particularly with regard to this third realm, medicine proper, public and professional preoccupation with uncertainty, error, and risk has increased (Fox, 1980). Medical interventions such as organ transplantations, prenatal diagnoses, carrier screening programs, or certain experimental therapies, all of which have stimulated public awareness and mass media coverage, seem to have awakened simultaneous attention to their potential for failure. Judgments about using diagnostic tools, making diagnoses, and selecting appropriate treatments all involve uncertainties on various levels. In many cases no probabilistic values exist for certain treatment alternatives; there will always be some uncertainty as to whether a particular patient matches the tested or personally experienced group of patients from whom applicable medical knowledge has been drawn; and uncertainty may exist regarding an individual physician's ignorance of collectively available knowledge.

Public management of health risks, like medicine proper, requires that risks be identified and assessed. Here, various nonobjective factors disrupt the illusion that value-free data are available to decision makers. Cultural, social, and political factors influence the selection of negativities, and the mass media play a significant role, often focusing on easily measurable kinds of harm. Serious problems, however, arise when those who function as risk managers—officials in public agencies or physicians in medical care—must understand and interpret epidemiological or care-related data. For instance, many practicing physicians make the important mistake of confusing the probability that, say, a particular laboratory test result proves disease (i.e., the test's predictive accuracy) with the probability that a diseased patient shows that particular test result (i.e., the test's retrospective accuracy); or, they gravely undervalue the predictive importance of the patient's so-called prior probability of being diseased, as determined by history, clinical symptoms, and so on (see Gigerenzer, 1993).

Public-policy risk managers, in turn, may overlook the fact that, due to the mathematical complexities involved, decisions concerning the kind and amount of evidence needed to estimate a risk are already highly value laden. Due to mathematical interrelations of (a) the probability that something is falsely called a risk, (b) the likelihood that risks of concern may go undetected, and (c) investigations that are too costly due to sample size, morally crucial trade-offs have to be made. Not one of these trade-offs (scientific accuracy in risk detection, meeting risk-preventive aims, and saving research costs) is, as such, adequate. But the chosen trade-offs must be made explicit so as not to give rise to dangerously uninformed risk management (Cranor, 1993). In addition, many experts warn against overestimating the advance measurability of risk (e.g., the real-world contamination of laboratory data) and against the tendency to make hard calculations with soft numbers.

Wherever disutilities are assessed and risk–benefit analyses are performed, heated moral debates are likely to occur (see MacLean, 1986; Mann, 1989) about unfair risk distribution or about loss of values due to the metricity requirement. Policies are sometimes accused of neglecting the relativity of negativities to individuals and contexts. Or policies are blamed because they "pater-

nalistically" prescribe a particular strategy in both risk taking (e.g., experimental drugs like Laetrile) and risk avoiding (e.g., debates on the safety of genetic engineering). The more, however, this criticism leads to abandoning the economic paradigm of risk analysis (remember the lotteries), where a dollar is simply a dollar or a (quality-adjusted) life year is just a (quality-adjusted) life year, the more difficult it gets to make risk calculation operational. If risk–benefit analysis is given up altogether, however, the result is likely to be intuitive, ad hoc decisions prone to producing otherwise avoidable harm. The moral trade-offs involved in managing risks, the political structures necessary to counterbalance those trade-offs, and the questions about alternative methods of risk assessment will certainly fuel ongoing debates on these issues.

Patient risk taking

Risk taking is part of almost all decisions about diagnostic or therapeutic interventions. Often, the risks at stake are both trivial and reversible, for example, the risk that a particular antibiotic treatment for a nonserious infection might fail and have to be replaced by some other treatment. But even in this example, some patient may wish to be informed and even draw conclusions from such knowledge (e.g., postpone an important appointment so as not to jeopardize it).

Both heightened public awareness of medicine's riskiness and a new "antipaternalistic" medical ethos have led to important changes in the understanding of informed consent (Faden et al., 1986). Informed consent includes not only an acceptance of kinds of possible or certain outcomes but also of their likeliness or uncertainty. The probabilistic nature of medical knowledge is just one more reason to insist that whenever possible patients ought to authorize their medical treatment. Debates on acceptable and overdone consent, on the locus and nature of proper decision making, and on conditions of waiver and criteria for incompetency (see Brody, 1992; Faden et al., 1986) all involve certain positions on how to communicate and handle risk and uncertainty in the context of medical decision making. Each patient should determine how much information he or she needs or wants; a patient's informed waiver in matters of risk information is as acceptable as in any other matter. The view, not uncommon among physicians, that it is never acceptable to express a bleak probability of life expectancy numerically, has not been proven to be common among the general population.

Some opponents of any detailed communication of risks claim that many patients are not able to understand what probabilities or uncertainties mean, with the effect that misunderstandings and unnecessary anxieties result in irrational and thus nonautonomous decisions. The difficulty here lies in differentiating between the merely unusual and the outright irrational decisions patients are said to make as a consequence of not understanding the very nature of risk (Brock and Wartman, 1990).

Evaluating harms and choosing from among high-risk, risk-neutral, or risk-aversive decision strategies involve irreducible personal biases. For instance, patients may rationally opt against some medically "indicated" therapy in making a personal decision for quality of life over longevity. Likewise, a physician and a patient, even though relying on the same research data, may estimate probabilities very differently, and it is by no means clear that in such cases patients' personal estimations of probabilities are less rational than those of their physicians.

Several effects in reporting and in understanding risk might compromise the risk taker's autonomy. The most widely discussed factor is the so-called framing effect, where patients tend to make different choices if some risk is formulated negatively (e.g., a 30 percent chance of death) rather than if it is formulated positively (e.g., a 70 percent chance of survival)—a behavior that, though understandable, is plainly unjustified (Tversky and Kahneman, 1981; Faden et al., 1986; Mann, 1989). Some physicians seem to use this effect intentionally to influence their patients. But a correct risk communication would require both formulations.

Other factors that may distort a patient's risk perception are unfamiliarity, remoteness in time, and low probability of risks as well as difficulties in understanding numerical expressions. All these influences cannot be recognized simply from the result of a patient's decision making; the various evaluative "ingredients" of a patient's coherent choice—albeit personal—must be gleaned from unhurried conversation and inquiry.

In any case, the fragility of patients' rationality in risk taking does not justify a return to paternalism; rather, it broadens physicians' professional and moral responsibilities to include aiding their patients in making rational choices that reflect the patients' personal evaluations of the risks they face. However, if competent patients ultimately insist on incoherent risk assessment, nonpaternalists would have to accept this as autonomous decision making. After all, we make irrational decisions throughout our lives.

There is always a danger that the probabilistic nature of medical knowledge itself might encourage a physician to treat the patient as part of a statistical collective rather than as an individual with very personal risk values (Wieland, 1986). Finally, as Jay Katz observes in his analysis of physicians' unjustifiable silence in risk matters, "patients' supposed intolerance of medical uncertainties may turn out to be significantly affected by a projection of physicians' intolerance onto patients" (Katz, 1984, p. 204).

Besides the daily problems in medical risk taking, there is the extremely difficult area of balancing risks and chances for incompetent patients such as newborns or patients with mentally handicapping conditions. Even with a conservative risk strategy, painstaking decisions that entail disproportionate risks and remote chances of benefit cannot always be prevented. Here, decision theory cannot even help to improve such deeply moral judgments. A somewhat related issue arises in the debate concerning medical futility and its bearing on professional responsibility and on patients' rights to claim such futile therapies (see Brody, 1992).

Yet another important issue is the question of just-risk distribution, specifically in (a) nontherapeutic research on humans; (b) mandatory testing for or immunization against infectious diseases; and (c) rationing in health care. With subjects who take research risks and uncertainties for the sake of future patients, both their consent and their compensability diminish but do not obviate the problem of one-sided burdens. Hence, there are generally considered to be limits to those risks that may be consented to. Research on children who cannot yet consent certainly requires a drastic further decrease of the threshold of risk acceptability, which ought to be subject to social consensus (see Freedman et al., 1993).

Mandatory immunization programs somehow have to balance the gainable increase in public safety against the specific harm to individuals being coerced. Once again, this decision ought to be made within a broader context of social policies and morality.

When searching for criteria for rationing medicine fairly, one aspect commonly viewed as significant consists of the very high risks for therapeutic failure faced by some patients. Take the paradigmatic triage case of two patients who are the same age and who have been waiting the same time for one organ transplant. Patient A is believed to have a 90 percent chance of organ survival; due to secondary illness, patient B has a bleak prognosis of only 2 percent probability of organ survival. Many may want to give the organ to patient A. However, when hypothetically decreasing the comparative differences in risks of organ failure between patients A and B, each of us may at some point favor some type of random selection, so as to give both patients a chance. It is questionable whether any further plausible justification could be found for the identification of this turning point.

Finally, the issue of just what degree of risk taking in medicine is acceptable is not confined to patients or research subjects. Controversies exist—and become more heated in times of infectious risks such as the human immunodeficiency virus (HIV)—as to whether and to what extent health-care workers have a duty to treat patients in spite of increased risks to their own health. The 1987 American Medical Association statemen' claims that such a duty does exist unconditionally; others, however, take the opposite position, denying any such duty at all. Defenders of a middle ground contend that physicians do indeed implicitly consent to taking some elevated risk of becoming infected by patients, although it should not exceed some standard level. The implicit or explicit consent of those involved is considered the main criterion for fair distribution of risks and benefits (see Daniels, 1991), just as it is primary to any ethically acceptable decision-making policy.

BETTINA SCHÖNE-SEIFERT
TRANSLATION ASSISTANCE BY IRENE SCHULTENS

Directly related to this entry are the entries ECONOMIC CONCEPTS IN HEALTH CARE; *and* HARM. *For a further discussion of topics mentioned in this entry, see the entries* BENEFICENCE; ETHICS, *articles on* NORMATIVE ETHICAL THEORIES, TASK OF ETHICS, *and* MORAL EPISTEMOLOGY; INFORMED CONSENT; JUSTICE; PATERNALISM; *and* VALUE AND VALUATION. *This entry will find application in the entries* ALTERNATIVE THERAPIES; ENDANGERED SPECIES AND BIODIVERSITY; ENVIRONMENTAL ETHICS; GENE THERAPY; GENETIC SCREENING, *especially the articles on* CARRIER SCREENING, *and* PREDICTIVE AND WORKPLACE TESTING; HAZARDOUS WASTES AND TOXIC SUBSTANCES; INJURY AND INJURY CONTROL; LIFESTYLES AND PUBLIC HEALTH; OBLIGATION AND SUPEREROGATION; ORGAN AND TISSUE TRANSPLANTS; PUBLIC HEALTH; RESEARCH POLICY, *especially the article on* RISK AND VULNERABLE GROUPS; *and* TRUST. *For a discussion of related ideas, see the entries* COMPETENCE; *and* PUBLIC POLICY AND BIOETHICS.

Bibliography

BROCK, DAN W., and WARTMAN, STEVEN A. 1990. "When Competent Patients Make Irrational Choices." *New England Journal of Medicine* 322, no. 22:1595–1599.

BRODY, HOWARD. 1992. *The Healer's Power.* New Haven, Conn.: Yale University Press.

BROOME, JOHN. 1991. *Weighing Goods: Equality, Uncertainty and Time.* Oxford: Basil Blackwell.

CRANOR, CARL F. 1993. *Regulating Toxic Substances: A Philosophy of Science and the Law.* Oxford: Oxford University Press.

DANIELS, NORMAN. 1991. "Duty to Treat or Right to Refuse?" *Hastings Center Report* 21, no. 2:36–46.

FADEN, RUTH R.; BEAUCHAMP, TOM L.; and KING, NANCY M. P. 1986. *A History and Theory of Informed Consent.* New York: Oxford University Press.

FOX, RENÉE C. 1980. "The Evolution of Medical Uncertainty." *Milbank Memorial Fund Quarterly Health and Society* 58, no. 1:1–49.

FREEDMAN, BENJAMIN; FUKS, ABRAHAM; and WEIJER, CHARLES. 1993. "In Loco Parentis: Minimal Risk as an Ethical Threshold for Research upon Children." *Hastings Center Report* 23, no. 2:13–19.

GÄRDENFORS, PETER, and SAHLIN, NILS-ERIC, eds. 1988. *Decision, Probability, and Utility: Selected Readings.* Cambridge: At the University Press.

GIGERENZER, GERD. 1993. "Die Repräsentation von Information und ihre Auswirkung auf statistisches Denken." In *Kognitive Täuschungen,* pp. 99–127. Edited by Walter Hell, Klaus Fiedler, and Gerd Gigerenzer. Heidelberg, Germany: Spektrum.

KATZ, JAY. 1984. *The Silent World of Doctor and Patient.* New York: Free Press.

MANN, RONALD D., ed. 1989. *Risk and Consent to Risk in Medicine.* Carnforth, U.K.: Parthenon.

MCLEAN, DOUGLAS, ed. 1986. *Values at Risk.* Totowa, N.J.: Rowman & Allanheld.

MOSER, PAUL K., ed. 1990. *Rationality in Action: Contemporary Approaches.* Cambridge: At the University Press.

NIDA-RÜMELIN, JULIAN. 1993. *Kritik des Konsequentialismus.* Munich: R. Oldenbourg.

NUSSBAUM, MARTHA C. 1986. *The Fragility of Goodness: Luck and Ethics in Greek Tragedy and Philosophy.* New York: Cambridge University Press.

RESCHER, NICHOLAS. 1983. *Risk: A Philosophical Introduction to the Theory of Risk Evaluation and Management.* New York: University Press of America.

TVERSKY, AMOS, and KAHNEMAN, DANIEL. 1981. "The Framing of Decisions and the Psychology of Choice." *Science* 211, no. 4481:453–458.

WIELAND, WOLFGANG. 1986. *Strukturwandel der Medizin und ärztliche Ethik.* Heidelberg, Germany: Carl Winter Universitätsverlag.

WILLIAMS, BERNARD. 1981. *Moral Luck: Philosophical Papers, 1973–1980.* New York: Cambridge University Press. See in particular the title essay.

RISK–BENEFIT

See RISK. *See also* ECONOMIC CONCEPTS IN HEALTH CARE; *and* TECHNOLOGY, *article on* TECHNOLOGY ASSESSMENT.

ROMAN CATHOLICISM

The Roman Catholic tradition has a long history of concern about the moral aspects of the physical and biological aspects of human life and various ways of dealing with the human body in health and disease. That long history has generated many theological and pastoral writings, as well as church teachings and practices. By the 1960s, when the modern interest in biomedical ethics might be said to begin, the Roman Catholic tradition could draw on these sources. Many books on medical ethics were in print in the major European languages (e.g., Bonnar, 1939; Healy, 1956; Kelly, 1958; Kenny,

1952; Niedermeyer, 1935; O'Donnell, 1956, 1976; Paquin, 1955; Payen, 1935; Pujiula, 1953; Scremin, 1954). Many periodicals devoted to medical morality were being published in many of the same countries, among them *Arzt und Christ, Cahiers Laënnec, Catholic Medical Quarterly, Linacre Quarterly,* and *Saint-Luc médicale.* The existence of a well-developed discipline of medical ethics in Roman Catholicism distinguishes this tradition from most others. This article will focus on the monolithic discipline of medical ethics that existed in Roman Catholicism before the 1960s. Specifically, the following aspects will be discussed: (1) the general context, (2) the historical development, (3) the specific characteristics, (4) the moral principles, and (5) the particular questions considered. A final section will summarize the significant developments that have occurred since 1960.

General context

The Christian tradition, rooted in both the Jewish and Christian scriptures, has always encouraged care for the sick. Sickness, in the Christian perspective, has a number of dimensions. God, as the author and giver of life, also heals. Sickness and death relate to the power of sin in the world, but sickness also comes from human weakness and fragility; human beings can and should try to heal and overcome sickness if possible, but ultimately all will die. In the suffering connected with sickness, the Christian tradition sees not only an evil to overcome, if possible, but also a mysterious sharing in the suffering, death, and resurrection of Jesus.

The church fostered different aspects of care for the sick corresponding to the multiple understandings of sickness. The spiritual care of the sick ultimately developed into the sacrament of anointing, one of the seven sacraments of the Roman Catholic church. Recently, the church has recognized a false emphasis in restricting that sacrament to the moment of death (generally known as the sacrament of extreme unction before the Second Vatican Council in the early 1960s), and has renewed the earlier emphasis on the sacrament as the anointing of the sick. The sacrament celebrates the presence of Jesus in the community as the healer of sickness and also as the Lord who through death and resurrection has transformed sin, sickness, suffering, and death itself.

Prayers for healing exist both in the sacrament of anointing and in the Christian life in general, but the believer knows that healing will not always come. Demonic possession and the rite of exorcism also recognize the relationship between sickness and sin. However, the church, while acknowledging the possibility both of miraculous cures by God and of possession by the devil, has generally been quite cautious because of the dangers of illusion and deception. By the same token, the church

has also been wary of the danger of magic and superstition in connection with healing.

The Christian tradition in general and the Catholic tradition in particular have emphasized that God usually works mediately, through secondary causes, and not immediately, without the help of human causes. Acceptance of this principle of mediation characterizes much of Roman Catholic theology and ethical thought. In the area of healing, human means of curing illness have been encouraged, for in that way the doctor is cooperating in God's work, although ultimately death will triumph. To relieve suffering and strive for healing involve working with God and do not constitute an offense to divine providence, since creaturely existence includes the responsibility to take care of one's life and health. While occasional tensions have erupted between medicine and the Roman Catholic church, on the whole the Roman Catholic tradition has fostered and encouraged the practice of medicine. Thus the Christian tradition encouraged medicine as well as prayer and fought against superstition and magic as opposed to both faith and reason.

The Christian church has fostered and sponsored the establishment of hospitals to care for the sick and the dying. Institutional involvement in hospitals and care for the sick has continued to be a vital aspect of the mission of the Catholic church. Communities of religious men and women within the church have dedicated themselves to the mission of caring for the sick and the dying. Similarly, the church has held in high regard vocations in the health-care field and commended such vocations to all its members.

Historical development

Many factors contributed to the growth of what ultimately became the discipline of medical ethics. Catholic theology stressed the importance of good works, for faith alone was not enough for salvation. The penitential practices of the Roman Catholic church emphasized the need to know whether certain actions were sinful or not. Casuistry focused discussion on the morality of particular acts. The discipline of canon law with its complete legislation on marriage, including such questions as sterility and impotence, called for a knowledge of biology and medicine. Great concern for the baptism of the endangered fetus still in the womb occasioned a heightened interest in embryology.

The historical development of medical ethics in the Roman Catholic tradition (Kelly, 1979) is closely connected with moral theology in general. Unfortunately, the definitive history of Catholic moral theology has not been written; but some helpful contributions exist (e.g., Häring, 1961–1966, vol. 1; Mahoney, 1987; Vereecke, 1986).

Early development.   The first six hundred years C.E. are generally referred to as the Patristic Age, because the principal writers were the Fathers of the Church. Specific moral teachings were developed and proposed in a pastoral rather than a systematic or academic perspective. Many subjects of interest to the later development of medical ethics were first discussed at that time. Clement of Alexandria (150–210), often called the founder of the first school of Christian theology, condemned contraception, because marital relations are justified only for the purpose of raising children (Noonan, 1986). From the earliest times Christian writers condemned abortion, although influential figures like Jerome and Augustine accepted a theory of delayed ensoulment, according to which the human soul entered the body some time after conception.

The most creative development in the period from the seventh to the twelfth century concerns the *libri poenitentiales* (penitential books) that came into existence with the new format of the sacrament of penance, involving confession of sins to a priest who made a judgment about their seriousness, prescribed a proportionate penance, and gave absolution in God's name. These penitentials consisted of an arrangement of sins by subject matter together with the prescribed penance the priest should give for every wrong act. In the midst of many other wrong acts, such as stealing, lying, cheating, and adultery, one finds abortion, contraception, and other matters connected with marriage and sexual behavior.

The twelfth century set the stage for the development of modern canon law in the Roman Catholic church. About 1140 Gratian, traditionally identified as an Italian Camaldolese monk, collected and put in order many of the various laws and norms that had evolved during the previous centuries. His work, known as the *Decretum* (Decree) of Gratian, was later accepted as the basis for church law. In 1234 Pope Gregory IX published an official collection of laws known as the *Decretals;* among other things they speak about medical examinations to determine sexual impotence as a condition to nullify marriage (*De probationibus*). In 1331 Pope John XXII formed a college of ecclesiastical judges, called the Roman Rota. In his decretal *Ratio iuris exigit*, he mentioned medical skills and knowledge that help the work of this tribunal. Thus the early stages in the development of canon law reveal the role and importance of biological and medical science, especially in the area of marriage.

The thirteenth century.   The thirteenth century witnessed the growth and development of Scholastic theology, which achieved its high point in Thomas Aquinas (d. 1274), whose philosophical and theological approach was later accepted as normative. Thomas proposed a highly systematic theology in his famous *Summa*

theologiae. In the second part of this work he treats the questions connected with the moral life of the Christian in the context of a threefold understanding—the human being related to God as ultimate end, the human being as an image of God insofar as he or she is capable of self-determination, and the humanity of Christ as the human way to God. The theory of natural law, the moral precepts derived by human reason through analysis of the basic tendencies of human nature, was elaborated by Thomas and became the characteristic approach of Roman Catholic moral theology.

The fourteenth to the eighteenth century.   In the fourteenth and fifteenth centuries penitential summas assumed the role of the earlier *libri poenitentiales*. These practical handbooks prepared the priest as confessor for dealing with the sins and problems of penitents. In the third tome of his four-volume *Summa* (1542), the archbishop of Florence, Saint Antoninus (d. 1459), considers the functions and obligations of different states in life—married people, virgins and widows, temporal rulers, soldiers, lawyers, doctors, merchants, judges, craft workers, and so on. The discussion of the functions and obligations of doctors extends for five folio pages and mentions medical competence; diligence in care of the patient; the obligation to tell the dying patient of the imminence of death; the legitimacy of accepting and caring for dying patients and receiving a fee from them; the proper fee or salary for the doctor (the doctor is bound to care for the sick when they cannot pay); the obligation not to prescribe as remedies actions, such as fornication or masturbation, which are against the moral law; and the question of abortion. Antoninus became a most important source, frequently cited by later theologians.

Beginning in 1621, Paolo Zacchia, a Roman doctor, published a multivolume work entitled *Quaestiones medico-legales,* which makes him the spiritual father of what would become the discipline of medical ethics. He treats many diverse subjects—age, birth, pregnancy, death, mental illness, poison, impotence, sterility, plagues, contagious diseases, virginity, rape, fasting, mutilation of parts of the body, and conjugal relations. Zacchia's work, which became quite influential, attempts to bridge the gap between theology, medicine, and law, and includes medical knowledge necessary for the pastor as well as the moral and legal issues facing the doctor. Michiel Boudewyns took a slightly narrower perspective in his *Ventilabrum medico-theologicum* (1666). This doctor of philosophy and medicine discussed the moral questions and cases most often faced by doctors. Catholic medical ethics in the twentieth century adopted the same scope and approach.

In his *De ortu infantium* (1637) Théophile Raynaud wrote about the morality of cesarean sections in the various circumstances that might arise in birth. In 1658 Girolamo Fiorentini published *Disputatio de ministrando baptismo*, in which he talks about the baptism of products of conception that are doubtfully human. Francesco Cangiamila (d. 1763), in his *Sacra embryologia*, discusses questions connected with embryology, such as the animation of the fetus and intrauterine baptism.

However, despite these significant developments in the seventeenth and eighteenth centuries, one still cannot speak of a well-developed and distinct discipline of pastoral medicine or medical ethics in Roman Catholic theology. In the same two centuries Catholic moral theology in general experienced the growth of the manuals known as the *institutiones theologiae moralis*, which came into existence in the late seventeenth century and continued to be the textbooks of moral theology until the Second Vatican Council (1962–1965). These textbooks briefly explain the more theoretical aspects of moral theology but concentrate on preparing the priest as confessor and judge in the sacrament of penance, often developing their material using the schema of the Ten Commandments and the sacraments. Questions pertaining to medical ethics are often discussed under the Fifth Commandment, which explicitly forbids killing and implicitly forbids mutilation, and under the sacrament of marriage. Books containing practical cases (*casus conscientiae*) supplemented the *institutiones theologicae moralis* and developed the method of casuistry (Jonsen and Toulmin, 1988). The manual and writings of Alphonsus Maria de Liguori (1789) carried great weight because he subsequently was declared a saint (1839), a doctor of the church (1871), and the patron of moral theology (1950).

The nineteenth and twentieth centuries: Pastoral medicine and medical ethics. Pastoral medicine emerged as a separate discipline in the nineteenth century. In the light of newer developments in biology and medical science, books with "pastoral medicine" in the title tried to bridge the gap between theology and pastoral practice, on the one hand, and medicine, on the other hand. In 1877 a German physician, Carl Capellmann, wrote the most influential of many such works; it was later translated into Latin (1879) and many modern languages. In his introduction Capellmann describes his purposes as providing the priest with the medical knowledge needed to carry out his ministry, and communicating to doctors the moral principles necessary to ensure that they act in accord with Christian morals. The chief areas covered by Capellmann are the Fifth Commandment, including questions of abortion, medical operations, and the use of medicine; the Sixth Commandment, including masturbation, pollution, and marriage; the commandments of the church, such as fasting and abstinence; the sacraments, particularly baptism, Communion, and extreme unction; impotence in marriage; and topics of lesser importance. Other signif-

icant books of the same type were published by Pierre Debreyne (1884), Alphons Eschbach (1884), and Giuseppe Antonelli (1906). These and additional books published in various modern languages at the end of the nineteenth and the beginning of the twentieth century created the new discipline called pastoral medicine.

The interest in theology and medicine continued and grew in the twentieth century. Ethical problems were still considered in general treatises on moral theology, but books on pastoral medicine, medical deontology (understood in light of the French word referring to professional obligations), and medical ethics flourished in all modern European languages. In Germany, Albert Niedermeyer published a multivolume work on pastoral medicine (1949–1952), which included a complete and updated treatment of the topics covered in the older works as well as material dealing with psychiatry and psychotherapy. In the twentieth century, especially in the United States, the discipline became known as medical ethics and focused on the moral issues and problems facing doctors, nurses, and Catholic hospitals. Many of these books served as texts for courses in Catholic medical schools and especially in Catholic nursing schools. Father Charles Coppens, who taught medical ethics at Creighton University in Omaha, Nebraska, at the turn of the century, published his lectures as *Moral Principles and Medical Practice* (1897). The Catholic Hospital Association's "Ethical and Religious Directives for Catholic Hospitals" were first formulated in 1949 and revised in 1955.

As the twentieth century progressed, more and more monographs appeared on subjects in medical ethics. Areas of medical ethics became favorite topics for doctoral dissertations in the area of Roman Catholic moral theology. And the journals in various languages published articles on the subject. Thus, by the 1950s there was a large body of literature and a distinct field in Roman Catholic theology generally known as medical ethics, although occasionally the more popular nineteenth-century term "pastoral medicine" was still used.

Specific characteristics

Roman Catholic medical ethics as it existed in the 1950s (e.g., Healy, 1956; Kelly, 1958; Kenny, 1952; McFadden, 1949; O'Donnell, 1956), like all Roman Catholic moral theology at that time, exhibited two distinctive characteristics: natural-law methodology and the role of authoritative church teaching.

Natural-law methodology. "Natural law" is a complex term involving a number of aspects. Catholic theology historically has recognized both faith and reason, Scripture and the natural law, as sources of ethical wisdom and knowledge for the Christian. The twentieth-century textbooks on medical ethics base their teaching primarily on natural law rather than on biblical texts.

The philosophical aspect of natural law concerns the precise meanings of human reason, human nature, and natural law itself. Roman Catholic textbooks in medical ethics, like all the Roman Catholic ethical considerations in the first part of the twentieth century, appealed to the teaching of Thomas Aquinas, especially as interpreted by the neo-Scholastic theologians and textbooks. According to neo-Scholastic theory, the eternal law is the plan of divine wisdom ordering all reality to its proper end. The eternal law is ultimately grounded in the very being of God.

The natural law is the participation of the eternal law in the rational creature. God directs all creatures to their ends in accord with their own natures. There are laws by which the physical universe is governed, such as the law of gravity. However, human beings are governed according to their rational nature. The human being is an image of God precisely insofar as he or she is endowed with reason, free will, and the power of self-determination. Through reason rational creatures direct their own activity toward their proper ends and thus are not merely passively directed to the ends by God. Right reason is able to recognize the threefold natural inclinations within human nature—the inclinations we share with all substances (the conservation of one's existence), the inclinations we share with animals (procreation and education of offspring), and the inclinations we have as rational beings (living in society). Thus the natural law is understood as human reason directing individuals to their own ends in accord with their natures.

The best of the Catholic tradition understood the natural law as an unwritten or unformulated law—the law of one's being as a rational creature. On the basis of the ontological structures of rational human nature, reason can arrive at universally valid principles or prescriptions of the natural law. The first principles of the natural law are known intuitively by human reason: Do good; avoid evil; act according to right reason. Human reason on the basis of the first principles can then deduce the secondary principles of the natural law, such as "Adultery is wrong" and "Stealing is forbidden."

The primary principles of the natural law are obligatory universally on all human persons, at all times and places. The secondary principles and the applications to particular cases are less universal, being open to some exceptions and modifications, as Aquinas stated, on rare occasions. However, the Roman Catholic moral theologians of the 1950s tended to take a more strict position, arguing that secondary principles rightly deduced from first principles have the same obligatory force, as do many applications. Thus such medical ethics questions as euthanasia, involving direct taking of human life, direct attacks on fetal life in abortion, and direct contraception and sterilization were considered absolutely wrong in all circumstances. Indirect killing or indirect sterilization could be justified according to the principle of double effect, discussed below.

Authoritative church teaching. A second distinctive characteristic of Roman Catholic medical ethics involves the authoritative teaching office of the church. The Roman Catholic church recognizes a special God-given hierarchical teaching function belonging to the pope and the bishops as well as to councils of the church, called the magisterium, charged with teaching the faithful in matters of faith and morals.

Early councils in the church as well as letters of popes and other bishops spoke about specific moral questions such as abortion and marriage. Mention has already been made of authoritative collections of canon law beginning in the twelfth century. The papal teaching office—especially the Congregation of the Holy Office (now known as the Congregation for the Doctrine of the Faith), which deals with faith and morals—made significant interventions in moral matters in the seventeenth and eighteenth centuries. Papal encyclicals addressed to all the bishops and faithful of the world and speaking on specific areas of faith or morals became prominent only in the nineteenth and twentieth centuries.

It is important to recognize the various grades or degrees of the hierarchical magisterium in the Roman Catholic Church. In the nineteenth century the distinction became formalized between infallible church teaching to which one owed the assent of faith, and the authoritative noninfallible teaching to which the faithful owed the religious assent of intellect and will. Catholic ethicists acknowledged in the 1950s that teaching in the area of medical ethics ordinarily does not fall under the category of infallible teaching, which in reality is very limited. Gradations also exist in the various forms of the ordinary noninfallible papal teaching office. However, Pius XII, in the encyclical *Humani generis* (1950), declared that whenever the pope goes out of his way to speak on a controverted subject, that subject is no longer open to free debate among theologians. In the light of such an understanding, any Roman pronouncement or decree both theoretically and practically ended debate about a specific question, but the papal teaching office recognized the need for theological input and advice.

The growth and development of medical ethics in the nineteenth and twentieth centuries corresponded to the greater emphasis on the papal teaching office in the Roman Catholic church. Between 1884 and 1902, for example, the Holy Office responded to a number of inquiries from bishops and theologians about abortion and eliminated some of the exceptions that had not been previously condemned. The Holy Office declared that one could not perform a craniotomy or directly kill the fetus to save the life of the mother, nor could one extract an ectopic pregnancy (Bouscaren, 1944). Encyclicals on marriage by Pope Pius XI (*Casti connubii*, 1930) and by Pope Paul VI (*Humanae vitae*, 1968) strongly reiterated the condemnation of artificial contraception.

Perhaps the most significant development in the matter of authoritative church teachings was the number of allocutions and addresses given by Pope Pius XII (1939–1958), very often dealing with questions of medical ethics. This corpus of papal teaching shows a wide-ranging interest in the problems of medical ethics as well as a penetrating knowledge of medicine and its problems. To various medical groups Pius XII spoke on such subjects as the duties of the medical profession, blood donation, artificial insemination, contraception, sterilization, abortion, the moral limits of medical research in experimentation, genetics, painless childbirth, transplants, death, and the various means necessary to preserve life. Obviously, the interest and concern of Pius XII sparked the growth and development of the discipline of medical ethics.

Moral principles

Since the method of natural law proceeded by first establishing the principles of natural law and then applying these principles to particular cases, Roman Catholic medical ethics developed a number of important principles. In fact, the textbooks of the 1950s often began their discussion with a brief summary of the more important principles governing medical ethics. These principles were generally accepted by all Catholic medical ethicists; only in the 1960s did the monolithic look of Catholic medical ethics begin to change.

The right to life. Both the gift of God and the natural law ground the right of the individual to life. Neither the state nor any human person can deny it. This natural right that belongs to all human beings is inalienable: It cannot be renounced by a person (such as someone who attempts suicide). However, the Roman Catholic ethical tradition recognized conflict situations and cases in which the life of another may be taken; for example, killing another as a necessary way of defending one's life, or just war, capital punishment, and accidental killing. The most precise formulation of the principle maintains that the direct killing of an innocent person on one's own authority is always wrong.

Right of use or stewardship. Much in the area of medical ethics follows from the moral principle that the individual as a rational creature possesses the right to use the faculties and powers of human nature in accord with their God-given and natural purpose. Since individuals are users and not proprietors, they do not have unlimited power to destroy or mutilate the body or

its functions. The principle of stewardship serves as the basis for the care individuals should take of their own bodies as well as the justification in general for surgery and other procedures.

Principle of totality. Thomas Aquinas pointed out that a member or part of the body exists for the good of the whole body; thus one may remove a diseased member if this is for the good of the whole. This principle was reaffirmed by Pius XII as the principle of totality, which maintains that the good of the whole body is the determining factor in regard to the part, and one can dispose of the part in the interest of the whole (Address to Congress on Histopathology, 1952). This principle justifies surgery that would otherwise constitute mutilation.

The pope and Roman Catholic moralists were very aware of the abuses of totalitarian governments in sacrificing individuals for the good of the state, so they carefully spelled out the meaning and limits of the principle of totality for medical ethics. Since the individual person does not exist totally for the good of the state, the individual cannot be totally subordinated to the state. The obvious example where the principle of totality applies concerns the individual organs and functions of the total bodily organism. Pope Pius XII stated that each single organ is subordinated not only to the good of the body but also to the spiritual good of the person (Address to College of Neuropsychopharmacology, 1958).

Principles regarding sexuality and procreation. In traditional Roman Catholic thought, the faculties and powers of human beings must be used according to the purpose for which God made them and nature intended them; for example, one perverts the finality of speech by using it to communicate to another what is directly contrary to one's thought. The sexual function and organs have a twofold purpose—procreation and the love union of husband and wife. Any use of sexual powers is immoral when it impedes the purpose for which God created these powers. As a result, contraception and contraceptive sterilization are wrong. The individual person may not positively interfere to thwart the sexual act of its God-given finality. According to this reasoning, the sexual organs and functions differ from other organs. The sexual organs exist not only for the good of the individual but also for the good of the species. Hence, one cannot invoke the principle of totality to sacrifice the species aspect of the sexual organs and functions for the good of the individual, as in the case of direct sterilization (Healy, 1956).

The principle of double effect. Catholic moral theology has recognized the possibility of conflict between values. What is the morality of actions that have two effects, one morally good and the other evil? Catholic medical ethics employed the principle of double effect to solve these dilemmas. It is morally permissible to perform an act with two effects, one good and one bad, if the following conditions are present: (1) the act must be good in itself or at least morally indifferent; (2) the good effect must follow as immediately from the cause as the evil effect, a condition that recognizes that the end does not justify the means; (3) the intention of the individual must be good; (4) there must be a proportionately grave reason for doing the action. This principle was used at times to justify the possibility of indirect abortion, indirect sterilization (e.g., removing a cancerous gravid uterus), or indirect killing (e.g., taking a painkiller that will also hasten death).

Cooperation and scandal. Especially in the work of doctors and nurses, questions arose about cooperation and scandal. Cooperation was generally defined as participation in the wrong or sinful act of another. Formal cooperation, described as intending the evil act, is always wrong. Immediate material cooperation, defined as participation in actually performing the wrong act, is likewise always wrong. Mediate material cooperation, which presupposes there is no intention to do evil and involves doing an act that is good or indifferent, may be permitted if there is a sufficient reason for so doing. In such a case the individual person neither intends nor does an immoral act. The morality of mediate material cooperation depends on the principle of the double effect, with special attention to the proportion between the cooperation (proximate or remote, necessary or unnecessary) in the wrong act of the other and the gravity of that wrong act. On the basis of these principles, it would be concluded that a physician should never perform an immoral operation, such as an abortion or sterilization, since this would be immediate material cooperation. A nurse who might be required to assist would be less guilty, or perhaps not guilty at all, since her cooperation is mediate.

Scandal is a sinful or seemingly sinful word, action, or omission that tends to incite or tempt another to sin. Direct scandal in which the sin of the other is intended is always wrong. Indirect scandal, in which the sin of the other is not intended but only permitted, may be allowed under two conditions: if the act giving scandal is in itself not morally wrong and if there is a sufficient reason for doing such an act. Much of the classic Roman Catholic literature of the 1950s employed these principles governing cooperation and scandal in their discussion of matters in medical ethics.

Specific questions

Obligations of physicians and rights of patients. The textbooks of medical ethics in the 1950s considered many of the questions originally posed by Antoninus of Florence more than five hundred years ago—professional competence, the obligation to attend patients, selection of remedies, correction of errors, fees, and newer additions such as "ghost" surgery and fee splitting. Important practical questions, such as the obligations of secrecy and truthfulness, especially informing the patient about death, received extended treatment. The professional secret, for example, may be divulged, but need not be, when the patient has become an unjust aggressor and is threatening harm to an innocent third party under the cover of professional secrecy.

Sexuality and the transmission of life. The natural purpose of the sexual organs and faculties and the limited stewardship that individuals have over them constitute the basis for the condemnation of contraception and contraceptive or direct sterilization. However, Roman Catholic teaching has accepted the basic principle of responsible parenthood: While always open to the gift of life, couples should have the number of children they can properly care for and educate as good Christians and human beings. Acceptance of responsible parenthood gradually appeared in formal Roman Catholic teaching. Pope Pius XII explicitly recognized that medical, eugenic, economic, and social indications can justify the limitation of the number of children (Address to Midwives, 1951). Official Roman Catholic teaching accepted rhythm, or the use of the infertile periods, because it involves no positive interference with the God-given purpose of the sexual faculty or act.

The Roman Catholic teaching on sexuality did not rest ultimately on the primacy of procreation but on an understanding of the sexual act as open to both procreation and expression of love union. Catholic teaching as illustrated by Pope Pius XII in 1956 opposed masturbation as a means of obtaining semen for fertility tests, even though procreation would thereby be facilitated. On three different occasions Pius XII spoke about and condemned artificial insemination, even with the husband's semen (AIH), because such an act goes against the nature and finality of the sexual act. Contraception interferes with the procreative aspect of the act; AIH does not recognize the love union aspect of the sexual act (Kenny, 1962).

The beginning of life and birth. Catholic theology acknowledges a theoretical doubt about when personal human life begins, but in practice all must act as if personal human life is present from the moment of conception. Since the fetus in the womb is defenseless, Catholic theology all the more feels the need to speak out in its defense. Direct abortion is always wrong. Indirect abortion is permitted for sufficient reasons. The two most often proposed examples of indirect abortion involve the removal of the cancerous uterus when the woman is pregnant and the removal of the fallopian tube or the cervix containing an ectopic pregnancy. Cesarean sections are still discussed in the textbooks of medical ethics. Premature delivery of a viable fetus is morally acceptable if there is a proportionate reason justifying the danger to the fetus involved in such a procedure. Inducement of labor follows the same general principle.

Care for health, surgery, and other procedures.   Rational human nature grounds the obligation to protect and promote one's well-being in general and one's health in particular. The patient has a right to use all moral means possible to overcome pain even though in some way all will know the meaning of suffering in human existence. However, the Catholic tradition recognizes the right of the person freely to accept pain as a form of participation in the redemptive suffering and death of Jesus. The danger of habit-forming drugs is often discussed in this context of using drugs to relieve pain.

The principle of totality justifies surgery and other procedures to suppress bodily organs and functions, provided they are for the proportionate good of the individual. Many Roman Catholic ethicists justified cosmetic surgery, but such an operation is less justifiable in relation to the danger it poses.

Organ transplants raised a problem, especially when the organ was taken from a living donor. Here the person is mutilated not for his or her own good but for the good of another. Pope Pius XII pointed out that the principle of totality cannot justify such transplants, because the mutilation is not for the good of the individual who is harmed (Address to Oculists, 1956). Some Roman Catholic moralists, therefore, considered organ transplants among the living as immoral, but others justified them on the basis of the principle of fraternal charity. However, even those allowing such transplants cautioned that the donors cannot gravely endanger their lives or seriously impair their functional integrity even for the sake of helping the neighbor (O'Donnell, 1976).

Death and dying.   On the basis of the teaching that the individual exercises only stewardship over life, Roman Catholic moral teaching rejects active euthanasia. However, painkillers may be given to the dying person even though an indirect effect of these drugs might be the hastening of the death of the patient.

Clearly distinct from euthanasia is the teaching that one does not have to use extraordinary means to preserve human life. The teaching arose in the context of the positive obligation to care for health. Positive obligations do not hold in the face of moral impossibility. By the sixteenth century there was much discussion in the moral literature about the means necessary to preserve life; moral theologians Domenico Soto and Domenico Banez offered the distinction between ordinary and extraordinary means of preserving life (McCartney, 1980). Generally speaking, an individual has no obligation to use extraordinary means to preserve life. A

well-accepted opinion views extraordinary means as all medicines, treatments, and operations that cannot be obtained or used without excessive expense, pain, or other inconvenience, or if used would not offer a reasonable hope of benefit (Kelly, 1958). From such an ethical perspective no moral difference exists between not using an artificial respirator to sustain life for a few hours or even days and shutting off a respirator already in use.

Even before recent discussions about the appropriate definition of the moment of death, Roman Catholic medical ethics treated the question. The traditional theological definition of death as the separation of the soul from the body lacks precision. To determine exactly when death occurs lies beyond the competence of the church or theology and belongs to the competence of medical science, as Pius XII stated (Address to Anesthesiologists, 1957).

Other questions.   Under the heading of the spiritual care of the patient, questions concerning informing the patient about impending death, and especially the administration of the sacraments of baptism, penance, and anointing of the sick (extreme unction), were considered. On the question of medical experimentation the textbooks generally followed the teaching of Pius XII in his address to the Eighth Congress of the World Medical Association, September 30, 1954, in distinguishing between experimentation for the good of the individual and experimentation in the strict sense for the good of others. For the good of the individual, experimentation is allowed, provided no certainly effective remedy is available, if the dubious treatment most likely to help the patient is chosen, and if the consent of the patient is at least reasonably presumed. Experimentation for the good of others (experimentation in the strict sense as opposed to therapy) may be permitted for the proportionate good of others and of science if the subject freely consents, if no experiment that directly inflicts grave injury or death is used, and if all reasonable precautions are taken to avoid even the indirect causing of grave injury or death. Later, theologians and ethicists would probe these criteria more deeply and apply them to the cases of children, prisoners, and others whose ability to consent is in some way diminished or lacking.

Current trends

Significant developments have occurred in Roman Catholic medical ethics since 1960. The newer technological and biomedical developments that have sparked such a broad interest in medical ethics today have had an impact on Roman Catholic medical ethics. Changes within the Roman Catholic church associated with the Second Vatican Council (1962–1965) have significantly affected medical ethics in the specific characteristics of authoritative church teaching and natural-law methodology.

In 1968 Pope Paul VI issued the encyclical *Humanae vitae*, reaffirming the condemnation of artificial contraception for married couples. For the first time in modern church history, many Catholic moral theologians publicly dissented from such teaching and affirmed the right of all Catholics to disagree in theory and in practice with such a noninfallible teaching. These theologians maintained that the specific moral teachings on complex issues depend primarily on human reasoning, do not involve the essence of the faith, and contain very specific judgments or applications that cannot claim absolute certitude. A presumption exists in favor of the authoritative teaching, but that presumption can be overturned by evidence or for serious reasons. Subsequently, many Roman Catholic theologians have proposed dissenting positions on many specific issues in medical ethics. The hierarchical teaching and pastoral office in the church seem to tolerate some dissent in practice, but in theory do not admit the legitimacy of such dissent and have taken disciplinary action against a few theologians because of their dissent. Some Roman Catholic medical ethicists strongly deny the legitimacy of such dissent from authoritative church teaching.

A number of criticisms have been directed against the concept of natural law as proposed in the manuals of theology and of medical ethics. A more historically conscious approach gives more emphasis to growth, development, and change, and likewise emphasizes the individual, the particular, and the contingent more than older natural-law theory did. A more inductive methodology remains more tentative about its conclusions than the former deductive method. Newer approaches put more emphasis on the personal and less on the (merely) "natural" and call for a greater stress on the uniqueness of individuals. A personalist perspective objects to basing morality only on the finality and purpose of distinct physical faculties viewed in isolation from the total person. Above all, revisionist Roman Catholic moral theologians disagree with the physicalism of the older approach, according to which the moral aspect of the human act is identified with the physical aspect of the act. The distinction is often proposed between physical or premoral evil, on the one hand, and moral evil, on the other. According to the theory of proportionalism, physical or premoral evil can be justified for a proportionate reason.

Feminist theory has been introduced into Roman Catholic bioethics (Farley, 1974), but its theoretical influence is less in this area than in other areas of Catholic thought. In practice the Sisters of Mercy (on sterilization) and some individual religious women (on abortion) have challenged the positions of the hierarchical magisterium. In the light of all these developments, one can no longer speak of a monolithic natural-law theory in Roman Catholic moral theology or medical ethics. A pluralism of methodological approaches now exists.

The revisionist ethicists (McCormick, 1981, 1984; Curran, 1978; Farley, 1974; Häring, 1973; Kelly, 1979; Maguire, 1974; Shannon and Cahill, 1988) do not necessarily form a single school or agree among themselves about specific issues. A good number of Roman Catholic moral theologians challenge the theory that bases morality on the purpose and finality of the sexual faculty viewed in itself and disagree with the absolute condemnations of contraception, sterilization, masturbation for seminal analysis, and AIH. A few even accept artificial insemination with a donor's semen in some circumstances. Many theologians reject the principle of double effect especially because of the condition that emphasizes the physical causality of the act by requiring that the good effect must be as immediate as the evil effect. To a lesser extent theologians have proposed differing positions on when truly individual human life begins and how this affects abortion decisions. Much discussion centers on withdrawing life-support systems from the dying, and disagreement exists about the role of quality-of-life considerations in such cases. A few ethicists (e.g., Maguire, 1974) argue for active euthanasia in some circumstances.

A smaller but strong number of Catholic medical ethicists (e.g., McFadden, 1976; O'Donnell, 1976) support the traditional natural-law theory or revise it in such a way (e.g., Grisez, 1970; Grisez and Boyle, 1979) as to better support the authoritative teachings of the hierarchical magisterium.

The hierarchical magisterium itself (including papal addresses, declarations and letters of the Congregation for the Doctrine of the Faith, documents of national conferences of bishops—such as "Ethical and Religious Directives for Catholic Health Care Facilities," approved as a national code for the United States by the National Conference of Catholic Bishops in 1971—and documents from committees of the National Conference of Catholic Bishops) continues to appeal directly and indirectly to the older monolithic natural-law methodology to support its teaching on the immorality of contraception, sterilization, abortion, euthanasia, in vitro fertilization, and questions associated with birth and dying. Significant official documents of the hierarchical magisterium on these questions include the *Humanae vitae* of Pope Paul VI (1968) and three documents from the Congregation for the Doctrine of the Faith whose purpose is to safeguard the truths of faith and morality—"Declaration on Procured Abortion" (1974), "Declaration on Euthanasia" (1980), and "Instruction on Respect for Human Life in Its Origin" (1987) (O'Rourke and Boyle, 1989; Verspieren, 1987). In the HIV/AIDS epidemic of the 1980s and 1990s, national hierarchies throughout the world have issued pastoral instructions repudiating the claim that AIDS is divine punishment for homosexuality and urging compassion and care for persons with AIDS. However, at the same time, they have reaffirmed, with greater or less emphasis, Catholic teaching on the immorality of homosexual practices and sexual prophylaxis.

Thus, on the contemporary scene Roman Catholic bioethics experiences tensions and pluralism concerning the role and binding force of the hierarchical magisterium, the methodology of bioethics, and the solution to many specific issues.

CHARLES E. CURRAN

Directly related to this entry is the entry ETHICS, *article on* RELIGION AND MORALITY. *Also directly related are the entries* EUGENICS AND RELIGIOUS LAW, *article on* CHRISTIANITY; POPULATION ETHICS, *section on* RELIGIOUS TRADITIONS, *article on* ROMAN CATHOLIC PERSPECTIVES; *and* REPRODUCTIVE TECHNOLOGIES. *For a further discussion of topics mentioned in this entry, see the entries* ABORTION; AIDS; DEATH; DOUBLE EFFECT; FEMINISM; FERTILITY CONTROL; LIFE; MARRIAGE AND OTHER DOMESTIC PARTNERSHIPS; NATURAL LAW; ORGAN AND TISSUE TRANSPLANTS; PASTORAL CARE; RESEARCH METHODOLOGY, *article on* CONCEPTUAL ISSUES; *and* SEXUAL ETHICS. *For a discussion of related ideas, see the entries* CASUISTRY; DEATH, *article on* WESTERN RELIGIOUS THOUGHT; DEATH, DEFINITION AND DETERMINATION OF, *article on* PHILOSOPHICAL AND THEOLOGICAL PESPECTIVES; DEATH AND DYING, *articles on* ETHICAL ISSUES, *and* HISTORICAL ASPECTS; *and* RIGHTS, *article on* RIGHTS IN BIOETHICS. *Other relevant material may be found under the entries* BENEFICENCE; HUMAN NATURE; MEDICAL ETHICS, HISTORY OF, *section on* EUROPE; *and* VALUE AND VALUATION. *See also the* APPENDIX (CODES, OATHS, AND DIRECTIVES RELATED TO BIOETHICS), SECTION II: ETHICAL DIRECTIVES FOR THE PRACTICE OF MEDICINE, ETHICAL AND RELIGIOUS DIRECTIVES FOR CATHOLIC HEALTH FACILITIES *of the* UNITED STATES CATHOLIC CONFERENCE; *and selections from the* HEALTH CARE ETHICS GUIDE *of the* CATHOLIC HEALTH ASSOCIATION OF CANADA.

Bibliography

For important church documents, in chronological order from the earliest times, see Denzinger and Schönmetzer, below. Official church documents since 1908 have been published in *Acta apostolicae sedis.* English translations of important papal declarations are in the serial *The Pope Speaks* (1954–). Textbooks of medical ethics often give references to the major addresses of Pius XII on these subjects (e.g., Kenny,

1962, p. 272). O'Rourke and Boyle, and Verspieren (see below) are the two best contemporary collections of the documents of the hierarchical magisterium.

ANTONELLI, GIUSEPPE. 1906. *Medicina pastoralis in usum confessariorum et curiarum ecclesiaticarum.* 2 vols. Rome: Frederico Pustet.

ANTONINUS [ARCHBISHOP OF FLORENCE]. 1983. [1477]. *Summa summarum.* 4 vols. Venice: Jenson.

AQUINAS, THOMAS. 1950–1952. *Summa theologiae: Cum texta ex recensione Leonina.* 4 vols. Turin: Marietti.

ASHLEY, BENEDICT M., and O'ROURKE, KEVIN D. 1989. *Health Care Ethics: A Theological Analysis.* 3d ed. St. Louis: Catholic Health Association.

BONNAR, ALPHONSUS. 1939. *The Catholic Doctor.* 2d ed. London: Burns, Oates and Washbourne.

BOUDEWYNS, MICHIEL. 1666. *Ventilabrum medico-theologicum quo omnes casus, tum medicos, cum aegros, aliosque concernentes eventilantur.* Antwerp: Cornelium Woons.

BOUSCAREN, TIMOTHY LINCOLN. 1944. *Ethics of Ectopic Operations.* 2d ed. Milwaukee: Bruce.

CANGIAMILA, FRANCESCO EMMANUELE. 1764. *Sacra embryologia, sive, de officio sacerdotum, medicorum, et aliorum circa aeternam parvulorum in utero existentium salutem libri quatuor.* Munich: J. F. X. Grätz.

CAPELLMANN, CARL FRANZ. 1879. *Medicina pastoralis.* 4th ed. Aachen: Rudolph Barth. Translated by William Dassel under the title *Pastoral Medicine.* New York: Frederico Pustet.

COPPENS, CHARLES. 1897. *Moral Principles and Medical Practice: The Basis of Medical Jurisprudence.* New York: Benziger Brothers.

CRONIN, DANIEL A. 1958. *The Moral Law in Regard to the Ordinary and Extraordinary Means of Conserving Life.* Rome: Pontificia Universitas Gregoriana.

CURRAN, CHARLES E. 1978. *Issues in Sexual and Medical Ethics.* Notre Dame, Ind.: University of Notre Dame Press.

CURRAN, CHARLES E., and MCCORMICK, RICHARD A., eds. 1988. *Dissent in the Church.* Readings in Moral Theology no. 6. Mahwah, N.J.: Paulist Press.

———. 1991. *Natural Law and Theology.* Readings in Moral Theology no. 7. Mahwah, N.J.: Paulist Press.

DEBREYNE, PIERRE J. C. 1884. *La Théologie morale et les sciences médicales.* 6th ed. Edited by Ange E. A. Ferrand. Paris: Poussielgue Frères.

DENZINGER, HEINRICH J. D., and SCHÖNMETZER, ADOLFUS. 1963. *Enchiridion symbolorum, definitionum et declarationum de rebus fidei et morum.* 32d ed. Barcelona: Herder.

ESCHBACH, ALPHONS. 1884. *Disputationes physiologico-theologicae de humanae generationis oeconomia, de embryologia sacra, de abortu medicali et de embryotomia, de colenda castitate.* Paris: Victor Palmé.

FARLEY, MARGARET A. 1974. "Liberation, Abortion, and Responsibility." *Reflection* 71 (May):9–13.

FIORENTINI, GIROLAMO [FLORENTINIUS]. 1658. *Disputatio de ministrando baptismo humanis foetibus abortivorum.* Lyons: Claudius Chancey.

FLOOD, PETER, ed. 1953–1960. *New Problems in Medical Ethics.* Translated by Malachy Gerard Carroll. 4 vols. Westminster, Md.: Newman Press. Published in French as *Cahiers Laënnec.* Paris: P. Lethielleux.

——. 1962–1963. *New Problems in Medical Ethics.* Nos. 1–4. Translated by Malachy Gerard Carroll. Cork, Ireland: Mercier Press. A series with content overlapping the Newman Press edition but arranged differently. In part published under the imprint of Divine Work Publications, Techny, Ill.

GRISEZ, GERMAIN G. 1970. *Abortion: The Myths, the Realities, and the Arguments.* New York: Corpus Books.

GRISEZ, GERMAIN G., and BOYLE, JOSEPH M., JR. 1979. *Life and Death with Liberty and Justice: A Contribution to the Euthanasia Debate.* Notre Dame, Ind.: University of Notre Dame Press.

HÄRING, BERNARD [BERNHARD]. 1961–1966. *The Law of Christ: Moral Theology for Priests and Laity.* Translated by Edwin G. Kaiser. 3 vols. Westminster, Md.: Newman Press.

——. 1973. *Medical Ethics.* Edited by Gabrielle L. Jean. Notre Dame, Ind.: Fides.

HEALY, EDWIN F. 1956. *Medical Ethics.* Chicago: Loyola University Press.

JONSEN, ALBERT R., and TOULMIN, STEPHEN. 1988. *The Abuse of Casuistry: A History of Moral Reasoning.* Berkeley: University of California Press.

KELLY, DAVID F. 1979. *The Emergence of Roman Catholic Medical Ethics in North America: An Historical-Methodological-Biographical Study.* 2d ed. New York: Edwin Mellen.

KELLY, GERALD A. 1958. *Medico-Moral Problems.* St. Louis: Catholic Hospital Association.

KENNY, JOHN P. 1952. *Principles of Medical Ethics.* Westminster, Md.: Newman Press.

——. 1962. *Principles of Medical Ethics.* 2d ed. Westminster, Md.: Newman Press.

LIGUORI, ALFONSUS MARIA DE. 1905–1912. [1789]. *Theologia moralis.* Vols. 1–4 of *Opera moralia Sancti Alphonsi Mariae de Ligorio.* Edited by Leonardi Gaude. Rome: Vatican.

MAGUIRE, DANIEL C. 1974. *Death by Choice.* Garden City, N.Y.: Doubleday.

MAHONEY, JOHN. 1987. *The Making of Moral Theology: A Study of the Roman Catholic Tradition.* Oxford: At the Clarendon Press.

MAY, WILLIAM E. 1977. *Human Existence, Medicine, and Ethics: Reflections on Human Life.* Chicago: Franciscan Herald Press.

MAZZOLINI, SILVESTRO [PRIERAS, SYLVESTER]. 1601. *Summa sylvestrinae que summa summarum merito nuncupatur pars 1–11.* Venice: Alexander Gryphius.

McCARTHY, JEREMIAH J., and CARON, JUDITH A. 1990. *Medical Ethics: A Catholic Guide to Healthcare Decisions.* Liguori, Mo.: Liguori.

McCARTNEY, JAMES J. 1980. "The Development of the Doctrine of Ordinary and Extraordinary Means of Preserving Life." *Linacre Quarterly* 47:215–220.

McCORMICK, RICHARD A. 1981. *How Brave a New World? Dilemmas in Bioethics.* Garden City, N.Y.: Doubleday.

——. 1984. *Health and Medicine in the Catholic Tradition: Tradition in Transition.* New York: Crossroad.

McFADDEN, CHARLES J. 1946. *Medical Ethics for Nurses.* Philadelphia: F. A. Davis.

——. 1949. *Medical Ethics.* Philadelphia: F. A. Davis. 2d edition of *Medical Ethics for Nurses.*

——. 1976. *The Dignity of Life: Moral Values in a Changing Society.* Huntington, Ind.: Our Sunday Visitor.

NIEDERMEYER, ALBERT. 1935. *Pastoralmedizinische Propädeutik. Einführung in die geistigen Grundlagen der Pastoral-Medizin und Pastoral-Hygiene.* Salzburg: A. Pustet.

——. 1949–1952. *Handbuch der speziellen pastoralmedizin.* 6 vols. Vienna: Herder.

NOONAN, JOHN THOMAS, JR. 1986. *Contraception: A History of Its Treatment by the Catholic Theologians and Canonists.* Enlarged ed. Cambridge, Mass.: Harvard University Press.

O'DONNELL, THOMAS JOSEPH. 1956. *Morals in Medicine.* Westminster, Md.: Newman Press.

——. 1976. *Medicine and Christian Morality.* New York: Alba House.

O'ROURKE, KEVIN D., and BOYLE, PHILIP. 1989. *Medical Ethics: Sources of Catholic Teachings.* St. Louis: Catholic Health Association.

PAQUIN, JULES. 1955. *Morale et médecine.* Montreal: L'Immaculée Conception.

PAYEN, GEORGES. 1935. *Déontologie médicale d'après le droit naturel: Devoirs d'état et droits de tout médecin.* New ed. Zi-ka-wei (near Shanghai): T'ou-se-we.

PUJIULA, JAIME. 1953. *De medicina pastorali: Recentiores quaestiones quaedam exponunter.* 2d ed. Turin: Marietti.

RAYNAUD, THÉOPHILE [THEOPHILUS RAYNAUDUS]. 1637. *De ortu infantium, contra naturam per sectionem caesaream tractatio.* Lyons: G. Boissat.

SANCHEZ, TOMÁS. 1606. *Disputationum de sancto matrimonii sacramento.* 3 vols. Venice: Jacob de Franciscis.

SCREMIN, LUIGI. 1954. *Dizionario de morale professionale per i medici.* 5th ed. Rome: Editrice Studium.

SHANNON, THOMAS A., and CAHILL, LISA SOWLE. 1988. *Religion and Artificial Reproduction: An Inquiry into the Vatican "Instruction on Respect for Human Life in Its Origin and on the Dignity of Human Reproduction."* New York: Crossroad.

SURBLED, GEORGES. 1891–1898. *La Morale dans ses rapports avec la médecine et l'hygiène.* 4 vols. Paris: Victor Retaux.

VEREECKE, LOUIS. 1986. *De Guillaume d'Ockham à Saint Alphonse de Liguori: Études d'histoire de la théologie morale moderne (1300–1789).* Rome: Collegium S. Alfonsi de Urbe.

VERSPIEREN, PATRICK. 1987. *Biologie, médecine, et éthique: Textes du Magistère catholique.* Paris: Le Centurion.

ZACCHIA, PAOLO. 1701. [1621]. *Quaestiones medico-legalium.* 3 vols. Lyons: Anisson and Joannis Posuel.

ROMANIA

See MEDICAL ETHICS, HISTORY OF, *section on* EUROPE, *subsection on* CONTEMPORARY PERIOD, *article on* CENTRAL AND EASTERN EUROPE.

RUSSIA

See MEDICAL ETHICS, HISTORY OF, *section on* EUROPE, *subsection on* CONTEMPORARY PERIOD, *article on* RUSSIA.